Applied Veterinary Clinical Nutrition

Applied Veterinary Clinical Nutrition

Second Edition

Edited by

Andrea J. Fascetti, VMD, PhD
Diplomate ACVIM (Nutrition and Small Animal Internal Medicine)
Board-Certified Veterinary Nutritionist®
Professor of Nutrition, Department of Molecular Biosciences,
School of Veterinary Medicine, UC Davis,
Davis, CA, USA

Sean J. Delaney, BS, DVM, MS
Diplomate ACVIM (Nutrition)
Board-Certified Veterinary Nutritionist®
Founder, Balance It®, A DBA of Davis Veterinary Medical Consulting, Inc.
Davis, CA, USA

Jennifer A. Larsen, DVM, MS, PhD
Diplomate ACVIM (Nutrition)
Board-Certified Veterinary Nutritionist®
Professor of Clinical Nutrition, Department of Molecular Biosciences,
School of Veterinary Medicine, UC Davis,
Davis, CA, USA

Cecilia Villaverde, BVSc, PhD
Diplomate ACVIM (Nutrition)
Board-Certified Veterinary Nutritionist®
Diplomate ECVCN
EBVS®, European Specialist in Veterinary and Comparative Nutrition
Consultant, Expert Pet Nutrition, Fermoy, County Cork, Ireland

WILEY Blackwell

Published by John Wiley & Sons, Inc., Hoboken, New Jersey.
Published simultaneously in Canada.

For general information on our other products and services or for technical support, please contact our Customer Care Department within the United States at (800) 762-2974, outside the United States at (317) 572-3993 or fax (317) 572-4002.

Wiley also publishes its books in a variety of electronic formats. Some content that appears in print may not be available in electronic formats. For more information about Wiley products, visit our web site at www.wiley.com.

Library of Congress Cataloging-in-Publication Data applied for
Hardback ISBN: 9781119375142

Cover Design: Wiley
Cover Images: Courtesy of Jennifer A. Larsen, Jonathan Stockman and Ady Gancz

Set in 9.5/12.5pt STIXTwoText by Straive, Pondicherry, India

SKY10061852_120523

Contents

List of Contributors

Robert C. Backus, MS, DVM, PhD
Diplomate ACVIM (Nutrition)
Board-Certified Veterinary Nutritionist®
Associate Professor and Director of the
Nestlé Purina Endowed Program in Small
Animal Nutrition
College of Veterinary Medicine
University of Missouri
Columbia, MO, USA

Joe Bartges, DVM, PhD
Diplomate ACVIM (Small Animal Internal
Medicine and Nutrition)
Board-Certified Veterinary Nutritionist®
Professor
Department of Small Animal Medicine
& Surgery
University of Georgia
Athens, GA, USA

Paul Brentson, BA, MBA
PB Consulting
Applegate, CA, USA

C.A. Tony Buffington, DVM, PhD
Diplomate ACVIM (Nutrition, retired)
Board-Certified Veterinary Nutritionist®
Clinical Professor
School of Veterinary Medicine
University of California–Davis
Davis, CA, USA
Emeritus Professor of Veterinary Clinical
Sciences
The Ohio State University
Columbus, OH, USA

Nick Cave PhD, MVSc, BVSc
Diplomate ACVIM (Nutrition)
Board-Certified Veterinary Nutritionist®
Associate Professor
Group Leader – Academic
School of Veterinary Science
Te Kunenga ki Pūrehuroa | Massey University
Palmerston North, New Zealand

Ronald J. Corbee, DVM, PhD
Diplomate ECVCN
EBVS®, European Specialist in Veterinary
and Comparative Nutrition
Professor
Department of Clinical Sciences
Universiteit Utrecht
Utrecht, Netherlands

Sean J. Delaney, BS, DVM, MS
Diplomate ACVIM (Nutrition)
Board-Certified Veterinary Nutritionist®
Founder, Balance It®, A DBA of Davis
Veterinary Medical Consulting, Inc.
Davis, CA, USA

David A. Dzanis, DVM, PhD
Diplomate ACVIM (Nutrition)
Board-Certified Veterinary Nutritionist®
CEO (retired), Regulatory Discretion, Inc.
Santa Clarita, CA, USA

Denise A. Elliott, BVSc (Hons), PhD
Diplomate ACVIM (Nutrition and Small
Animal Internal Medicine)
Board-Certified Veterinary Nutritionist®

Global Vice President
Research & Development
Royal Canin
Aimargues, Occitanie, France

Andrea J. Fascetti, VMD, PhD
Diplomate ACVIM (Nutrition and Small
Animal Internal Medicine)
Board-Certified Veterinary Nutritionist®
Professor of Nutrition
Department of Molecular Biosciences
School of Veterinary Medicine
University of California–Davis
Davis, CA, USA

Lisa M. Freeman, DVM, PhD
Diplomate ACVIM (Nutrition)
Board-Certified Veterinary Nutritionist®
Professor, Department of Clinical Sciences &
Agriculture, Food and Environment
Cummings School of Veterinary Medicine
Tufts University
North Grafton, MA, USA

Herman Hazewinkel, DVM, PhD
Diplomate European College of Veterinary
Surgeons
Diplomate ECVCN
EBVS®, European Specialist in Veterinary
and Comparative Nutrition
Emeritus Professor Companion Animal
Orthopaedics
Dept of Clinical Sciences and
Companion Animals
Utrecht University,
Utrecht, Netherlands

Marta Hervera, BVSc, PhD
Diplomate ECVCN
EBVS®, European Specialist in Veterinary
and Comparative Nutrition
Co-founder and Consultant
Expert Pet Nutrition
Zurich, Switzerland

Richard C. Hill, VetMB, PhD
Diplomate ACVIM (Nutrition and Small
Animal Internal Medicine)

Board-Certified Veterinary Nutritionist®
Associate Professor
Small Animal Clinical Sciences
University of Florida
Gainesville, FL, USA

**Aarti Kathrani, BVetMed (Hons), PhD,
FHEA, MRCVS**
Diplomate ACVIM (Nutrition and Small
Animal Internal Medicine)
Board-Certified Veterinary Nutritionist®
Senior Lecturer in Small Animal Internal
Medicine
Department of Clinical Science and Services
Royal Veterinary College
Hatfield, Herts, UK

Elizabeth Koutsos, PhD
President, EnviroFlight, LLC
Apex, NC, USA

Jennifer A. Larsen, DVM, MS, PhD
Diplomate ACVIM (Nutrition)
Board-Certified Veterinary Nutritionist®
Professor of Clinical Nutrition
Department of Molecular Biosciences
School of Veterinary Medicine
University of California–Davis
Davis, CA, USA

Stanley L. Marks, BVSc, PhD
Diplomate ACVIM (Nutrition,
Small Animal Internal Medicine
and Oncology)
Board-Certified Veterinary Nutritionist®
Board-Certified Veterinary Oncologist®
Professor
Department of Medicine & Epidemiology
University of California–Davis
Davis, CA, USA

Isabel Marzo
Agricultural Engineer
Senior Consultant in animal feed and
veterinary medicines
Costa-Marzo Consulting, SLU
Barcelona, Spain

Glenna E. Mauldin, DVM, MS
Diplomate ACVIM (Oncology and Nutrition)
Board-Certified Veterinary Nutritionist®
Director of Clinical Research
Thrive Pet Healthcare and PetCure Oncology
Austin, TX, USA

Kathryn E. Michel, BA, DVM, MS, MSED
DACVIM (Nutrition)
Board-Certified Veterinary Nutritionist®
Professor of Nutrition and Associate
Dean of Education, School of Veterinary
Medicine, University of Pennsylvania,
Philadelphia, PA, USA

Catherine A. Outerbridge, DVM, MVSc
Diplomate, ACVD
Board-Certified Veterinary Nutritionist®
Diplomate ACVIM (Small Animal Internal
Medicine)
Professor of Clinical Dermatology
Department of Medicine and Epidemiology
School of Veterinary Medicine
University of California–Davis
Davis, CA, USA

Tammy J. Owens, DVM, MS
Diplomate ACVIM (Nutrition)
Board-Certified Veterinary Nutritionist®
Assistant Professor
Small Animal Clinical Sciences
Western College of Veterinary Medicine –
University of Saskatchewan
Saskatoon, SK, Canada

Sally C. Perea, DVM, MS
Diplomate ACVIM (Nutrition)
Board-Certified Veterinary Nutritionist®
Veterinary Nutritionist, Research &
Development
Royal Canin, A division of Mars, Inc.
Lewisburg, OH, USA

Olivia A. Petritz, DVM
Diplomate ACZM
Assistant Professor
Department of Clinical Sciences
North Carolina State University
Raleigh, NC, USA

Yann Queau, DVM
Diplomate ACVIM (Nutrition)
Board-Certified Veterinary Nutritionist®
Discover Vet Pillar Team Manager
Research & Development
Royal Canin
Montpellier, Occitanie, France

Jon J. Ramsey, PhD
Professor
Department of Molecular Biosciences
School of Veterinary Medicine
University of California–Davis
Davis, CA, USA

John E. Rush, MS, DVM
Diplomate ACVIM (Cardiology)
Board-Certified Veterinary Cardiologist®
Diplomate ACVECC
Board-Certified Veterinary Specialist in
Veterinary Emergency and Critical Care®
Professor, Department of Clinical Sciences
Cummings School of Veterinary Medicine
Tufts University
North Grafton, MA, USA

Brian Speer, DVM
Diplomate ABVP (Avian Practice)
Diplomate ECZM (Avian)
Director
Medical Center for Birds
Oakley, CA, USA

Jonathan Stockman, DVM
Diplomate ACVIM (Nutrition)
Board-Certified Veterinary Nutritionist®
Assistant Professor
Department of Clinical Veterinary Sciences
Long Island University
Brookville, NY, USA

Cecilia Villaverde, BVSc, PhD
Diplomate ACVIM (Nutrition)
Board-Certified Veterinary Nutritionist®
Diplomate ECVCN
EBVS®, European Specialist in Veterinary and
Comparative Nutrition
Consultant, Expert Pet Nutrition
Fermoy, County Cork, Ireland

Preface

We envision this text to be a resource not only for the veterinary practitioner but also for students and residents of multiple disciplines. Many veterinary schools and universities are now teaching a course in small animal clinical nutrition, and this text will make a nice complement to such lecture material. (From the first edition)

We have been very fortunate to have the first edition fulfill its original vision. This is largely thanks to its widespread promotion and adoption by our colleagues in industry and academia.

Like many sciences and specialties, nutrition knowledge evolves, and it became clear that an update was needed. We also saw an opportunity to enhance the text's international applicability to better support its use outside of North America and translation into multiple languages.

With this edition, we have astoundingly maintained all but one now retired contributor and added many more contributors to give additional depth as well as to add international perspective and species expertise outside of dogs and cats, including avian and small mammalian species. To quote the first edition again, "We consider our contributors to be the experts in their fields, so we are extremely fortunate that they have been willing to share their knowledge and experience through their respective chapters" and now sidebars. This sentiment remains even more true with this second edition.

We have kept the structure and approach similar in this new version. Notably, one will continue to find heavy use of citations wherever possible. These references provide additional opportunities for further reading and enrichment, especially in areas where controversy may exist or our understanding is not yet complete.

With this edition, two new co-editors have been added from two previous contributors and colleagues, Drs. Jennifer Larsen and Cecilia Villaverde. Dr. Larsen brings an unrivaled degree of clinical experience teaching veterinary students and residents. Dr. Villaverde, as a board-certified veterinary nutritionist in both North America and Europe with extensive teaching experience in South America, provides unparalleled international expertise. Their generosity in the midst of many other commitments made this second edition possible.

With so many necessary updates, additions, and contributors and a multiyear life-altering pandemic, our publisher Wiley has shown an impressive and unwavering commitment to this text and by extension veterinary nutrition. We are indebted to their team's guidance and patience, especially from Erica Judisch, Merryl Le Roux, Susan Engelken, Sally Osborn, Simon Yapp, ETC.

It is the four co-editors' collective hope that this second edition will further the practice of veterinary nutrition in small animals globally and serve you, the reader, as a ready and accessible resource to help your understanding, students, residents, clients, and/or patients.

Acknowledgments

I would like to welcome and thank Dr. Jennifer Larsen and Dr. Cecilia Villaverde for agreeing to assist in completing the second edition of the textbook with Dr. Sean Delaney and me.

I am also appreciative of all of our collaborators from around the world who worked so hard in bringing their expertise to this book. It is only through their tireless efforts that we have a second edition.

I remain truly grateful for the continuous support from my immediate family, my husband Greg, sons Noah and Ari, and our dog Holly.

Andrea J. Fascetti, VMD, PhD
Diplomate ACVIM (Nutrition and Small Animal Internal Medicine)
Board-Certified Veterinary Nutritionist®
Professor of Nutrition
Department of Molecular Biosciences
School of Veterinary Medicine
University of California–Davis
Davis, CA, USA

In the first edition, I acknowledged my teachers/mentors, veterinary nutrition colleagues, co-editor, family, and personal animal companions in detail. I remain very grateful to them all, especially my wife Siona, and daughters Maya and Ruby. For this second edition, I would like to concisely acknowledge my two new co-editors, co-workers, past students, residents, referring veterinarians and veterinary specialists, clients, customers, and patients. I am forever better for having crossed paths with these tens of thousands of beings over the last three decades. These interactions have given me the frequent and great privilege to see people at their most humane. I hope this text helps to give a little back as a way to show my sincere appreciation for this gift.

Sean J. Delaney, BS, DVM, MS
Diplomate ACVIM (Nutrition)
Board-Certified Veterinary Nutritionist®
Founder, Balance It®, A DBA of Davis Veterinary Medical Consulting, Inc.
Davis, CA, USA

I would like first to express my thanks and appreciation to my co-editors. I am grateful to be a part of this project, which represents the collective experience, knowledge, and wisdom of each contributor. This text resource is a valuable contribution to our discipline, and I also thank each author for sharing their efforts with us.

Jennifer A. Larsen, DVM, MS, PhD
Diplomate ACVIM (Nutrition)
Board-Certified Veterinary Nutritionist®
Professor of Clinical Nutrition
Department of Molecular Biosciences
School of Veterinary Medicine
University of California–Davis
Davis, CA, USA

I would like to thank my co-editors for inviting me to participate in this unique project in the area of companion animal nutrition, and all the authors for sharing their knowledge and expertise so generously.

Cecilia Villaverde, BVSc, PhD
Diplomate ACVIM (Nutrition)
Board-Certified Veterinary Nutritionist®
Diplomate ECVCN
EBVS®, European Specialist in Veterinary and Comparative Nutrition
Consultant, Expert Pet Nutrition
Fermoy, County Cork, Ireland

1

Integration of Nutrition into Clinical Practice

Sean J. Delaney, Andrea J. Fascetti, Jennifer A. Larsen, and Paul Brentson

Introduction

While some veterinarians enjoy the various complex aspects of owning and managing a clinical practice, many more take on these roles out of necessity rather than preference. In either case, this results in many clinical approaches being at least partially viewed through a "fiscal filter." Although this filter should not be fine enough to strain out appropriate medical decisions, it certainly requires that the economics associated with certain medical practices be considered. Therefore, this introductory chapter will discuss the "business" of nutrition in clinical practice, as an understanding of these basics will enable the practitioner to afford to implement the knowledge contained in the rest of this textbook.

Average Revenue from Food Sales and the Potential

In 2017, the average food revenue was static compared to 2015 at 3.5% of total veterinary practice revenue in the United States (range 2.8–4.3%; AAHA 2019). At the same time, average total revenue earned by practices in 2017 was US$1 271 402. The therapeutic food revenue-to-expense ratio has remained fairly static over time at 1.3, and is consistent across practice types (with regard to number of full-time clinicians, revenue level, years at current location, and American Animal Hospital Association [AAHA] member status). Practices with higher ratios may be managing expenses more efficiently (including consideration of costs related to inventory control) or have higher markups. Lower ratios may reflect undercharging relative to the cost of managing food inventory. Revenue from therapeutic diet sales, while relatively significant on average, can be higher, as practices that focus more on the large compliance gap with therapeutic food recommendations (this gap includes both veterinarians who do not actively recommend medically needed foods and clients who do not choose to feed them) can easily double gross profits from food sales with minimal additional effort or expenditures.

Theoretically, there is much opportunity for growth in revenues and profits if practices can successfully identify and correct barriers to care both for wellness and for chronic and acute disease management (Volk et al. 2011). In large part, the longevity and success of any given practice model will depend on the ability to remain flexible and responsive to changing client demographics, the impacts of the economic climate, and the continued growth in internet resources for both information and products. For some clients, the accessibility

Applied Veterinary Clinical Nutrition, Second Edition. Edited by Andrea J. Fascetti, Sean J. Delaney, Jennifer A. Larsen, and Cecilia Villaverde.

Box 1.1 Dietary Recommendations to Maximize Patient Outcome and Ensure Practice Sustainability

Few recommendations hold as much weight with clients about what to feed their animal companion as a veterinarian's recommendation. Many pet food companies are aware of this and invest heavily in the veterinary community, vying for the veterinarian's awareness of their products and, ideally, for their recommendation. Unfortunately, the resulting influx of generous support is increasingly viewed by some as creating a conflict of interest for veterinarians and resulting in a bias in dietary recommendations. This perception is increased by veterinarians who have limited recommendations beyond the products, brands, and/or companies they stock. Therefore, the goal of this chapter is to assist the veterinarian in methods to ensure they can afford to provide the best medical care for their patients and clients by fully integrating nutrition into their clinical practice.

---

and cost of veterinary care and products are a challenge, and the practitioner must effectively communicate the value of services and facilitate convenience in order not just to achieve compliance, but also to maximize both medical outcomes and revenue (Box 1.1). In fact, profits could be increased more than fivefold based on the low compliance found in a study by the AAHA, which includes sales of therapeutic pet foods (AAHA 2003).

Strategies to Increase Product Sales

Recommending an Effective Therapeutic Food

The surest way to increase compliance and therapeutic pet food sales is to recommend an effective one. This sounds simple enough, but can be quite challenging in practice. To start, one must make the correct diagnosis and select a food that can produce measurable improvement in the animal companion's condition or disease management. For example, clients feeding a "weight loss" food that does not result in weight loss are likely to stop feeding the ineffectual food. Similarly, trying to sell food that an animal companion will not eat is unlikely to be successful. Therefore, establishing expectations, performing a nutritional assessment to guide more informed food recommendations, monitoring the patient response, and providing a variety of options are vital for client compliance.

Establishing Expectations

Many clients choose not to start feeding a recommended therapeutic food, or choose to stop feeding one, because they do not clearly understand what is expected from the food. Expectations are built on the client's understanding of the purpose and mechanism of the food. For example, clients who understand that higher dietary phosphorus can cause progression of chronic kidney disease, and that most dietary phosphorus comes from protein-rich ingredients, are more likely to feed an appropriately lower protein- or phosphorus-containing food. Not surprisingly, human patients have better retention of medical information when verbal information is accompanied with written information (Langdon et al. 2002). Therefore, in the veterinary setting, client handouts can be a very useful adjunct to verbal client education. Equally helpful can be reinforcement of key points by veterinary staff at checkout or discharge. Veterinary staff can play an instrumental role in drafting these materials, as they are often aware of common questions and issues that should be addressed. Staff involvement is expected to enhance their investment in effective transmission of this information to clients, and helps maintain a unified approach to communication.

Performing a Nutritional Assessment

An evaluation of the patient's medical status as well as lifestyle, life stage, weight trends, body composition, appetite, and diet history is a critical step to inform a confident food recommendation. The process of collecting this information, and assessing it in the context of the patient's clinical presentation, provides valuable data to the healthcare team. In some cases this may help achieve a diagnosis, while in other cases a specific treatment plan can be more confidently justified. For example, the clinician may need to discuss specific risk factors in the case of clients who feed raw meat to their omnivore or carnivore. Similarly, a different approach may need to be considered for a feline patient with recurrent constipation that has only ever eaten foods with high fiber content.

Monitoring Patient Response

Although therapeutic foods can be quite effective, not all foods work for every patient. A food's failure may be simply due to a patient being unwilling to eat the food. Therefore, monitoring both acceptance and response to a newly recommended food is crucial to improving compliance. Initially, the greatest risk to compliance is food refusal. Often this can be managed with appropriate recommendations for transitioning to the new food, as well as planned and periodic follow-up in the form of an email, phone call, or in-person office visit to address any issues that arise. Follow-up is equally important to reinforce the importance of the dietary recommendation. Recommendations that have no follow-up are more likely to be perceived as not being as crucial or important. Finally, checking on progress provides an opportunity to discuss and select an alternative but still appropriate food if the first recommendation is not successful. At times there can be a reluctance to perform follow-up since it often is "nonbillable" time; however, follow-up can be tiered or bundled, and veterinary support staff can be leveraged to assist. Many outbound calls can be conducted by veterinary staff, with elevation to veterinarians as needed. This "triaging" of sorts can increase efficiency, and often is welcomed by staff members who feel both entrusted and empowered.

Providing a Variety of Options

Since no food will work in every situation, it is important to have additional options for the client. A ready and specific alternative recommendation should reduce the likelihood that the client may choose a food by themselves, resulting in the potential for an inappropriate food to be selected and the possible loss of a medically justified sale. The tendency to stock only one "house brand" – while convenient from an inventory management perspective – decreases the ability to readily offer alternatives and can lead to a perception that there is only one option, or, worse yet, that the recommendation is made solely on the basis that the particular brand is all the veterinarian sells. Certainly, carrying every therapeutic food available (which now number in the hundreds for small animals) is not feasible in most practice settings. A selection of those foods most often used for the management of diseases seen frequently at the practice, along with a willingness to special order or even identify direct delivery options for clients, is probably the best approach.

Additionally, stocking more smaller bags can help increase the variety of foods offered without substantially increasing the "carrying cost of inventory." Small bags also can be useful for a trial, and if successful, a standing order for that patient in larger sizes can be created. Such standing orders then help to increase the number of inventory turns, thereby improving cash management. This "small bag" approach might also assist with reducing the labor involved in stocking larger bags as well as increasing the storage capacity of a facility. Some foods are also available in sample packs or starter kits, which are more cost effective and lower the commitment for clients who may be skeptical of acceptance or efficacy. In addition, most therapeutic food manufacturers will accept return not just of foods under a "satisfaction guarantee," but also of inventory that has expired. For those manufacturers where that is not the case, carrying smaller package sizes and fewer of them can minimize "perishable shrink" by reducing the cost of any expired bag that cannot be returned.

The greatest value of carrying and recommending a variety of products for the same condition can be increasing options to account for co-morbidities or other individualized needs. In addition, clinical experience with more products increases the likelihood of making the best initial recommendation, as well as increasing options for alternative products in case the initial recommendation proves unsuccessful.

Recommending Therapeutic Treats

A growing category within veterinary product offerings is therapeutic treats. These treats often pair with a "matching" therapeutic food to give the client a nutritionally appropriate treat option. Treats generally do not offer anything novel to the nutritional management of the condition or disease, but rather assist with compliance by encouraging the patient's interest in the new dietary approach while preventing the use of potentially inappropriate treats. The same process as outlined earlier should be used when recommending an effective therapeutic food.

Recommending Nutraceuticals and Dietary Supplements

For more discussion on this subject, see Chapter 5.

From a financial perspective, stocking certain dietary supplements should be considered. Although the margin on such products can vary greatly, they generally take up much less shelf space than food and treats. Typically, products that are only sold through veterinarians should be considered, unless carrying nonexclusive products adds overall value for the client due to convenience. Caution should be used when recommending or offering products for sale at a premium if comparable human supplements of equal or even greater quality or potency are available for a similar or lower price. If such products are available from other retailers, whether "brick and mortar" or online, it is in the best interest of solid client relations to refer clients to that retailer, while being sure to give a specific product and retailer recommendation for clarity and convenience. If a product is widely available only online, then clients are generally willing to purchase such products directly from the veterinarian, who may be able to compete on the basis of reduced delivery time and cost.

Creating or Increasing Revenue from Nutritional Advice

Veterinarians' time is limited for both their own continuing education and client education. Therefore, there is an "opportunity cost" associated with spending time on nutrition. If a veterinarian earns more income from learning about and performing surgery, for example, than learning about and advising on nutrition, there is a financial incentive to focus on surgery and a disincentive to focus on nutrition. Certainly the generalist cannot pick and choose only the aspects of veterinary medicine that are most profitable, but recognizing the potential for fiscal disparity provides context for a discussion on nutritional advice revenue.

The value of a veterinarian's nutritional advice can also be diluted by the perception that they lack the expertise to make nutritional recommendations. There is no shortage of such claims, especially from online sources, which are often used to dismiss or minimize expert opinion in order to promote alternative ideas or products. The perception of veterinary ignorance about nutrition can be increased by the appearance of bias for a particular brand or company's food in one's recommendation(s), as already discussed, or by a variety of compounding factors. Another factor is the belief that nutrition is not a real science or that it is not learned in veterinary school. These assertions are untrue, of course, since nutrition is such a key aspect of the management of many companion animal diseases. Thus, nutritional concepts are inherent in the veterinary curriculum, whether as distinct courses or rotations, or integrated into many other disciplines. In addition, continuing education and other resources related to nutrition are widely available to practicing veterinarians. Unfortunately, clients are not always aware that veterinarians who recommend a particular therapeutic food may choose to do so because such recommendations are based on scientifically proven strategies or have, in fact, actually been tested for the condition or disease in question. Certainly many therapeutic veterinary foods are in need of additional clinical study (Roudebush et al. 2004); however, they are largely based on very sound science.

Clients may also believe that nutrition is simple, after all, as they likely have successfully fed themselves for most of their lives. However, many people neglect to consider that many human foods are fortified with essential nutrients to address common gaps in intake, and that poor nutritional status in various human populations is not uncommon. Additionally, in circumstances where adequate intake is crucial, a carefully balanced diet (similar to pet food) is provided, such as in the intensive care unit, for baby formula, and when humans go into space or are involved in military operations. Finally, the field of nutrition is also beset by self-proclaimed "nutritionists" who have little, if any, medical or nutritional training, yet they still promote the idea that only they are experts in this discipline. Combined with the barrage of sometimes misleading and aggressive marketing used to promote a huge and growing number of pet food products, these factors have led to a level of discomfort for many on the subject, rather than the expertise or mastery they may feel on other veterinary medical topics. Thus, a climate exists where veterinarians acquiesce in the nutritional management of their patient, or at least fail to take a very active role unless intervention is absolutely necessary, such as in cases

of hepatic lipidosis or food allergy. Therefore, the following recommendations are intended to encourage practitioners to take an active role in the management of all their patients' diets.

Nutritional Advice for Healthy Patients

The number one obligation of the veterinarian when advising clients about an appropriate diet for a healthy animal companion is to ensure that it maintains an ideal body condition (see Chapter 9 on the nutritional management of body weight). Keeping dogs lean is the only proven intervention to increase both the quantity and quality of life (Kealy et al. 2002). Although yet to be proven in cats or many other companion animal species, caloric restriction has repeatedly been shown to extend lifespan in mammals (Sohal and Weindruch 1996; Barja 2004). Therefore, avoidance of overweight and obesity should be a goal for the feeding of every patient.

In addition to weight management, an appropriate food should have an appropriate nutritional adequacy statement for the patient. This means that the food is appropriate for the patient's species, age, and reproductive status if the patient is a reproducing female. As would be expected, many foods meet these criteria, and further discrimination should be based on both client and patient preference. For a client, convenience, cost, and personal nutritional philosophy may be important in deciding which foods they select. For patients, ingredients and their associated impact on palatability, along with texture (i.e. dry, wet, semi-moist) and macronutrient distribution (e.g. protein, fat, and carbohydrate percentages), play key roles in the foods they consume when given a choice. Recognizing that no one food can meet all of these preferences and needs underscores why so many brands and varieties exist and what needs to be considered when advising clients about food options.

It can often be useful to have the client select a few foods they like and review these products with them during wellness visits. This method helps to narrow down the very wide field of foods to consider, and typically provides an opportune time to exhibit some expertise, as well as an openness to discuss nutrition. If the client has no preconceived notions, then recommendations should favor companies that manufacture their own food and employ nutritionists. Such companies are more likely to have the technical expertise to address any issues that might arise, as well as the knowledge to make nutritionally sound and safe products.

From a fiscal perspective, such a review of potential foods or nutritional recommendations should not result in a unique charge for the client, but rather should be captured in the office visit fee. This assumes that any requested review does not require additional research and analysis outside the office visit. In cases where this becomes necessary, time should be charged either on an agreed flat rate or on a per-unit of time basis up to some pre-established maximum. Clients who do not wish to pay for the

veterinarian's time should be advised that the evaluation is accordingly limited. Some veterinarians find it difficult to charge for researching an issue, but if the research is specific to a patient, most clients will accept that it is appropriate when the point is raised with confidence and the resolve that one's professional time is of value. In addition, consultation with a variety of specialists is increasingly available to other clinicians, and asking for input from a board certified veterinary nutritionist® can be a valuable tool as well (Box 1.2). It should be noted that a veterinarian's review frequently involves dietary supplements, and the variety and number of novel and often unconventional supplements greatly exceed those of pet foods, which are, in practice, more closely regulated.

At times, veterinarians have difficulty distinguishing the continuing self-study required as a veterinary medical professional and the work involved in researching unique supplements or foods. The best way to distinguish this in one's

---

Box 1.2   What Is a Board Certified Veterinary Nutritionist®?

A board certified veterinary nutritionist® is a licensed veterinarian who has undergone additional education and training in the field of veterinary nutrition. This typically involves additional graduate coursework and/or graduate degrees in nutrition, along with residency training at the secondary or tertiary referral level under the supervision of a board certified veterinary nutritionist®. In addition to clinical residency training and publication of animal nutrition-related research in peer-reviewed scientific journals, candidates for certification also complete formalized clinical case benchmark exercises to demonstrate mastery of the discipline. To complete certification, candidates must also pass a rigorous, multipart general examination that covers advanced physiology, pharmacology, and disease-related topics. Candidates must also pass a more focused, intensive specialty examination that covers advanced metabolism and biochemistry as well as basic, applied, and

clinical nutrition. Candidates who successfully achieve all of the requirements can refer to themselves as board certified veterinary nutritionists® or "diplomates." There are currently two veterinary nutrition specialty colleges in the world, the American College of Veterinary Internal Medicine (nutrition is one of the six specialties of ACVIM, which is also the basis for most of the summary of requirements above) and the European College of Veterinary Comparative Nutrition (ECVCN). Members of the ACVIM Nutrition Specialty can be found in North America, the Caribbean, the United Kingdom, Europe, and Australasia, while most ECVCN diplomates are found in Europe. The majority of diplomates are employed in academia, industry, private practice, or the government. Attending veterinarians and specialists in other disciplines typically refer cases to diplomates of the ACVIM Nutrition Specialty or ECVCN in academia or at large referral hospitals.

own mind is that the veterinarian is not charging for the knowledge of how to interpret and find information, but rather for the act of applying their critical thinking and scientific knowledge to the patient's and/or client's specific products and/or needs. An analogy might be that one does not charge for the time it takes to learn a surgical procedure, but rather charges for using the resulting skills and knowledge to perform the surgery on particular patients.

Nutritional Advice for Unhealthy Patients

Most, if not all, diseases and conditions can be affected by diet. In some cases, this may simply be related to the adverse effects of inadequate caloric intake associated with illness-related hyporexia or anorexia. For many other diseases, there are specific nutritional management interventions that are the subject of most of the rest of this textbook. For these sick patients, both improved outcomes and revenue generation are more likely to occur through the use of veterinary therapeutic foods, treats, and/or parenteral solutions, or through procedures such as feeding tube placement, compared to specific nutritional guidance and/or advice involved in

their selection. However, it should be noted that consultation with a board certified veterinary nutritionist® on specific cases will generate justified fees for such advice, and the primary veterinarian will need in turn to communicate this to the client. It is recommended that when a board certified veterinary nutritionist® needs to be consulted, the referring veterinarian charges for their time specifically if they act as the "conduit" for the consultation, similar to how clinical pathology reports may be handled.

A veterinarian should not hesitate to charge for their time, or to set up an office visit specifically to address an unhealthy patient's nutritional needs and educate the client accordingly. The veterinarian should be able to realize adequate revenue through nutritional counseling, product sales, and nutrition-related procedures, to justify the full integration of nutrition into clinical practice to the benefit of healthy and unhealthy patients. It is expected that the reader of the rest of this textbook should be better able to advise clients about the nutritional management of unhealthy patients and recognize when consultation with or direct referral to a board certified veterinary nutritionist® is indicated.

References

AAHA (2003). *The Path to High-Quality Care*. Lakewood, CO: American Animal Hospital Association Press.

AAHA (2019). *Financial & Productivity Pulsepoints*, 10e. Lakewood, CO: American Animal Hospital Association Press.

Barja, G. (2004). Aging in vertebrates, and the effect of caloric restriction: a mitochondrial free radical production-DNA damage mechanism? *Biol. Rev. Camb. Philos. Soc.* 79 (2): 235–251.

Kealy, R., Lawler, D., Ballam, J. et al. (2002). Effects of diet restriction on life span and age-related changes in dogs. *J. Am. Vet. Med. Assoc.* 220 (9): 1315–1320.

Langdon, I., Hardin, R., and Learmonth, I. (2002). Informed consent for total hip arthroplasty: does a written information sheet improve recall by patients? *Ann. R. Coll. Surg. Engl.* 84 (6): 404–408.

Roudebush, P., Allen, T., Dodd, C. et al. (2004). Application of evidence-based medicine to veterinary clinical nutrition. *J. Am. Vet. Med. Assoc.* 224 (11): 1765–1771.

Sohal, R.S. and Weindruch, R. (1996). Oxidative stress, caloric restriction, and aging. *Science* 273 (5271): 59–63.

Volk, J.O., Felsted, K.E., Thomas, J.G. et al. (2011). Executive summary of the Bayer veterinary care usage study. *J. Am. Vet. Med. Assoc.* 238 (10): 1275–1282.

2

Basic Nutrition Overview

Sean J. Delaney and Andrea J. Fascetti

While the vast majority of this text is focused on the application of veterinary nutrition in clinical practice, this chapter centers around basic nutrition. Although the chapter is not exhaustive, it should provide enough depth to enable the applied veterinary clinical nutrition portion of the text to be used with a strong understanding of key underlying nutrition principles.

Energy

After oxygen and water, the next most important component for any animal to gain from its environment is energy. Energy is available from the macronutrients of protein, fat, and carbohydrate, each providing a specific amount of energy that can be measured or estimated. Currently the most commonly used unit for measuring energy is the pre-International System (SI) metric unit, kilocalories (kcal), which is equal to "Calories" (with an uppercase "C") seen on human food labels in certain countries like the United States (1000 kcal is often written as "Mcal," the abbreviation for Megacalorie). The less commonly used SI unit for energy, kiloJoule (kJ), is converted from kilocalorie or Calorie by multiplying by 4.185 (1 kcal or Calorie = 4.185 kJ).

In pet food, both the energy content of the food and the requirements of the animal are expressed as metabolizable energy, which is the energy available to be used after fecal and urinary losses are accounted for. The amount of metabolizable energy is determined by knowing the mass of the macronutrient in a food or diet and the corresponding energy conversion factor. Energy conversion factors are standardized values for the amount of energy available from a gram of the specified macronutrient. For pet foods, the energy conversion factors that are used are referred to as modified Atwater factors: 3.5, 8.5, and 3.5 kcal/g for protein, fat and carbohydrate, respectively. These values are slightly lower than those used for human foods (i.e. 4 kcal/g for protein, 9 kcal/g for fat, and 4 kcal/g for carbohydrate) due to the typically lower digestibility of pet food (assumed average apparent digestibility for protein is 80%, 90% for fat, and 84% for carbohydrate). There are other equations to estimate the metabolizable content of pet food. For example, in Europe, the metabolizable energy content of commercial pet foods must be estimated using the equation provided by the National Research Council (NRC) (2006b), based on protein, fat, carbohydrate, and fiber.

Dietary energy is used to create adenosine triphosphate (ATP) through phosphorylation as ATP is the "energy currency" of the body. For protein (which is made up of amino acids) this means conversion to glucose via gluconeogenesis with ATP generation via glycolysis and the Krebs or tricarboxylic acid (TCA) cycle during cellular respiration. Gluconeogenesis is the metabolic pathway by which glucogenic amino acids (lysine and leucine excluded) are converted to glucose. Glucose is then converted to pyruvate during glycolysis, which produces ATP and the potential for more ATP if pyruvate enters the TCA cycle. For fat (which contains fatty acids), ATP is typically produced via beta oxidation where ATP is produced from acetyl coenzyme A (acetyl-CoA) in the TCA cycle. Generated glucose or glucose from the breakdown of glycogen or starch and from sugars in the diet can be used to generate ATP via glycolysis and the TCA cycle as well. It should be noted that the TCA cycle produces substantially more ATP than glycolysis, which solely generates pyruvate, but the TCA cycle cannot occur in the absence of oxygen, and thus the importance of breathing and the intake of oxygen in the production of energy by the body. However, lactic acid produced during anaerobic glycolysis (typically in muscle) can be converted to glucose by the liver in the Cori cycle.

It is worth noting that any protein consumed in excess of needs for anabolic pathways such as protein synthesis will be converted to glucose or fat and used or stored in those forms as a source of energy, as there is no body store for amino acids (as opposed to fat, which will be stored in adipose tissue, and glucose, which can be stored as glycogen). The energy provided by protein, fat, and carbohydrate that exceeds energy needs will end up being stored as adipose tissue. Unlike glycogen, theoretically there is no limit in the amount of energy that can be stored in adipose tissue, although there may be adverse health consequences with extreme levels of storage as seen with obesity.

Energy Requirements

Dogs and cats eat to meet their energy needs. Unlike some species that have "specific hungers" for certain nutrients (e.g. ruminants for certain minerals), dogs and cats will not seek out certain foods or nutrients in the face of specific nutrient deficiencies. This makes sense teleologically for a carnivore like the cat or a species that has some carnivorous roots or tendencies like the dog. From an evolutionary perspective, there was (or is) no penalty for the inability to seek out specific nutrients, as the search for and consumption of specific evolutionary prey species should inherently provide the right balance and types of essential nutrients. The only risk for deficiency is really related to inadequate consumption of prey. Therefore, determining a dog's or cat's energy requirement is very important.

Pet foods are generally formulated with a certain amount of nutrient per unit of energy. This ensures that essential nutrients are provided to the dog or cat at appropriate levels when fed to meet the pet's energy requirement. Consequently, this means that pets that are fed such foods below their energy requirement are in danger of nutritional deficiencies. Pets fed above their energy requirement are in danger of receiving excessive amounts of nutrients (this latter case really only represents a risk of obesity or potentially urolithiasis). For further discussion on determining a dog's or cat's energy requirement as well as different energy terms such as gross energy, digestible energy, metabolizable energy, and net energy, the reader is referred to Chapter 3 on energy requirements.

Essential Nutrients

Essential nutrients are organic compounds and non-organic elements that cannot be produced by the body but are needed to support life. Essentiality is different for different species, although for mammalian species such as the dog and the cat there are many similarities in what is essential; differences are mainly in the amount needed. In addition, there are nutrients that are required only at certain times or under the right circumstances. These nutrients are referred to as "conditionally essential nutrients." An example of a conditionally essential nutrient that also exemplifies interspecies differences is the amino acid taurine. In premature human infants, taurine, which is essential for cats but not dogs, is conditionally essential. Premature neonates are not metabolically mature enough to produce adequate amounts of taurine from the normal sulfur amino acid precursors, methionine and cystine.

Cysteine is a good example of another category of nutrients that are called "sparing." Sparing nutrients are able to decrease the amount of essential nutrients needed in the diet. Methionine is an essential sulfur amino acid, and one of its main roles is to synthesize cysteine (a non-essential amino acid). Thus, directly including cysteine in the diet decreases by up to 50% the amount of methionine needed in the diets of both dogs and cats. Methionine itself is sparing for choline, as it can also serve as a source of methyl groups. Therefore, methionine is both an essential and a sparing nutrient. The other commonly encountered sparing nutrient is tyrosine, which spares the amino acid phenylalanine and has been shown to be important in maximal melanin synthesis in black cats (Yu et al. 2001).

As cited in Box 2.1, the cat as a true carnivore requires nutrients that the dog as an omnivore does not. The following is a list of the cat's unique metabolics:

- Unable to convert carotenoids to adequate vitamin A/retinol.
- Inadequate synthesis of vitamin D (even if hairless and exposed to sunlight/ultraviolet [UV] radiation). The dog is also unable to synthesize all required vitamin D.
- Unable to use tryptophan for niacin synthesis.
- Unable to synthesize adequate amounts of taurine from sulfur amino acids, methionine, and cysteine.
- Unable to synthesize citrulline (needed for the urea cycle; as a result, a single

arginine-free but protein-containing meal can cause death).
- Glutamic acid (high in plants and low in animal tissues) intolerance.
- Reduced ability to conserve nitrogen.
- Reduced ability to desaturate long-chain polyunsaturated fatty acids (PUFAs), therefore need arachidonic acid, since cats are unable to make it from its precursor, linoleic acid.
- Metabolically adapted to low-carbohydrate diet (e.g. less activity of enzymes involved in glucose metabolism like glucokinase, which is the enzyme needed for the first step in deriving ATP from glucose).

Protein and Amino Acids

Protein provides nitrogen and amino acids in the diet. Amino acids are either essential or non-essential (or dispensable). Essential amino acids for dogs and cats include arginine, which is not essential for humans. In addition cats require taurine, unlike dogs and humans who can make adequate amounts from sulfur amino acid precursors. In commercial pet foods, taurine, like several other commonly limiting amino acids, can be supplied as a purified amino acid. Essential amino acids (except taurine) can potentially come in two isoforms: L-amino acids and D-amino acids. L-amino acids are the commonly encountered form, while D-amino acids are less common and at times less available or unavailable for use by the body. For example, D-lysine cannot be used by dogs and cats the way L-lysine can be. However, D-methionine can be used to meet up to 50% of the methionine requirement. Therefore, one should not see a dog or cat food supplemented with D-lysine, but can see one supplemented with DL-methionine.

Methionine can be added for urine acidification and is also used in pet foods that derive a large portion of their protein content from legumes such as soy, which are limiting in sulfur amino acids. Limiting means that the particular essential amino acid in that

---

Box 2.1   List of Essential Nutrients for Dogs and Cats by Group

Protein

- Amino acids
  - Arginine
  - Histidine
  - Isoleucine
  - Leucine
  - Lysine
  - Methionine (spared by cystine)
  - Phenylalanine (spared by tyrosine)
  - Threonine
  - Tryptophan
  - Valine
  - Taurine (cat, not dog)

Fat

- Linoleic acid
- Arachidonic acid (cat, not dog)
- +/– Eicosapentaenoic acid (EPA) and doco-sahexaenoic acid (DHA)

Minerals

- Macrominerals (required at ≥100 mg/Mcal, or approx. ≥400 ppm)
  - Calcium (Ca)
  - Phosphorus (P)
  - Magnesium (Mg)
  - Sodium (Na)
  - Potassium (K)
  - Chloride (Cl)

- Trace minerals or microminerals (required at <100 mg/Mcal, or approx. <400 ppm)
  - Iron (Fe)
  - Copper (Cu)
  - Zinc (Zn)
  - Manganese (Mn)
  - Selenium (Se)
  - Iodine (I)

Vitamins

- Fat-soluble vitamins
  - Vitamin A, retinol
  - Vitamin D3, cholecalciferol
  - Vitamin E, α-tocopherol
  - +/– Vitamin K3, menadione (also vitamin K1, phylloquinone) (cat, not dog)

- Water-soluble vitamins
  - Thiamin, vitamin B1
  - Riboflavin, vitamin B2
  - Pyridoxine, vitamin B6
  - Niacin, vitamin B3
  - Pantothenic acid, vitamin B5
  - Cobalamin, vitamin B12
  - Folic acid, vitamin B9
  - Biotin, vitamin H or B7
  - Choline

---

ingredient/formulation is closest to the requirement of the species. Therefore, when the species' requirement for that essential amino acid is met, all other essential amino acids the protein provides are in excess of the requirement. Thus, it can be more cost effective for a pet food manufacturer to add a single limiting amino acid in its purified form (likely to be a DL-amino acid where available to reduce cost) than to simply increase the amount of protein-rich ingredients to meet a single amino acid requirement. In addition to sulfur amino acids that are limiting in legumes, lysine is typically limiting in grains. Ancestral peoples recognized this in a limited way and combined legumes and grains (e.g. "rice and beans") in meals to ensure a complete and balanced amino acid profile.

There are several ways to assess an ingredient's or a food's protein content. The typically required and reported crude protein value does not give any indication of how well a food will meet a dog's or cat's protein or amino acid requirements, although higher crude protein values are often perceived as better. In fact, crude protein does not even represent protein content directly, but rather nitrogen content times 6.25 (assuming that all nitrogen is from protein and that protein contains 16% nitrogen). Therefore, crude protein is really an indirect measurement of protein quantity and does not provide any information about quality. Ideally, a measure of protein quality should provide some insight as to how well a particular source of protein meets the protein and amino acid requirements of a particular species, which depends on amino acid profile and bioavailability. Values for protein quality include the following:

- Protein efficiency ratio (PER) is the gain in body mass or weight for a subject fed a particular food divided by the mass of the protein intake; higher values mean the protein quality is higher.
- Biological value (BV) is the mass of nitrogen incorporated into the subject's body divided by the mass of nitrogen from protein in the food times 100. A value of 100% (sometimes given to fresh chicken egg protein by convention) means all of the dietary protein eaten and absorbed becomes protein in the body; thus 100% is the absolute maximum, with lower values indicating lower quality.
- Net protein utilization (NPU) is the ratio of amino acids converted to protein to the amino acids provided by the food; a value of 1 is the highest value possible and is given to fresh chicken eggs.
- Protein digestibility corrected amino acid score (PDCAAS) is mg of limiting amino acid (for humans) in 1 g of test protein/mg of the same amino acid in 1 g of reference protein times true digestibility percentage (fecal); values up to 1 can be achieved, and the closer to 1 the higher the protein quality.

All of these methods have flaws, but generally they predict how well a particular protein-rich food will meet an animal's or human's protein and/or amino acid needs. Unfortunately, these values are not reported for pet foods or for many protein-rich ingredients used in pet foods.

Fat

Besides energy provision, fats facilitate fat-soluble vitamin absorption and provide essential and important fatty acids that have multiple roles in the body, including structural (main components of cell membranes) and eicosanoid production. Essential fatty acids are polyunsaturated and from the omega 6 and 3 families, depending on the location of the first double bond counting from the omega (methyl) end. Linoleic acid (LA) is essential for both the dog and cat and is 18 carbons long with two double bonds, and can be referred to as "18:2(n-6)" where the "18" is the carbon chain length, the "2" is for the number of double bonds and the "n" denotes the family. Similarly, arachidonic acid (AA; sometimes abbreviated ARA, especially on human infant formula and to distinguish it from the abbreviation for amino acid) is essential for cats, and can be referred to as "20:4(n-6)" since it has more carbon (20) and double bonds (4). Dogs can synthesize AA from LA. Good sources of LA are vegetable oils (such as corn, walnut, or sunflower) or fats from animals raised predominantly on plants rich in LA such as corn-fed chickens. Good sources of AA are animal fats, although gamma-linolenic acid (GLA or 18:3(n-6); note the second "n" in linolenic that is not present in linoleic acid or LA) from borage oil and evening primrose oil can be used as a precursor in cats that cannot derive AA or ARA from LA as humans and dogs can.

The n-3 or omega-3 fatty acids are thus named because their "first" double bond is at the third carbon from the "omega" end. Terrestrial plants such as flaxseed (or linseed) can be rich sources of n-3 fatty acids in the form of alpha-linolenic acid (ALA or 18:3(n-3)), but its shorter carbon chain cannot be efficiently elongated to the more "beneficial" (see later) long-chain n-3 fatty acids, eicosapentaenoic (EPA, 20:5(n-3)) and docosahexaenoic (DHA, 22:6(n-3)) acids. Therefore, marine oils such as algal oil, krill oil, and fish oil are preferred as sources of n-3 fatty acids. Generally, species closest on the food chain to phytoplankton (which can efficiently synthesize the longer-chain n-3 fatty acids) are selected to avoid the concurrent issue of bioaccumulation of pollutants. It is worth noting that there is debate about the importance of the ratio of n-6 to n-3 fatty acids versus the total dietary amount of long-chain n-3 fatty acids (NRC 2006b). It would seem that the increased production of the less inflammatory eicosanoids from long-chain n-3 fatty acids would be greatest when the least amount of alternative n-6 fatty acid precursors is available.

Carbohydrates

Although carbohydrates are not essential, they are included here as they provide energy. In addition, carbohydrate-rich ingredients or foods are also the source of dietary fiber, which can be important for normal gastrointestinal (GI) function and health. Also, fiber is often used in the nutritional management of diabetes mellitus to reduce postprandial hyperglycemia, and in weight management to decrease energy density (i.e. kcal per can or cup) and potentially promote satiety.

The measure of fiber typically reported on pet food labels is crude fiber. This analytic method does not capture all forms of fiber and largely reports the insoluble portion. A better value used for human foods is total dietary fiber, which includes both soluble and insoluble fibers. Soluble fiber has the ability to hold water and generally makes feces softer. Common sources of soluble fiber are fruits and gums, with gums more commonly used in pet food as they are frequently employed to improve canned food texture. Insoluble fiber generally increases fecal bulk, but does not soften feces as it does not have the ability to absorb water. Insoluble fiber generally comes from grains in the diet (although fiber from whole grains is typically mixed, including both soluble and insoluble fibers) and can be added in the form of cellulose. Many fiber types used for supplementation are mixed

fibers. The best example of a mixed fiber type is psyllium fiber, found in products like Metamucil® (Procter & Gamble, Cincinnati, OH, USA). It is also worth noting that many soluble fibers are fermentable to different degrees. Fermentable fibers can be used by normal gut bacteria as an energy source and in the process produce short-chain fatty acids that have many roles, including being an energy source for enterocytes and colonocytes. Fermentable fibers that promote the growth of beneficial bacteria are sometimes referred to as prebiotics (for more discussion about fiber and microflora, see Chapter 12).

Minerals

Macrominerals
Minerals that are needed by dogs and cats in amounts of 100 mg/Mcal or more are generally considered macrominerals. These minerals (e.g. calcium, phosphorus, magnesium, sodium, potassium, and chloride) are commonly provided in intravenous fluids. Typical dietary sources for calcium are bone or calcium salts. Phosphorus comes from protein-rich foods, plants, and bones, and is often supplied in adequate levels in pet foods that use "meals," which can have a significant amount of bone and thus phosphorus. Magnesium, sodium, potassium, and chloride can often be found in the form of salts in pet food.

The form of the mineral salt affects its bioavailability (for both macro- and microminerals). Although this can be the case either due to a truly higher bioavailability or due to a higher potency (i.e. more elemental mineral per unit of mass of salt due to molecular formula differences), most of these differences can be overcome by simply providing more of the salt so that an equivalent amount of the essential element is delivered. However, it should be noted that some mineral salts, such as oxides, are poorly available, and therefore care should be taken that selected salts provide a known percentage of available element(s).

Trace Minerals (Microminerals)

Microminerals are elements that are generally needed by dogs and cats in amounts less than 100 mg/Mcal. These trace minerals are generally provided from the consumption of liver or entire prey in nature, but supplementation in the form of salts is more common in commercial pet food. Inorganic salts are common, but chelated forms bound to amino acids and peptides do exist. These chelated forms are typically (but not always) more bioavailable and may be better tolerated than certain inorganic forms (e.g. iron proteinate vs. iron sulfate) in some cases.

Vitamins

Water Soluble

For dogs and cats, the only essential water-soluble vitamins are B vitamins, because unlike humans they are able to synthesize vitamin C from glucose. Sources of B vitamins include internal organs, the germinal portion of grains, and yeasts. Vitamin B12 is the exception because it must come from animal sources. Since B vitamins can generally be eliminated in urine, they are considered very safe and there are generally no set maximums or safe upper limits (SULs), although high doses of niacin can cause "flushing" due to prostaglandin-induced vasodilation.

Vitamin C is commonly used in natural pet foods as an antioxidant for potential benefits within the body, as well as being a component in natural preservation systems to recycle mixed tocopherols used to prevent fat oxidation/rancidity. Excessive dietary vitamin C is raised as a concern in patients with a history of calcium oxalate urolithiasis, since it can increase urinary oxalate excretion (Baxmann et al. 2003). Vitamin C is mainly provided in a purified form, but rich natural sources include fruits and vegetables.

Fat Soluble

For dogs and cats, the fat-soluble vitamins A, D, and E are essential. They are stored in the body and can be potentially toxic, particularly vitamins A and D, therefore they have described SULs. Vitamin K, although essential, can typically be provided in adequate amounts by gut microbial synthesis. An exception to this is when a diet high in fish is consumed by cats (Strieker et al. 1996). The exact mechanism by which a vitamin K deficiency is created is unknown, but Dr. James Morris, professor emeritus at the University of California–Davis, has suggested that it could be due to the high levels of vitamin E in fish (personal communication), which could delay oxidation of vitamin K hydroquinone, or act as a competitive inhibitor of vitamin K. Cat foods rich in fish (>25% fish on a dry matter basis) are currently required by states that adopt Association of American Feed Control Officials (AAFCO) guidelines (see Chapter 5) to add vitamin K3 or menadione, and not the natural form vitamin K1 or phylloquinone found in foods such as green leafy vegetables. Occasionally, the safety of oral menadione supplementation is raised as a concern, but the basis of these concerns is not fully supported by the published literature (National Research Council (NRC) 2006b).

Vitamin A can be produced from carotenoids such as beta-carotene present in orange- or red-colored fruits and vegetables such as carrots as well as in green leafy vegetables. Cats, however, are unable to efficiently perform this conversion, so their diet must contain active vitamin A or retinol. Hypervitaminosis A can occur when large amounts of liver are consumed (as discussed later in this chapter).

In contrast to humans, dogs and cats cannot synthesize sufficient vitamin D and it is therefore a dietary essential (Hazewinkel et al. 1987; Morris 1999). Typically vitamin D3 (cholecalciferol) is supplemented in pet food and is usually derived from lanolin from sheep's wool. Vitamin D3 is inactive as it is unhydroxylated; the hydroxylated active form is called calcitriol (1,25-dihydroxyvitamin D3). The richest natural sources of vitamin D are fatty fishes.

Vitamin E is a family of eight antioxidants (four tocopherols and four tocotrienols), each of which has several isomers, all with differing activities. The natural form is D-alpha-tocopherol, and pet food often includes a synthetic form (DL-alpha-tocopherol). These are usually provided esterified (e.g. as acetate) to protect from oxidation during storage. On the other hand, "mixed tocopherols," which contain different isomers, are used in commercial pet foods to protect against oxidative damage to dietary fat during storage and are not included to provide vitamin E activity to the animal. They do not provide the same relative activity as alpha-tocopherol or what is frequently referred to as "vitamin E" (i.e. beta 1/2, delta 1/10, gamma 1/10 the activity of alpha). Therefore, any guarantees for vitamin E (which is really a family of eight antioxidants) amounts should be representative of the biologically active portion of all "tocopherols" and "tocotrienols" present. Occasionally, "natural" vitamin E is suggested as being superior for supplementation, which is based on the fact that D-alpha-tocopherol has about twice the biological activity of synthetic DL-alpha-tocopherol. Obviously, this difference in biological activity can be corrected for by making adjustments in dosing when using synthetic versus natural alpha-tocopherol. Good natural sources are seeds, the germ portion found in whole grains, vegetable oils, and green leafy vegetables.

Storage Pools for Essential Nutrients

Unfortunately, malnutrition can affect veterinary patients. As such, it is important to briefly discuss the concept of nutrient storage pools. The body's main focus for storage is energy in the form of glycogen, which is rapidly depleted within a matter of hours, and fat, which can last patients days to weeks depending on adiposity. Along with fat, fat-soluble vitamins can be deficient in a patient's diet for weeks to months without clinically identifiable consequences, assuming that a good plane of nutrition was maintained prior to the deficient diet or the lack of access to food. Some of the macrominerals, specifically calcium and phosphorus, have stores in the form of bone, and it can take long periods (i.e. months to even years in the case of calcium) to recognize clinical manifestations of a deficient diet in an adult dog or cat. Deficiencies in water-soluble vitamins and several electrolytes like potassium can be more rapidly recognized given the lack of body storage pools. Similarly, there is no storage pool for protein or amino acids, and so deficient diets result in a breakdown of body tissues such as muscle. Therefore, incomplete and unbalanced diets that are deficient in protein, electrolytes, and B vitamins are much more likely to result in clinically identifiable problems in previously appropriately fed adults than those diets that do not have adequate amounts of fat, fatty acids, fat-soluble vitamins, and calcium, at least in the short to medium term. This explains the lack of apparent consequences often seen in adult patients fed diets of just cottage cheese/chicken/meat and enriched rice (enriched in B vitamins). In the authors' clinical experience, diets deficient in thiamin and calcium that clinically present to veterinarians in practice (e.g. neurologic and skeletal, respectively) are most likely to be identified in adults. Many nutritional deficiencies will appear more rapidly in growing dogs and cats fed a deficient diet due to the high demand for nutrients during this period. A more comprehensive list of nutrient deficiencies, their clinical signs, and the methods for diagnosing follows.

Essential Nutrient Deficiency Signs and Clinically Available or Relevant Methods of Assessing Nutrient Status

For detailed information the reader is referred to the *Nutrient Requirements of Dogs and Cats* from the National Research Council published by the United States National Academies in 2006.

Protein

Weight loss (or lack of weight gain if a puppy or kitten), hypoalbuminemia (albumin has a half-life of approximately 20–21 days, so it may take a while for this marker to become low), and poor coat quality may also be recognized; plus any of the clinical signs associated with specific amino acid deficiencies, especially those associated with the limiting amino acids, often methionine, lysine, and tryptophan for both dogs and cats.

RECOMMENDED TESTING: Albumin and potentially analyze diet sample for crude protein with a commercial food laboratory. If a large portion of nitrogen is suspected not to be from protein, amino acid analysis, as well as evaluation using commercial formulation software if nutrient data are available.

Amino Acids

Arginine

In dogs, vomiting, ptyalism, and muscle tremors are seen with arginine-free diets; simply deficient diets have resulted in cataracts in puppies (orotic aciduria has also been reported, but there is no readily available commercial laboratory test available). In cats, diarrhea, weight loss, food refusal, and hyperammonemia; if completely devoid (only experimentally possible, but deficiency possible with human enteral products that may be used in veterinary critical care patients) death may result.

RECOMMENDED TESTING: Fasted plasma amino acid sample and potentially analyze a diet sample, as well as evaluate using commercial formulation software if nutrient data are available.

Histidine

In dogs, weight loss, decreased hemoglobin and albumin concentrations, food refusal, lethargy. In cats, cataracts and decreased hemoglobin.

RECOMMENDED TESTING: Hemoglobin and fasted plasma amino acid sample and potentially analyze a diet sample, as well as evaluate using commercial formulation software if nutrient data are available.

Isoleucine

Clinical signs have only been reported for growing dogs and cats; in puppies, poor food intake and weight gain; in kittens, reddish-purple tinted crusty material around eyes, nose, and mouth, desquamation on paw pads, and incoordination.

RECOMMENDED TESTING: Fasted plasma amino acid sample and potentially analyze a diet sample, as well as evaluate using commercial formulation software if nutrient data are available.

Leucine

Clinical signs have only been reported for growing dogs and cats: in puppies, weight loss and decreased food intake; in kittens, weight loss.

RECOMMENDED TESTING: Fasted plasma amino acid sample and potentially analyze a diet sample, as well as evaluate using commercial formulation software if nutrient data are available.

Lysine

Clinical signs have only been reported for growing dogs and cats: in puppies, decreased food intake and weight loss; in kittens, weight loss (in other species, graying of hair has been noted, but this has not been recognized in dogs and cats).

RECOMMENDED TESTING: Fasted plasma amino acid sample and potentially analyze a diet sample, as well as evaluate using commercial formulation software if nutrient data are available.

Methionine (Spared by Cystine)

In dogs, pigment gallstones and dilated cardiomyopathy (DCM) secondary to taurine deficiency, and in puppies, weight loss, swelling and reddening of the skin, necrotic and hyperkeratotic front foot pads with ulceration; in cats, severe perioral and footpad lesions, and in kittens weight loss, lethargy, and abnormal ocular secretions.

RECOMMENDED TESTING: Fasted plasma amino acid sample and potentially analyze a diet sample, as well as evaluate using commercial formulation software if nutrient data are available; imaging, especially for DCM, as well as whole blood and plasma taurine in dogs.

Phenylalanine (Spared by Tyrosine)

In dogs, reddish-brown hair coat in black dogs, and in puppies, decreased food intake and weight loss; in cats, abnormal, uncoordinated gait with the tail bending forward, ptyalism, vocalizing and hyperactivity, and in kittens, weight loss and reddish-brown hair in black cats.

RECOMMENDED TESTING: Fasted plasma amino acid sample; potentially analyze a diet sample, as well as evaluate using commercial formulation software if nutrient data are available; close inspection of any black hairs for reddish-brown tint.

Threonine

Clinical signs have only been reported for growing dogs and cats: in puppies, decreased food intake and weight loss; in kittens, decreased food intake and weight loss and cerebellar dysfunction with slight tremors, ataxia, jerky head and leg movements, and difficulty maintaining equilibrium.

RECOMMENDED TESTING: Fasted plasma amino acid sample and potentially analyze a diet sample, as well as evaluate using commercial formulation software if nutrient data are available.

Tryptophan

Clinical signs have only been reported for growing dogs and cats, although additional tryptophan has been reported to reduce territorial aggression (DeNapoli et al. 2000); in puppies, decreased food intake and weight loss; in kittens, decreased food intake and weight loss.

RECOMMENDED TESTING: Fasted plasma amino acid sample and potentially analyze a diet sample, as well as evaluate using commercial formulation software if nutrient data are available

Valine

Clinical signs have only been reported for growing dogs and cats: in puppies, decreased food intake and weight loss; in kittens, weight loss.

RECOMMENDED TESTING: Fasted plasma amino acid sample and potentially analyze a diet sample, as well as evaluate using commercial formulation software if nutrient data are available.

Taurine

This amino acid is required only in cats; feline central retinal degeneration and blindness, DCM and heart failure, deafness, poor reproduction with congenital defects including hydrocephalus and anencephaly can result when it is deficient; in dogs, taurine can become depleted due to insufficient dietary precursor(s), methionine (and cystine), DCM, and poor reproduction.

RECOMMEND TESTING: Fasted plasma amino acid sample and whole blood sample; potentially analyze a diet sample, as well as evaluate using commercial formulation software if nutrient data are available; fundic examination and echocardiogram; review breeding program and health status of breeding animals to rule out other causes of poor reproductive performance.

Fat

Linoleic Acid

In puppies, greasy pruritic skin with keratinization with parakeratosis; in cats, dry, lusterless hair, dandruff, behavioral infertility, and hepatic lipid infiltrates. No dog or kitten clinical signs have been reported but are likely an amalgamation of the signs seen in puppies and cats.

RECOMMENDED TESTING: Potentially analyze a diet sample, as well as evaluate using commercial formulation software if nutrient data are available; consider LA-rich oil supplementation if only a dull coat with scaling or dandruff presents; monitor for resolution for confirmation of likely LA deficiency.

Arachidonic Acid (Cat, Not Dog)

AA is not required in dogs as they have adequate activity of delta-6-desaturase to convert LA to AA, unlike cats; in cats, reproductive failure with congenital defects and low kitten viability, and deficiency may manifest only after one or two successful litters.

RECOMMENDED TESTING: Potentially analyze a diet sample, as well as evaluate using commercial formulation software if nutrient data are available; review breeding program and health status of breeding animals to rule out other causes of poor reproductive performance.

Minerals

Macrominerals (Typically Required at ≥100 mg/Mcal)

Calcium

In dogs and puppies, nutritional secondary hyperparathyroidism (see Chapter 10); in kittens, bone rarefaction, especially of the pelvis and lumbar vertebrae; in cats, decreased bone density; in cats and kittens, nutritional secondary hyperparathyroidism.

RECOMMENDED TESTING: Potentially analyze a diet sample, as well as evaluate using commercial formulation software if nutrient data are available; whole body radiographs ensuring that mandibular, vertebral, and pelvic bones are imaged; serum calcium concentrations are likely maintained within normal reference intervals; however, ionized calcium, parathyroid hormone (PTH), and vitamin D measurements may be useful.

Phosphorus

In dogs, hypophosphatemia and, if severe, anemia may be present; and in puppies, poor growth and hypophosphatemia (remember to compare to reference intervals for growing dogs, as adults inherently have lower P concentrations).

RECOMMENDED TESTING: Serum phosphorus concentrations and potentially analyze a diet sample, as well as evaluate using commercial formulation software if nutrient data are available.

Magnesium

In dogs, hypomagnesemia, and in puppies, lameness and hyperextension of carpi; in cats, hypomagnesemia, and in kittens, poor growth, hyperextension of metacarpi, muscular twitching, and convulsions.

RECOMMENDED TESTING: Serum ionized magnesium concentrations and potentially analyze a diet sample, as well as evaluate using commercial formulation software if nutrient data are available.

Sodium

In dogs, hyponatremia, and in puppies, dry, tacky mucous membranes, restlessness, and increased heart rate, hematocrit, and hemoglobin (likely hemoconcentration), as well as polyuria and polydipsia; in cats, hyponatremia, and in kittens, anorexia, poor growth, polyuria, polydipsia, hemoconcentration.

RECOMMENDED TESTING: Serum sodium concentrations and potentially analyze a diet sample, as well as evaluate using commercial formulation software if nutrient data are available.

Potassium

In dogs, hypokalemia and hypotension; in puppies, poor growth, restlessness, ventroflexion of the head, rear leg paralysis, and generalized weakness; in cats, hypokalemia and elevation in serum creatinine; in kittens, anorexia, poor growth, ventroflexion of the head, ataxia, and muscular weakness leading to the inability to walk.

RECOMMENDED TESTING: Serum potassium concentrations and potentially analyze a diet sample, as well as evaluate using commercial formulation software if nutrient data are available.

Chloride

Clinical signs have only been reported for growing dogs and cats; in puppies, hypochloremia, hypokalemia, and metabolic alkalosis, poor growth, weakness, ataxia (potentially due to concurrent potassium deficiency); in kittens, hypokalemia.

RECOMMENDED TESTING: Serum chloride and potassium concentrations and potentially analyze a diet sample, as well as evaluate using commercial formulation software if nutrient data are available.

Microminerals (Typically Required at <100 mg/Mcal)

Iron

In dogs, microcytic hypochromic anemia and a low-percentage saturation of plasma transferrin, and in puppies, low hemoglobin concentrations and hematocrit, poor growth, pale mucous membranes, lethargy, weakness, diarrhea, hematochezia, and melena.

RECOMMEND TESTING: Complete blood count and total iron-binding capacity (TIBC) and, if available, plasma ferritin along with percent saturation; reticulocyte indices may also be worth exploring, even though there is some debate about their value and they may not be clinically available (Steinberg and Olver 2005; Fry and Kirk 2006); potentially analyze a diet sample, as well as evaluate using commercial formulation software if nutrient data are available.

Copper

In dogs, no clinical signs reported, and in puppies, loss of hair pigmentation and hyperextension of the distal phalanges; in cats, increased time to conception in queens, and in kittens, fading coat color, hindlimb ataxia, twisted limbs, and curled tails.

RECOMMENDED TESTING: Liver biopsy is considered the gold standard, but if it is not practical, consider serum or plasma copper in dogs (not reflective of status in cats); potentially analyze a diet sample, as well as evaluate using commercial formulation software if nutrient data are available. If the sole source of copper supplementation is cupric oxide, this may increase suspicion as this form has very poor bioavailability.

Zinc

In dogs, skin lesions, and in puppies, very poor growth rates, skin lesions starting at contact or wear points like foot pads (also see Chapter 11); in cats, no clinical signs reported, and in kittens, poor growth and skin lesions.

RECOMMENDED TESTING: Plasma zinc and analyze a diet sample, as well as evaluate using commercial formulation software if nutrient data are available.

Manganese

In dogs and cats, there are no reports of clinical signs seen with manganese deficiency (there are reports in other species suggesting bone and joint abnormalities).

RECOMMENDED TESTING: Consider whole blood manganese analysis; analyze a diet sample, as well as evaluate using commercial formulation software if nutrient data are available.

Selenium

In dogs, cats, and kittens, there are no reports of clinical signs; in puppies, anorexia, depression, dyspnea, and coma.

RECOMMENDED TESTING: Consider erythrocyte GPx activity and selenoprotein P analysis (be prepared to provide normal control samples) or serum selenium; analyze a diet sample, as well as evaluate using commercial formulation software if nutrient data are available.

Iodine

In dogs and puppies, goiter/enlarged thyroid gland, alopecia, dry coat, weight gain, and sometimes reduced thyroid hormone; in cats and kittens, no clinical signs have been seen, but at necropsy enlarged thyroid tissue has been seen.

RECOMMENDED TESTING: Thyroid hormones (not conclusive) or urinary iodine excretion and analyze a diet sample, as well as evaluate using commercial formulation software if nutrient data are available.

Vitamins

Fat-Soluble Vitamins

Vitamin A

Retinol only in cats; if vitamin A is needed in dogs, they can convert beta-carotene to vitamin A. In dogs and puppies, anorexia, weight loss, ataxia, xerophthalmia ("dry eyes"), conjunctivitis, corneal opacity and ulceration (likely due to xerophthalmia), skin lesions, and deafness; in cats, conjunctivitis, xerosis (specifically dry conjunctiva) with keratitis and vascularization of the cornea (likely due to the xerosis), photophobia, delayed papillary response to light, cataracts, abortions and premature birth; in kittens, the signs seen in cats, plus hairlessness and cleft palates.

RECOMMENDED TESTING: Schirmer tear test (not conclusive); plasma retinol (laboratory availability unknown); analyze a diet sample, as well as evaluate using commercial formulation software if nutrient data are available.

Vitamin D

In dogs and cats, there are no reports of clinical signs; in puppies, lethargy, poor muscle tone, large swellings at the epiphyseal ends of bones, bending of long bones, and osteopenia on radiographs; in kittens, reluctance to move, progressive caudal paralysis, sometimes enlargement of the metatarsal joints, poor food intake, weight loss, hypocalcemia, elevated PTH.

RECOMMENDED TESTING: Serum 25-OHD, PTH, serum calcium and ionized calcium (in kittens); radiographs (consistent with "rickets," see Chapter 10); analyze a diet sample, as well as evaluate using commercial formulation software if nutrient data are available.

Vitamin E

In dogs and puppies, dermatosis, degeneration of skeletal muscles, muscle weakness, reproductive failure, retinal degeneration, subcutaneous edema, anorexia, depression, dyspnea, and coma; in cats (and presumably kittens), depression, anorexia, hyperesthesia on palpation of the ventral abdomen and nodular adipose tissue (also known as steatitis or yellow fat disease).

RECOMMENDED TESTING: Physical examination (plus biopsy of nodules); plasma alpha-tocopherol (laboratory availability unknown; possibly dialuric acid hemolysis assay but likely clinically unavailable); analyze a diet sample, as well as evaluate using commercial formulation software if nutrient data are available.

Vitamin K

In dogs and puppies, prolongation of clotting times and excessive bleeding only achievable with the use of anticoagulants (e.g. coumarin, a vitamin K antagonist); in cats and kittens, excessive bleeding, prolonged clotting times, increased proteins induced by vitamin K antagonism or absence (PIVKAs); high-fish diets can induce a vitamin K deficiency, as noted earlier in this chapter. (Note: the Devon Rex breed can have a genetic defect that causes a deficiency of all vitamin K-dependent blood coagulation factors.)

RECOMMENDED TESTING: Prothrombin time (PT); partial thromboplastin time (PTT); PIVKA test; possibly analyze a diet sample, as well as evaluate using commercial formulation software if nutrient data are available.

Water-Soluble Vitamins

Thiamin, Vitamin B1

In puppies (and presumably in dogs), inappetence, failure to grow, weight loss, coprophagia, neurologic signs (e.g. central nervous system [CNS] depression, sensory ataxia, paraparesis, torticollis, circling, tonic–clonic convulsions, muscular weakness, recumbency), and sudden death; in cats, bradycardia, anorexia, neurologic signs (i.e. posture changes, short tonic convulsive seizures), progressive weakness prostration, and death; in kittens, mydriasis, ataxia, and erect tails; ventroflexion of the head and bradycardia have also been reported. It should be noted that along with taurine and calcium deficiency, this is the other common nutritional deficiency that the authors have recognized in multiple clinical patients in a tertiary referral setting.

RECOMMENDED TESTING: Erythrocyte transketolase activity; thiamine phosphorylated esters in plasma (reported to be more sensitive than erythrocyte transketolase, laboratory unknown); CNS imaging (i.e. magnetic resonance, although the use of computed tomography has been reported in humans; Swenson and Louis 2006); analyze a diet sample, as well as evaluate using commercial formulation software if nutrient data are available.

Riboflavin, Vitamin B2
In dogs (presumably puppies as well), anorexia, weight loss, muscular weakness, ataxia, ocular lesions described as opacity of the corneas, sudden collapse to a semicomatose state, and death; in cats (presumably kittens as well), anorexia, weight loss, periauricular alopecia, cataracts, and testicular atrophy.

RECOMMENDED TESTING: Erythrocyte glutathione reductase activity coefficient (EGRAC; laboratory availability unknown) and analyze a diet sample, as well as evaluate using commercial formulation software if nutrient data are available.

Pyridoxine, Vitamin B6
In dogs, convulsions, muscle twitching, and microcytic hypochromic anemia, and in puppies, anorexia, weight loss, and death; in cats (presumably kittens as well), growth depression, mild microcytic hypochromic anemia, convulsive seizures, and calcium oxalate crystalluria.

RECOMMENDED TESTING: Complete blood count (CBC); urinalysis; plasma tyrosine (it can be elevated, as the first enzyme for tyrosine degradation can be depressed); analyze a diet sample, as well as evaluate using commercial formulation software if nutrient data are available.

Niacin, Vitamin B3
In dogs (presumably puppies as well), anorexia, weight loss, reddening of the inside of the upper lip that progresses to inflammation and ulceration, vermilion bands on the lips, ptyalism with thick blood-stained saliva, bloody diarrhea, and eventually death (historically described as "black tongue" and compared to pellagra in humans); in cats and kittens, anorexia, fever, fiery red tongue with ulceration (not always), weight loss, respiratory disease, and death.

RECOMMENDED TESTING: Nicotinamide loading test (laboratory unknown); analyze a diet sample, as well as evaluate using commercial formulation software if nutrient data are available.

Pantothenic Acid, Vitamin B5
In dogs and puppies, poor food intake, sudden prostration or coma, tachypnea, tachycardia, convulsions, gastroenteritis, and intussusceptions; in cats, no reports; in kittens, poor growth.

RECOMMENDED TESTING: Analyze a diet sample, as well as evaluate using commercial formulation software if nutrient data are available.

Cobalamin, Vitamin B12
In dogs and puppies, inappetence, neutropenia with hypersegmentation and megaloblastic anemia; in cats, no obvious clinical signs have been reported; in kittens, anorexia and "wet" hair coat (cobalamin deficiency has been reported secondary to inflammatory bowel disease and bacterial overgrowth; deficiency is also possible if the ileum has been resected, as that is the site of absorption).

RECOMMENDED TESTING: Serum cobalamin; CBC; analyze a diet sample, as well as evaluate using commercial formulation software if nutrient data are available.

Folic Acid, Vitamin B9

In dogs and puppies, cleft palates (in Boston terrier puppies), decreased growth rate, decreased hemoglobin and hematocrit; in cats, no reports; in kittens, decreased growth rate.

RECOMMENDED TESTING: Serum folate; CBC (the formiminoglutamic or "FIGLU" test has been used in research environments); analyze a diet sample, as well as evaluate using commercial formulation software if nutrient data are available.

Biotin, Vitamin H or B7

In dogs, hyperkeratosis; in cats, no reports; in kittens, accumulation of salivary, nasal, and lachrymal secretions, alopecia, loss of hair pigment, weight loss, and diarrhea.

RECOMMENDED TESTING: Dietary history of feeding raw eggs or egg whites (containing the protein "avidin," which binds biotin), as this appears to be the only way to create a deficiency.

Choline

In dogs, weight loss, hypocholesterolemia, vomiting, fatty liver, and death; in kittens, decreased food intake, and decreased growth rate.

RECOMMENDED TESTING: Plasma choline and phosphatidylcholine; analyze diet sample for all methyl group donors (i.e. choline, betaine, and methionine in excess of the amino acid requirement); evaluate using commercial formulation software if nutrient data are available.

Benefits of Dietary Omega-3 Fatty Acids—Courtesy John E. Bauer

Dietary omega-3 fatty acids are incorporated into cell membranes such as neutrophils, heart, kidney, skin, and joint tissues. They compete with omega-6 fatty acids (namely arachidonic acid) as substrates for the production of important cell mediators including those associated with inflammation. Because inflammation characterizes many chronic progressive disorders, provision of dietary long-chain omega-3 fatty acids (i.e. docosahexaenoic acid and eicosapentaenoic acid; DHA and EPA) are currently thought to be beneficial. However, the shorter-chain omega-3 fatty acids from vegetable sources, such as alpha-linolenic acid (ALA) from flaxseed, are inefficiently converted to the longer-chain fatty acids, which are better able to modify inflammatory and immune responses (i.e. EPA and DHA from marine sources).

It should be noted that omega-3 dosages indicated on product labels are those suggested for health maintenance of normal animals or to help optimize dietary intake.

These amounts may be sufficient to help alleviate low-level inflammatory states by balancing omega-6 and omega-3 intakes. For both dogs and cats, low concentrations of long-chain omega-3 fatty acids (expressed as DHA plus EPA) are considered essential for all life stages by the National Research Council (NRC), and should be included in diets formulated for growth and reproduction according to the guidance of both the Association of American Feed Control Officials (AAFCO) and the European Pet Food Industry Federation (FEDIAF). Dosages are often expressed on a metabolic body weight (MBW) basis, since many nutrients as well as energy requirements vary relative to this parameter. MBW is expressed as kg of body weight, with an exponent of 0.75 for dogs and 0.67 for cats.

Therapeutic Use in Dogs
Therapeutic dosages for dogs are based on studies involving skin, cardiovascular, renal,

Table 2.1 Daily long-chain omega-3 fatty acid doses (in mg of combined EPA plus DHA) calculated on a metabolic body weight basis for adult dogs.

Disorder	Dosage
Idiopathic hyperlipidemia	$120\,mg/kg^{0.75}$
Kidney disease	$140\,mg/kg^{0.75}$
Cardiovascular disorders	$115\,mg/kg^{0.75}$
Osteoarthritis	$310\,mg/kg^{0.75}$
Inflammatory/immune (atopy, inflammatory bowel disease)	$125\,mg/kg^{0.75}$
National Research Council (NRC) recommended allowance	$30\,mg/kg^{0.75}$
NRC safe upper limit	$370\,mg/kg^{0.75}$

Source: Adapted from Bauer (2011).

and lipid disorders, and osteoarthritis. Recommended amounts of EPA plus DHA use MBW multiplied by factors ranging from 115 to 310 (Table 2.1). These recommendations are intended as a starting point for therapy under veterinary supervision and are below the canine safe upper limit (NRC 2006a).

Therapeutic Use in Cats

Less is known about the use of omega-3 fatty acids in cats, although effects on skin and orthopedic health do appear to exist. Given the known limited ability of cats to synthesize longer-chain fatty acids, similar benefits in this species to those in dogs are expected. Studies to date have fed dosages from 100 to 750 mg EPA+DHA/day. However, untoward effects on certain immune parameters at the higher end of this range have been reported (Chew et al. 2000; Bauer 2011). Therapeutic dosages in the order of those used for skin disorders of dogs (but using the cat exponent; i.e. 125 mg EPA+DHA/kg$^{0.67}$) are likely to be safe, but individual differences may exist. Until further studies are conducted, long-term daily dosages exceeding 75 mg EPA+DHA/kg$^{0.67}$ should be monitored under veterinary supervision.

Sources of Long-Chain Omega-3 Fatty Acids

Although several sources of omega-3 fatty acids exist, companion animal studies have typically used fish oils containing both EPA and DHA. These products are primarily composed of triglyceride forms, the digestion and absorption of which are well known. Other sources include krill oil containing phospholipids, algae-based triglyceride forms, green-lipped mussel oil extracts containing some unique fatty acids, and esterified omega-3 fatty acids. The relative efficacy of the various forms has not been established. However, the triglyceride form is the most extensively studied in both animal and human health. As such, recommendations are based on triglyceride sources.

Other Metabolic Benefits of Long-Chain Omega-3 Fatty Acids

DHA and Puppy Development

Feeding fish oil to puppies results in significant DHA incorporation into the cells of the canine eye (Delton-Vandenbroucke et al. 1998). Diets enriched in fish oil provided during gestation, lactation, and after weaning showed statistically significant improvement in visual function at 12 weeks compared to controls (Heinemann et al. 2005). Another trial also evaluated visual function and cognitive and learning ability in puppies fed DHA (Zicker et al. 2012). In that study, DHA-enriched diets were initiated at weaning, a period in which puppies have lost the ability to convert DHA from precursors (Heinemann et al. 2005). Again, strong correlations between dietary DHA and improved visual performance were observed. In addition, enhanced cognitive function was reported in DHA-fed puppies compared to controls, including fewer errors for learning to run through a maze setup (Zicker et al. 2012).

Cognition and Healthy Aging

In humans, DHA may support healthy aging, and low DHA has been correlated with cognitive impairment. The effects of aging on cognitive function in older dogs have been reported using client-owned animals and various questionnaires. Objective assessments with canine models of aging have also contributed to our understanding of these phenomena. A number of dog studies examining foods enriched with mixtures of antioxidants and mitochondrial cofactors reported improvements in learning and memory (reviewed in Roudebush et al. 2005). With respect to DHA, subsequent studies employing either whole cell algae at 0.1% diet DHA (Hadley et al. 2017) or fish oil at 0.24% diet DHA (Pan et al. 2018) resulted in improved cognitive performance and visual processing, as measured using a contrast discrimination task. It should be noted that the whole cell algae diet also contained small amounts of antioxidants and the fish oil diet contained both antioxidants and mitochondrial cofactors as well. In contrast, a placebo-controlled study in older dogs that employed a diet rich in porcine sphingolipids and DHA (approx. 0.4% diet DHA) demonstrated improved cognitive performance using measures typically impaired in canine aging; however, dietary concentrations of antioxidants or other cofactors were not reported (Araujo et al. 2022). Finally, one investigation in middle-aged and older cats compared diets with or without a blend of fish oil (0.28% diet DHA), B vitamins, antioxidants, and arginine, and reported that supplemented cats performed significantly better on standardized behavioral measures of cognitive function (Pan et al. 2013).

In summary, omega-3 fatty acids, most notably DHA, appear to play a role in healthy canine and feline aging and cognition. Further controlled dietary studies will be needed to better understand the interplay among the various dietary cofactors involved in this complex process.

Newly Described Metabolites from Omega-3 Fatty Acid Precursors

In addition to direct competition of long-chain omega-3 for inflammatory mediator synthesis, EPA and DHA are also precursors for other health-supporting metabolites, including resolvins and protectins (Serhan and Petasis 2011). Resolvins appear to have the capacity to help resolve the inflammatory responses, while protectins may protect neurologic function. Preliminary findings indicate that these compounds may afford additional support for skin conditions as well as nerve and eye functions. These metabolites are an important target for future studies.

Fatty Acid Ratios

It is important to distinguish which specific fatty acids are used in calculating the omega-6: omega-3 ratio, since ALA and EPA+DHA have differential metabolic effects and are present in foods and supplements in variable concentrations and proportions. In addition, ALA cannot be efficiently elongated to EPA before exerting its eicosanoid-mediated biological effects. As such, a ratio calculated using all major types of omega-3 (i.e. ALA, EPA, and DHA) is not metabolically equivalent to one where only EPA and DHA is used (even when the concentrations are equal). However, any ratio may be useful when considered as a way to help minimize a potential overabundance of the omega-6 fatty acid linoleic acid (LA) in a particular food (Dunbar et al. 2010). For example, a ratio of LA : ALA of 3 : 1 to 5 : 1 will typically accomplish this goal (Dunbar et al. 2010). Regardless, consideration of the concentrations and proportions of all relevant fatty acids from all dietary and supplement sources is recommended to help assure metabolic balance in healthy animals as well as when aiming for therapeutic benefits.

Diagnostic and Food Analysis Laboratories and Diet Computer Analysis

As can be seen from the earlier list, samples may need to be submitted to laboratories for the diagnosis of certain nutritional deficiencies. The most common nutrients analyzed in veterinary patients are taurine, calcium/ vitamin D, electrolytes (i.e. phosphorus, sodium, potassium, magnesium, chloride), iron (via TIBC), vitamin K (via PIVKA), thiamin, cobalamin (vitamin B12), and folate. Many of these nutrients may be analyzed in the normal course of working up a case and may be familiar to the veterinary practitioner. Others may be more exotic or available only through a research laboratory. For the reader's convenience the following laboratories are suggested (note these are all in the United States given the authors' geography and are current as of 2022):

- Eurofins Scientific, Des Moines, IA, +1 (515) 265 1461, http://www.eurofinsus.com/food-testing/laboratories/eurofins-nutrition-analysis-center, for food analysis.
- Midwest Laboratories, Omaha, NE, +1 (402) 334 7770, https://midwestlabs.com, for food analysis.
- UC Davis Amino Acid Laboratory, Davis, CA, +1 (530) 752 5058, https://www.vetmed.ucdavis.edu/labs/amino-acid-laboratory, for amino acid and trace mineral analysis from patients and diets (run by one of the authors, AJF).
- Michigan State University Diagnostic Center for Population and Animal Health (DCPAH), Lansing, MI, +1 (517) 353 1683, https://cvm.msu.edu/vdl, for vitamin D metabolites and PTH in patients.
- Texas A&M GI Lab, College Station, TX, +1 (979) 862 2861, https://vetmed.tamu.edu/gilab, for cobalamin and folate.

Other tests may be available via national commercial veterinary diagnostic laboratories such as IDEXX Laboratories and ANTECH Diagnostics.

As some tests may not be available, analysis of a diet via computer analysis may be useful, particularly in patients consuming a homemade diet. Any such analysis is only as good as the nutrient database that is used. Certain nutrients of interest are not always reported or there can be large variations in the range of values seen with foods; therefore, such analyses must be used as supportive or suggestive only. Commercial formulation software used by pet food companies (e.g. Concept 5 Formulation System, www.agri-data.com) is typically too complex and expensive for even veterinary academicians and does not come with preloaded nutrient data for foods or ingredients. Software used for livestock (e.g. Dalex Livestock, www.dalex.com) is generally too cumbersome to adapt to dogs and cats from swine modules. Three software programs, Food Processor (available at www.esha.com for a fee), Diet Check Munich (available at www.dietcheckmunich.com for a fee), and Balance It® (available at www.balance.it for free), are known to the authors as being used by veterinary nutritionists and veterinarians. The latter two programs are designed specifically for veterinary use, and Balance It was created by one of the authors (SJD). These programs rely heavily on reference databases like that of the US Department of Agriculture (USDA) at FoodData Central (https://fdc.nal.usda.gov/fdc-app.html#/), which has an extensive database of human foods. However, certain nutrients of interest such as taurine, chloride, iodine, and vitamin D are typically or often not available. Therefore, "deficiencies" in these nutrients suggested by computer analysis when compared to reported nutrient requirements for dogs and cats may be the result of a lack of available data rather than a real deficiency (this can also be true of choline, which is not routinely reported by USDA).

Nutrient Requirements

Nutrient requirements are available from three main references, the annually published *Official Publication* of the Association of AAFCO and the European FEDIAF nutritional guidelines, whose assembled experts largely base the "AAFCO nutrient profiles" or guidelines on the *Nutrient Requirements of Dogs and Cats* from the National Research Council (commonly referred to as the NRC), published by the US National Academies, and published data. The most recent NRC requirements were published in 2006. Most existing nutrient requirements were not vastly changed with the publication of the 2006 NRC, but the NRC suggested requirements for several omega-3 fatty acids (e.g. EPA, DHA, and ALA), and there were a few amino acid and mineral shifts.

Nutrient requirements from AAFCO are provided as "minimum" and "maximum" levels for "growth and reproduction" and "adult maintenance" on both a dry matter basis and a "per 1000 kcal ME," or energy basis. The nutrient profile on a dry matter basis presumes a specific energy density (i.e. 4000 kcal ME/kg food for AAFCO). Higher energy density formulations must be corrected for energy density with this approach. FEDIAF guidelines utilize requirements on an amount of energy per kilogram body weight to the three-quarter power. Both account for energy in requirements to ensure that adequate amounts of nutrients are consumed, since dogs and cats eat to their calorie needs, as discussed earlier in the chapter. The profile on a dry matter basis essentially ensures that if an animal is eating a less energy-dense diet, the volume of food it will need to eat to meet its nutrient requirements is physically possible. Certain nutrient minimums also change depending on the food. Different recommendations are provided for copper and taurine for foods that are extruded versus canned. The recommendations for vitamin K are higher if the product has a high fish content. Maximums are provided for select nutrients and are the same regardless of life stage.

The NRC provides separate requirements for growing and reproducing dogs and cats. Additionally, three different "minimal" requirements are provided instead of just one as with the AAFCO profiles, along with an SUL, which is potentially different for every life stage (unlike with AAFCO). The three

different minimal requirements in the NRC are minimal requirement (MR), adequate intake (AI), and recommended allowance (RA). The MR is defined as "the minimal concentration or amount of a bioavailable nutrient that will support a defined physiological state." This requirement assumes that 100% of the nutrient is available; therefore, it does not account for, say, a lower digestibility or antagonisms that can frequently occur with amino acids, minerals, and fat-soluble vitamins. The AI is defined as "the concentration in the diet or amount required by the animal of a nutrient that is presumed to sustain a given life stage when no MR has been demonstrated." This value is used when graded studies were not available or when comparative data had to be relied on. The RA is defined as "the concentration or amount of a nutrient in a diet formulated to support a given physiological state." This requirement is most analogous to the AAFCO minimum, as both requirements attempt to insert a safety factor to the MR or AI to account for uncertain bioavailability. The NRC also uses an additional unit not used by AAFCO: amount per kilogram body weight raised to the three-quarter power (i.e. amt/kg $BW^{0.75}$), which is more analogous to the "dosing" of medications. This third method of expressing requirements is not as commonly used by nutritionists, who generally think about the nutrient concentrations needed in foods rather than a "dose" for a particular patient. However, when a very low energy intake is expected or suggested, this third method may be used. The reader is directed to Chapter 6 for further discussion on units for expressing nutrient levels and comparing values provided in different units.

Key Clinical Nutritional Excesses and Signs

Beyond calcium and vitamin D excess and related orthopedic or renal consequences (covered later in the text), the main nutrient excesses of clinical significance are vitamin A and methionine. Hypervitaminosis A can occur clinically when an all-liver diet (or a mainly liver diet) is fed to kittens that leads to extensive osseocartilaginous hyperplasia of the first three cervical vertebrae. These changes restrict movement and result in an unkempt coat as the affected cat will not groom itself. Methionine excess can result in a hemolytic anemia with methemoglobinemia with Heinz body formation. However, the risk appears to be associated with purified amino acid supplementation, not with the consumption of intact dietary protein. From NRC 2006a,b: "and it would be predicted that peptide-bound methionine in protein would be less toxic than that provided in the free form. Thus, it is unlikely that cats eating natural prey would exceed the SUL for methionine." The authors have not recognized methionine toxicity in cats that eat essentially all-meat diets, even when the protein content was quite high (at 50% protein calories). Several other nutrients have maximum values set by AAFCO due to concerns of antagonism, but these are generally clinically less important, with the exception of zinc excess, which is discussed in Chapter 13 regarding the management of copper storage disease.

Additional Education on Nutrition

Inherently this chapter's coverage of basic nutrition is limited; therefore, readers with a greater interest in basic nutrition as well as nutrition in general are referred to the following resources (roughly listed in increasing level of intensity or depth):

- American Academy of Veterinary Nutrition (AAVN) Listserv (www.aavnutrition.org, annual membership fee required).
- General nutrition or biochemistry texts.
- Veterinary medical school/college coursework (often available to the public through "open campus" or "extension" programs).
- Continuing education: Diplomates of the American College of Veterinary Internal Medicine (Nutrition) – DACVIM (Nutrition) – actively present at regional, national, and international meetings (e.g. United States, Canada, United Kingdom, Australia, New Zealand), as do Diplomates of the European College of Veterinary and Comparative Nutrition, DECVCN.
- Internship/externship (available with numerous DACVIMs).
- Fellowships (some universities host veterinarians, such as UC Davis through the Donald G. Low-CVMA Practitioner Fellowship).
- Graduate courses in nutrition (aimed at Master's and/or PhD students; may require enrollment).
- Veterinary nutrition residency training (see the American College of Veterinary Internal Medicine at acvim.org); these two- to four-year programs are currently available at a variety of veterinary medical institutions.

Readers are encouraged to explore these additional resources to build on their knowledge of nutrition, and it is hoped that this text will play a supportive role if any of these additional learning opportunities are undertaken.

References

Araujo, J.A., Segarra, S., Mendes, J. et al. (2022). Sphingolipids and DHA improve cognitive deficits in aged Beagle dogs. *Front Vet Sci* 9: 646451.

Bauer, J.E. (2011). Therapeutic use of fish oils in companion animals. *J. Am. Vet. Med. Assoc.* 239: 1441–1451.

Baxmann, A.C., de Mendonça, O.G., and Heilberg, I.P. (2003). Effect of vitamin C supplements on urinary oxalate and pH in calcium stone-forming patients. *Kidney Int.* 63 (3): 1066–1071.

Chew, B.P., Park, H.J., Park, J.S. et al. (2000). Role of omega-3 fatty acids on immunity and inflammation in cats. In: *Recent Advances in Canine and Feline Nutrition. Vol III. Iams Nutrition Symposium Proceedings* (ed. G.A. Reinhart and D.P. Carey), 55–67. Wilmington, OH: Orange Frazer Press.

Delton-Vandenbroucke, I., Maude, M.B., Chen, H. et al. (1998). Effect of diet on the fatty acid and molecular species composition of dog retina phospholipids. *Lipids* 33: 1187–1193.

DeNapoli, J.S., Dodman, N.H., Shuster, L. et al. (2000). Effect of dietary protein content and tryptophan supplementation on dominance aggression, territorial aggression, and hyperactivity in dogs. *J. Am. Vet. Med. Assoc.* 217 (4): 504–508.

Dunbar, B.L., Bigley, K.E., and Bauer, J.E. (2010). Early and sustained enrichment of serum n-3 long chain polyunsaturated fatty acids in dogs fed a flaxseed supplemented diet. *Lipids* 45: 1–10.

Fry, M.M. and Kirk, C.A. (2006). Reticulocyte indices in a canine model of nutritional iron deficiency. *Vet. Clin. Pathol.* 35: 172–181.

Hadley, K.B., Bauer, J.E., and Milgram, N.W. (2017). The oil-rich alga Schizochytrium sp. as a dietary source of docosahexaenoic acid improves shape discrimination learning associated with visual processing in a canine model of senescence. *Prostaglandins Leukot. Essent. Fatty Acids* 118: 10–18.

Hazewinkel, H.A.W., How, K.L., Bosch, R. et al. (1987). Inadequate photosynthesis of vitamin D in dogs. In: *Nutrition, Malnutrition and Dietetics in the Dog and Cat, Proceedings of an International Symposium* (ed. A.T. Edney). London: British Veterinary Association & Waltham Centre for Pet Nutrition.

Heinemann, K.M., Waldron, M.K., Bigley, K.E. et al. (2005). Long-chain (n-3) polyunsaturated fatty acids are more efficient than α-linolenic acid in improving electroretinogram response of puppies exposed during gestation, lactation, and weaning. *J. Nutr.* 135: 1960–1966.

Morris, J.G. (1999). Ineffective vitamin D synthesis in cats is reversed by an inhibitor of 7-dehydrocholesterol-delta7-reductase. *J. Nutr.* 129: 903–909.

National Research Council (2006a). Nutrient requirements and dietary nutrient concentrations. In: *Nutrient Requirements of Dogs and Cats*, 359. Washington, DC: National Academies Press.

National Research Council (NRC) (2006b). *Nutrient Requirements of Dogs and Cats*. Washington, DC: National Academies Press.

Pan, Y., Araujo, J.A., Burrows, J. et al. (2013). Cognitive enhancement in middle-aged and old cats with dietary supplementation with a nutrient blend containing fish oil, B vitamins, antioxidants and arginine. *Br. J. Nutr.* 110: 40–49.

Pan, Y., Kennedy, A.D., Jönsson, T.J. et al. (2018). Cognitive enhancement in old dogs from dietary supplementation with a nutrient blend containing arginine, antioxidants, B vitamins and fish oil. *Br. J. Nutr.* 119: 349–358.

Roudebush, P., Zicker, S.C., Cotman, C.W. et al. (2005). Nutritional management of brain aging in dogs. *J. Am. Vet. Med. Assoc.* 227: 722–727.

Serhan, C.N. and Petasis, N.A. (2011). Resolvins and protectins in inflammation-resolution. *Chem. Rev.* 111: 5922–5943.

Steinberg, J.D. and Olver, C.S. (2005). Hematologic and biochemical abnormalities indicating iron deficiency are associated with decreased reticulocyte hemoglobin content (CHr) and reticulocyte volume (rMCV) in dogs. *Vet. Clin. Pathol.* 34: 23–27.

Strieker, M.J., Morris, J.G., Feldman, B.F. et al. (1996). Vitamin K deficiency in cats fed commercial fish-based diets. *J. Small Anim. Pract.* 37 (7): 322–326.

Swenson, A.J. and Louis, E.K.S. (2006). Computed tomography findings in thiamine deficiency-induced coma. *Neurocrit. Care* 5 (1): 45–48.

Yu, S., Rogers, Q.R., and Morris, J.G. (2001). Effect of low levels of dietary tyrosine on the hair colour of cats. *J. Small Anim. Pract.* 42 (4): 176–180.

Zicker, S.C., Jewell, D.E., Yamka, R. et al. (2012). Evaluation of cognitive, learning, memory, psychomotor, immunologic, and retinal functions in healthy puppies fed foods fortified with docosahexaenoic acid-rich fish oil from 8 to 52 weeks of age. *J. Am. Vet. Med. Assoc.* 241: 583–594.

3

Determining Energy Requirements

Jon J. Ramsey

Determining the energy requirements of an individual patient is a challenge for any nutritionist or veterinarian. Animals require a very specific amount of energy to maintain a given body weight, and even slight deviations from this requirement can induce weight gain or loss. To determine the amount of food required by an animal, it is necessary to know the animal's energy requirement and the energy content of the foods offered to the animal. There are a number of equations available to predict either energy requirements or the amount of energy in foods. However, a number of assumptions typically need to be made when using these equations, and it is important to realize the limitations of commonly used equations. It should be stressed that predicted energy requirements should be viewed as an "educated guess" at the animal's true energy requirement. These equations should be used as a tool to provide a starting point for selecting the amount of food to give an animal, and adjustments should be made based on any observed changes in body weight. The purpose of this chapter is to provide the background necessary to estimate energy requirements for dogs and cats and calculate the energy content of foods.

Units

Energy is frequently defined as the capacity to do work. In the United States, the most common unit of energy used in nutrition is the calorie. A calorie is defined as the amount of heat required to increase the temperature of water from 14.5 to 15.5 °C. This is sometimes referred to as the "15 °C calorie," "small calorie," or "gram-calorie." A calorie is a very small unit of energy, and the unit typically used in nutrition is the kilocalorie. A kilocalorie (kcal) is equivalent to 1000 cal, and it is sometimes called the "kilogram-calorie," "big calorie," or "Calorie" (written with an uppercase C). This last term is commonly used in human nutrition, including on labels for human foods. The kilocalorie is the energy unit primarily used in dog and cat nutrition, although the megacalorie (Mcal), equivalent to 1 000 000 cal or 1000 kcal, is also occasionally used.

Although the kilocalorie is still widely used in the United States, the joule is actually the designated SI unit of energy. Conversion between calories and joules can easily be accomplished using the following equation:

$$1 \text{ calorie} = 4.184 \text{ joules}$$

Applied Veterinary Clinical Nutrition, Second Edition. Edited by Andrea J. Fascetti, Sean J. Delaney, Jennifer A. Larsen, and Cecilia Villaverde.
© 2024 John Wiley & Sons, Inc. Published 2024 by John Wiley & Sons, Inc.

A joule (J) is a small amount of energy, and therefore the kilojoule (kJ, equal to 1000 J) and megajoule (MJ, 1 000 000 J or 1000 kJ) are the units most commonly used in animal nutrition.

Animal energy requirements are given as an amount of energy per unit of time, and energy requirements for dogs and cats are often given as kcal/day or kJ/day.

The energy content of food is generally expressed as the amount of energy per unit of weight or volume. Energy per unit of weight is typically used in equations for calculating diet energy content (grams or kilograms), as it is more accurate than volume. Conversions are best accomplished by weighing a given volume of the specific food, since there is no standard equation for converting volume to weight. The weight of a volume of food will depend on the density of the food, which can be highly variable.

Basic Concepts and Terminology

The laws of thermodynamics form the foundation for the study of energy metabolism. In particular, the first law of thermodynamics is central to all systems for predicting animal energy requirements. This law indicates that energy can neither be created nor destroyed, but can simply change from one form to another (Haynie 2001). Thus, energy metabolism in animals can be viewed as an accounting exercise, since the energy consumed by the animal must appear in tissue macromolecules (i.e. fat, protein, or glycogen) or leave the body as energy expenditure or excreta. Animal energy requirements are often described in terms of energy balance.

Energy balance is defined as the mathematical difference between energy intake and energy expenditure. An animal is in a state of energy balance (i.e. body energy stores are constant) if the amount of energy consumed matches the amount of energy expended by the animal. If energy intake exceeds energy expenditure, the animal enters a state of positive energy balance and net retention of energy leads to an increase in body weight. Similarly, if energy intake is less than energy expenditure, the animal enters a state of negative energy balance and net loss of body energy leads to weight loss.

The maintenance energy requirement (MER) is the amount of energy required to maintain an animal in a state of energy balance, or in other words the amount of energy needed to maintain an animal at its current weight (and body composition). It is typical to predict the MER for a dog or cat and then make adjustments to this value if weight loss or weight gain is desired.

As a first step toward determining energy requirements, it is important to understand the terminology that is commonly used in energy metabolism. A number of terms are used to describe the energy intake and energy expenditure of an animal (Wenk et al. 2001). The following terms describe the energy available to the animal after accounting for various sources of energy loss (Figure 3.1).

Gross energy (GE) is the amount of heat that is released from a given amount of food following complete combustion in a bomb calorimeter. GE is a physical rather than biological measure and represents the maximum energy of a diet or feedstuff. Another term for

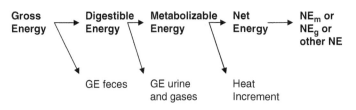

Figure 3.1 Energy terms and sources of energy loss in animal nutrition.

GE is "heat of combustion." GE gives little information about the energy available to the animal, since foods are not entirely digested and energy is lost in feces, urine, and as heat produced during the digestion and assimilation of dietary nutrients. Digestible energy (DE) is the energy remaining after subtracting the GE of feces from the GE of food:

$$DE = GE_{food} - GE_{feces}$$

DE energy is a measure of the "apparent" digestible energy, since the feces contains energy from products other than food (e.g. digestive enzymes, sloughed cells from the gut, mucus, etc.). Energy requirements for horses are given as DE, but this term is rarely used in dog and cat nutrition. Metabolizable energy (ME) is the energy remaining after subtracting the GE of urine and the GE of gaseous products of fermentation from DE:

$$ME = DE - GE_{urine} - GE_{gas}$$

Energy requirements for dogs and cats are primarily given in terms of ME. Net energy (NE) is the energy remaining after subtracting the heat increment (heat production associated with the consumption of food) from ME:

$$NE = ME - \text{heat increment}$$

NE includes energy that may be used for either maintenance of the animal or production (i.e. growth, lactation, reproduction). Energy requirements for agricultural species are often given in terms of NE, and there is currently not sufficient information to accurately provide energy requirements for dogs or cats in terms of NE.

Energy expenditure at maintenance is composed of four basic components: (i) resting energy expenditure, (ii) activity-related energy expenditure, (iii) heat increment, and (iv) facultative thermogenesis. Energy requirements can be determined by measuring energy expenditure, and energy requirements are often given in relation to resting (or basal) energy expenditure, with adjustments made for other components of total energy expenditure. Resting energy expenditure is typically the largest component of total energy expenditure and frequently accounts for greater than 50% of energy expenditure. The following terms are frequently used to describe this component of energy expenditure.

Basal metabolic rate or basal energy expenditure is a term that applies primarily to human nutrition and physiology, because the conditions required to measure basal metabolic rate are so stringent that it is virtually impossible to complete these measurements in animals. Basal metabolic rate is energy expenditure measured in a postabsorptive state under thermoneutral conditions (i.e. no additional energy expenditure is required specifically to maintain body temperature), with the subject lying but awake and in complete muscular repose. The subject should also be free from emotional stress.

Because it is difficult to have an animal cooperate with all of these conditions, the term resting energy (or resting metabolic rate) is more often used in animal nutrition. Resting energy expenditure is measured in animals that are lying down. Resting energy expenditure is often measured in animals that are not fasting, and therefore it may contain some energy associated with the digestion of food.

Fasting energy expenditure (or fasting heat production) is measured in animals that are denied access to food. These measurements are generally completed in animals that have been fasted for a sufficient duration to ensure that no food remains in the gastrointestinal tract. Many of the original equations for predicting MERs were derived from measures of fasting energy expenditure. These measurements were completed using calorimetry systems that allowed limited movement for the animals, and thus these measures are generally only slightly higher than basal energy expenditure.

Activity-related energy expenditure is the energy expenditure associated with muscular exercise. The energy expenditure associated with physical activity is highly variable both between animals (working dog vs. a sedentary apartment-dwelling dog) and within the animal (day of intense work vs. day of rest). A rough measure of physical activity can be obtained by dividing 24-hour energy expenditure by resting energy expenditure. For a sedentary animal these values will be similar, and the ratio will be less than 1.5, while for an active athlete this ratio will be 2.0 or greater.

Heat increment is the energy expenditure associated with ingestion, digestion, assimilation, and metabolism of food. Heat increment is also called the thermic effect of feeding, diet-induced thermogenesis, or meal-induced thermogenesis. Heat increment is responsible for 10–15% of total daily energy expenditure in many simple-stomached animals (Blaxter 1989), and it likely contributes a similar percentage to energy expenditure in dogs and cats. The magnitude of heat increment is dependent on both meal size and the nutrient composition of the meal. As expected, heat increment is zero in fasted animals, and it tends to increase in proportion to the amount of energy consumed in a meal. Heat increment is greatest for dietary protein followed by carbohydrate and fat. The high heat increment of protein is sometimes given as one of the reasons for including relatively high amounts of protein in weight-loss diets.

Facultative thermogenesis is a term used to describe the increase in energy expenditure associated with cold or heat stress (and occasionally other forms of stress). This is the energy expenditure required to maintain body temperature when an animal is outside its thermoneutral zone (the temperature range where the previously mentioned components of energy expenditure are sufficient to maintain body temperature). The thermoneutral zone for adult dogs has been reported to lie between 20 and 25°C and 30 and 35°C (NRC 2006), although the exact thermoneutral zone for a given dog will depend on breed, coat length, and adaptation time to a particular ambient temperature. For cats, the thermoneutral zone is not entirely known, although it has been estimated to lie between 30 and 38°C

(NRC 2006). Facultative thermogenesis will be increased in dogs and cats exposed to temperatures either above or below their thermoneutral zones, and it is often considered to be a relatively small component of energy expenditure in animals that live indoors and do not experience prolonged exposure to very cold or warm temperatures. However, facultative thermogenesis can be a major contributor to energy expenditure in dogs or cats that live outdoors and experience temperatures well outside their thermoneutral zone.

Energy requirements for dogs and cats are typically given as metabolizable energy at maintenance. The terms described in the preceding paragraphs are occasionally mentioned when it is necessary to adjust maintenance energy requirements for changes in ambient temperature or physical activity.

Diet Records or History

An accurate diet record or history is the best way to determine the ME requirement for an animal that is weight stable and maintaining a constant body condition score (BCS). This reflects the fact that the animal is currently selecting (or the owner is feeding) the appropriate amount of energy needed to maintain constant body weight. The task now becomes to determine the amount of ME being consumed from the information supplied by the owner. To accomplish this task, it is essential to have detailed and accurate information about all food sources being offered to the animal. To estimate ME intake, a diet record should contain the following information:

- The type of food consumed by the animal (i.e. brand and product information for commercial diets, food ingredients for home-cooked diets, etc.).
- The amount of food offered to the animal (preferably given in weight, but from a practical standpoint this information is more often available as volume of food).

- The type and amount of treats offered to the animal (i.e. brand and product information for commercial treats, human foods used as treats, and amount of each food treat typically consumed).
- The type and amount of nutritional supplements given to the animal.
- The type and amount of "table scraps" commonly given to the animal.

A diet record should also provide information on the daily variation in energy intake. For animals that consume the same diet each day, estimates of ME intake can be made from information provided for a typical day. In contrast, information from several days to over a week may be required to reasonably estimate ME intake in an animal that experiences daily variation in the type and amount of food that it consumes.

In addition to information about the composition and amount of food consumed, it is also important that the diet record include information that will determine the ability of the owner to properly monitor and control the animal's energy intake. This information should include:

- The feeding strategy used with the animal. Is the animal given free-choice consumption of food or is it given food in discrete meals?
- The number of other pets in the household. Does the animal eat alone or does it have access to food offered to other pets? Do other pets have access to the animal's diet?
- The number of people feeding the animal. Does only one person feed the animal or do multiple people give the animal food, including treats?
- The housing conditions for the animal. Does the animal live indoors or does it spend some time outside? If the animal is outside, does it have access to food or people who may offer it food?

The inclusion of this information on the diet record will help determine if a reasonable estimate of ME intake is possible. While diet records provide the best way to determine the ME requirement for maintenance in a dog or cat, there are also several key limitations that need to be considered when calculating ME from diet records. First, it has been noted that many owners are not particularly accurate when reporting food intake for their pets (Hill 2006). This is not surprising, since it has been widely reported that human volunteers tend to underestimate their own energy intake when using diet records. Second, owners often use measures of volume to quantify the amount of food offered to their pets, while measures of weight are more accurate and are generally used for calculating ME. Whenever possible, food scales should be used to help assign a weight to the volume of food given to the animal. Third, all owners do not use uniform measuring devices for determining the amount of food given to their animals. What one owner considers a "cup" may be very different from what another owner uses as a cup. The use of weight, rather than volume, removes this source of error. Fourth, owners may not always be precise in measuring the volume of food given to the animal. A heaping cup may be listed as a cup on a diet record, and accuracy needs to be stressed when completing a diet record.

Despite the limitations of diet records, an attempt should be made to estimate ME intake at maintenance using diet records prior to calculating MERs using standard equations. Accurate diet records are still the best method available to calculate the MERs of an individual animal.

Calculating the Energy Content of a Diet

It can be a challenge to determine the energy content of dog and cat foods. Most commercial dog and cat foods (including treats) that are sold in the United States and subject to the model laws suggested by the Association of American Feed Control Officials (AAFCO) are required to disclose calorie content on the label. This must be provided as ME, both in units of kcal per kg and in kcal per unit of common measure (such as cup, can, or piece). Manufacturers also must specify how the calorie content was determined: calculated or fed (measured). Certain types of treats such as pig ears and bully sticks are exempt from this rule. Also, dogs and cats may be fed human foods for which energy information is not readily available. Thus, some knowledge of basic energy calculations is needed to provide an estimate of the energy content of specific foods or complete diets. Energy calculations are used to convert the measures of food intake included in a diet record into values of energy intake (kcal or kJ per day). This information may then be used to calculate the ME requirement for an animal. Energy calculations are also used to simply estimate the energy content of a diet and allow comparisons of energy content between diets.

There are several ways in which the energy content of a food or diet can be either determined or calculated. One way is simply to determine if the food comes in packaging that contains energy information. Packaged human foods are required to contain energy information, and most commercial pet foods and treats also will have this information on the label. In the case of human foods, the United States Department of Agriculture (USDA) FoodData Central database (https://fdc.nal.usda.gov) may also be searched for energy information of foods when labels that contain energy information are not readily available.

All energy information provided on labels, websites, or databases is obtained either from direct experiments or from calculations using standard values for energy. Experiments that measure the energy content of diets are the most accurate way to determine energy, but also the most expensive and time consuming. Some companies use feeding experiments to determine the ME content of their diets, and AAFCO publishes details for animal protocols (AAFCO 2022) that need to be followed if a company wishes to report ME values on a "fed" basis. Similarly, AAFCO provides equations and calculation procedures for determining the "calculated" ME. A typical animal protocol for determining diet ME includes the following steps:

1) GE (kcal or kJ per gram) is determined for the diet by bomb calorimetry.
2) The animal is adapted to the diet and the environment where the experiment will be completed. In the AAFCO protocol (AAFCO 2022), the animal is fed the diet for at least five days prior to the start of feces (and possibly urine) collection. During this time, it is important to make certain that the animal is consuming an appropriate amount of food to maintain weight.
3) All feces (and possibly urine) are collected and weighed over at least a five-day period. Food intake is also carefully determined during this time. The collected feces are pooled and mixed, and a representative sample is taken for determination of GE by bomb calorimetry. If urine is collected, the urine is combined and an aliquot is taken for determination of GE by bomb calorimetry.
4) ME is calculated using one of the following equations:

Equation A: used when both feces and urine are collected.

$$ME(kcal/kg)$$
$$= \frac{\left(FI \times GE_{food}\right) - \left(F \times GE_{feces}\right) - \left(U \times GE_{urine}\right)}{FI} \times 1000$$

FI = food intake (g)
GE_{food} = gross energy of the diet/food (kcal/g)
F = amount of feces collected (g)
GE_{feces} = gross energy of feces (kcal/g)
U = amount of urine collected (ml)
GE_{urine} = gross energy of urine (kcal/ml)

The following example demonstrates the use of this equation:

$FI = 1000\,g$
$GE_{food} = 4.2\,kcal/g$
$F = 410\,g$

$GE_{feces} = 1.8\,\text{kcal/g}$
$Urine = 950\,\text{ml}$
$GE_{urine} = 0.3\,\text{kcal/ml}$

$$ME = \frac{(1{,}000\,\text{g} \times 4.2\,\text{kcal/g}) - (410\,\text{g} \times 1.8\,\text{kcal/g}) - (950\,\text{ml} \times 0.3\,\text{kcal/ml})}{1000\,\text{g}} \times 1000$$

ME = 3180 kcal/kg

Equation B: used when urine is not collected. It is common to use standard equations for the GE lost in urine rather than collect urine during the experiment. Under normal physiologic conditions, energy lost in urine is associated primarily with the excretion of nitrogen, and thus it is the amount of protein in the diet that determines the GE of urine.

$$ME(\text{kcal/kg}) = \frac{(FI \times GE_{food}) - (F \times GE_{feces}) - \left[(P_{food} - P_{feces}) \times c\right]}{FI} \times 1000$$

FI = food intake (g)
GE_{food} = gross energy of the diet/food (kcal/g)
F = amount of feces collected (g)
GE_{feces} = gross energy of feces (kcal/g)
P_{food} = amount of protein in the food (g)
P_{feces} = amount of protein in the feces (g)
c = correction factor for energy lost from protein through the excretion of urinary nitrogen. This factor is 1.25 kcal/g of protein for dogs and 0.86 kcal/g of protein for cats (AAFCO 2022).

The following example demonstrates the use of this equation:

$FI = 1000\,\text{g}$
$GE_{food} = 4.2\,\text{kcal/g}$
$F = 410\,\text{g}$
$GE_{feces} = 1.8\,\text{kcal/g}$
$P_{food} = 280\,\text{g}$
$P_{feces} = 50\,\text{g}$
$c = 1.25\,\text{kcal/g}$

$$ME = \frac{(1{,}000\,\text{g} \times 4.2\,\text{kcal/g}) - (410\,\text{g} \times 1.8\,\text{kcal/g}) - [(280\,\text{g} - 50\,\text{g}) \times 1.25\,\text{kcal/g}]}{1000\,\text{g}} \times 1000$$

ME = 3175 kcal/kg

It should be noted that by definition ME equals DE minus the GE of both urine and combustible gases. However, dogs and cats produce relatively little combustible gas from fermentation in the gastrointestinal tract. Thus, it is common practice to consider the GE of combustible gases as negligible in dogs and cats, and the GE of gases is generally ignored in experiments measuring ME.

Data from experiments that measured ME have been used to develop factors for calculating ME from diet nutrient composition. Calculating ME through the use of standard factors is the most common way of obtaining an ME value for a particular diet. It is also the fastest and easiest way to predict ME content. Although the factors used to calculate ME were derived from experiments, assumptions about the GE of nutrients and nutrient digestibility had to be made to develop equations that could widely be applied to diets. To illustrate where these assumptions occur and to demonstrate how the ME equations were obtained, it is a useful exercise to work through the calculation of GE, DE, and ME for a sample diet. For this purpose, a diet with the following nutrient composition will be used:

Crude Fat = 12.0%
Crude Protein = 22.0%
Carbohydrate by difference (also called "nitrogen-free extract") = 46.0%
Crude Fiber = 3.0%
Ash = 7.0%
Moisture = 10.0%

GE is calculated by multiplying each nutrient by a standard GE value for that nutrient. The GE values for triglycerides range from 6.5 to 9.9 kcal/g (depending on fatty acid chain length and degree of unsaturation), proteins range from 4.0 to 8.3 kcal/g (depending on amino acid composition), and carbohydrates range from 3.7 to 4.3 kcal/g (Livesey and Elia 1988; Elia and Livesey 1992). Standard GE values of 9.4, 5.65, and 4.15 are routinely used for fats, proteins, and carbohydrates, respectively. These values are in good agreement with the measured GE of pet food ingredients (Kienzle et al. 2002). The GE of a diet can be estimated using the following equation:

$$GE\,(kcal/kg) = 10[(9.4\,kcal/g \times \%\;crude\;fat)$$
$$+ (5.65\,kcal/g \times \%\;crude\;protein)$$
$$+ (4.15\,kcal/g \times \%\;nitrogen\text{-}free\;extract)$$
$$+ (4.15\,kcal/g \times \%\;crude\;fiber)]$$

Using values from the sample diet the following result is obtained:

$$GE\,(kcal/kg) = 10[(9.4\,kcal/g \times 12)$$
$$+ (5.65\,kcal/g \times 22)$$
$$+ (4.15\,kcal/g \times 46)$$
$$+ (4.15 \times 3)]$$

$$GE\,(kcal/kg) = 4404.5$$

Neither water (moisture) nor ash is combustible in a bomb calorimeter, and thus these dietary components have a GE of 0 kcal/g, and they are not included in the equation. Also, it is assumed that crude fiber has a GE value similar to that of starch and, with the exception of lignin, the data do support the idea that the GE values of various fibers are not greatly different from starch (Kienzle et al. 2002). The primary assumption with the use of this equation is that the GE values used are representative of the energy values of the nutrients in the diet. The values used are representative of mixed triglycerides, proteins, and carbohydrates found in conventional foods, and it is unlikely that these values will produce large errors unless the diet is high in medium-chain triglycerides, monosaccharides, or possibly other ingredients that deviate substantially from the standard values.

DE is calculated by multiplying the GE of each nutrient by the digestibility of the nutrient. Digestibility coefficients of 0.90 for crude fat, 0.80 for crude protein, 0.85 for carbohydrates (nitrogen-free extract), and 0 for crude fiber are often used for commercial dog and cat

foods. The DE of a diet can be estimated using the following equation:

$$DE\,(kcal/kg) = 10[(9.4\,kcal/g$$
$$\times \%\;crude\;fat \times dig.coeff.fat) + (5.65\,kcal/g$$
$$\times \%\;crude\;protein \times dig.coeff.protein)$$
$$+ (4.15\,kcal/g \times \%\;nitrogen\text{-}free\;extract$$
$$\times dig.coeff.nitrogen\text{-}free\;extract)$$
$$+ (4.15\,kcal/g \times \%\;crude\;fiber$$
$$\times dig.coeff.fiber)]$$

Using values from the sample diet the following result is obtained:

$$DE\,(kcal/kg) = 10[(9.4\,kcal/g \times 12 \times 0.9)$$
$$+ (5.65\,kcal/g \times 22 \times 0.8)$$
$$+ (4.15\,kcal/g \times 46 \times 0.85)$$
$$+ (4.15\,kcal/g \times 3 \times 0)]$$

$$DE\,(kcal/kg) = 3632.3$$

The major assumption with the use of this equation is that the digestibility coefficients for each nutrient will truly reflect the digestibility of these nutrients in the diet. This is the primary source of error in calculating the energy content of a diet. The digestibility coefficients used in the equation were determined on commercial pet foods available in the late 1970s and early 1980s (NRC 2006), and the digestibility of some current foods on the market may differ from these values. In particular, the digestibility of crude fiber and the influence of fiber on the digestibility of other nutrients are ignored in the equation. Nonetheless, the digestibility factors used in this equation still reflect reasonably well the digestibility of many pet foods on the market (Kienzle 2002). Also, these digestibility factors form the foundation for equations that are still routinely used to predict the ME content of diets.

ME is calculated using the same equation as given for DE, except the GE value for protein is corrected for the energy lost in urine with the excretion of nitrogen. Thus, if a correction factor of 1.25 kcal/g of protein is used for loss of energy in urine, then the GE value of protein becomes 4.40 kcal/g ($GE_{protein} = 5.65\,kcal/g - 1.25\,kcal/g$).

The corrected protein GE of 4.40 kcal/g is routinely used for both dogs and cats, even though the actual value for protein in cat foods is likely higher. The ME of a diet can be estimated using the following equation:

$$ME\,(kcal/kg) = 10[(9.4\,kcal/g \times \%\,crude\,fat$$
$$\times dig.coeff.fat) + (4.40\,kcal/g$$
$$\times \%\,crude\,protein$$
$$\times dig.coeff.protein) + (4.15\,kcal/g$$
$$\times \%\,nitrogen\text{-}free\,extract$$
$$\times dig.coeff.nitrogen\text{-}free\,extract)]$$

Using values from the sample diet the following result is obtained:

$$ME\,(kcal/kg) = 10[(9.4\,kcal/g \times 12 \times 0.9)$$
$$+ (4.40\,kcal/g \times 22 \times 0.8)$$
$$+ (4.15\,kcal/g \times 46 \times 0.85)]$$

$$ME\,(kcal/kg) = 3412.3$$

The ME equation relies primarily on the same assumptions as used for the DE equation. In other words, assumptions made about digestibility coefficients generally have the greatest influence on both DE and ME calculations. ME values are similar to those calculated for DE, and ME is approximately 93% of DE for dog and cat foods.

Practical Equations for Predicting the Metabolizable Energy Content of Dog and Cat Foods

Two equations (the Atwater and the modified Atwater, sometimes called the AAFCO equation) are routinely used to predict the ME values of diets for dogs and cats. These equations contain factors that include energy values corrected for digestibility and loss of energy in urine. Thus, these equations are relatively simple and involve multiplying the amount of a particular nutrient by only one factor. The Atwater equation was developed over 100 years ago to predict the energy content of human diets (Atwater 1902). It is still used in human nutrition, and it provides a reasonable estimate

for the ME value of human foods fed to dogs (and possibly cats). The Atwater equation may also be appropriate for highly digestible commercial pet foods. It is as follows:

$$ME\,(kcal/kg) = 10[(9\,kcal/g \times \%\,crude\,fat)$$
$$+ (4\,kcal/g \times \%\,crude\,protein)$$
$$+ (4\,kcal/g \times \%\,nitrogen\text{-}free\,extract)]$$

Using values from a diet containing 12% crude fat, 22% crude protein, and 46% nitrogen-free extract, the following result can be obtained with the Atwater equation:

$$ME\,(kcal/kg) = 10[(9\,kcal/g \times 12)$$
$$+ (4\,kcal/g \times 22)$$
$$+ (4\,kcal/g \times 46)]$$

$$ME\,(kcal/kg) = 3800$$

The modified Atwater equation was developed by AAFCO (AAFCO 2022) to produce an equation that would better reflect the fact that the digestibility of commercial pet foods tends to be lower than the digestibility of typical human foods. Under AAFCO regulations, the modified Atwater equation may be used to determine the ME values included on pet food labels. The modified Atwater equation is as follows:

$$ME\,(kcal/kg) = 10[(8.5\,kcal/g \times \%\,crude\,fat)$$
$$+ (3.5\,kcal/g \times \%\,crude\,protein)$$
$$+ (3.5\,kcal/g \times \%\,nitrogen\text{-}free$$
$$extract)]$$

Using values from a diet containing 12% crude fat, 22% crude protein, and 46% nitrogen-free extract, the following result can be obtained with the modified Atwater equation:

$$ME\,(kcal/kg) = 10[(8.5\,kcal/g \times 12)$$
$$+ (3.5\,kcal/g \times 22)$$
$$+ (3.5\,kcal/g \times 46)]$$

$$ME\,(kcal/kg) = 3400$$

Both the Atwater and modified Atwater equations contain assumptions about the GE and digestibility of nutrients and therefore should always be viewed simply as providing an estimate of the ME value of the diet. It is best if measured or average values of nutrient composition, rather than guaranteed analysis, are used for these equations. It is important to realize that the guaranteed analysis provides only upper limits of moisture, fiber, and ash content, and lower limits of protein and fat content. Thus, the guaranteed analysis does not provide a precise measure of the absolute amount of specific nutrients in the diet. It has been reported that differences between measured nutrient composition and guaranteed analysis of pet foods result in an average underestimation of ME of 230 kcal/kg when using the modified Atwater equation (Hill et al. 2009). Thus, it is important to keep in mind that the ME value obtained using the guaranteed analysis from the pet food label will likely be at least slightly lower than the true ME value of the diet. It is also important to note when using the guaranteed analysis from pet food labels that values for ash and carbohydrate (nitrogen-free extract) are not required to be listed on the label. Thus, to roughly estimate the ME content of a diet, it is typically necessary to determine carbohydrate by difference (carbohydrate = 100 − % crude protein − % crude fat − % crude fiber − % moisture − % ash) by estimating the ash content of the diet. Ash values of 2.5% for canned and 8% for dried diets may be used to provide a rough estimate of carbohydrate. However, it should be noted that there can be large variations in ash content between different diets and that use of an assumed ash value can lead to over- or underestimates of carbohydrate.

With the development of a wide range of pet foods that differ in digestibility, there has been debate about whether the modified Atwater equation still adequately predicts the ME value of diets. It has been reported that the equation predicts the ME content of average pet foods with reasonable precision (Kienzle 2002), and the equation provides adequate estimates of the ME content of dry dog foods and canned cat foods (Laflamme 2001). The modified

Atwater equation tends to underestimate the ME value of cat foods with a high ME content and overestimate the value for cat foods with a low ME content (Kienzle 2002). Thus, the Atwater equation may be more appropriate for diets with high energy values and high digestibility. There is also some question about whether the same equation should be used for dog and cat foods, since it has been shown that the digestibility of fat tends to be lower in cats than in dogs (Kendall et al. 1982). Nonetheless, it is common to use the same equations for both dog and cat foods and these equations seem to work reasonably well for providing estimates of the ME contents of many diets. The Atwater and modified Atwater equations are easy to memorize and use, and they provide quick estimates of the ME contents of diets.

Major assumptions are made about nutrient digestibility for all of the equations presented in this section. In particular, the influence of crude fiber on digestibility has been ignored. There has been interest in developing equations that use dietary crude fiber to better estimate the ME content of commercial dog and cat foods. The National Research Council (NRC) has recently recommended separate equations for dog and cat foods using crude fiber to better predict the ME content of diets (NRC 2006). The equation for dog food is:

Step 1: GE (kcal) = (5.7 × g protein) + (9.4 × g fat) + [4.1 × (g nitrogen-free extract + g fiber)]

Step 2: % energy digestibility = 91.2 − (1.43 × % crude fiber in dry matter)

Step 3: DE (kcal) = GE × (% energy digestibility/100)

Step 4: ME (kcal) = DE − (1.04 × g protein)

Similarly, the equation for cat food is:

Step 1: GE (kcal) = (5.7 × g protein) + (9.4 × g fat) + [4.1 × (g carbohydrate + g fiber)]

Step 2: % energy digestibility = 87.9 − (0.88 × % crude fiber in dry matter)

Step 3: DE (kcal) = GE × (% energy digestibility/100)

Step 4: ME (kcal) = DE − (0.77 × g protein)

For example, the ME value for a dog food containing 12% crude fat, 22% crude protein, 46% carbohydrate, 3% crude fiber, 7% ash, and 10% moisture may be calculated as:

Step 1: GE (kcal) = (5.7 × 0.22) + (9.4 × 0.12) + [4.1 × (0.46 + 0.03)] = 4.39

Step 2: % energy digestibility = 91.2 − (1.43 × 3.3[a]) = 86.48

Step 3: DE (kcal) = 4.39 × (86.48/100) = 3.80

Step 4: ME (kcal) = 3.80 − (1.04 × 0.22) = 3.57

[a] Crude fiber on a dry matter basis is calculated as fiber (DM) = fiber (as fed)/(DM/100).

These equations take into consideration the influence of crude fiber on digestibility. They also take into consideration differences in digestibility and urinary energy loss between dogs and cats. The equations may be difficult to memorize or use when quickly obtaining an estimate of ME in conditions when access to references is not readily available, and they may not offer substantial improvement over the modified Atwater equation for average pet foods. However, these equations currently appear to do the best job at predicting ME value over the wide range of pet foods currently on the market. Figure 3.2 provides a summary of the methods used to estimate the ME content of a diet.

Calculating Energy Requirement from Body Weight

Methods of Determining Energy Expenditure and Energy Requirements

The energy requirements of an animal can be determined by accurately measuring either energy intake or energy expenditure. These measurements are the only ways to precisely determine the energy requirement of an individual animal. Data from these measurements have been used to develop equations for predicting animal energy requirements.

As discussed in the diet history section of this chapter, measuring energy intake in a weight-stable animal is the best way to determine the MER of the animal. A standard way, especially in growing animals, to determine MERs has been to feed animals over a range of energy intakes and measure change in body weight. Energy intake may then be plotted against change in body weight and regression equations can be used to fit a line or curve through the data points. The point where change in body weight equals zero is the MER. In contrast to this method, studies in dogs and cats often simply measure energy intake in adult animals that are weight stable or adjust energy intake until weight stability is achieved. The MER is then taken as the amount of energy consumed by the weight-stable dog or cat. The primary advantage of this method is that it does not require expensive laboratory equipment, and only balances are needed to weigh the food and the animal. The major disadvantage of this method is that it can be time consuming, since measurements need to be completed over a sufficient amount of time to make certain that the animal is truly weight stable.

Direct calorimetry has also been used as a method to determine energy requirements. Direct calorimetry measures heat production by the animal to determine energy expenditure and energy requirements. Direct calorimetry works because at maintenance, energy consumed is expended and released as heat (no net gain in body energy). Modern direct calorimeters consist of a chamber surrounded by temperature probes or a thermal jacket that absorbs heat. The rate of temperature change by the thermal jacket (or probe) is proportional to the heat production by the animal. This can be expressed as kcal or kJ per unit of time and equals the energy expenditure and energy requirement for the animal. These calorimetry systems can be very accurate, but the systems are expensive, and they require considerable

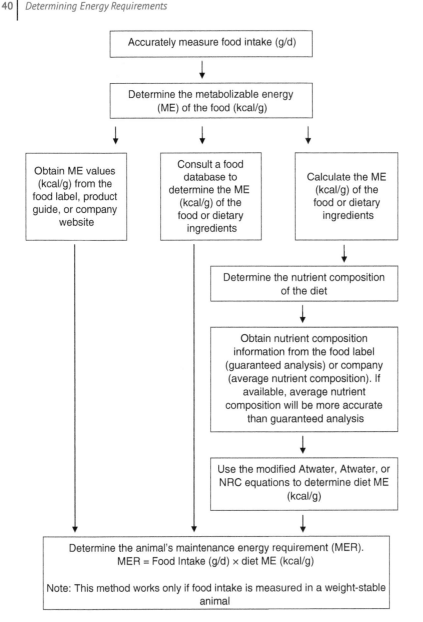

Figure 3.2 A summary of the steps required to estimate the metabolizable energy (ME) content of a diet.

expertise for proper use. Also, the measurements must be made in a calorimeter, and the environment in the calorimeter can be very different from normal housing conditions for the animal. Direct calorimetry also assumes no energy or heat storage in the animal and that all energy transferred from the animal occurs as heat. There are relatively few large animal direct calorimeters, and this method has not been commonly used to determine energy requirements in dogs and cats.

Indirect respiration calorimetry is a method that has frequently been used to measure energy expenditure in both dogs and cats. Indirect respiration calorimetry measures oxygen consumption and/or carbon dioxide production and energy expenditure is calculated from these values. Indirect respiration calorimetry works because the heat released (kcal or kJ) during the oxidation of a particle nutrient/substrate is constant. The ratio of carbon dioxide produced to oxygen consumed (CO_2/O_2) is termed the respiratory quotient (RQ), and this indicates which substrates are being oxidized and the amount of heat released per liter of oxygen consumed and per liter of carbon dioxide produced. The following values are standard numbers used for RQ and heat equivalents of oxygen and carbon dioxide (Blaxter 1989):

Lipids = 0.71 RQ, 4.71 kcal/l O_2 consumed, 6.64 kcal/l CO_2 produced

Proteins = 0.81 RQ, 4.59 kcal/l O_2 consumed, 5.69 kcal/l CO_2 produced

Carbohydrates = 1.0 RQ, 5.07 kcal/l O_2 consumed, 5.07 kcal/l CO_2 produced

RQ is important not only because it provides information about the substrates being oxidized by the animal, but also because it can provide information about energy expenditure. The energy expenditure (or heat production) per liter of O_2 or CO_2 is unique for each value of RQ. Thus, energy expenditure can be calculated from either gas if a reasonable estimate of the expected RQ of the animal can be made. Alternatively, information about the heat production associated with the oxidation of specific substrates has been used to develop equations that allow for the very accurate calculation of energy expenditure if oxygen consumption, carbon dioxide production, and urinary nitrogen can be measured. An example is the Weir equation (Weir 1949):

$$\text{Energy Expenditure (kcal)} = 3.94\,(\text{L } O_2)$$
$$+ 1.11(\text{L } CO_2)$$
$$- 2.17(\text{g } N^a)$$

[a]N refers to grams of urinary nitrogen.

Three methods are commonly used for indirect respiration calorimetry: the calorimetry chamber, face mask, and doubly labeled water methods. The calorimetry chamber method involves placing the animal in a sealed chamber. The rate of air flow through the chamber is carefully regulated and the O_2 and CO_2 content of the inlet and outlet air are measured. Consumption of O_2 and production of CO_2 are calculated from these measures of air flow (l/min) and differences in the concentration of O_2 and CO_2 between the air entering and leaving the chamber.

The face mask method involves placing a sealed mask over the mouth and nostrils of the animal. Air flow through the mask and the gas content of the air flowing into and out of the mask are measured.

The doubly labeled water method involves administering a dose of $^2H_2^{18}O$ to the animal (usually as an injection). Urine or blood samples are collected at some later time to determine differences in the concentration of the two isotopes ($^2H_2$ and ^{18}O). The isotope ^{18}O may be lost from the body as either CO_2 or water, while $^2H_2$ is lost from the body as water only. The difference in the concentration of the two isotopes thus gives a measure of CO_2 production. Energy expenditure may then be calculated from this measure of CO_2 production using an assumed RQ.

The advantages of indirect respiration calorimetry include the fact that these methods can provide a very accurate measure of energy expenditure, and consequently energy requirements for maintenance. The measurements, at least in the case of the doubly labeled water method, can also be completed in the animal's home environment. Indirect respiration calorimetry can provide a measure of energy expenditure over a short period of time, and resting energy expenditure values can be obtained from properly adapted animals in a matter of minutes or hours. The primary disadvantage of the indirect respiration calorimetry method is that the equipment (i.e. gas analyzers, chambers, flow meters, mass spectrometer for doubly labeled water) required for these measurements is expensive and requires some expertise to operate. Thus, while indirect respiration calorimetry is widely used in laboratory settings for measuring energy expenditure and determining energy requirements, this method has not yet found widespread use in veterinary clinics and hospitals.

Methods of Calculating Energy Expenditure and Energy Requirements

Body weight is the primary component used in all equations for calculating MERs. Larger animals have a greater overall energy expenditure (kcal or kJ/day) than small animals. However, when energy expenditure is divided by body weight (kcal or KJ/kg/day), large animals have a lower energy expenditure than small animals. In other words, large animals consume less food and produce less heat per unit of mass than do small animals. For example, a rat weighing 1 lb will eat 72 kcal/day. If this same energy intake were directly extrapolated to an 80 lb dog, the dog would consume 5760 kcal per day!

The relationship between energy expenditure and body weight has been studied by many groups. In the nineteenth century, scientists proposed that energy expenditure was related to body surface area. Equations were developed that showed that in bodies that are geometrically similar, surface area is related to weight by the function $kg^{0.67}$ (Blanc et al. 2003; Hill and Scott 2004). Thus, small animals have a greater surface area for their body weight than do large animals. Rubner (1883) proposed that energy expenditure is constant at 1000 kcal/m^2 body surface area, and other studies have suggested that weight is related to energy expenditure by the mass exponent $kg^{0.67}$. The mass exponent $kg^{0.67}$ is still frequently used today to normalize energy expenditure for differences in body weight.

In the 1930s, Brody at the University of Missouri plotted basal energy expenditure against body weight in animals ranging in size from mice and canaries to elephants, and determined that the curve running through the data points was best represented by the following equation (kg BW = body weight in kilograms) (Brody and Procter 1932; Brody et al. 1934):

$$Basal\ metabolism\,(kcal/day) = 70 \times kg\,BW^{0.734}$$

At the same time, Kleiber at the University of California–Davis was also comparing basal energy expenditure and body weight data from adult animals covering a wide range of body sizes and determined that $BW^{0.75}$ fit the energy expenditure data as well as $BW^{0.73}$ (Kleiber 1961). The equation proposed by Kleiber has remained the standard equation for predicting basal energy expenditure in adult animals. Although Brody and Kleiber used the term "basal metabolism" with their equations, the conditions used to measure energy expenditure in the animals studied may best be described as resting energy expenditure under fasting conditions, since the stringent requirements for measuring basal metabolic rate were not likely met in many of the measurements. Thus, it can be considered that Kleiber's equation predicts resting energy expenditure. The equation is:

$$Resting\ energy\ expenditure\,(kcal/day) = 70 \times kg\,BW^{0.75}$$

Resting energy requirements (RER) calculated for adult dogs and cats using this equation are provided in Tables 3.1 and 3.2, respectively.

Energy Requirements for Maintenance

It has been common to assume that resting energy expenditure is responsible for 50% of total energy expenditure in the typical adult animal. Therefore, multiplying 70 in the previous equation by a factor of 2 provides the following equation to estimate MERs in adult animals:

$$Maintenance\,(kcal/day) = 140 \times kg\,BW^{0.75}$$

Table 3.1 Resting and maintenance energy requirements (kcal/day) of adult dogs.

Body weight (kg)	Body weight (lb)	RER[a]	MER[b] active pet dogs	MER[c] young dogs	MER[d] inactive dogs	MER[e] active old dogs
1	2.2	70	130	140	95	105
2	4.4	118	219	235	160	177
3	6.6	160	296	319	217	239
4	8.8	198	368	396	269	297
5	11	234	435	468	318	351
6	13.2	268	498	537	364	403
7	15.4	301	559	602	409	452
8	17.6	333	618	666	452	499
9	19.8	364	675	727	494	546
10	22	394	731	787	534	590
11	24.2	423	785	846	574	634
12	26.4	451	838	903	613	677
13	28.6	479	890	958	650	719
14	30.8	507	941	1013	688	760
15	33	534	991	1067	724	800
16	35.2	560	1040	1120	760	840
17	37.4	586	1088	1172	795	879
18	39.6	612	1136	1223	830	918
19	41.8	637	1183	1274	865	956
20	44	662	1229	1324	898	993
21	46.2	687	1275	1373	932	1030
22	48.4	711	1321	1422	965	1067
23	50.6	735	1365	1470	998	1103
24	52.8	759	1410	1518	1030	1139
25	55	783	1453	1565	1062	1174
26	57.2	806	1497	1612	1094	1209
27	59.4	829	1540	1658	1125	1244
28	61.6	852	1582	1704	1156	1278
29	63.8	875	1625	1750	1187	1312
30	66	897	1666	1795	1218	1346
31	68.2	920	1708	1839	1248	1379
32	70.4	942	1749	1884	1278	1413
33	72.6	964	1790	1928	1308	1446
34	74.8	986	1830	1971	1338	1478
35	77	1007	1871	2015	1367	1511
36	79.2	1029	1911	2058	1396	1543
37	81.4	1050	1950	2100	1425	1575

(Continued)

Table 3.1   (Continued)

Body weight (kg)	Body weight (lb)	RER[a]	MER[b] active pet dogs	MER[c] young dogs	MER[d] inactive dogs	MER[e] active old dogs
38	83.6	1071	1990	2143	1454	1607
39	85.8	1092	2029	2185	1483	1639
40	88	1113	2068	2227	1511	1670
41	90.2	1134	2106	2268	1539	1701
42	92.4	1155	2145	2310	1567	1732
43	94.6	1175	2183	2351	1595	1763
44	96.8	1196	2221	2392	1623	1794
45	99	1216	2259	2432	1651	1824
46	101.2	1236	2296	2473	1678	1855
47	103.4	1257	2334	2513	1705	1885
48	105.6	1277	2371	2553	1732	1915
49	107.8	1296	2408	2593	1759	1945
50	110	1316	2444	2632	1786	1974
51	112.2	1336	2481	2672	1813	2004
52	114.4	1356	2517	2711	1840	2033
53	116.6	1375	2554	2750	1866	2063
54	118.8	1394	2590	2789	1892	2092
55	121	1414	2626	2827	1919	2121
56	123.2	1433	2661	2866	1945	2149
57	125.4	1452	2697	2904	1971	2178
58	127.6	1471	2732	2942	1997	2207
59	129.8	1490	2767	2980	2022	2235
60	132	1509	2803	3018	2048	2264
61	134.2	1528	2838	3056	2074	2292
62	136.4	1547	2872	3093	2099	2320
63	138.6	1565	2907	3131	2124	2348
64	140.8	1584	2942	3168	2150	2376
65	143	1602	2976	3205	2175	2404
66	145.2	1621	3010	3242	2200	2431
67	147.4	1639	3044	3279	2225	2459
68	149.6	1658	3078	3315	2250	2486
69	151.8	1676	3112	3352	2274	2514
70	154	1694	3146	3388	2299	2541
71	156.2	1712	3180	3424	2324	2568
72	158.4	1730	3213	3460	2348	2595
73	160.6	1748	3247	3496	2373	2622
74	162.8	1766	3280	3532	2397	2649

Table 3.1   (Continued)

Body weight (kg)	Body weight (lb)	RER[a]	MER[b] active pet dogs	MER[c] young dogs	MER[d] inactive dogs	MER[e] active old dogs
75	165	1784	3313	3568	2421	2676
76	167.2	1802	3346	3604	2445	2703
77	169.4	1820	3379	3639	2469	2729
78	171.6	1837	3412	3675	2493	2756
79	173.8	1855	3445	3710	2517	2782
80	176	1872	3477	3745	2541	2809

[a] RER = resting energy requirement = $70 \times kg\ BW^{0.75}$.
[b] MER = maintenance energy requirement for active pet dogs or kennel dogs = $130 \times kg\ BW^{0.75}$.
[c] MER = maintenance energy requirement for active young adult dogs = $140 \times kg\ BW^{0.75}$.
[d] MER = maintenance energy requirement for inactive dogs = $95 \times kg\ BW^{0.75}$.
[e] MER = maintenance energy requirement for older active dogs e = $105 \times kg\ BW^{0.75}$.

Table 3.2   Resting and maintenance energy requirements (kcal/day) of adult cats.

Body weight (kg)	Body weight (lb)	RER[a]	MER[b] lean cats	MER[c] overweight cats
1	2.2	70	100	130
1.5	3.3	95	131	153
2	4.4	118	159	172
2.5	5.5	139	185	188
3	6.6	160	209	202
3.5	7.7	179	231	215
4	8.8	198	253	226
4.5	9.9	216	274	237
5	11	234	294	247
5.5	12.1	251	313	257
6	13.2	268	332	266
6.5	14.3	285	350	275
7	15.4	301	368	283
7.5	16.5	317	386	291
8	17.6	333	403	299
8.5	18.7	348	419	306
9	19.8	364	436	313
9.5	20.9	379	452	320
10	22	394	468	327

[a] RER = resting energy requirement = $70 \times kg\ BW^{0.75}$.
[b] MER = maintenance energy requirement for lean cats = $100 \times kg\ BW^{0.67}$.
[c] MER = maintenance energy requirement for obese cats = $130 \times kg\ BW^{0.40}$.

It is important to note that the exponent 0.75 used in these equations was simply determined from the regression equation that best fit the energy expenditure and body weight data, and the physiologic meaning of this exponent is still the subject of considerable debate. The 0.75 exponent was derived from comparisons across species, and this exponent may not be appropriate for some comparisons within a species.

For dogs and cats, there have generally been two approaches to calculating MERs.

The first approach has been to calculate resting energy expenditure using Kleiber's equation ($70 \times kg\ BW^{0.75}$) or a linear equation such as resting energy expenditure (kcal/g) $= 70 + (30 \times kg\ BW)$ (Thatcher et al. 2010). The same equations for calculating MERs are commonly used for both dogs and cats. MERs are then multiplied by a factor that takes into account the age, activity, or physiologic condition of the animal (Box 3.1).

Box 3.1   Feline Maintenance Energy Requirements

Neutered adult	= 1.2 – 1.4 × RER
Intact adult	= 1.4 – 1.6 × RER
Inactive/obese prone	= 1.0 × RER
Weight loss	= 0.8 × RER
Senior	= 1.1 – 1.4 × RER
Elderly cat	= 1.1 × 1.6 × RER
Critical care	= 1.0 × RER
Weight gain	= 1.2 – 1.8 × RER

Feline Gestation

- Cats gain weight linearly during gestation.
- Calorie intake should be increased to 1.6 × RER at time of breeding.
- Calorie intake should be increased to 2 × RER at time of parturition.

Feline Lactation

- 2–6 × RER is recommended, but the number of kittens must also be taken into consideration.
- The following can be used to estimate the MER of lactating queens:
  - Weeks 1–2   = RER + 30%/kitten
  - Week 3   = RER + 45%/kitten
  - Week 4   = RER + 55%/kitten
  - Week 5   = RER + 65%/kitten
  - Week 6   = RER + 90%/kitten

Kittens are usually introduced to the dam's food somewhere between 6 and 7 weeks of age. This timeline is influenced by the number of kittens the queen is nursing.

In general, energy intake of growing kittens should be approximately RER × 2.5. These authors recommend free-choice feeding in growing kittens.

Canine Maintenance Energy Requirements

Neutered adult	= 1.6 × RER
Intact adult	= 1.8 × RER
Inactive/obese prone	= 1.2 – 1.4 × RER
Weight loss	= 1.0 × RER
Critical care	= 1.0 × RER
Weight gain	= 1.2 × 1.8 × RER

Work

Light work	= 1.6 – 2.0 × RER
Moderate work	= 2.0 – 5.0 × RER
Heavy work	= 5.0 – 11.0 × RER

Gestation

During the first two-thirds of gestation, feed the bitch as a normal dog

For the last third of gestation, feed 3 × RER. Check body condition routinely to ensure that the bitch is consuming enough food. In some cases, dogs may require less or more food to maintain body condition.

Lactation

Lactation is the most demanding life stage, so experts suggest that nursing dogs be fed free choice. Lactation requirements are influenced by the number of puppies the bitch has thrown. The following recommendations can be used to estimate the MER of a lactating dog:

Number of Puppies	RER
1	$3.0 \times RER$
2	$3.5 \times RER$
3–4	$4.0 \times RER$
5–6	$5.0 \times RER$
7–8	$5.5 \times RER$
9	$\geq 6 \times RER$

Growth

Maintenance energy intake should be $3 \times RER$ from weaning until 4 months of age. Thereafter energy intake should be reduced to $2 \times RER$ until the puppy reaches adult size.

Source: Adapted from Thatcher et al. 2010.

Example Calculation

What would be the predicted MER for a neutered, adult cat with a body weight of 6 kg?

$$\text{ME at maintenance (kcal/day)} = 1.2 \times 70 \times (6)^{0.75}$$

$$= 322 \text{ kcal/day}$$

The primary advantage of these factorial calculations is that the calculations give the veterinarian or nutritionist the flexibility to select or devise a factor that they feel will best predict the energy needs of the animal. However, the disadvantages of the factorial approach are that it is often unclear how the factors were derived and that the factors have not been rigorously tested to determine if they predict energy requirements better than other equations. Also, the large number of factors can sometimes make it difficult to determine which factor is most appropriate for an individual animal.

- Calculation of MER – this requirement is based on RERs modified by a factor to account for normal activity (i.e. gestation, lactation). RER is a function of metabolic body size. RER is calculated by raising the animal's body weight (in kg) to the 0.75 power.
- These energy requirements are only guidelines and estimates/starting points for individual requirements.

- It is imperative that animals be assessed frequently, and calorie intake modified when indicated to maintain ideal body condition score.

The second approach has been to use an equation that was developed specifically to predict MERs. MERs calculated for adult dogs and cats using this approach are provided in Tables 3.1 and 3.2, respectively. The NRC uses the following equation to predict MER for kennel dogs or active pet dogs (NRC 2006):

$$\text{ME at maintenance} = 130 \text{ kg} \times BW^{0.75} \text{ kcal/day}$$

Equations using different multipliers are recommended for groups of dogs that have been reported to have higher or lower energy requirements than those obtained from the standard MER equation. Rather than use 130 in the previous equation, it is recommended that the following multipliers are used for the indicated groups of dogs (NRC 2006):

Young, active dogs	140 (i.e. ME at maintenance $= 140$ kg $BW^{0.75}$)
Active Great Danes	200
Active terriers	180
Inactive dogs	95
Newfoundlands	105
Older active dogs	105

Example Calculation

What would be the predicted MER for an active mixed-breed dog with a body weight of 30 kg?

$$\text{ME at maintenance (kcal/day)} = 130 \times (30\,\text{kg})^{0.75}$$
$$= 1666\,\text{kcal/day}$$

In some cases, there is an advantage to having an equation that can easily be calculated without using exponents of body weight. The following linear equation is provided by the NRC and gives results comparable to the previous equation using $W^{0.75}$ for dogs weighing 8–20 kg (NRC 2006):

$$\text{ME at maintenance} = 358 + (39 \times \text{kg BW})$$

The NRC equations for predicting MERs in cats are as follows (NRC 2006):

Lean domestic cats[a]: ME at maintenance (kcal/day) = 100 kg BW$^{0.67}$

Overweight cats[b]: ME at maintenance (kcal/day) = 130 kg BW$^{0.40}$

[a] "Lean" refers to cats with a BCS of less than or equal to five on a nine-point scale.

[b] "Overweight" refers to cats with a BCS of greater than or equal to six on a nine-point scale.

Example Calculation

What would be the predicted MER for a 4 kg lean cat?

$$\text{ME at maintenance} = 100 \times (4\,\text{kg})^{0.67}$$
$$= 253\,\text{kcal/day}$$

A linear equation was used to calculate MERs for cats in the 1986 NRC. This equation overestimated the energy requirements for large cats and led to the recent development of equations for lean and overweight cats. Nonetheless, the linear equation may still be useful for a quick estimate of energy requirements, without the need to calculate exponents of body weight. The cat linear equations are as follows (NRC 1986):

Active cats: ME at maintenance (kcal/day) = 80 × kg BW

Inactive cats: ME at maintenance (kcal/day) = 70 × kg BW

Figure 3.3 shows a comparison of MERs calculated using either an exponential or linear equation. The steps for calculating MERs for both dogs and cats are summarized in Figure 3.4.

It is important to note that prediction equations provide only a rough estimate of energy requirements for individual animals (they predict the requirements for the "average" animal). There is considerable variation in energy requirements between animals, and the true energy requirements of an individual animal may differ by as much as 50% from predicted values. Therefore, the equations simply provide a starting point for determining how much to feed an animal. Assuming weight stability is the goal for an individual, energy intake would clearly need to be adjusted if the predicted MERs caused either an increase or decrease in body weight. The best equation to use for predicting the MER of an individual animal is somewhat of an academic argument, since none of the equations accounts for the tremendous amount of individual variability that is observed in the energy requirements of dogs and cats. The equations simply allow the user to take an educated guess at the MERs of a particular animal. It is important for a veterinarian or nutritionist to tell clients that it is not currently possible to precisely predict the energy requirement of an individual animal, that energy calculations simply provide a starting point, and that adjustments may be required to find the animal's true MER.

Energy Requirements for Growth

The requirement for energy is higher during growth compared to adult maintenance. During this process, some energy is deposited in tissue, and some energy is expended in the process of building new tissue:

Energy Intake → Maintenance Energy Expenditure
    + Energy Expenditure Associated with
        Tissue Synthesis
    + Energy Deposited in Tissue

Efficiency of energy use in maintenance and growth differs because the energy costs of anabolic and catabolic pathways differ. In general,

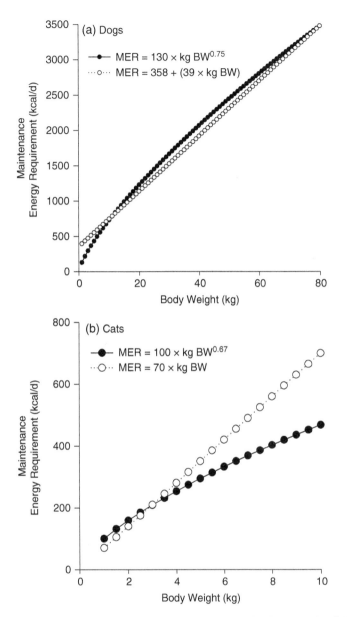

Figure 3.3 Comparisons of maintenance energy requirements (MERs) for dogs (panel A) and cats (panel B) using linear or exponential equations. BW, body weight.

efficiency of energy use in growth is low. Therefore, on a per-unit weight basis, the energy requirement for growth is greater than that for maintenance.

Growing puppies require approximately twice as much energy per gram of body weight as adult dogs (Arnold and Elvehjem 1939). However, energy requirements change as a dog grows from weaning to adult body weight. Predicted energy requirements are approximately 2.5 times maintenance requirements at weaning and requirements decrease to approximately 1.5 times maintenance requirements by the time the dog reaches 60% of maximal mature weight. A factorial approach may be used to calculate energy requirements for growth by multiplying formulas for predicting MERs by these factors.

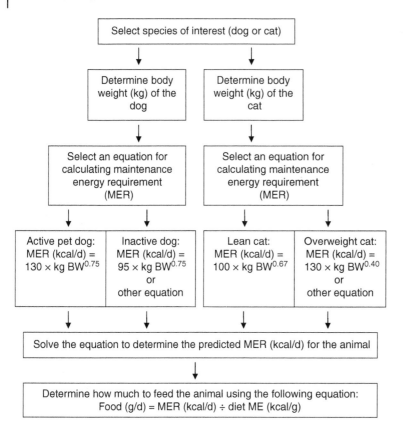

Figure 3.4 A summary of the steps required to estimate the maintenance energy requirements for dogs or cats. BW, body weight; ME, metabolizable energy.

The energy requirements for growth in dogs can be predicted using the following equation (NRC 2006):

$$ME\ (kcal/day) = 130 \times BW_c^{0.75} \times [3.2 \times (e^{-0.87p} - 0.1)]$$

where:

BWc = current body weight in kg
e = base of natural log (i.e. 2.71828...)
p = current body weight divided by expected mature body weight

Notice that the first part of the equation ($130 \times BW_c^{0.75}$) simply calculates MERs. All animals have an MER, and energy required for growth, reproduction, or other physiologic processes occurs in addition to this maintenance requirement. The second part of the equation $[3.2 \times (e^{-0.87p} - 0.1)]$ includes the energy required for growth.

Example Calculation

What is the daily energy requirement for a 3-month-old golden retriever puppy that weighs 11 kg and has an expected mature body weight of 30 kg?

$$MC\ (kcal/day) = 130 \times 11 kg^{0.75}$$
$$\times 3.2 \times (e^{-0.87(11/30)} - 0.1)$$
$$= 130 \times 6.04 \times 3.2$$
$$\times (e^{-0.319} - 0.1)$$
$$= 2512.64 \times 0.627$$
$$= 1575\ kcal/day$$

For dogs, the equations for predicting energy requirements for growth should simply serve as a starting point for determining how much to feed puppies. Puppies should always be fed to promote optimal growth rather than maximal growth. Optimal growth requires monitoring BCS and adjusting energy intake as needed. For purebred dogs, puppy weights can be compared to growth standards for the breed, and energy intake should be adjusted if the puppies deviate from ideal body condition. It has been shown that Newfoundland puppies require less energy (kcal/kg body weight) than Great Dane puppies, despite the fact that they grow at the same rate (Legrand-Defretin 1994). Labrador puppies also appear to require less energy (kcal/kg body weight) than briard puppies (Legrand-Defretin 1994), and this further supports the point that purebred puppies should be fed to support the appropriate growth rate for their breed and to maintain an ideal body condition score.

Similar to dogs, a detailed equation has been developed to predict the energy requirements for growth in kittens (NRC 2006):

$$ME\ (kcal/day) = 100 \times BW_c^{0.67}$$
$$\times 6.7 \times (e^{-0.189p} - 0.66])$$

where:

BW_c = current body weight in kg
e = base of natural log (i.e. 2.718 28. . .)
p = current body weight divided by expected mature body weight

To allow kittens to meet their energy requirements, it is generally recommended that they be provided with ad libitum access to food. The NRC equation provides an estimate of the expected energy intake of kittens and offers a quantitative way to see how energy requirements change as an animal approaches adult body weight. However, given the risks of neutering on the development of obesity, body condition should be closely monitored in spayed and castrated kittens.

Energy Requirements for Pregnancy and Lactation

Similar to growth, the energy requirements during both pregnancy and lactation are greater than maintenance because of the energetic cost of fetal growth or milk production. In bitches, no increase in energy intake is required until 4–5 weeks after mating (Case et al. 2010; NRC 2006). At this time, and until parturition, energy requirements will increase by 25% to over 60% depending on the size of the bitch (the percentage increase in energy requirements during pregnancy tends to be greater for large-breed bitches). The following equation is used to predict energy requirements in bitches during late gestation (NRC 2006):

$$ME\ (kcal/day) = 130 \times kg\ BW^{0.75}$$
$$+ (26 \times kg\ BW)$$

Notice that the first part of the equation ($130 \times kg\ BW^{0.75}$) is simply the MER of the bitch, and the second part of the equation ($26 + kg\ BW$) is the energy required for weight gain during gestation.

Queens should be fed to encourage a 40–50% increase in body weight during pregnancy (Loveridge 1986). In general queens gain in a linear fashion, and energy requirements increase by approximately 40% during pregnancy. The following equation has been used to predict energy requirements in queens during pregnancy (NRC 2006):

$$ME\ (kcal/day) = 140 \times kg\ BW^{0.67}$$

However, it is common practice to allow queens ad libitum access to food during pregnancy to promote weight gain, which is needed to subsequently support lactation.

Lactation represents the greatest energy demand on the animal. It can often be difficult for the female to consume enough energy to meet this great demand, and thus it is common practice to allow bitches and queens ad libitum access to food through at least the first several weeks of lactation. The energy cost of lactation will vary depending on the number of offspring, and the amount of solid food that is given to the offspring. Puppies and kittens are often weaned by 8 weeks of age, and solid food should be offered to puppies and kittens by 3–4 weeks of age (Case et al. 2010). Energy requirements are typically increased by 2–4 times maintenance requirements during lactation in bitches or queens. Energy requirements during lactation in bitches may be calculated using the following equation (NRC 2006):

$$ME\ (kcal/day) = 145 \times kg\,BW^{0.75} + [kg\,BW\,(24n + 12m) \times L]$$

where:

kg BW = body weight of the dog in kg
n = number of puppies between 1 and 4
m = number of puppies between 5 and 8
L = correction factor for stage of lactation (week 1 = 0.75, week 2 = 0.95, week 3 = 1.1, week 4 = 1.2)

Example Calculation
What is the daily energy requirement of a 35 kg Labrador retriever in the second week of lactation nursing five puppies?

$$ME\ (kcal/day) = 145 \times 35^{0.75} + 35[(24 \times 4) + (12 \times 1)] \times 0.95$$

$$ME\ (kcal/day) = 2086.5 + 35(96 + 12) \times 0.95\ ME\,(kcal/day)$$

$$= 2086.5 + 3780 \times 0.95$$
$$= 2086.5 + 3591$$
$$= 5678\,kcal/day$$

Energy requirements during lactation in cats may be calculated using the following equations (NRC 2006):

Fewer than three kittens: $ME\,(kcal/day)$
$$= 100 \times kg\,BW^{0.67} + (18 \times BW\,kg \times L)$$

Three to four kittens: $ME\,(kcal/day)$
$$= 100 \times kg\,BW^{0.67} + (60 \times BW\,kg \times L)$$

More than four kittens: $ME\,(kcal/day)$
$$= 100 \times kg\,BW^{0.67} + (70 \times BW\,kg \times L)$$

where:

kg BW or BW kg = body weight of the cat in kg
L = correction factor for stage of lactation (week 1 = 0.9, week 2 = 0.9, week 3 = 1.2, week 4 = 1.2, week 5 = 1.1, week 6 = 1.0, week 7 = 0.8)

It is important for the user of these equations to understand that the multipliers are only a starting point. It is vital that the veterinarian repeatedly assess the patient's body condition and adjust food intake accordingly.

Neutered adult male dog, 7 kg, BCS 6/9, with an adverse food reaction
For an overweight, obese-prone dog, a lower multiplier of 1.2–1.4 is indicated:

$$RER = 7\,kg^{0.75} \times 70 = 301\,kcal/day$$

$$MER = 1.2 \times 301\,kcal$$

$$MER = 361\,kcal/day$$

Intact female dog, 20 kg, BCS 5/9, in second third of gestation that is about to enter lactation
Bitches in the first two trimesters of gestation should be fed to maintain a normal adult body condition. In the third trimester, bitches are often free fed to support lactational needs or initially three times their RER:

$$RER = 20\,kg^{0.75} \times 70 = 622\,kcal/day$$

$$3 \times 662 = 1986\,kcal/day$$

6-month-old, intact male Great Dane puppy, 31 kg, BCS 4/9
Energy requirements for puppies are approximately three times the RER until 4 months of age:

$$RER = 31\,kg^{0.75} \times 70 = 920\,kcal/day$$

$$RER \times 3 = 920 \times 3 = 2760\,kcal/day$$

Then two times the RER for the remainder of growth after 4 months of age, so for a 6-month-old that would be:

$$2 \times 920 = 1840\,kcal/day$$

Recently weaned kitten

Young, recently weaned kittens should be fed ad libitum. After neutering, body condition should be monitored and food intake is likely to require reduction.

8-year-old overweight female spayed dog, 7 kg, BCS, 8/9, with uroliths

For an obese animal the initial multiplier if current intake is unknown is 1:

$$7 \text{kg}^{0.75} \times 70 = 301 \text{kcal/day}$$

10-year-old spayed cat, 3.5 kg, BCS 4/9, with IRIS Stage 2 chronic kidney disease

The multiplier for an underweight senior neutered cat can be in the range of 1.2–1.6:

$$\text{RER} = 3.5 \text{kg}^{0.75} \times 70 = 179 \text{kcal/day}$$

$$\text{RER} \times 1.4 = 179 \times 1.4 = 251 \text{kcal/day}$$

Calculating Energy Requirements in States of Disease

It can be a challenge to determine the energy requirements of injured or ill animals. However, the proper energy intake is essential for recovery or to stabilize the illness. Energy intakes that are too low can lead to accelerated loss of lean tissue mass, which could induce further complications. In contrast, energy intakes that are too high can lead to hyperglycemia, hyperlipidemia, and hyperammonemia (Burkholder 1995). High energy intakes may also cause hepatomegaly and hyperbilirubinemia (Lowry and Brennan 1979), which may prevent proper recovery from the injury or illness. Therefore, it is important to provide an appropriate amount of dietary energy to promote recovery and prevent the development of further complications.

Unfortunately, there have been relatively few studies that have measured energy expenditure in dogs and cats with injury or illness. Some studies have used indirect respiration calorimetry using a face mask system to measure energy in dogs with osteosarcoma (Mazzaferro et al. 2001), lymphoma (Ogilvie et al. 1993), non-hematologic tumors (Ogilvie et al. 1996), surgery (O'Toole et al. 2004), or trauma (O'Toole et al. 2004). However, there are two key limitations with these studies. First, the face mask system of indirect respiration calorimetry requires training to ensure that the animal does not become stressed by wearing the face mask. Thus, it is only possible to obtain reliable data in well-adapted animals. One study, which completed indirect respiration calorimetry measurements over a 16-minute period repeated four times during the day, found that the most reliable measures of energy expenditure using the face mask system were obtained without the first two measurements of the day (O'Toole, et al. 2001). This at least suggests that adaptation to the face mask was occurring with repeated measurements. In hospitalized patients, it may be difficult to adequately adapt the animals to the face mask. Second, the indirect respiration calorimetry measurements using the face mask system are completed only in animals at rest and thus provide information only about the influence of injury or illness on resting energy expenditure. The influence of injury and illness on total energy expenditure will determine the animal's energy requirement, and measures of only resting energy expenditure do not provide information about physical activity or total energy expenditure. Currently there is very limited information about the energy expenditure and energy requirements of sick or injured dogs and cats.

Because of the limited information on energy requirements in companion animals with disease, it has been necessary to use human data to devise equations for estimating energy requirements in hospitalized dogs and cats. Early studies investigating the influence of disease on energy requirements in humans often measured resting energy expenditure in patients during periods of peak hypermetabolism and then used these data to calculate energy requirements (Weekes 2007). It was often assumed that the increase in measured resting energy expenditure would translate into increases in total energy expenditure. Equations were then developed that predicted that injury and illness would cause increases in energy requirements above those of a healthy animal at maintenance. Human equations were adopted for use in veterinary medicine with factors that predicted increases in MERs of up to twofold, depending on the injury (Donoghue 1989). However, it is now considered that injury and illness do not generally increase overall MERs and often may actually decrease it. In particular, there is relatively little information about the influence of many diseases on physical activity-related energy expenditure (Kulstad and Schoeller 2007), despite the fact that this is a major contributor to MERs.

The use of the doubly labeled water method combined with measures of resting energy expenditure, nonetheless, has allowed physical activity to be measured in human patients with diseases. Data from these studies indicate that most chronic and acute diseases produce a considerable decrease in physical activity-related energy expenditure (Elia 2005). While resting energy expenditure is typically increased with acute disease (Elia 2005) and injury (Frankenfield 2006), the decrease in physical activity-related energy expenditure may negate the changes in resting energy expenditure and produce a net decrease in total energy expenditure (and MERs). Decreases in total energy expenditure may also be exacerbated by medications such as sedatives and analgesics, which may make the animal drowsy and limit voluntary physical activity. Cage confinement can also limit movement and contribute to decreases in energy expenditure.

Based on current information (mostly from human studies), it is prudent to be conservative in predicting the energy requirements for dogs and cats with disease or injury. Starting at RER helps ensure tolerance of the specific diet and the feeding method. Body weight should be monitored, and the amount fed should be adjusted as needed to initially maintain weight. If gain is desired, this can then be gradually implemented. Weight loss is never a goal during treatment and recovery from trauma and

critical illness. Rather, a weight-loss plan is a longer-term goal that can be instituted at home once the animal is recovered and stable. It should rarely be necessary to feed injured or ill cats and dogs above the predicted energy requirement for a healthy animal at maintenance. A series of factors for calculating energy requirements with disease and injury have been developed for use in hospitalized human patients. These factors are multiplied by RERs to determine the energy requirements for individuals with disease or injury. Energy requirements are generally equal to 1.1–1.8 times resting energy expenditure, depending on the disease or severity of injury (Barndregt and Soeters 2005; Newton and Heimburger 2006).

The following equations have been proposed for predicting energy requirements in injured or ill dog and cats (Remillard and Thatcher 1989) or humans (Lagua and Claudio 2004):

Surgery: $ME (kcal/day) = 1.1–1.3 \times (70 \text{ kg BW}^{0.75})$

Cancer: $ME (kcal/day) = 1.2–1.5 \times (70 \text{ kg BW}^{0.75})$

Trauma: $ME (kcal/day) = 1.3–1.4 \times (70 \text{ kg BW}^{0.75})$

Multiple trauma, head trauma: $ME (kcal/day) = 1.5–2.3 \times (70 \text{ kg BW}^{0.75})$

Sepsis: $ME (kcal/day) = 1.8–2.0 \times (70 \text{ kg BW}^{0.75})$

Burns, <40% of body: $ME (kcal/day) = 1.2–1.8 \times (70 \text{ kg BW}^{0.75})$

Burns, >40% of body: $ME (kcal/day) = 1.8–2.0 \times (70 \text{ kg BW}^{0.75})$

Respiratory/renal failure: $ME (kcal/day) = 1.2–1.4 \times (70 \text{ kg BW}^{0.75})$

Fractures, long bone or multiple: $ME (kcal/day) = 1.2–1.3 \times (70 \text{ kg BW}^{0.75})$

Infections, mild to moderate: $ME (kcal/day) = 1.1–1.4 \times (70 \text{ kg BW}^{0.75})$

Infections, severe: $ME (kcal/day) = 1.5–1.7 \times (70 \text{ kg BW}^{0.75})$

These factors have not been extensively tested in dogs and cats, and use of these equations assumes that dogs and cats will have similar energetic responses to disease and injury to humans. Without additional information on changes in total energy expenditure in response to illness and injury in companion animals, it seems reasonable to target energy requirements for most sick or injured dogs and

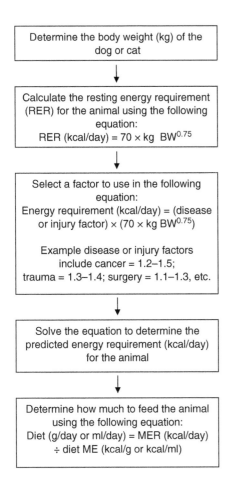

Figure 3.5 A summary of the steps required to determine how much to feed a dog or cat that has an injury or illness. BW, body weight; ME, metabolizable energy; MER, maintenance energy requirement.

cats initially at RER, followed by adjustments based on individual progress. Veterinarians or nutritionists should be ready to make adjustments in the energy given to the animal based on the response of the patient. A summary of the steps involved in determining how much to feed an injured or ill animal is provided in Figure 3.5.

Summary

- An accurate diet record is the best way to determine the MER of an animal that is weight stable.

- The energy requirements of dogs and cats are given in units (kcal or kJ) of metabolizable energy (ME).

- The energy content of a diet may be calculated using factors that contain assumptions about the gross energy and digestibility of the diet components. The modified Atwater equation (crude protein = 3.5 kcal/g; crude fat = 8.5 kcal/g; carbohydrate = 3.5 kcal/g) is commonly used in dog and cat nutrition, although this equation may underestimate the ME content of high-energy diets and overestimate the ME content of low-digestible, high-fiber diets.

- The RER of dogs, cats, and other mammals may be predicted using the equation RER (kcal/day) = $70 \times$ kg $BW^{0.75}$.

- The MER of dogs and cats can be predicted using one of several equations derived specifically for determining MER or by multiplying RER by factors for the activity, age, or physiologic status of the animal. Because of the large variation in MER between animals, prediction equations can only provide a rough estimate of the MER for an individual animal. It is important to realize that these equations provide a starting point for determining how much to feed an animal and that adjustments in energy intake may be needed to find the animal's true MER.

- Growth, pregnancy, and lactation all cause increases in energy requirements above maintenance. Increases of more than double MER occur during early growth and lactation.

- Injury and illness often cause an increase in RER but a decrease in physical activity-related energy expenditure. Overall, total energy expenditure is often not changed, or is even decreased, with injury and disease. The energy requirements of hospitalized animals are often predicted by multiplying RER by a factor that adjusts for the specific disease or injury. In general, most animals with injury or disease are fed somewhere between the RER and the MER of healthy animals.

References

AAFCO (2022). *Official Publication*. Oxford, IN: Association of American Feed Control Officials.

Arnold, A. and Elvehjem, C.A. (1939). Nutritional requirements of dogs. *J. Am. Vet. Med. Assoc.* 95: 187–194.

Atwater, W.O. (1902). Principles of nutrition and nutritive value of food. In: *Farmer's Bulletin No. 142*. Washington, DC: US Department of Agriculture.

Barndregt, K. and Soeters, P. (2005). Nutritional support. In: *Clinical Nutrition* (ed. E.J. Gibney, M. Elias, O. Ljungquist and J. Dowsett), 115–131. Ames, IA: Blackwell.

Blanc, S., Schoeller, D., Kemnitz, J. et al. (2003). Energy expenditure of rhesus monkeys subjected to 11 years of dietary restriction. *J. Clin. Endocrinol. Metab.* 88 (1): 16–23.

Blaxter, K. (1989). *Energy Metabolism in Animals and Man*. Cambridge: Cambridge University Press.

Brody, S. and Procter, R.C. (1932). *Growth and Development with Special Reference to Domestic Animals. Further Investigations of Surface Area in Energy Metabolism*, 116. University of Missouri Agricultural Experiment Station Research Bulletin.

Brody, S., Procter, R.C., and Ashworth, U.S. (1934). *Basal Metabolism, Endogenous Nitrogen, Creatinine and Neutral Sulphur Excretions as Functions of Body Weight*. University of Missouri Agricultural Experiment Station Research Bulletin, 220.

Burkholder, W.J. (1995). Metabolic rates and nutrient requirements of sick dogs and cats. *J. Am. Vet. Med. Assoc.* 206 (5): 614–618.

Case, L.P., Daristotle, L., Hayek, M.G., and Raasch, M.F. (2010). *Canine and Feline Nutrition*, 3e. St. Louis, MO: Mosby.

Donoghue, S. (1989). Nutritional support of hospitalized patients. *Vet. Clin. N. Am. Small Anim. Pract.* 19 (3): 475–495.

Elia, M. (2005). Insights into energy requirements in disease. *Public Health Nutr.* 8 (7A): 1037–1052.

Elia, M. and Livesey, G. (1992). Energy expenditure and fuel selection in biological systems: the theory and practice of calculations based on indirect calorimetry and tracer methods. In: *Metabolic Control of Eating, Energy Expenditure and the Bioenergetics of Obesity* (ed. A.P. Simopoulos), 68–131. Basel: Krager.

Frankenfield, D. (2006). Energy expenditure and protein requirements after traumatic injury. *Nutr. Clin. Pract.* 21 (5): 430–437.

Haynie, D.T. (2001). *Biological Thermodynamics*. Cambridge: Cambridge University Press.

Hill, R.C. (2006). Challenges in measuring energy expenditure in companion animals: a clinician's perspective. *J. Nutr.* 136 (7 Suppl): 1967S–1972S.

Hill, R.C. and Scott, K.C. (2004). Energy requirements and body surface area of cats and dogs. *J. Am. Vet. Med. Assoc.* 225 (5): 689–694.

Hill, R.C., Choate, C.J., Scott, K.C., and Molenberghs, G. (2009). Comparison of the guaranteed analysis with the measured nutrient composition of commercial pet foods. *J. Am. Vet. Med. Assoc.* 234 (3): 347–351.

Kendall, P.T., Holme, D.W., and Smith, P.M. (1982). Comparative evaluation of net digestive and absorptive efficiency in dogs and cats fed a variety of contrasting diet types. *J. Small Anim. Pract.* 23 (9): 577–587.

Kienzle, E. (2002). Further developments in the prediction of metabolizable energy (ME) in pet food. *J. Nutr.* 132 (6): 1796S–1798S.

Kienzle, E., Schrage, I., Butterwick, R., and Opitz, B. (2002). Calculation of gross energy in pet foods: do we have the right values for heat of combustion? *J. Nutr.* 132: 1799S–1800S.

Kleiber, M. (1961). *The Fire of Life*. New York: Wiley.

Kulstad, R. and Schoeller, D.A. (2007). The energetics of wasting diseases. *Curr. Opin. Clin. Nutr. Metab. Care* 10 (4): 488–493.

Laflamme, D.P. (2001). Determining metabolizable energy content in commercial pet foods. *J. Anim. Physiol. Anim. Nutr.* 85 (7–8): 222–230.

Lagua, R.T. and Claudio, V.S. (2004). *Nutrition and Diet Therapy Reference Dictionary*. Oxford: Blackwell.

Legrand-Defretin, V. (1994). Energy requirements of cats and dogs—what goes wrong? *Int. J. Obes.* 18 (Suppl 1): S8–S13.

Livesey, E. and Elia, M. (1988). Estimation of energy expenditure, net carbohydrate utilization, and net fat oxidation and synthesis by indirect calorimetry: evaluation of errors with special reference to the detailed composition of fuels. *Am. J. Clin. Nutr.* 47 (4): 608–628.

Loveridge, G.G. (1986). Body weight changes and energy intakes of cats during gestation and lactation. *Anim. Technol.* 37: 7–15.

Lowry, S.F. and Brennan, M.F. (1979). Abnormal liver function during parenteral nutrition: relation to infusion excess. *J. Surg. Res.* 26 (3): 300–307.

Mazzaferro, E.M., Hackett, T.B., Stein, T.P. et al. (2001). Metabolic alterations in dogs with osteosarcoma. *Am. J. Vet. Res.* 62 (8): 1234–1129.

National Research Council (NRC) (1986). *Nutrient Requirements of Cats*. Washington, DC: National Academy Press.

National Research Council (NRC) (2006). *Nutrient Requirements of Dogs and Cats*. Washington, DC: National Academy Press.

Newton, L.E. and Heimburger, D.C. (2006). *Handbook of Clinical Nutrition*. Philadelphia, PA: Mosby Elsevier.

Ogilvie, G.K., Fettman, M.J., Salman, M.D., and Wheeler, S.L. (1993). Energy expenditure in dogs with lymphoma fed two specialized diets. *Cancer* 71 (10): 3146–3152.

Ogilvie, G.K., Walters, L.M., Salman, M.D., and Fettman, M.J. (1996). Resting energy expenditure in dogs with nonhematopoietic malignancies before and after excision of tumors. *Am. J. Vet. Res.* 57 (10): 1463–1467.

O'Toole, E., McDonnell, W.N., Wilson, B.A. et al. (2001). Evaluation of accuracy and reliability of indirect calorimetry for the measurement of resting energy expenditure in healthy dogs. *Am. J. Vet. Res.* 62 (11): 1761–1767.

O'Toole, E., Miller, C.W., Wilson, B.A. et al. (2004). Comparison of the standard predictive equation for calculation of resting energy expenditure with indirect calorimetry in hospitalized and healthy dogs. *J. Am. Vet. Med. Assoc.* 225 (1): 58–64.

Remillard, R.L. and Thatcher, C.D. (1989). Parenteral nutritional support in the small animal patient. *Vet. Clin. N. Am. Small Anim. Pract.* 19 (6): 1287–1306.

Rubner, M. (1883). Ueber die einfluss der körpergrösse auf Stoff und Kraftwechsel. *Zietschrift fur Biologie* 19: 535–562.

Thatcher, C.D., Hand, M.S., and Remillard, R.L. (2010). Small animal clinical nutrition: an iterative approach. In: *Small Animal Clinical Nutrition*, 5e (ed. M.S. Hand, C.D. Thatcher, R.L. Remillard and P. Roudebush), 3–21. Topeka, KS: Mark Morris Institute.

Weekes, C.E. (2007). Controversies in the determination of energy requirements. *Proc. Nutr. Soc.* 66 (3): 367–377.

Weir, J.B.V.d. (1949). New methods of calculating metabolic rate with special reference to protein metabolism. *J. Physiol.* 109 (1–2): 1–9.

Wenk, C., Colombani, P.C., van Migen, J., and Lemme, A. (2001). Glossary: terminology in animal and human energy metabolism. In: *Energy Metabolism in Animals* (ed. A. Chwalibog and K. Jakobsen), 409–421. Wageningen Pers: Wageningen.

4

Nutritional and Energy Requirements for Performance
Richard C. Hill

The purpose of this chapter is to provide practical advice regarding the feeding of dogs that undertake different types of exercise. This advice is based on the review of the effect of physical exercise and climate on the nutrition of dogs and cats published by the National Research Council (NRC 2006) and subsequent, relevant peer-reviewed studies that have been published since the last edition of this text. The reader should turn to the NRC for a more detailed explanation of most of the recommendations in this chapter and for the references on which they are based, as well as this second edition's added references.

How Much Should Exercising Dogs Be Fed?

It is not possible to make an accurate recommendation of how much to feed an individual exercising dog. Theoretically, it should be possible to divide the daily metabolizable energy (ME) requirement in kcal/day by the ME density of the diet in kcal/g to obtain the amount to feed in g/day. Nevertheless, individual variation about the mean has always proved to be substantial when energy utilization has been measured in groups of dogs of similar body weight (BW) undertaking similar amounts of exercise. Thus, any calculation of the ME

requirements based on mean energy requirements can provide no more than an uncertain estimate of the true requirements of any individual animal. It is best, therefore, not to rely on a calculation to determine how much to feed an exercising dog, but instead to adjust the amount fed to ensure that the dog maintains an ideal body condition.

The ideal body condition for exercising dogs has not been determined, but some studies suggest that dogs live longer and perform better when they are fed less food and consequently weigh slightly less than they would if they were given free access to food. For example, Labrador retrievers that undertook modest amounts of activity in kennels with runs died a median of two years earlier and required treatment for arthritis a median of three years earlier when fed 25% more than paired retrievers (Kealy et al. 2002). The dogs fed less food were lean, with a mean body condition score (BCS) of 4.6 on a 9-point scale, whereas control dogs fed more were only modestly overweight, with a mean BCS of 6.7 on the same scale. Interestingly, in this same breed the consumption of a lower-fat (14% fat calories) diet compared to a higher-fat (41% fat calories) diet over a 30-day period had no effect on resting energy expenditure or body composition (Yoo et al. 2006). However, this study was only short term and both groups were fed to maintain BW. In another study,

Applied Veterinary Clinical Nutrition, Second Edition. Edited by Andrea J. Fascetti, Sean J. Delaney, Jennifer A. Larsen, and Cecilia Villaverde.

Table 4.1 Approximate daily metabolizable energy (ME) requirements of exercising dogs expressed relative to metabolic body weight[a] and "resting energy expenditure (REE)."[b]

Activity	Daily ME requirement[c]		Amount required by 25 kg dog[c]	
	kcal ME/kg BW$^{0.75}$	Ratio to REE	kcal ME	g[d]
Basal metabolic rate	76 (48–114)	1.1 (0.7–1.6)	850 (540–1280)	190 (120–280)
Resting fed metabolic rate[e]	84 (53–125)	1.2 (0.8–1.8)	935 (590–1410)	210 (130–310)
Companion dogs (depends on activity, breed, etc.)	(50–200)	(0.7–3)	(560–2240)	(120–500)
Laboratory dogs in kennels with runs	130 (80–170)	1.9 (1.1–2.4)	1450 (890–1900)	320 (200–420)
Racing greyhounds	140 (120–160)	2 (1.7–2.3)	1560 (1340–1790)	350 (300–400)
Hunting dogs	240 (200–280)	3.4 (3–4)	2680 (2240–3130)	600 (500–700)
Sled dogs racing long distances in the cold	1050 (860–1240)	15 (12–18)	11 700 (9600–9613 900)	2600 (2100–3100)

[a] Metabolic body weight = (BW in kg)$^{0.75}$ where BW = body weight.
[b] Resting energy expenditure in kcal calculated as $70 \times$ (body weight in kg)$^{0.75}$ or using an approximation of $30 + (70 \times$ (body weight in kg)) for medium–sized dogs. REE calculated in this way is less than the value obtained by averaging reported values for basal metabolic rate in dogs shown in the table.
[c] Values are means with ranges in parentheses.
[d] Assumes a high-fat dry diet containing 4.5 kcal/g as is.
[e] Resting fed metabolic rate is the energy required by dogs confined to a cage and includes an additional 10% energy for assimilation of food above basal metabolic rate.

trained greyhounds racing over a distance of 500 m ran on average 0.7 km/h faster when weighing 6% less and being fed 15% less food than when they were fed free choice (Hill et al. 2005). These trained racing greyhounds had a median BCS (3.75 on a 9-point scale) when fed free choice, but were leaner, with a median BCS of 3.5, when fed 15% less food.

Being overweight also has disadvantages for dogs running longer distances. When BW increased 20% and fat mass increased from 17% to 20% in beagles, water loss increased 50% during a 50-minute run on a treadmill at 6 km/h (Young 1960). The respiratory quotient (RQ) also increased from 0.85 to 0.97 during a run when these dogs became overweight, suggesting that more energy was derived from carbohydrate (RQ = 1.0) and less from fat (RQ = 0.7). Increased use of glucose may limit stamina. Conversely, slight weight loss associated with five days of food deprivation

increased endurance in beagles running on a treadmill (Young 1959).

Thus, for optimum performance and long-term health, exercising dogs should not be fed free choice. An initial estimate of how much to feed can be obtained from the mean daily ME requirements of dogs undertaking different amounts of exercise (Table 4.1). The amount should then be adjusted to ensure that dogs maintain a lean body condition for that breed; that is, a BCS of 4–5 on a 9-point scale for most breeds, and a BCS of 3.5 on the same scale for greyhounds and other sighthounds.

Energy Requirements for Performance and Work

There is a misconception among the general public that a dog, such as a greyhound, that runs fast requires more energy than a dog that runs more slowly. On the contrary, whereas energy is expended more rapidly when a dog runs more rapidly, it is expended for a shorter period of time. The total energy expended relative to distance traveled does not change with speed of running, because dogs, like other animals, adjust their gait to minimize energy expenditure (Blaxter 1989).

For a greater appreciation of this concept, it is necessary to consider the various parts of the energy budget for exercise. When a dog is lying down awake having not eaten for a while in a thermoneutral environment (in which it does not have to expend energy to keep itself warm), the dog still expends energy to maintain itself. This basal energy (76 kcal/kg $BW^{0.75}$ daily or 13 kcal/kg $BW^{0.75}$ hourly for an average dog; NRC 2006) is also required to maintain basic body functions during exercise. In addition, energy expenditure increases 50% when an animal stands. This energy continues to be expended all the time the dog stands for exercise, irrespective of the speed of travel. Energy is expended to support horizontal motion, but this energy expenditure for horizontal movement is proportional to distance traveled (approximately 1 kcal/kg BW for each horizontal km traveled for a dog of more than 10 kg BW and 1.5 kcal/kg BW for each horizontal km traveled for a dog of less than 10 kg; NRC 2006).

Thus, an average 30 kg dog with a basal metabolic rate of 41 kcal/h (970 kcal daily) will require an additional 20 kcal/h when it stands and another 90 kcal if it runs slowly at 3 km/h for 3 km. Surprisingly, however, an average 30 kg dog that stands and runs at twice the rate at 6 km/h over those 3 km, and thus completes the distance in half the time, but then lies down for the remaining half hour would require less energy overall! The faster animal remains standing for only half the time and so uses less energy for standing (only 10 kcal), whereas both animals expend the same amount of energy for covering the ground (90 kcal) and the same 41 kcal for basal energy over the hour. Similarly, a more excitable dog, say a terrier, that stands up all day and is in constant motion around a house at low speed will require more energy relative to its weight than a more mellow dog, say a greyhound, that lies down most of the day and runs around rapidly for 30 seconds in the yard two or three times daily.

In addition to the energy required for standing and horizontal motion, additional energy is needed to support the change in kinetic energy associated with acceleration. Thus, a greyhound requires three times as much energy for acceleration during the first few seconds of a race than it does while maintaining its pace during the rest of the race; that is, approximately 3 kcal/kg BW for each horizontal km as it accelerates up to almost 70 km/h, but only 1 kcal/kg BW for each km traveled while it continues to run at more than 40 km/h. This latter value of 1 kcal/kg BW is the same amount of energy required by dogs of similar BW that run more slowly (NRC 2006).

Dogs in jumping trials probably require the same amount of energy for acceleration as greyhounds during the few seconds before takeoff, but this need for increased energy is very brief. Agility dogs will require extra energy for acceleration several times during a trial, but on each occasion the increased energy will be required only briefly, and the size of the increase is likely to be more modest because agility dogs do not accelerate to such high speeds as greyhounds. Thus, dogs undertaking short-distance sprint exercise over distances less than 2 km, such as racing greyhounds, retrieving gun dogs, agility dogs, and jumping dogs, require relatively little energy to support activity, whereas dogs undertaking endurance exercise for many hours over long distances, such as sled dogs or hunting dogs, require much more energy.

Dogs also require additional energy as they gain potential energy running uphill. The energy required by dogs to overcome gravity on a slope of up to 20% has been variously measured to be between 5 and 14 kcal/kg BW for each vertical km in height gained (NRC 2006). Then dogs are able to recoup some of that potential energy as they run downhill again. If muscle were perfectly efficient, then dogs would be able to recoup all the extra energy for climbing when they ran downhill again, but dogs are less than 40% efficient in converting muscle energy, so increased energy is needed for running uphill and downhill. Dogs are even less efficient at recouping potential energy when running down a steep slope (20% or more), so the increase in energy requirements for traveling uphill and downhill is greater when the terrain is steep.

Energy requirements also increase proportionately with the work required when carrying or pulling a load. For a dog carrying a load, energy expenditure increases in proportion to the increase in body mass, so that a load that increases body mass by 10% requires a 10% increase in energy expenditure. The energy required for pulling a load has not been measured, but is probably three times the work of traction, as muscle is 30% efficient in most species (Blaxter 1989).

In addition, energy is required for running over rough terrain, for overcoming wind resistance, and for undertaking other activities such as swimming, jumping, playing, stretching, grooming, eating, and drinking, but the energy requirements for those activities have not been determined. Furthermore, dogs become extremely excited at the prospect of exercise (greyhound heart rates increase fivefold before a race), which will increase energy utilization. Body temperature also increases during exercise, so dogs have to expend energy after a race to lose body heat by panting.

Theoretically, therefore, it should be possible to estimate the energy required for activity by multiplying the energy required for each activity by the duration of each activity. The duration and intensity of activity are difficult to measure, however. Accelerometers, pedometers, and heart rate monitors might be used to measure activity intensity and duration in dogs or cats, but even should the energetic equivalency of heart rate or accelerometer readings be determined, the individual variation in energy required for those activities is likely to be large. Any energy required for activity must be added to basal energy requirements, which are also extremely variable among individuals. The energy requirements of an individual exercising dog will therefore not be determined by calculation in the near future.

For the time being, an estimate of ME requirements and the amount to feed to provide that ME can only be made based on the mean field metabolic rate of free-living dogs undertaking comparable amounts of exercise (Table 4.1; Figure 4.1). The amount fed must then be adjusted so that a dog maintains a lean BCS. When making this estimate, however, it is important to consider the duration of any activity, the distance traveled, the terrain, and the load that the dog is pulling or carrying, and not the speed of travel. It is also important not to rely on classifications such as working dog or canine companion. Activity varies in all dogs, regardless of background, with the degree of confinement, time of day, ambient temperature, extent of human and canine contact, and among dogs of different sizes, ages, and breeds. Both working dogs and companion dogs tend to be inactive or asleep for more than 60% of each day, and some working dogs and most companion dogs undertake very little additional exercise. Such dogs require little more than basal amounts of energy plus energy for the assimilation of food (approximately 10% increase) for a total of approximately $84\,kcal/kg\,BW^{0.75}$ daily (NRC 2006). On the other hand, many working dogs and some companion dogs are active for many hours daily, and sled dogs may even require over 10 times that amount of energy daily during a long-distance race (Loftus et al. 2014). Training does not alter the energy required to maintain any speed, so estimates based on the values in Table 4.1 can be used in untrained dogs. Training does increase stamina, however, so untrained dogs are likely to be less active and the intensity of exercise undertaken by an untrained dog will be limited.

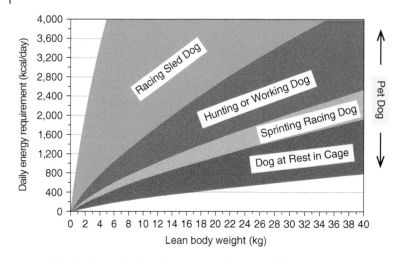

Figure 4.1   Daily metabolizable energy requirements of dogs undertaking different types of activity. The requirements are represented as ranges for each body weight to reflect the great individual variation shown by dogs of similar weight that undertake similar amounts of activity. The energy requirements of "pet" or companion dogs encompass a wide range because the duration of companion dog activity varies widely. Dogs that spend most of each day lying down require less energy than dogs that are always active. Sprinting dogs running short distances need less energy than working dogs running longer distances more slowly.

Types of Exercise and Nutrient Requirements

The dietary protein, fat, and carbohydrate requirements of dogs *are* affected by the speed of running *and* the degree of training. Thus, dogs that run very rapidly over a short distance using mostly anaerobic metabolism have different requirements than dogs that run more slowly over long distances using primarily aerobic metabolism. The requirements of untrained companion dogs that only exercise occasionally also differ from those of athletic dogs that undertake intense exercise many times weekly. To understand these differences, it is necessary to understand where an animal obtains energy to support activity.

Initially, energy comes from the high-energy phosphate bond of adenosine triphosphate (ATP) within muscle buffered by the high-energy phosphate bond of creatine phosphate. The energy from these high-energy phosphate bonds is immediately available, but stores are small, and the energy of ATP has to be constantly replenished either from the

anaerobic metabolism of carbohydrate or the aerobic metabolism of carbohydrate and fat. Unfortunately, the rapidity with which energy can be made available from glucose (stored as glycogen) and from fat is inversely proportional to the size of the energy store available (Hultman et al. 1994). Thus, the anaerobic metabolism of glucose can generate energy relatively rapidly, but provides only two molecules of ATP from each molecule of glucose and generates lactic acid in the process. Access to oxygen increases the yield of ATP from glucose up to 19 times, but provides energy less rapidly, and glycogen can become exhausted at the end of a long run because stores of glycogen are limited. Fat provides an almost inexhaustible source of energy, but can deliver energy only at a slow rate, which limits the speed of run that can be sustained. Thus, the duration of the ability to run fast (stamina) is limited by the availability of glycogen. Both people and animals are unable to accelerate at the end of a long-distance race because muscle glycogen is no longer available to support more intense activity.

Dogs differ from human beings in that dogs are adapted for long-distance running using the aerobic metabolism of fat, and derive twice as much energy from fat oxidation both at rest and during exercise compared to human beings (McLelland et al. 1994; de Bruijne et al. 1981; de Bruijne and de Koster 1983). Dog muscle does not contain the anaerobic, easily fatigued type IIb fast-twitch fibers found in animals such as cats, which are adapted to sprinting. Dog muscle contains only fibers with a high aerobic capacity that are fatigue resistant; that is, type I slow-twitch fibers that rely more on aerobic than anaerobic metabolism and type IIa fast-twitch fibers that rely more on anaerobic than aerobic metabolism (Gunn 1978). Dogs store more glycogen and fat in muscle and also can supply more fatty acids to the tissues, because albumin binds more free fatty acids in dogs than in less aerobic species (McLelland et al. 1994).

Dogs at rest derive energy almost equally from the oxidation of fat and glucose, but when trained dogs start to walk and run, glucose oxidation increases only slightly and most of the increased energy comes from fat oxidation. Then, as the intensity of exercise increases, the supply of oxygen becomes limiting and lactic acid is produced, which increases the concentration of lactic acid and limits utilization of fat. Thus, trained dogs that undertake exercise below the maximum rate of oxygen utilization (VO_2 max), so-called submaximal exercise, rely more on the oxidation of fat, whereas dogs undertaking exercise above their VO_2 max, so-called supramaximal exercise, rely to a greater extent on the anaerobic and aerobic metabolism of glucose.

Racing greyhounds undertake supramaximal exercise (see Figure 4.2). They develop a marked lactic acidosis (24–34 mmol/l) after running for less than a kilometer at speeds of over 40 km/h for less than a minute (NRC 2006). Almost all other exercising dogs perform submaximal exercise because very few dogs can be persuaded to perform supramaximal exercise when running on a flat surface (Seeherman et al. 1981). Lactic acid production does increase slightly in dogs running submaximally, but lactic acid utilization also increases so that concentrations in the blood at the end of a run remain unchanged (approximately 1 mmol/l) or increase only slightly (approximately 3 mmol/l). This modest change in lactic acid concentrations after exercise has been

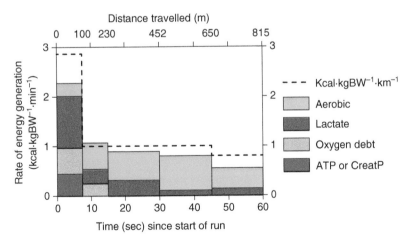

Figure 4.2 Sources of energy for a greyhound during sprint exercise. High-energy phosphate bonds in ATP and creatine phosphate (CreatP), alactacid oxygen debt (Oxygen debt), and anaerobic metabolism of glucose to lactate (Lactate) deliver energy rapidly to support the high-energy requirements for acceleration during the first 100 m of a run. Subsequently aerobic metabolism (Aerobic) provides most of the energy for the rest of the race when anaerobic sources of energy have been exhausted. *Source:* Adapted from Staaden 1984 as described in National Research Council (2006).

demonstrated in dogs running on a treadmill, undertaking a sled dog race or an agility trial, or retrieving (Seeherman et al. 1981; Matwichuk et al. 1999; Rovira et al. 2007; Young et al. 1959; Hinchliff et al. 1993). Rather than becoming acidotic, dogs undertaking submaximal exercise tend to become alkalotic because they have to pant to maintain body temperature.

Protein and amino acid synthesis and catabolism increase in exercising dogs to support the anatomic changes associated with training and also to support gluconeogenesis in dogs undertaking long-distance submaximal exercise. Dogs initially use glycogen as a source of glucose during submaximal exercise, but increase gluconeogenesis from protein after about 30 minutes (Wasserman et al. 1992). Dogs running for more than 30 minutes, therefore, require much more protein in their diet than dogs such as greyhounds, which run for much shorter periods of time (Reynolds et al. 1999; Hill et al. 2001).

Terms such as "sprint," "marathon," "short distance," and "long distance" are not helpful in this context because such terms mean very different distances and speeds for greyhounds or sled dogs. Greyhounds never race for more than a kilometer and indulge in supramaximal exercise in both "sprint" and "marathon" races, whereas sled dogs race over many kilometers and indulge in submaximal exercise in both "sprint" and "long-distance" races. When deciding how to feed an athletic dog; therefore, it is more important to consider whether it is undertaking anaerobic supramaximal exercise or aerobic submaximal exercise. As a general rule, most dogs should be considered to perform submaximal exercise. Only racing sighthounds or dogs running on a steep slope or pulling heavy loads are likely to approach or exceed their VO_2 max and be performing supramaximal exercise.

The Importance of Training

Most nutritional studies of exercising dogs have used dogs that have undergone some form of training for the exercise that they are required to perform. In contrast, most companion dogs are not trained and often only undertake intense exercise intermittently on weekends. Training is more efficient than diet change to increase exercise performance. Training does not affect energy requirements but has marked effects on stamina (Musch et al. 1985). Training increases heart size so that heart rate is decreased during exercise while blood flow to the tissues is increased. Untrained dogs have a 30% lower VO_2 max and produce more lactic acid, which limits the use of fat as an energy source and increases the rate of decline in blood glucose during exercise (Paul and Holmes 1975). Thus, the improvement in stamina associated with feeding more fat to trained dogs may not occur in untrained dogs.

Training also increases olfactory acuity and reduces free radical formation and may reduce the risk of injury (NRC 2006). Interestingly, one study looking at different dietary fat concentrations failed to show any significant differences in detecting three different explosives in trained detection dogs, but suggested that a lower-protein diet with a higher omega 6:3 ratio of 18.2 led to better performance than a higher-protein diet with a lower ratio of 8.4, but with a similar total omega-6 concentration (Angle et al. 2014).

Nutritional Recommendations for Dogs Undertaking Different Types of Exercise

The minimum requirement of a nutrient has been defined by the NRC as "the minimal concentration or amount of a bioavailable nutrient that will support a defined physiological state" (NRC 2006). To determine the minimum requirement, performance, health, or some other suitable measure of well-being must be measured as the amount of a nutrient is gradually increased in the diet. Unfortunately, no minimum requirements have been established for exercising dogs, because the effect of

Table 4.2 Adequate intakes[a] for dogs that undertake long-distance aerobic exercise and short-distance primarily anaerobic exercise.

Nutrient	Long-distance aerobic	Short-distance mostly anaerobic
Protein	90 g/Mcal (40% as is[b])	60 g/Mcal (27% as is)
Fat	59 g/Mcal (27% as is)	36 g/Mcal (16% as is)
Carbohydrate	0	105 g/Mcal (47% as is)
Water[c]	2.4 L/Mcal	2.4 L/Mcal
Sodium	1 g/Mcal	1 g/Mcal
Potassium	1 g/Mcal	1 g/Mcal
Calcium	3 g/Mcal	3 g/Mcal
Phosphorus	3 g/Mcal	3 g/Mcal

[a] Diets containing these adequate intakes or more have been reported to sustain trained dogs repetitively undertaking the type of exercise described, but lower amounts may also sustain satisfactory performance.
[b] % as is: the equivalent adequate intake in % as is shown in parentheses assuming the diet is a dry high-fat diet containing 4.5 kcal/g as is.
[c] Average requirements are 1.2 L/Mcal, but some dogs consume twice that amount.

gradually increasing nutrient density on performance or health has not been assessed for any nutrient in active dogs. Most studies have only compared two concentrations of nutrient or else the differences between nutrient concentrations have been too large to accurately establish a minimum requirement. Thus, any recommendation for an exercising dog (Table 4.2) only represents an adequate intake, which has been defined by the NRC as the lowest concentration or amount of a nutrient that published studies report has sustained trained dogs (usually sled dogs or racing greyhounds) that undertake regular exercise. It is quite possible, however, that lower concentrations than those listed could support exercising dogs, especially if the type of exercise is less intense than that performed by sled dogs and racing greyhounds. Furthermore, nutrient intake will increase with caloric intake meeting energy

needs. Requirements for some nutrients may not increase in parallel with energy requirements as exercise increases, so it is possible that lower concentrations of a nutrient than those recommended for the maintenance of dogs that undertake more modest amounts of exercise may maintain a more active dog that consumes increased amounts of food to meet its increased energy needs. Conversely, sedentary dogs may need to consume more nutrient-dense foods than are required for maintenance of modestly active dogs.

There are no studies of the nutrient requirements of untrained dogs that exercise, so a recommendation cannot be made for untrained active dogs. Nevertheless, most companion dogs are untrained and only exercise infrequently on weekends. Their stamina will be low, so companion dogs are unlikely to undertake much more activity than laboratory-housed dogs. As most nutrient requirements for dogs have been determined based on studies using untrained, laboratory-housed dogs that are only moderately active, nutrient requirements established for growing and adult dogs should provide adequate nutrition for most untrained companion dogs. Human companions of dogs that perform more exercise than a laboratory-housed dog in a kennel with a run should train their dogs by gradually increasing the frequency and intensity of exercise. Training is likely to improve performance and health more than any change in diet. Then, once a dog is trained, recommendations made in this chapter will become relevant.

Long-Distance Submaximal Aerobic Exercise

Dogs running long distances have more stamina when adapted to very high-fat diets because they use muscle glycogen more slowly when fed a higher-fat diet (Reynolds et al. 1995). In trained dogs only running at 12.5 km/h for 30 min on a 2.5% inclined treadmill, the addition of 53.9 g corn oil/Mcal (corn oil is rich in the long-chain omega-6 fatty acid linoleic acid), resulting in a diet with a lower-protein, higher-fat caloric distribution of 18% ME protein, 57% ME fat, and 25% ME carbohydrate, has been shown to slightly lower core and rectal temperatures post exercise (Ober et al. 2016). Fatty acid composition of any added fat may be important depending on the outcome measurement. One pilot study has shown a reduced marker for inflammation in a subset of dogs from one single sled dog team fed 8% krill meal, rich in long-chain omega-3 fatty acids (Burri et al. 2018), while 12 weeks of 54 mg fish oil (also rich in omega-3) per kg metabolic weight per day added to a complete and balanced commercial food when slightly lowered trained dogs' heart rates after twice-weekly 30-min sessions on a treadmill set at 8 km/h at a 7.5% slope (Pellegrino et al. 2019). This contrasts with human long-distance athletes, whose stamina increases when they consume a high-carbohydrate diet. Dogs undertaking long-distance exercise also develop "sports anemia" and suffer more injuries unless fed a high-protein diet containing an adequate balance of amino acids (Reynolds et al. 1999). The source of this protein must be very digestible to limit the amount of undigested protein entering the large intestine. Excess protein or fermentable carbohydrate entering the large intestine will be fermented to short-chain fatty acids and can cause an osmotic diarrhea (Taylor et al. 1959; Orr 1966).

Dogs running long distances do not require digestible carbohydrate provided there is enough dietary protein to support gluconeogenesis. It is unclear, however, whether there is a need for indigestible carbohydrate. Short-chain fatty acids produced by anaerobic fermentation support colonic mucosal health, but it has not been established whether soluble fiber is needed in the diet in addition to undigested protein and undigested starch as a substrate for that fermentation. Large amounts of dietary fiber are not desirable, however, because increased fiber increases the weight of the colon and water loss in the feces.

Guaranteed Analysis

Crude Protein	26.0%	minimum
Crude Fat	18.0%	minimum
Crude Fiber	3.0%	maximum
Moisture	10.0%	maximum
Ash	5.5%	maximum

Figure 4.3 Typical guaranteed analysis on the label of a higher-protein, higher-fat commercial dry/extruded dog food suitable for feeding an active companion dog. Note that this food does not contain enough protein and fat for a working or hunting dog running long distances daily over many hours. Such dogs should be fed a high-protein, high-fat canned/retorted diet. Compare the guarantees on different canned diets to find a canned diet that contains the most fat and protein for the same moisture percentage. Do not compare the guarantee on dry/extruded and canned/retorted diets. Dry diet guaranteed percentages are inherently "inflated" compared to canned diet guaranteed percentages because dry diets contain less water, but they also contain less protein and fat when the difference in water content is taken into account.

Therefore, for most active dogs that undertake moderate amounts of activity, a high-protein, high-fat, dry commercial diet should provide sufficient protein and fat (see Figure 4.3). Dog owners should select a dry/extruded diet with the highest guarantee on the label for both protein and fat. As the frequency and duration of exercise increase, however, dry diets may not provide enough protein and fat, so a high-protein, high-fat canned diet should be added to provide the extra energy the dog will need as well as the extra protein.

Short-Distance Supramaximal Anaerobic Exercise

Dogs such as racing greyhounds undertaking sprint exercise do not require as much protein or fat as dogs undergoing long-distance submaximal exercise. Performance has decreased when dietary protein has increased in substitution for dietary carbohydrate (Hill et al. 2001). When the duration of exercise is short, glycogen stores are unlikely to be depleted, and protein is not needed to support gluconeogenesis. Both lower and very high amounts of dietary fat have been associated with reduced performance too, but the ideal amount of fat and carbohydrate to include in the diet has not been established (NRC 2006). Currently, a diet is recommended that contains only typical maintenance amounts of protein (60–70 g protein/ Mcal ME) and fat (36–50 g fat/Mcal kcal ME), but the amount of fat may need to be adjusted for optimum performance. Both canned and dry diets exist that meet this specification.

Fluid and Electrolyte Requirements, Hydration, and "Sports Drinks"

Dogs require unlimited and frequent supplies of water before, during, and after exercise, but do not require extra sodium or other electrolytes or vitamins. Dogs do not sweat. Sports drinks designed for humans that contain sodium and electrolytes are not recommended for dogs that exercise and they can reduce performance (Young et al. 1960). Some glucose may be added to the water after exercise to replenish glycogen stores, but the exact amount to add is uncertain. There is also no evidence that other, so-called ergogenic nutrients have any benefit.

Adequate hydration is essential for optimum athletic dog performance. Body temperature increases during exercise and limits activity in dogs (Kozlowski et al. 1985). Very high body temperatures can result in tissue damage, especially damage to the intestine and kidneys, that can be life threatening and should be avoided at all costs. Keeping dogs cool by using cold packs and exercising dogs in cold ambient temperatures allows dogs to exercise for longer periods of time (Kozlowski et al. 1985; Kruk et al. 1985). Dehydration increases the rate of increase of body temperature during exercise and reduces the duration and intensity of exercise of which dogs are capable (NRC 2006). Maintaining hydration improves stamina, therefore, and reduces the risk of life-threatening hyperthermia.

Water loss by evaporation for cooling increases during exercise with increased ambient temperature. Urine production also increases as food intake increases to support the energy needs of exercise in proportion to the amount of salt and urea (from protein) that must be excreted. Average water requirements increase from 0.5 ml/kcal at cold ambient temperatures to 0.6–1.2 ml/kcal at room temperature (depending on the amount of sodium and protein in the diet) and 1.8 ml/kcal in obese dogs (NRC 2006). Dogs should be offered twice these mean amounts, however, because individual dogs may require double the average amount.

Dogs become dehydrated intermittently over time because water is lost continuously in urine and by evaporation, but dogs drink water only intermittently. Sedentary dogs do not usually anticipate the need to drink and only drink after losing about 0.5% of BW, but dogs will maintain their hydration during exercise by drinking regularly if given the opportunity (O'Connor 1975). Thus, water should be made available to dogs before exercise, at intervals during, and shortly after exercise.

Because dogs lose water but little sodium during exercise, their blood becomes hyperosmolar. Drinking water without any solute corrects this hyperosmolality immediately, whereas drinking water containing salt or glucose will not correct the hyperosmolality, and dogs will continue to wish to drink more (Ramsay and Thrasher 1991). It is best, therefore, to correct dehydration during exercise with water containing no solute, and to provide glucose-containing water after exercise to facilitate replenishment of glycogen stores.

Commercial sports drinks sold for human athletes should not be offered to exercising dogs. Dogs do not sweat except on their footpads. The increase in salt loss when dogs pant and drool during exercise is small, so there is little increase in a dog's requirement for salt during exercise. Any salt consumed in drinking water will have to be excreted in the urine, which will increase the rate of water loss and may exacerbate dehydration. The adequate intake for both sodium and potassium recommended by the NRC for exercising dogs is 1 g/ Mcal. One recent study suggested that 1.2 g of sodium/Mcal may be ideal in sled dogs undergoing a 1600 km race (Ermon et al. 2014).

Most commercial diets will provide sufficient sodium and potassium without the need for supplementation.

Antioxidants

Oxidation occurs as a normal process within mitochondria as energy is made available during exercise. More oxidation occurs as the amount of energy required increases, but regular exercise also increases the antioxidant defense mechanisms within the body. Antioxidant nutrients, such as vitamin E, are an essential component of the diet of exercising dogs, and thus should minimize oxidation during exercise. Requirements for antioxidant vitamins also increase with the amount of dietary fat and with the amount of polyunsaturated fatty acids in all diets, especially if the food is to be stored for any length of time. It remains to be determined, however, whether dogs that exercise require any more antioxidant nutrients than sedentary dogs. Antioxidant requirements for dogs that exercise regularly may even be less than for sedentary dogs that only exercise intermittently on weekends, and it is better to exercise dogs more regularly than to recommend any increase in antioxidant vitamins in the diet.

Other Vitamins, Trace Minerals, and Other Essential Nutrients

Requirements for some B vitamins, such as thiamin, are likely to increase and decrease in proportion to energy requirements, whereas requirements for vitamin B6 (pyridoxine) tend to vary with protein intake. Most commercial diets contain an excess of B vitamins to compensate for losses during processing. Furthermore, intake of these vitamins will increase and decrease proportionally as food intake varies with energy requirements. It is unlikely, therefore, that B vitamins will be deficient in most commercial diets, and supplementation with these vitamins above that already present in the diet is almost certainly unnecessary.

It is also almost certainly true that the requirements for calcium, phosphorus, and other minerals do not increase directly in proportion to energy requirements, so the amount of minerals in the diet of sedentary dogs should be adequate for exercising dogs. Thus, on the contrary, there is a potential for excess intake of calcium and trace minerals by dogs that take in large amounts of food because of their very high energy requirements. The amount of trace minerals in the diet of dogs undertaking large amounts of exercise should be kept close to the minimum requirement and should probably not be increased as the amount of fat is increased in the diet, but this is an unstudied area in dogs.

Other Nutritional Supplements

There is currently very limited experimental evidence that so-called ergogenic nutrients improve the performance of exercising dogs. Adding creatine to the diet of dogs has not been shown to increase the amount of creatine in muscle or performance. Dimethylglycine and diisopropylammonium dichloroacetic acid reduced the race time of greyhounds (Gannon and Kendall 1982), but this beneficial effect was probably due to dichloroacetic acid, which reduces lactic acidosis. Addition of dichloroacetic acid to the diet is not recommended, however, because dichloroacetic acid is toxic to dogs in small doses (Cicmanec et al. 1991). Glucosamine and other nutrients designed to moderate the effects of osteoarthritis may be of benefit in exercising dogs with this condition, but there is currently no evidence that such nutrients prevent osteoarthritis. One uncontrolled/non-randomized study suggested that a proprietary supplement of "yeast, betaine, magnesium, L-carnitine, sodium bicarbonate, biotin, niacin, pantothenic acid, pyridoxine, and cyanocobalamin" helped the performance of five dogs coyote tracking (Huntingford et al. 2014).

Two other reports support the potential benefit of daily L-carnitine supplementation at a dose of 125 mg in trained sled dogs, weighing on average 29 kg, to reduce measures of muscle tissue degradation or damage 1 h after a 24.2 km endurance run (Varney et al. 2017, 2020).

Time of Feeding

Food deprivation does not compromise the performance of dogs undertaking endurance exercise (Young 1959). However, dogs fed a morning meal have been shown to search more accurately than when fasted (Miller and Bender 2012). Glucose given before or during exercise minimizes the decline in blood glucose concentrations during exercise and minimizes the increase in body temperature during exercise, whereas glucose given after exercise promotes the repletion of muscle glycogen. The amount of glucose that should be administered is uncertain, however, because the amounts of glucose given to dogs have varied widely from 1.5 mg to 1.5 g/kg BW (Reynolds et al. 1997; Wakshlag et al. 2002). In one relevant diet study, supplementation after a first pull series with 5% dextrose, 32.4% maltodextrin, and 16% whey/soya protein did not statistically improve weight-pulling in dogs during a second pull series conducted within 180 minutes of the first pull series (Frye et al. 2017). In another study, feeding dogs a supplemental "bar" with 37.4% of the rapidly digestible carbohydrates, maltodextrin plus dextrin, and 25% protein immediately after exercise increased blood nutrient concentrations for glycogen and protein synthesis, compared with control dogs (Zanghi et al. 2015).

Dogs should not be fed food containing fat immediately before or during intense exercise. Consumption of food directs blood toward the intestine and can compromise performance while exercise compromises intestinal function. Ideally, dogs should be fed shortly *after* intense exercise when the dog's excitement has abated.

Summary

- Regular exercise training more than any change in diet will improve the performance of an exercising dog.
- Active dogs should be fed enough food to maintain a lean body condition.
- Dogs mostly perform aerobic exercise.
- Dogs exercising for more than 30 min require extra protein in their diet.
- Dogs undertaking long-distance exercise require extra fat in their diet.
- Commercial high-protein, high-fat dry dog foods should provide enough protein and fat for most active dogs.
- Working or hunting dogs should have the extra energy they require supplied by commercial high-protein, high-fat canned diets containing little carbohydrate.
- Active dogs should always have free access to water to maximize performance.
- Water given to active dogs may contain some glucose but not other nutrients such as salt or electrolytes.
- Dogs should not be given human sports drinks.
- Feeding of a higher-carbohydrate treat to non-sled dogs after exercise may be beneficial.

References

Angle, C.T., Wakshlag, J.J., Gillette, R.L. et al. (2014). The effects of exercise and diet on olfactory capability in detection dogs. *J. Nutr. Sci.* 3: e44.

Blaxter, K. (1989). *Energy Metabolism in Animals and Man*. Cambridge: Cambridge University Press.

Burri, L., Wyse, C., Gray, S.R. et al. (2018). Effects of dietary supplementation with krill meal on serum pro-inflammatory markers after the Iditarod sled dog race. *Res. Vet. Sci.* 121: 18–22.

Cicmanec, J.L., Condie, L.W., Olson, G.R. et al. (1991). 90 day toxicity study of dichloroacetate in dogs. *Fundam. Appl. Toxicol.* 17 (2): 376–389.

De Bruijne, J.J., Altszuler, N., Hampshire, J. et al. (1981). Fat mobilization and plasma hormone levels in fasted dogs. *Metabolism* 30 (2): 190–194.

De Bruijne, J.J. and de Koster, P. (1983). Glycogenolysis in the fasting dog. *Comp. Biochem. Physiol. B* 75 (4): 553–555.

Ermon, V., Yazwinski, M., Milizio, J.G. et al. (2014). Serum chemistry and electrolyte alterations in sled dogs before and after a 1600 km race: dietary sodium and hyponatraemia. *J. Nutr. Sci.* 3: e26.

Frye, C.W., VanDeventer, G.M., Dinallo, G.K. et al. (2017). The effects of a post-exercise carbohydrate and protein supplement on repeat performance, serum chemistry, insulin and glucagon in competitive weight-pulling dogs. *J. Nutr. Sci.* 6: e27.

Gannon, J.R. and Kendall, R.V. (1982). A clinical evaluation of N,N-dimethylglycine (DMG) and diisopropylammonium dichloroacetate (DIPA) on the performance of racing greyhounds. *Canine Pract.* 9 (6): 7–13.

Gunn, H.M. (1978). Differences in the histochemical properties of skeletal muscles of different breeds of horses and dogs. *J. Anat.* 127 (3): 615–634.

Hill, R.C., Lewis, D.D., Randell, S.C. et al. (2005). Effect of mild restriction of food intake on the speed of racing greyhounds. *Am. J. Vet. Res.* 66 (6): 1065–1070.

Hill, R.C., Lewis, D.D., Scott, K.C. et al. (2001). Effect of increased protein and decreased carbohydrate in the diet on performance and body condition in racing greyhounds. *Am. J. Vet. Res.* 62 (3): 440–447.

Hinchcliff, K.W., Olson, J., Crusberg, C. et al. (1993). Serum biochemical changes in dogs competing in a long-distance sled race. *J. Am. Vet. Med. Assoc.* 202 (3): 401–405.

Hultman, E., Harris, R.C., and Spriet, L.L. (1994). Work and exercise. In: *Modern Nutrition in Health and Disease*, 8e (ed. M.E. Shils, J.A. Olson and M. Shike), 663–685. Philadelphia, PA: Lea & Febiger.

Huntingford, J.L., Kim, B.N., Cramer, K. et al. (2014). Evaluation of a performance enhancing supplement in American foxhounds during eventing*. *J. Nutr. Sci.* 3: e24.

Kealy, R.D., Lawler, D.F., Ballam, J.M. et al. (2002). Effects of diet restriction on life span and age-related changes in dogs. *J. Am. Vet. Med. Assoc.* 220 (9): 1315–1320.

Kozlowski, S., Brzezinska, Z., Kruk, B. et al. (1985). Exercise hyperthermia as a factor limiting physical performance: temperature effect on muscle metabolism. *J. Appl. Physiol.* 59 (3): 766–773.

Kruk, B., Kaciuba-Uscilko, H., Nazar, K. et al. (1985). Hypothalamic, rectal, and muscle temperatures in exercising dogs: effect of cooling. *J. Appl. Physiol.* 58 (5): 1444–1448.

Loftus, J.P., Yazwinski, M., Milizio, J.G. et al. (2014). Energy requirements for racing endurance sled dogs. *J. Nutr. Sci.* 3: e34.

Matwichuk, C.L., Taylor, S., Shmon, C.L. et al. (1999). Changes in rectal temperature and hematologic, biochemical, blood gas, and acid-base values in healthy Labrador retrievers before and after strenuous exercise. *Am. J. Vet. Res.* 60 (1): 88–92.

McLelland, G., Zwingelstein, G., Taylor, C.R. et al. (1994). Increased capacity for circulatory fatty acid transport in a highly aerobic mammal. *Am. J. Phys.* 266: R1280–R1286.

Miller, H.C. and Bender, C. (2012). The breakfast effect: dogs (Canis familiaris) search more accurately when they are less hungry. *Behav. Process.* 91 (3): 313–317.

Musch, T.I., Haidet, G.C., Ordway, G.A. et al. (1985). Dynamic exercise training in foxhounds. I. Oxygen consumption and hemodynamic responses. *J. Appl. Physiol.* 59 (1): 183–189.

National Research Council (NRC) (2006). *Nutrient Requirements of Dogs and Cats.* Washington, DC: National Academy Press.

Ober, J., Gillette, R.L., Angle, T.C. et al. (2016). The effects of varying concentrations of dietary protein and fat on blood gas, hematologic serum chemistry, and body temperature before and after exercise in Labrador retrievers. *Front Vet. Sci.* 3: 59.

O'Connor, W.J. (1975). Drinking by dogs during and after running. *J. Physiol.* 250 (2): 247–259.

Orr, N.W.M. (1966). The feeding of sledge dogs on Antarctic expeditions. *Br. J. Nutr.* 20 (1): 1–12.

Paul, P. and Holmes, W.L. (1975). Free fatty acid and glucose metabolism during increased energy expenditure and after training. *Med. Sci. Sports* 7 (3): 176–183.

Pellegrino, F.J., Risso, A., Relling, A.E. et al. (2019). Physical response of dogs supplemented with fish oil during a treadmill training programme. *J. Anim. Physiol. Anim. Nutr.* 103 (2): 653–660.

Ramsay, D.J. and Thrasher, T.N. (1991). Regulation of fluid intake in dogs following water deprivation. *Brain Res. Bull.* 27 (3–4): 495–499.

Reynolds, A.J., Carey, D.P., Reinhart, G.A. et al. (1997). Effect of postexercise carbohydrate supplementation on muscle glycogen repletion in trained sled dogs. *Am. J. Vet. Res.* 58 (11): 1252–1256.

Reynolds, A.J., Fuhrer, L., Dunlap, H.L. et al. (1995). Effect of diet and training on muscle glycogen storage and utilization in sled dogs. *J. Appl. Physiol.* 79 (5): 1601–1607.

Reynolds, A.J., Reinhart, G.A., Carey, D.P. et al. (1999). Effect of protein intake during training on biochemical and performance variables in sled dogs. *Am. J. Vet. Res.* 60 (7): 789–795.

Rovira, S., Munoz, A., and Benito, M. (2007). Hematologic and biochemical changes during canine agility competitions. *Vet. Clin. Pathol.* 36 (1): 30–35.

Seeherman, H.J., Taylor, C.R., Maloiy, G.M. et al. (1981). Design of the mammalian respiratory system. II. Measuring maximum aerobic capacity. *Respir. Physiol.* 44 (1): 11–23.

Taylor, R.J.F., Worden, A.N., and Waterhouse, C.E. (1959). The diet of sledge dogs. *Br. J. Nutr.* 13 (1): 1–16.

Varney, J.L., Fowler, J.W., Gilbert, W.C. et al. (2017). Utilisation of supplemented l-carnitine for fuel efficiency, as an antioxidant, and for muscle recovery in Labrador retrievers. *J. Nutr. Sci.* 6: e8.

Varney, J.L., Fowler, J.W., McClaughry, T.C. et al. (2020). L-carnitine metabolism, protein turnover and energy expenditure in supplemented and exercised Labrador retrievers. *J. Anim. Physiol. Anim. Nutr.* 104 (5): 1540–1550.

Wakshlag, J.J., Snedden, K.A., Otis, A.M. et al. (2002). Effects of post-exercise supplements on glycogen repletion in skeletal muscle. *Vet. Ther.* 3 (3): 226–234.

Wasserman, D.H., Lacy, D.B., Bracy, D. et al. (1992). Metabolic regulation in peripheral tissues and transition to increased gluconeogenic mode during prolonged exercise. *Am. J. Phys.* 263: E345–E354.

Yoo, S., Ramsey, J.J., Havel, P.J. et al. (2006). Resting energy expenditure and body composition of Labrador retrievers fed high fat and low fat diets. *J. Anim. Physiol. Anim. Nutr.* 90 (5–6): 185–191.

Young, D.R. (1959). Effect of food deprivation on treadmill running in dogs. *J. Appl. Physiol.* 14 (6): 1018–1022.

Young, D.R. (1960). Effect of body composition and weight gain on performance in the adult dog. *J. Appl. Physiol.* 15 (3): 493–495.

Young, D.R., Mosher, R., Erve, P. et al. (1959). Energy metabolism and gas exchange during treadmill running in dogs. *J. Appl. Physiol.* 14 (5): 834–838.

Young, D.R., Schafer, N.S., and Price, R. (1960). Effect of nutrient supplements during work on performance capacity in dogs. *J. Appl. Physiol.* 15 (6): 1022–1026.

Zanghi, B.M., Middleton, R.P., and Reynolds, A.J. (2015). Effects of postexercise feeding of a supplemental carbohydrate and protein bar with or without astaxanthin from Haematococcus pluvialis to exercise-conditioned dogs. *Am. J. Vet. Res.* 76 (4): 338–350.

5

Pet Food and Supplement Regulations: Practical Implications

David A. Dzanis and Isabel Marzo

US Regulation

Commercial foods for pets are subject to regulation in the US at both the federal and state levels. The category of "pet food" includes not only complete and balanced products, but also therapeutic diets, treats, toppers, chews, and nutritional supplements, as well as the components of such products. However, the specific means by which a given subcategory of pet food is regulated may vary.

The application of the law as it pertains to pet supplements is particularly convoluted. For dietary supplements intended for human consumption, federal law provides for the inclusion of ingredients that normally would not be permitted for foods in conventional form. More explicit claims in terms of health benefits are also allowed for supplements as opposed to foods in general. Importantly, though, those legal provisions do not apply to animal products. As a result, ingredients and claims that are acceptable by law in regard to a human dietary supplement may not necessarily be OK with respect to a pet product. That said, it is quite evident that the marketplace is replete with pet supplements that, in fact, do not wholly comply with the applicable law.

There are also "exceptions to the rule" when it comes to therapeutic pet diets. While it is helpful for the veterinarian to have a basic understanding of the regulation of pet foods in general, it is especially important to be aware of the issues pertaining to both supplements and therapeutic diets so as to provide for their most appropriate use in practice.

US Regulation of Pet Foods and Supplements

Definitions, Abbreviations, and Acronyms

- *AAFCO*: Association of American Feed Control Officials. A nongovernmental organization (whose members must be state, federal, or foreign government employees) that establishes model animal feed laws, regulations, and ingredient definitions, which then may be adopted by individual state agencies responsible for regulatory oversight of animal feed.
- *CVM*: Center for Veterinary Medicine. Part of the Food and Drug Administration (FDA) responsible for interstate regulation of animal foods and drugs.
- *Dietary supplement*: As defined in part by the Dietary Supplement Health and Education Act (DSHEA), a product (other than tobacco) that is intended to supplement the diet that bears or contains one or more of the following dietary ingredients: a vitamin, a mineral, a herb or other botanical, an amino acid, a dietary substance for use by humans to

Applied Veterinary Clinical Nutrition, Second Edition. Edited by Andrea J. Fascetti,
Sean J. Delaney, Jennifer A. Larsen, and Cecilia Villaverde.
© 2024 John Wiley & Sons, Inc. Published 2024 by John Wiley & Sons, Inc.

supplement the diet by increasing the total daily intake, or a concentrate, metabolite, constituent, extract, or combinations of these ingredients (Title 21 United States Code Sec. 321(ff)(1)).

- *Drug*: As defined in part by the Federal Food, Drug, and Cosmetic Act (FFDCA), an article intended for use in the diagnosis, cure, mitigation, treatment, or prevention of disease in humans or other animals; and articles (other than food) intended to affect the structure or any function of the body of humans or other animals (Title 21 United States Code Sec. 321(g)(1)).
- *DSHEA*: Dietary Supplement Health and Education Act of 1994.
- *FDA*: United States Food and Drug Administration. The federal agency responsible for the regulation of foods and drugs in interstate commerce.
- FFDCA: Federal Food, Drug, and Cosmetic Act of 1938.
- *Food*: As defined in part by FFDCA, articles used for food or drink for humans or other animals (Title 21 United States Code 321(f)).
- *Food additive*: As defined in part by FFDCA, any substance the intended use of which results or may reasonably be expected to result, directly or indirectly, in its becoming a component or otherwise affecting the characteristics of any food if such substance is not generally recognized as safe (GRAS); except that such term does not include a dietary supplement (Title 21 United States Code Sec. 321(s)).
- *FSIS*: Food Safety and Inspection Service. Part of USDA responsible for the inspection of meat and poultry products intended for human consumption.
- *GRAS*: "Generally Recognized As Safe." As defined in part by FFDCA, a substance generally recognized, among experts qualified by scientific training and experience to evaluate its safety, as having been adequately shown through scientific procedures (or, in the case of a substance used in food prior to January 1, 1958, through either scientific

procedures or experience based on common use in food) to be safe under the conditions of its intended use (Title 21 United States Code Sec. 321(s)).

- *NASC*: National Animal Supplement Council. A trade organization comprising manufacturers of dietary supplements for companion animals (and associated industries).
- *PDP*: Principal display panel. The part of the label most likely to be displayed to the purchaser under typical conditions of sale.
- *USDA*: United States Department of Agriculture.

US Regulatory Oversight

FDA, under the authority of FFDCA, has jurisdiction over all animal feeds (including pet foods) in interstate commerce (Dzanis 2018). Meat and poultry products, which when intended for human consumption are regulated by the US Department of Agriculture's Food Safety and Inspection Service (USDA-FSIS), are instead under the oversight of FDA when intended for animal consumption. Within FDA, CVM has primary responsibility for enforcement of the regulations codified under Title 21, Parts 500–599 of the Code of Federal Regulations (Government Publishing Office 2020). These include regulations to address the safety and utility of ingredients, the imposition of requirements for manufacturers to follow current Good Manufacturing Practices (cGMPs), as well as basic labeling rules for animal feeds in general.

Most states also exercise jurisdiction over pet foods sold within their respective borders. Individual state laws do differ, but to mitigate inconsistencies between them, the majority of states participate in the activities of AAFCO. AAFCO is a nongovernmental body, but its members must be government officials charged with the oversight of animal feeds. AAFCO fosters uniform interpretation and enforcement between states, largely though the establishment of model laws and regulations, ingredient definitions, and other guidelines and policies that constitute a consensus as to how feed should be regulated. The regulations specific to the labeling of pet foods include aspects that go beyond those required by FDA. These requirements along with other information are published annually in the AAFCO *Official Publication* (AAFCO 2022). Although this information is subject to copyright and there is a fee for purchase of the publication, access to the ingredient definitions is available to the public at no charge (www.aafco.org).

Importantly, it must be noted that AAFCO does not regulate, inspect, test, approve, or certify pet food in any way, and the AAFCO model regulations have no power of law in and of themselves. However, a majority of states have incorporated (directly or by reference) much of the AAFCO language into their own rules, at which time these become fully enforceable at the individual state level. For all intents and purposes, then, AAFCO serves as the national standard where FDA regulations are silent.

General Labeling Requirements

Considering both FDA and AAFCO regulations, mandatory components of a pet food label include the following.

Product Name

AAFCO has very extensive rules regarding the callout of ingredients in the product name depending on their percentage inclusion. For example, "Chicken" requires 95% inclusion of the named ingredient (excluding water for processing), while "Chicken Recipe" and "With Chicken" require notably less (25% and 3%, respectively). A pet food with the declaration "Chicken Flavor" may not necessarily contain any chicken at all, provided that a discernible source of that flavor is present (e.g. chicken meals, byproducts, digests).

Statement of Identity/Intended Species

FDA regulations require a succinct description of the contents in common terms on the PDP. Similarly, AAFCO requires that the PDP identify the intended species in words.

Verbiage such as "dog food" or "snacks for cats" is typically sufficient, but a graphic depiction of a dog or cat alone would be inadequate.

It is important to note that through AAFCO's Pet Food Labeling Modernization initiative, new model regulations are being contemplated to require more explicit identification of intended purpose on the PDP. While details have not been finalized, it is expected that the statement will expressly include in prescribed words and format the type of food (e.g., "complete," "treat," "supplement") as well as any appropriate life stage and size designation.

Ingredient Declaration

Both FDA and AAFCO regulations require that each ingredient (with some exceptions for incidental additives, etc.) in a pet food must be declared in descending order of predominance by weight. Many if not most ingredients incorporated into pet foods are expressly defined by AAFCO, though the means by which demonstration of safety and utility is established to provide for their inclusion may vary (e.g. Food Additive Petition, GRAS Notification, AAFCO Feed Ingredient Definition Petition). Regardless of the procedures utilized, CVM works closely with AAFCO in the process before a definition (including any identifying characteristics, specifications, or limitations of use) appears in the AAFCO *Official Publication*.

Some ingredients common in pet food may be universally understood by the public as "food" (e.g. apples, spinach), so in those instances no official approval or other sanction is required. Historically, these types of ingredients have not been expressly defined by AAFCO so have not appeared in the publication. However, AAFCO intends to publish a "Common Food Index" in the near future to document its interpretation of what food ingredients fit in this category.

Guaranteed Analysis

Information regarding the nutrient content of a pet food is not addressed in FDA regulations,

However, AAFCO rules do require the pet food label to bear guarantees for components of nutritional importance. For most pet foods that would include values for minimum percentages of crude protein and crude fat, and maximum percentages of crude fiber and moisture on an as-is basis. Additional guarantees may be added voluntarily or in the case where a specific nutrient content claim appears on the label, as needed to support the claim. For example, "with calcium" requires that the label include a minimum percentage calcium guarantee, while a "low fat" claim requires a maximum percentage crude fat guarantee in addition to the minimum.

Although a complete and balanced product making a general claim for vitamin and mineral content does not need to guarantee individual vitamins/minerals, a product represented to be a vitamin or mineral supplement must provide guarantees for each and every added vitamin and/or mineral in the product. On the other hand, some pet products may be exempt from certain guarantees, such as where the pet food does not provide appreciable amounts of that nutrient (e.g. crude protein and fiber guarantees on a liquid fish oil supplement label).

Required guarantees on dog and cat food labels are expected to change as AAFCO's Pet Food Labeling Modernization efforts are implemented. It is anticipated that "crude fiber" will be replaced with "dietary fiber," a more nutritionally meaningful value equivalent to that used for human foods. Also, a calculation of the maximum percentage of total carbohydrate content likely will be included in the guarantees.

Also in the future, the appearance of the guaranteed analysis itself is expected to be altered dramatically once proposed amendments to the AAFCO model regulations are promulgated. The guarantees, along with calorie content information and the nutritional adequacy statement, likely will be combined to form a more easily located and identifiable "Pet Nutrition Facts" box. The new format is intended to emulate (though is decidedly

different from) the nutrition information presently required on human food labels under FDA regulations,

Calorie Content Statement

AAFCO requires that labels of all dog and cat foods (including treats, toppers, nutritional supplements, etc.) bear a statement of calorie content in terms of kilocalories (kcal) of metabolizable energy (ME) per kilogram as is. In addition, this information must be presented in terms of kcal per unit of product consistent with the feeding directions (e.g. per can, cup, biscuit, or tablespoon) as well. The method used to determine calorie content must be specified: "calculated" for estimates derived from employment of the modified Atwater formula using analytic values for crude protein, crude fat, crude fiber, moisture, and ash; and "fed" for estimates determined through feeding tests. Future regulations likely will require that caloric distribution information (i.e. contributions of calories from protein, fat, and carbohydrate) also appear on the label.

Nutritional Adequacy Statement

All dog and cat foods labeled as "complete," "balanced," or by words of similar intent must bear a statement attesting to the food's nutritional suitability for its intended use. Precise verbiage is required, citing either conformance with the AAFCO Dog or Cat Food Nutrient Profiles or the successful passage of feeding trials following AAFCO protocols as the basis for substantiation. Each method has its pros and cons in terms of ensuring nutritional adequacy (Dzanis 2003). Arguably the least reliable method of ensuring adequacy is for products that were neither feeding trial tested directly nor necessarily formulated to meet the profiles, but rather were deemed to be a member of a "Product Family" by virtue of their nutritional similarity to a lead member that did pass the feeding trial. Such products can bear the same "Animal feeding tests substantiate" statement that appears on the labels of products that were directly tested by feeding trial, as long as the calorie content was determined by in vivo feeding trials. If calorie content was determined by calculation and assumptions of macronutrient digestibility, the family member products statement must specify that the product "is comparable in nutritional adequacy to a product which has been substantiated using AAFCO feeding tests." Most often, manufacturers will conduct the short-term (10-day) calorie feeding trial rather than the much longer (up to 6 months) nutritional adequacy trial, so that the statement that appears on the label for the product family member is indistinguishable from that for the lead member.

Any limitations as to the specific life stage or size of animal must be included in the statement. Dog and cat products that do not meet either means of substantiation but are not conspicuously identified as a "Snack," "Treat," or "Supplement" on the PDP must bear the statement "This product is intended for intermittent or supplemental feeding only." It is expected with future changes to the regulations that all labels for foods that are not complete and balanced must bear this statement without exception.

Feeding Directions

All complete and balanced dog and cat foods (including some treat products) must bear quantitative feeding directions, at minimum "Feed ___ per ___ pounds daily." AAFCO does not stipulate the means by which feeding directions are determined, however.

Although not explicitly called out in the AAFCO model regulations, nutritional supplements and value-added treats/toppers (those with added vitamins or other trace nutrients, but not complete and balanced) generally need sufficient directions on the label to provide for safe and appropriate feeding. On the other hand, words such as "feed as a snack or reward" may be sufficient for those treats where explicit quantitative directions are not deemed to be necessary.

Name and Address of Manufacturer or Distributor

The name of the party responsible for state registration of the product for distribution of the pet food (the "guarantor," in AAFCO-speak) must appear on the label. Words such as "manufactured for" or "distributed by" must accompany the name when the guarantor is not the actual manufacturer. Also required are the city, state, and ZIP code of the responsible party. The physical street address of the principal place of business must also appear, unless that information is easily accessible to the public elsewhere.

Net Contents

Both FDA and AAFCO regulations require a quantity statement on the PDP. Most often this is expressed in terms of net weight (weight of product without packaging), but it can be in terms of volume for liquid products, or on occasion by count (e.g. "XX tablets"). Extensive FDA rules dictate the size, placement, units, terms used, and degree of conspicuousness. Also, Federal Trade Commission (FTC) regulations (enforceable by FDA) require that the declaration be provided in terms of both avoirdupois units (pound/ounce) and their metric equivalents.

Country of Origin

By US Customs and Border Protection (CBP) regulations (enforceable by FDA), the labels of all imported products must bear a country-of-origin statement, for example "Made in [Country]" or "Product of [Country]." However, if the imported materials are materially transformed within the USA by mixing with other ingredients and/or further processing (i.e. more than simply cleaned or repackaged), labels are not required to declare country of origin regardless of the origin of the component ingredients.

"Made in USA" or similar statements on domestically manufactured product labels are not required by law. However, when such claims do appear on the label, FTC guidance requires that "all or virtually all" the ingredients must be of US origin as well. For products that do not meet that burden, the claim must be further qualified to adequately inform the consumer of the presence of more than negligible foreign content, e.g. "Made in USA with ___from ___," "Made in USA from domestic and imported ingredients."

Labeling Claims

Where space permits on the label, manufacturers will often include "romance copy," which may incorporate claims extolling the benefits of the product, its ingredients, nutrient content, or other qualities of the food. Only a few regulations address specific claims. However, under the general provisions of the law all copy on the label must be truthful and not misleading or the product may face enforcement action.

Descriptive Terms

AAFCO requires that a dog or cat food labeled as "lite," "low calorie," or by words of similar intent should not exceed specified calorie limits, depending on species and moisture content. For example, a "low calorie" dry dog food cannot exceed 3100 kcal ME/kg as is, whereas a canned cat food must contain no more than 950 kcal ME/kg as is. Products that fail to meet that restriction may still make a comparative claim, e.g. "XX% less calories than [product of comparison]."

Similar AAFCO rules are in place for claims such as "low" or "less fat." In those cases a maximum percentage crude fat, in addition to the mandatory minimum percentage, must appear in the guaranteed analysis. "Low carb" claims are not allowed by AAFCO, but a comparative claim for carbohydrate content can be made provided that maximum percentage guarantees for both dietary starch and sugars appear on the label.

"Natural" Claims

As per AAFCO, all ingredients in a "natural" pet food must be of natural origin (plant, animal, or mined sources only). Certain processing is allowed (e.g. physical or heat processing, fermentation), but any ingredient or component that is derived by chemically synthetic means or

contains synthetic additives would invalidate the claim. However, an exception is made in the case of added trace nutrients. In that case, the presence of these chemically synthetic components must be disclaimed, for example "natural with added vitamins."

Essentially, most macroingredients are "natural" as AAFCO defines it, so the term largely indicates the absence of artificial preservatives, flavors, or colors. In fact, some preservatives of natural origin are not as effective as synthetic antioxidants (Gross et al. 1994), which has practical impacts. For example, degraded fats as a result of poor preservation may impact palatability and affect the degree of oxidative stress on the animal.

Negative Claims

There are no applicable regulations with respect to claims regarding the absence of an ingredient or class of ingredients, such as "made without chicken" or "grain free." As generally interpreted by regulators, the claim most often indicates the lack of intentional addition of the ingredient(s) to the food. However, as a practical matter, in the typical course of manufacturing there is a significant chance of cross-contact with these unwanted ingredients due to shared equipment during transport, storage, and manufacturing. Hence, trace amounts of these presumably excluded ingredients may remain in the final product.

"Human-Grade" Claims

A conflict in authority between FDA and USDA has made substantiation of the veracity of "human-grade" claims difficult over the years. Under USDA regulations, meat and poultry products that have not been subject to FSIS inspection and deemed suitable for human consumption are "inedible" by definition. Further, FSIS will not and does not inspect pet products (with a minor exception for "certified" animal foods under regulations that are rarely if ever employed). As a result, essentially all pet foods containing meat and poultry cannot meet the human edible standard, even if the component meat and poultry ingredients have passed FSIS inspection.

To help remedy this conundrum, AAFCO has been working with another facet of USDA (the Agricultural Marketing Service, AMS) to establish a means by which pet food companies are voluntarily inspected/audited by the AMS to ensure conformance with AAFCO's standard for "human grade." Essentially, under the standard all ingredients going into the pet food must be suitable for human consumption, and the final pet product must be produced in a facility that is appropriately licensed to manufacture human food (under either FDA or USDA authority). As a result, in addition to the need to meet specified processes and practices, many ingredients commonly used in pet food formulations (e.g. meat and poultry meals, byproducts) are not allowed. However, a "human-grade" designation is not necessarily indicative of higher standards for quality or nutritional value.

Drug Claims

Perhaps the claims of greatest concern to regulators are "drug claims." Under the law, the distinction between a "food" and a "drug" largely depends on what claims are associated with the product; that is, for what purpose the product is intended by the manufacturer or distributor. While the statutory definition of "food" is admittedly vague, a precedent-setting court ruling established a "common-sense" definition, as an item consumed "primarily for taste, aroma, or nutritive value" (*NutriLab, Inc.* v. *Schweiker*, 713F.2d 335 (7th circa 1983)).

On the other hand, the statutory definition of a "drug" includes any article *intended* to treat or prevent disease or to affect the structure or function of the body in a manner distinct from the provision of qualities normally ascribed to food, such as nutritive value. As a result, any product, even one containing only common food ingredients, can be subject to regulation as a drug under the law if the claims associated with the commercial distribution of

the product indicate or imply an intent to offer it as a drug.

The regulatory category into which a substance is placed affects its requirements for legal distribution. A drug is held to a higher standard and with only a few exceptions must be proven by the manufacturer to be safe and effective for its intended use prior to marketing. On the other hand, foods do not require pre-market clearance from FDA. Because the food product bearing a drug claim was not approved by FDA as a drug, the food becomes subject to enforcement action as an "adulterated drug" under FDA law.

For example, a perfectly acceptable feed ingredient, such as calcium carbonate, may be safely added to a pet food for its nutritive value. A claim to "help support healthy bone growth and development in puppies" is within the realm of acceptable food claims, as that is the recognized nutritional function of calcium. However, a promise to "cure bone deformations" is a drug claim. Similarly, ginger may be added to a pet food for flavor, but not to "soothe upset tummies." Even a claim to "boost" function or "increase health" of a body structure (as opposed to "maintain" or "support health") may be an implied drug claim and potentially actionable.

Supplements

It is estimated that from 10% to 33% of the companion animals (dogs, cats, and horses) in the USA receive a daily dietary supplement, with approximately 90% of practicing veterinarians dispensing supplements in their practice (Freeman et al. 2006; Bookout and Khachatoorian 2007; NRC 2009). Historically, use of supplements was mostly limited to essential dietary nutrients such as vitamins and minerals, generally meant to augment or balance a poor-quality, incomplete, or otherwise inadequate diet. Even with the advent of "complete and balanced" pet foods (circa the 1960s), sales of dietary supplements continued. However, it was not until recent decades that greatly increased numbers and types of dietary supplements for animals have been available. This followed a similar increase in the availability of human dietary supplements following passage of the Dietary Supplement Health and Education Act of 1994 (DSHEA).

Briefly, DSHEA dramatically impacted the regulatory framework under which dietary supplements may be distributed in the USA. Under FFDCA, a food ingredient has to be explicitly or implicitly GRAS or approved as a food additive, or the product containing it may be subject to regulation as an adulterated food. However, DSHEA changed FFDCA to allow for a broad use of substances in dietary supplements not normally acceptable for use in foods in conventional form. Thus, in addition to vitamins, minerals, and so on, supplements may now contain herbs and botanicals, metabolites, antioxidants, chondroprotective agents, and many other substances. Further, DSHEA provides for claims relating to effect on the structure or function of the body beyond recognized nutritional precepts. These would normally be construed as "drug claims" if made for food in general.

Importantly, DSHEA was never intended for, nor does it apply to, animal products (FDA 1996). Rather, the aforementioned restrictions on ingredients and claims for foods in general are still enforceable when it comes to pet supplements. Nutritional supplements for pets must meet the FDA and AAFCO regulations like any other animal feed. However, many other pet supplement products that contain other substances simply do not wholly meet these requirements. Non-nutritive supplements may contain substances for which safety and utility have not been established, or their labels may bear poorly supported if not totally unsubstantiated claims.

Why is this allowed? In play at many times, especially in the case of pet supplements, is the concept of "enforcement discretion." This is when a recognized violation is overlooked by regulators under certain conditions, either because it is of relatively low priority or to provide for uniform enforcement. NASC, a trade organization representing many manufacturers of pet supplement products, has developed its own system of oversight that has helped alienate many concerns of regulators. For example, to help address safety of products, members of NASC are subject to audits and must participate in a mandatory adverse event reporting system.

For non-nutritive supplements, NASC has coined a new term that is not in the regulatory lexicon: "dosage form animal health product." From a regulatory perspective, these products are generally afforded informal status as "unapproved drugs of low regulatory priority" by CVM, which allows for federal oversight and requires that certain conditions be met, albeit much less than is required for approved drugs. Assuming that the product is not represented as a food, these products escape scrutiny by state feed control officials. However, they are still required to be registered in those few states that enforce "animal remedy" laws.

NASC has also developed a labeling format for pet supplements that do not meet FFDCA as a food so that they are distinct from the labeling required by FDA/AAFCO for nutritional supplements (Bookout and Khachatoorian 2007). Examples of how labels of products in these two categories differ are shown in Figures 5.1 and 5.2. Realizing that the non-nutritive supplements are not subject to the same regulatory scrutiny as either nutritional supplements or approved drugs, it is prudent for the practitioner to consider the type of supplement when evaluating the product (see Sidebar 5.1).

Therapeutic Pet Foods

Fundamentally, therapeutic dog and cat foods are "drugs" under FFDCA. They do not contain drugs as the term is typically contemplated by the public, but rather are intentionally formulated to exert an effect on a disease or condition by virtue of manipulation of common feedstuffs to alter nutrient content (e.g. controlled protein/phosphorus for management of chronic kidney disease). Still,

Melanie's 5H Formulas

For Happy, Healthy, Hale 'n' Hearty Hounds

Healthy Bones & Teeth Formula

Beef-flavored vitamin and mineral supplement for dogs and puppies

Net wt 15 oz (425 g)

Ingredients
Dicalcium Phosphate, Tapioca Starch, Magnesium Oxide, Natural Beef Flavor, Zinc Amino Acid Complex, Thiamine Mononitrate, Caramel (color), Silicon Dioxide, Vitamin A Palmitate, Copper Proteinate, dl-Alpha Tocopherol Acetate. Riboflavin, Citric Acid (preservative), Cholecalciferol, Vitamin B$_{12}$ Supplement.

Guaranteed Analysis	Calorie Content ME
Moisture (max)..................... 2%	(calculated)
Calcium (min)................... 15%	928 kcal/kg
Phosphorus (min)........... 13.5%	20 kcal/tsp
Magnesium (min)............... 1.2%	
Copper (min)................45 mg/kg	**Feeding Directions**
Zinc (min)................ 210 mg/kg	1 teaspoon per 10 pounds
Vitamin A (min).........6500 IU/kg	body weight daily, mixed
Vitamin D$_3$ (min).........479 IU/kg	with food. Double daily
Vitamin E (min)...........260 IU/kg	amount for puppies and
Thiamine (min).......... 150 mg/kg	nursing mothers.
Riboflavin (min)........... 70 mg/kg	
Vitamin B$_{12}$ (min).......015 mg/kg	

Contact Us!
Distributed by Melanie's 5H Formulas, San Angeles, CA 90298
Toll free: 800-555-4959
www.melanies5Hformulas.com

See Best Before date on bottom of container

Figure 5.1 Example of a label for a nutritional supplement in conformance with AAFCO Model Regulations for Pet Food and Specialty Pet Food.

Melanie's 5H Formulas

For Happy, Healthy, Hale 'n' Hearty Hounds

Advanced Hip & Joint Formula

Beef Flavor
for dogs and puppies

Net wt 15 oz (425 g)

Product Facts
ACTIVE INGREDIENTS PER TEASPOON

Glucosamine HCl (shellfish)	375 mg
Chondroitin Sulfate (poultry)	200 mg
Proprietary Blend (Ginger Root, Boswellia, Turmeric)	75 mg
Ascorbic Acid (Vitamin C)	20 mg
Magnesium (as Magnesium Citrate)	5 mg

INACTVE INGREDIENTS: Tapioca Starch, Natural Beef Flavor, Caramel (color), Silicon Dioxide, Citric Acid (preservative).
CAUTIONS: Safe use in pregnant or nursing animals has not been proven. If lameness worsens, discontinue use and contact your veterinarian. Administer during or after the animal has eaten to reduce incidence of gastrointestinal upset.
FOR USE IN DOGS ONLY
RECOMMENDED TO SUPPORT HEALTHY JOINT FUNCTION
DIRECTIONS FOR USE: Give 1 teaspoon per 10 pounds body weight daily for initial loading dose (3-4 weeks). For maintenance, give 1/2 teaspoon per 10 pounds daily. Double doses above for puppies.
WARNINGS: For animal use only. Keep out of reach of children and pets. In case of accidental overdose, contact a health professional immediately.
CONTACT US! Distributed by Melanie's 5H Formulas, San Angeles, CA 90298 Toll free: 800-555-4959
www.melanies5Hformulas.com

See Best Before date on bottom of container

Figure 5.2 Example of a label for a non-nutritive supplement in the format developed by the National Animal Supplement Council.

because these foods are expressly intended for the treatment, prevention, or mitigation of disease, they can be construed to be unapproved drugs under the law and theoretically subject to enforcement action.

In recognition of these products' potential value to the practice of veterinary medicine, regulators generally have exercised enforcement discretion with regard to them. Historically, oversight of therapeutic diets has

Sidebar 5.1   Use of Foods and Supplements in Practice

As with all elements of practice, veterinarians may be legally or ethically liable for adverse events that may stem from using, dispensing, or recommending foods or supplements for their patients. Depending on the exact wording of the state's veterinary practice act under which the veterinarian practices, use of these products may or may not be considered a component of recognized veterinary practice, hence this may impact how a claim against a veterinarian is handled (Scoggins 1998). Thus, it behooves the veterinarian to critically evaluate the merits of a product prior to use and closely monitor outcomes, particularly for those products that do not wholly meet regulatory requirements for their intended uses (e.g. therapeutic pet foods and non-nutritive supplements) (see Table 5.1).

Table 5.1   Steps and key considerations for assessment of veterinary food and supplement products.

Step	Key considerations
Assess need	Sound basis for use
	Reliable source of recommendation
	Accurate diagnosis
Assess supportive data	Manufacturer studies
	Literature search
	Ranking of study strengths
Assess commercial source	Regulatory status (food or drug?)
	Human vs. animal supplement
	Company history/reputation
Assess outcomes	Keep consistent, searchable records
	Periodically evaluate outcomes

The veterinarian should establish a sound rationale for use of a food or supplement before it is administered to the patient. Principles underlying therapeutic use of some supplements, such as herbs, may diverge from conventional veterinary practice (Ramey 2007). For example, a vague indication for use, such as "to detoxify the liver," may or may not mean the product is appropriate for all cases of hepatic disease, and in fact it may be contraindicated for some animals. Recommendations or opinions from qualified experts and published papers in peer-reviewed journals may be more reliable than those from self-proclaimed authorities on the internet or elsewhere. Potential conflicts of interest, such as the proponent's financial connection to the company that markets the product, also should be considered.

The decision by the veterinarian to use a food or supplement to address a particular disease or condition should demand ample scientific evidence to show that it is both efficacious and safe for its intended use. As indicated earlier, current regulatory policies do not require that data to support use of therapeutic pet foods be submitted to a regulatory authority prior to distribution. Similarly, supplements that fall out of the regulatory rubric for foods most often are not critically evaluated by FDA or state feed control officials. The manufacturer may cite studies to support use of the product in advertising or on its website. Practitioners should not be shy in asking the manufacturer for access to the studies cited. In addition, the veterinarian should seek other sources of information for assurances of appropriate use, including the scientific and medical literature.

The regulatory category under which the commercial supplement is marketed may offer valuable insight to the veterinarian. An animal supplement product that is not labeled in accordance with AAFCO/FDA requirements for pet foods most likely has not been subject to scrutiny by CVM or state feed control officials. It may contain ingredients that have not been duly evaluated for safety and utility for its intended use. Also, claims for benefits that go beyond the provision of nutrients to help maintain or support healthy structure or function of the body should be suspect, as their veracity most likely has not been verified by an authoritative body.

Finally, in choosing a food or supplement for use in practice, the manufacturer's history and reputation should be considered. Is the brand widely known? Is the company willing to answer questions? Does it freely provide technical information on its products, manufacturing controls, or other areas of concern? Have colleagues had experience with the product or company? For therapeutic diets, does the company conform to CVM/AAFCO guidance (or, for example, does it sell outside the veterinarian–client–patient relationship)? The veterinarian should proceed only when comfortable with the answers.

If the practitioner proceeds to use the product on patients, careful observation of the response of animals, positively or negatively, to administration is paramount to the decision of whether or not to continue using it in other clinical cases. Ideally, the supplement, and only the supplement, would be the sole treatment, so that the effects of other modalities would not obscure or interfere with the observations. However, in a practical situation this is likely to be the exception rather than the norm.

Because a clinical or adverse response to a dietary supplement may not be as speedy or apparent as that to an approved drug, a product may have to be used on multiple patients over an extended period before a valid assessment of the outcomes can be conducted. As a fundamental component of the practice of evidence-based medicine, procedures to appropriately record clinical outcomes for later evaluation are detailed elsewhere (Faunt et al. 2007). Briefly, computerized records are preferred, in that they allow for easier search and capture of relevant clinical outcome information. Consistent use of standardized nomenclature in records helps ensure that all sought data are found. Establishing "best practice" treatment protocols that are followed by everyone in the practice enables outcome data for all patients to be compared equally.

Once appropriate data on outcomes are collected, a systematic evaluation can be revealing. Obviously, finding evidence of clinical improvement in the majority of patients compared to similar treatment without the supplement suggests that continued use of the supplement may be warranted. Just as importantly, a pattern of adverse effects may be discerned by comparing outcomes of treatments with or without the supplement. Adverse effects may include direct toxic effects, allergic reactions, or interactions with other drugs or treatments (Ramey 2007). Indirect effects – that is, the potential consequences of delaying or replacing known effective conventional treatments with dietary supplements – should also be considered.

not been a high regulatory priority. Rather, CVM has generally allowed therapeutic pet foods to remain on the market provided that manufacturers abided by certain (albeit unwritten) conditions. In 2016, FDA formalized these conditions with release of guidance to identify the circumstances under which the agency is less likely to initiate enforcement action (FDA 2016). Recently AAFCO has developed very similar guidelines.

Under this guidance, mitigation of the risk of enforcement action by CVM or states stipulates that the therapeutic pet food must be made available only through veterinarians or on the order of a veterinarian. While not a "prescription" in the legal sense of the term, this stipulation encourages the use of products only where a valid veterinarian–client–patient relationship exists.

Further, promotional materials available to the veterinarian may include discussion of the product's therapeutic intent and provide a rationale for that distinction (i.e. make "drug claims"). However, labeling and other materials intended for the animal owner, in print or electronic form, cannot bear any indications of therapeutic use. This discourages diagnoses and treatment without adequate veterinary supervision.

In addition, the product must contain only acceptable pet food ingredients (no drugs or unapproved food additives). Finally, the therapeutic diet must be otherwise compliant with all labeling and other regulatory requirements for pet food.

Frankly, not all products on the market today meet all these criteria, particularly with regard to the inclusion of drug claims in promotional materials intended for the consumer. Regardless, the most important aspect for the veterinarian to recognize is that while regulatory bodies do have the authority to take action against improperly formulated or otherwise unsafe products, the criteria discussed here do not include premarket review of data sufficient to demonstrate safety and utility by an authoritative body. In other words, it is left to the practitioner to read the available information, assess its merits and limitations, and monitor patient outcomes while using or dispensing the product to the client (see Sidebar 5.1).

Dog Chews

By AAFCO policy, rawhide, pig ears, pizzles, and similarly specified chew products are exempt from state registration and labeling requirements, provided that they are not labeled in a manner that implies nutritive value (e.g. "high protein"). Importantly, they are still "food" under the law, and so regulators still can take appropriate action against adulterated or misbranded products. Also, all chews must wholly abide by FDA labeling requirements. So, for example, a chew label would need an ingredient list, but typically would not bear a guaranteed analysis or calorie content statement. Many products on the market are labeled by count (e.g. "10 chew sticks"), but a recent decision by the National Conference on Weights and Measures requires that all such products declare contents in terms of net weight; that is, numerical count alone is no longer sufficient.

Summary

The federal and state regulations pertinent to pet foods sold in the USA are extensive and complex. They are primarily designed to help ensure safe, wholesome, and properly labeled products on the market. For the veterinarian who uses, dispenses, or recommends pet foods to clients, understanding of and appreciation for the regulatory scrutiny these products must face are helpful in practice. This is particularly true in the cases of pet supplements and therapeutic diets.

European Union Regulation

Nutritional products targeted at pets have greatly evolved in the last years and continue diversifying to meet the demands for food and complements, which are more and more specialized. Pet caregivers and veterinarians have access to a wide range of nutritional products for pets in the market, which are marketed for dogs and cats of different breeds, ages, physiologic stages, or specific characteristics. In fact, many advances in human nutrition are adapted to pet food. It is logical to think that owners want to offer to their pets the benefits of these advances in nutrition, as they want to use them for themselves.

This pet food vision has led to the development of many complete feed options for pets, as well as a great variety of supplements or complementary feeds, which are sometimes also intended to manage metabolic diseases that could be treated with medications.

From the legislative point of view, it is important to know the limits of nutritional products with specific claims. Since these products are not medications, they cannot include any therapeutic claims.

In fact, the line between some complementary feed and veterinary medications is very thin. Within this section, some references will be provided for a better understanding of the complexity of this issue, which is directly linked to European Union (EU) legislation.

Definitions, Abbreviations, and Acronyms

- *Complementary feed*: compound feed that has a high content of certain substances but that, by reason of its composition, is sufficient for a daily ration only if used in combination with other feeds.
- *Complete feed*: compound feed that, by reason of its composition, is sufficient for a daily ration.
- *Compound feed*: a mixture of at least two feed materials, whether or not containing feed additives, for oral animal feeding in the form of complete or complementary feed.
- *Daily ration*: the average total quantity of feedingstuffs, calculated on a moisture content of 12%, required daily by an animal of a given species, age category, and yield to satisfy all its needs.
- *EFSA*: European Food Safety Authority. A European agency funded by the EU that operates independently of the European legislative and executive institutions (Commission, Council, Parliament) and EU Member States. Its main function is to provide independent nonbinding scientific advice (including advice on nutrition and animal feed) to policymakers to promote safety within the food chain.
- *FEDIAF*: European Pet Food Industry Federation. FEDIAF is the trade body representing the European pet food industry that has developed Nutritional Guidelines and a Code of Good Labelling Practice for Pet Food.

- *Feed (or feedingstuff)*: any substance or product, including additives, whether processed, partially processed, or unprocessed, intended to be used for oral feeding to animals.
- *Feed additives*: substances, microorganisms, or preparations, other than feed material and premixtures, which are intentionally added to feed or water in order to perform, in particular, one or more of the functions mentioned in Article 5(3) of EC Regulation No. 1831/2003.
- *Feed intended for particular nutritional purposes*: feed that can satisfy a particular nutritional purpose by virtue of its particular composition or method of manufacture, which clearly distinguishes it from ordinary feed. Feed intended for particular nutritional purposes does not include medicated feedingstuffs.
- *Feed materials*: products of vegetable or animal origin, whose principal purpose is to meet animals' nutritional needs, in their natural state, fresh or preserved, and products derived from the industrial processing thereof, and organic or inorganic substances, whether or not containing feed additives, which are intended for use in oral animal feeding either directly as such, or after processing, or in the preparation of compound feed, or as a carrier of premixtures.
- *Mineral feed*: complementary feed containing at least 40% crude ash.
- *Non-food-producing animals*: any animal that is fed, bred, or kept but that is not used for human consumption, such as fur animals, pets, and animals kept in laboratories, zoos, or circuses.
- *Particular nutritional purpose or PARNUT*: the purpose of meeting the specific nutritional needs of animals whose process of assimilation, absorption, or metabolism is, or could be, temporarily or irreversibly impaired and who can therefore benefit from the ingestion of feed appropriate to their condition.
- *Pet food*: Any product produced by a pet food manufacturer, whether processed, partially

processed, or unprocessed, intended to be ingested by pet animals after placing on the market. Regulations sometimes uses "feed" or "feedingstuff" as synonyms.

- *Pet or pet animal*: any non-food-producing animal belonging to species fed, bred, or kept, but not normally used for human consumption in the EU.
- *Placing on the market*: the holding of food or feed for the purpose of sale, including offering for sale or any other form of transfer, whether free of charge or not, and the sale, distribution, and other forms of transfer themselves.
- *Premixtures*: mixtures of feed additives or mixtures of one or more feed additives with feed materials or water used as carriers, not intended for direct feeding to animals.
- *OJEU*: *Official Journal of the European Union*. This is the publication in which all tenders from the public sector that are valued above a certain financial threshold, according to EU legislation, must be published.

General Pet Food Regulations

European food and feed legislation is based on Regulation (EC) N°178/2002 (2002), which lays down the general principles and requirements of food law. In 2002, and after a serious crisis due to bovine spongiform encephalopathy (BSE, or "mad cow disease"), a new regulation was needed. Within the context of food law, it was appropriate to include requirements for production and use of feed intended for food-producing animals, and expanding later to encompass all animals, including pets.

EFSA offers scientific advice in the areas that influence the safety of food and feed. Among other functions, it must evaluate the additives used in the feeding of animals, and the proposals of new particular nutritional purposes (dietary supplements), and it offers assessment of food risks.

To better understand how different types of food are classified, Regulation (EC) N° 767/2009 (2009), on the placing on the market and use of

feed, should be consulted. According to this regulation, "the distinction between feed materials, feed additives, and other products such as veterinary drugs has implications for the conditions for the placing of such products on the market. Feed materials are primarily used to meet animals' needs, for example for energy, nutrients, minerals, or dietary fibres. They are usually not chemically well-defined except for basic nutritional constituents. Effects which can be justified by scientific assessment and which are exclusive to feed additives or veterinary drugs should be excluded from the objective uses of feed materials."

Regulation (EC) N° 1831/2003 (2003) on additives for use in animal nutrition establishes the conditions for feed additives and their mixtures, called premixtures, in order for them to be used in animal feed. It also defines the process of requesting and authorizing the marketing of feed additives. This process is very complex and requires extensive documentation, as well as effectiveness and safety studies, so that the feed additive can be authorized.

On the other hand, and to guarantee the conditions of manufacture of all products intended for animal feed, Regulation (EC) N° 183/2005 (2005) lays down the requirements for feed hygiene. Other legislation establishes specific regulations for the use of products of animal origin, undesirable substances, and feed materials that can be used for animal feed. It is important to note Regulation (EU) N° 2020/354 (2020), which establishes a list of intended uses of animal feedingstuffs for particular nutritional purposes and regulates complementary pet food, colloquially called "dietary supplements"

The aforementioned framework legislation (Figure 5.3) is only part of the many regulations, perhaps hundreds, that can affect the production and marketing of pet food in the EU. In addition, these regulations are subject to continuous review, as they must adapt to scientific and technological advances.

It is important to note that the term "food" is always dedicated to products intended for

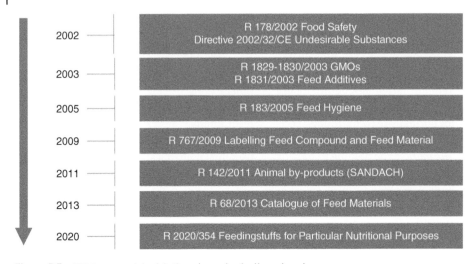

Figure 5.3 EU framework legislation chronologically ordered.

human consumption and the only exception is for pets, where the term "pet food" instead of "feed" has been legally accepted precisely to recognize the social perception of proximity of pets to the environment of humans.

As a general principle, a substance that is intended for animal feed is a feed material or a feed additive, no other options. Feed material mixtures with or without feed additives result in compound feeds, while mixtures of feed additives, which can also contain feed materials as a carrier, are premixtures. Obviously, this is a simple approach that can be greatly complicated depending on the nature of the products, their use, and the influence of other regulations. The European legislation is extremely complex and pet food is a highly regulated product to achieve the highest standards of hygiene, safety, and quality.

Complementary Pet Food: Composition, Uses, and Labeling

The term "compound feed" has been defined as a mixture of at least two feed materials (see the list of definitions). In turn, a compound feed is divided into:

- *Complete pet food*, which, by reason of its composition, is sufficient for a daily ration.

- *Complementary pet food*, which has a high content of certain substances but which, by reason of its composition, is sufficient for a daily ration only if used in combination with another pet food.

Complementary pet foods are very diverse, with different uses and covering a wide range of products that include the following:

- Products intended to be mixed with other food components. They are often mixed at home, in varying proportions, to form a complete diet for pets. They provide considerable energy content and also macronutrients such as protein, calcium, phosphorus, etc.
- Treats and snacks that are normally given during training. These products can have a high energy value, but in fact their function is not strictly nutritional, although it can have an impact on the daily total energy intake, so the instructions for use must be well defined so as not to supply excessive amounts.
- Vitamin and trace element supplements, which would also be classified as complementary pet food. They are typically marketed to consumers as extra contributions of these components in certain periods (convalescence, training, etc.) or, less commonly, as a means to balance a homemade diet. It

should be noted that these supplements cannot exceed certain limits of some vitamins and trace elements for which the legislation of additives has set a maximum limit on the daily complete food.

- Mineral pet food or macromineral supplements (calcium, phosphorus, magnesium, etc.). These are often marketed for uses such as for pets that may require an extra supply of minerals, such as in a decalcification process or other similar problems. To be classified as mineral pet food it must contain at least 40% of crude ash.
- Other products that do not have a significant energy value but provide some special features (fatty acids, amino acids, etc.), which are still marketed as complementary pet food because of the current definition.

Feed Additives

Feed additives must be authorized before use and there must be a regulation that sets the characteristics of the additive and also the conditions of its use: target species, maximum content in the food in some cases, and other recommendations. Additives are divided into five categories: technological, sensory, nutritional, zootechnical, and coccidiostats/histomonostats. Each of these is included in functional groups that describe the activity and effect that the additive has on the food or on the animal when it is ingested (Table 5.2).

It is important to note that all the additives are in the revision phase. Since 2010, the European authorities have been evaluating all the additives that already existed in the market (approximately 1400 additives), in addition to requests for new products. The practical consequence is the continuous publication of regulations that often change their name, identification number, maximum levels, or other restrictions on use. For this reason, it is important that the legislation is always consulted, directly from the website edited by the European Commission. The list of additives is exclusive; that is to say, only the authorized additives listed in the Register of Feed Additives (European Commission 2022) can be used.

It is important to note that this current version of the register has no legal value, but should be consulted to check if additives are approved by referring to the authorizing legal act.

Claims

As for food for humans, both functional declarations and nutritional claims can be made (e.g. low in sodium, with high content in omega-3, etc.). It is Regulation (EC) N° 767/2009 (2009) that establishes that labeling and the presentation of feed materials and compound feed may draw particular attention to the presence or absence of a substance in the feed, to a specific nutritional characteristic or process, or to a specific function related to any of these. The claim should be objective, verifiable by the competent authorities, and understandable by the user of the feed.

When requested by the authorities, the manufacturer or the person responsible for the product in the market must demonstrate the claims that they have indicated on the label through scientific references or their own studies. This may create some distortion in the market, since not all operators will use exactly the same criteria to label their products with nutritional claims.

Labeling

The legislation establishes mandatory minimum declarations on complementary pet food that are very well defined. The label must identify the manufacturer, the company responsible for commercialization, the date of manufacture and durability of the product, the batch number, and weight or net volume.

The type of feed must always be identified: "Complementary pet food." Other products should indicate "complete pet food" if they meet daily needs and it can be the only food the animal consumes.

Regarding the declarations of analytical components, Table 5.3 indicates the values that must be declared in pet food (complete or

Table 5.2 Classification of feed additives: categories and functional groups, as written in current legislation.

Additive groups: categories and functional groups	
1. Technological additives	
a Preservatives	Substances or, when applicable, micro-organisms which protect feed against deterioration caused by micro-organisms or their metabolites
b Antioxidants	Substances prolonging the storage life of feedingstuffs and feed materials by protecting them against deterioration caused by oxidation
c Emulsifiers	Substances that make it possible to form or maintain a homogeneous mixture of two or more immiscible phases in feedingstuffs
d Stabilisers	Substances which make it possible to maintain the physico-chemical state of feedingstuffs
e Thickeners	Substances which increase the viscosity of feedingstuffs
f Gelling agents	Substances which give a feedingstuff texture through the formation of a gel
g Binders	Substances which increase the tendency of particles of feedingstuffs to adhere
h Substances for control of radionucleide contamination	Substances that suppress absorption of radionucleides or promote their excretion
i Anticaking agents	Substances that reduce the tendency of individual particles of a feedingstuff to adhere
j Acidity regulators	Substances which adjust the pH of feedingstuffs
k Silage additives	Substances, including enzymes or microorganisms, intended to be incorporated into feed to improve the production of silage
l Denaturants	Substances which, when used for the manufacture of processed feedingstuffs, allow identification of the origin of specific food or feed materials
m Substances for reduction of the contamination of feed by mycotoxins	Substances that can suppress or reduce the absorption, promote the excretion of mycotoxins or modify their mode of action
n Hygiene condition enhancers	Substances or, when applicable, microorganisms which favourably affect the hygienic characteristics of feed by reducing a specific microbiological contamination
2. Sensory additives	
a Colourants	Substances that add or restore colour in feedingstuffs
	Substances which, when fed to animals, add colours to food of animal origin
	Substances which favourably affect the colour of ornamental fish or birds
b Flavouring compounds	Substances the inclusion of which in feedingstuffs increases feed smell or palatability

Table 5.2 (Continued)

Additive groups: categories and functional groups	
3. Nutritional additives	
a Vitamins, pro-vitamins, and chemically well-defined substances having similar effect	
b Compounds of trace elements	
c Amino acids, their salts and analogs	
d Urea and its derivatives	
4. Zootechnical additives	
a Digestibility enhancers	Substances which, when fed to animals, increase the digestibility of the diet, through action on target feed materials
b Gut flora stabilisers	Microorganisms or other chemically defined substances which, when fed to animals, have a positive effect on the gut flora
c Substances which favourably affect the environment	Substances which favourably affect the environment, that is to say reduce ammonia or methane
d Other zootechnical additives	Substances which favourably affect the performance and growth of healthy animals
5. Coccidiostats and histomonostats	

Table 5.3 Analytical constituents that should be declared.

Feed	Analytical constituents	Target species
Complete feed	Crude protein	Cats, dogs, and fur animals
	Crude fibers	Cats, dogs, and fur animals
	Crude oils and fats	Cats, dogs, and fur animals
	Crude ash	Cats, dogs, and fur animals
	Moisture if >14%	Cats, dogs, and fur animals
Complementary feed – mineral	Calcium	All species
	Sodium	All species
	Phosphorus	All species
Complementary feed – other	Crude protein	Cats, dogs, and fur animals
	Crude fibers	Cats, dogs, and fur animals
	Crude oils and fats	Cats, dogs, and fur animals
	Crude ash	Cats, dogs, and fur animals

complementary) when the target species are cats, dogs, and fur animals.

If amino acids, vitamins, and/or trace elements are indicated under the heading of analytical constituents, they must be declared, along with the total amount thereof.

If the energy value and/or protein value are indicated, such an indication should be in accordance with the EU method, if available, or with the respective official national method in the Member State where the feed is placed on the market, if available.

The ingredients that are part of the complementary feed should be declared indicating the name of the feed material or the name of the category to which the feed materials belong, for instance "Corn" declared as feed material or "Cereal grains" declared as category. Both forms of declaration are correct and it is not mandatory to indicate the percentage of inclusion in the label. However, the name and percentage by weight of a feed material should be indicated if its presence is emphasized on the labeling in words, pictures, or graphics.

As for additives, they are notifiable in the following cases:

- Additives where a maximum content is set for any kind of target species (e.g. vitamin A, vitamin D).
- Additives belonging to the category of "zootechnical additives" (e.g. enzymes or microorganisms).
- Additives of the functional groups preservatives, antioxidants, or colorants, where only the functional group in question needs to be indicated.

However, a free telephone number or other appropriate means of communication should be indicated on the label of the pet food product in order to allow the purchaser to obtain information in addition to the mandatory particulars on other feed additives contained in the pet food and feed materials contained therein that are designated by category.

Dietetic Pet Food

Particular nutritional purposes (PARNUTs), also known as dietetic pet food, define those situations in which it is considered that the animal needs a series of nutritional modifications to try to prevent or diminish the effects of certain physiologic states, deficiencies, or imbalances. The use of dietetic pet food is also justified for animals whose metabolism is temporarily or irreversibly impaired.

Once again, we are at the limit of nutritional products, almost entering into the field of veterinary medicines. Precisely because of the thin separation between one and the other, particular nutritional purposes have been regulated through Regulation (EU) N° 2020/354 (2020), establishing a list of intended uses of animal feedingstuffs for PARNUTs.

The list includes the following data:

- Particular nutritional purpose.
- Essential nutritional characteristics.
- Species or category of animals.
- Labeling declarations.
- Recommended length of time.
- Other provisions.

Table 5.4 lists all the PARNUTs that are currently authorized specifically for dogs, cats, and horses. Only the PARNUTs, essential nutritional characteristics, and species or category of animals as summarized information are included in the table. Given that it is a positive list, only the products that meet the requirements established for any of these purposes, already published in the regulations, can be classified as a PARNUT product. Any other advance or dietary supplement that has been proven effective in studies cannot be labeled and therefore cannot be advertised as a PARNUT product until it has been requested, evaluated by the authorities, and included in the list.

A dietary complementary pet food has some special characteristics, so it must contain in its labeling all the general information of a complementary pet food that has already been referenced, plus the additional requirements established by the list of the PARNUTs Regulation.

Usually, the following sentence is stated on the label of a dietary supplement: "It is recommended that advice from a veterinarian be sought before use and before extending the period of use." However, this is not mandatory and consumers can purchase dietetic foods (complete or complementary) without the input of a veterinary professional.

It is important to note that the established list may be modified, where appropriate,

Table 5.4 Particular nutritional purposes that are currently authorized specifically for dogs, cats, and horses.

Particular nutritional purpose	Essential nutritional characteristics (GP1)	Species or category of animal
Support of renal function in case of chronic renal insufficiency	High-quality proteins and phosphorus ≤5 g/kg complete feed with a moisture content of 12% and crude protein ≤220 g/kg complete feed with a moisture content of 12%	Dogs
	Reduced phosphorus absorption by means of incorporation of lanthanum carbonate octahydrate	Adult dogs
	High-quality proteins and phosphorus ≤6.5 g/kg complete feed with a moisture content of 12% and crude protein ≤320 g/kg complete feed with a moisture content of 12%	Cats
	Reduced phosphorus absorption by means of incorporation of lanthanum carbonate octahydrate	Adult cats
	High density of energy with more than 8.8 MJ/kg feed with a moisture content of 12%	Equines
	Highly digestible and highly palatable sources of starch	
	Restricted protein level: ≤106 g crude protein/kg feed with a moisture content of 12%	
	Level of sodium: 2 g/100 kg body weight (BW)/d	
	High level of sum of eicosapentaenoic acid and docosahexaenoic acid ≥0.2 g/kg $BW^{0.75}$/d	
Reduction of oxalate stones formation	Low level of calcium, low level of vitamin D, and urine alkalizing properties	Dogs and cats
Regulation of glucose supply (diabetes mellitus)	Total sugars (mono- and disaccharides) ≤62 g/kg complete feed with a moisture content of 12%	Dogs and cats
Reduction of ingredient and nutrient intolerances	Selected and limited number of protein source(s) and/or Hydrolyzed protein source(s) and/or Selected carbohydrate source(s)	Dogs and cats
Reduction of cystine stones formation	Urine alkalizing properties and crude protein ≤160 g/kg complete feed with a moisture content of 12% or Proteins selected for a limited cystine and cysteine content (e.g. casein, pea protein, soy protein) and crude protein ≤220 g/kg complete feed with a moisture content of 12%	Dogs
Nutritional restoration, convalescence	Highly digestible ingredients with energy density ≥3520 kcal and crude protein ≥250 g/kg complete feed with a moisture content of 12%	Dogs
	Highly digestible ingredients with energy density ≥3520 kcal and crude protein ≥270 g/kg of complete feed with a moisture content of 12%	Cats

(Continued)

Table 5.4 (Continued)

Particular nutritional purpose	Essential nutritional characteristics (GP1)	Species or category of animal
Reduction of urate stones formation	Crude protein ≤130 g/kg complete feed with a moisture content of 12% or Crude protein ≤220 g/kg complete feed with a moisture content of 12% and selected protein sources	Dogs
	Crude protein ≤317 g/kg complete feed with a moisture content of 12%	Cats
Dissolution of struvite stones	Urine undersaturating properties for struvite and/or Urine acidifying properties and Magnesium ≤1.8 g/kg complete feed with a moisture content of 12%	Dogs and cats
Reduction of struvite stone recurrence	Complete feed with urine undersaturating or metastabilizing properties for struvite and/or Diet with urine acidifying properties and Magnesium ≤1.8 g/kg complete feed with a moisture content of 12%	Dogs and cats
Compensation for maldigestion	Highly digestible diet: apparent digestibility of low-fiber feed (crude fiber ≤44 g/kg of complete feed with a moisture content of 12%): crude protein ≥85%, crude fat ≥90% or fiber-enhanced feed (crude fiber >44 g/kg of complete feed with a moisture content of 12%): crude protein ≥80%, crude fat ≥80%	Dogs and cats
Reduction of intestinal absorptive disorders	Highly digestible diet: apparent digestibility of low-fiber feed (crude fiber ≤44 g/kg of complete feed with a moisture content of 12%): crude protein ≥85%, crude fat ≥90% or fiber-enhanced feed (crude fiber >44 g/kg of complete feed with a moisture content of 12%): crude protein ≥80%, crude fat ≥80% and Sodium ≥1.8 g/kg of complete feed with a moisture content of 12% and Potassium ≥5 g/kg of complete feed with a moisture content of 12%	Dogs and cats

Table 5.4   (Continued)

Particular nutritional purpose	Essential nutritional characteristics (GP1)	Species or category of animal
Reduction of acute intestinal absorptive disorders	Increased level of electrolytes: Sodium ≥1.8% Potassium ≥0.6% and Highly digestible carbohydrates ≥32%	Dogs and cats
Support of lipid metabolism in the case of hyperlipidemia	Fat ≤110 g/kg complete feed with a moisture content of 12%	Dogs and cats
Support of liver function in a case of chronic liver insufficiency	Moderate level of protein: Crude protein ≤279 g/kg complete feed with a moisture content of 12% for dogs Crude protein ≤370 g/kg complete feed with a moisture content of 12% for cats and Selected protein sources and Recommended dietary protein digestibility ≥85%	Dogs and cats
	Low level of protein but of high-quality and highly digestible carbohydrates	Equines
Support of heart function in the case of chronic cardiac insufficiency	Restricted level of sodium: Sodium ≤2.6 g/kg complete feed with a moisture content of 12%	Dogs and cats
Reduction of excessive body weight	Metabolizable energy <3060 kcal/kg complete feed with a moisture content of 12% or Metabolizable energy <560 kcal/kg complete feed with a moisture content of 85%	Dogs
	Metabolizable energy <3190 kcal/kg complete feed with a moisture content of 12% or Metabolizable energy <580 kcal/kg complete feed with a moisture content of 85%	Cats
Support of skin function in the case of dermatosis and excessive loss of hair	Linoleic acid ≥12.3 g/kg and sum of eicosapentaenoic acid and docosahexaenoic acid ≥2.9 g/kg of complete feed with a moisture content of 12%	Dogs and cats
	Linoleic acid ≥18.5 g/kg and sum of eicosapentaenoic acid and docosahexaenoic acid ≥0.39 g/kg of complete feed with a moisture content of 12%	Dogs
	Linoleic acid ≥18.5 g/kg and sum of eicosapentaenoic acid and docosahexaenoic acid ≥0.09 g/kg of complete feed with a moisture content of 12%	Cats

(Continued)

Table 5.4 (Continued)

Particular nutritional purpose	Essential nutritional characteristics (GP1)	Species or category of animal
Support of the metabolism of joints in the case of osteoarthritis	Total omega-3 fatty acids ≥29 g/kg and eicosapentaenoic acid ≥3.3 g/kg complete feed with a moisture content of 12% and Adequate levels of vitamin E	Dogs
	Total omega-3 fatty acids ≥10.6 g/kg complete feed with a moisture content of 12% and docosahexaenoic acid ≥2.5 g/kg complete feed with a moisture content of 12% and Increased levels of methionine and manganese Adequate levels of vitamin E	Cats
Reduction of copper in the liver	Restricted level of copper: copper ≤8.8 mg/kg complete feed with a moisture content of 12%	Dogs
Reduction of iodine levels in feed in a case of hyperthyroidism	Restricted level of iodine: iodine ≤0.26 mg/kg complete feed with a moisture content of 12%	Cats
Support in stressful situations, which will lead to the reduction of associated behavior	1–3 g trypsin-hydrolyzed bovine casein/kg complete feed with a moisture content of 12%	Dogs
Support preparation for estrus and reproduction	High level of selenium and a minimum content of vitamin E/kg complete feed with a moisture content of 12% for pigs of 50 mg, rabbits of 35 mg, for dogs, cats, mink of 88 mg; a minimum content of vitamin E/animal/d for ovines of 100 mg, cattle of 300 mg, horses of 1100 mg or High level(s) of vitamins A and/or vitamin D and/or a minimum content of beta-carotene of 300 mg/animal/d The complementary feed may contain selenium and vitamins A and D in a concentration higher than 100 times the relevant fixed maximum content in complete feed	Mammals
Support the regeneration of hooves, trotters, and skin	High level of zinc The complementary feed may contain zinc in a concentration higher than 100 times the relevant fixed maximum content in complete feed	Horses, ruminants, and pigs
Support weaning	Minimum supply via the dietetic feed of selenium: 0.1 mg/kg complete feed with a moisture content of 12%	Mammals
Support the preparation for and recovery from sporting effort	High level of selenium and a minimum content of 50 mg vitamin E/kg complete feed with moisture content of 12% The complementary feed may contain compounds of selenium in a concentration higher than 100 times the relevant fixed maximum content in complete feed	Equidae

Table 5.4 (Continued)

Particular nutritional purpose	Essential nutritional characteristics (GP1)	Species or category of animal
Compensation of electrolyte loss in cases of heavy sweating	Must contain sodium chloride and should contain potassium chloride. Low levels of magnesium, calcium, and phosphorus The inclusion of other electrolyte salts is optional	Equines
Support of energy metabolism and of the muscle function in a case of rhabdomyolysis	Starch and sugar not more than 20% of available energy Crude fat more than 20% of available energy Minimum of 350 IU vitamin E/kg complete feed with a moisture content of 12%	Equines
Compensation for chronic digestive disorders of large intestine	Starch content to provide <1 g/kg BW/meal (<0.5 g/kg BW/meal, if diarrhea present) Cereal grains processed via a hydrothermal treatment, such as extrusion, micronization, expansion, or flaking, to improve small intestinal starch digestion Additional supply of water-soluble vitamins and adequate mineral/electrolyte levels Additional supply of oil if no diarrhea	Equines
Compensation for chronic insufficiency of small intestinal function	Highly digestible fibers High-quality protein sources and lysine >4.3% of crude protein Total sugar and starch to provide a maximum of 0.5 g/kg BW/meal Cereal grains processed via a hydrothermal treatment, such as extrusion, micronization, expansion, or flaking, to improve prececal digestion	Equines
Stabilization of the physiologic digestion	Feed additives of the functional group "Gut flora stabilizer" as referred to in Annex I to Regulation (EC) No 1831/2003 or, pending the reauthorization procedure as referred to in Article 10 of Regulation (EC) N° 1831/2003 (2003), feed additives of the group "microorganisms"	Animal species for which the gut flora stabilizer or microorganism is authorized

Note: In most cases, the nutrient concentrations are based on a diet with a dry matter energy density of 4000 kcal metabolizable energy (ME)/kg (calculated using the equation described in the FEDIAF (2019) Nutritional Guidelines; nutrient values shall be adapted accordingly if the energy density deviates from 4000 kcal ME/kg dry matter). The exceptions are for "Support of lipid metabolism in the case of hyperlipidaemia" (based on a diet with a dry matter energy density of 3500 kcal ME/kg) and "Reduction of excessive body weight" where the particular nutritional purpose defines the recommended maximum ME content. See also FEDIAF (2019) Code of good labelling practice for pet food for more information.

following developments in scientific and technical knowledge. Since the list is subject to constant changes or modifications, the current list of European legislation should always be consulted (Regulation (EU) N° 2020/354 (2020)).

Practical Implications

European legislation is very extensive and limits the uses to which a product intended for pets can be put and the publicity that can be contained in its labeling. First of all, it is important to emphasize that the word "nutraceutical" does not exist in the European legislation, so products that are denominated under this general name and in a colloquial way in the market should always be labeled as complementary pet food, with all the obligations and restrictions that have been detailed in this chapter, or, if they strictly comply with any of the PARNUTs, may be identified as such in their labeling. This label as a "dietary" product is already entering a field very close to that of veterinary medicines. In fact, it is "recommended," although not required, to be used under the supervision of a veterinarian or a specialist.

It is important that any product that is recommended or marketed comes from an authorized operator. This is vital in terms of responsibility.

Although European regulations are very broad, certain components such as botanical extracts or some products used in human food may not be clearly classified. The person responsible for the product's compliance with the regulations is the operator (company) that appears on the label.

Complementary pet foods are products that are usually sold with great marketing support. Sometimes, statements that do not strictly comply with the regulations can be found on a label, and frequently it is difficult to know to what extent there are commercial arguments on the label that are not well justified. That would be the case for "claims" that do not have to be justified, unless the authorities request the manufacturer to do so. Close attention

must be paid to products labeled "dietetic." Only those that meet all the requirements of a PARNUT found on the list in Regulation (EU) N° 2020/354 (2020) can be named and marketed as such.

The authorities control, in a random way, the products that are in the market and also, in a specific way, the manufacturers and operators that commercialize the products destined for animal feeding. But it is evident that they cannot control absolutely everything, for which reason it is important to know the regulations in order to be able to detect to what extent the declarations or advertising of a product are true and rigorous and, if they are proven not to be, to consider purchasing other products that deserve greater confidence.

Summary

European legislation regulates and controls all products intended for animal pet food. There is specific legislation for complementary feeds and there is also a list that clearly establishes what kind of particular nutritional purposes can be considered as such because they have been authorized.

The legislation is often modified, both for feed additives, currently under review, and for the list of particular nutritional purposes (dietary supplements), currently under expansion, so it is very important to consult the legislation to know, at any time, what can be marketed and under what conditions.

References

AAFCO (2022). *Official Publication*. Champaign IL: Association of American Feed Control Officials.

Bookout, W. and Khachatoorian, L.B. (2007). Regulation and quality control. In: *Veterinary Herbal Medicine* (ed. S.G. Wynn and B.J. Fougère), 99–119. St. Louis, MO: Mosby.

Dzanis, D.A. (2003). Ensuring nutritional adequacy. In: *Petfood Technology* (ed. J.L. Kvamme and T.D. Phillips), 62–67. Mt. Morris, IL: Watt Publishing.

Dzanis, D.A. (2018). Veterinary products. In: *An Overview of FDA Regulated Products* (ed. E. Pacifici and S. Bain), 181–198. London: Elsevier.

European Commission (2022). European union register of feed additives. https://food.ec.europa.eu/safety/animal-feed/feed-additives/eu-register_en (accessed 19 December 2022).

Faunt, K., Lund, E., and Novak, W. (2007). The power of practice: harnessing patient outcomes for clinical decision making. *Vet. Clin. North Am. Small Anim. Pract.* 37 (3): 521–532.

FEDIAF (2019). Code of good labelling practice for pet food. https://europeanpetfood.org/self-regulation/labelling (accessed 19 December 2022).

Food and Drug Administration (1996). Inapplicability of the dietary supplement health and education act to animal products. *Fed. Regist.* 61 (78): 17706–17708.

Food and Drug Administration (2016). Compliance policy guide Sec. 690.150 Labeling and marketing of dog and cat food diets intended to diagnose, cure, mitigate, treat, or prevent disease. https://www.fda.gov/media/83998/download (accessed 19 December 2022).

Freeman, L.M., Abood, S.K., Fascetti, A.J. et al. (2006). Disease prevalence among dogs and cats in the United States and Australia and proportions of dogs and cats that receive therapeutic diets or dietary supplements. *J. Am. Vet. Med. Assoc.* 229 (4): 531–534.

Government Publishing Office (2020). Title 21 Food and drugs; Subchapter E – Animal, drugs, feeds and related products, §500–599. In: *Electronic Code of Federal Regulations*. Washington, DC: National Archives https://www.ecfr.gov/cgi-bin/text-idx?SID=c878763823816300568cc1852626d0bc&mc=true&tpl=/ecfrbrowse/Title21/21cfrv6_02.tpl#0.

Gross, K., Bollinger, R., Thawnghmung, P., and Collings, G. (1994). Effect of 3 different preservative systems on the stability of extruded dog food subjected to ambient and high temperature storage. *J. Nutr.* 124: 2638S–2642S.

National Research Council (2009). *Safety of Dietary Supplements for Horses, Dogs and Cats.* Washington, DC: National Academies Press.

Ramey, D.W. (2007). A skeptical view of herbal medicine. In: *Veterinary Herbal Medicine* (ed. S.G. Wynn and B.J. Fougère), 121–135. St. Louis, MO: Mosby.

OJEU, (2002). Regulation (EC) N°178/2002 of 28 January 2002, laying down the general principles and requirements of food law, establishing the European Food Safety Authority and laying down procedures in matters of food safety. OJ L 31, 1. https://eur-lex.europa.eu/legal-content/AUTO/?uri=CELEX:02002R0178-20220701&qid=1667582302943&rid=1 (accessed 19 December 2022).

OJEU, (2003). Regulation (EC) N° 1831/2003 of 22 September 2003 on additives for use in animal nutrition. (Consolidated text). OJ L 268, 29. https://eur-lex.europa.eu/legal-content/AUTO/?uri=CELEX:02003R1831-20210327&qid=1667582379056&rid=1 (accessed 19 December 2022).

OJEU, (2005). Regulation (EC) N° 183/2005 of 12 January 2005 laying down requirements for feed hygiene (Consolidated text). OJ L 35, 1. https://eur-lex.europa.eu/legal-content/AUTO/?uri=CELEX:02005R0183-20220128&qid=1667582414860&rid=1 (accessed 19 December 2022).

OJEU, (2009). Regulation (EC) N° 767/2009 of 13 July 2009 on the placing on the market and use of feed (Consolidated text) OJ L 229, 1. https://eur-lex.europa.eu/legal-content/AUTO/?uri=CELEX:02009R0767-20181226&qid=1667582451006&rid=1 (accessed 19 December 2022).

OJEU, (2020). Regulation (EU) N° 2020/354 of 4 March 2020 establishing a list of intended uses of animal feedingstuffs for particular nutritional purposes and repealing Directive 2008/38/EC. OJ L 67, 1. https://eur-lex.europa.eu/legal-content/AUTO/?uri=CELEX:32020R0354&qid=1667582511367&rid=1 (accessed 19 December 2022).

Scoggins, G.A. (1998). Legal issues in holistic veterinary practice. In: *Complementary and Alternative Veterinary Medicine: Principles and Practice* (ed. A.M. Schoen and S.G. Wynn), 743–751. St. Louis, MO: Mosby, Inc.

6

Using Pet Food Labels and Product Guides

Sean J. Delaney and Andrea J. Fascetti

Pet food packaging and supportive product brochures or guides can be useful to the veterinary practitioner assessing a food. This chapter highlights the clinically useful information available from these materials.

"Reading" a Pet Food Label

Overview of Regulatory Oversight

Packaging is governed by several groups or bodies (see Chapter 5 for more insight into pet food regulatory bodies). At the highest level is the federal or national regulatory body such as the US Food and Drug Administration (FDA) and US Department of Agriculture (USDA), followed by more localized governance at the state level. In the United States, most of the regulation and enforcement of pet food labels come at the state level, with state feed control officials ensuring that labels are in compliance with guidelines published in the then-current *Official Publication* of the Association of American Feed Control Officials (AAFCO), which is generally adopted by state legislatures as law. Therefore, most of the rules governing a pet food label in the United States, and in many countries that adopt or adapt AAFCO guidelines, can be found in AAFCO's annually published *Official Publication*; the reader is encouraged to purchase a copy if further

insight into pet food labeling in the United States is desired (see www.aafco.org for purchasing information). In the rest of this section on pet food labels, the rules that will be covered apply to those established by AAFCO. Readers in other countries are encouraged to contact their local government to identify the rules that apply to their particular region. The second part of this chapter on using product guides, as well as sections on common calculations or conversions, should still be of use to all readers regardless of geography.

Principal Display Panel or Front Display Panel

Inherently, all front-facing portions of pet food labels and packages attempt to communicate the nature of the product and how it should be used, as well as draw the attention of the consumer. From a regulatory perspective, the main consumer-facing portion of the label must contain only three elements: the product name, the intended species, and the net quantity of product within the package. Other elements that might assist with the other goals of the label, such as company or distributor name, endorsements, comparative statements, or product highlights and images, are optional. However, anything appearing on the label must be both truthful and substantiated.

Applied Veterinary Clinical Nutrition, Second Edition. Edited by Andrea J. Fascetti, Sean J. Delaney, Jennifer A. Larsen, and Cecilia Villaverde.

Product Name

The name of the product is strictly regulated, and a product that says it consists of 100% of something must be exclusively that ingredient. This type of product is rare and is almost without exception incomplete and unbalanced, as typically these products are all meat without any minerals or vitamins added. Products that have meat and just enough minerals and vitamins to be complete and balanced typically fall under the 95% rule. If the 95% rule is used, then all 95% of the ingredients listed must be from an animal; therefore, a food labeled as "95% lamb & rice" would not be allowed, but "95% lamb & beef" would be. It is worth noting that a little over half of the weight of the fresh meat typically found in such canned foods is from water, which counts toward the total inclusion percentage.

Most pet foods fall under the 25% rule, which states that at least 25% of the food must be made up of the indicated ingredients, with the first listed ingredient being the largest among the ingredients included in the product's name. In addition, the product name must include a descriptor such as "dinner," "formula," "entrée," or "recipe." With this rule, "25%" does not need to appear on the packaging, unlike the "100% rule" and "95% rule" where the percentages must generally appear (i.e. higher percentages than 95% could be listed). With the 25% rule, plant-derived ingredients may be included in the name. Therefore, "lamb & rice dinner" could be used and would mean that at least 25% of the food is lamb and rice and that the lamb is either equal to or greater than the amount of rice in the food (equal, as the company can choose which to list first if the inclusion amount is the same).

There is also a "with" or "3% rule," which means that any food "with" a separately identified ingredient (outside of the ingredient declaration) must have at least 3% of the ingredient (unless followed by the term "flavor," as discussed later). Unlike the 25% and 95% rules, this is not an additive rule. Thus, if one says "with lamb and rice" there needs to be 3% lamb and 3% rice. This rule does not apply to added minerals, vitamins, and trace nutrients that may appear in support of a food that is stating that it is "natural" (e.g. saying "natural pet food with added vitamins, minerals, and trace nutrients" does not mean, nor is it required to mean, that the food has 3% vitamins, 3% minerals, and 3% trace nutrients).

Finally, the last rule is the flavor rule, which is the vaguest and simply means that the food contains a source of the flavor that is "detectable."

Therefore, awareness of naming rules can help to better understand the potential inclusion concentrations of named or highlighted ingredients and explain, for instance, why a largely chicken- and corn-based food could be named "lamb & rice dinner," or how a pet food company can afford to sell an inexpensive food "with Angus beef." Interestingly, unlike the term "natural," which is defined by AAFCO, other commonly used terms like "premium," "super premium," and "organic" ("organic" is defined by the USDA National Organic Program) are not defined by AAFCO. Other descriptors such as "light," "lite," "low calorie," "lean," and "low fat" are defined and have specific cutoffs as to energy density or fat content that foods must meet to use these terms, unlike the "comparative" terms such as "less calories," "reduced calories," "less fat," and "reduced fat," which are only defined by the concentrations found in the product that is being compared. Thus, one cannot easily tell the caloric or fat content of a food described with a comparative term.

Back Panel

The most useful information on a package is located on the "back panel," as this is where information about nutritional adequacy, ingredients, nutrient concentrations, the company's contact information, and feeding amounts can be found, as well as (at times) calorie content information.

Nutritional Adequacy

Nutritional adequacy statements indicate for which species and for what life stage the food is appropriate. The term "all life stages" means that the food can be fed to gestating or lactating females, growing animals, and adults.

Adequacy can be established in three ways. The first way is by computer formulation to a specific nutritional profile established by AAFCO. The second method is with a feeding trial or protocol, where the specific food has been fed to animals in a controlled setting with monitoring following a defined protocol. The last method, which cannot be determined from the label, is via the "family product rule." This rule allows foods that are similar in ingredients and that have been tested to match or exceed key nutrient concentrations of another food that has passed a feeding trial or protocol to claim that the unfed "family member" food passed a feeding trial or protocol for the same life stage. If a food is not complete and balanced, it must be labeled as a treat, snack, or supplement, or state that it is for "intermittent and supplemental feeding only." Unfortunately, this statement is very short and often not easily seen, and in the authors' experience results in clinical cases of nutritional deficiencies.

Ingredient Declaration

Ingredients used in a food must be listed on the packaging and in descending order of inclusion before any cooking or drying takes place. Therefore, the first ingredient listed must have the greatest mass of all the ingredients in the formula or recipe. At times, companies will make formulation choices based on the resulting order of the ingredient declaration. The most commonly employed technique to change the ingredient declaration order is referred to as "ingredient splitting." In this method, an ingredient that may be perceived by the consumer as less desirable (such as corn) is "fractionated" into different components such as corn, corn meal, or corn gluten, in part so that the individual inclusion concentrations are less than the more desirable

animal protein source like chicken or chicken meal. At times, it will also be raised that a dried product like "chicken meal" will provide more chicken protein than chicken, given the higher moisture and often higher fat content of the fresh ingredient. This is typically true for equal inclusion concentrations, but really is an argument about marketing strategies as much as anything else. In addition to listing ingredients by predominance, ingredients must be defined by AAFCO or the FDA to be used and must be the generic name (i.e. no brand or trade names). Often the veterinary practitioner will be asked what certain ingredient terms mean, like "by-product" or "meal." The reader is encouraged to purchase a copy of the AAFCO *Official Publication* for examples of "by-products" and "meal" as defined by the AAFCO (as of 2011):

9.14 **Poultry By-Products** must consist of non-rendered clean parts of carcasses of slaughtered poultry such as heads, feet, viscera, free from fecal content and foreign matter, except in such trace amounts as might occur unavoidably in good factory practice. If the product bears a name descriptive of its kind, the name must correspond thereto. (Proposed 1963, Adopted 1964, Amended 2000.)

9.71 **Poultry Meal** is the dry rendered product from a combination of clean flesh and skin with or without accompanying bone, derived from the parts of whole carcasses of poultry or a combination thereof, exclusive of feathers, heads, feet, and entrails. It shall be suitable for use in animal food. If it bears a name descriptive of its kind, it must correspond thereto. (Proposed 1988, Adopted 1992.)

Also, references "to the quality, nature, form, or other attributes of an ingredient shall be allowed when the designation is not false or misleading; [and] the ingredient imparts a distinctive characteristic to the pet food because it possesses that attribute; [and] a reference to quality or grade of the ingredient does not appear in the ingredient statement." Thus, one cannot say "USDA Choice beef" in the ingredient declaration or list.

Nutrient Concentrations or Guaranteed Analysis

The guaranteed analysis must provide minimal nutrient information as follows:

- minimum percentage of crude protein
- minimum percentage of crude fat
- maximum percentage of crude fat (if using "lean" or "low fat")
- maximum percentage of crude fiber
- maximum percentage of moisture

Other guarantees must follow in the order they appear in the AAFCO profile and, if not listed in the AAFCO profile, must have the disclaimer "not recognized as an essential nutrient by the AAFCO dog [or cat] food nutrient profiles." As the reader will note, ash and carbohydrate percentages are not required. The absence of at least one of these two nutrients makes calculating the calorie content of a food more challenging and less precise, as will be discussed later. All guarantees must be for a nutrient, although a frequent exception is for "direct-fed microbials" or probiotics, which are currently required to have a guarantee but are not nutrients. Also, all guarantees must be either a minimum or maximum value, as averages or ranges cannot be used.

It should be highlighted that the values listed are minimums or maximums, and although they may closely match the actual amount in the food, there can be some significant discrepancies. Therefore, if a particular nutrient concentration is important, the company should be contacted to ascertain the average nutrient concentration. One can quickly determine likely nutrient concentration minimums based on the nutritional adequacy statement. If a food is formulated to meet a nutrient profile for a particular life stage, nutrient concentrations should be equal to or greater than the nutrient profile's minimums and equal to or less than the nutrient profile's maximums. Since a food can pass a feeding trial without meeting a nutrient profile's values, one cannot

make assumptions on the nutrient values of foods that meet nutritional adequacy via a feeding trial. This knowledge can be useful to explain why no complete and balanced over-the-counter food that has been formulated to meet an AAFCO nutrient profile is low enough in phosphorus for the management of renal disease, as no phosphorus minimum in the AAFCO profiles is low enough.

Company's Contact Information

The company must provide its mailing address, although a street address can be omitted if it is listed in a city directory or phone book. Unfortunately, a telephone number is not required but is very important in the authors' opinion, as it enables any information that is unclear or unavailable on a label to be asked directly.

Feeding Directions or Guidelines

Feeding guidelines must be provided on packaging and must include at least "feed (weight/unit of product) per (weight only) of dog (or cat)," along with the frequency of the feeding. The exception is for veterinary foods, which can state "use only as directed by your veterinarian."

Calorie Content

Only recently have calorie content statements been required on pet food bags, cans, and other types of food containers. This information is intended to help veterinarians and pet owners determine how much to feed the animal they are caring for. Long term this mandate may help reduce overweight and obesity in cats and dogs.

Estimating Calorie Content

One can use the required guaranteed analysis values to determine a food's calorie content or energy density. Unfortunately, as mentioned earlier, companies are not required to provide an ash or carbohydrate concentration, and actual values can vary greatly from the minimum and maximum values provided. Thus, the value that is generated is only an estimate (it is also only an estimate if actual concentrations for protein, fat, and carbohydrate are known, given the variability of digestibility that can affect the amount of energy these three macronutrients provide).

Step 1: Estimate carbohydrate content (this step can be skipped if the carbohydrate percentage for the food is provided). By subtracting the crude protein minimum percentage (CP %), crude fat minimum percentage (CF %), crude fiber maximum percentage (Fib %), moisture maximum percentage (M %), and ash maximum percentage (A %; if not reported, estimate between 2% and 10% using higher values with dry, higher-protein foods) from 100, one can estimate the percentage of carbohydrate (CHO %). Written as an equation:

$$CHO\% = 100 - (CP\% + CF\% + Fib\% + M\% + A\%)$$

Step 2: Estimate the calories from the macronutrients. By multiplying standard energy conversion factors (see Chapter 2; the example uses the modified Atwater factors) by the percentages for the minimum crude protein, minimum crude fat, and calculated carbohydrate, one can estimate the number of Calories coming from protein, fat, and carbohydrate. Written as equations:

$$Calories\ from\ protein = CP\% \times 3.5\ kcal/g$$

$$Calories\ from\ fat = CF\% \times 8.5\ kcal/g$$

$$Calories\ from\ carbohydrate = CHO\% \times 3.5\ kcal/g$$

Step 3: Estimate the total calories. By adding the Calories from protein, fat, and carbohydrate, one can estimate the total Calories available in 100 g of food as fed. The Calories are from 100 g, as the percentage used for the earlier calculation is the same as gram of macronutrient per 100 g food as fed. If the amount per kilogram is desired, the result can be multiplied by 10 since $10 \times 100\ g = 1000\ g$ or $1\ kg$. Written as equations:

$$\begin{aligned} Total\ Calories/100\ g\ food \\ = Calories\ from\ protein \\ + Calories\ from\ fat \\ + Calories\ from\ carbohydrate \end{aligned}$$

$$\begin{aligned} Total\ Calories/kg\ food \\ = Total\ Calories/100\ g\ food \times 10 \end{aligned}$$

A useful estimate for the amount of calories per 8 fl oz cup is to assume that this volume of food weighs 100 g; therefore, 1 cup of dry food is roughly equal to the "Total Calories/100 g food" value.

Caloric Distribution Calculation

The best method to compare concentrations of protein, fat, and carbohydrate is based on caloric distribution, which is simply the percentages of the total calories that come from the three macronutrients. This enables direct comparisons to be made without concerns about varying moisture or fiber concentrations, which can vary greatly and impact other units of comparison. To calculate the Calories from protein, fat, or carbohydrate as determined earlier, one divides one of these values by the Total Calories per 100 g of food and multiples by 100. Written as equations:

$$\begin{aligned} Percent\ Calories\ from\ protein \\ = (Calories\ from\ protein/ \\ Total\ Calories\ per\ 100\ g\ food) \times 100 \end{aligned}$$

$$\begin{aligned} Percent\ Calories\ from\ fat \\ = (Calories\ from\ fat/ \\ Total\ Calories\ per\ 100\ g\ food) \times 100 \end{aligned}$$

$$\begin{aligned} Percent\ Calories\ from\ carbohydrate \\ = (Calories\ from\ carbohydrate/ \\ Total\ Calories\ per\ 100\ g\ food) \times 100 \end{aligned}$$

The three resulting values are referred to as the caloric distribution. These values are most useful for comparing and determining if a food is truly lower or higher in a particular macronutrient. Given their utility, they are provided in the product guides provided by manufacturers of veterinary therapeutic foods.

Using Product Brochures and Guides

Product brochures and product guides can be an excellent repository of useful information about foods. They generally provide all the key nutritional information found on packaging, such as the ingredient list and guaranteed analysis (but generally not the nutritional adequacy statement), as well as available sizes and suggested uses along with highlighting features and benefits. For veterinary product guides, indications and contraindications are typically provided, as are caloric distributions as well as key nutrients in units beyond those on an as fed basis. Typically, the nutrients are provided in these guides on

both a dry matter (dm) basis and a per 100 kcal or per 1000 kcal or Mcal (energy) basis. Generally, comparing nutrient concentrations on a dm basis has fallen out of favor, with the preference being to compare nutrients on a per unit of energy basis. If calorie density is not taken into account, one can derive the wrong conclusions when comparing foods based on dry matter alone. Therefore, it is important to be able to calculate the amount of the nutrient on a per unit of energy basis. This can be best illustrated with the example in Box 6.1.

Converting Nutrient Concentrations to a Dry Matter Basis

To calculate a food's content on a dry matter basis, the percent moisture is subtracted from 100 and then divided by 100, and the resulting value is used to divide the "as fed" value of interest (units are not important as they do not change with the conversion) to get the dry matter value. For example, for a food with 25%

Box 6.1 Increasing Comparison Accuracy Using an Energy Instead of Dry Matter Basis

If one has a food with 3000 kcal/kg as fed, 10% moisture, and 1% calcium, and a second food with 4750 kcal/kg as fed, 10% moisture, and 1.1% calcium, the practitioner may be led to believe that their patient is getting more calcium from the second food as it has more calcium on a dry matter (DM) basis: 1.11% dm versus 1.22% [1/(1−0.1) = 1.11% dm versus the second food with 1.1/(1−0.1) = 1.22%]. However, patients eat to meet their energy requirement (see Chapter 2); therefore, let us say the patient consumes 1000 kcal/day. On the first food, the patient will get 3.3 g calcium/day:

1% × 1000 g/kg = 10 g calcium/kg

10 g /3000 kcal/kg = 0.0033 g/kcal

0.0033 × 1000 = 3.3 g/1000 kcal or 3.3 g/ Mcal or 3.3 mg/kcal

1000 kcal × 3.3 mg/kcal = 3300 mg/d or 3.3 g/d

And on the second food, the patient will get 2.316 g calcium per day:

1.1% × 1000 g/kg = 11 g calcium/kg

11 g /4750 kcal/kg = 0.0023 g/kcal

0.0023 × 1000 = 2.3 g/1000 kcal or 2.3 g/ Mcal or 2.3 mg/kcal

1000 kcal × 2.3 mg/kcal = 2300 mg/d or 2.3 g/d

This means that the patient eating the second food will consume 30% less calcium than on the first food. If the practitioner had just looked at the information on a dry matter basis, they would have thought that the patient was getting less calcium with the first food.

protein as fed and 10% moisture, the equation and the result would be:

$$25\% \text{ protein as fed } / [(100-10)/100]$$
$$= 25/0.9 = 27.78\% \text{ protein dm}$$

Since most dry foods have ~10% moisture and canned foods ~75% moisture, one can simply divide by 0.9 or 0.25 for dry and canned foods, respectively, to convert to a rough estimate of the dry matter value when the moisture is unknown but the format of the food is.

Converting Nutrient Concentrations to an Energy Basis

To convert or calculate the amount of a nutrient on an energy basis (typically written as "mass/1000 kcal" or "mass/Mcal"), one needs to know the kcal/kg amount (see earlier for how to estimate this value from the label if unavailable). If the nutrient is provided as a percentage, it will need first to be converted to a mass (gram is the easiest and the most common unit of mass used; other units such as milligram (mg), microgram (µg), and International Units (IU) do not need to be converted, as the starting unit will be kept) per kilogram of food on an as fed basis. For example, if the food has 2% calcium, one can divide the percentage by 100 and then multiply the result by 1000 to get the grams of calcium per kilogram of food as fed. Thus, $(2/100) \times 1000 = 20 \text{ g}$ calcium/kg of food as fed. With the kcal/kg as fed value and the mass of nutrient per kg as fed, one simply divides the nutrient mass by the kcal/kg value and multiplies the result by 1000. Thus the equation for a food with 3000 kcal/kg as fed and 20 g calcium/kg is:

$$(20 \text{ g calcium}/3000 \text{ kcal/kg food as fed})$$
$$\times 1000 = 6.67 \text{ g calcium per Mcal}$$

Converting to Other Units

Occasionally one will encounter other units, and the reader is encouraged to use the method whereby unwanted units are canceled by using known conversion factors. For example, if one wishes to convert 50 IU of vitamin A to micrograms of retinol, one can perform this conversion by knowing that 1 IU vitamin A = 0.3 µg retinol and then canceling units by putting like units opposite like units in the numerator or denominator of equations, as in the following:

$$50 \text{ IU vitamin A} \times (0.3 \text{ µg retinol}/$$
$$1 \text{IU vitamin A}) = 15/1 = 15 \text{ µg retinol}$$

In this equation, note how one IU value is a numerator (i.e. 50 IU vitamin A = 50 IU vitamin A/1, thus the "50 IU" is the numerator) and one IU value is a denominator (i.e. "1 IU"). This enables the units to be canceled, as the numerator and denominator are multiplied by each other and the numerator product is divided by the denominator product. Other encountered conversions are 40 IU vitamin D3 = 1 µg cholecalciferol; 1 IU vitamin E = 1 mg all-*rac*-alpha-tocopheryl acetate; 1 kg = 1000 g; 1 g = 1000 mg; and 1 mg = 1000 µg. As noted elsewhere in the text (see Chapter 3), 1 Calorie = 4.185 kJ.

Product Guide Recommendations for Conditions and Diseases

With the tools described here to determine a food's caloric distribution and nutrient amounts per megacalorie, the reader should be better equipped to make comparisons among foods. These tools can be best employed to compare and contrast approaches and recommendations for the management and treatment of different conditions and diseases as found in veterinary product guides and online (websites can often be more up to date as formulation changes may occur more frequently than the release of brochure/guide reprints). One will find that for many conditions and diseases there is general agreement about the best strategies for nutritional management. However, the reader is strongly encouraged to confirm that these general recommendations apply to the specific needs of particular patients. For others there can be varying philosophies, and the reader is encouraged to use the remainder of this text to aid them in exploring these approaches and recognizing when and where product guide recommendations may vary or differ. Finally, the authors recommend that veterinarians request product guides (paper or electronic) from their sales representative for use in their practice. Having product guides available, even if their practice does not carry every company's diets, provides veterinarians with the ability to compare and contrast products. Having access to all the guides permits access to a wider range of diets, often resulting in a better recommendation for the patient.

Summary

- Packaging and product guides provide required and at times useful nutritional information about foods.

- The information provided can be used to determine a food's energy density and caloric distribution, as well as nutrient amounts on a dry matter and energy basis.
- Nutrient amounts, ingredient lists, feeding guidelines, and product guide recommendations can all be useful in selecting the best food for patients.

Recommended Resources

Official Publication of the Association American Feed Control Officials, available for purchase at www.aafco.org

US Food and Drug Administration, Center for Veterinary Medicine websites (as of August 2022):

https://www.fda.gov/animal-veterinary
https://www.fda.gov/animal-veterinary/animal-food-feeds/pet-food

7

Feeding the Healthy Dog and Cat

Andrea J. Fascetti and Sean J. Delaney

Both dogs and cats are members of the biological order Carnivora. Scientific observation and research support that differences in their metabolism and nutritional requirements exist. The differences in nutritional requirements likely correlate with the evolution of these two species. Nutritionally and metabolically, dogs and other members of *Canidae* are generally considered omnivores, whereas cats and other members of the family *Felidae* are regarded as carnivores. However, there exist nutritional and metabolic examples that are not consistent with the view that the cat is a strict carnivore and the dog is simply an omnivore.

The only member of the family *Felidae* whose nutritional requirements have been studied extensively is the domestic cat (*Felis catus*). Scientific research has shown that cats have obligatory requirements for nutrients that are not essential for many other mammals. The high protein requirement of cats is due to their high requirement for nitrogen. This appears to be because cats have a limited ability to control the activity of their aminotransferases and urea cycle enzymes (Rogers et al. 1977; Green et al. 2008). Conversely, cats are able to control the activity of enzymes in the first irreversible step of essential amino acid degradation to some extent, explaining why they do not have a high requirement for essential amino acids (Rogers and Morris 1980). The lack of downregulatory control over aminotransferases and urea cycle enzymes renders cats immediately able to metabolize and use amino acids for gluconeogenesis and as an energy source. Additional benefits of this ability are realized in times of starvation; carnivores are better able to immediately maintain blood glucose concentrations compared to omnivorous species (Morris 2002).

There are five other nutrients considered essential in feline diets that are not recognized as essential in most other species due to the low activities of enzymes in their synthetic pathways (Table 7.1). Two of these nutrients are the amino acids arginine and taurine. The low activities of ornithine aminotransferase and pyrroline-5-carboxylate result in the minimal production of citrulline in the gastrointestinal tract (Costello et al. 1980; Rogers and Phang 1985). As a result, the cat is completely dependent upon dietary arginine to meet its needs for this amino acid (Figure 7.1).

The endogenous synthesis of taurine is limited by the low activities of cysteine dioxygenase and cysteine sulfinic acid decarboxylase (Figure 7.2; Park et al. 1999). The low activity of these enzymes in the synthetic pathway, coupled with the low affinity of N acyltransferase for glycine for bile acid synthesis, results in the depletion of body taurine stores.

The remaining three nutrients are niacin, vitamin A, and vitamin D. The cat has a dietary requirement for niacin and vitamin D because

Applied Veterinary Clinical Nutrition, Second Edition. Edited by Andrea J. Fascetti,
Sean J. Delaney, Jennifer A. Larsen, and Cecilia Villaverde.
© 2024 John Wiley & Sons, Inc. Published 2024 by John Wiley & Sons, Inc.

Table 7.1 Idiosyncrasies of the carnivorous cat in comparison to the omnivorous dog and rat.

	Cat	Dog	Rat
Requires arginine?	Yes	Yes	No
Glucokinase activity?	No	Yes	Yes
Makes sufficient taurine?	No	Yes	Yes
Bile acid conjugation	Taurine	Taurine	Taurine or glycine
Converts beta-carotene to vitamin A?	No	Yes	Yes
Makes vitamin D from skin?	No	No	Yes
Makes niacin?	No	Yes	Yes

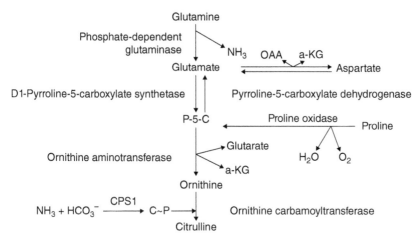

Figure 7.1 Arginine.

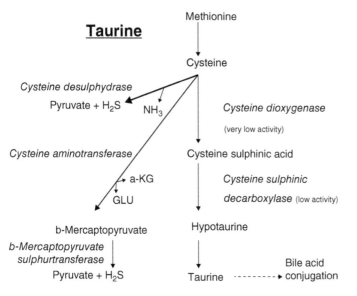

Figure 7.2 Taurine.

of the high activity of the enzymes picolinic carboxylase (Sudadolnik et al. 1957; Ikeda et al. 1965) and 7-dehydrocholesterol-Δ^7-reductase (Morris 1999), respectively, which results in the degradation of precursors for their synthesis. Vitamin A must be supplied preformed in the diet, presumably because cats lack or have reduced activity of the enzyme β,β-carotene 15,15′–dioxygenase, needed to cleave beta-carotene (NRC 2006).

Consistent with their classification as obligate carnivores, cats have a reduced number of carbohydrate-metabolizing enzymes compared to omnivores. Cats lack glucokinase in their livers (Washizu et al. 1999). However, in contrast to certain other carnivores, and not at all consistent with the cat being a strict carnivore, cats can efficiently digest cooked starch (Morris et al. 1977; Kienzle 1993).

Nutritionally and metabolically, many consider the dog an omnivore. However, there are nutritional and metabolic characteristics that the dog shares with the cat. One veterinary nutritionist (D. Kronfeld) has suggested the term "adaptive carnivore" when referring to the dog. In contrast to the cat, and similar to other omnivores, the dog has the ability to make taurine from the sulfur amino acid precursors methionine and cysteine (Hayes 1988), as well as vitamin A from beta-carotene (Turner 1934). However, unlike many other omnivores and more like the cat, the dog conjugates bile acids only with taurine (Haslewood 1964) and cannot make vitamin D, an animal product (How et al. 1994, 1995; NRC 2006). Like cats, dogs require a source of dietary arginine to maintain nitrogen balance in adults and puppies (Ha et al. 1978; Czarnecki and Baker 1984). The dog's requirement for arginine is less than that of the cat but greater than that of the rat (NRC 2006), positioning it between carnivores and other omnivores nutritionally.

Over time, evolution rendered some of the metabolic pathways and enzymes present in omnivores redundant in the cat. These pressures likely resulted in changes in biochemical pathways and nutritional requirements more suited to the cat's metabolism (Morris 2002). Although the nutritional requirements of the cat differ from those of the dog, scientific findings and observations are not fully consistent with the cat being a strict carnivore and the dog a simple omnivore.

Feeding the Healthy Dog and Cat

Healthy animals normally eat sufficient food to satisfy their energy requirements. It is one of the jobs of the nutritionist to ensure that all other nutrient needs have been met when animals stop eating because they have met their energy needs. The greatest metabolic demands occur during growth, gestation, and lactation, and this is when a marginal diet is most likely to result in nutritional problems. The majority of commercial pet foods are formulated to ensure adequate intake of all required nutrients based on energy intake, as long as consideration is given to the manufacturer's life-stage recommendation.

How Much to Feed

Ideally, the amount of food to feed an animal should be determined based on a diet history correlated with weight trends (Figure 7.3). Diet history forms should be obtained and updated for every patient in your practice at every visit. Information that should be included in every diet history form includes the specific product name, form (i.e. dry, canned, or semi-moist), and manufacturer of the pet's diet, quantitative data on how much the pet is consuming daily, details regarding names and amounts of snacks and treats, information about who feeds the pet, and the setting in which the pet consumes its food. It is also a good idea to ask how the food is stored and more details regarding additional animals in the household and potential access to other food sources. In instances where owners are home-preparing the pet's meals, detailed information on the ingredients and supplements as well as

DIET HISTORY FORM

Provided by **Veterinary TECHNICIAN**

Content courtesy of the
Nutrition Support Center
University of California–Davis
Veterinary Medical Teaching Hospital

UCDAVIS
UNIVERSITY OF CALIFORNIA

TO BE COMPLETED BY CLIENT

Client Information

Name:_____ Date: _____

Address: _____

City:_____ State:_____ Zip:_____

Telephone (home):_____ (other): _____

Email address: _____

Patient Information

Name:_____ Species:_____ Breed:_____

Age:_____ Sex: ❑ Male ❑ Female ❑ Neutered/spayed

1. Where is your pet housed? ❑ Indoors ❑ Outdoors ❑ Both ❑ Outside mainly for walks or exercise

2. Please describe your pet's activity level (i.e., type, duration, frequency): _____

xx _____

xx _____

3. Do you have other pets? ❑ Yes ❑ No If so, please list: _____

xx _____

4. Is your pet fed in the presence of other animals? ❑ Yes ❑ No If yes, please describe: _____

xx _____

5. Is food left out for your pet during the day or taken away after the meal? _____

xx _____

6. Does your pet have access to other, unmonitored food sources (e.g., treats fed by neighbor, food left for outdoor cats)?

xx❑ Yes ❑ No If yes, please describe: _____

xx _____

xx _____

7. Who typically feeds your pet? _____

Figure 7.3 Diet history form. *Source:* Used with permission from *Veterinary Technician Magazine,* January 2008.

DIET HISTORY FORM

8. How do you store your pet's food? _____

_____

9. Please list your pet's current and past medical problems, if any, and whether they have been resolved:

_____

_____

10. Please list all the medications your pet is currently receiving and any that have been administered over the past 3 months:

_____

_____

11. Please indicate whether your pet has experienced any of the following problems before today's visit:

Recent involuntary or unintended ❑ Weight gain ❑ Weight loss How many pounds? _____

Over what time period? _____

❑ Vomiting _____ times/day _____ times/week ❑ Diarrhea _____ times/day _____ times/week

12. Have you observed changes in any of the following?

❑ Urination ❑ Drinking What was the specific change? _____

Since when? _____

❑ Defecation What was the specific change? _____

Since when? _____

❑ Appetite What was the specific change? _____

Since when? _____

13. Does your pet have any of the following? ❑ Allergies ❑ Difficulty chewing ❑ Difficulty swallowing

If so, please describe: _____

Current and Previous Diets and Supplements

Below, please list the brand or product names (if applicable) and amounts of all foods, snacks, and treats your pet *currently* eats. This description should provide enough detail so that anyone could go to the store and purchase the same food. It should include human foods given as treats or at the table. Three examples are given in italics.

Brand/Product/Food	Form	Amount Fed per Meal	No. of Meals	Fed Since
EXAMPLES:				
Brand X Dog Food	*Dry*	*1½ cups*	*Twice a day*	*5/00*
Brand A Dog Treats	*Treats*	*1/day*	*—*	*8/01*

Figure 7.3 (Continued)

DIET HISTORY FORM

Boneless chicken (white meat)	*Boiled*	*2 ounces*	*3 times a week*	*6/98*

Please list other diets your pet has received in the past, indicating the approximate time period when they were fed. Two examples are given in italics.

Brand/Product/Food	Form	Amount Fed per Meal	Time Period Fed	No. of Meals	Reason Stopped
EXAMPLES:					
Brand Y Puppy Food	*Can*	*6½ ounces*	*6/99 to 12/99*	*Twice a day*	*Became an adult*
Brand Z Puppy Food	*Dry*	*1½ cups*	*6/99 to 3/00*	*Twice a day*	*Became an adult*

Please list the name of each additional supplement your pet receives, and indicate how much and how often your pet receives it (i.e., herbal product, fatty acid, vitamin or mineral supplement):

Patient Dietary Preferences

Please complete this section *only* if a home-cooked diet formulation is being requested or may be needed. If the diet formulation is needed due to an adverse reaction to certain foods, please provide protein and carbohydrate options that are both *palatable* and *tolerated* by your pet. This will need to be determined before submitting this consult.

Protein Sources

❑ Beef   ❑ Salmon
❑ Chicken   ❑ Tofu
❑ Cottage Cheese   ❑ Tuna
❑ Crab   ❑ Turkey
❑ Egg   ❑ Whitefish
❑ Lamb   Other _____
❑ Pork   Other _____

Carbohydrate Sources

❑ Barley   ❑ Quinoa
❑ Millet   ❑ Rice, Brown
❑ Oatmeal   ❑ Rice, White
❑ Pasta, Spaghetti   ❑ Tapioca
❑ Peas, Green   Other _____
❑ Potato, Sweet   Other _____
❑ Potato, White   Other _____

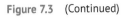

Figure 7.3 (Continued)

preparation methods should be requested and entered into the record. When the animal is in an ideal body condition, weight stable, and otherwise healthy, these authors recommend feeding the amount of food the animal is currently consuming provided that an accurate and detailed diet history is available.

If the exact number of calories to feed is difficult to determine with certainty, in some cases it can be approximated. Although many animals are fed free choice, owners should still be able to provide an estimate of how much food the animal receives daily. The estimated number of calories currently consumed can then be compared to the required maintenance requirements based on calculation. This information should be considered in light of the animal's body condition score and any history of recent weight loss or gain when arriving at a final decision regarding the appropriate amount of calories to feed.

Determining the amount of calories to feed becomes more difficult if a diet history is unavailable. Many pet foods provide guidelines on the product label, and these can be used as a starting point. It is important to understand that these guidelines are limited, however, due to the variation of efficiency of food utilization among animals and individual differences in physical activity, metabolism, body condition, and environment.

Controlled studies have demonstrated that energy requirements may vary significantly among similar animals housed in similar conditions (NRC 2006). Therefore, the calculated food dosage should be considered as a starting point that will most likely have to be adjusted. The authors recommend determining the animal's maintenance energy requirement (MER) by using the resting energy requirement (RER) equation and then multiplying by the factor for the appropriate life stage rather than using the single MER equation. In many cases the single MER equation overestimates the animal's energy needs (Lewis and Morris 1987a). However, it is imperative to remember that the calculated amount to feed

is only an educated guess (or a starting point) and that this amount may vary by as much as 50%, particularly for dogs (NRC 2006). The animal's weight and body condition score should be monitored frequently and the caloric intake adjusted accordingly.

When and How to Feed

There are basically three types of feeding regimens that humans use to feed their dog or cat. It is also not uncommon to see more than one of these in the same animal.

Free-Choice (Ad Libitum, Self-Feeding)

This approach ensures that there is a surplus of food available at all times, and it is often the method of choice for the queen or bitch during lactation. Ad libitum feeding relies upon the animal regulating its daily caloric intake. This type of feeding allows cats to consume small multiple meals throughout the day, closely mimicking their natural feeding behavior (Kane et al. 1981). This method of feeding provides the least amount of work on behalf of the owner. Free-choice feeding may be advantageous for animals who tend to consume small multiple meals, or for picky or slow eaters that cannot consume enough calories in one meal. Furthermore, there may be an advantage concerning energy balance due to meal-induced energy loss. In a kennel situation, this method helps to minimize the noise associated with feeding and may relieve boredom. Free-choice feeding helps to ensure that the subordinate animals in multiple-pet households have the opportunity to eat. The disadvantages associated with an ad libitum feeding schedule include the likelihood of overlooking medical problems, anorexia, or the denial of food to subordinate animals when food intake is not closely monitored. Most importantly, this style of feeding increases the probability that an animal will become overweight. It has been suggested that 30–40% of dogs and cats will overeat if food is available at all times (NRC 2006). Dry food is the only type of pet food that can be fed in this manner. Canned food, some semi-moist food, and dry food combined with water should not be left out in the environment for extended periods of time.

Time-Restricted Meal Feeding

Similar to the free-choice style of feeding, this method relies upon the animal's ability to regulate its daily caloric intake. At meal time a surplus of food is given, and the pet is allowed to eat for a set period of time. This form of feeding is most applicable to dogs but not practical for cats. Most dogs will learn to consume their energy requirements in a 5–15-minute time period. Proponents of this manner of feeding recommend a twice-a-day schedule to minimize begging. The major advantages of this method are that it does not require much effort on behalf of the owner and may be used with any type of pet food. It also permits some monitoring of the dog's food intake. This form of feeding may not be appropriate for fastidious animals that are not able to consume enough food in the allotted time period to meet their caloric needs. Meal feeding may also encourage gluttony and aerophagia.

Portion-Controlled Feeding

With portion-controlled feeding the dog or cat is given a specific amount of food, often divided into two meals per day. This method of feeding is considered by many experts to be the best approach for both dogs and cats in all life stages. The advantage of this method is that it allows the owner to carefully monitor their pet's food intake. This may ultimately result in a lower probability of the development of obesity. This method of feeding also alerts an owner much sooner to any medical problems or anorexia. The biggest disadvantage of portion-controlled feeding is that it requires more of a time commitment and effort on behalf of the owner.

Snacks and Treats

One study reported that 56.8% of dogs and 26.1% of cats receive a treat at least once daily (Laflamme et al. 2008). Offering a treat or sharing food with one's pet is an important part of the human–animal bond and should be included in a diet plan for every patient. The authors recommend that the energy intake from snacks or treats not exceed 10% of the animal's total daily calories. Intakes above this amount increase the risk of creating a nutritional imbalance in the animal's diet. Some commercial treats are formulated to support various life stages, so the utilization of such products will reduce that risk. Regardless of which approach to treats an owner chooses, they should be advised to avoid treats that are extremely high in fat. High-fat treats may incite gastrointestinal problems or pancreatitis in susceptible populations and are very calorie dense, thereby limiting the amount that can be fed daily. Human foods can also be used as treats. The US Department of Agriculture's (USDA) FoodData Central database (https://fdc.nal.usda.gov) is a very useful resource to determine the calorie content of human foods.

Feeding Behavior, Food Preferences, and Finicky Eaters

C. A. Tony Buffington

The feeding behavior of pet dogs and cats is an important aspect of clinical nutrition. It arguably may be even more important to primary care clinicians than the nutrient, ingredient, or diet aspects of nutrition, for at least two reasons. First, feeding behavior may provide a window into the quality of the home environment from the pet's point of view, and second, we may be able to modify feeding behavior in ways that benefit the health and well-being of the pet.

Feeding Behavior

John Bradshaw reviewed the evolutionary basis for domestic cat and dog feeding behavior (2006). Cats evolved as solitary hunters ("ambush predators") of small prey: rodents, birds, reptiles, and insects. Because individual prey contains fewer nutrients than a cat's daily needs, cats needed to hunt multiple times each day, whenever prey was available. This diet also resulted in a variety of anatomic and metabolic adaptations, resulting in cats being described as "hypercarnivorous" (Eisert 2011), although modern cat foods accommodate these adaptations. Cats retain many of their predecessor's feeding behaviors to the present time (leading one to question just how "domesticated" they really are; Clutton-Brock 1999).

Dogs evolved as social hunters of larger prey. In contrast to cats, however, their domestication by humans (possibly because of their social hunting behavior) and the intense selection pressure that followed has caused many dogs' feeding behavior to diverge from that of their canid ancestors. Some dogs have retained the primeval feeding behavior of gorging (consuming large meals rapidly), which might promote excess weight gain if access to food is not controlled. Other reasons for gorging in both cats and dogs include high food palatability (the "holy grail" of the pet food industry), competition or perception of threat from other animals (McMillan 2013), and possibly early life experiences in food-limited environments (Rinaudo and Wang 2012).

Food Preferences

Like other species, cats and dogs appear to have individual food preferences, likely the result of variable combinations of genetics and experience (Bradshaw 2006). Preferences for (unpredictable) particular smells, tastes, and "mouth feels" occur, which can only be determined for unfamiliar foods by offering them as choices. Moreover, in safe environments, pets tend to be neophilic, preferring new foods. In threatening environments, however, the situation seems more complex: pets become more neophobic, eating more of familiar ("comfort") foods initially, and less as the threat potential increases (McMillan 2013; Morton et al. 2014).

Finicky Eaters

Finicky or "picky" eaters occasionally cause concern to their owners. Interestingly, this behavior also commonly occurs in children (Cole et al. 2017). Some causes of finicky eating appear to include the pet learning that they can "hold out" for something better by waiting out their owner, and the perception of threat (Stella et al. 2011).

Some Suggestions

Most of the pets seen in our community practice are captive animals that can adapt to a wide range of diets and feeding schedules – in a sufficiently enriched environment. I recommend that owners choose diets that accommodate their preferences, and then offer a selection of them to their pet so that it can express *its* preferences. Keeping feeding times as naturalistic and consistent as possible often benefits confined pets, although the amount fed need not be the same at each meal. For example, feeding a larger meal later in the day after a play-about to cats that wake their owners up to be fed too early in the morning may be tried, with a smaller morning meal fed before the owner leaves for the day. Smaller meals in the morning may also result in fewer "accidents" by crated dogs. For cats fed from a bowl, locating the bowl in a safe, quiet place away from machinery that could come on unexpectedly and scare the cat, or where the cat could be startled (or trapped) by other animals (including humans), helps the cat feel safe while eating. For dogs, feeding in a safe, uncompetitive situation may be helpful.

Food puzzles are an interesting recent development for feeding confined pets. These devices offer the opportunity for both physical and mental stimulation. Many examples of these are available, as an internet search for "cat (or dog) food puzzles" will reveal. A variety of puzzles can be purchased or made for pets, and both dry and canned (by freezing it in the feeder) food can be fed using them. Animals have an intrinsic drive to eat, so food puzzles can be a powerful form of environmental enrichment for confined pets.

I recommend that food puzzles be introduced to pets at mealtime, with a portion of the usual meal in the feeder, which is placed next to the usual food source. Owners can choose to make or purchase a puzzle they like from a local pet store or website, and introduce it at mealtime on a day when they can stay around the home to observe the pet's reaction to the puzzle. For owners concerned about leaving food particles around the house, the puzzle can be "confined" to a single room with an uncarpeted floor (like the kitchen or bathroom), or placed in a bathtub or large sweater box (for cats) to restrict its access to the rest of the home. We and others (e.g. Dantas et al. 2016; Delgado and Dantas 2020) have described the health and well-being benefits of using puzzles rather than bowls to deliver food to confined cats and dogs.

Feeding can be an enrichment opportunity regardless of whether a bowl or feeder is used, and we can help owners provide environments their pet(s) can thrive in, which I imagine will permit many of the current concerns attributed to diets to recede into the background – where they belong.

Jerky Treats and Fanconi Syndrome in Dogs

Fanconi syndrome is an inherited disease that affects the proximal renal tubule and causes abnormalities in sodium, glucose, calcium, phosphate, and amino acid resorption, sometimes leading to fatal disturbances in acid–base balance (Bovee et al. 1978). To date, this disease has been described in dogs, but not in cats. Fanconi syndrome is well recognized in basenjis and has been seen in other canine breeds with increased frequency, but it may also be acquired. The mode of inheritance and specific nature of the hereditary defects have not yet been identified. Amino acid resorption abnormalities vary from one animal to the next, but generally include an increased excretion of cystine (cysteine bound to another cysteine via a disulfide bond). Dogs with Fanconi syndrome will often resorb as little as 50% of urinary amino acids compared to unaffected dogs. Screening urine for a general aminoaciduria is one test used to help arrive at a diagnosis.

There are multiple causes of Fanconi syndrome, including kidney infection, medications such as antibiotics or chemotherapy, and liver disease. Clinical signs include increased water consumption, increased urination, dehydration, and weight loss. While the signs of Fanconi syndrome are not specific, one often sees urinary loss of glucose, phosphate, sodium, potassium, uric acid, and amino acids.

The US Food and Drug Administration (FDA) began releasing statements in 2007 to caution owners about the potential association of chicken jerky treat consumption and the development of renal disease and Fanconi syndrome (FDA 2018). As time progressed, the illnesses associated with jerky treats were not only confined to chicken, but included other animal protein sources. Jerky containing everything from duck to sweet potato has also been implicated.

As of the end of 2015, the FDA had received approximately 5200 complaints of illness associated with consumption of chicken, duck, or sweet potato jerky treats (FDA 2018). Many of these treats had China as the country of origin. The complaints received by the FDA involved dogs of different breeds, sizes, and ages. Approximately 60% of the reports were for gastrointestinal signs, with 30% reporting kidney or urinary tract signs. The remaining 10% of complaints reported varied clinical signs including convulsions, tremors, hives, and skin irritation.

As of 2015, the FDA had confirmed 214 dogs as positive for Fanconi syndrome out of 263 cases. A majority of the dogs testing positive survived. Their Fanconi syndrome resolved after the jerky treats were eliminated from the diet. These dogs also received supportive care (FDA 2018).

Recently an abstract was published hypothesizing that consumption of commercial dried meat treats potentially results in excessive intake of highly available phosphorus, which can result in disruption of calcium and phosphorus homeostasis and adversely impact renal function (Fleeman et al. 2021).

Suspected cases can be further evaluated by sending a urine sample for quantitative amino acid analysis, such as the one run by one author (AJF; e.g. UC Davis Amino Acid Laboratory) or to a lab that offers testing for Fanconi syndrome (e.g. Penn Vet PennGen).

The mechanism of how jerky treats can lead to Fanconi syndrome in some dogs remains elusive. Practitioners who suspect Fanconi syndrome in one of their patients associated with jerky treat consumption are encouraged to contact the FDA to report their case and suggest that the client stop feeding the jerky treat.

What to Feed

"What is the best diet for my pet?" is one question the authors are often asked. The answer is: "There is no one diet that is best for every cat or dog. Cats and dogs are individuals, and the best diet will vary from animal to animal." That being said, it is helpful to clients to provide some guidelines for choosing a diet for their healthy animal, and even more helpful if one can give them a few specific recommendations. When considering the appropriate response to this question, it is important that the clinician consider three factors: (i) the animal in question; (ii) the variety of external factors that may influence how and what the animal is fed; and finally (iii) the product itself.

There are many factors related to the animal that will influence your suggestions. One must consider not only the animal's signalment (i.e. age, species, breed, and sexual status) but its body condition, activity levels, and food or texture preferences. It is also helpful to know if the animal is a normal or finicky eater.

External factors can have a strong influence on your final dietary recommendations for the pet. Knowing the owner's budget can help narrow your recommendations to products that meet their price range. The diet and how the animal is fed may be influenced by its environment, which includes, but is not limited to, the number and type of the animals in the household, where the animal is housed (i.e. indoors versus outdoors), the human inhabitants of the house (i.e. a household with small children, elderly individuals, or adults only), and the feeding philosophies of the owner. Some owners follow a particular dietary philosophy for themselves (e.g. vegetarian, organic, locally sourced food, etc.) and want to apply that approach to their animals as well.

After assessing your patient and reviewing the external factors in that animal's environment, consideration needs to be given to the product itself. It is important to select a diet that supports the life stage of the patient that one is feeding and a lean body condition when fed an appropriate amount. The authors recommend feeding foods produced by larger manufacturers, so that if there is a problem with a particular diet it will likely be detected sooner. Strong consideration should be given to companies that employ animal nutritionists and support research in an effort to continually improve foods and the knowledge about dog and cat nutrition. When making specific recommendations, the authors prefer foods that have undergone and passed feeding trials in accordance with the guidelines of the Association of American Feed Control

Officials (AAFCO; see Chapter 6). It is unfortunate that the current court of public opinion seems to view such feeding trials negatively and as generally yielding few useful data. This opinion is often expressed by well-intentioned individuals with little understanding of the process or dog and cat nutrition. While such trials do have limitations with respect to catching long-term nutritional problems, all life-stage feeding trials can pick up concerns before a food is marketed (Q.R. Rogers and A.J. Fascetti, personal communication). Many critics are also unaware of the fact that even though a product states it is formulated to meet an AAFCO nutrient profile, that does not mean it will pass a feeding trial for the life stage it is designed to support. Nonetheless, even many reputable companies are no longer conducting feeding trials in an effort to appease their customers, so it makes it harder to say that every food should undergo a feeding trial in order to recommend it to a client.

The authors are comfortable recommending foods that have not undergone feeding trials when they are produced by larger companies that have a long history of making foods and a good working knowledge of their ingredients. While not necessarily conducting an official AAFCO trial, many of these companies still have current knowledge on how their products perform by continually feeding their diets to dogs and cats in a controlled setting. There is less confidence in foods from newer or smaller companies that have not conducted any feeding trials and may not have any historical data on how their formulations or ingredients perform, and/or they may not have maintained animals for years on their foods. Special concern is warranted with regard to products that employ newer feeding approaches, such as raw food, especially when largely unsupplemented with essential minerals and vitamins. Data from the controlled feeding of these diets are virtually non-existent, so pets eating these foods are in essence the test animals if the manufacturer has not tested the food prior to release into the market.

Feeding Guidelines for Different Life Stages

Gestation and Lactation

For mammals, the period of pregnancy puts a significant nutritional demand on both the dam and the fetus. Both mother and offspring are in a positive energy and nitrogen balance. Given the nutritional demands of this life stage, it is important that the diet be one that supplies all the energy and nutrients needed to meet the maintenance requirements of the queen or bitch, in addition to supplying all the energy and nutrients required to support fetal growth and development and milk demands during lactation (Wills 1996).

Cats

Queens that are significantly under- or overweight should not be bred until their body condition is closer to ideal (5 out of 9 on a 9-point scale). Malnourished queens are more likely not to conceive or to have kittens that are underweight and perform poorly during lactation (personal communication, A.J. Fascetti). It has been reported that obese cats have a higher incidence of dystocia (Lawler and Monti 1984).

Weight gain in cats is unlike other mammals such as humans and dogs, where most weight is gained in late pregnancy (Wills 1996). Cats, like pigs, show a different pattern characterized by a linear gain throughout pregnancy that is independent of the number of fetuses (Loveridge 1986; Wichert et al. 2009). Energy intake parallels this linear weight gain. It has been estimated that energy requirements increase approximately 25–50% above maintenance to between 90 and 100 kcal/kg body weight/day (Loveridge and Rivers 1989).

Just prior to and immediately following parturition, food intake is reduced, but quickly increases driven by the need for energy to meet the demands of lactation (Legrand-Defretin and Munday 1993). Following parturition, approximately 40% of the weight gained during gestation is lost, and by the time the kittens are weaned from the queen she should have returned to her pre-breeding weight (Loveridge and Rivers 1989). However, a recent study found that most queens were heavier than their breeding weight two weeks following weaning (Wichert et al. 2009). The retention of some weight allows the queen to maintain a body fat reserve to use as energy during lactation (Wills 1996). This may be because it is difficult for the queen to consume enough energy through her diet alone to meet this demand.

Lactation is considered to be the most demanding life stage with regard to energy and nutrient needs. It has been suggested that the actual energy and protein requirements of lactating queens may in fact exceed current National Research Council (NRC) recommendations (Wichert et al. 2009). During lactation, energy demands peak at about the seventh week, although peak milk production typically occurs at week 3 (Munday and Earle 1991). This discrepancy occurs because energy intake at week 7 not only includes the calories consumed by the queen, but also those eaten by the kittens that are consuming a portion of their intake from the queen's diet at this time (Munday and Earle 1991).

Because cats begin to increase their energy intake shortly after conception, it is recommended that queens be fed a diet designed to support gestation and lactation prior to breeding and continue with this food until weaning. The diet should be concentrated in terms of its energy density, and be highly digestible and palatable. Such a diet will assist in meeting the queen's high energy demands without volume restriction. To further assist with this goal, queens should be fed free choice throughout these two life stages. Following the weaning of their kittens, queens can be returned to their normal maintenance ration.

Dogs

Like cats, it has been recommended that dogs be fed a complete and balanced diet and be in an ideal body condition prior to breeding.

While supportive studies are lacking, one could speculate that malnourished bitches will have lower conception rates and perform poorly during lactation. It has been reported that puppies born to malnourished dogs have reduced birth weights, are prone to hypoglycemia, and have poor survival rates (Schroeder and Smith 1994). Bitches that are obese prior to breeding have lower ovulation rates, smaller litter sizes, and perform poorly during lactation (Bebiak et al. 1987; Debraekeleer et al. 2010).

Unlike cats, the bitch's energy requirements will not increase until the last third of gestation. In general the average bitch will gain anywhere from 15% to 25% of her pre-breeding weight prior to whelping (Legrand-Defretin and Munday 1993). Energy requirements for gestation peak anywhere between 30% and 60% of the pre-breeding requirements depending upon the litter size (Romsos et al. 1981; Debraekeleer et al. 2010). Energy requirements continue to increase following whelping and into lactation, peaking at approximately 3–5 weeks. At this point, energy requirements can fall between two and four times the adult maintenance requirement (Ontko and Phillips 1958; Legrand-Defretin and Munday 1993).

It is recommended that all breeding bitches be in an ideal body condition prior to conception. A diet designed to support the life stages of gestation and lactation should be selected and started prior to breeding and fed to maintain an ideal body condition. As the need for extra energy and nutrients is relatively small, a gradual increase in the amount of energy offered can be started during the second half of gestation. Every animal should be fed on an individual basis, but one suggestion is to consider beginning to increase the amount of calories offered by 10–15% each week around the fifth week of gestation until whelping (Wills 1996). This approach results in an overall increase of approximately 40–60% compared to the food intake at the time of breeding. In many cases offering two meals per day during the last few weeks of gestation is sufficient for the dam to meet her energy needs. However, some giant-breed dogs and bitches with large litters may need to be fed free choice due to volume limitations (Mosier 1977; Debraekeleer et al. 2010). During lactation, with the exception of when a bitch only has one or two surviving puppies, most dogs should be fed free choice or small, multiple meals throughout the day to allow them to meet their energy needs and produce adequate milk for their offspring. The amount of calories offered can be reduced as the weaning process is started; this helps reduce the amount of milk the bitch is producing. Once weaning has been completed, the bitch should be fed the same amount of calories as her pre-breeding intake.

There is some controversy regarding the need for carbohydrates in diets fed to bitches during gestation and lactation. Romsos et al. (1981) reported smaller litter sizes in beagles fed a diet containing 26% of the calories from protein and 74% from fat. A second study fed a carbohydrate-free diet containing 42% of the calories from protein and 58% from fat (Kienzle et al. 1985). In that study, litter sizes, birth weights, and puppy survival rates were comparable to control dogs consuming a diet with carbohydrates. These data indicate that although pregnant and lactating bitches do not require a dietary source of carbohydrate, they have an increased protein requirement when a carbohydrate-free diet is fed (NRC 2006). That being said, there are some data to support that the lactose content of the milk is higher when a diet containing some carbohydrate is fed (Kienzle et al. 1985). The recommendations from that study are that diets for lactation provide at least 10–20% of the energy from digestible carbohydrates (Kienzle et al. 1985).

Supplementation during Gestation and Lactation

Some breeders regularly supplement their bitch's or queen's diet with calcium or calcium-containing foods such as cottage cheese throughout gestation or lactation. This stems from the theory that the added minerals will ensure healthy fetal development, prevent eclampsia, and aid in milk production. This practice is not necessary as long as the dam is consuming a commercial ration designed to support gestation/lactation. In fact, some experts feel that excess supplements during pregnancy may adversely affect skeletal development, result in fetal deformities or problems during growth, and actually increase the likelihood of eclampsia (Linde-Forsberg 2010). The higher calcium needs that result during gestation and lactation are met by increasing energy consumption from a diet that is nutritionally adequate for gestation and lactation.

Assessment

Assessment of the suitability of the feeding plan for the queen or bitch should be conducted routinely throughout gestation and lactation. This is done primarily by observation and determination of the health and body condition score of the dam. The nutritional adequacy of the mother's diet will also be reflected in the health and vitality of the kittens or puppies. Poor or inadequate milk production during lactation may be reflected in high neonatal mortality rates, poor growth rates, and continuous vocalization indicating hunger in the offspring. If the body condition of the dam drops below 4–5 out of 9, consideration should be given to adjusting the amount or type of food offered (preferably more energy dense and/or more palatable) after other causes of weight loss have been eliminated.

Growth

Orphan Kittens and Puppies

Ideally kittens and puppies will be raised uneventfully by their mother and weaned to an appropriate growth diet. Occasionally they are orphaned and other feeding approaches are required. If a nursing queen or bitch is available, it is ideal to try to foster the orphaned offspring to that dam. In the event that is not possible, then they will need to be hand-raised with either tube feeding in very young or debilitated neonates, or bottle feeding in older and healthier ones. Bottle feeding is safest and easiest, but can be time consuming, especially if one is managing a large litter. Tube feeding can be mastered by most clients with a little training and is a faster, albeit riskier, method to deliver nutrition.

It is recommended that a commercial milk replacer be used, as many home-prepared formulas are not adequate to meet the needs of a growing kitten or puppy. If using a home-prepared formulation, it should be reviewed and balanced if necessary by a board-certified veterinary nutritionist® to ensure adequacy for growth. Cow's and goat's milk does not contain as much fat, protein, or calories as milk from queens and bitches and therefore should be avoided (Wills and Morris 1996).

Most commercial formulas contain approximately 1 kcal/ml, although there is some variation, and dilution with water will reduce the caloric density. Recommendations for feeding are variable, but range from 13 to 18 ml/100 g body weight (using a formula with a caloric density of approximately 1 kcal/ml) to begin with and then gradually increasing as the orphan gains weight (Gross et al. 2010; Hoskins 2010). Every feeding should be followed with anogenital stimulation by using a cotton swab or warm cloth to encourage urination and defecation.

Assessment

The feeding program should be re-evaluated frequently by assessing the health, appearance, and weight gain of the orphans. Weight gain should approximate that of nursing kittens and puppies. Nursing kittens gain approximately 18–20 g/d (Wills and Morris 1996). Nursing puppies gain approximately 1 g of body weight per 2–5 g of milk intake during the first five weeks following birth, or 2–4 g/d/kg of anticipated adult weight for the first five months of their lives (Lewis et al. 1987b; Debraekeleer et al. 2010). Kittens and puppies should be active and responsive to their environment. Chronic vocalization or whimpering may be a sign of discomfort or alternatively

hunger, and should be an indication to re-evaluate the feeding program.

Weaning to Adult

All kittens and puppies should be encouraged to start eating the food fed to the dam when they are 3–4 weeks of age, regardless of whether they were nursed by the dam or hand reared. This diet should be mixed with enough water to form a thick gruel. At weaning, every growing animal should be fed a complete and balanced diet designed, and preferably tested, for growth or all life stages.

Kittens

Kittens normally weigh between 90 and 110 g at birth and should gain 50–100 g until they are 5 or 6 months of age (Wills and Morris 1996). In kittens, excessive growth rates do not invoke the same consequences as in dogs; however, obesity can become a problem. Often kittens are fed free choice, so monitoring is essential to catch and eliminate any excessive weight gain. Kittens should be fed a diet that meets the nutrient and energy requirements for growth or all life stages.

Puppies

Puppies should gain between 2 and 4 g/d/kg of anticipated adult weight for the first five months of life (Lewis et al. 1987b). If the dog should weigh 20 kg as an adult, the puppy should gain between 40 and 80 g/d. Excessive feeding during growth can lead to obesity and in larger-breed dogs can result in skeletal problems (Hedhammar et al. 1974; Lavelle 1989; Kealy et al. 1992). Studies have demonstrated that controlled meal feeding of pups leads to a slower growth rate and fewer skeletal problems, but does not decrease the final mature body size compared to pups fed free choice (Hedhammer et al. 1974). Refer to Chapter 10 for a more extensive discussion of this topic.

"How much should I feed my puppy?" is one of the more challenging questions for the practitioner to answer. In order to address this question, one should start by getting a complete diet history on the dog, including the name and amount of diet it is currently being fed. The nutritional adequacy statement should be checked to ensure that it is appropriate for growth or all life stages and the number of calories consumed daily should be calculated. Assuming the puppy is in an ideal body condition, the current amount fed is likely appropriate, and the owners should be instructed to continue their feeding regime, increasing food intake gradually as the puppy grows. Alternatively, one can calculate the number of calories the dog should be eating using an equation for growth (see Chapter 3). However, this method may significantly under- or overestimate the actual energy requirement (NRC 2006). An easier approach to get an estimate is to start with the feeding directions from the food the client is feeding. Because feeding directions are designed to provide enough calories for all the dogs receiving a particular diet, there is a tendency for them, at times, to overestimate calorie needs. Regardless of which approach is chosen, both are only an approximation of the dog's actual caloric needs and will require frequent monitoring and adjustment as the puppy grows to maintain an ideal body condition.

Portion-controlled feeding is recommended for puppies in order to prevent obesity and the skeletal developmental disorders that are linked to overnutrition, especially in large- to giant-breed dogs. Puppies should be fed at least twice daily, and some may require three or more meals. Some individuals suggest using a time-limited feeding approach to assist with housebreaking, but one study reported that some dogs may consume more with this approach than if they were fed free choice (Toll et al. 1993). In addition, these dogs gained more weight and body fat compared to dogs receiving the same diet ad libitum (Toll et al. 1993).

Neutering and the Prevention of Weight Gain in Kittens and Puppies

Multiple studies have shown that intact adult pets generally weigh less than neutered animals of the same breed and size (Root 1995; Duch et al. 1978; Houpt et al. 1979; Flynn et al. 1996; Fettman et al. 1997). This is probably a combination of physiologic and environmental factors. Owners are generally encouraged to neuter their pets between 6 and 12 months of age. This time period corresponds to a natural decrease in the animal's growth rate and energy needs. If owners are not aware of this change, and continue to feed their pet the same amount of food, excess weight gain will result. Increasing age and a change in sexual status are also associated with a decrease in voluntary physical activity. Recent studies have demonstrated that ovariohysterectomy and castration in cats lead to an increase in food intake and weight gain (Fettman et al. 1997; Martin et al. 2001; Kanchuk et al. 2003; Nguyen et al. 2004).

Recently, early-age neutering (at 8–16 weeks of age) has become more common. One concern has been the potential of early-age neutering to influence a pet's tendency to become obese. However, a study evaluating metabolic rates and obesity development in cats neutered at 7 weeks of age, 7 months of age, or left intact found no difference between cats neutered between 7 weeks and 7 months of age (Root 1995). These results indicate that early-age neutering presents the same level of risk of weight gain as does neutering at the traditional age of 6–9 months (Root 1995).

Given the strong link between weight gain and neutering, it would make sense that this milestone is a good time to discuss the risk of obesity and the opportunity for prevention in the client's pet. There are several steps that an owner can take to prevent weight gain in their pet following neutering. Changing from an ad libitum feeding approach to one in which the food is offered in carefully controlled meals may prevent weight gain. Alternatively, one can consider feeding a diet with a lower energy density. A recent study demonstrated a reduction in weight gain in neutered cats that were fed a low-fat, low–energy density diet compared to neutered cats fed a higher-fat and more energy-dense diet (Nguyen et al. 2004).

Assessment

It is important to monitor kittens and puppies frequently during the growth process. This monitoring is facilitated by the fact that they are visiting the veterinary office frequently during this life stage for check-ups and vaccinations. Puppies and kittens should be weighed and body condition scored at every visit and the diet history form updated. Owners should also be asked about appetite and food intake (i.e. amount and enthusiasm for eating) to ensure that they are meeting their energy and nutrient needs without significant difficulty. In addition to the routine examination, one should evaluate the animal to ensure that its coat quality is good and that the puppy or kitten is bright, curious, and active. If there is excessive weight gain or a body condition score greater than 5 out of 9, owners should be directed to feed 10% fewer calories (or more if indicated based on the animal's weight, body condition, and calorie intake). Alternatively, if the animal is not growing normally or is underweight and metabolic causes have been eliminated, consideration should be given to increasing the amount of food fed by 10%. Regardless of the problem, the animal should come back for a weight and body condition score check within 2–3 weeks to ensure that it is returning to an ideal body condition and growing normally.

Adult Cats and Dogs

In addition to feeding a diet that is nutritionally formulated to meet the nutrient needs of dogs and cats, probably the most important feeding recommendation for this life stage is to keep animals in a lean body condition. The maintenance of a lean body condition has been proven to increase both the quantity and quality of life in dogs (Kealy et al. 2002). Currently there is no similar data in cats. Obesity has been linked to diabetes mellitus, lameness, and skin disease (Scarlett and Donoghue 1998), and it is a risk factor for hepatic lipidosis in anorexic cats (Biourge et al. 1994). One might

surmise that by avoiding conditions that contribute to early mortality by maintenance of a lean body condition, one will secondarily contribute to life extension in cats as well.

There exists some controversy regarding whether it is better to feed cats dry compared to moist diets. Proponents of canned food cite the documented increase in water consumption in cats consuming such products (Kane et al. 1981), the possible prevention of urinary tract problems, and the potential voluntary reduction in food intake and consequent reduction in calories, all helping to prevent weight gain in cats. Proponents of dry food cite the dental health benefits and the ability to feed ad libitum, thereby more appropriately mimicking the natural pattern of food intake in the cat (Kane et al. 1981), and the esoteric pleasure of consuming food that is crunchy and requires chewing. Consideration should be given to these variables and the animal's preferences when recommending one type of food over another. However, the authors recommend exposing young cats to the different food formats to prevent texture preferences that might otherwise limit future diet options.

Assessment

Adult cats and dogs should be seen routinely for a medical evaluation. Success of the feeding program can be evaluated based on the animal's maintenance of a lean body condition and an active lifestyle. A diet history should be updated at every visit to maintain historical records on the types and amount of calories fed, in case conditions requiring dietary modification occur in the future. Frequent alterations in the diet or a significant increase or decrease in food intake may be an early indicator to the practitioner of an underlying problem.

Senior Dogs and Cats

Although the concept of aging is difficult to define, most experts agree that aging is not a disease. Aging has been defined as "a complex biologic process resulting in progressive reduction of an individual's ability to maintain homeostasis under physiologic and external environmental stresses, thereby decreasing the individual's viability and increasing its vulnerability to disease, and eventually causing death" (Goldston 1989). It is difficult to define old age in dogs and cats. As with humans, the aging process varies tremendously from individual to individual. The aging process is influenced by an animal's breed, size, genetics, nutrition, environment, and other factors. As a general rule, larger breeds have a shorter life expectancy than smaller breeds, and mixed-breed dogs live longer than purebreds of a similar size. A survey of veterinarians revealed that clinicians believe the term "geriatric" is appropriate when applied to small dogs (<20 lb [<9.1 kg]) at 11.5 years, medium dogs (21–50 lb [9.5–22.7 kg]) at 10 years, large breeds (51–90 lb [23.1–40.8 kg]) at 9 years, and giant-breed dogs (>90 lb [>40.8 kg]) at 7.5 years (Goldston 1989; Allen and Roudebush 1990). Other authors suggest that a dog or cat is aged when it completes 75–80% of its expected life span, or reaches 5–7 years of age (Maher and Rush 1990; Moser 1991; Laflamme 1997). While the definition of when a dog or cat becomes "mature" has not been agreed upon, there are data to suggest that our dog and cat population is getting older. Over a 10-years

period, the number of pet cats over 10 years of age has increased by 15%, and the percentage of cats over the age of 15 years has increased from 5% to 14% of the population (Stratton-Phelps 1999). It has also been reported that more than 35% of dogs in the United States are older than 7 years (Lund et al. 1999). One might speculate that with earlier and more advanced care, those numbers have likely increased since those surveys were published.

Physiological Changes Associated with Aging

Rather than relying on chronologic age to categorize a patient (Box 7.1), older animals should be assessed as individuals using functional and physiologic changes that commonly occur as the pet gets older.

Energy Requirement

In many dogs, RERs and MERs decrease as they age (Kienzle and Rainbird 1991; Speakman et al. 2003). Multiple studies examining a variety of breeds estimated an 18–24% reduction in MERs compared to those of younger dogs (Finke 1991; Kienzle and Rainbird 1991; Taylor et al. 1995; Harper 1997). The change in energy requirements is also related to changes in body composition. It has been reported that there is a highly significant, negative linear correlation between age and

---

Box 7.1 Aging and Nutrition

The following principles should be kept in mind when considering the interaction of aging and nutrition:

- Chronological age is not a reliable indicator of functional age. Changes in body composition, organ function, physical performance, and mental alertness are age related, but there is great individual variability. Within a particular individual, various organs may age at different rates.
- Nutrient requirements for older dogs and cats have not been adequately determined, but most likely vary from individual to individual because of genetic, health, and environmental influences.
- Elderly dogs and cats are more variable than any other age group (e.g. puppies or kittens).
- The incidence of chronic disease increases with age.
- A properly administered geriatric nutrition program is one in which dietary recommendations are made on an individual basis, with modifications secondary to re-evaluation at regular intervals.

Source: Moser, E.A. 1991 / Public Domain.

the lean-to-fat ratios in dogs (Meyer and Stadtfeld 1980; Harper 1998b).

One interesting exception to a general decline in energy needs with aging was reported in a study looking at working versus pet border collies in the United Kingdom (Harper 1998a). Border collies that were maintained as pets had a similar decline in energy requirements as reported in previous studies. However, working border collies experienced no change in energy needs with aging, supporting the author's hypothesis that dogs that remain active do not display a change in their MERs over time.

The degree of decline in energy requirements appears to be breed and size related based on models of energy expenditure over the lifetime of the dog (Speakman et al. 2003). It has been hypothesized that the decline in metabolic rates with age is a consequence of the declining force of selection with aging, and that older animals have lower metabolic rates because they invest less in defense and repair mechanisms (Speakman et al. 2003).

The situation appears to be somewhat different in cats. Previous evidence suggested that MERs remained constant throughout adult life (Anantharaman-Barr et al. 1991; Taylor et al. 1995; Harper 1998a). These findings were supported by additional work that did not document a change in the lean-to-fat ratio in cats with age (Munday and Earle 1991; Harper 1998b). However, more recent studies suggest that MERs decrease in mature cats compared to younger cats, but increase again when the cats become older at approximately 10–12 years of age (Cupp et al. 2004; Perez-Camargo 2004; Laflamme 2005). This increase was not linear, but rose dramatically between the ages of 12 and 15 years (Perez-Camargo 2010). These same researchers also reported that cats that lose body fat, lean mass, and bone mass are at a greater risk for earlier mortality (Perez-Camargo 2010).

Digestion and Absorption

Changes in the alimentary system may contribute to inadequate food intake, decreased appetite, and systemic disease. As animals age,

there is an increased incidence of dental calculus, periodontal disease, periodontitis, and tooth loss. These alterations, combined with a reduction in the amount of functional saliva, will often contribute to a decline in food intake.

Age-related changes in digestive physiology, hormones, and gut microbiota may directly or indirectly reduce digestive capacity (Fahey et al. 2008). Unlike in humans, structural changes in the canine digestive tract are not very pronounced during aging, and atrophy and fibrosis are rarely seen (Mundt 1991). Nevertheless, on histologic examination, changes are evident in the salivary glands, small intestine, liver, and pancreas of older dogs (Mundt 1991). Despite these changes, advancing age does not reduce apparent nutrient digestibility in dogs (Lloyd and McCay 1954, 1955; Sheffy et al. 1985; Buffington et al. 1989; Taylor et al. 1995). In fact, several studies reported higher apparent digestibility coefficients for protein and fat (Lloyd and McCay 1954; Sheffy et al. 1985) and energy (Sheffy et al. 1985), although explanations for why this occurred are not provided.

Morphologic changes, transit times, and the secretory capacity in the feline gastrointestinal tract have not been as well studied. Several studies have demonstrated no significant difference in orocecal transit times in young compared to older cats (Papasouliotis et al. 1996; Peachey et al. 2000). Nonetheless, several studies have reported reductions in the digestibility of protein, fat, and starch in older cats (Taylor et al. 1995; Peachey et al. 1999; Patil and Cupp 2010; Teshima et al. 2010). One study reported a positive correlation between fat digestibility and serum vitamin E concentrations (Patil and Cupp 2010). This same study also reported a positive correlation between fat and protein digestibility and plasma vitamin B12 concentrations (Patil and Cupp 2010).

Integument and Musculoskeletal System

Multiple changes are visible in the integument and musculoskeletal system of older dogs and cats. The skin loses elasticity and becomes less pliable (Markham and Hodgkins 1989). Loss of elasticity is often accompanied by hyperkeratosis of the skin and follicles. Follicles typically atrophy, resulting in hair loss. Loss of pigment results in the production of white hairs, often seen around the muzzle of older dogs and cats. Along with a decline in lean body mass, there is a reduction in bone mass. The cortices of the long bones become thinner and more brittle (Case et al. 1995). This may be due to the reduced absorption of calcium from the intestine of some older pets (Case et al. 1995). Arthritis is a common occurrence in older animals and may affect the pet's desire (or ability) to eat. Obesity can compound the effects of arthritis, or, conversely, arthritic pets may experience a reduction in appetite leading to severe weight loss.

Renal System

Renal failure is a major cause of illness and mortality in geriatric cats, and of one of the three leading causes of death in older dogs (Morris Animal Foundation 1998). Despite this statistic, little is known about renal function in the general population of geriatric companion animals (Brown 1997). It is important to remember that gradual renal senescence with normal aging is opposed by the tremendous reserve capacity of the kidneys. Studies have shown that dogs and cats have 10–20 times more renal tissue than is required to sustain normal life (Brown et al. 1991). Studies have suggested that normal kidney aging may lead to nephron loss of up to 75% before clinical or biochemical signs occur in older animals (Cowgill and Spangler 1981). Therefore, practice approaches that assume inadequate renal function in geriatric patients may have adverse effects.

Immune Response

Alterations in the immune system associated with aging are well recognized (Cowan et al. 1998). These changes may contribute to the increased incidence of infectious diseases and tumors (Meydani and Hayek 1995). Older dogs and cats have reduced blood CD4$^+$ T cells, elevations in the CD8$^+$ subset, and reductions in the CD4 : CD8 ratio (Day 2010). The cutaneous delayed-type hypersensitivity response is reduced, while humoral immune responses are not significantly impacted by age (Day 2010). Serum and salivary immunoglobulin (Ig)A production increases, and IgG concentration remains unaltered (Day 2010). Little is known about "inflammaging," which is defined as the effect of cumulative antigenic exposure and onset of late-life inflammatory disease in dogs and cats (Day 2010).

Sensory

The aging process results in a general reduction in the sensations of vision, hearing, taste, and smell. These changes occur in humans and companion animals alike (Markham and Hodgkins 1989; Harper 1996). Involution of nervous tissue is believed to be responsible for the diminution of taste and smell responses (Markham and Hodgkins 1989). These may contribute to a reduction in the desire to eat and result in weight loss in older animals. Geriatric animals often experience a decreased sensitivity to thirst, which has the potential to contribute to a state of dehydration. Patil and Cupp (2010) reported no difference in fecal water losses between adult cats (1–7 years) and geriatric cats (>12 years). However, urine volumes were significantly higher in the older cats. They hypothesized that this may be the result of a decreased ability for the aged kidneys to concentrate urine even in the absence of renal insufficiency. Aging also diminishes an animal's thermoregulatory capacity and subsequent tolerance to heat or cold (Markham and Hodgkins 1989).

Behavior

Behavioral changes are common in older pets and are a frequently overlooked physiologic alteration that may affect the animal's ability or desire to obtain adequate nutrition. Behavioral changes can be the result of many disorders, including systemic illness, organic brain disease, true behavioral problems, or cognitive dysfunction syndrome (CDS) (Neilson et al. 2001; Gunn-Moore et al. 2007). CDS is a term applied to age-related deterioration of cognitive abilities, characterized by behavioral changes, where no medical cause can be determined (Gunn-Moore et al. 2007). Animals that are suffering from chronic pain may become irritable and reluctant to eat properly, if at all. Changes in the home environment, such as the loss of another pet or the owner or the introduction of a new animal or person, can induce an alteration in eating behavior or a state of anorexia (Houpt and Beaver 1981).

Nutrient Requirements of Older Pets

Elderly pets have the same nutrient needs as their younger counterparts (NRC 2006). However, the quantities per unit of body weight may change, and the way they are provided may require modification. Feeding recommendations for this life stage are not unlike any other life stage, in that each animal should be treated as an individual and as a consequence will vary from patient to patient.

Energy

If an animal's energy needs decrease without a reduction in caloric intake, obesity will develop. Some diets for mature dogs and cats are designed with higher fiber levels to combat this problem by decreasing the food's energy density. However, not all animals will gain weight as they age; many remain weight stable and a large number will experience varying degrees of weight loss. This population of pets may benefit from more energy-dense, palatable diets to help them maintain or gain weight. Similar to other life stages, dogs and cats should be fed to maintain a lean body condition through their senior years.

Protein

The decline in lean body mass that occurs with aging results in a loss of protein "reserves" in the body, frequently required to combat stress

and disease. Results from one study suggest that older dogs have higher protein requirements than adult dogs (Wannemacher and McCoy 1966). The investigators of this study found that older dogs required up to 50% more protein than young dogs to maintain labile protein. A more recent study examined 8-year-old pointers fed either 16.5% or 45% protein calories over a two-year period (Kealy 1999). Both groups had a reduction in lean body mass. Even the group consuming a higher percentage of their calories from protein lost 3.5% of their lean body mass. While neither of these studies provides definitive recommendations for protein requirements in older dogs, they do suggest that the amount of protein in the diet is important and may impact health and body condition.

Similarly, recommendations regarding protein requirements for older cats are lacking. One study reported maintenance of lean body mass in adult cats consuming 36% protein on a dry matter (DM) basis (Hannah and Laflamme 1996). Cats consuming lower amounts of protein (22% and 28% DM) maintained nitrogen balance but lost lean body mass (Hannah and Laflamme 1996). This study suggests that the amount of protein consumed may impact lean body mass. A second study looking at the impact of dietary protein concentrations on the preservation of lean body mass following neutering also reported a loss of lean body mass on average of 1.2% when cats were fed a diet containing 30% protein DM (Nguyen et al. 2004). When the cats were fed 53% protein DM, they reported an average accumulation of 4.2% of lean body mass.

The quality of protein is an important consideration. To reduce bacterial metabolites, the protein should have a high biological value and a high pre-cecal digestibility. Most commercial pet foods are formulated to exceed minimum requirements, so adequate protein is usually not a concern. However, if energy intake is reduced secondary to a decreased metabolic rate or food intake, the protein-to-calorie ratio may need to be adjusted to meet the protein requirement. Furthermore, some high-energy foods with reduced protein concentrations, such as products designed to address renal or liver failure, do not provide as high a level of protein, especially if food intake is reduced.

There is a great deal of controversy concerning the restriction of protein in elderly animals as a measure to prevent renal disease. Although there is evidence that protein restriction is effective in minimizing the clinical signs of renal failure once disease is present (Elliott et al. 2000; Jacob et al. 2002), there is no evidence that protein restriction is of any benefit to healthy older dogs and cats. Considering that older dogs may have an increased protein requirement, that there is loss of lean body mass in both dogs and cats with advancing age, and that a decline in protein digestibility exists in older cats, the authors do not recommend protein restriction in older dogs and cats unless indicated by an underlying disease. In some cases, other dietary changes, such as phosphorus restriction with renal disease, may be a more important strategy. The strategy of restricting dietary phosphorus, but not protein, is one that is present in early-stage renal diets for cats. This strategy also permits a slow reduction in protein intake and may help adjust cats in getting used to consuming less protein over time, thereby being more accepting of a low-protein, low-phosphorus diet. Care may be needed to avoid an excessive calcium-to-phosphorus ratio and resulting hypercalcemia (Schauf et al. 2021).

Fat

Fat is necessary in every animal's diet to provide essential fatty acids, energy, a vehicle for fat-soluble vitamin absorption, and enhancement of palatability. Fat increases the energy density of food. In animals prone to obesity this can pose a problem. A slight reduction in dietary fat may be necessary to aid in the prevention of weight gain. On the other hand, in underweight animals a diet with a high energy density may be beneficial.

Supplementation with Antioxidants and Fatty Acids

Recently there has been the advent of diets on the market enhanced with antioxidants to support immune function. The implication is that such enhancement will extend (or reverse) the aging process and prevent or reduce the likelihood of disease. A number of these studies were conducted in young animals, but a few have looked at the effects on older dogs and cats. Dietary supplementation of vitamin E at 250 IU/kg in the diet stimulated lymphocyte genesis in young and old cats (Hayek et al. 2000). Beta-carotene supplementation restored immune response in older dogs when compared to their age-matched controls and younger counterparts (Massimino et al. 2003). Another study examined the effect of n-3 and n-6 fatty acids on immune parameters in young and old dogs. Supplementation with n-3 fatty acids (n-6 : n-3 ratio of 5 : 1) did not affect interleukin (IL)-1, IL-6, or tumor necrosis factor (TNF)-α production, but did reduce malondialdehyde concentrations in older dogs, an indicator of antioxidant status (Kearns et al. 2000).

A second area of product development has focused on addressing canine cognitive dysfunction disorder. Recent research has provided some support for the use of docosahexaenoic acid (DHA) in the improvement of memory and health status (Araujo et al. 2005) and medium-chain triglycerides in improving performance in cognitive testing in dogs (Pan et al. 2010). Medium-chain triglycerides may help with this condition by providing the brain with ketones as an alternate energy source (Pan et al. 2010). It is unclear if these fats may also aid in the prevention of cognitive dysfunction disorder; further research is needed.

The addition of medium-chain triglycerides to the diet has been investigated as a treatment for cognitive dysfunction in dogs (Pan et al. 2010) and dogs with epilepsy. A six-month prospective, randomized, double-blinded, placebo crossover dietary trial was conducted in dogs with idiopathic epilepsy. The investigators reported that seizure frequency and monthly seizure days were significantly lower in dogs finishing the test diet than those eating the placebo diet (Law et al. 2015). Another approach to treating canine cognitive dysfunction has been the development of diets that incorporate antioxidants and mitochondrial co-factors. One diet has been shown to improve canine cognitive dysfunction in both laboratory and clinical trials (Head 2007). The goals of the diet are to use antioxidants and mitochondrial co-factors to reduce the production of reactive oxygen species (ROS) and facilitate their clearance from the body, to slow the progression of age-related pathologies and cognitive decline by reducing oxidative damage (Christie et al. 2010).

Despite documented alterations in immune and antioxidant parameters in dogs and cats, as well as clinical improvement in cognitive function in dogs, existing studies do not address the possible preventive or long-term effects of these supplements and diets, and whether animals consuming them will live longer or have a lower incidence of disease. Long-term studies are necessary to address some of these questions. However, the lack of data in some cases is not a fatal flaw, although it does necessitate careful evaluation of the food and its claims and supportive research. In many cases the diets or supplements are unlikely to be harmful, but may not help in all animals.

Feeding Recommendations for Mature Dogs and Cats

The major objectives of a feeding program designed for an older pet should include the maintenance of health and an optimal body weight, the slowing or prevention of chronic disease, and the improvement of clinical signs of diseases that may already be present. When determining dietary recommendations for older pets, it is important to complete a thorough nutritional evaluation of the animal. A thorough evaluation includes evaluation of the pet, diet, and feeding management program. Evaluation of the animal includes a complete medical history and thorough physical examination (including body weight and body condition score).

Elderly dogs or cats that are healthy, in a lean body condition, and eating an appropriate

diet do not need to be changed to another diet simply based on their age. It is not appropriate in many cases (especially in dogs) to feed older animals ad libitum, as this predisposes them to obesity. Owners should be instructed to monitor their animal's food intake, as alterations may indicate the presence of an underlying disease process. Proper care of the pet's teeth and gums is essential to prevent a reduction in food intake secondary to dental problems. Based on the animal's physical condition, regular and sustained periods of exercise should be recommended for all patients. Regular exercise helps maintain muscle tone and optimal body weight, and enhances circulation. If a dietary change is necessary, it can be done gradually over a period of at least a week.

Once it has been determined how much to feed, feeding management should also be discussed with the owner. Dividing the number of calories into small multiple meals throughout the day will help minimize hunger and begging, as well as possibly increase the metabolic rate. Treats and snacks are important to the human–animal bond and should not be eliminated. It is important, however, that the calories contributed by treats be accounted for. As with all life stages, treats and snacks should never make up more than 10% of the animal's daily calorie intake.

Weight Loss

In contrast to obese animals, geriatric dogs and cats may have the problem of unintended weight loss, and this may often be overlooked. This weight loss may be associated with an increase or decrease in food intake. If the animal is consuming more food secondary to a recent change to a food with a lower caloric density, this response could be normal. Less energy-dense pet foods may be inappropriate for an animal with unusually high energy needs or an active lifestyle. Alternatively, an underlying metabolic process may be present.

A decline in food intake may occur for many reasons. In human geriatric medicine they use the mnemonic of nine "Ds" to describe the common causes of weight loss in their patients: dentition, dysgeusia (distortion of taste), diarrhea, disease, depression, dementia, dysfunction, drugs, and "do not know" (Masoro 1994). Most of these nine Ds can be applied to our veterinary patients as well. If a specific cause for unintended weight loss cannot be determined, symptomatic treatment for weight loss should be instituted. Feeding an energy-dense, nutrient-dense, highly palatable food more frequently would be appropriate. Examples include, but are not limited to, diets designed for growth, critical care formulas, or offering cat food to dogs.

Feeding and environmental modifications may be helpful as well. Food intake can be stimulated by serving fresh food, moistening dry food, warming food to body temperature, and having the client encourage the pet during eating. Feeding the animal away from the other household pets in a noise- and stress-free environment may also be helpful. One should make sure that the pet's nasal passages are clear, as dogs and cats rely on olfaction to select food. Bowls for cats should be wide and shallow so they do not touch their whiskers, as that can decrease food intake.

Assessment

Recently experts have been recommending that an appointment for an elderly pet include blood, fecal, and urine analyses on a routine basis (Fortney 2010). Although many of these tests are not sensitive indicators of nutritional status, they may indicate the presence of a subclinical process that may be nutrient responsive. Similar to other life stages, senior dogs and cats should maintain a lean body condition. In cases where animals are gaining weight, action should be taken promptly by implementing calorie restriction. Alternatively, previously healthy animals that begin to experience unintended weight loss or loss of lean body mass should receive a thorough examination and diagnostic workup. Nutritional strategies to address any underlying conditions or that encourage an increase in food intake should be instituted immediately.

Summary

- A complete diet history should be obtained and updated at every visit for every patient.
- The best diet will vary from animal to animal. Each dog and cat should be evaluated as an individual.
- Careful consideration should be given to the animal, the diet, and the animal's environment when making a dietary recommendation.
- Dietary recommendations should be appropriate for the animal's life stage.
- Treats and snacks are an important part of the human–animal bond and should be included in a feeding program. The amount of energy provided from snacks and treats should never exceed more than 10% of the patient's daily calorie intake.
- Regardless of life stage, all dogs and cats should be fed to maintain a lean body condition.
- Each patient's feeding program should be assessed at every visit and adjustments made as indicated based on the animal's body condition, life stage, and general health.

References

Allen, T. and Roudebush, P. (1990). Canine geriatric nephrology. *Compend. Contin. Educ. Pract. Vet.* 12 (7): 909–917.

Anantharaman-Barr, H.G., Gicquello, P., and Rabot, P. (1991). The effect of age on digestibility of macronutrients and energy in the cat" (abstract). In: *Proceedings of the British Small Animal Veterinary Association Congress*, 164.

Araujo, J.A., Studzinski, C.M., Head, E. et al. (2005). Assessment of nutritional interventions for modification of age-associated cognitive decline using a canine model of human aging. *Age* 27: 27–37.

Bebiak, D.M., Lawler, D.F., and Reutzel, L.F. (1987). Nutrition and management of the dog. *Vet. Clin. N. Am. Small Anim. Pract.* 17: 505–533.

Biourge, V.C., Groff, J.M., Munn, R.J. et al. (1994). Experimental induction of hepatic lipidosis in cats. *Am. J. Vet. Res.* 55: 1291–1302.

Bovee, K.C., Joyce, T., Reynolds, R., and Segel, S. (1978). Spontaneous Fanconi syndrome in the dog. *Metabolism* 1978 (27): 45–52.

Bradshaw, J.W. (2006). The evolutionary basis for the feeding behavior of domestic dogs (Canis familiaris) and cats (Felis catus). *J. Nutr.* 136: 1927S–1931S.

Brown, S.A. (1997). Kidney function and aging. *Proceedings from the Fifteenth Annual Veterinary Medical Forum*, Lake Buena Vista, FL (22 May). American College of Veterinary Internal Medicine.

Brown, S.A., Finco, D.R., Crowell, W.A. et al. (1991). Dietary protein intake and the glomerular adaptations to partial nephrectomy in dogs. *J. Nutr.* 121: S125–S127.

Buffington, C.A., Branam, J.E., and Dunn, G.C. (1989). Lack of effect of age on digestibility of protein, fat and dry matter in beagle dogs. In: *Nutrition of the Dog and Cat* (ed. I.H. Burger and J.P.W. Rivers), 397. Cambridge: Cambridge University Press.

Case, L.P., Carey, D.P., and Hirakawa, D.A. (1995). Feeding management throughout the life cycle. In: *Canine and Feline Nutrition* (ed. L.P. Case, D. Daristotle, M.G. Hayek and M. Raasch), 209–270. St. Louis, MO: Mosby-Year Book.

Christie, L., Pop, V., Landsberg, G.M. et al. (2010). Cognitive dysfunction in dogs. In: *Small Animal Clinical Nutrition* (ed. M.S. Hand, C.D. Thatcher, R.L. Remillard, et al.), 715–730. Topeka, KS: Mark Morris Institute.

Clutton-Brock, J. (1999). *A Natural History of Domesticated Animals*, 2e. Cambridge: Cambridge University Press.

Cole, N.C., An, R., Lee, S.-Y. et al. (2017). Correlates of picky eating and food neophobia in young children: a systematic review and meta-analysis. *Nutr. Rev.* 75 (7): 516–532.

Costello, M.J., Morris, J.G., and Rogers, Q.R. (1980). Effect of dietary arginine level on urinary orotate and citrate excretion in growing kittens. *J. Nutr.* 110: 1204–1208.

Cowan, L.A., Kirk, C.A., McVey, S. et al. (1998). Immune status in old vs. young adult cats" (abstract). In: *Proceedings of the Sixteenth Annual Veterinary Medical Forum*, 734. San Diego, CA: American College of Veterinary Internal Medicine.

Cowgill, L.D. and Spangler, W.L. (1981). Renal insufficiency in geriatric dogs. *Vet. Clin. N. Am. Small Anim. Pract.* 11: 727–749.

Cupp, C., Perez-Camargo, G., Patil, A., and Kerr, W. (2004). Long-term food consumption and body weight changes in a controlled population of geriatric cats. *Compend. Contin. Educ. Pract. Vet.* 26 (Suppl 2A): 60.

Czarnecki, G.L. and Baker, D.H. (1984). Urea cycle function in the dog with emphasis on the role of arginine. *J. Nutr.* 114: 581–590.

Dantas, L.M., Delgado, M.M., Johnson, I. et al. (2016). Food puzzles for cats: feeding for physical and emotional wellbeing. *J. Feline Med. Surg.* 18: 723–732.

Day, M.J. (2010). Ageing, immunosenescence and inflammaging in the dog and cat. *J. Comp. Pathol.* 142 (Suppl 1): S60–S69.

Debraekeleer, J., Gross, K.L., and Zicker, S.C. (2010). Feeding reproducing dogs. In: *Small Animal Clinical Nutrition* (ed. M.S. Hand, C.D. Thatcher, R.L. Remillard, et al.), 281–294. Topeka, KS: Mark Morris Institute.

Delgado, M. and Dantas, L. (2020). Feeding cats for optimal mental and behavioral well-being. *Vet. Clin. North Am. Small Anim. Pract.* 50: 939–953.

Duch, D.S., Chow, F.H.C., Hamar, D.W. et al. (1978). The effect of castration and body weight on the occurrence of feline urological syndrome. *Feline Pract.* 8: 35–40.

Eisert, R. (2011). Hypercarnivory and the brain: protein requirements of cats reconsidered. *J. Comp. Physiol. B* 181: 1–17.

Elliott, J., Rawlings, J.M., Markwell, P.J. et al. (2000). Survival of cats with naturally occurring chronic renal failure: effect of dietary management. *J. Small Anim. Pract.* 41: 235–242.

Fahey, G.C., Barry, K.A., and Swanson, K.S. (2008). Age-related changes in nutrient utilization by companion animals. *Annu. Rev. Nutr.* 28: 424–445.

FDA (2018). FDA investigates animal illnesses linked to jerky pet treats. https://www.fda.gov/AnimalVeterinary/NewsEvents/ucm360951.htm (accessed November 11 2021).

Fettman, M.J., Stanton, C.A., Banks, L.L. et al. (1997). Effects of neutering on body weight, metabolic rate and glucose tolerance of domestic cats. *Res. Vet. Sci.* 62: 131–136.

Finke, M.D. (1991). Evaluation of the energy requirements of adult kennel dogs. *J. Nutr.* 121: S22–S28.

Fleeman, L., Dobenecker, B., and Foster, S.F. (2021). Is glucosuria in dogs fed jerky treats associated with excessive intake of soluble phosphorus? Abstract. 2021 ACVIM Forum research abstract program. *J. Vet. Intern. Med.* 35 (6): 2943–3079.

Flynn, M.F., Hardie, E.M., and Armstrong, P.J. (1996). Effect of ovariohysterectomy on maintenance energy requirement of cats. *J. Am. Vet. Med. Assoc.* 209: 1572–1581.

Fortney, W.D. (2010). Declining physiological reserves: defining aging. In: *Proceedings from the Companion Animal Nutrition Summit, Focus on Gerontology* (26–27 March), 1–6. FL: Clearwater Beach.

Goldston, R.T. (1989). Preface to geriatrics and gerontology. *Vet. Clin. N. Am. Small Anim. Pract.* 19 (1): ix–x.

Green, A.S., Ramsey, J.J., Villaverde, C. et al. (2008). Cats are able to adapt protein oxidation to protein intake provided their requirement for dietary protein is met. *J. Nutr.* 138 (6): 1053–1060.

Gross, K.L., Becvarova, I., and Debraekeleer, J. (2010). Feeding nursing and orphaned kittens from birth to weaning. In: *Small Animal Clinical Nutrition* (ed. M.S. Hand, C.D. Thatcher, R.L. Remillard, et al.), 415–427. Topeka, KS: Mark Morris Institute.

Gunn-Moore, D.A., Moffat, K., Christie, L.A. et al. (2007). Cognitive dysfunction and neurobiology of aging cats. *J. Small Anim. Pract.* 48: 456–553.

Ha, H.Y., Milner, J.A., and Corbin, J.E. (1978). Arginine requirements in immature dogs. *J. Nutr.* 108: 203–210.

Hannah, S.S. and Laflamme, D.P. (1996). Effect of dietary protein on nitrogen balance and lean body mass in cats. *Vet. Clin. Nutr.* 3: 30.

Harper, E.J. (1996). The energy requirements of senior cats. *Waltham Focus* 6: 32.

Harper, E.J. (1997). The energy requirements of senior dogs. *Waltham Focus* 7: 32.

Harper, E.J. (1998a). Changing perspectives on aging and energy requirements: aging and energy intakes in humans, dogs and cats. *J. Nutr.* 128: 2623S–2626S.

Harper, E.J. (1998b). Changing perspectives on aging and energy requirements: aging, body weight and body composition in humans, dogs and cats. *J. Nutr.* 128: 2627S–2631S.

Haslewood, G.A. (1964). The biological significance of chemical differences in bile salts. *Biol. Rev.* 39: 537–574.

Hayek, M.G., Massimino, S.P., Burr, J.R., and Kearns, R.J. (2000). Dietary vitamin E improves immune function in cats. In: *Recent Advances in Canine and Feline Nutrition* (ed. G.A. Reinhart and D.P. Carey), 555–564. Wilmington, OH: Orange Frazer Press.

Hayes, K.C. (1988). Taurine nutrition. *Nutr. Res. Rev.* 1: 99–113.

Head, E. (2007). Combining an antioxidant fortified diet with behavioral enrichment leads to cognitive improvement and reduced brain pathology in aging canines: strategies for healthy aging. *Ann. N. Y. Acad. Sci.* 1114: 398–406.

Hedhammar, A., Wu, F., Krook, L. et al. (1974). Overnutrition and skeletal disease: An experimental study in growing great Dane dogs. *Cornell Vet.* 64 (Suppl 5): 11–160.

Hoskins, J.D. (2010). Neonatal and pediatric nutrition. In: *Textbook of Veterinary Internal Medicine* (ed. S.J. Ettinger and E.C. Feldman), 666–668. St. Louis, MO: Saunders.

Houpt, K.A. and Beaver, B. (1981). Behavioral problems in geriatric dogs and cats. *Vet. Clin. N. Am. Small Anim. Pract.* 11: 643–652.

Houpt, K.A., Coren, B., Hintz, H.F. et al. (1979). Effect of sex and reproductive status on sucrose preference, food intake and body weight of dogs. *J. Am. Vet. Med. Assoc.* 174: 1083–1085.

How, K.L., Hazewinkel, H.A.W., and Mol, J.A. (1994). Dietary vitamin D dependence of cat and dog due to inadequate cutaneous synthesis of vitamin D. *Gen. Comp. Endocrinol.* 96: 12–18.

How, K.L., Hazewinkel, H.A.W., and Mol, J.A. (1995). Photosynthesis of vitamin D in the skin of dogs, cats, and rats. *Vet. Q.* 17 (suppl 1): 26–29.

Ikeda, M.H., Tsuji, H., Nakamura, S. et al. (1965). Studies on the biosynthesis of nicotinamide adenine dinucleotides. II. Role of picolinic carboxylase in the biosynthesis of NAD from tryptophan in mammals. *J. Biol. Chem.* 240: 1395–1401.

Jacob, F., Polzin, D.J., Osborne, C.A. et al. (2002). Clinical evaluation of dietary modification for treatment of spontaneous chronic renal failure in dogs. *J. Am. Vet. Med. Assoc.* 220: 1163–1170.

Kanchuk, M., Backus, R.C., Calvert, C.C. et al. (2003). Weight gain in gonadectomized normal and lipoprotein lipase-deficient male domestic cats results from increased food intake and not decreased energy expenditure. *J. Nutr.* 133: 1866–1874.

Kane, E., Rogers, Q.R., Morris, J.G. et al. (1981). Feeding behavior of the cat fed laboratory and commercial diets. *Nutr. Res.* 1: 499–507.

Kealy, R.D. (1999). Factors influencing lean body mass in aging dogs. *Compend. Contin. Educ. Pract. Vet.* 21: 34–37.

Kealy, R.D., Olsson, S.E., Monti, K.L. et al. (1992). Effects of limited food consumption on the incidence of hip dysplasia in growing dogs. *J. Am. Vet. Med. Assoc.* 201: 857–863.

Kealy, R., Lawler, D., Ballam, J. et al. (2002). Effects of diet restriction on life span and age-related changes in dogs. *J. Am. Vet. Med. Assoc.* 220 (9): 1315–1320.

Kearns, R.J., Hayek, M.G., Turek, J.J. et al. (2000). Effect of age, breed and dietary omega-6 (n-6) and omega-3 (n-3) fatty acid ratio on immune function, eicosanoid production, and lipid peroxidation in young and aged dogs. *Vet. Immunol. Immunopathol.* 69: 165–183.

Kienzle, E. (1993). Carbohydrate metabolism of the cat 2. Digestion of starch. *J. Anim. Physiol. Anim. Nutr.* 69: 102–114.

Kienzle, E. and Rainbird, A. (1991). Maintenance energy requirement of dogs: what is the correct value for the calculation of metabolic body weight in dogs? *J. Nutr.* 121 (11 Suppl): S39–S40.

Kienzle, E., Meyer, H., and Lohrie, H. (1985). Effect of differing protein/energy ratios in carbohydrate-free diets for breeding bitches on development and vitality of puppies and milk composition. *Adv. J. Anim. Physiol. Anim. Nutr.* 16: 73–99.

Laflamme, D.P. (1997). Nutritional management. *Vet. Clin. N. Am. Small Anim. Pract.* 6: 1561–1579.

Laflamme, D.P. (2005). Nutrition for aging cats and dogs and the importance of body condition. *Vet. Clin. N. Am. Small Anim. Pract.* 35: 713–742.

Laflamme, D.P., Abood, S.K., Fascetti, A.J. et al. (2008). Pet feeding practices of dog and cat owners in the United States and Australia. *J. Am. Vet. Med. Assoc.* 232 (5): 687–694.

Lavelle, R. (1989). The effect of overfeeding of a balanced complete diet to a group of growing Great Danes. In: *Nutrition of the Dog and Cat* (ed. I.H. Burger and J.P.W. Rivers), 303–315. Cambridge: Cambridge University Press.

Law, T.H., Davies, E.S., Pan, Y. et al. (2015). A randomised trial of a medium-chain TAG diet as treatment for dogs with idiopathic epilepsy. *Br. J. Nutr.* 114: 1438–1447.

Lawler, D.F. and Monti, K.L. (1984). Morbidity and mortality in neonatal kittens. *Am. J. Vet. Res.* 45: 1455–1459.

Legrand-Defretin, V. and Munday, H.S. (1993). *Feeding dogs and cats for life. In: The Waltham*

Book of Companion Animal Nutrition (ed. I.H. Burger), 57–68. Oxford: Pergamon Press.

Lewis, L.D., Morris, M.L. Jr., and Hand, M.S. (1987a). Nutrients. In: *Small Animal Clinical Nutrition III*, 1-9-1-10. Topeka, KS: Mark Morris Associates.

Lewis, L.D., Morris, M.L. Jr., and Hand, M.S. (1987b). Dogs—feeding and care. In: *Small Animal Clinical Nutrition III*, 3-1-3-32. Topeka, KS: Mark Morris Associates.

Linde-Forsberg, C. (2010). Abnormalities in canine pregnancy, parturition, and the periparturient period. In: *Textbook of Veterinary Internal Medicine* (ed. S.J. Ettinger and E.C. Feldman), 1890–1901. St. Louis, MO: Elsevier Saunders.

Lloyd, L.E. and McCay, C.M. (1954). The use of chromic oxide indigestibility and balance studies in dogs. *J. Nutr.* 53: 613–621.

Lloyd, L.E. and McCay, C.M. (1955). The utilization of nutrients by dogs of different ages. *J. Gerontol.* 10: 182–187.

Loveridge, G.G. (1986). Bodyweight changes and energy intake of cats during gestation and lactation. *Ani. Tech.* 37 (1): 7–15.

Loveridge, G.G. and Rivers, J.P.W. (1989). Bodyweight changes and energy intakes of cats during pregnancy and lactation. In: *Nutrition of the Dog and Cat* (ed. I.H. Burger and J.P.W. Rivers), 113–132. Cambridge: Cambridge University Press.

Lund, E.M., Armstrong, P.J., Kirk, C.A. et al. (1999). Health status and population characteristics of dogs and cats examined at private veterinary practices in the United States. *J. Am. Vet. Med. Assoc.* 214: 1336–1341.

Maher, E.W. and Rush, J. (1990). Cardiovascular changes in the geriatric dog. *Compend. Contin. Educ. Pract. Vet.* 12 (7): 921–931.

Markham, R.W. and Hodgkins, E.M. (1989). Geriatric nutrition. *Vet. Clin. N. Am. Small Anim. Pract.* 19: 165–185.

Martin, L., Siliart, B., Dumon, H. et al. (2001). Leptin, body fat content and energy expenditure in intact and gonadectomized adult cats: a preliminary study. *J. Anim. Physiol. Anim. Nutr.* 85 (7–8): 195–199.

Masoro, E.J. (1994). Energy intake and the aging process. *Nutr. MD.* 1994. 20 (6): 1–2.

Massimino, S., Kearns, R.J., Loos, K.M. et al. (2003). Effects of age and dietary beta-carotene on immunological variables in dogs. *J. Vet. Intern. Med.* 17 (6): 835–842.

McMillan, F.D. (2013). Stress-induced and emotional eating in animals: a review of the experimental evidence and implications for companion animal obesity. *J. Vet. Beha. Clin. Appl.* 8: 376–385.

Meydani, S.N. and Hayek, M.G. (1995). Vitamin E and aging immune response. *Clin. Geriatr. Med.* 11 (4): 567–576.

Meyer, J. and Stadtfeld, G. (1980). Investigation on the body and organ structure of dogs. In: *Nutrition of the Dog and Cat* (ed. R.S. Andersen), 15–30. Oxford: Pergamon Press.

Morris, J.G. (1999). Ineffective vitamin D synthesis in cats is reversed by an inhibitor of 7-dehydrocholosterol-_7-reductase. *J. Nutr.* 129: 903–908.

Morris, J.G. (2002). Idiosyncratic nutrient requirements of cats appear to be diet-induced evolutionary adaptations. *Nutr. Res. Rev.* 15: 153–168.

Morris Animal Foundation (1998). *Animal Health Survey*. Denver, CO: Morris Animal Foundation.

Morris, J.G., Trudell, J., and Pencovic, T. (1977). Carbohydrate digestion by the domestic cat (*Felis catus*). *Br. J. Nutr.* 37: 365–373.

Morton, G.J., Meek, T.H., and Schwartz, M.W. (2014). Neurobiology of food intake in health and disease. *Nat. Rev. Neurosci.* 15: 367–378.

Moser, E.A. (1991). Dietetics for geriatric dogs. *Compend. Contin. Educ. Pract. Vet.* 13: 1762–1765.

Mosier, J.E. (1977). Nutritional recommendations for gestation and lactation in the dog. *Vet. Clin. N. Am. Small Anim. Pract.* 7: 683–693.

Munday, H.S. and Earle, K.E. (1991). Energy requirements of the queen during lactation and kittens from birth to 12 weeks. *J. Nutr.* 121: S43–S44.

Mundt, H.C. (1991). Nutrition of old dogs. *J. Nutr.* 121: S41–S42.

National Research Council (NRC) (2006). *Nutrient Requirements of Dogs and Cats*. Washington, DC: National Academies Press.

Neilson, J.C., Hart, B.L., Cliff, K.D. et al. (2001). Prevalence of behavioral changes associated with age-related cognitive impairment in dogs. *J. Am. Vet. Med. Assoc.* 218: 1787–1791.

Nguyen, P.G., Dumon, H.J., Siliart, B.S. et al. (2004). Effects of dietary fat and energy on body weight and composition after gonadectomy in cats. *Am. J. Vet. Res.* 65: 1708–1713.

Ontko, J.A. and Phillips, P.H. (1958). Reproduction and lactation studies with bitches fed semipurified diets. *J. Nutr.* 65: 211–218.

Pan, Y., Larson, B., Araujo, A.A. et al. (2010). Dietary supplementation with medium-chained TAG has long-lasting cognition-enhancing effects in aged dogs. *Br. J. Nutr.* 103 (12): 1746–1754.

Papasouliotis, K., Sparkes, A.H., Gruffydd-Jones, T.T. et al. (1996). Breath hydrogen assessment of orocaecal transit time in cats: the effect of age. In: *Proceedings from the Fourteenth Annual Veterinary Medical Forum*, 775. San Antonio, TX: American College of Veterinary Internal Medicine.

Park, T., Rogers, Q.R., and Morris, J.G. (1999). High dietary protein and taurine increase cysteine desulfhydration in kittens. *J. Nutr.* 129: 2225–2230.

Patil, A.R. and Cupp, C.J. (2010). Addressing age-related changes in feline digestion. In: *Companion Animal Nutrition Summit, Focus on Gerontology*, (26–27 March), 55–61. FL: Clearwater Beach.

Peachey, S.E., Dawson, J.M., and Harper, E.J. (1999). The effect of ageing on nutrient digestibility by cats fed beef tallow-, sunflower oil- or olive oil-enriched diets. *Growth Dev. Aging* 63 (1–2): 61–70.

Peachey, S.E., Dawson, J.M., and Harper, E.J. (2000). Gastrointestinal transit times in young and old cats. *Comp. Biochem. Physiol.* 126 (1): 85–90.

Perez-Camargo, G. (2004). Cat nutrition: What's new in the old? *Compend. Contin. Educ. Pract. Vet.* 26 (Suppl 2A): 60.

Perez-Camargo, G. (2010). Feline decline in key physiological reserves has implications for mortality. In: *Companion Animal Nutrition Summit, Focus on Gerontology*, (26–27 March), 5–11. FL: Clearwater Beach.

Rinaudo, P. and Wang, E. (2012). Fetal programming and metabolic syndrome. *Annu. Rev. Physiol.* 74: 107–130.

Rogers, Q.R. and Morris, J.G. (1980). Why does the cat require a high protein diet? In: *Nutrition of the Dog and Cat* (ed. R.S. Anderson), 45–66. Oxford: Pergamon Press.

Rogers, Q.R. and Phang, J.M. (1985). Deficiency of pyrroline-5-carboxylate synthase in the intestinal mucosa of the cat. *J. Nutr.* 115: 146–150.

Rogers, Q.R., Morris, J.G., and Freedland, R.A. (1977). Lack of hepatic enzymatic adaptation to low and high levels of dietary protein in the adult cat. *Enzyme* 22: 348–356.

Romsos, D.R., Palmer, H.J., Muiruri, K.L. et al. (1981). Influence of a low carbohydrate diet on performance of pregnant and lactating dogs. *J. Nutr.* 111: 678–689.

Root, M. (1995). Early spay-neuter in the cat. *Vet. Clin. Nutr.* 2: 132–134.

Scarlett, J.M. and Donoghue, S. (1998). Associations between body condition and disease in cats. *J. Am. Vet. Med. Assoc.* 212 (11): 1725–1731.

Schauf, S., Coltherd, J.C., Atwal, J. et al. (2021). Clinical progression of cats with early-stage chronic kidney disease fed diets with varying protein and phosphorus contents and calcium to phosphorus ratios. *J. Vet. Intern. Med.* 35 (6): 2797–2811.

Schroeder, G.E. and Smith, G.A. (1994). Food intake and growth of German shepherd puppies. *J. Small Anim. Pract.* 35: 587–591.

Sheffy, B.E., Williams, A.J., Zimmer, J.F. et al. (1985). Nutrition and metabolism of the geriatric dog. *Cornell Vet.* 75: 324–347.

Speakman, J.R., van Acker, A., and Harper, E.J. (2003). Age-related changes in the metabolism and body composition of three dog breeds and their relationship to life expectancy. *Aging Cell* 5: 265–275.

Stella, J.L., Lord, L.K., and Buffington, C.A. (2011). Sickness behaviors in response to unusual external events in healthy cats and cats with feline interstitial cystitis. *J. Am. Vet. Med. Assoc.* 238: 67–73.

Stratton-Phelps, M. (1999). AAFP and AFM panel report of feline senior health care. *Compend. Contin. Educ. Pract. Vet.* 21: 531–539.

Sudadolnik, R.J., Stevens, C.O., Dechner, R.H. et al. (1957). Species variation in the metabolism of 3-hydroxyanthranilate to pyridinecarboxylic acids. *J. Biol. Chem.* 228: 973–982.

Taylor, E.J., Adams, C., and Neville, R. (1995). Some nutritional aspects of aging in dogs and cats. In: *Proc. Nutr. Soc.*, vol. 54, 645–656.

Teshima, E., Brunetto, M.A., Vasconcellos, R.S. et al. (2010). Nutrient digestibility, but not mineral absorption, is age-dependent in cats. *J. Anim. Physiol. Anim. Nutr.* 94: e251–e258.

Toll, P.W., Richardson, D.C., Jewell, D.E. et al. (1993). The effect of feeding method on growth and body composition in young puppies" (abstract). In: *Waltham Symposium on the Nutrition of Companion Animals, Abstract Book*, (23–25 September), 33. Adelaide, Australia.

Turner, R.G. (1934). Effect of prolonged feeding of raw carrots on vitamin a content of liver and kidneys of dogs. In: *Proc. Soc. Exp. Biol.*, vol. 31, 866–868.

Wannemacher, R.W. and McCoy, J.R. (1966). Determination of optimal dietary protein requirements of young and old dogs. *J. Nutr.* 88: 66–74.

Washizu, T., Tanaka, A., Sako, T. et al. (1999). Comparison of the activities of enzymes related to glycolysis and gluconeogenesis in the liver of dogs and cats. *Res. Vet. Sci.* 67: 203–204.

Wichert, B., Schade, L., Gebert, S. et al. (2009). Energy and protein needs of cats for maintenance, gestation and lactation. *J. Feline Med. Surg.* 11: 808–815.

Wills, J.M. (1996). Reproduction and lactation. In: *Manual of Companion Animal Nutrition & Feeding* (ed. N. Kelly and J. Wills), 47–51. Ames, IA: Iowa State University Press.

Wills, J.M. and Morris, J.G. (1996). Feeding puppies and kittens. In: *Manual of Companion Animal Nutrition & Feeding* (ed. N. Kelly and J. Wills), 52–61. Ames, IA: Iowa State University Press.

8

Commercial and Home-Prepared Diets

Andrea J. Fascetti and Sean J. Delaney

Introduction

According to a recent industry organization survey, 90.5 million American households (70%) have an animal companion (American Pet Products Association 2021–2022). According to an AVMA survey in 2020, there were 83.7 million dogs and 60 million cats. Advice regarding what and how much to feed is one recommendation every dog and cat caretaker should receive from their veterinarian. The discussion regarding what to feed an individual animal companion can be somewhat overwhelming as there are so many pet foods on the market. Many clients wish their veterinarian would recommend a specific diet (Crane et al. 2010), and in a study veterinarians were the most frequently cited source for information about pet food (Laflamme et al. 2008). While it helps to have specific recommendations on hand for clients after reviewing their animal companion's diet history, many clients may still want to discuss foods or feeding approaches that are unfamiliar to the veterinary practitioner. There are numerous pet food manufacturers in the United States, so it is impossible for the practitioner to be familiar with every company and its products. Regardless, one should have a working understanding of the variety of feeding practices and food types available to one's

client to facilitate conversations. This chapter will review the various types and market segments of commercial pet foods, including considerations related to their formulation, home-prepared diets, and special considerations with respect to feeding raw food.

Commercial Diets

According to one study, 93.2% and 98.8% of dogs and cats, respectively in the United States and Australia consume more than half of their daily calories from commercial pet foods (Laflamme et al. 2008). Commercial pet foods are available in four basic forms: dry, moist (retorted and cooked, frozen), semi-moist, and raw. Understanding the general characteristics and the potential advantages and disadvantages of each food type is helpful for client communication and diet recommendations.

Types of Pet Foods

Dry Food
Dry foods were the most common type of pet food fed to dogs in one animal caretaker survey (Laflamme et al. 2008). Dry pet foods on average contain between 3% and 11% moisture and more than 89% dry matter. This is the food type of choice for free feeding. In general, dry pet

Applied Veterinary Clinical Nutrition, Second Edition. Edited by Andrea J. Fascetti,
Sean J. Delaney, Jennifer A. Larsen, and Cecilia Villaverde.
© 2024 John Wiley & Sons, Inc. Published 2024 by John Wiley & Sons, Inc.

foods are the most economical form of food to feed due to lower packaging, raw material storage, and freight costs (Kratzer et al. 2022). Some, but not all, dry pet foods may offer dental hygiene advantages. Dry foods may be less palatable to some dogs and cats. This characteristic can be an advantage in patients that are overweight or obese, but a disadvantage in finicky eaters. In some (but not all) cases, manufacturers may use harsh and improper cooking and drying techniques that can result in a loss of nutrients (poor-quality foods may have low digestibility and therefore a reduction in nutrient availability).

Moist Foods

Historically, moist diets were often referred to as "canned" products, and their moisture content ranges anywhere from 60% to 87% (Crane et al. 2010). The term "canned" may no longer be appropriate given the wide variety of products that now contain a similar water content, such as pet food in trays and tubes (the latter frequently referred to as "chubs") or sealed in pouches and frozen, so the term "moist" will be used instead. Cats are significantly more likely to receive half of their diet from moist food compared to dogs (Laflamme et al. 2008).

Moist diets generally have a high level of palatability and contain high concentrations of meat and/or meat by-products. Compared to dry or semi-moist products they are often higher in fat, sodium, and phosphorus (Crane et al. 2010). These diets usually have a very long shelf life as they are produced using heat sterilization and vacuum preservation or are frozen. Moist products often have a lower energy density than dry or semi-moist foods on an as-fed basis. The higher water content and lower energy density may be useful in providing satiety and reducing calorie intake, which may be helpful in preventing obesity. Moist foods also are recommended as a method to deliver more water to a patient with urinary tract health concerns. A lower energy density, combined with the costs of production, creates a situation where moist products often have a

higher price per calorie compared to dry and semi-moist diets (Crane et al. 2010). This can be a major disadvantage for some clients if they are feeding moist food exclusively. The perceived advantage of being less energy dense can actually become a disadvantage if the animal is a finicky eater or underweight. Many clients do not like the odor and messiness of moist products and unused food must be stored in the refrigerator or freezer. Another potential concern can be seen in dogs and cats being exclusively fed some of the gourmet moist foods or chubs. While often very palatable, in some cases these foods are not nutritionally balanced or complete. Furthermore, such feeding practices can also encourage some cats and dogs to develop fixed food preferences so they will not eat another diet.

Semi-Moist Foods

Most semi-moist foods contain 15–35% water. These products are softer in texture than dry pet foods, contributing to their acceptability and palatability. The inclusion of organic acids and humectants such as simple sugars, glycerol, or corn syrup binds water molecules in the food and makes them unavailable for use by microorganisms. This processing technique helps to control water activity (the amount of water available to microorganisms) and reduces the growth of molds (Crane et al. 2010). Over the years there has been a reduction in semi-moist products on the market, but it is still not uncommon to find them as inclusion pieces in dry foods or as treats. Semi-moist foods generally have a high level of palatability, and feeders find them convenient because they are often packaged in single serving portions. Some clients also favor semi-moist foods because they lack the odor and mess associated with moist products and come in shapes similar to foods they consume (burgers, vegetables, etc.). Semi-moist foods can be expensive and will become dry if allowed to sit out for several hours. The high palatability of these foods can be an advantage in picky eaters or underweight animals. This advantage becomes a disadvantage in obesity-prone patients. These products should not be used in diabetics if they use a large amount of sugar or syrup.

Raw

These diets are often referred to by the acronym "BARF," which stands for "bones and raw food" or "biologically appropriate raw food" diet. It is unclear how many people are feeding their pets raw food diets; however, based on the growing number of commercially available raw food diets, one can surmise the number is growing, but likely they are still fed to only a small percentage of dogs and cats.

There are two forms of commercial raw foods on the market. The first are commercially available, "complete" foods, intended to be the sole source of nutrition, like any other commercial diet. These products are supplied in several forms. The most common include fresh raw food; frozen raw food, which the feeder thaws before serving; or freeze-dried raw food that can be rehydrated with water upon serving if the feeder so desires. Combination diets are the second type of commercial raw food diet commonly used. With this approach the client purchases a supplement mix that is then combined with raw meat that they purchase themselves to yield a nutritionally complete diet. The supplement may or may not contain carbohydrates. This approach is designed to allow the humans to rotate protein sources or choose protein sources with particular characteristics (e.g. organic, locally grown, etc.) for their animal companions. Proponents of raw food diets proclaim many health benefits associated with this feeding regime, stating that dogs and cats are carnivores and as such they evolved eating raw food. However, there have been no studies to date to support that this feeding approach has any long-term health benefits compared to feeding other types of pet food. Potential disadvantages will vary with individual raw diets, but may include the risk of nutritional imbalances, cracked or fractured teeth, gastrointestinal obstructions and perforations, bacterial contamination, and other potential zoonotic diseases (such as parasites). These concerns are discussed later in this chapter.

Terminology

Deciphering some of the terminology and descriptors used on pet food labels or in advertising and product-associated literature can be challenging. A full discussion of pet food labels is provided in Chapter 6, but some of the terminology associated with marketing and used to categorize pet foods is discussed here.

It is difficult for veterinarians and consumers alike to know which marketing terms and descriptors such as organic, natural, holistic, human (food) grade, premium, and super premium are regulated terms and which are solely marketing. Currently, only the terms "natural," "organic," and "human (food) grade" have regulatory guidelines associated with their use.

The Association of American Feed Control Officials (AAFCO) defines the term "natural" as:

> A feed or ingredient derived solely from plant, animal, or mined sources, either in its unprocessed state or having been subject to physical processing, heat processing, rendering, purification, extraction, hydrolysis, enzymolysis, or fermentation, but not having been produced by or subject to a chemically synthetic process and not containing any additives or processing aids that are chemically synthetic except in amounts as might occur unavoidably in good manufacturing practices. (AAFCO 2022)

Natural pet foods are sometimes marketed with the claim that they contain no artificial ingredients. This may or may not be true depending upon the company. One of the common additives that purchasers are concerned about are fat preservatives such as butylated hydroxytoluene (BHT), butylated hydroxyanisole (BHA), and ethoxyquin.

Products that do not contain a fat preservative will have a decreased shelf life because of problems with rancidity. The definition of "natural" includes ingredients that are subject to traditional processing methods such as rendering and extraction. Human purchasers are often unaware that "natural preservatives" such as vitamin E or mixed tocopherols, vitamin C, or rosemary extract may also be processed and/or extracted. The term "natural" also permits a disclaimer clause for products that contain synthetic components in order to assure nutritional adequacy, such as "with added vitamins and minerals." "Trace nutrients" may also be added to this disclaimer when purified amino acids such as taurine are added. Finally, veterinarians and their clients also must be cautious of products that contain natural additives such as herbs, because the safety of many of these compounds has not been tested.

According to AAFCO, the term "organic" has been defined as:

> A formula feed or a specific ingredient within a formula feed that has been produced or handled in compliance with the requirements of the USDA National Organic Program (Title 7, Part 205 of the Code of Federal Regulations). (AAFCO 2022)

Under these guidelines, a food may carry the following organic designations (United States Government Printing Office 2010):

- 100% organic: must have 100% organic ingredients and additives, including processing aids.
- Organic: at least 95% of the content is organic by weight.
- Made with organic: at least 70% of the content is organic, and the front product panel may display the phrase "Made with Organic" followed by up to three specific ingredients.
- Less than 70% of the content is organic: may list only those ingredients that are organic

on the ingredient panel with no mention of organic on the main panel.

Only the first two categories are entitled to use the USDA seal on their packaging.

The terms "human grade" and "human quality" are being used with increasing frequency these days on food labels and marketing materials. Very few pet foods could be considered officially "human edible" or "human-grade" or food grade. The United States Department of Agriculture (USDA) defines products fit for human consumption to be officially "edible." These foods have to undergo processing and inspection, and pass manufacturing regulations. The regulations are designed to assure safety for human consumption. For a foodstuff to be deemed edible for humans, all ingredients must be edible by humans and the product must be produced, packed, and held in accordance with federal regulations in the Code of Federal Regulations (CFR PART 117). If the conditions in CFR 117 are met for a pet food, human-grade claims are permitted. Products not meeting these conditions are listed with an unqualified claim and the product is considered to be misbranded. AAFCO provides guidelines for Human Grade Claims (AAFCO 2022). More information about AAFCO Human Grade Standards for Pet Products can be found at the following link: https://www.agriculture.nh.gov/publications-forms/documents/aafco-human-grade-pet-products-standards.pdf.

Other terms that have no legal definition include "premium," "super premium," "gourmet," and "holistic." These labels are used on a variety of foods with different nutrient profiles, ingredients, and quality. They can even appear on foods intended for supplemental feeding only. A client who is relying on these terms to select a diet may unknowingly choose a food that if fed solely could result in a nutritional deficiency in the long term. Further concern has been expressed about the term "holistic," as it may imply a therapeutic benefit when none may exist (Crane et al. 2010).

Market Segments

Pet foods are sold through a variety of market segments, and many clients will judge the quality of a food based on where it is purchased and how much money it costs (known as the Veblen effect). It is incorrect to assume that the amount of money spent on a diet will always equate to the quality of the food. The bottom line is that the quality among any group of diets sold in a particular outlet, whether it be a grocery store or an exclusive pet store, is going to be variable. Quality pet foods that can support all the life stages of dogs and cats can be found in all market segments or channels. A detailed discussion on how to evaluate pet foods and recommend diets to clients is provided in Chapters 1 and 7.

Commercial Dog and Cat Diet Formulation and Considerations

Commercially prepared diet formulation is often the most challenging work that an animal nutritionist can undertake. There are many considerations, which include several related but diverse fields such as agriculture, economics, analytical chemistry, statistics, computer science, food technology, engineering, veterinary medicine, microbiology, marketing, sales, and law. These areas all interact when formulating a scalable, commercially prepared food that may be fed to up to millions of dogs and cats as their sole source of nutrition. While the challenges can be daunting, the ability to impact the health of animal companions regularly and positively is unique, with few, if any, comparable opportunities for the animal healthcare provider. Given the brevity of this section, this should not be considered a primer, but rather a short outline of things to consider when formulating diets based on one author's (SJD) past experience working with various commercial animal companion food manufacturers.

At the top of the list of considerations for veterinarians considering evaluation (including any endorsement or "approval") and/or formulation of commercially prepared animal companion food should be the pursuit of advanced, structured training. This should include a graduate degree (i.e. Master's or PhD) in nutrition from an accredited university, a residency in veterinary nutrition approved by a formally recognized certifying body, and a mentorship/apprenticeship with a seasoned formulator. Failure to pursue this path can, put bluntly, lead to potential bias (see the Dunning–Kruger effect) that can harm not only one's profession and reputation, but also the very animal companions one has dedicated one's life to helping.

Ingredient Database Population

Ingredient Safety and Legality First

The world is filled with thousands of potential food ingredients. Most can provide wholesome nutrition while some may be toxic to certain species. Novelty can be a compelling marketing tool, but care must be taken to ascertain both the safety and the nutrient impact of any ingredient used in a commercially prepared diet. Apparent successful feeding of an ingredient in an uncontrolled and often limited sample size (e.g. "people feed this to their dog as a treat and they seem fine") is not adequate evidence to support its inclusion. To help keep the consumer safe, regional and country-specific regulations govern what foods or ingredients can be used in commercial products (see Chapter 5 for more details based on North American and European regulations). The regulatory approval process establishes animal feed ingredient definitions and assesses if an ingredient is generally recognized as safe (GRAS) or is an acceptable, with restrictions, food additive. Use of unapproved ingredients makes a commercially prepared food "adulterated" by definition and illegal to sell. This regulatory oversight can be very important as species variations exist, as is seen with common human foods such as garlic, onion, chocolate, grapes/raisins, macadamia nuts, kabocha squash, and so on being toxic to certain species like dogs and cats. Once an ingredient is determined to be safe and can be legally used in a commercially prepared food for the targeted species, one can then decide to further explore its feasibility based typically on availability, cost, and/or nutrient profile.

Ingredient Regulatory Considerations

Given the importance and cost of developing an accurate nutrient profile for ingredients one wishes to formulate with, the regulatory status of an ingredient should first be considered. In most jurisdictions, there are regulations and/or laws about what ingredients can be used in food and feed. Approval of new ingredients can be byzantine and seemingly glacial; however, that should not lead one to underappreciate its importance. As already noted, some ingredients can be toxic at concentrations tolerated in other species. To determine safety, expert panels may need to be formed and often these panels are composed of volunteers with other responsibilities. Marketing excitement can sometimes lead to impatience, but using an unapproved ingredient in a food can result in the inability to sell the product when regulators issue a stop-sale order. Some very small or "fly-by-night" companies may unintentionally or intentionally, respectively, "fly under the radar," and release products into the market with (an) unapproved ingredient(s). However, ignorance of or ignoring regulations comes with its own peril, including to the animal nutritionist professional's reputation. Being associated with an ingredient that is illegal to use or, worse yet, harmful is ill-advised. One must ascertain that an ingredient is legal for use in the species of interest and in the jurisdiction of sale. Relying on an ingredient being acceptable for use in human food is no guarantee that the same will be true for an animal companion. If the definition or status of an ingredient is unclear, reaching out to consultants and regulators is advised.

Ingredient Availability and Cost

The availability of an ingredient is a frequent initial consideration when exploring its utility. Seasonality of some foods can present several challenges. It can prevent the regular use of a food and discourage or prevent the use of a fixed formulation. In some cases, the nutrient composition may change with the season or over time (see the next section on nutrient profiles). Even without considering cost, if the likely demand exceeds the supply then an ingredient cannot be used. In many facilities, there can also be limits to the number of raw materials that can be properly and readily stored and handled. Consequently, if an ingredient's availability for procurement misaligns with production schedules, then it cannot be used as there may not be room to store it, or it could spoil following harvest and before it can be used. It may not be worth the effort to validate an ingredient and develop a new product offering using it if it can only be used at limited times or in restricted amounts. In addition, an ingredient may be expensive, especially if it is subject to a fad, and its concentration must be kept dilute to minimize costs. This minimal use can still have value from a marketing, if not a nutritional, perspective, as will be discussed later. Such an ingredient's low inclusion amount will be reflected in the ingredient declaration or by naming convention (i.e. it would be cited as a flavor).

Qualifying reliable sources for certain ingredients can also present a challenge. Companies that follow current good manufacturing practices (cGMPs) require extensive qualification processes for suppliers and raw materials. This means that it may not be feasible to use an ingredient if in order to meet demand, multiple suppliers and their version of the ingredient must be qualified. This can result in very novel ingredients being used first by small-scale manufacturers who need minimal quantities and are willing to expend more effort qualifying ingredients in exchange for a marketing distinction. Conversely, larger manufacturers may avoid very novel ingredients not due to a lack of innovative spirit/capability, conspiracy, or "profit over nutrition" as some commentators may suggest, but rather solely due to pragmatic concerns over sourcing.

Establishing Reliable Nutrient Profiles for Ingredients

The higher the amount of an ingredient included or the greater the reliance on an ingredient to meet a limiting nutrient, the greater the importance of an accurate nutrient profile for that ingredient. Nutrient variation needs to be accounted for using repeated and ongoing nutrient testing (as well as formulations with some flexibility to account for likely fluctuations). Testing methodology must be suitable for complex matrices to ensure accurate extraction, and adjustments need to be made for anticipated or known bioavailability or degradation from storage or processing (e.g. oxidation, Maillard reaction products). Nutrient concentrations that may need to be tightly controlled should be carefully assayed. As an example, one may need to reduce the concentration of sulfur amino acids from legumes, pulses, or beans by about 50% to address bioavailability due to ingredient interactions and the range of values obtained by laboratory analysis (Sarwar et al. 1989; Rafii et al. 2020; Reilly et al. 2020). Another common example is in long-chain omega-3 fatty acid variations between farmed marine fish and wild-caught fish. All nutrients present in each ingredient must be considered and accounted for. For example, one may be selecting a marine fish for its fatty acid profile and concurrently relying on its amino acid contribution; however, its potentially high vitamin D3 (cholecalciferol) concentration must also be assessed and accounted for, especially if formulating for dogs that are relatively vitamin D intolerant. Variations in nutrient concentrations can also

occur due to seasonality (wild-caught species only being available during the fishing season) as well as regional differences in soil conditions, rainfall, and the amount of light that can affect the nutrient profile of crops.

Given the potential variability of key or limiting nutrients, repeated analysis of representative test lots will be needed prior to final formulation. Modeling for worst-case nutrient concentrations (minimums and maximums) must be performed, as that can have a profound effect on ingredient inclusion and overall finished product cost. For instance, if data suggest a potential minimum concentration for a limiting nutrient that is 30% below the mean or average, one cannot formulate using the mean value and hope for the best, but rather the minimum value must be used unless a rejection specification is set and agreed to (unlikely) by the vendor/supplier when the mean is not met. This means the real cost of the ingredient in this example would become at least 30% higher given the potential requirement to include an overage for safety and to make sure finished product is never deficient in the limiting nutrient. If this potential ingredient cost increase is unacceptable, then a separate, purified source of this limiting nutrient could be sought and used. Consequently, the additional cost of a second source/supplier would need to be factored in.

Overall, any nutrient that is limiting or is regulated (for marketing or legal reasons) should be regularly assayed in a statistically significant way. Assays are typically done for raw materials and then for finished products. Because nutrient concentration outliers in raw materials can affect finished products, statistically representative sampling may be inadequate, and each lot may need to be assayed and a certificate of analysis (COA) obtained from the vendor or supplier. The COA will be used to verify that the limiting nutrient is within a pre-defined specification. The raw material is rejected if the specifications are not met. Failure to develop reliable raw material rejection specifications and testing/assaying protocols of raw materials and finished product can be a leading cause for finished products having deficiencies or excesses (e.g. thiamine deficiency with retorted cat food; vitamin D excess in extruded dog food).

Extrapolation of nutrient concentration data from generic reference databases can be a helpful start, but it remains just that, a starting point. In one of the author's (SJD) experiences, many entrepreneurial and newer companies are initially reluctant to make the investment in conducting nutrient analysis and in the time needed to await test results. However, the importance of not solely relying on a vendor's or supplier's sales materials, and verifying the nutrient concentrations oneself and at one's own expense, cannot be emphasized enough. For animal nutritionists, a large red flag against a potential formulation client would be resistance to nutrient analysis and/or inability to analyze raw materials (a thought-provoking analogy: would you be willing to be an architect for a building contractor who is unsure about the tolerances and grades of their construction materials?).

Ingredient Procurement

Sustainability

The selection of ingredients goes beyond establishing reliable nutrient profile data and legal/regulatory status. One must also determine whether it is a sustainable ingredient. This is not initially about environmental sustainability (although that can be important and related), but rather whether an ingredient's supply will be consistently available. Unique ingredients that are only novelties may not be worth developing. Transiently popular/available ingredients may require additional marketing and/or nutritional impact assessments as their inclusion may need to be very low due to the limited amount of material available. Additionally, one must be cautious about accepting what is seemingly the same ingredient from a different vendor or supplier if alternative vendors or suppliers are not thoroughly qualified. Unfortunately, vendors and suppliers can sometimes be opaque and take purchase orders for ingredients that they do not yet have full confidence in being able to procure themselves. Certainly, considerations of sustainability should include market forecasts as well as environmental issues. Logistics should also be sustainable as initially cited pricing may be free on board (aka FOB) at the origin and not include any shipping costs. Lastly, storage costs for ingredients that require temperature and/or humidity control may need to be factored in as well as the feasibility of necessary storage space depending on the facility/location.

Consistency

Ingredient variability is typically inversely proportional to how much ingredients are processed. Processing, whether by fractionating or purifying ingredient components, allows for specific nutrient or component targets to be hit. For example, a crude protein target should be easier to meet with the grain/milling fraction than with the whole grain itself. This extends to other ingredients and nutrients. Isolation of nutrient-rich components can also often be accompanied by drying or heating that may also improve shelf stability. Drying ingredients may be cost favorable as energy costs for transport, storage, and at the time of manufacturing (e.g. extruded diets) can be reduced. Ingredients that are stable in average ambient conditions are usable where specialized storage conditions (e.g. refrigeration) are not available or cost-effective.

In general, the less complex and varied the nutrient profile of an ingredient is, the easier it is to formulate as it avoids concurrent nutrient enrichment and/or dilution when trying to change a single nutrient concentration. An example of this may be a meat meal that has been defatted. One can increase overall crude protein concentration without also increasing dietary fat. For ingredients viewed as less favorable in the marketplace, dehydration can "benefit" ingredient order as one can then add less mass when dried compared to when raw or hydrated (see the next section).

Ingredient Declaration

A key marketing strategy is controlling the ingredient order on packaging. Ingredients must be listed in order of decreasing mass as added. Ingredient order can be manipulated by using fractionated ingredients, use of similar but varied or separately defined ingredients, and water balance. A commonly known strategy is to use fractions of a grain rather than the whole grain as this splits the mass across multiple ingredients that can be separately listed. As noted earlier, fractions can also make formulation easier and resulting finished products more consistent. The use of similar but distinct ingredients such as multiple grains, tubers, or legumes instead of just one kind, allows for them collectively to appear lower in the ingredient declaration (aka list). This diversity can also be seen as favorable to address perceptions of monotony as well to provide "more" nutrients.

A less well-known strategy is the potential ability to reconstitute spray-dried or similar shelf-stable and dehydrated animal flesh. Reconstitution during extrusion or during retorting allows a potentially more favorably perceived ingredient to move higher in the order, and also to be labeled as unprocessed animal flesh without terms or adjectives that indicate additional processing. The cost and quality of these dried animal flesh ingredients are higher, but can provide significant benefits from formulating, manufacturing, and marketing perspectives. It can be hard, if not impossible, as a purchaser to determine if this is being done to ingredients in a finished product without visible inclusions (where actual pieces of an ingredient can be seen in the finished product). Consequently, there are significant concerns that this practice could intentionally be misleading and disingenuous.

Although ingredients that weigh more need to appear higher on ingredient declarations, ingredients of the same weight can be listed in whatever order the manufacturer wishes. Thus, top-listed ingredients may be used in exactly equal amounts to allow for more favorable ingredients to appear first and less favorable ingredients, typically with lower cost, to be listed lower. Considerable effort can be put into ingredient order and formulation efforts can be largely focused on optimization at the least cost while still meeting nutrient profile targets. Very low inclusion concentrations may also be used for highly favorable but expensive and/or hard to handle/utilize/source ingredients more to be attractive to the purchaser than for any nutritional impact of the ingredient. As a result, some ingredients highlighted in product advertisements or on packaging may only appear near other very low-inclusion supplements such as flavoring or minerals. Sometimes the inclusion is so low that they may appear among vitamins or, in extreme cases, after vitamins, suggesting that only a trivial amount is added. The value of these types of ingredients is almost exclusively limited to marketing.

Formulation Software

Options

There are hundreds of variables that must be calculated when formulating a commercially prepared food. This includes not just the nutrient profile but also the desired ingredient declaration order and overall cost. It is impossible to do these calculations and iterations to the needed depth without specialized software. Commonly used homemade companion animal food formulation software like Balance It® (https://balance.it; co-owned by one author, SJD) does not assist with ingredient reordering or consider least cost; however, formulation software like Concept5 (https://cfctech.com/products/concept5/default.aspx) or MixitWin (http://www.mixitwin.com/mixitwin) does. These commercial software options can be quite expensive to license (thousands to tens of thousands of dollars) and not all come with a food database of nutrient profiles. None of these programs offers full optimization for ingredient order. Because of these limitations, there are ongoing attempts to create software that fully explores ingredient order and cost simultaneously. One author (SJD) successfully developed a computer cluster and specialized algorithms and software to do just that for a medium-sized, private pet food company over a decade ago. This software was able to identify significant cost savings for multiple formulations without impacting order or nutrient profile. It is anticipated that, as computing costs increase and machine learning (ML) becomes more widely used, formulation software will become increasingly more powerful and able to explore thousands of possible iterations automatically and unaided by a human technical expert. Current least-cost formulation software has a steep learning curve and involves additional elements that may be initially foreign to a recent animal nutritionist graduate (related to water balance and specific equipment considerations like flow rate) as will be discussed in a later section.

Limitations

Given the potentially infinite number of variations, most least-cost formulation software solutions may control for only a handful of nutrients and nutrient relationships while determining the least-cost option with available/selected ingredients. This means that formulating a solution for more than 40 targeted nutrients and their ranges is not possible with available least-cost formulation software. Instead, for example, macronutrients and possibly macrominerals may be the focus and then one fills in the remainder of the nutrients with purified supplements/premixes based on limiting nutrient(s) to meet the overall desired nutrient profile. This can, however, result in significant overages for some nutrients. This approach along with software limitations can make the formulation of therapeutic foods challenging, especially in instances where very narrow acceptable ranges for numerous nutrients exist.

Equipment

The processing equipment that will be used for a specific formulation must be known and its effects on ingredients, nutrients, and food should be well understood.

Extruder

For extruded food, one must know if a preconditioner is used and what its capabilities are. Preconditioners can add "functionality" to some ingredients by heating and/or pre-cooking ingredients before they enter the barrel of the extruder. The degree of preconditioning can have effects on the overall settings used during extrusion. Heating of higher-fat ingredients may change their flow characteristics (e.g. congealed fat versus liquid fat or oil viscosity). Residence time or transit time through the extruder can be reduced if some starches are partially gelatinized by cooking in the preconditioner. If this preconditioning is unavailable, use of pre-gelatinized starches may be needed to limit energy inputs or, at times, to get the necessary binding for the kibble matrix to stick together and avoid unacceptable amounts of "fines" (e.g. crumbs found at the bottom of a bag of kibble) or "re-work" (e.g. extruded material that must be re-ground and re-extruded to attain the desired kibble shape and structure, leading to additional thermal processing and affecting bioavailability and reduction in facility yield). Higher inclusions of materials that do not bind well can be improved or harmed through preconditioning. The extrusion line operator may also need to be consulted as energy inputs and yields can be improved with some line settings that may not be beneficial to the finished product and overall "cook" (i.e. percent gelatinization).

There are different types of extruders, and some rely more on thermal processing versus mechanical forces/friction to achieve "cook." This can have a significant effect on what is referred to as "flow rate." Flow rate generally refers to the ratio of "slurry" (or homogenized wet ingredients) to dry ingredients that can be used with a specific extruder. Basically, the greater the flow rate, the higher the slurry inclusion can be. If the flow rate goes beyond the extruder's capability, the kibble coming off the die will not hold its shape or stay intact during conveyance and drying. Certain conveyance systems can better help hold desired shapes than others, which then allows for some increase in flow rate. Kibble coming off the extruder still needs to be dried and is moldable until it is dried.

Flow-rate limits have a direct effect on formulations as one will be limited on how much fresh or higher-moisture ingredients can be used. This can be of great importance depending on marketing, ingredient declarations, and other claims that are desired. It can also trigger the use of sprayed dried animal flesh, which can be considered by some as reconstituted, during the injection of adequate steam by the extruder or added processing water in other cooking methods/steps. When this is done, careful calculation of water balance is needed. The manufacturing team may also be concerned about the effect on yield (or tons per hour rates) and energy costs if significant amounts of water must be removed, or on stability if water activity is raised. Overall, there can be important considerations for ingredient selection based on the specific extrusion line used.

Canning/Retorting Line

Canning or retorting presents additional challenges especially as it relates to desired consistency and final finished product appearance. Whether visible inclusions of ingredients like vegetables and/or meat cuts and gravy are desired, or for a pâté or loaf-type product, one needs to consider the types of available equipment and adjust ingredients to ensure that adequate gelling agents like soluble fibers are used.

Availability of Pilot Plant or Line

There are many variables involved and numerous unique interactions can happen during extrusion or retorting. Consequently, the availability of a pilot plant or line can be very useful for testing new products and processes. When one is not available, the importance of close monitoring and active adjustments when first producing a new formulation on production equipment cannot be overemphasized, especially for extrusion. Material that binds too much can clog the extruder die or even the barrel. This can lead to processing down time that is far longer than desired or scheduled for a test run. In addition, test runs on production lines can be very expensive as they are often set up to run using larger volumes of material resulting in higher raw material costs for each test run. However, there is no substitute for producing a formulation to verify feasibility. This allows for gathering needed data including percentage of gelatinization, water activity, nutrients, oxidation rate, and so on. If an adequate amount of test product is produced, digestibility trials to more accurately predict calorie content can be conducted. One can also determine stool quality and palatability compared to a previous formula iteration of the same product or as compared to a competitive product. This may provide needed insight for adjusting purified vitamins, preservatives/antioxidants, "natural flavors," added palatines, or dietary fiber concentrations (typically insoluble fiber if increased stool firmness is desired). Costly production runs that may need to be completely reworked or scrapped as waste can be avoided by using test runs, because, even with experienced formulators and operators, the unforeseen can happen, and any means to limit losses and delays will be helpful.

Guaranteed Analysis Target

When formulating, one begins with the target percentages for the macronutrients, protein, fat, and carbohydrate by difference (i.e. 100% − protein % + fat % + moisture % + ash % + crude fiber % = carbohydrate by difference). This directly drives the guaranteed analysis minimums and maximums. These targets are typically first driven by the nutrient requirements of the target species and its life stage. Once nutrient needs are met, further adjustments or refinements to the targets are made based on an analysis of competitive products. Although "specmanship" can be considered a fool's errand, it can still be important for marketing. One may wish to have a comparable or a higher concentration for a macronutrient that is perceived as beneficial (e.g. protein). In addition, fat may need to be increased to hit a desired calorie content or energy density which may convey that a product is higher quality or provides more value (e.g. less backyard cleanup) to some purchasers.

Ingredient Declaration Order

After setting the guaranteed analysis targets, formulators will often have a concurrent request from the marketing team to have a certain ingredient declaration order. As noted previously, this order is based on mass with the highest-mass ingredient appearing first and the lowest last. However, if ingredient masses are identical, the manufacturer can order ingredients as it prefers. This typically means that ingredients with the lowest cost-to-calorie ratio are maximized and then the exact same amount of higher cost-to-calorie ratio ingredients (that may be perceived as superior) are added. This allows for ingredients that are perceived to be more favorable/desirable to be listed first or higher in the declaration order. One must also consider the regulations governing the ability to reconstitute dehydrated ingredients and then use the added water as part of the ingredient's total mass especially if that water is later removed during further processing, as with drying post extrusion (see more earlier about this practice).

Functionality

Some ingredients may be selected over others based on their "functionality," as discussed in the equipment (i.e. preconditioning) section. This can have non-nutritive impacts, but especially applies to binding ability as most commercially prepared pet foods are homogenized and then are required to hold a shape. This may be a kibble shape when extruded, or cuts/pieces or pâté/loaf shape/texture for retorted foods. There can also be a need during production to control functionality to prevent clogging the extruder barrel and to enable conveyance during kibble drying. In addition to holding a shape, there may be a desired finished product color as well as a mouth feel or texture. Certain colors and textures may not be achievable with ingredients that meet other requirements like macronutrient percentages or ingredient declaration order. Ideally, ingredients should meet all the requirements simultaneously. For example, one might want a green finished product and use more plant-based ingredients that are green to do so.

Shelf Life

Shelf life is the result of a combination of water activity, fat rancidity, and vitamin degradation control or mitigation.

To protect the food from spoiling, retorted products rely on their packaging, whether that be a can, carton, pouch, or tray. This is achieved by making the product essentially sterile and then ensuring that the package creates a complete water and oxygen barrier. Because of this, no preservatives are required or typically used in retorted products. In contrast, extruded foods reduce moisture and add preservatives, which are mainly antioxidants to protect against fat rancidity. The reduction of moisture lowers the "water activity" to a point where microbes (i.e. bacterial and fungal) cannot grow due to a lack of free water (i.e. unbound water). Semi-moist products, mainly treats on the market now, can also use humectants to lower water activity and prevent microbial growth. The humectants used may be common ingredients, like salt and sugar, when making animal flesh jerky, or they can be chemicals like propylene glycol. However, care should be taken as some of these humectants can be toxic at high enough doses in some species (e.g. cats and propylene glycol).

Frozen foods use low temperature to prevent microbial growth and may or may not use antioxidants. Unfortunately, the most potent antioxidants are artificial or chemically produced and are less favored by purchasers for that reason (e.g. ethoxyquin, BHA, BHT, etc.). Consequently, naturally derived mixed tocopherols with varying vitamin E biological activity can also be used. These tocopherols, however, are not as effective and care must be taken with their use given the potential to impact vitamin K status (Delaney and Dzanis 2018).

Vitamin degradation naturally occurs over time. Natural forms of vitamins generally degrade more rapidly and are more subject to heat degradation. Adding chemical moieties to vitamins makes them less heat labile and protects against oxidation. This results in synthetic vitamins that can fortify and withstand heating processes and oxidation being used in products that are not in retortable packaging. While these modifications can make the vitamin source less friendly sounding on an ingredient declaration to some purchasers, it allows for products that will not spoil in days or weeks but rather over many months. Attempts can be made to solely use increased overages to meet vitamin guarantees, but there are few practical overages or purified sources of natural vitamins that will allow this without at least being cost prohibitive (the exception may be natural vitamin E). The marketing value of using natural vitamin E to meet the nutrient need when varied and artificial stereoisomers are also present in a product from mixed tocopherols added for preservation is likely low.

Palatability

Ultimately, commercially prepared food must be palatable to be viable as a product. As reductions in water activity and oxidation (generally) reduce palatability, the use of concentrated "natural flavors" is often seen with extruded foods. Retorted and frozen foods often rely on higher fat concentrations to improve palatability. Natural flavors are mainly digests of animal liver as well as familiar palatants such as salt, sugar, and some amino acids including monosodium glutamate. For formulators, one must thoughtfully consider palatants' inclusion not only due to high cost but also for any "free-from" marketing claims. Most notably, one must consider whether an ingredient is to be free from grains or animal-origin ingredients (aka vegan). For example, soy sauce, as a component in a "natural flavor" or palatant, cannot be used in a grain-free product, as it is made from wheat. Similarly, animal digests cannot be used in a vegetarian or vegan food. Some manufacturers of palatants are reluctant to share the full scope of ingredients used in their proprietary palatants due to concerns about industrial espionage and loss of competitive advantages, but for the reasons cited, formulators must know what is used when making formulations that must increasingly support "free-from" claims.

Least Cost

Once a formulator has determined the available ingredients with known nutrient profiles, guaranteed analysis targets, life stage/nutrient requirements, key ingredient declaration order, limits based on processing line, any functionality requirements, specific purified vitamins, moisture targets, overages to address shelf life given planned packaging, and palatability enhancers, one can attempt to formulate a least-cost formulation using specialized software. Least-cost formulations often need to be calculated to the fourth decimal point when pricing in US dollars. Many iterations should be attempted, as a few cents per pound (or kilogram) of finished product difference can mean savings of hundreds of thousands of dollars over time even for smaller pet food companies.

Although the goal is to develop a fixed formulation, one must be careful not to paint oneself into a corner or cut things too closely. This means that optimizing a formulation to the point where any foreseeable supplier or ingredient change results in one or more key finished product specifications not being met is not ideal. There should be some resilience to changes or, if there is a linchpin, specifications should be established to protect against failure. If a very narrow nutrient range must be hit, then key raw materials that provide that nutrient should be assayed for said nutrient on every lot for it to be either accepted or rejected. A COA with that specification may be required, and one can create a receiving procedure to verify that the COA meets the pre-determined specification. Understanding and tracing sources for these types of key nutrients are also vital to establishing specifications for raw materials.

Stool Quality and Digestibility

As previously mentioned, hopefully a pilot plant or test run is possible to produce enough food to conduct studies on stool quality and digestibility (or less commonly a life-stage feeding trial) depending on the intended claims. Palatability may also be tested so that adjustments can be made to the palatant used and to the inclusion concentration(s) based on performance. For more novel products, accelerated shelf-life studies (usually accomplished by increasing storage temperatures to higher than typical) can also be conducted. This allows any antioxidant preservative concentrations to be fine-tuned based on measures of fat rancidity and for vitamin overages to be increased, if insufficient, to avoid missing finished product vitamin minimum guarantees at the end of shelf life.

Labeling

Marketing claims should have been established early so that a formulation can support desired claims. One notable early consideration given its impact on timeline is the calorie content claim. Claims of superior digestibility may be dependent on calorie content claims. Calorie content claims are based solely on standard modified Atwater or energy conversion factors in most jurisdictions, unless the product is actually fed in a controlled digestibility trial. Digestibility trials must await at least a pilot-plant or test-run food, and packaging artwork and printing plates cannot be finalized until after digestibility trial data are available. Lastly, there can be a potential need to change antioxidant and vitamin concentrations based on accelerated shelf-life testing, which can result in increased launch lead times even with extrapolation.

Continuous Improvement

Formulations are never truly final and should always be subject to the concept of continuous improvement. This can take many forms and may be triggered by experience with ingredient sourcing and testing, additional production, nutrient analysis of finished product, market performance, and so on. Reformulations should be embraced by the formulator as opportunities to address any area that is not optimal and to look for opportunities for the formulation to be improved. Do not assume that performance with a newer formulation in actual animals fed the food will be comparable to the previous version without fresh testing. A classic example of the potential drift to inferior performance is with palatability. Often a two-pan preference test is used, and the performance of two foods is compared. If one food is a well-performing food and the other is a reformulation suspected to have potentially reduced palatability, there may be no significant difference. However, if in the next test the previously new formulation/food is compared to a third iteration, the difference may once again be insignificant, but would be significant if the third iteration were compared directly to the first iteration. Thus, controls like a competitor's food may need to be incorporated in testing to ensure that one is achieving continuous improvement and not continuous change instead.

Home-Prepared Diets

With the advent of complete and balanced commercial pet foods, the use of home-prepared diets has declined. However, over the past decade and a half there has been a growing segment of clients who are electing to home-cook diets for their dogs and cats; home preparation of food can include cooked or raw food feeding. A telephone survey of 1104 dog and cat caretakers in the United States and Australia found that fewer than 3% of dogs and cats received at least 50% of their daily diet from home-prepared foods (Laflamme et al. 2008). On the other hand, 30.6% of dogs and 13.1% of cats received "non-commercial" foods (home-prepared foods, leftovers, and table scraps) as part of their main meal. In this study, 17.4% of dogs and 6.2% of cats received over one-quarter of their daily diet from these non-commercial foods. While this number may seem low to some, it is important to note that this survey was conducted prior to the major pet food recall of 2007. Many nutritionists feel that this number has increased since that time.

There are many reasons why clients wish to prepare meals at home for their dogs and cats. Some of the more common ones include the negative press against commercial pet foods, the belief that home-prepared foods are closer to the natural diets of ancestral dogs and cats, the feeling of a stronger bond between the human and animal companions, and the ability to avoid undesired ingredients such as additives and preservatives or to use desired ingredients like raw ingredients (Laflamme et al. 2008). Many clients wish to follow philosophies that they incorporate into their personal approach to eating and apply those to their animal companion (e.g. vegetarian, low

cholesterol, organic, etc.) or believe that home preparing a diet is cheaper than purchasing a commercial product.

Most nutritionists agree that it is in the animal's best interest to eat a commercially available food if at all possible. A very important point to remember is that home-prepared diets have not typically undergone animal feeding trials or even laboratory analysis to confirm that they support the life stage for which they were designed. However, there are a number of medically appropriate reasons to institute a home-prepared diet in some patients. The major indication for placing an animal on a home-prepared diet is a medical condition that has special nutritional concerns not addressed in a commercial or veterinary therapeutic diet. One of the more common conditions where home-prepared diets have been extremely useful is in managing adverse food reactions. By feeding a home-prepared diet one can select a protein and carbohydrate source not available in commercial foods, avoid additives and preservatives, and maintain control over the type and amounts of ingredients used. In addition, home-prepared diets are often the only option for animals with multiple medical conditions. By selecting a commercial diet to treat one condition, the practitioner may be feeding in a method that is contraindicated for another. A common example is an animal with hyperlipidemia, a history of severe recurrent pancreatitis, and renal disease. Home-prepared diets are also useful for patients with medical conditions that necessitate the use of a veterinary therapeutic diet, but the diet is not well accepted by the patient for any number of reasons.

Nutritional Adequacy

Nutritional adequacy should be the first concern of every practitioner who has a patient that consumes a home-prepared diet. Only 16 of 54 human companions who were feeding their dogs and cats a home-prepared diet in one survey were using a recipe designed for dogs or cats (Laflamme et al. 2008). Eight were obtained from a veterinarian, three from the internet, and five from other sources (Laflamme et al. 2008).

The practitioner should be concerned about where clients obtain their recipes. Frequently, the recipes selected are from unknown or questionably reputable sources. In one survey, 89% and 93% of home-prepared elimination diets used for initial testing in dogs and cats, respectively, were not complete and balanced for adult maintenance (Roudebush and Cowell 1992). Nutritionally adequate home-prepared elimination diets for long-term use were only recommended 65% and 46% of the time in dogs and cats, respectively (Roudebush and Cowell 1992). A second prospective study recruited humans to home-prepare their dogs' food for a 30-day period. The home-prepared diets were evaluated and compared to the AAFCO's nutrient profile recommendations (Streiff et al. 2002). Of the diets, 35 fell below AAFCO recommendations with respect to calcium, phosphorus, potassium, zinc, copper, and vitamins A and E. These nutrients were not compared to NRC recommendations, but closer inspection of the results suggests that in some cases nutrient concentrations would have exceeded NRC minimums (NRC 2006). A more recent study specifically evaluated 49 maintenance and 36 growth diets for dogs and cats (Lauten et al. 2005). These diets were obtained from books that are frequently used by veterinarians recommending home-prepared recipes for their patients. Compared to AAFCO requirements for the respective life stage, 55% were found to be inadequate in protein or amino acids, 64% were inadequate in vitamins, and 86% were inadequate in minerals. These same diets were then compared to 1985/1986 NRC Nutrient Requirements of Dogs and Cats, respectively. In this case 34% were deficient in amino acids (taurine in all cases), 45% in vitamins, and 21% in minerals. Stockman et al. in 2013 reported on 200 recipes:

obtained from 34 sources (133 recipes were obtained from 2 veterinary textbooks and 9 pet care books for owners, and 67 recipes were obtained from websites). Of these, 129 (64.5%) were written by veterinarians, whereas the remaining 71 (35.5%) were written by nonveterinarians.

They added:

Only 3 recipes provided all essential nutrients in concentrations meeting or exceeding the NRC RA, and another 2 recipes provided all essential nutrients in concentrations meeting or exceeding the NRC MR; all 5 of these recipes were written by veterinarians. Nine recipes provided all essential nutrients in concentrations exceeding the AAFCO nutrient profile minimums for adult dogs; 4 of these also met or exceeded the NRC RA or NRC MR. Of these 9 recipes, 8 were written by veterinarians. Overall, most (190/200 [95%]) recipes resulted in at least 1 essential nutrient at concentrations that did not meet NRC or AAFCO guidelines, and many (167 [83.5%]) recipes had multiple deficiencies.

Concerns with regard to nutritional adequacy apply to raw home-prepared diets as well. One study evaluated the nutritional adequacy of five raw food diets. Two were commercial products, the remaining three home-prepared. All five diets had essential nutrients that were analyzed to be below AAFCO minimum recommendations (Freeman and Michel 2001). The home-prepared diets had excessive concentrations of vitamins D and E, as well as inappropriate calcium to phosphorus ratios.

More and more reports are beginning to appear in the literature with respect to the clinical consequences of feeding home-prepared diets that are not nutritionally adequate for the animal's life stage. Growth is one period where concerns are frequently reported, as this is one of the most nutritionally demanding life stages, and deficiencies and excesses are manifested quite rapidly (Tomsa et al. 1999; McMillan et al. 2006) (see Box 8.1 for an example). However, some of the published cases are in adults, thereby underscoring the risk involved for individuals at any life stage. Reports in younger animals are frequently related to inadequate calcium or improper calcium to phosphorus ratios

---

Box 8.1   Nutritional secondary hyperparathyroidism due to a home-prepared growth diet

The authors managed a case in a litter of feral kittens rescued by a local organization. One 2½-month-old female intact kitten was presented for evaluation. The client acquired the kitten at approximately 7–10 days of age (also fostering three other kittens of similar age). All kittens received a commercial colostrum and milk replacement formula (powder form). The kittens were weaned onto a home-prepared diet consisting of approximately 60% store-bought ground meat (beef, chicken, or turkey), and 40% fresh seasonal vegetables (carrots, green leafy vegetables, broccoli, kale, and/or celery root). Cooked bone meal (ground bones from the store) was also fed intermittently.

The first symptoms of lameness developed at approximately 2½ months of age when the kitten could not use her hind legs. She appeared to have feeling in her legs, could move them a little without bearing weight, and had normal bowel control. The following day another kitten in the household started to display similar signs with a hind limb lameness, and approximately one week later a third kitten began to show similar signs with a front limb lameness. The lameness varied in each cat, affecting different limbs, and varying in severity from day to day. The kittens all had good appetites and energy levels. The client reported that they still played (although they did not move their legs) and would drag themselves to the litter box.

On presentation, the kitten was bright and alert, with a body condition score of 4 out of 9. Physical examination revealed pain and a probable fracture in the left femur as well as pain in the lumbosacral area. The remainder of the physical and neurological examination was normal. With the exception of a high alkaline phosphatase (expected in a kitten of this age), the blood work was all within normal limits. Radiographic evaluation reported severe generalized decreased bone opacity with thin cortices. There was a mid-diaphyseal folding fracture of the left femur, a fracture of the left ileum, and possible compression of several of the sacral vertebrae; additional radiographs were recommended for further evaluation. Bone fragments were noted in the gastrointestinal tract (Figure 8.1).

A computer evaluation of a sample meal from the diet history was completed and revealed deficiencies in all the essential minerals and vitamins. The authors noted that while bone chips appeared in the gastrointestinal tract on the radiographs, the availability of calcium from that bone had to be questionable given the clinical signs. Based on the history, examination findings, and diet evaluation, a diagnosis of nutritional secondary hyperparathyroidism was made.

Due to financial concerns, no additional radiographs and diagnostics were performed. The caretaker was instructed to cage rest all of the kittens and to place them on a commercial kitten diet that had undergone and passed feeding trials for growth. Concerns about feeding nutritionally inadequate and raw food diets were also discussed.

The same kitten returned approximately one month later. She had grown and her behavior had returned to normal. Repeat radiographs reported a normalized bone density and repair of the fractures (Figure 8.2).

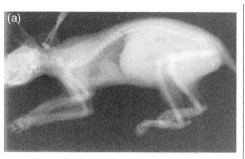

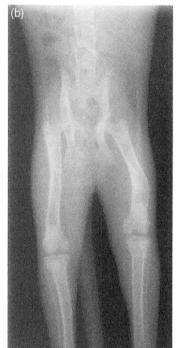

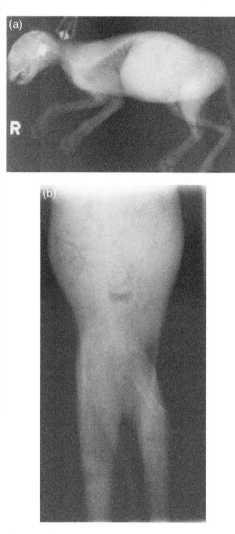

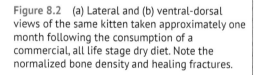

Figure 8.1 (a) Lateral and (b) ventral-dorsal views of a 2½-month-old kitten fed an unbalanced, raw home-prepared diet. Note the generalized decreased bone opacity and thin cortices, mid-diaphyseal folding fracture of the left femur, fracture of the left ilium, and possible compression of several of the sacral vertebrae.

Figure 8.2 (a) Lateral and (b) ventral-dorsal views of the same kitten taken approximately one month following the consumption of a commercial, all life stage dry diet. Note the normalized bone density and healing fractures.

(Tomsa et al. 1999; McMillan et al. 2006), leading to lesions or fractures in the long bones. Comparatively, clinical signs secondary to calcium deficiency in adults are frequently manifested as rubber jaw syndrome with resorption of the mandible or maxilla (De Fornel-Thibaud et al. 2007). While most reports are related to major mineral deficiencies or imbalances, other nutritional problems can occur. There is an interesting case series of growing and juvenile cats with pansteatitis associated with the consumption of high levels of unsaturated fatty acids in fish or pork brain–based diets (Niza et al. 2003).

Managing Patients Using Home-Prepared Diets

A diet history should be obtained on every patient, each time they are seen in one's practice. If a client mentions that they are preparing food at home for their animal, it is recommended that a copy of the detailed recipe (including the source) be obtained from the client and entered into the patient's permanent medical record. The client should also be asked about their reasons for opting to prepare food at home rather than purchasing a diet for their animal. This will help the practitioner understand the client's motivations, and such knowledge may be useful in directing them to a more appropriate alternative if necessary.

As the primary care provider, the practitioner is the first line of defense with respect to identifying and stopping feeding practices that are nutritionally inadequate. Chemical analysis of the home-prepared diet is one of the best methods of evaluating the adequacy of a particular recipe. However, it is cost prohibitive for most clients. It is virtually impossible to determine if a recipe meets a patient's nutrient needs by inspection alone; however, one can often identify areas of concern based on a quick overview. This type of review can provide a foundation for the practitioner's recommendation to have the diet evaluated and revised by a board-certified veterinary nutritionist® or evaluated by the veterinarian themselves using a nutritional software program. One online software program available to veterinarians for free is Balance It (see earlier), which has been shown to be "highly predictive of deficiencies or excesses of nutrients as measured via laboratory methods" (Stockman et al. 2013).

During initial inspection of the diet, one should try to identify the protein, fat, carbohydrate, vitamin, and mineral (especially calcium) sources. The absence of any one of these is an immediate indication that the diet should be evaluated further.

Protein and Amino Acids

When evaluating the dietary source of protein and amino acids, it is important to consider a multitude of factors. Is the protein source of animal or plant origin? Animal-based protein sources are recommended for both dogs and cats due to their pattern of essential amino acids. However, it is not unusual to see plant proteins as the major or sole protein source in a canine diet. Plant proteins can be used for feline diets, but are not recommended by these authors as it is often difficult to meet the cat's nitrogen and amino acid requirements using plant proteins, and diet palatability is typically poor. Plant proteins are also frequently limited in the essential amino acids methionine, lysine, and tryptophan.

Most plant proteins do not contain taurine, an essential amino acid for cats, and under some circumstances possibly a conditionally essential amino acid in dogs. Even when animal-based protein sources are used, these authors prefer to see supplemental taurine in every feline diet.

The taurine content in animal proteins can vary significantly, with muscle generally containing less taurine than organ meats (Spitze et al. 2003). Cooking also influences taurine concentrations, and it can be lost to a significant extent when using cooking methods that expose proteins to water, thereby leaching the taurine from the food (Spitze et al. 2003). These findings imply that if one does not cook the protein source, taurine deficiency is less of a concern; however, the literature does not support this thinking. Taurine deficiency has been recognized in cats that consume home-prepared diets using raw protein. One research update reported dilated cardiomyopathy associated with taurine deficiency in a group of growing cats fed a diet consisting solely of ground raw rabbit (Glasgow et al. 2002). A second study evaluated plasma taurine concentrations in sand cats (*Felis margarita*) fed either a commercial feline kibble or a raw food diet (Crissey et al. 1997). Despite a 15% increase in digestibility and a 40% increase in taurine content compared to the kibble diet, cats consuming the raw food diet had significantly lower plasma taurine concentrations. Although the plasma taurine concentrations were not below the point at which clinical taurine deficiency would be seen, they were reduced by approximately 25% during the 12-day study period. While arguably this is a crude estimate at best, if one were to project the continued rate of decline, plasma taurine would fall below the concentration where the clinical signs of taurine deficiency are frequently noted at approximately day 20 of raw food consumption. These effects would likely be more pronounced under the conditions of a more demanding life stage than maintenance, such as during growth or reproduction.

The exact mechanism of how raw diets can potentiate taurine deficiency is unknown at this time. The amount of taurine available to the cat from its diet is dependent upon a number of factors including the quality and quantity of dietary protein, as well as how that protein is processed (Hickman et al. 1990; Backus et al. 1994; Kim et al. 1996a, 1996b). These factors in turn influence gastrointestinal microbial numbers and/or species that can cause taurine loss by accelerating turnover of bile acids conjugated with taurine and decrease recycling of taurine by the enterohepatic route. These factors may influence changes in bacteria that favor those populations that degrade taurine. In addition to these factors, low levels of vitamin E in a diet can cause meat to lose taurine when it is processed and ground (Lambert et al. 2001).

Specific recommendations should be provided regarding the cut and fat content of the protein source for animal proteins. The fat content of a diet can vary considerably if different cuts of meat or poultry are used. The inclusion or absence of skin should be noted in the recipe and if using ground meat or ground poultry, the percentage of fat in the product should be specified.

Fatty Acids

Dogs and cats require linoleic acid (18:2 n-6) (NRC 2006). While animal fats contain some linoleic acid, an additional source is often necessary to meet the dog's or cat's requirement. Many common vegetable oils can be used as a dietary source of linoleic acid including corn, walnut, safflower (high oleic), sunflower, and soybean oil. Corn and walnut oils have the highest concentration of linoleic acid so one of them is needed in the least amount to meet the requirement. This can be very helpful if one is trying to limit the overall amount of fat in the diet. Many clients want to use olive oil since they are using it in their own diets to combat coronary artery disease. However, while olive oil is high in monounsaturated fatty acids, it is a poor source of linoleic acid, thereby requiring large amounts to meet the animal's requirement. In addition, dogs and cats do not develop clinically significant atherosclerosis leading to myocardial infarctions and death, likely due to differences in lipoproteins and life span compared to humans. Therefore, the use of olive oil is not often recommended. Cats also require arachidonic acid, found in high concentrations in animal fats and not in vegetable-based fats. This adds another layer of complexity in trying to meet the nutrient requirements of cats using vegetarian diets. Borage, blackcurrant, and evening primrose oils may be used, as these can supply gamma linolenic acid, a precursor for arachidonic acid.

Emerging evidence suggests that omega-3 fatty acids may provide some health benefits to dogs and cats, especially during growth and development (Bauer 2006). Specifically, benefits may be derived from docosahexaenoic (DHA, 22:5 n-3) and eicosapentaenoic (EPA, 20:5 n-3) acids. While alpha-linolenic acid (18:3 n-3) is often supplied in products by ingredients such as flaxseed or canola oil, dogs and cats cannot efficiently convert alpha-linolenic acid to EPA and DHA, so fish, krill, or algal oil sources are required (NRC 2006).

Carbohydrates

While carbohydrates are not required in dogs and cats (NRC 2006), one should note their presence or absence in the diet. Their absence, while not nutritionally essential, is noteworthy as the diet will then be one that is high in protein and/or fat. There are four carbohydrate groups from a functional perspective: absorbable (monosaccharides); digestible (disaccharides, certain oligosaccharides, and non-structural polysaccharides); fermentable (lactose, certain oligosaccharides, dietary fiber, and resistant starch); and non-fermentable (certain dietary fibers) carbohydrates (NRC 2006). While many view carbohydrates negatively (especially those in the absorbable and digestible categories) due to their high digestible starch content and the belief that such products are bad for dogs and cats (unsubstantiated scientifically), they often overlook the other nutrients supplied. For example, oatmeal can supply a significant amount of protein and fat to a diet. Carbohydrates also provide fermentable and non-fermentable carbohydrates in the form of dietary fiber. Soluble fibers are generally better energy substrates for gastrointestinal microorganisms than insoluble fibers due to their increased rate and extent of fermentation (NRC 2006). Prebiotics are one form of soluble fiber that may stimulate the growth and well-being of bacteria in the gastrointestinal tract, thereby supporting overall health.

Vitamin and Mineral Supplements

An obvious vitamin and mineral supplement should be readily apparent in every recipe. Many clients prefer to try to address their dog's or cat's vitamin and mineral needs using whole foods such as liver or bone rather than a manufactured supplement. Such an approach is very difficult to do and can heighten the risk of a nutritional deficiency or excess in the diet. Natural foods have tremendous variability in their vitamin and mineral content based on how and where the food source was raised, feeding or fertilizing methods, the part of the animal or plant used, and how the source is prepared. For these reasons, the authors recommend using a distinct vitamin and mineral supplement.

Some veterinary nutritionists and clients prefer to use a patented all-in-one veterinary supplement (Balance It brand, founded by one of the authors, SJD), which limits the number of ingredients added to the diet, whereas others prefer to use supplements designed for the human market to meet the vitamin and mineral needs of the patient. With this latter approach the number of ingredients that must be measured and added to the diet will increase significantly. This approach generally necessitates a calcium/phosphorus supplement; a multivitamin/multimineral supplement; a taurine supplement (for cats and occasionally dogs); iodized salt or light salt to provide iodine, sodium, potassium, and chloride; choline if methionine is limited in the diet (i.e. vegetarian diets); and then often additional zinc and/or vitamin B12, as many human vitamin/mineral supplements have lower concentrations of these nutrients. In some cases, however, this latter approach must be used if additional nutrient restriction is required beyond what an all-in-one veterinary supplement provides due to an underlying disease process. A common example includes dogs (and also cats) with chronic kidney disease requiring potassium restriction secondary to life-threatening hyperkalemia (Segev et al. 2010).

General Considerations

After reviewing the recipe for nutrient categories and specific ingredients, consideration should be given to the calories the recipe provides on a daily basis as well as the percentage of calories coming from each of the major nutrients: protein, fat, and carbohydrate. Home-prepared diets can be very energy dense depending on their ingredient composition. They are highly digestible in most cases and very palatable. This combination can predispose animals that consume them to weight gain and obesity if they are receiving too many calories a day and not being closely monitored.

The percentage of calories coming from protein, fat, and carbohydrate should be considered in light of the animal's signalment and health status. It is important that the nutrient distribution be appropriate if an animal is receiving a home-prepared diet to manage a disease. In some cases, this may also include the micronutrients. For example, in an animal with renal disease, one is not only concerned about the protein content but also phosphorus, sodium, and potassium. In the authors' experience if a recipe has not been formulated by a board-certified veterinary nutritionist, it is often very difficult to determine the calorie content, the percentage of calories supplied by protein, fat, and carbohydrate, and the micronutrient composition. The absence of any of this information is an indicator that the diet should be evaluated further.

One should inspect the recipe with regard to the instructions. In the ingredient list it should specify if units of measure are of cooked or raw material. Specifying gram units in addition to traditional volume measures (i.e. cups or teaspoons) is very helpful because often the required amounts of some nutrients fall outside or below the units available on common measuring equipment in the average kitchen. The authors recommend that clients who wish to home prepare their dogs' or cats' diets purchase a kitchen scale, as weighing the ingredients is much more accurate than volume measures. Very clear cooking instructions and ingredient preparation guidelines should be provided. For example: Should the meat be pan fried (with or without added fat), baked, boiled, or braised? How should the rice be prepared (with or without added salt)? Should the skin be left on potatoes?

Specific brand names should be provided with respect to vitamin and mineral supplements as there is tremendous variability in the market with regard to the nutrient content and amounts provided in such products. Furthermore it is not uncommon for many recipes to simply state "add a vitamin and mineral supplement to meet the patient's requirements." Such guidelines are very poor advice as they provide no information and require that a client with no nutritional training decide what supplement to give and how much. Guidelines with respect to how the supplements are added and handled should also be provided. Many vitamins can be destroyed by heating, which can occur if they are added during the cooking process.

Lastly, because many clients like to prepare their pet's food in large batches, it is very helpful if instructions are provided for them to do so. How and when should vitamin and mineral supplements be added to batches? Can the recipe be prepared in one pot/vessel or in a "closed system" or separately to ensure shifts in fat and water are accounted for? Can the batch of food be refrigerated or frozen? In some cases, defrosting and reheating instructions may be necessary as well.

Many veterinary practitioners successfully use home-prepared diets in the management of their patients. It is important to obtain home-prepared diet recipes from reputable sources, formulated by properly trained individuals. While there are a number of recipes in the veterinary literature, in textbooks, and referred publications, studies suggest that they may not always be nutritionally adequate (Lauten et al. 2005; Stockman et al. 2013). Be extremely cautious of recipes obtained from the internet if the site is not maintained by a veterinary nutritionist, or from publications designed for use by the general public. A better option is to have a diet specially formulated for one's patient or to formulate one for one's patient using commercially available formulation software such as Balance It (https://balance.it), esha RESEARCH (esha.com), Feedsoft®, or Mixit (www.agriculturalsoftwareconsultants.com). A custom-formulated diet accounts for the patient's specific needs and medical problems, using ingredients the patient likes. Contact the veterinary teaching college/hospital in one's area/region to see if their clinical veterinary nutritionist(s) provides this service. There are also a number of veterinary nutritionists in the private sector who will custom-formulate diets. Board-certified veterinary nutritionists® may be located through the American College of Veterinary Internal Medicine (https://vetspecialists.com).

Assessment while on a Home-Prepared Diet

It is recommended that any animal receiving a home-prepared diet be checked by a veterinarian at least every six months (animals with a concurrent medical condition may need to be seen more frequently, e.g. every three months or less, as indicated by their problem). The physical examination should include an assessment of body condition, body weight, and, if indicated, diagnostic tests such as blood work and urinalysis. A retinal examination should be performed on every cat. This visit also allows the inclusion of specific diagnostic tests to determine how well the patient is responding to its medical and/or nutritional management.

The patient's diet history should also be updated at every visit; this will help alert the practitioner to any changes in the prescribed recipe. It can also be helpful to have the client provide a diet record of exactly how much and what the animal ate for the past week. If changes from the prescribed feeding plan are noted, often occurring in the form of ingredient substitutions (referred to as "diet drift") or the exclusion of an ingredient (often the vitamin and mineral supplements), it is important to determine why the client implemented these changes. In some cases the client may simply not understand the importance of the ingredient. Often what may appear to be a simple substitution can drastically alter the nutrient profile of the overall diet. In animals with an underlying medical condition, such innocent adjustments may potentiate advancement of their animal companion's disease. In other cases, perhaps the patient does not find the diet to be palatable. The dog or cat may also be having an adverse response to the formulation or one of the ingredients,

or it may be experiencing a progression of its disease process. Recheck visits allow the practitioner to educate the client, make adjustments, or pursue a reformulation of the diet if needed.

Raw Food Feeding

Concerns regarding nutritional adequacy not only apply to home-prepared raw diets but to commercial raw diets that do not inherently undergo any cooking/kill step or an alternative high-pressure processing step as well. One study that looked at the nutritional adequacy of home-prepared raw food also looked at the nutritional adequacy of several commercial raw food diets (Freeman and Michel 2001). Both commercial raw diets had nutrient concentrations that fell below minimum AAFCO recommendations. Similarly, clinical case reports of problems in animals consuming commercial raw food diets are now beginning to appear in the literature (Taylor et al. 2009). Commercially produced raw diets fall under the same AAFCO labeling guidelines with respect to reporting nutrient content, ingredients, and nutritional adequacy statements. AAFCO recommendations for nutrient minimums and maximums exist to guide and protect against nutritional concerns in commercially produced foods. While some of these recommendations are based on studies using semi-purified diets, there are also many studies using extruded or moist diets. On the other hand, there is still a paucity of data concerning nutritional requirements, bioavailability, and the effect of raw food on gastrointestinal microbial populations in dogs and cats. It is well known that nutrient requirements can vary depending on the type of diet (i.e. taurine requirements are almost double for canned products compared to extruded diets). Therefore, one can speculate that similar examples may exist for dogs and cats that consume raw diets and that further research is needed.

There are concerns that the consumption of bones can cause oral and dental trauma as well as esophageal and gastrointestinal foreign bodies. The use of raw bones (compared to cooked) may reduce the risk of splintering and tooth fractures, but sharp fragments can still occur and puncture the mucosa at any point along the gastrointestinal route. Grinding bones may help reduce the risk of trauma and obstruction, but the availability of the calcium from these sources is unknown (see Box 8.1).

The veterinarian's job is not only to care for the health and well-being of their animal patients, but also those who are the guardians of these animals as well. From this perspective concerns regarding pathogenic bacteria in raw diets and subsequent environmental contamination are paramount.

There is growing evidence to support these concerns. Evidence for the possible transmission of food-borne pathogenic bacteria from dogs to humans exists (Gutman et al. 1973; Morse et al. 1976; Sato et al. 2000). In Alberta, Canada, 9 of 12 case patients with *Salmonella infantis* infection had been exposed to pig ear treats, and *Streptococcus infantis* was isolated from a pig ear treat collected from one of the case patients. The isolate recovered from the pig ear was indistinguishable from *S. infantis* isolates recovered from fecal samples obtained from humans with salmonellosis (Laboratory Centre for Disease Control 2000; Finley et al. 2006).

Potential human pathogens have been isolated in both commercial and home-prepared raw diets (Chengappa et al. 1993; Freeman and Michel 2001; Joffe and Schlesinger 2002; Weese et al. 2005; Strohmeyer et al. 2006; Leonard et al. 2010). Animals fed raw diets have been reported to shed the same viable organisms that were isolated in their food (Finley et al. 2007). There have been reports of racing greyhounds, sled dogs, guard dogs, and cats with *Salmonella* infections due to consumption of contaminated raw meat (Caraway et al. 1959; Cantor et al. 1997; Stone et al. 1993; Stiver et al. 2003; Morley et al. 2006).

Arguably, while many animals never become ill while consuming raw food diets, they still pose a risk to humans and other animals through environmental shedding (Finley et al. 2006, 2007). Individuals preparing raw diets are also at risk by handling contaminated meat and egg products. Those greatest at risk are the very young and old, in addition to the immunocompromised.

There is no documented evidence that feeding raw meat has any health or nutritional advantages over cooked foods. The US Food and Drug Administration (FDA) does not advocate the feeding of raw meat, poultry, or seafood to pets (FDA 2007). However, recognizing that some clients will continue this practice, it provides a set of recommendations regarding the safe handling of raw foods for clients to follow.

As veterinarians, it is important to discuss with clients the risks associated with feeding raw diets not only to the animal, but also to those who share the environment with that animal. In many cases, safer alternatives can be offered that will often address the underlying motivations that lead the client to try this feeding approach initially. There are numerous commercial diets on the market that provide similar nutrient profiles to raw diets or do not contain grains or offer natural ingredients and preservatives. If the client still wishes to prepare food at home, a home-prepared, cooked diet formulated by a board-certified veterinary nutritionist is an excellent option.

In some cases, despite understanding all of the risks, a client may wish to continue to feed a raw diet. Practitioners should refer their clients to the FDA's website and go over safe handling and preparation of food, as well as cleaning practices. It has been shown that simple routine washing may not be enough to eliminate potential food-borne pathogens in the animal companion's food bowl and environment (Weese and Rousseau 2006). It is also important to document any discussions one has on this subject, as there may be legal ramifications (LeJeune and Hancock 2001).

Summary

- Each type of commercial pet food – dry, moist, semi-moist, and raw – has potential advantages and disadvantages. It is important for the practitioner to understand these in order to recommend the best diet to their patient.
- There are good-quality commercial diets in every segment of the market, and the price of a pet food does not always equate to the quality of the diet.
- The major indication for placing an animal on a home-prepared diet is a medical condition that requires special nutritional modifications not addressed in a commercial or veterinary therapeutic diet.
- All home-prepared diet recipes should be reviewed by the practitioner and entered into the patient's medical record. Recipes that are obtained from books, lay publications, or the internet should be evaluated for adequacy by a board-certified veterinary nutritionist (if not already the origin) or the practitioner using available evaluation software.
- Raw food diets pose many potential risks including nutritional excesses or deficiencies, dental injury, gastrointestinal obstructions and perforations, bacterial contamination, and other zoonotic diseases. Clients should be educated by their veterinarian with respect to these risks.

References

American Pet Products Association (2022). Industry statistics & trends. In: *American Pet Products Association 2021–2022 National Pet Owners Survey*. http://www.americanpetproducts.org/press_industrytrends.asp.

Association of American Feed Control Officials (AAFCO) (2022). Official feed terms. In: *Official Publication of the Association American Feed Control Officials*, 351. Champaign, IN: AAFCO.

Backus, R.C., Rogers, Q.R., and Morris, J.G. (1994). Microbial degradation of taurine in fecal cultures from cats given commercial and purified diets. *J. Nutr.* 124: 2540S–2545S.

Bauer, J.E. (2006). Facultative and functional fats in dogs and cats. *J. Am. Vet. Med. Assoc.* 229 (5): 680–684.

Cantor, G.H., Nelson, S. Jr., Vanek, J.A. et al. (1997). *Salmonella* shedding in racing sled dogs. *J. Vet. Diagn. Invest.* 9: 447–448.

Caraway, C.T., Scott, A.E., Roberts, N.C. et al. (1959). Salmonellosis in sentry dogs. *J. Am. Vet. Med. Assoc.* 135: 599–602.

Chengappa, M.M., Staats, J., Oberst, R.D. et al. (1993). Prevalence of *salmonella* in raw meat used in diets of racing greyhounds. *J. Vet. Diagn. Invest.* 5: 372–377.

Crane, S.W., Cowell, C.S., Stout, N.P. et al. (2010). Commercial pet foods. In: *Small Animal Clinical Nutrition* (ed. M.S. Hand, C.D. Thatcher, R.L. Remillard, et al.), 157–190. Topeka: Mark Morris Institute.

Crissey, S.D., Swanson, J.A., Lintzenich, B.A. et al. (1997). Use of a raw meat-based diet or a dry kibble diet for sand cats (Felis margarita). *J. Anim. Sci.* 75: 2154–2160.

De Fornel-Thibaud, P., Blanchard, G., Escoffier-Chateau, L. et al. (2007). Unusual case of osteopenia associated with nutritional calcium and vitamin D deficiency in an adult dog. *J. Am. Anim. Hosp. Assoc.* 43 (1): 52–60.

Delaney, S.J. and Dzanis, D.A. (2018). Safety of vitamin K, and its use in pet foods. *J. Am. Vet. Med. Assoc.* 252 (5): 537–542.

Finley, R., Reid-Smith, R., and Weese, J.S. (2006). Human health implications of salmonella-contaminated natural pet treats and raw pet food. *Clin. Infect. Dis.* 42: 686–691.

Finley, R., Ribble, C., Aramini, J. et al. (2007). The risk of salmonellae shedding by dogs fed *salmonella*-contaminated commercial raw food diets. *Can. Vet. J.* 48 (1): 69–75.

Food and Drug Administration, Center for Veterinary Medicine (2007). FDA tips for preventing food-borne illness associated with pet food and pet treats. http://www.fda.gov/AnimalVeterinary/NewsEvents/CVMUpdates/ucm048030.htm

Freeman, L.M. and Michel, K.E. (2001). Evaluation of raw food diets for dogs. *J. Am. Vet. Med. Assoc.* 218 (5): 705–709. Correction in *J. Am. Vet. Med. Assoc.* 218(10): 1582.).

Glasgow, A.J., Cave, N.J., Marks, S.L. et al. (2002). Role of diet in the health of feline intestinal tract and in inflammatory bowel disease. Center for Companion Animal Health, University of California Davis, School of Veterinary Medicine. http://www.vetmed.ucdavis.edu/CCAH/local-assets/pdfs/Role_of_diet_feline%20 health_Glasgow.pdf

Gutman, L., Ottesen, E., Quan, T. et al. (1973). An inter-familial outbreak of yersinia entercolitica enteritis. *N. Engl. J. Med.* 288: 1372–1377.

Hickman, M.A., Rogers, Q.R., and Morris, J.G. (1990). Effect of processing on fate of dietary [14C]taurine in cats. *J. Nutr.* 120: 995–1000.

Joffe, D.J. and Schlesinger, D.P. (2002). Preliminary assessment of the risk of *salmonella* infection in dogs fed raw chicken diets. *Can. Vet. J.* 43: 441–442.

Kim, S.W., Rogers, Q.R., and Morris, J.G. (1996a). Maillard reaction products in purified diets induce taurine depletion which is reversed by antibiotics. *J. Nutr.* 126: 195–201.

Kim, S.W., Rogers, Q.R., and Morris, J.G. (1996b). Dietary antibiotics decrease taurine loss in cats fed a canned heat-processed diet. *J. Nutr.* 126: 509–515.

Kratzer, G.R., Shepherd, M., Delaney, S.J. et al. (2022). Home-cooked diets cost more than commercially prepared dry kibble diets for dogs with chronic enteropathies. *J. Am. Vet. Med. Assoc.* 260 (S3): S53–S60.

Laboratory Centre for Disease Control (2000). Human health risk from exposure to natural dog treats—preliminary report. *Can. Commun. Dis. Rep.* 26: 41–42.

Laflamme, D.P., Abood, S.K., Fascetti, A.J. et al. (2008). Pet feeding practices of dog and cat owners in the United States and Australia. *J. Am. Vet. Med. Assoc.* 232 (5): 687–694.

Lambert, I.H., Nielsen, J.H., Andersen, H.J. et al. (2001). Cellular models for induction of drip loss in meat. *J. Agric. Food. Chem.* 49 (10): 2225–2230.

Lauten, S.D., Smith, T.M., Kirk, C.A. et al. (2005). Computer analysis of nutrient sufficiency of published home-cooked diets for dogs and cats (abstract). *J. Vet. Intern. Med.* 19: 476.

LeJeune, J.T. and Hancock, D.D. (2001). Public health concerns associated with feeding raw meat diets to dogs. *J. Am. Vet. Med. Assoc.* 219 (9): 1222–1225.

Leonard, E.K., Pearl, D.L., Finley, R.L. et al. (2010). Evaluation of pet-related management factors and the risk of *salmonella* spp. carriage in pet dogs from volunteer households in Ontario (2005–2006). *Zoonoses Public Health* 58: 140–149.

McMillan, C.J., Griffon, D.J., Marks, S.L. et al. (2006). Dietary-related skeletal changes in a Shetland sheepdog. *J. Am. Anim. Hosp. Assoc.* 42 (1): 57–64.

Morley, P.S., Strohmeyer, R.A., Tankson, J.D. et al. (2006). Evaluation of the association between feeding raw meat and salmonella enterica infections at a greyhound breeding facility. *J. Am. Vet. Med. Assoc.* 228 (10): 1524–1532.

Morse, E.V., Duncan, M.A., Estep, D.A. et al. (1976). Canine salmonellosis: a review and report of dog to child transmission of *salmonella* enteritidis. *Am. J. Public Health* 66: 82–84.

Niza, M.M., Vilela, C.L., and Ferreira, L.M. (2003). Feline pansteatitis revisited: hazards of unbalanced home-made diets. *J. Feline Med. Surg.* 5: 271–277.

National Research Council (NRC) (2006). *Nutrient Requirements of Dogs and Cats.* Washington, DC: National Academies Press.

Rafii, M., Pencharz, P.B., Ball, R.O. et al. (2020). Bioavailable methionine assessed using the indicator amino acid oxidation method is greater when cooked chickpeas and steamed rice are combined in healthy young men. *J. Nutr.* 150 (7): 1834–1844.

Reilly, L.M., von Schaumburg, P.C., Hoke, J.M. et al. (2020). Macronutrient composition, true metabolizable energy and amino acid digestibility, and indispensable amino acid scoring of pulse ingredients for use in canine and feline diets. *J. Anim. Sci.* 98 (6): skaa149.

Roudebush, P. and Cowell, C.S. (1992). Results of a hypoallergenic diet survey of veterinarians in North America with a nutritional evaluation of homemade diet prescriptions. *Vet. Dermatol.* 3: 23–28.

Sarwar, G., Peace, R.W., Botting, H.G. et al. (1989). Digestibility of protein and amino acids in selected foods as determined by a rat balance method. *Plant Foods Hum. Nutr.* 39 (1): 23–32.

Sato, Y., Mori, T., Koyama, T. et al. (2000). Salmonella virchow infection in an infant transmitted by household dogs. *J. Vet. Med. Sci.* 62 (7): 767–769.

Segev, G., Fascetti, A.J., Weeth, L.P. et al. (2010). Correction of hyperkalemia in dogs with chronic kidney disease consuming commercial renal therapeutic diets by a potassium-reduced home prepared diet. *J. Vet. Intern. Med.* 24 (3): 546–550.

Spitze, A.R., Wong, D.L., Rogers, Q.R. et al. (2003). Taurine concentrations in animal feed ingredients; cooking influences taurine content. *J. Anim. Physiol. Anim. Nutr.* 87 (7–8): 251–262.

Stiver, S.L., Frazier, K.S., Mauel, M.J. et al. (2003). Septicemic salmonellosis in two cats fed a raw meat diet. *J. Am. Anim. Hosp. Assoc.* 39 (6): 538–542.

Stockman, J., Fascetti, A.J., Kass, P.H. et al. (2013). Evaluation of recipes of home-prepared maintenance diets for dogs. *J. Am. Vet. Med. Assoc.* 242 (11): 1500–1505.

Stone, G.G., Chengappa, M.M., Oberst, R.D. et al. (1993). Application of polymerase chain reaction for the correlation of *salmonella* serovars recovered from greyhound feces with their diet. *J. Vet. Diagn. Invest.* 5: 378–385.

Streiff, E.L., Zwischenberger, B., Butterwick, R.F. et al. (2002). A comparison of the nutritional adequacy of home-prepared and commercial diets for dogs. *J. Nutr.* 132: 1698S–1700S.

Strohmeyer, R.A., Morley, P.S., Hyatt, D.R. et al. (2006). Evaluation of bacterial and protozoal contamination of commercially available raw meat diets for dogs. *J. Am. Vet. Med. Assoc.* 228 (4): 537–542.

Taylor, M.B., Geiger, D.A., Saker, K.E. et al. (2009). Diffuse osteopenia and myelopathy in a puppy fed a diet composed of an organic premix and raw ground beef. *J. Vet. Med. Assoc.* 234 (8): 1041–1048.

Tomsa, K., Glaus, T., Hauser, B. et al. (1999). Nutritional secondary hyperparathyroidism in six cats. *J. Small Anim. Pract.* 40 (11): 533–539.

United States Government Printing Office (2010). Electronic Code of Federal Regulations. Title 7: Agriculture, Part 205, National Organic Program. http://ecfr. gpoaccess.gov/cgi/t/text/textidx?type=simple; c=ecfr;cc=ecfr;sid=4163ddc3518c1ffdc539675 aed8ee33;region=DIV1;q1=national%20 organic%20program;rgn=div5;view=txt;idno =7;node=7%3A3.1.1.9.31.

Weese, J.S. and Rousseau, J. (2006). Survival of salmonella Copenhagen in food bowls following contamination with experimentally inoculated raw meat: effects of time, cleaning, and disinfection. *Can. Vet. J.* 47 (9): 887–889.

Weese, J.S., Rousseau, J., and Arroyo, L. (2005). Bacteriological evaluation of commercial canine and feline raw diets. *Can. Vet. J.* 46: 513–516.

9

Nutritional Management of Body Weight

Kathryn E. Michel and Robert C. Backus

Animals become overweight as a consequence of maintaining a state of positive energy balance, which results when they consume calories in excess of their caloric expenditure. Weight gain can be rapid if the caloric excess is large. However, even a modest chronic excess in caloric intake can result in significant weight gain over the long term. For example, a cat that consumes a mere 10 kcal above its daily energy requirement every day will accumulate about a pound of adipose tissue in the course of a year. For the typical domestic shorthaired cat, that would be equivalent to 10% of its ideal weight, not at all an insignificant weight gain.

Obesity has been defined as an accumulation of excessive energy storage in the form of adipose tissue sufficient to contribute to disease (National Institutes of Health 1985). For humans, both overweightness and obesity have been clearly defined using anthropometric criteria. Epidemiologic data from the past few decades have revealed that increasing numbers of people in developed and developing regions of the world are overweight or obese (Ogden et al. 2006; Flegal et al. 2015). The impact of overweightness and obesity on human health has also been extensively investigated, and it is estimated that in the United States alone these conditions result in up to $147 billion in direct healthcare costs each year (Hammond and Levine 2010).

There seems to be general agreement that excess weight gain is the most common nutrition-related disorder seen in companion animals today. While compared to human studies there have been relatively few large investigations of the prevalence of overweightness and obesity in pet dogs and cats, estimates range from 24% to 44% of the adult population (Scarlett and Donoghue 1996; Lund et al. 2005, 2006; Mao et al. 2013; Chiang et al. 2022a, b). The survey of the body condition of pet dogs and cats that examined the largest and most geographically diverse cohort obtained body condition scores (BCSs) from private veterinary practices throughout the United States. These investigators found that 28.7% of 8159 adult cats were classified as overweight and 6.4% as obese (Lund et al. 2005). Of 21 754 dogs seen at these same practices, 29.0% were deemed overweight and 5.1% obese (Lund et al. 2006). When the data for only middle-aged pets (between the ages of 5 and 11 years) were analyzed, 44% of the cats and 42% of the dogs were scored as overweight or obese, percentages that approach those reported for people living in the United States (Lund et al. 2005, 2006; Ogden et al. 2006).

Applied Veterinary Clinical Nutrition, Second Edition. Edited by Andrea J. Fascetti, Sean J. Delaney, Jennifer A. Larsen, and Cecilia Villaverde.

The Health Consequences of Overweightness and Obesity

In comparison to the scientific literature regarding the adverse effects of excess weight gain on human health, our knowledge of the impact of this condition on the health of pet dogs and cats is more limited. Not too long ago the potential sequelae of weight gain, as discussed in the veterinary literature, were mostly matters of speculation based on data from human patients. However, there are now a number of published investigations that document an association between overweightness and obesity and increased risk of disease and decreased longevity in both cats and dogs. The best evidence to date documents the association between obesity and orthopedic disease in dogs, and between obesity and diabetes mellitus in cats.

Obesity as a Risk Factor for Canine Orthopedic Disease

One of the first large-scale epidemiologic studies on overweightness and obesity in dogs was performed in the United Kingdom, and it found that 2.9% of a sample of 8268 dogs seen at 11 different veterinary clinics were classified as grossly overweight (Edney and Smith 1986). This subset of dogs had an increased prevalence of circulatory and articular/locomotor diseases. However, this finding was confounded by the fact that in this population these disorders were also highly associated with old age. This was consistent with a larger study of 40 038 dogs presented to an academic institution, which reported an overall prevalence of overweight and obesity of 41.3% and a significantly increased risk of orthopedic disease (adjusted odds ratio 1.57; Chiang et al. 2022b).

In a 14-year longitudinal study of pair-fed Labrador Retriever littermates, one member of the pair was fed 25% less food than the other throughout life (Kealy et al. 2002). On average the limit-fed dogs maintained an optimal BCS (4.6 ± 0.2/9), while their respective full-fed pairs were moderately overweight (6.7 ± 0.2/9). Significantly fewer of the limit-fed dogs developed osteoarthritis than the full-fed dogs, and those that did had less severe disease with a later onset in life. This finding was particularly dramatic in light of the relatively modest difference in body condition between the limit-fed and full-fed dogs.

There is also evidence that overweight dogs with pre-existing orthopedic disease benefit from weight loss. One prospective study found that when nine pet dogs with radiographic and clinical signs of coxofemoral joint osteoarthritis underwent a successful weight-reduction program, all dogs experienced a significant decrease in severity of clinical signs based on subjective evaluation (Impellizeri et al. 2000). Other investigations of the impact of weight loss on dogs with documented osteoarthritis have reported similar findings, with dogs showing significant improvement of lameness as documented by force plate and kinetic gait analysis after a successful weight-loss program (Burkholder et al. 2001; Marshall et al. 2010).

Obesity as a Risk Factor for Feline Diabetes Mellitus

The association between obesity and type II diabetes mellitus in people is well documented (Hu et al. 2001). Obesity promotes insulin resistance, which in turn leads to increased insulin secretion by the pancreatic beta cells, with the consequence over time of beta-cell destruction through one or more proposed mechanisms, including islet amylin deposition, beta-cell exhaustion, and glucose toxicity (Rossetti et al. 1990). Abnormal insulin secretion and abnormal glucose tolerance have been documented in both overweight dogs and cats. Both species have been shown to develop glucose intolerance and hyperinsulinemia with weight gain, which resolves if the animal returns to normal body condition (Mattheeuws et al. 1984; Fettman et al. 1998).

The form of diabetes that affects the majority of dogs most closely resembles human type I diabetes. Feline diabetes mellitus, however, resembles human type II diabetes in several key respects, including islet amylin deposition and an association with an overweight body condition (Yano et al. 1981; Panciera et al. 1990). One investigation found that overweight cats had a fourfold greater risk of becoming diabetic than normal-weight cats (Scarlett and Donoghue 1998). However, a larger study of 9062 cats presented to an academic institution reported that only 107 of 232 cats with diabetes mellitus were overweight or obese, resulting in no significant association (Chiang et al. 2022a). Differences in patient population might underlie the apparent inconsistency. Among cats presented to primary-care veterinary practices in the United Kingdom (n = 193 435), risk for diabetes mellitus reportedly increases substantially with increasing body weight, where disease odds ratio exceeds 10 to 1 when body weight is greater than 6 kg (O'Neill et al. 2016).

Additional Health Risks of Obesity in Dogs and Cats

Other investigations have shown excess body weight to be a risk factor for a number of other health problems seen in companion animals. Overweight cats have been found to be at greater risk for lower urinary tract diseases, non-allergic dermatitis, oral disease, lameness, feline idiopathic hepatic lipidosis, and a range of other disease categories (Burrows et al. 1981; Scarlett and Donoghue 1998; Lund et al. 2005; Chiang et al. 2022a). Overweight dogs have been found to be at increased risk for pancreatitis, hyperlipidemia, endocrine diseases, renal pathology, and respiratory and dermatologic diseases (Hess et al. 1999; Finco et al. 2001; Chiang et al. 2022a, b). There is also epidemiologic evidence that neoplasia is associated with an overweight body condition in both dogs and cats (Lund et al. 2005, 2006; Chiang et al. 2022a, b), although one study suggested that such associations in dogs are likely cancer type specific (Weeth et al. 2007). In general,

obesity can compromise an animal's ventilatory capacity ("Pickwickian syndrome") and thus affect tolerance of exercise, heat, and anesthesia.

It has become increasingly evident that adipose tissue, long viewed simply as an energy depot, actively produces both hormones that are involved in energy homeostasis (e.g. leptin and resistin) and cytokines, some of which are important modulators of inflammation (e.g. tumor necrosis factor [TNF]-alpha, interleukin [IL]-1) (Miller et al. 1998; Gayet et al. 2004; Barić et al. 2017). Consequently, obesity is now recognized as a state of chronic low-grade inflammation, a condition that may prove to play a role in the pathogenesis of some of the diseases for which overweight individuals are at risk, including osteoarthritis and diabetes mellitus. This inflammatory state is shown to be reversible with loss of body weight in dogs (German et al. 2009; Wakshlag et al. 2011).

As previously noted, there is evidence that overweight dogs and cats experience decreased longevity. In the study involving the pair-fed Labrador retrievers, a significant difference in median lifespan was found: 13 years for the limit-fed dogs compared to 11.2 years for the control (full-fed) dogs (Kealy et al. 2002). With regard to cats, in an investigation of over 2000 adult cats seen at veterinary clinics in the mid-Atlantic region of the United States, multivariate statistical analysis controlled for age found that middle-aged obese cats had greater risk of mortality than cats at optimal body weight (Scarlett and Donoghue 1996).

Increasing Awareness of Overweightness and Obesity

Given the evidence that excessive weight gain can have significant health consequences for pet dogs and cats, why are so many pets overweight? Since most pets do not obtain food on their own, it would seem a relatively simple task for the caregiver to feed adequate but not excessive amounts and avoid inappropriate weight gain. In order to do this, however, the caregiver must be able to distinguish what constitutes an optimal weight for the pet.

Targeting Optimal Weight

Basing a pet's feeding management on maintaining a target body weight has disadvantages, particularly in the case of dogs. Weight tables similar to available human height–weight tables would be impractical and difficult to develop for dogs and cats due to the variation in conformation among and within breeds and the large number of mixed-breed pets. Furthermore, most people do not have ready access to an accurate scale that would accommodate a dog or a cat. There have been attempts to develop zoometric techniques for dogs and cats similar to the anthropometric techniques used in humans (Stanton et al. 1992; Witzel et al. 2014a, b). However, while these

techniques might be useful in a research or clinical setting, they are again impractical as a means of assessing a pet on a day-to-day basis. Body condition scoring, on the other hand, requires no special equipment, is simple to learn, and can be used to assess and modify feeding practices in the home setting.

Body Condition Scoring

Several different scoring systems for dogs and cats have been developed. A nine-point system is described in Tables 9.1 and 9.2 and illustrated in Figures 9.1 and 9.2. Applying the system involves both visual assessment of the pet and palpation to assess body fat over the ribs, abdomen, lumbar area, and tail base. The combination of the description and illustrations clarifies the distinctions between scores and makes the system simple to apply. This system has been validated for use with dogs and

Table 9.1 The nine-point body condition scoring system for dogs.

Too Thin	
1	Ribs, lumbar vertebrae, pelvic bones, and all bony prominences evident from a distance; no discernible body fat; obvious loss of muscle mass.
2	Ribs, lumbar vertebrae, and pelvic bones easily visible; no palpable fat; some evidence of other bony prominence; minimal loss of muscle mass.
3	Ribs easily palpated and may be visible with no palpable fat; tops of lumbar vertebrae visible; pelvic bones becoming prominent; obvious waist and abdominal tuck.
Ideal	
4	Ribs easily palpable, with minimal fat covering; waist easily noted, viewed from above; abdomen tucked up when viewed from side.
5	Ribs palpable without excess fat covering; waist observed behind ribs when viewed from above; abdomen tucked up when viewed from side.
Too Heavy	
6	Ribs palpable with slight excess fat covering; waist is discernible viewed from above but is not prominent; abdominal tuck apparent.
7	Ribs palpable with difficulty; heavy fat cover; noticeable fat deposits over lumbar area and base of tail; waist absent or barely visible; abdominal tuck may be present.
8	Ribs not palpable under very heavy fat cover, or palpable only with significant pressure; heavy fat deposits over lumbar area and base of tail; waist absent; no abdominal tuck; obvious abdominal distension may be present.
9	Massive fat deposits over thorax, spine, and base of tail; waist and abdominal tuck absent; fat deposits on neck and limbs; obvious abdominal distension.

Source: Reproduced with permission from the Nestlé Purina PetCare Company.

Table 9.2 The nine-point body condition scoring system for cats.

Too Thin

1	Ribs visible on shorthaired cats; no palpable fat; severe abdominal tuck; lumbar vertebrae and wings of the ilia easily palpated.
2	Ribs easily visible on shorthaired cats; lumbar vertebrae obvious with minimal muscle mass; pronounced abdominal tuck; no palpable fat.
3	Ribs easily palpable with minimal fat covering; lumbar vertebrae obvious; obvious waist behind ribs; minimal abdominal fat.
4	Ribs palpable with minimal fat covering; noticeable waist behind ribs; slight abdominal tuck; abdominal fat pad absent.

Ideal

5	Well proportioned; observe waist behind ribs; ribs palpable with slight fat covering; abdominal fat pad minimal.

Too Heavy

6	Ribs palpable with slight excess fat covering; waist and abdominal fat pad distinguishable but not obvious; abdominal tuck absent.
7	Ribs not easily palpable with moderate fat cover; waist poorly discernible; obvious rounding of abdomen; moderate abdominal fat pad.
8	Ribs not palpable with excess fat covering; waist absent; obvious rounding of abdomen with prominent abdominal fat pad; fat deposits present over lumbar area.
9	Ribs not palpable under heavy fat cover; heavy fat deposits over lumbar area, face, and limbs; distension of abdomen with no waist; extensive abdominal fat deposits.

Source: Reproduced with permission from the Nestlé Purina PetCare Company.

cats both in terms of reproducibility between trained observers and body composition as measured by dual energy X-ray absorptiometry (Laflamme 1997a, b). Each increment in BCS is approximately equivalent to 10–15% additional weight due to body fat. A score of 4–5 is considered optimal for dogs and reflects a body fat level of 15–20%. For cats, a BCS of 5 is considered optimal and in this species reflects a level of 25% body fat. Recently validated BCS systems are notably applicable for assigning body condition in extremely obese dogs and cats (Witzel et al. 2014a, b). The systems are useful for estimating percentage body fat excess over a wider range than the nine-point system.

In practice, once a person was familiarized with the system and was able to recognize what constituted ideal body condition, they could use it to adjust how their pet was fed. The caregiver would assess the pet's BCS on a routine basis (such as monthly) and increase or decrease accordingly the amount of food offered to the pet. However, despite the simplicity of this approach, several studies have found that people's perception of their pet's body condition is often at odds with the assessment of a trained observer. Most investigations suggest that people are likely to underestimate their pet's BCS. A study involving 201 dogs found that while the expert scored 79% of the dogs as overweight or obese, only 28% of the caregivers scored their dogs above ideal (Singh et al. 2002). Another study of cats living in New Zealand found that overall, people underestimated their cat's BCS only 25% of the time; however, people underestimated BCS in 60% of the cats that were overweight or obese (Allan et al. 2000).

This misperception is compounded if the attending veterinarian neglects to identify and call attention to overweight and obese patients. In a large survey of US veterinary practices, approximately 28% of the canine and feline

⊞ Nestlé PURINA
BODY CONDITION SYSTEM

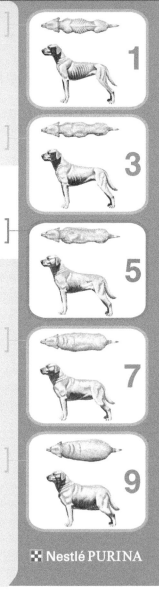

TOO THIN

1 Ribs, lumbar vertebrae, pelvic bones and all bony prominences evident from a distance. No discernible body fat. Obvious loss of muscle mass.

2 Ribs, lumbar vertebrae and pelvic bones easily visible. No palpable fat. Some evidence of other bony prominence. Minimal loss of muscle mass.

3 Ribs easily palpated and may be visible with no palpable fat. Tops of lumbar vertebrae visible. Pelvic bones becoming prominent. Obvious waist and abdominal tuck.

IDEAL

4 Ribs easily palpable, with minimal fat covering. Waist easily noted, viewed from above. Abdominal tuck evident.

5 Ribs palpable without excess fat covering. Waist observed behind ribs when viewed from above. Abdomen tucked up when viewed from side.

TOO HEAVY

6 Ribs palpable with slight excess fat covering. Waist is discernible viewed from above but is not prominent. Abdominal tuck apparent.

7 Ribs palpable with difficulty; heavy fat cover. Noticeable fat deposits over lumbar area and base of tail. Waist absent or barely visible. Abdominal tuck may be present.

8 Ribs not palpable under very heavy fat cover, or palpable only with significant pressure. Heavy fat deposits over lumbar area and base of tail. Waist absent. No abdominal tuck. Obvious abdominal distention may be present.

9 Massive fat deposits over thorax, spine and base of tail. Waist and abdominal tuck absent. Fat deposits on neck and limbs. Obvious abdominal distention.

The BODY CONDITION SYSTEM was developed at the Nestlé Purina Pet Care Center and has been validated as documented in the following publications:

Mawby D, Bartges JW, Moyers T, et. al. *Comparison of body fat estimates by dual-energy x-ray absorptiometry and deuterium oxide dilution in client owned dogs.* Compendium 2001; 23 (9A): 70

Laflamme DP. *Development and Validation of a Body Condition Score System for Dogs.* Canine Practice July/August 1997; 22:10-15

Kealy, et. al. *Effects of Diet Restriction on Life Span and Age-Related Changes in Dogs.* JAVMA 2002; 220:1315-1320

Call 1-800-222-VETS (8387), weekdays, 8:00 a.m. to 4:30 p.m. CT

⊞ Nestlé PURINA

Figure 9.1 Illustration of the nine-point body condition scoring system for dogs. *Source:* Used with permission from Nestlé Purina PetCare Company.

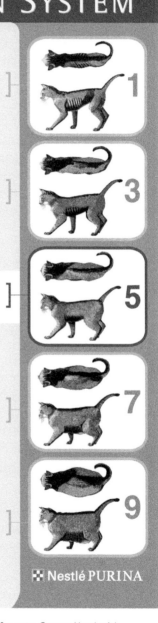

Nestlé PURINA
BODY CONDITION SYSTEM

TOO THIN

1 Ribs visible on shorthaired cats; no palpable fat; severe abdominal tuck; lumbar vertebrae and wings of ilia easily palpated.

2 Ribs easily visible on shorthaired cats; lumbar vertebrae obvious with minimal muscle mass; pronounced abdominal tuck; no palpable fat.

3 Ribs easily palpable with minimal fat covering; lumbar vertebrae obvious; obvious waist behind ribs; minimal abdominal fat.

4 Ribs palpable with minimal fat covering; noticeable waist behind ribs; slight abdominal tuck; abdominal fat pad absent.

IDEAL

5 Well-proportioned; observe waist behind ribs; ribs palpable with slight fat covering; abdominal fat pad minimal.

TOO HEAVY

6 Ribs palpable with slight excess fat covering; waist and abdominal fat pad distinguishable but not obvious; abdominal tuck absent.

7 Ribs not easily palpated with moderate fat covering; waist poorly discernible; obvious rounding of abdomen; moderate abdominal fat pad.

8 Ribs not palpable with excess fat covering; waist absent; obvious rounding of abdomen with prominent abdominal fat pad; fat deposits present over lumbar area.

9 Ribs not palpable under heavy fat cover; heavy fat deposits over lumbar area, face and limbs; distention of abdomen with no waist; extensive abdominal fat deposits.

Call 1-800-222-VETS (8387), weekdays, 8:00 a.m. to 4:30 p.m. CT

Nestlé PURINA

Figure 9.2 Illustration of the nine-point body condition scoring system for cats. *Source:* Used with permission from Nestlé Purina PetCare Company.

patients were scored as overweight or obese, but only 2% had weight recorded as an issue (Lund et al. 1999). Likewise, in one study of 8739 cats assigned to various disease categories, 41.6% were assigned an overweight or obese BCS, but only 5.6% were given that specific diagnosis in the medical record (Chiang et al. 2022a). A similar finding was reported for a large study of dogs, in that only 9.9% of those assigned an overweight or obese BCS were given that specific diagnosis in the medical record (Chiang et al. 2022b). The findings were also similar in investigations conducted in the United Kingdom, which found that veterinarians discussed weight status and body condition with fewer than 2% of owners of overweight dogs (German and Morgan 2014; Rolph et al. 2014).

The best practice is to record a body weight and a BCS for each patient on every visit, to recognize overweightness and obesity as distinct diseases, and to discuss the finding with the owner. The BCS puts the body weight in context for monitoring trends and is useful when more than one clinician is caring for the patient. Scoring body condition during an office visit also provides opportunities to ensure that the pet's caregiver is properly instructed in this technique and to initiate a discussion about weight control when indicated.

Understanding the Risk Factors for Weight Gain

Genetic background, growth rate, and many aspects of how companion animals are housed and fed can predispose a dog or cat to weight gain. Recognizing these risks and educating the pet's caregiver could help prevent a pet from becoming overweight in the first place.

Varying prevalence of obesity among dog breeds has compelled a few candidate gene studies into genetic predispositions for excessive accumulation of adipose tissue (Stachowiak et al. 2016). Exemplary of this research are studies correlating overweight body condition in Labrador retrievers with a deletion mutation of the pro-opiomelanocortin (*POMC*) gene (Raffan et al. 2016; Mankowska et al. 2017). The *POMC* gene encodes brain peptides that are important to food intake control and possibly food reward.

Several studies have implicated feeding calorically dense commercial foods as a contributing factor for weight gain in cats (Scarlett et al. 1994; Robertson 1999; Lund et al. 2005; Rowe et al. 2015). Interestingly, with one exception, the studies that have looked at frequency of feeding (free choice vs. meal fed) have not found this factor to be associated with risk for becoming overweight, although clearly pets that are fed free choice are at liberty to consume excess calories, particularly when they are fed energy-dense, palatable foods (Robertson 1999; Allan et al. 2000; Russell et al. 2000). Dietary fat contributes largely to the caloric density of commercial foods. Unfortunately, fat is preferred by dogs among the macronutrient sources of dietary calories (Roberts et al. 2018).

Lack of exercise has also been cited as a contributing factor in obesity for humans and pets alike (Scarlett et al. 1994; Colditz 1999; Robertson 1999; Lund et al. 2005; Rowe et al. 2015). The physical environment where increasing numbers of people, along with their pets, are residing lacks the space and infrastructure (e.g. parks, sidewalks) to facilitate physical activity. Many cats, and increasingly some dogs, are confined indoors. Large numbers of dogs rely on a caregiver to exercise them by leash walking or taking them to a protected open space to run, endeavors that require time, commitment, and accessibility.

Another major contributing factor for weight gain in companion animals is neutering. A number of investigations have shown that neutering can affect feline and canine energy balance (Root et al. 1996; Fettman et al. 1998; Hoenig and Ferguson 2002; Kanchuk et al. 2003; Jeusette et al. 2006). Upon neutering, cats will increase food intake within days of the procedure, an effect possibly mediated by increased circulating ghrelin, a gastric orexigenic peptide (Kanchuk et al. 2003). Accelerometry observations indicate that neutering significantly decreases physical activity in female cats (Belsito et al. 2009), but not clearly in dogs (Morrison et al. 2014). There is also some evidence to suggest that neutering results in a decrease in energy requirements (Bermingham et al. 2010, 2014). However, normalization by body weight and/or fat-free mass after post-neutering weight gain confounds interpretation of this evidence. Supporting these findings on neutering, which implicate neutering as a factor predisposing to weight gain, are the epidemiologic studies that have found neutered dogs and cats to be at greater risk of being overweight or obese (Edney and Smith 1986; Scarlett et al. 1994; Lund et al. 2005, 2006; McGreevy et al. 2005; Weeth et al. 2007; Courcier et al. 2010; Lefebvre et al. 2013; Chiang et al. 2022a, b).

Rapid post-natal growth rate, even while maintaining lean body condition, is correlated with overweight body condition in adulthood (Serisier et al. 2013; Leclerc et al. 2017). Because growth rate is impacted by food availability, feeding puppies and kittens to precociously attain a large body size may increase risk for later obesity.

Accurate Accounting of Caloric Intake

The first step for developing a weight-loss program is to perform a complete physical exam and obtain a thorough dietary history. The physical exam findings will help identify underlying conditions that may have contributed to the weight gain, or that may need to be taken into account when formulating the weight loss plan, such as those that could limit the pet's ability to exercise. It will also verify that the pet's weight gain is indeed attributable to an increase in adiposity and not another condition such as ascites. The physical exam may prompt further diagnostic testing for conditions that could predispose to weight gain,

including hypothyroidism or hyperadrenocorticism. While it is likely that a minority of overweight pets have an underlying endocrinopathy, it will be necessary to diagnose those cases and manage them appropriately in order to have success with the weight-loss program.

An absolutely key step for formulating a successful weight-loss plan is performing a thorough dietary history (see Box 9.1). This process has several objectives, the first of which is to obtain an accurate accounting of all foods fed to a pet on a typical day. However, a properly executed diet history goes beyond simply counting up calories. This is also an opportunity to evaluate all the ways that food is involved in interactions between the pet and the other members of its household. The caregivers should be given the opportunity to offer their viewpoints regarding the pet's need for weight loss and the proposition of

---

Box 9.1   Checklist for a Diet History

- Who lives in the household?
- People
- Other pets
- Who feeds the pet?
- How is the pet fed?
- Free choice vs. meals
- How is the fed portion measured?
- What is the pet's feeding behavior?
- Can the pet hunt or scavenge for food?
- What is fed?
- Specific varieties and amounts of commercial pet foods
- Table foods or scraps
- Home-prepared diets
- Treats
- Products for chewing and dental hygiene
- Chewable medications such as heartworm preventives and non-steroidal anti-inflammatory drugs
- Dietary supplements
- Food used to give medications or supplements

modifying their feeding practices. It has to be absolutely clear from the start that the caregivers perceive that the pet is overweight, that they understand why weight loss is being recommended for their pet, and that they are willing to address the problem. Thus, in addition to detailing what and how much the pet is being fed, the dietary history will also reveal potential pitfalls and obstacles in advance and allow the weight-loss plan to be tailored to the individual's circumstances, all of which should improve the chances for a successful outcome.

First it should be determined who lives in the household, including other pets, particularly those to whose food the patient might have access. Ask whether one or multiple persons regularly feed the patient. Inquire about the feeding methods. Is the patient offered food free choice or is it fed at specified meal times? Is the feeding portion measured, and what type of device is used to measure the food? Never assume that a "cup" of food means an 8 fl oz (236.6 ml) measuring cup. Inquire about the patient's feeding behavior. Is this individual a greedy eater or does it prefer to graze on its food throughout the day? Does the patient beg for food between meals? Does the patient share feeding bowls with other pets? Is this pet allowed unsupervised time outdoors when it may hunt or scavenge food?

Obtain the precise names of any commercial pet foods and treats that the patient receives and the specific amounts fed. Often the caregiver will not be able to provide this information accurately by recall alone and will need to check labels and measure feeding portions. Specify that dry pet foods be measured with a standard 8 fl oz. measuring cup or, if possible, with a gram scale.

When inquiring about treats, specifically ask about products that are used to promote chewing and dental hygiene. People do not always consider such things treats, and many are high in calories. Ask about the kinds and amounts of table foods or scraps that are given to the patient and, if a home-prepared diet is being used, request a detailed recipe. Inquire

as to whether the pet routinely receives any supplements or medications that are disguised with food, since these are often high-value items such as cheese, lunch meats, or peanut butter, which can be high in fat and calories. Some supplements (e.g. fatty acids) can also contain a significant number of calories. It may be indicated to arrange for the caregiver to go home and keep a food diary for a few days so they can accurately answer all of these questions. In some cases, it may be impossible to quantify the pet's energy intake from the information obtained, especially when a pet is receiving significant amounts of table foods and treats or is fed a highly variable diet. However, discovering that such feeding practices exist in a household in advance will reveal the issues that must be addressed in order to implement a successful weight-loss program.

Formulation of the Weight-Loss Plan

Ideally, the diet history will have provided an accurate accounting of the patient's daily caloric intake. If this is the case, weight reduction may be achieved simply by restricting the current calorie intake by 20–40%. Unfortunately, an accurate diet history is not always obtainable and in that circumstance, the first step in formulating a weight-loss plan is to establish the patient's weight-loss goal (Box 9.2). This should be informed by how overweight the pet is, as well as the presence of any obesity-related diseases that are impacting quality of life. It can be more important to set a reasonable goal and accomplish it than to set an overly ambitious goal and have the pet's caregiver become discouraged and abandon the program. It may be necessary to repeat a program several times for an individual animal in order to reduce it to an optimal body weight.

The second step is to estimate the patient's maintenance energy requirement (i.e. the caloric intake necessary to maintain the patient

---

Box 9.2   Formulating a Weight-Loss Program

- Perform a physical examination, including body condition score and any indicated diagnostic workup such as a biochemistry panel.
- Obtain a thorough diet history.
- Weigh the patient on an accurate scale and set the weight-loss goal.
- Estimate the patient's optimal body weight.
- Estimate the patient's current maintenance energy requirement from the diet history or its optimal body weight and activity level.
- Set the level of caloric restriction.
- Choose the diet and calculate the food dosage.
- Tailor a program to meet the needs and preferences of the patient and its caregiver. Include recommendations for feeding management, increasing physical activity, and behavior modification.
- Recheck the patient at 2–4-week intervals for weigh-ins on the same scale and to solicit feedback from the caregiver. Adjust feeding amounts as needed to achieve the target weight loss rate of 1–2% of body weight/week and address any problems or caregiver concerns.

---

at its current weight). As previously mentioned, ideally this information would be obtained from the dietary history and serial body weight assessments. However, if it is not possible to quantify an individual pet's caloric intake accurately because feeding portions are not measured, because it is fed with other pets, or because the types and amounts of foods offered to the pet vary from day to day, the maintenance energy requirement must be estimated (see Chapter 3).

The patient's resting energy requirement (RER) should be calculated using an estimate of its optimal body weight (RER $= 70 \times BW_{kg}^{0.75}$).

This is because the RER reflects the energy needs of metabolically active tissues such as the cardiac muscle and the central nervous system. Adipose tissue does not contribute greatly, relatively speaking, to the RER, but does account for almost all of the excess body mass in overweight individuals. The maintenance energy requirement is then estimated by applying an activity coefficient to the calculated RER. The typically recommended activity factor for adult maintenance is 1.6; however, overweight and obese pets are often sedentary, and their activity level may be more accurately represented by a lower coefficient.

The third step is to calculate how many calories the pet should receive each day to achieve adequate caloric restriction for weight loss. Typically the recommendation is to restrict the pet to 60–70% of the calories it would normally require to maintain its current weight. The final step is to calculate a food dosage for the patient based on the pet foods that it will be receiving, so that the caregivers have clear and specific feeding directions. The veterinary technician has an important role in this process (Box 9.3).

Dietary Considerations

There are a large number of commercial therapeutic diets formulated for weight loss. In general, these foods have a reduced caloric density that is achieved by lowering the fat content and/or increasing the fiber and/or water content. A major advantage of using these foods over conventional maintenance diets is that they contain increased amounts of protein, vitamins, and minerals relative to calories in order to compensate for caloric restriction and possible decreased bioavailability of these nutrients when fiber content is increased. Maintenance foods in general are likely not fortified enough in essential nutrients to be safely used for the caloric restriction necessary for active weight loss. Furthermore, increasing dietary protein may help preserve lean body mass during weight loss in both dogs and cats

---

Box 9.3   The Role of the Veterinary Technician in the Prevention and Treatment of Obesity in Companion Animals

Prevention

- Teaching pet owners how to properly give a body condition score (BCS) to their pets.
- Teaching pet owners about the calorie needs of dogs and cats and the calorie content of pet foods, treats, and table foods.
- Teaching pet owners about proper feeding management of companion animals and how to adjust food portions to maintain an optimal BCS.

Treatment

- Obtaining an accurate diet history.
- Collecting calorie information for pet foods, treats, and table foods.
- Helping tailor weight-loss protocols to the pet and its household.
- Overseeing weight-loss protocols:
  - Follow-up phone calls.
  - Recheck visits for weigh-ins.
  - Troubleshooting.

(Hannah and Laflamme 1998; Laflamme and Hannah 2005).

Along with decreasing caloric density, the addition of fiber to a pet food may enhance satiety. In two separate investigations, dogs decreased voluntary food intake when offered free-choice access to dry foods supplemented with fiber compared to their intake while eating a lower-fiber diet (Jewell and Toll 1996; Jackson et al. 1997). Another study found that a dry diet with both high protein and high fiber had a greater influence on satiety than either a high-protein or a high-fiber dry diet, even when food intake was limited analogous to what would be done to promote weight loss (Weber et al. 2007). However, another study, where overweight dogs were fed canned diets and their intake was restricted to promote weight loss, did not find any satiety effect from fiber supplementation (Butterwick and Markwell 1997). Hence, it is likely that the impact of fiber on satiety could vary from patient to patient. Feeding canned foods, which are high in moisture content, or adding water to a pet's food is another means of reducing caloric density. Caloric intake in cats in particular appears to be moderated by volume, so that calorie intake decreases with increasing the volume in which the calories are contained (Stoll and Laflamme 1995; Wei et al. 2011).

Therefore, switching from dry to canned food could improve satiety in cats in addition to enhancing portion control, given the perishable nature of high-moisture foods.

There has been speculation that lower-carbohydrate diets may be more suitable for promoting optimal body weight in cats (Zoran 2002). This is based on the assumption that cats as carnivores are naturally insulin resistant and as such when high dietary carbohydrate is consumed, hyperinsulinemia results and adipose fat storage is increased. However, evidence to date does not support that high carbohydrate intake induces increased adiposity (Laflamme et al. 2022), and diets low in carbohydrate have not been investigated in controlled studies of weight-loss programs. One investigation found that total caloric intake, but not carbohydrate content, determined weight loss or gain in group-housed cats (Michel et al. 2005). Similarly, no significant effect on body weight was reported in young adult, sexually intact cats, free fed purified diets with similar protein content and a carbohydrate content ranging from 24% to 64% of metabolizable energy. However, the diet highest in fat and lowest in carbohydrate induced overconsumption and weight gain (Backus et al. 2007). Dietary fat's importance over carbohydrate in promoting gain in body fat of cats also was reported in prospective studies during which commercial diets were fed ad libitum (Nguyen et al. 2004; Coradini et al. 2014).

Many other nutrients or dietary supplements have been proposed for weight-loss effects in dogs and cats, although most have not been critically evaluated. Table 9.3 lists a number of these compounds that are available as supplements, some of which also have been incorporated into commercial and therapeutic pet foods.

Table 9.3 Nutrients and dietary supplements that have been proposed as aids for weight reduction.

Compound	Investigations in companion animals	Comments
L-carnitine A metabolite involved in mitochondrial transport of long-chain fatty acids	Dogs and cats	May increase the rate of weight loss while promoting retention of lean body mass in companion animals during caloric restriction. Effects are modest and inconsistent (Sunvold et al. 1999; Center et al. 2000; Gross et al. 2000).
Conjugated linoleic acid (CLA) Isomers of the omega-6 fatty acid linoleic acid	Dogs and cats	Effects on weight loss in human studies are inconsistent. No effects reported on body weight and body composition in one study of normal cats and two studies of dogs on weight loss regimens (Bierer and Bui 2004; Jewell et al. 2006; Leray et al. 2006).
Chromium An essential trace element	Dogs only	Purported to enhance weight loss and reduction in body fat when used in conjunction with caloric restriction, but no companion animal study to date has shown any benefit from supplementation (Gross et al. 2000).
Dehydroepiandrosterone (DHEA) A metabolite involved in steroidogenesis	Dogs only	Supplementation has enhanced weight loss in dogs during caloric restriction; however, there are undesirable side effects from increased sex-hormone production (MacEwen and Kurzman 1991; Kurzman et al. 1998).
Pyruvate A non-essential metabolite of carbohydrate metabolism	Dogs only	Supraphysiologic supplementation in humans may enhance weight loss and reduction in body fat; however, a single study involving dogs on a weight-loss regimen reported no effect of supplementation (Zhang et al. 2004).
Omega-3 fatty acids Essential and non-essential polyunsaturated fatty acids	Dogs only	May increase energy expenditure through the upregulation of mitochondrial uncoupling protein. Supplementation-enhanced weight loss in one preliminary study of dogs during caloric restriction (Ishioka et al. 2004).
Diacylglycerol (DAG) oil A non-essential fat	None	Human studies suggest that substitution of DAG oil for other fats in food may enhance weight loss and reduction in body fat; however, there are no studies in companion animals to date.
Amylase inhibitors Enzyme inhibitors of plant origin	None	Impair carbohydrate digestion; however, no clinical efficacy has been demonstrated in human weight-loss trials, and the one report in dogs that exists suffers from study design concerns.

Exercise

While caloric restriction is the cornerstone of a weight-reduction plan for a dog or cat, increasing physical activity to affect energy expenditure is another way to achieve a negative energy balance. Cats and dogs are inactive for much of the time, but will have short bouts of activity typically associated with feeding and other human interaction. Mildly increasing physical activity in the least active individuals reduces compulsion for overeating by humans (Shook et al. 2015). Increasing physical activity is easier said than done, however, as it will generally require a greater commitment on the part of the caregiver, and may be contraindicated due to pre-existing health conditions in some individuals.

Little is known about the duration and intensity of activity necessary to promote weight loss in companion animals compared to the human literature, as there have been few investigations that have objectively assessed the range of activity typical of pet dogs and cats or the contribution of increased exercise to successful weight loss in overweight companion animals. One investigation found in a cohort of dogs undergoing a weight-loss regimen that the dogs classified as "active" (based on pedometer data) consumed more calories than their "inactive" counterparts while achieving the same rate of weight loss (Wakshlag et al. 2012). Other research showed that treadmill sessions three times a week in a weight-loss plan for dogs resulted in a modest decrease in body fat and a gain in lean mass (Vitger et al. 2016). Furthermore, some preliminary studies indicate that physical therapy techniques, such as exercise on an underwater treadmill, can be useful adjuncts in weight-loss programs for dogs (Mlacnik et al. 2006; Chauvet et al. 2011). Caregivers can be coached on ways to increase their pet's activity level even in the absence of data on which to base clear-cut recommendations. At the very least, such strategies can help refocus both the pet and the owner on activities other than the feeding ritual.

Tailoring the Program to the Patient

While the basic design of a weight-loss program is to induce a negative energy balance by restricting caloric intake through dietary modification and increasing caloric expenditure through the promotion of physical activity, there are many ways to go about achieving this goal. To be successful, the program should be tailored as much as possible to fit the lifestyle of the patient's household. Caregivers are unlikely to embrace proposed radical changes in behavior such as a ban on treats or an ambitious exercise program. Obtaining a thorough dietary history will reveal the needs and the preferences of both the caregiver and the patient. Table 9.4 lists some considerations to address when designing a weight-loss program.

Table 9.4 Considerations for the design of a weight-loss program.

Multipet households
  Can the pets be fed separately?
  To what lengths is the caregiver willing to go to feed the pets separately?

Feeding methods
  Can the patient be fed portion-restricted meals?
  Can the caregiver's lifestyle accommodate meal feeding?

Diet
  Will the patient tolerate a change in diet?
  Is the caregiver willing to change the patient's diet?
  Will the patient tolerate reduced portions?
  Is the caregiver willing to reduce feeding portions?

Treats
  If the patient receives excessive amounts of food as treats, will the caregiver accept modifications of the kinds and amounts of treats offered?

Exercise
  How active is the patient and can it tolerate an increase in activity level?
  Can the caregiver's lifestyle accommodate measures for increasing the patient's activity level?

Household
  Will all the people in the household cooperate with the program?

Assessment of the Weight-Loss Plan

The success of a weight-loss program hinges on follow-up. In fact, monitoring and appropriate intake adjustments are arguably more important than the exact starting point for caloric restriction. Through the entire program the patient should be monitored on a regular basis (every 2–4 weeks) in order to assess whether weight loss is occurring at an appropriate rate and whether there are barriers to adherence to the plan. Soliciting any concerns of the caregiver ensures that the plan can be modified as necessary. Maintaining contact throughout the program is the only way to ensure that the patient achieves the targeted weight-loss goal.

The pet should be weighed on the same scale during each visit. It is not uncommon to have to make adjustments to the feeding recommendations in order to achieve and then maintain the target rate of weight loss (1–2% of body weight per week – see Box 9.4). One investigation that examined weight loss in dogs on different degrees of caloric restriction found, as one would expect, that those dogs that were the most calorically restricted lost weight the most rapidly (Laflamme and Kuhlman 1995). However, these same dogs were the ones most predisposed to regain the weight when they came off the diet.

During follow-up visits, inquiring whether anyone in the household has been experiencing difficulties in implementing the weight-reduction plan may reveal unforeseen issues. The patient may not accept the recommended changes in diet or feeding management and may begin to exhibit unacceptable behaviors such as stealing food or breaking into the trash. The human members of the household may have difficulties adhering to the program because of the pet's behavior, their own time constraints, or feelings of guilt over withholding food or treats from their companion. Undetected problems that go unresolved can result in the caregivers becoming discouraged with the program and giving up.

Box 9.4   Estimating Time Needed to Achieve a Weight-Loss Goal

The time it will take to achieve the weight-loss goal can be estimated by multiplying the kilograms of weight the pet needs to lose by 7700 kcal/kg. Dividing the resulting number by the daily caloric deficit provides an estimate of how long it will take to lose the weight (e.g. a cat that needs to lose 1 kg and is being restricted by 100 kcal/day below its maintenance energy requirement will need to be on the diet for approximately 77 days or 11 weeks). Alternatively, one can use the rate of weight loss and body condition score (BCS) to estimate how long the plan will take. A BCS indicating that the pet is 15% overweight coupled with a weight-loss rate of 1% will mean the pet will take at least 15 weeks to lose the needed weight, assuming no plateaus or regressions.

Safety and Efficacy of Weight-Loss Programs for Companion Animals

There have been published studies evaluating the efficacy of weight-loss programs for dogs and cats. A number of these studies, some conducted in a controlled setting such as a kennel and some conducted as clinical trials, have reported excellent results (Laflamme and Kuhlman 1995; Watson et al. 1995; Center et al. 2000; Impellizeri et al. 2000; Burkholder et al. 2001). However, success in other clinical settings is challenging. Investigations evaluating weight-loss programs in pet dogs report significant dropout rates of 37–60% (Yaissle et al. 2004; German et al. 2012; Flanagan et al. 2017). Further, even when a weight-loss program is successful, there is a significant risk of rebound weight gain. Studies of overweight companion animals have reported that 48% of dogs and 46% of cats rebound after successful weight loss (German et al. 2012; Deagle et al. 2014). One reason may be that energy requirements are reduced due to energy restriction and/or to weight loss compared to prior to initiation of the weight-loss program, as has been demonstrated in cats (Villaverde et al. 2008). For dogs it has been observed that weight regain is less likely if the patient continues to be fed the same therapeutic diet used during the weight-loss phase as opposed to switching back to a maintenance diet (German et al. 2012). The numerous challenges of achieving successful long-term weight loss in companion animals underscore the need for greater focus of effort on prevention of obesity.

Most investigations of weight-reduction programs for companion animals have found them to be safe. The greatest concern over the safety of aggressive food restriction is particular to cats and involves the risk of inducing hepatic lipidosis. Investigations where overweight cats were restricted from 25% to 60% of normal maintenance energy requirement found that the cats lost weight while maintaining their appetite without any changes in serum chemistry (Armstrong et al. 1992; Watson et al. 1995). While weekly rate of body weight loss was not reported, these findings suggest that the risks of inducing feline idiopathic hepatic lipidosis by a weight-reduction regimen in an otherwise healthy cat are minimal for this range of caloric restriction. However, caregivers of cats who undertake a weight-loss plan should be familiar with the signs of hepatic lipidosis and should be instructed to seek medical attention for their cat if it becomes anorexic. Body weight losses no greater than of 2% per week are recommended for cats (Michel and Scherk 2012).

Adjustment of the Weight-Loss Plan

When a patient is not losing weight at the anticipated rate, the first step is to review the feeding plan with the caregiver to determine whether all aspects of the plan are being adhered to and whether any problems have arisen. If the caregiver adhered to the plan, then in most cases it will be necessary to modify the amount of calories as necessary (a 10% adjustment is a reasonable place to start) to achieve the targeted rate of weight loss. Many patients who successfully lose weight will reach a plateau in their rate of weight loss after a period of time, which may be a consequence of reduced metabolic rate due to several factors including metabolic adaptations and the inevitable loss of some lean body mass (Villaverde et al. 2008).

Even when care has been taken to tailor a weight-reduction plan to an individual household, problems can arise. There are a variety of tactics that can be used to motivate the caregiver toward success (Table 9.5).

Table 9.5 Weight-loss program troubleshooting tips.

Food-seeking behavior
   Use a therapeutic weight-loss diet
   Switch to canned food or add water to the food
   Add vegetables low in starch and calories to the meal
   Feed the daily food portion in multiple small meals (including one shortly before bedtime)
   Substitute other forms of attention (e.g. grooming, play, walks) for treats
   Give the caregiver a daily treat allowance
   Keep pets out of the kitchen during food preparation or the dining areas during meals
   Serve the meal in a food puzzle toy
   Environmental enrichment

Multipet households
   Meal feed in separate rooms
   Feed on a raised surface (cats)
   Construct or purchase a creep feeder or smart bowl (cats or small dogs)

Sedentary pets
   Feeding puzzles
   Food-motivated play
   Environmental enrichment
   Start a walking program or hire a dog walker (dogs)
   Physical therapy

One common concern is lack of satiety, and most owners have a low tolerance of their pets behaving as if they are very hungry. There may also be undesirable behaviors such as stealing food, coprophagia, and consumption of other non-food items. There are a number of ways in which this situation can be addressed. If the patient is not already consuming an appropriate therapeutic diet with reduced calorie density and strategies to promote satiety, this should be suggested. Switching to a food with a lower caloric density will permit feeding of larger portions. In particular, feeding canned rather than dry food, or adding water to any food, will increase meal volume and may be more satisfying for some pets. As previously discussed, there is evidence that cats do not readily compensate for the reduced caloric density of canned foods, and studies of human subjects have shown that adding water to foods to decrease caloric density (e.g. eating soup rather than a casserole) has a satiating effect (Rolls et al. 1999). Another tactic to increase meal volume is to add vegetables that are low in calories but that provide more moisture and fiber, such as carrots, cabbage, or green beans.

Feeding the pet three or four small meals a day rather than one or two large ones can also be helpful. Having part of the daily food ration available to feed throughout the day should help decrease the temptation to "cheat" by giving treats when the pet begs for food. For cats this approach will help to mimic the more natural feeding pattern of the species. Also, more calories are expended in digesting and assimilating nutrients from multiple small meals than from one or two large ones (Leblanc and Diamond 1986).

The diet history will reveal the households where feeding the pet is a bonding activity. Giving family members a prescribed treat allowance can help in these cases. Most people are familiar with counting calories, so a treat allowance will give the household some flexibility in how they give treats from day to day. Set the allowance at no more than 10% of the pet's targeted daily caloric intake, and provide caregivers with information about the caloric content of the pet treats they use, and with some low-calorie alternatives such as appropriate fruits and vegetables. The calorie content of most commercial pet treats can be obtained from the label or calling the manufacturer if necessary.

Because food is commonly used for bonding with a pet, there is often a behavioral component to begging in addition to hunger. Ignoring these behavioral aspects of feeding will doom a program to failure. The caregiver can be counseled to substitute play, walks, or grooming, in addition to lower-calorie treats, as alternatives to feeding calorically dense foods and treats for bonding. Another tip to help curtail begging behavior is to keep the pet out of the kitchen during food preparation or away from dining areas during meals.

Using food puzzles or some other type of ploy to make a pet work for its food may also help to decrease begging. This approach and other forms of environmental enrichment may have an added benefit of increasing the pet's energy expenditure (Clarke et al. 2005).

Multipet households present their own challenges, as it can be difficult to restrict portions for the pet on the weight-reduction diet when food for other pets is available. Ideally all the pets in the household would be separately meal fed. It can be difficult for some caregivers to transition to meal feeding, as well as to make certain that the dieting pet does not have access to the other pets' food. Sometimes feeding the pets in separate rooms will be the solution. With cats, feeding on a counter or other raised surface will keep food away from a dog or an overweight cat that is not able to jump or climb. It is also possible to construct or purchase feeders that have openings that will permit a thin pet access to the food, but exclude the overweight one. There is a growing array of microchip feeders and similar technology that limits access to food bowls and can help manage multipet households by controlling which pet can consume specific amounts of specific foods.

One final challenge is increasing activity level for sedentary pets. As already discussed, this will generally require a greater commitment from the caregiver than changes in feeding management. Some things that can be tried are using feeding puzzles or moving food bowls throughout the house. Food can be used to motivate the pet to climb, jump, and run, especially if the pet's environment is enriched with objects to facilitate these activities. The services of a pet walker can be used if the caregiver is unable to exercise the pet themselves. And if the caregiver has access to a veterinary physical therapy facility, regular use of a swimming pool or underwater treadmill can be incorporated into the program. This approach should be of particular benefit for dogs with orthopedic disease. For cats, addition of water to food reportedly increases physical activity, but the long-term effect on caloric balance is not known (Alexander et al. 2014; Hooper et al. 2018).

Summary

- Many companion animals are overweight or obese and, as a consequence, are at risk of impaired health and reduced longevity.
- To address this problem, pet caregivers must learn how to apply BCSs to their pets and be able to recognize when a pet is not in optimal condition.
- When veterinarians perceive that a pet is overweight, they must bring it to the attention of that pet's caregiver.
- A successful weight-reduction program begins with a thoroughly conducted diet history and should be tailored to the individual household to increase the likelihood of adherence and help ensure success.
- Follow-up visits are absolutely essential for monitoring the patient's progress and adjusting the plan as necessary, thereby ensuring the success of the program.

References

Alexander, J.E., Colyer, A., and Morris, P.J. (2014). The effect of reducing dietary energy density via the addition of water to a dry diet, on body weight, energy intake and physical activity in adult neutered cats. *J. Nutr. Sci.* 3: e21.

Allan, F.J., Pfeiffer, D.U., Jones, B.R. et al. (2000). A cross-sectional study of risk factors for obesity in cats in New Zealand. *Prev. Vet. Med.* 46 (3): 183–196.

Armstrong, P.J., Hardie, E.M., Cullen, J.M. et al. (1992). L-Carnitine reduces hepatic fat accumulation during rapid weight reduction in cats. In: *Proceedings of the 10th American College of Veterinary Internal Medicine Forum*, San Diego, CA, 810, 28–31 May, 1992.

Backus, R.C., Cave, N.J., and Keisler, D.H. (2007). Gonadectomy and high dietary fat but not high dietary carbohydrate induce gains in body weight and fat of domestic cats. *Br. J. Nutr.* 98 (3): 113–119.

Barić Rafaj, R., Kuleš, J., Marinculić, A. et al. (2017). Plasma markers of inflammation and hemostatic and endothelial activity in naturally overweight and obese dogs. *BMC Vet. Res.* 13 (1): 13.

Belsito, K.R., Vester, B.M., Keel, T. et al. (2009). Impact of ovariohysterectomy and food intake on body composition, physical activity, and adipose gene expression in cats. *J. Anim. Sci.* 87 (2): 594–602.

Bermingham, E., Thomas, D., Morris, P., and Hawthorne, A. (2010). Energy requirements of adult cats. *Br. J. Nutr.* 103 (8): 1083–1093.

Bermingham, E.N., Thomas, D.G., Cave, N.J. et al. (2014). Energy requirements of adult dogs: a meta-analysis. *PLoS ONE* 9 (10): e109681.

Bierer, T.L. and Bui, L.M. (2004). High protein, low carbohydrate diets enhance weight loss in dogs. *J. Nutr.* 134 (8 Suppl): 2087S–2089S.

Burkholder, W.J., Taylor, L., and Hulse, D.A. (2001). Weight loss to optimal body condition increases ground reactive force in dogs with osteoarthritis. *Compend. Contin. Educ. Pract. Vet.* 23 (9(A) Suppl): 74.

Burrows, C.F., Chiapella, A.M., and Jezyk, P. (1981). Idiopathic feline hepatic lipidosis: the syndrome and speculations on its pathogenesis. *Florida Vet. J.* 18 (Winter): 18–20.

Butterwick, R.F. and Markwell, P.J. (1997). Effect of amount and type of dietary fiber on food intake in energy restricted dogs. *Am. J. Vet. Res.* 58 (3): 272–276.

Center, S.A., Harte, J., Watrous, D. et al. (2000). The clinical and metabolic effects of rapid weight loss in obese pet cats and the influence of supplemental oral L-carnitine. *J. Vet. Intern. Med.* 14 (6): 598–608.

Chauvet, A.J.L., Elliott, D.A., and German, A.J. (2011). Incorporation of exercise, using an underwater treadmill, and active client education into a weight management program for obese dogs. *Can. Vet. J.* 52 (5): 491–496.

Chiang, C.-F., Villaverde, C., and Chang, W.-C. (2022a). Prevalence, risk factors, and disease associations of overweight and obesity in cats that visited the veterinary medical teaching Hospital at the University of California, Davis from January 2006 to December 2015. *Top. Companion Anim. Med.* 47: *100620*.

Chiang, C.-F., Villaverde, C., and Chang, W.-C. (2022b). Prevalence, risk factors, and disease associations of overweight and obesity in dogs that visited the veterinary medical teaching Hospital at the University of California, Davis from January 2006 to December 2015. *Top. Companion Anim. Med.* 47: 100620.

Clarke, D.L., Wrigglesworth, D., Holmes, K. et al. (2005). Using environmental and feeding enrichment to facilitate feline weight loss. *J. Anim. Physiol. Anim. Nutr. (Berl.)* 89: 427.

Colditz, G.A. (1999). Economic costs of obesity and inactivity. *Med. Sci. Sports Exerc.* 31 (11, Suppl): S663–S667.

Coradini, M., Rand, J.S., Morton, J.M., and Rawlings, J.M. (2014). Metabolic determinants of body weight after cats were fed a low-carbohydrate high-protein diet or a high-carbohydrate low-protein diet ad libitum for 8 wk. *Domest. Anim. Endocrinol.* 49: 70–79.

Courcier, E.A., O'Higgins, R., Mellor, D.J., and Yam, P.S. (2010). Prevalence and risk factors for feline obesity in a first opinion practice in Glasgow, Scotland. *J. Feline Med. Surg.* 12 (10): 746–753.

Deagle, G., Holden, S.L., Biourge, V. et al. (2014). Long-term follow-up after weight management in obese cats. *J. Nutr. Sci.* 3: e25.

Edney, A.T.B. and Smith, P.M. (1986). Study of obesity in dogs visiting veterinary practices in the United Kingdom. *Vet. Rec.* 118 (14): 391–396.

Fettman, M.J., Stanton, C.A., Banks, L.L. et al. (1998). Effects of weight gain and loss on metabolic rate, glucose tolerance, and serum lipids in domestic cats. *Res. Vet. Sci.* 64 (1): 11–16.

Finco, D.R., Brown, S.A., and Cooper, T.A. (2001). Effects of obesity on glomerular filtration rate (GFR) in dogs. *Compend. Contin. Educ. Pract. Vet.* 23 (9(A) Suppl): 78.

Flanagan, J., Bissot, T., Hours, M.A. et al. (2017). Success of a weight loss plan for overweight dogs: the results of an international weight loss study. *PloS ONE* 12 (9): e0184199.

Flegal, K.M., Kruszon-Moran, D., Carroll, M.D. et al. (2015). Trends in obesity among adults in the United States, 2005 to 2015. *JAMA* 315 (21): 2284–2291.

Gayet, C., Bailhache, E., Dumon, H. et al. (2004). Insulin resistance and changes in plasma concentration of TNFa, IGF1, and NEFA in dogs during weight gain and obesity. *J. Anim. Physiol. Anim. Nutr. (Berl.)* 88 (3–4): 157–165.

German, A.J. and Morgan, L.E. (2014). How often do veterinarians assess the body weight and body condition of dogs? *Vet. Rec.* 163 (17): 503–505.

German, A.J., Hervera, M., Hunter, L. et al. (2009). Improvement in insulin resistance and reduction in plasma inflammatory adipokines after weight loss in obese dogs. *Domest. Anim. Endocrinol.* 37 (4): 214–226.

German, A.J., Holden, S.L., Morris, P.J., and Biourge, V. (2012). Long-term follow-up after weight management in obese dogs: the role of diet in preventing regain. *Vet. J.* 192 (1): 65–70.

Gross, K.L., Wedekind, K.J., Kirk, C.A. et al. (2000). Dietary chromium and carnitine supplementation does not affect glucose tolerance in obese dogs during weight loss. *J. Vet. Intern. Med.* 14 (3): 345.

Hammond, R.A. and Levine, R. (2010). The economic impact of obesity in the United States. *Diabetes Metab. Syndr. Obes.* 3 (7): 265–295.

Hannah, S.S. and Laflamme, D.P. (1998). Increased dietary protein spares lean body mass during weight loss in dogs. *J. Vet. Intern. Med.* 12 (3): 224.

Hess, R.S., Kass, P.H., Shofer, F.S. et al. (1999). Evaluation of risk factors for fatal acute pancreatitis in dogs. *J. Am. Vet. Med. Assoc.* 214 (1): 46–51.

Hoenig, M. and Ferguson, D.C. (2002). Effects of neutering on hormonal concentrations and energy requirements in male and female cats. *Am. J. Vet. Res.* 63 (5): 634–639.

Hooper, S.E., Backus, R., and Amelon, S. (2018). Effects of dietary selenium and moisture on the physical activity and thyroid axis of cats. *J. Anim. Physiol. Anim. Nutr.* 102 (2): 495–504.

Hu, F.B., Manson, J.E., Stampfer, M.J. et al. (2001). Diet, lifestyle, and the risk of type 2 diabetes mellitus in women. *N. Engl. J. Med.* 345 (11): 790–797.

Impellizeri, J.A., Tetrick, M.A., and Muir, P. (2000). Effect of weight reduction on clinical signs of lameness in dogs with hip osteoarthritis. *J. Am. Vet. Med. Assoc.* 216 (7): 1089–1091.

Ishioka, K., Sagawa, M., Okumura, M. et al. (2004). Treatment of obesity in dogs through increasing energy expenditure by mitochondrial uncoupling proteins. *J. Vet. Intern. Med.* 18 (3): 431.

Jackson, J.R., Laflamme, D.P., and Owens, S.F. (1997). Effects of dietary fiber content on satiety in dogs. *Vet. Clin. Nutr.* 4 (4): 130–134.

Jeusette, I., Daminet, S., Nguyen, P. et al. (2006). Effect of ovariectomy and ad libitum feeding on body composition, thyroid status, ghrelin and leptin plasma concentrations in female dogs. *J. Anim. Physiol. Anim. Nutr. (Berl.)* 90 (1–2): 12–18.

Jewell, D.E. and Toll, P.W. (1996). Effects of fiber on food intake in dogs. *Vet. Clin. Nutr.* 3 (4): 115–118.

Jewell, D.E., Azain, M.J., Edwards, M.J. et al. (2006). Fiber but not conjugated linoleic acid influences adiposity in dogs. *Vet. Ther.* 7 (2): 78–85.

Kanchuk, M.L., Backus, R.C., Calvert, C.C. et al. (2003). Weight gain in gonadectomized normal and lipoprotein lipase-deficient male domestic cats results from increased food intake and not decreased energy expenditure. *J. Nutr.* 133 (6): 1866–1874.

Kealy, R.D., Lawler, D.F., Ballam, J.M. et al. (2002). Effects of diet restriction on life span and age-related changes in dogs. *J. Am. Vet. Med. Assoc.* 220 (9): 1315–1320.

Kurzman, I.D., Panciera, D.L., Miller, J.B., and MacEwen, E.G. (1998). The effect of dehydroepiandrosterone combined with a low-fat diet in spontaneously obese dogs: a clinical trial. *Obes. Res.* 6 (1): 20–28.

Laflamme, D.P. (1997a). Development and validation of a body condition score system for dogs: a clinical tool. *Canine Pract.* 22: 10–15.

Laflamme, D.P. (1997b). Development and validation of a body condition score system for cats: a clinical tool. *Feline Pract.* 25 (5–6): 13–18.

Laflamme, D.P. and Hannah, S.S. (2005). Increased dietary protein promotes fat loss and reduces loss of lean body mass during weight loss in cats. *Int. J. Appl. Res. Vet. Med.* 3 (2): 62–68.

Laflamme, D.P. and Kuhlman, G. (1995). The effect of weight loss regimen on subsequent weight maintenance in dogs. *Nutr. Res.* 15 (7): 1019–1028.

Laflamme, D.P., Backus, R.C., Forrester, S.D., and Hoenig, M. (2022). Evidence does not support the controversy regarding carbohydrates in feline diets. *J. Am. Vet. Med. Assoc.* 260 (5): 506–513.

Leblanc, J. and Diamond, P. (1986). Effect of meal size and frequency on postprandial thermogenesis in dogs. *Am. J. Physiol.* 250: E144–E147.

Leclerc, L., Thorin, C., Flanagan, J. et al. (2017). Higher neonatal growth rate and body condition score at 7 months are predictive factors of obesity in adult female Beagle dogs. *BMC Vet. Res.* 13 (1): 104.

Lefebvre, S.L., Yang, M., Wang, M. et al. (2013). Effect of age at gonadectomy on the probability of dogs becoming overweight. *J. Am. Vet. Med. Assoc.* 243 (2): 235–243.

Leray, V., Dumon, H., Martin, L. et al. (2006). No effect of conjugated linoleic acid or *Garcinia cambogia* on fat-free mass and energy expenditure in normal cats. *J. Nutr.* 136 (7 Suppl): 1982S–1984S.

Lund, E.M., Armstrong, P.J., Kirk, C.A. et al. (1999). Health status and population characteristics of dogs and cats examined at private veterinary practices in the United States. *J. Am. Vet. Med. Assoc.* 214 (9): 1336–1341.

Lund, E.M., Armstrong, P.J., Kirk, C.A., and Klausner, J.S. (2005). Prevalence and risk factors for obesity in adult cats from private U.S. veterinary practices. *Int. J. Appl. Res. Vet. Med.* 3 (2): 88–96.

Lund, E.M., Armstrong, P.J., Kirk, C.A., and Klausner, J.S. (2006). Prevalence and risk factors for obesity in adult dogs from private U.S. veterinary practices. *Int. J. Appl. Res. Vet. Med.* 4 (2): 177–186.

MacEwen, E.G. and Kurzman, I.D. (1991). Obesity in the dog: role of the adrenal steroid dehydroepiandrosterone (DHEA). *J. Nutr.* 121 (11 Suppl): S51–S55.

Mankowska, M., Krzeminska, P., Graczyk, M., and Switonski, M. (2017). Confirmation that a deletion in the POMC gene is associated with body weight of Labrador Retriever dogs. *Res. Vet. Sci.* 112: 116–118.

Mao, J., Xia, Z., Chen, J., and Yu, J. (2013). Prevalence and risk factors for canine obesity surveyed in veterinary practices in Beijing, China. *Prev. Vet. Med.* 112 (3–4): 438–432.

Marshall, W.G., Hazewinkel, H.A., Mullen, D. et al. (2010). The effect of weight loss on lameness in obese dogs with osteoarthritis. *Vet. Res. Commun.* 34 (3): 241–253.

Mattheeuws, D., Rottiers, R., Kaneko, J.J., and Vermeulen, A. (1984). Diabetes mellitus in dogs: relationship of obesity to glucose intolerance and insulin resistance. *Am. J. Vet. Res.* 45 (1): 98–103.

McGreevy, P.D., Thomson, P.C., Price, C. et al. (2005). Prevalence of obesity in dogs examined by Australian veterinary practices and the risk factors involved. *Vet. Rec.* 156 (22): 695–702.

Michel, K. and Scherk, M. (2012). From problem to success: feline weight loss programs that work. *J. Feline Med. Surg.* 14 (5): 327–336.

Michel, K.E., Bader, A., Shofer, F.S. et al. (2005). Impact of time-limited feeding cat foods of differing carbohydrate content on weight loss in group-housed cats. *J. Feline Med. Surg.* 7 (6): 349–355.

Miller, C., Bartges, J., Cornelius, L. et al. (1998). Tumor necrosis factor-α levels in adipose tissue of lean and obese cats. *J. Nutr.* 128 (12S, Suppl): 2751S–2752S.

Mlacnik, E., Bockstahler, B.A., Müller, M. et al. (2006). Effects of caloric restriction and a moderate or intense physiotherapy program for treatment of lameness in overweight dogs with osteoarthritis. *J. Am. Vet. Med. Assoc.* 229 (11): 1756–1760.

Morrison, R., Penpraze, V., Greening, R. et al. (2014). Correlates of objectively measured physical activity in dogs. *Vet. J.* 199 (2): 263–267.

National Institutes of Health (1985). Health implications of obesity: National Institutes of Health consensus development conference statement. *Ann. Intern. Med.* 103 (6): 1073–1077.

Nguyen, P.G., Dumon, H.J., Siliart, B.S. et al. (2004). Effects of dietary fat and energy on body weight and composition after gonadectomy in cats. *Am. J. Vet. Res.* 65 (12): 1708–1713.

Ogden, C.L., Carroll, M.D., Curtin, L.R. et al. (2006). Prevalence of overweight and obesity in the United States, 1999–2004. *JAMA* 295 (13): 1549–1555.

O'Neill, D.G., Gostelow, R., Orme, C. et al. (2016). Epidemiology of diabetes mellitus among 193,435 cats attending primary-care veterinary practices in England. *J. Vet. Intern. Med.* 30 (4): 964–972.

Panciera, D.L., Thomas, C.B., Eicker, S.W., and Atkins, C.E. (1990). Epizootiologic patterns of diabetes mellitus in cats: 333 cases (1980–1986). *J. Am. Vet. Med. Assoc.* 197 (11): 1504–1508.

Raffan, E., Dennis, R.J., O'Donovan, C.J. et al. (2016). A deletion in the canine POMC gene is associated with weight and appetite in obesity-prone Labrador Retriever dogs. *Cell Metab.* 23 (5): 893–900.

Roberts, M.T., Bermingham, E.N., Cave, N.J. et al. (2018). Macronutrient intake of dogs, self-selecting diets varying in composition offered ad libitum. *J. Anim. Physiol. Anim. Nutr.* 102 (2): 568–575.

Robertson, I.D. (1999). The influence of diet and other factors on owner-perceived obesity in privately owned cats from metropolitan Perth, Western Australia. *Prev. Vet. Med.* 40 (2): 75–85.

Rolls, B.J., Bell, E.A., and Thorwart, M.L. (1999). Water incorporated into a food but not served with a food decreases energy intake in lean women. *Am. J. Clin. Nutr.* 70 (4): 448–455.

Rolph, N.C., Nobel, P.J.M., and German, A.J. (2014). How often do primary care veterinarians record the overweight status of dogs? *J. Nutr. Sci.* 3: e58.

Root, M.V., Johnston, S.D., and Olson, P.N. (1996). Effect of prepuberal and postpuberal gonadectomy on heat production measured by indirect calorimetry in male and female domestic cats. *Am. J. Vet. Res.* 57 (1): 371–374.

Rossetti, L., Giaccari, A., and DeFronzo, R.A. (1990). Glucose toxicity. *Diabetes Care* 13 (6): 610–630.

Rowe, E., Browne, W., Casey, R. et al. (2015). Risk factors identified for owner-reported feline obesity at around one year of age: dry diet and indoor life style. *Prev. Vet. Med.* 121 (3–4): 273–281.

Russell, K., Sabin, R., Holt, S., and Harper, E.J. (2000). Influence of feeding regimen on body condition in the cat. *J. Small Anim. Pract.* 41 (1): 12–18.

Scarlett, J.M. and Donoghue, S. (1996). Obesity in cats: prevalence and prognosis. *Vet. Clin. Nutr.* 3 (4): 128–132.

Scarlett, J.M. and Donoghue, S. (1998). Associations between body condition and disease in cats. *J. Am. Vet. Med. Assoc.* 212 (11): 1725–1731.

Scarlett, J.M., Donoghue, S., Sadia, J., and Wills, J. (1994). Overweight cats: prevalence and risk factors. *Int. J. Obes. (Lond)* 18 (Suppl 1): S22–S28.

Serisier, S., Feugier, A., Venet, C. et al. (2013). Faster growth rate in ad libitum-fed cats: a risk factor predicting the likelihood of becoming overweight during adulthood. *J. Nutr. Sci.* 23 (2): e11.

Shook, R.P., Hand, G.A., Drenowatz, C. et al. (2015). Low levels of physical activity are associated with dysregulation of energy intake and fat mass gain over 1 year. *Am. J. Clin. Nutr.* 102 (6): 1332–1338.

Singh, R., Laflamme, D.P., and Sidebottom-Nielsen, M. (2002). Owner perceptions of canine body condition score. *J. Vet. Intern. Med.* 16 (3): 362.

Stachowiak, M., Szczerbal, I., and Switonski, M. (2016). Genetics of adiposity in large animal models for human obesity-studies on pigs and dogs. *Prog. Mol. Biol. Transl. Sci.* 140: 233–270.

Stanton, C.A., Hamar, D.W., Johnson, D.E., and Fettman, M.J. (1992). Biolelectrical impedance and zoometry for body composition analysis in domestic cats. *Am. J. Vet. Res.* 53 (2): 251–257.

Stoll, J.A. and Laflamme, D.P. (1995). Effect of dry vs. canned rations on food intake and bodyweight in cats. *Vet. Clin. Nutr.* 2 (4): 145.

Sunvold, G.D., Vickers, R.J., Kelley, R.L. et al. (1999). Effect of dietary carnitine during energy restriction in the canine. *Fed. Am. Soc. Exp. Biol. J.* 13: A268.

Villaverde, C., Ramsey, J.J., Green, A.S. et al. (2008). Energy restriction results in a mass-adjusted decrease in energy expenditure in cats that is maintained after weight regain. *J. Nutr.* 138: 858–860.

Vitger, A.D., Stallknecht, B.M., Nielsen, D.H., and Bjornvad, C.R. (2016). Integration of a physical training program in a weight loss plan for overweight pet dogs. *J. Am. Vet. Med. Assoc.* 248 (2): 174–182.

Wakshlag, J.J., Struble, A.M., Levine, C.B. et al. (2011). The effects of weight loss on adipokines and markers of inflammation in dogs. *Br. J. Nutr.* 106 (Suppl 1): S11–S14.

Wakshlag, J.J., Struble, A.M., Warren, B.S. et al. (2012). Evaluation of dietary energy intake and physical activity in dogs undergoing a controlled weight-loss program. *J. Am. Vet. Med. Assoc.* 240 (4): 413–419.

Watson, T.D.G., Butterwick, R.F., and Markwell, P.G. (1995). Effects of weight reduction on plasma lipid and lipoprotein metabolism in obese cats. *J. Vet. Intern. Med.* 9 (3): 214.

Weber, M., Bissot, T., Servet, E. et al. (2007). A high-fiber, high-protein diet designed for weight loss improves satiety in dogs. *J. Vet. Intern. Med.* 21 (6): 1203–1208.

Weeth, L.P., Fascetti, A.J., Kass, P.H. et al. (2007). Prevalence of obese dogs in a population of dogs with cancer. *Am. J. Vet. Res.* 68 (4): 389–398.

Wei, A., Fascetti, A.J., Villaverde, C. et al. (2011). Effect of water content in a canned cat food on voluntary food intake and body weight in cats. *Am. J. Vet. Res.* 72 (7): 918–923.

Witzel, A.L., Kirk, C.A., Henry, G.A. et al. (2014a). Use of a novel morphometric method and body fat index system for estimation of body composition in overweight and obese cats. *J. Am. Vet. Assoc.* 244 (11): 1285–1290.

Witzel, A.L., Kirk, C.A., Henry, G.A. et al. (2014b). Use of a novel morphometric method and body fat index system for estimation of body composition in overweight and obese dogs. *J. Am. Vet. Assoc.* 244 (11): 1279–1284.

Yaissle, J.E., Holloway, C., and Buffington, C.A.T. (2004). Evaluation of owner education as a component of obesity treatment programs for dogs. *J. Am. Vet. Med. Assoc.* 224 (12): 1932–1935.

Yano, B.L., Hayden, D.W., and Johnson, K.H. (1981). Feline insular amyloid: association with diabetes mellitus. *Vet. Pathol.* 18 (5): 621–627.

Zhang, P., Jackson, J.R., Roos, M. et al. (2004). Evaluation of pyruvate supplementation on body weight and fat loss in overweight dogs. *Compend. Contin. Educ. Pract. Vet.* 26 (2(A) Suppl): 78.

Zoran, D.L. (2002). The carnivore connection to nutrition in cats. *J. Am. Vet. Med. Assoc.* 221 (11): 1559–1567.

10

Nutritional Management of Orthopedic Diseases

Herman Hazewinkel

The percentage of patients with orthopedic (i.e. non-traumatic) disease has been reported to be around 10%, although this figure varies depending upon the type of veterinary clinic and its location. The percentage of some orthopedic diseases is higher in large dogs (LaFond et al. 2000), with particular breeds more at risk. The popularity of these at-risk large-breed dogs can differ considerably between countries; for instance, Bernese mountain dogs are in the top 10 among popular breeds in some countries, whereas in other states they rank much lower. Historically, orthopedic diseases are less well recognized in cats than in dogs, but this is changing as specialization in feline medicine increases.

Nutrition plays a role in skeletal growth and development, may have an influence on the occurrence of skeletal diseases, and can be applied to support treatment of orthopedic patients. This chapter will discuss the relevant nutritional aspects in all three roles after a short overview to facilitate the understanding of the particular role of nutrition.

Bone Composition and Calciotropic Hormones

Skeletal growth can be divided into three inter-related processes: (i) endochondral ossification, which includes growth, maturation, and apoptosis of chondrocytes followed by bony replacement of cartilage; (ii) periosteal growth, including lamellar new bone formation; and (iii) remodeling, including the removal of newly formed metaphyseal bone to adapt the shape of the bone, the removal of bone at the endosteal site of long bones and in tunnel-like structures around growing soft tissues, and the remodeling of lamellar bone into Haversian structures. Endochondral ossification takes place in primary and secondary ossification centers around birth and in growth plates between the epiphyses and metaphyses, as well as in the cartilage layer covering the epiphyses during the growth phase. Cancellous bone remains in the metaphyses and epiphyses of long bones as well as in vertebral bodies, and is easily accessible by bone-removing cells. Periosteal growth takes place in the diaphyseal area of the long bones and in flat bones like the pelvis, ribs, and skull. Remodeling is especially seen at the endosteum and the metaphyseal areas and in vertebral and nutritional canals.

The cell types involved in bone growth and remodeling are chondrocytes forming the cartilage matrix, chondroclasts removing that matrix after its mineralization, and osteoblasts forming osteoid on the cartilage template (in case of endochondral ossification in ossification centers and metaphyses) or directly on the periosteum to stimulate its mineralization by alkaline phosphatase secretion. Osteoclasts are able to resorb mineralized osteoid with the aid

Applied Veterinary Clinical Nutrition, Second Edition. Edited by Andrea J. Fascetti, Sean J. Delaney, Jennifer A. Larsen, and Cecilia Villaverde.

Table 10.1 Content and ratio of calcium, phosphorus, and magnesium in dogs.

	Calcium	Phosphorus	Magnesium
% of adult body weight	1–1.5%	0.5–0.8%	~0.25%
% present in skeleton	98%	80%	50%
Absorption	Active (vitamin D regulated) and passive diffusion	Active (vitamin D regulated) and passive diffusion	Facilitated and passive diffusion
Octocalciumphosphate $Ca_8(HPO_4)_2(PO_4)_4 \cdot 5H_2O$	8	6	N/A
Whitlockite $Ca_9Mg(HPO_4)(PO_4)_6$	9	7	1
Sodium-containing apatite $Ca_{8.5}Na_{1.5}(PO_4)_{4.5}(CO_3)_{2.5}$	17	9	N/A
Carbonated apatite $Ca_9(PO_4)_{4.5}(CO_3)(OH)_{1.5}$	18	9	N/A
Hydroxyapatite $C_{10}(PO_4)_6(OH)_2$	10	6	N/A

N/A, not available.

of acid phosphatase, and osteocytes are able to communicate with peripheral osteoblasts via their canalicular system and resorb bone locally. The skeleton provides a solid framework for muscles and a harness for delicate structures, but is also a depot for minerals (Table 10.1), of which calcium is the most biologically important element, playing a vital role in blood clotting, muscle contraction, and enzymatic processes. More than 98% of the body's calcium is stored in the skeleton as stable crystals (including hydroxyl apatite) and in labile calcium compounds (including calcium phosphate and calcium bound to plasma albumin), which can quickly be mobilized. Of the remaining 1%, half of it is in the extracellular fluid as the biologically active, ionized form. Of the body's phosphorus, 80% is stored in the skeleton and is of major importance in the formation of calcium salts and thus mineralization of newly formed cartilage and osteoid.

Chemical Composition of Bone

After musculature (40–57% of body weight [BW]), the skeleton makes up the largest part of the body weight of an adult dog (8–13%),

whereas it is 10% in newly born puppies (Meyer and Zentek 2005). The composition of an adult dog by weight includes 1–1.5% calcium, 0.5–0.8% phosphorus, and 0.25% magnesium, of which 98%, 80%, and 50%, respectively, is present as mineral in the skeleton (Meyer and Zentek 2005). Whole bone, including marrow and periosteum, consists of 33% organic components (including 95% collagen, 5% glycoproteins and sulfated glycosaminoglycans), 17% water, and 48% inorganic material, primarily calcium, phosphate, carbohydrate, and magnesium (Jee et al. 1970; Kincaid and Van Sickle 1983). The various skeletal locations reveal marked differences in composition. Lumbar vertebrae can contain twice the amount of water, depending on the amount of cancellous bone. Trabecular bone has more water and less ash than cortical bone, and it has slightly less organic material, although this also can differ considerably: the ash percentage in vertebrae is 50% and in mandibles only 7% of the bone weight.

Minerals in bone are formed in different phases, starting with octacalcium phosphate and whitlockite, followed by sodium-containing apatite, carbonated apatite, and eventually hydroxyapatite in the adult skeleton. Mineral complexes other than apatite are of interest for ionic exchange. The grams of calcium per cm^3 of bone increases with advancing age: in beagles from 0.468 and 0.536 g at 6 weeks to 0.512 and 0.612 g at 11 years of age, in low- and high-density areas, respectively. Not only age but also mineral composition of the diet may influence the mineral composition of bone (Hazewinkel and Schoenmakers 1995; Jee et al. 1970).

Mineral Composition During Growth

Joint cartilage has a high heterogeneity of chondrocyte types and arrangements within the matrix, with its collagen fibers encored in the calcified zone with hydroxyapatite salts (Table 10.2) (Poole et al. 2001).

In one study, seven growing miniature poodles were raised on the same food

Table 10.2 Biochemical composition of cartilage.

	Chemical content of cartilage in the extracellular matrix
Water	66–79%
Collagen Mainly collagen II Also collagen XI, III, V, VI, X, XII, XIV	60% (% of dry weight)
Proteins	8–15%
Glycosaminoglycan	14–23%
Hyaluronate	<1%
Lipid	<1%
Inorganic (ash)	2%

formulated according to the 1985 National Research Council (NRC) guidelines. Partial weaning was started at 3 weeks of age and completed by 6 weeks of age.

Magnesium content was higher in rib biopsies at 11 weeks than at 21 weeks of age in these miniature poodles (Table 10.3) (Huis in 't Veld et al. 2001). When maturation proceeds, firmer calcium-phosphate crystals are formed, reducing the magnesium content. It is also possible that whitlockite is exchanged for other apatites during growth (Driessen 1980). The increase in the calcium-to-phosphorus ratio, as reported in ruminants (Chicco et al. 1973), was also seen in the dogs of this study.

Comparison with an identical study in Great Danes, raised on the same food and investigated according to the same procedure, revealed that the calcium-to-phosphorus ratio did not increase in this time period (1.570 vs. 1.527 at 11 and 21 weeks, respectively). This finding was probably due to the slower skeletal maturation in giant-breed dogs when compared to small-breed dogs. There was also a decrease in whitlockite content (0.302 mmol/cm^3 at 11 weeks vs. 0.238 mmol/cm^3 at 21 weeks of age) (Huis in 't Veld et al. 2001). Excessive calcium intake will increase the calcium content and decrease the magnesium content in the bones of young dogs (Hazewinkel and Schoenmakers 1995). However, when excess vitamin D was given to Great Dane dogs starting at partial weaning (i.e. 10 or 100 times the recommended dietary content), the ratio of calcium to phosphorus increased, but the amount of whitlockite decreased at the same rate as in the controls (Hazewinkel and Tryfonidou 2002; Huis in 't Veld et al. 2001).

Table 10.3 Mineral composition of rib biopsies at 11 and 21 weeks of age in miniature poodles.

	Calcium (mg ± SD/cm³)	Phosphorus (mg ± SD/cm³)	Magnesium (mg ± SD/cm³)	Calcium-to-phosphorus ratio	Whitlockite (mmol/cm³)
11 weeks	377 ± 74	183 ± 35	7 ± 0.42	1.658	0.304
21 weeks	368 ± 11	177 ± 5	6.5 ± 0.3	1.697	0.272

SD, standard deviation.

In addition to age and food composition, skeletal location influences bone composition. In low-density areas, 1.02–1.28 g of hydroxyapatite was found per cm^3 of bone in adult beagles. In the high-density bone areas, this was 1.23–1.54 g hydroxyapatite, without any effect on breaking stress in healthy dogs (Jee et al. 1970).

These analyses illustrate the role of the skeleton as a buffer for excess minerals, as well as an organ with biomechanical functions and its related architecture and composition.

Hormonal Regulation of Calcium

A constant extracellular concentration of ionized calcium is of importance to maintain a variety of physiologic processes, which can be life-threatening when they do not occur properly due to a deficiency or excess of this element. The uncontrolled input of calcium (i.e. passive diffusion of calcium through the intestinal wall) takes place only in the immature dog and especially in cases of a positive gradient (Tryfonidou et al. 2002). The uncontrolled excretion of calcium via the glomerulus could be as high as 60% of the circulating calcium, being the ultrafilterable amount. Calcium deposition in the skeleton (i.e. in newly formed cartilage and osteoid) is largely a physicochemical process and will take place especially in growing individuals. These uncontrolled processes do not guarantee a constant and sufficiently high extracellular calcium level. Hormonal regulation is necessary to accomplish this, adapted to different life stages and environmental influences. There are mainly three hormones involved in the homeostasis of calcium.

Sudden changes in extracellular calcium concentration, especially lowered concentrations, can be life-threatening due to calcium's function in nerve conduction, muscle contracture, enzymatic activity, and as co-factor in the blood coagulation cascade; therefore extracellular calcium concentrations are kept between narrow limits. The extracellular calcium concentration is maintained at its optimal concentration by physicochemical-driven processes, the combined action of the calciotropic hormones parathyroid hormone (PTH), calcitonin (CT), and vitamin D, and controlled by calcium sensors, keeping the calcium concentration in dogs constant; that is, between 2.0 and 3.0 mmol/l in adult dogs. Changes in calcium concentration have consequences for the coupling of calcium to receptors (i.e. calcium sensors) as present on the cell wall of parathyroid chief cells, CT-producing C cells, kidney cells, osteoclasts, and osteoblasts, but also present in the placenta, intestine, brain, and lung, with presumably different second messenger systems involved with events following the sensing of changes in extracellular calcium concentration. Plasma Ca^{2+} concentrations are PTH related: when PTH is expressed as a percentage of its maximum value reached at very low Ca^{2+} levels, the actual Ca^{2+} levels correspond with the actual PTH levels in a reversed S-shape curve, with over a narrow range of plasma calcium concentrations a linear segment in this relationship. This linear segment includes at its midpoint the calcium concentration that inhibits 50% of the maximum value of PTH, defined as the "Ca^{2+} setpoint for PTH secretion." This calcium setpoint is close to the Ca^{2+} concentration that is maintained under normal circumstances (Cloutier et al. 1993).

The relationship between plasma Ca^{2+} and plasma PTH concentration was determined in two groups of Great Dane dogs (both n = 9) raised on food with 1.04 g Ca/100 g dry matter (DM; diet 1) or 3.11 g Ca/100 g DM (diet 2) from 3 to 17 weeks of age for each diet and diet 1 for both groups thereafter; the Ca^{2+} setpoint for PTH secretion in the dogs raised on the high-calcium diet till 17 weeks and diet 1 thereafter revealed a significant (P < 0.10) increase in the Ca^{2+} setpoint for PTH secretion at week 27 when compared with the control dogs (raised solely on diet 1). What is remarkable is that the basal plasma concentrations for calcium and PTH did not differ, but stimulation of secretion with standardized ethylenedinitrilotetraacetic acid disodium salt dihydrate (Na-EDTA) infusion demonstrated this altered

PTH secretion pattern in the diet 2 dogs, reflecting a chronic relatively hypocalcemic state, which may have consequences for the coordinated osteoclast and -blast activity later in life and thus skeletal integrity (Schoenmakers et al. 1999b). In a study in Great Dane pups (n = 7) from bitches either on a diet with 1.14 g Ca/100 g DM or on 3.27 g Ca/100 g dm during the second half of the gestation period, no differences in Ca^{2+} setpoint for PTH secretion could be found, leading to the conclusion that excessive calcium intake during late pregnancy in the bitch, unlike what has been demonstrated in the offspring from maternal sheep at high calcium intake (Corbellini et al. 1991), has no deleterious effects on hormonal calcium homeostasis and skeletal integrity of the pups during their first half year of life (Schoenmakers et al. 2001). Ergocalciferol, vitamin D2, and cholecalciferol, vitamin D3, appear to have similar potencies in the dog, but not in the cat, where vitamin D3 is metabolized more efficiently than vitamin D2 (Morris 2002b; Stockman et al. 2021).

During the evolution of terrestrial mammals living in a calcium-deprived environment, PTH became the most important of these calciotropic hormones. Its role is to increase plasma calcium concentration when it decreases. PTH executes this role by increasing re-absorption of calcium from the pre-urine and by activating osteoclasts to resorb bone (i.e. freeing calcium and phosphorus from bone minerals). Under the influence of PTH, the renal threshold for phosphorus will be lowered, with a subsequent increase in phosphaturia. In addition, PTH stimulates the synthesis of another calciotropic hormone, calcitriol. Dogs as omnivores are able to convert ergocalciferol to calcitriol (25OHvitD) and to cholecalciferol, whereas cats as obligate carnivores use ergocalciferol less efficiently (Morris 2002b; Zafalon et al. 2020b).

The product of cholecalciferol (vitamin D) hydroxylation in the liver is 25-hydroxycholecalciferol (25OHvitD), and it is the most abundant metabolite of vitamin D in plasma. PTH stimulates the synthesis of an enzyme present in the kidney, 1α-hydroxylase, which is responsible for the hydroxylation of 25OHvitD into calcitriol (1,25(OH)₂vitD). In addition, other hormones and minerals influence vitamin D metabolism, causing significant differences in vitamin D metabolism under different circumstances, and even in dogs of different breeds raised under the same circumstances (Hazewinkel and Tryfonidou 2002) (Table 10.4). In miniature poodles receiving supraphysiologic doses of growth hormone (GH; 0.5 IU GH/kg BW/d), the plasma insulin-like growth factor (IGF-1) levels and the (1,25(OH)₂D) production both increased, whereas 24,25(OH)₂vitD decreased. As a result, the plasma concentrations of the vitamin D metabolites resembled those of Great Danes (Tryfonidou and Hazewinkel 2004).

The primary function of calcitriol is to mineralize cartilage and newly formed osteoid.

Table 10.4 Similar plasma mineral levels with significant differences in vitamin D metabolites in different breeds. Mean (± standard error of the mean, SEM) of plasma concentrations in nine Great Danes and eight miniature poodles, 3 months of age, raised on a diet with 0.94 g Ca, 0.75 g P, and 1.14 µg vitamin D per 100 g dry matter at twice maintenance.

	Calcium mmol/l	Phosphorus mmol/l	Parathyroid hormone (ng/l)	25(OH)vitD nmol/l	24,25(OH)₂vitD nmol/l	1,25(OH)₂vitD pmol/l
Great Dane	2.8±0.1	2.7±0.1	62±6.5	14.7±2.8	39.9±3.2	250±9
Miniature poodle	2.8±0.2	2.6±0.1	70±5.0	50±2.0	140±6.0	190±10

Source: Tryfonidou et al. (2003b) / with permission of Elsevier.

Calcitriol performs this role by increasing re-absorption of calcium from the pre-urine, by acting as a permissive factor for PTH (thus stimulating osteoclast activity), and by increasing the process of active absorption of calcium and phosphorus from the food in the intestine. This hormonally regulated, active absorption is of special importance in growing dogs due to their high calcium requirement in case of low dietary calcium content (Hazewinkel and Tryfonidou 2002; Parker et al. 2017).

When the calcium concentration of the intestinal contents is high, calcium will diffuse between the intestinal cells by non-saturable, paracellular passive diffusion. In addition to calcitriol, another vitamin D metabolite is formed: $24,25(OH)_2$vitD, which has long been seen as a waste product of 25OHvitD in order to avoid providing too much of the biologically active $1,25(OH)_2$vitD. However, an important role for $24,25(OH)_2$vitD was demonstrated in endochondral ossification: $24,25(OH)_2$vitD stimulates maturation of chondrocytes and increases the responsiveness of these chondrocytes to $1,25(OH)_2$vitD for further differentiation and matrix mineralization (Wu et al. 2006). In addition, $24,25(OH)_2$vitD increases the bone mineral content (Mortensen et al. 1993) together with reducing osteoclast activity – that is, reduced bone turnover – in contrast to $1,25(OH)_3$vitD (Norman et al. 2002). Minimal recommendations for cholecalciferol for growing dogs are given by NRC (2006) as 110–136 IU, FEDIAF (2021) as 125–138 IU, and AAFCO (2022) as 125 IU per Mcal. Dietary vitamin D can be provided from animal origin (vitamin D3, ergocalciferol) or from vegetable ingredients (vitamin D2, ergocalciferol), or as a purified additive (vitamin D3). Vitamins D2 and D3 appear to have similar potencies in the dog, but not in the cat, where vitamin D3 is metabolized more efficiently than vitamin D2 (Morris 2002b; Stockman et al. 2021). Recently it has been reported that in plant-based pet food, vitamin D is among the most commonly found insufficiencies, whereas vitamin D3 and not only D2 could be analyzed in some of these North American plant-based foods (Zafalon et al. 2020a).

CT is the third calciotropic hormone, which is of special biological importance in animals living in a calcium-rich environment, such as saltwater fish. In mammals the release of CT, which is mainly formed in the thyroid glands, can be caused by an acute rise in plasma calcium concentration as well as in gastrin concentration. A correcting decrease of plasma calcium concentration in mammals occurs mainly via the reduction of osteoclast activity; the ruffle borders of the osteoclasts are retracted instantly under the influence of CT. CT has many more functions and effects, including activation of the satiety center (Tryfonidou et al. 2010).

GH is not a calciotropic hormone per se, but one of the major hormones responsible for the longitudinal and periosteal growth of the skeleton. GH stimulates the formation of IGF-I in the liver and in target cells, including osteoblasts. GH stimulates intestinal calcium absorption by hypertrophy of intestinal cells and directly, or via an increase in IGF-I level, by stimulating $1,25(OH)_2$vitD and suppressing $24,25(OH)_2$vitD production, respectively. IGF-I synthesis can also be stimulated by PTH and by the ingestion of nutritional factors such as protein and energy. IGF-I stimulates bone and collagen synthesis, as well as chondrocyte cell proliferation (and thus longitudinal growth), and to a lesser extent chondrocyte differentiation, and it can suppress GH synthesis and release from the pituitary gland (Tryfonidou and Hazewinkel 2004).

In addition to calcium and phosphorus, other minerals also play a role in bone formation. Magnesium (Mg) is an important stabilizer of DNA, RNA, and ribosomes, is a co-factor in many enzymes, and influences bone mineral formation. It is regulated by PTH and vitamin D, and not, importantly, by CT. Magnesium absorption is not active but facilitated by vitamin D and takes place by diffusion. Magnesium absorption increases with increasing dietary vitamin D and decreases in cases of excess dietary calcium, phosphorus, or long-chain triglycerides. PTH decreases renal losses of magnesium. In addition, magnesium excess will be reflected in the plasma and lead to increased magnesium content in the bone. Magnesium stimulates 1α-hydroxylation of 25OHvitD and will increase bone turnover. Magnesium deficiency also causes muscular weakness, but not clinical abnormalities of the skeleton (Dobenecker et al. 2006).

The Role of Nutrition During Skeletal Growth and Development

Energy

Energy, provided by carbohydrate, protein, and fat, is the driving force behind food intake. Dietary carbohydrates have not been recognized to be essential for growth in dogs (Meyer 1983), and there are no reports on the relationship between carbohydrate deficiency and skeletal disease. In the case of malnutrition, there is often a deficiency of both protein and energy. Low protein intake will coincide with growth retardation and finally growth cessation and weight loss (Sheffy 1979). Plasma albumin will decrease, especially when protein intake is inadequate in the face of sufficient energy intake (Lunn and Austin 1983; Nap et al. 1993c). Low energy and protein intake will cause a decrease in hepatic IGF-I production and thus a decrease in skeletal growth.

Beagles raised from 6 to 25 weeks on a diet with 12% protein (as a percentage of metabolizable energy [ME]) never reached normal body weight, even after being fed a food with 25% (ME) free choice thereafter (Sheffy 1979). Great Danes raised from 7 to 20 weeks of age on a balanced food with 13% (ME) protein developed hypoalbuminemia and a lower body weight, but had no abnormalities in size or skeletal development when compared to controls raised on a diet containing 21% protein (ME) (Nap et al. 1991). Research dogs raised on food with a calcium content of 3.11 g/100 g

(DM (vs. 1.04 g for controls), starting at the time of partial weaning (3 weeks of age), developed significant hypercalcemia (3.64 vs. 2.94 mmol/l) together with a decreased calcium absorption percentage (25% vs. 54%) and decreased voluntary food intake (900 kJ/kg$^{0.75}$ vs. 1300 kJ/kg$^{0.75}$). Adult mixed-breed dogs fed the same food revealed a slight increase in plasma calcium concentration (2.70 vs. 2.63 mmol/l) without decreased energy intake (645 kJ/kg$^{0.75}$) when compared with control food (Schoenmakers 1999), thus revealing that the palatability of the food itself did not decrease food intake in the young dogs, but demonstrating that the voluntary lowering of the food intake of unbalanced food is the ultimate mechanism of the young dog to prevent further hypercalcemia. From cancer-associated studies of hypercalcemia it is known that hypercalcemia goes together with decreased appetite and nausea (Kohart et al. 2017). Hypercalcemia influences directly or indirectly (i.e. via increased plasma concentrations of CT) the satiety center and thereby food intake (Tryfonidou et al. 2010). Low energy intake is not a common clinical problem (Richardson et al. 2010), and therefore in cases where animals are small for their age the clinician should also consider a biological variation in body size or growth rate, metabolic diseases such as GH deficiency, hypothyroidism, liver shunt, or skeletal abnormalities like chondrodystrophy (in breeds where it is not part of the breed standard) or rickets.

Excess energy intake is much more common in today's clinical practice. Diets containing an excess of protein (>30 g/100 g DM) will be metabolized, although in some cases one can document an increase in plasma albumin or blood urea nitrogen, reflecting the increased deamination of protein and not a malfunction of the kidneys (Romsos et al. 1976). In a study in growing Great Danes, raised on a diet with 29% protein (ME), except for an increase in plasma albumin and blood urea nitrogen concentrations, no differences were found in plasma total protein, growth rate, calcium metabolism, or skeletal development (Nap et al. 1993b).

Excess fat cannot only predispose an animal to excessive calorie consumption, thereby increasing body weight, but can also decrease the intake of essential nutrients when these are not adapted to the high energy content of the food. Dietary fat is very readily absorbed and converted more efficiently into body fat than dietary carbohydrates or proteins, without affecting the growth in lean body mass (Romsos et al. 1976). When the fat content of the food was increased from 8% to 24% of dry matter in a diet with 22% protein, 10% ash, and no fiber added, the ME increased by 22.5%. This resulted in a higher percentage of body fat and an increase in body weight when fed free choice compared to control dogs raised on an 8% fat (DM) diet (Richardson et al. 2010).

There are a variety of studies demonstrating the deleterious effects of overnutrition on skeletal development (Alexander et al. 1988; Hedhammar et al. 1974; Lavelle 1989), causing osteochondrosis and poor hip conformation and resulting in secondary osteoarthritis in multiple joints (Kealy et al. 1992) (Table 10.5). Since overnutrition often includes providing an excess of all nutrients, it is not obvious whether the causative role of excess calories is a matter of overweightness alone. Since excess minerals (Hazewinkel 1985; Schoenmakers et al. 2000) and vitamin D (Tryfonidou et al. 2003b), but not protein or carbohydrate (Nap and Hazewinkel 1994), disturb skeletal development severely, and excessive fat intake has no influence on calcium metabolism (Hallebeek and Hazewinkel 1998), a deleterious role for specific nutrients is to be expected (see Figure 10.1). Therefore, the most relevant nutrients in clinical practice will be discussed in the following sections.

Calcium, Phosphorus, and Vitamin D

Calcium Deficiency

Calcium is required for biological processes and for skeletal mineralization. The calcium requirement for growing dogs ranges between 0.33% and 1.2% of calcium on a dry matter basis (Table 10.5). In rapidly growing animals, the daily calcium requirement is much higher than in slower-growing animals. In rapidly growing Great Danes, the daily calcium deposition in the skeleton can be as high as 225–900 mg Ca/kg BW, whereas in miniature poodles the daily deposition of calcium in the skeleton sufficient for undisturbed skeletal mineralization was 140 mg Ca/kg BW (Nap et al. 1993a).

These findings are comparable with the results of the study published by Atwal et al. (2021) in adult beagles (age 1.4–4.4 years) on a control diet and a test diet containing 5× the calcium and 4× the phosphorus content of the test food for a period of 40 weeks. The apparent calcium digestibility did not differ from controls (32%), except for the dogs on the test diet at 8 weeks, which coincided with significantly lowered $1,25OH_2vitD$ levels and increased ionized plasma calcium levels. In comparison with Labradors on 2.6% Ca dm (Stockman et al. 2017), these beagles consumed 50% more energy and had therefore a higher calcium intake per $kg/BW^{0.75}$ (Atwal et al. 2021). However, neither the Labradors nor the beagles in these studies fed a diet with high calcium and phosphorus content for a 40-week period revealed any effect on blood chemistry, bone health, or kidney function (Atwal et al. 2021; Stockman et al. 2017).

In pregnant Great Danes fed a control diet (Ca 1.14 and P 0.89 g/100 g dm) or a test diet (Ca 3.27 and P 1.11 g/100 g dm), the basal plasma concentrations of Ca, P, PTH, 25OHvitD, and $24,25OH_2vitD$ did not differ between groups during the second half of gestation, and only $1,25OH_2vitD$ tended to decrease when on the test diet (20–37 ng/l vs. 40–44 ng/l when fed the control food), with a true calcium absorption of 3.8–4.4 mmol on the control diet and 3.8–8.3 mmol on the test diet due to decreased (29–50%) calcium absorption on high calcium and phosphorus when fed the control diet in comparison with this

Table 10.5 Investigations of the influence of excess or deficiencies on skeletal development. Breeds of research dogs and dietary composition with their variables are summarized for different studies together with the clinical and radiologic findings (see references for further details).

	Hedhammar et al. (1974)	Lavelle (1989)	Hazewinkel (1991)	Nap et al. (1991)	Nap et al. (1993b)	Schoenmakers et al. (1999b)	Tryfonidou et al. (2002)
Breed of research dog	Great Dane	Great Dane	Great Dane	Great Dane	Miniature poodle	Great Dane	Great Dane
Food composition per 100 g (dm)							
ME in kcal (kJ)	501 (2094)	431 (1802)	402 (1680)	359 (1500)	359 (1500)	N/A	450 (1884)
Crude protein	36	29.6	21	21	21	21	27
Crude fat	13.7	14.4	9.9	9.7	9.9	10.2	15
Calcium	2.05	2.3	1.1	1.0	1.0	1.04	0.95
Phosphate	1.44	1.6	0.9	0.9	0.9	0.82	0.75
Vitamin D (in µg)	N/A	N/A	2.77	2.77	2.77	2.76	1.14
Variables in study	Ad lib or restricted to 66%	Ad lib or restricted to 60%	Ca 0.55%, 1.1%, or 3.3% (dm)	Proteins: 31, 23, or 14% (dm)	Calcium: 0.05%, 0.33%, 1.1% and 3.3% (dm)	Calcium: 1.1% and 3.3% calcium starting at different ages	Vitamin D content: 1.14, 10.0, and 135 µg/100g (dm)
Clinical, radiologic, and pathologic findings	Ad lib group had higher rates of osteochondrosis, radius curvus syndrome, poor hip conformation, and wobbler syndrome	No differences in skeletal problems between the groups	Pathologic fractures in 0.55% Ca group; severe osteochondrosis, radius curvus, and wobbler syndrome in the 3.3% Ca group	No differences in skeletal problems between groups	Pathologic fractures in 0.05% Ca group; no clinical pathology in 0.33% Ca, 1.1% Ca, or 3.3% Ca group	3.3% Ca from 3 to 6 weeks only: panosteitis at 4 mo. 3–17 weeks: Hypophosphatemic rickets 6–26 weeks: severe osteochondrosis and radius curvus	1.14 µg vitamin D/kg food: normal endochondral ossification; at 10 µg and 135 µg vitamin D/kg food: slight and severe osteochondrosis

dm, dry matter; ME, metabolizable energy; N/A, not available.

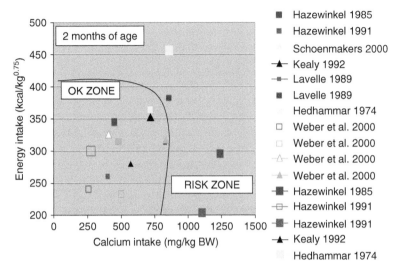

Figure 10.1 Potential deleterious effects in skeletal development in large-breed puppies raised on controlled calcium and energy intake. The graph depicts the calcium intake (in mg Ca/kg body weight [BW]) provided together with the energy intake (expressed as kcal/kg$^{0.75}$) for different studies in large-breed dogs (e.g. Labradors, German shepherds, Newfoundlands, Great Danes) of 2 months of age, with special attention to the development of skeletal diseases (including osteochondritis dissecans, retained cartilage cone with radius curvus syndrome, and hip dysplasia). The area left of the curved line represents the calcium intake with no or minimal skeletal abnormalities, whereas right of the curved line is the potentially deleterious zone. The various studies referenced are included in the reference list. *Source:* Modified from Hazewinkel and Mott (2006), with acknowledgment to Dr. M. Weber.

absorption when fed the control diet (75–97%). The calcium balance in both groups of pregnant bitches did not differ significantly (3.3–4.3 mmol Ca/kg BW/day), without any adverse effects reflected in blood chemistry, serious bone health disturbance, or kidney function, either in the bitches or in their offspring till the age of 27 weeks (Schoenmakers et al. 2001).

In a meta-analysis of repetitive calcium balance studies in growing dogs of different breeds, apparent calcium absorption as the true intestinal absorption of calcium was included from 271 calcium balance studies with the aid of ^{45}calcium, as performed in 67 Great Danes (207 studies) and 23 miniature poodles (64 studies), raised on uniform diets only differing in calcium salts content, resulting in a range of 0.55–3.3 g Ca/100 g dm for Great Danes and 0.33–3.3 g Ca/100 g dm for miniature poodles, between the age of 6 and 27 weeks. A curvilinear relationship between calcium intake (mg Ca/kg BW/d) and true absorption (= absorption minus endogenous fecal excretion) was demonstrated for both Great Danes (r = 0.832) and miniature poodles (r = 0.927; P < 0.01), whereas the fractional absorption of the ingested amount (= true absorption/intake) was inversely related (r = −0.450 and −0.444, respectively) to the amount of calcium intake (Tryfonidou et al. 2002). This indicates the presence of both an active and a passive calcium absorption mechanism in these immature dogs. The model in which the two mechanisms can be discerned demonstrates that active calcium absorption (mainly present at low calcium intake levels) changes with age, whereas passive absorption (at higher calcium intake levels) remains constant at approximately 53% of the ingested amount of calcium. The intestinal mechanisms did not differ between these two breeds with extreme body size.

In a calcium study in two other breeds, young beagles and Labrador crossbred dogs received either 1.1 or 3.6 g Ca/100 g dm and apparent calcium absorption (as the difference between calcium intake and its fecal excretion) was determined, demonstrating a retention (intake minus fecal and urinary calcium excretion) in beagles on the control and supplemented diet of 72% and 70% at 12 weeks of age and of 51% and 54% at 18 weeks of age, respectively, whereas in the crossbreds this was 48% and 40% at 12 weeks and 41% and 28% at 18 weeks, respectively (Dobenecker 2004). This confirmed that at a young age the absorption percentage is not so much influenced by the amount of dietary calcium and decreases with age, but that there might be breed differences in calcium absorption ability. Miniature poodles raised on a diet with 1.1% calcium on a dm basis revealed in calcium kinetic studies with use of the ^{45}calcium isotope a true intestinal absorption coefficient for calcium of 27% (i.e. true calcium absorption of 100 mg/kg BW/d) at the age of 24 weeks (Nap et al. 1993a), and 53% (i.e. true calcium absorption of 132 mg/kg BW/d) for beagles of that age (Hallebeek and Hazewinkel 1998) and 60% (i.e. 320 mg/kg BW/d) in Great Danes of that age (Schoenmakers et al. 1999a), thus covering the mineralization of the skeleton at different growth rates to the adult body weight of 6, 20, and 70 kg, respectively.

A meta-analysis of 34 published, classic digestion trials (i.e. apparent calcium absorption as the difference between calcium intake and its fecal excretion) in adult dogs revealed a linear relationship (P < 0.0001) between calcium intake and calcium excretion, suggesting the absence of a systematic quantitative adaptation mechanism in calcium absorption in these adult dogs. The calcium digestibility in adult dogs did not differ significantly in different diets with different calcium-to-phosphorus ratios (Mack et al. 2015). These findings were supported by Stockman et al. (2017), who found no difference in calcium digestibility (approximately 20%) and total calcium balance (not significantly different from 0 g/d for both groups) in mature Labradors fed 4.2 the

amount of calcium (and phosphorus) as the control group of comparable sex and age. It revealed that the high calcium intake was well tolerated for a period of 40 weeks without any adverse effects.

These studies illustrate the lack of effect of normal or elevated calcium intake on the skeleton in mature dogs, due to the low bone turnover. This may be different in cases of prolonged calcium deficiency, which can result in calcium mobilization of the skeleton (Mack and Kienzle 2016), especially in case of gravitation and/or lactation.

Dietary calcium deficiency can be caused by feeding meat-based, home-prepared diets with insufficient supplementation of calcium salts, unbalanced commercially prepared diets as might be present in the Bones and Raw Food (BARF) diet (Mack and Kienzle 2016), commercial vegan foods (Zafalon et al. 2020a), or poor-quality diets with an excess of phytates that bind intestinal calcium as insoluble and non-absorbable complexes. If there is a decrease in body growth, the mineralization of the skeleton will have a tendency to result in a decrease in plasma calcium levels and will induce hyperparathyroidism. As a result, there will be an increase in bone resorption by activated osteoclasts and osteocytes. In cases of chronic calcium deficiency, calcium resorption from bone and calcium accretion (i.e. skeletal mineralization) are both significantly increased (Hazewinkel 1991; Nap et al. 1993b), with a subsequent increase in plasma alkaline phosphatase levels. Thus bone turnover is significantly increased in animals with dietary-induced hyperparathyroidism.

This explains the radiologic and pathologic findings in the skeleton of growing dogs: long bones reveal normal growth in length, together with excessively increased osteoclastic bone removal, especially in the endosteum (resulting in a wide intramedullary cavity) and in the areas of cancellous bone. The cortex can become so thin that it cannot withstand normal muscle contracture or the body weight of the animal, leading to pathologic fractures (i.e. greenstick and compression fractures) (Figure 10.2). Compression fractures of vertebrae can cause paralysis and can worsen the prognosis of the animal. The PTH-induced increase in 1,25(OH)$_2$vitD$_3$ plasma levels explains

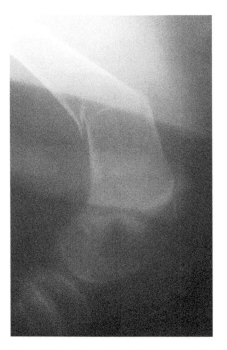

Figure 10.2 Young dog with hyperparathyroidism due to calcium-deficient diet, causing folding fractures in the long bones ("greenstick fractures") due to the narrowing of the cortex. Notice the poor contrast difference between bone and soft tissues, and the growth plate of normal width with adjacent white area of mineralized cartilage.

the normal mineralization of the growth plate cartilage, visible as a white area bordering the growth plates of normal width. This finding is important to aid in the differentiation between alimentary secondary hyperparathyroidism and hypovitaminosis D (see the section on Rickets). In mature dogs, chronic calcium deficiency will not cause clinical signs due to the low bone turnover. However, pregnancy and lactation might cause massive demineralization of the skeleton, first at sites of high bone turnover; that is, cancellous bone in the vertebrae and metaphyseal area. Compression fractures of the vertebrae will cause severe back pain and possibly even paralysis.

In growing dogs the diagnosis of nutritionally induced hyperparathyroidism can be made by taking a diet history, careful radiologic interpretation (poor contrast between bone and soft tissues, greenstick and compression fractures, wide medulla, bended flat bones, normal growth plates) (Figure 10.2), and in some cases measurement of plasma PTH concentrations. In most cases, plasma concentration of calcium will be kept in the physiologic range (although at the lower end) by the calciotropic hormones, with phosphorus plasma levels normal to slightly above normal combined with increased urine levels of phosphorus (Table 10.6). Analysis of plasma calcitriol concentration will reveal elevated levels compared to normal dogs of the same breed and

Table 10.6 Plasma levels of calcium, phosphorus, and the major vitamin D metabolites in 3-month-old small-breed dogs raised under normal circumstances (on a balanced food with Ca 1.1%, P 0.9% [dry matter, dm], vitamin D 500 IU/kg food), or on a diet deficient in calcium ("hyperparathyroidism": Ca 0.05%, P 0.9% (dm), vitamin D 500 IU/kg food) or vitamin D ("hypovitaminosis D": Ca 1.0%, P 0.9% (dm), vitamin D not added to semi-synthetic food). *Source:* Based on Hazewinkel and Tryfonidou (2002).

	Calcium (mmol/l)	Phosphorus (mmol/l)	Parathyroid hormone (ng/l)	25OHvitD (nmol/l)	1,25(OH)$_2$vitD (pmol/l)	24,25(OH)$_2$vitD (nmol/l)
Normal	2.8±0.1	2.7±0.1	20±2	50±5	95±5	169±44
Hyperparathyroidism	2.7±0.1	2.7±0.1	30±1[a]	77±22	494±87[a]	45±29[a]
Hypovitaminosis D	2.7±0.1	2.0±0.3[a]	>35[a]	6.2±0.2[a]	65±5[a]	1.4±0.5[a]

[a] Significantly different from normal.

age. Bone biopsies will demonstrate thin cortices and thin cancellous bone spiculae, no unmineralized osteoid, an increased amount of multinucleated osteoclasts within Howship's lacunae reflecting their high activity, and growth plates that are normally mineralized and of normal width (Figure 10.3a,b). The most practical approach for confirming the diagnosis based on clinical and radiologic investigation is to institute treatment and re-evaluate the skeletal status after three weeks. Differential diagnoses are rickets (see later), osteogenesis imperfecta (a rare hereditary disease with abnormal bone collagen), and renal hyperparathyroidism (see Chapter 15).

Therapy includes strict cage rest to prevent more damage and normalization of the diet. Cage rest should be started immediately to prevent other bones from fracturing, especially vertebral collapse and subsequent spinal cord damage, as well as to prevent further skeletal malformations. Normalization of the diet can be accomplished by changing the food to a complete and balanced diet and extra calcium carbonate (50 mg Ca/kg BW/d) can be supplemented for three weeks. Injections of calcium are not indicated; the amount of circulating calcium is sufficient to prevent cardiac abnormalities. Extra vitamin D is not indicated in a case of pure alimentary secondary hyperparathyroidism, since the endogenous $1,25(OH)_2vitD_3$ is increased by the high level of PTH (see Table 10.6). Therefore, calcium absorption is very efficient – that is, up to 100% of the amount of calcium in the food – and extra vitamin D is contraindicated to increase osteoclast activity (Nap et al. 1993b). The bone is too thin to consider orthopedic treatment of the fractures other than rest; even splints cannot be applied, since the bone will break at the proximal margin of the splint. After mineralization of the skeleton, which is completed within a month, corrective surgery can be considered when indicated. The prognosis depends on the severity of secondary spinal cord damage and the severity of skeletal malformation, especially narrowing of the pelvic canal with disturbed passage of the feces.

Phosphorus Deficiency

An absolute deficiency of dietary phosphorus rarely occurs in companion animals; however, a relative deficiency may occur in extreme cases. When providing a food with very high calcium content to puppies less than 2 months of age, insoluble and thus non-absorbable calcium-phosphorus salts are formed in the intestinal tract. Due to the excess of dietary calcium, there is hypercalcemia with negative feedback on PTH synthesis and thus decreased $1,25(OH)_2vitD$ synthesis. The increased calcium absorption in these young dogs consuming diets with excessive calcium (Schoenmakers et al. 2000) will cause hypercalcemia. Both the hypophosphatemia and the lack of $1,25(OH)_2vitD$ will cause a disturbance in skeletal mineralization, resulting in wide growth plates and thin cortices evident on radiographs.

The diagnosis can be made from the diet history, radiologic investigation, and laboratory findings. Hypercalcemia and hypophosphatemia together with hypoparathyroidism and decreased hydroxylation of vitamin D will coincide with the radiologic signs seen in rickets (Schoenmakers et al. 2000), commonly referred to as hypophosphatemic rickets (Figure 10.4).

Vitamin D Deficiency (Rickets or Hypovitaminosis D)

The ability to synthesize cholecalciferol in the skin under the influence of ultraviolet light has been developed in amphibians, reptiles, birds, herbivores, and omnivores, but not in dogs, cats (How et al. 1994), and other carnivorous species (Corbee et al. 2015b). The cutaneous level of the vitamin D_3 precursor 7-dehydrocholesterol (7-DHC) is low due to a high level of 7-DHC reductase, an enzyme with a high activity that converts 7-DHC into cholesterol (Morris 1999). Thus dogs and cats are solely dependent on dietary sources to meet their vitamin D requirement. Animal fat has high levels of vitamin D; vegetarian food

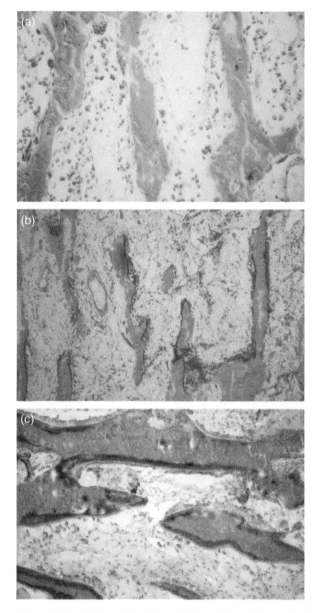

Figure 10.3 (a) Cancellous bone of the epiphyseal area of a 6-month old dog. (b) Cancellous bone in the corresponding area of a 6-month-old dog with nutritional secondary parathyroidism due to low calcium content of the food (0.55% Ca on a dry matter basis). Notice the large number of osteoblasts and osteoclasts causing high bone turnover, active in new bone formation and bone resorption, respectively, responding to the hypocalcemia-induced high parathyroid hormone (PTH) level. Thinned bone will break (greenstick fracture) and collapse (compression fracture). (c) Cancellous bone of a 6-month-old dog with hypovitaminosis D. Notice the red seams of osteoid (equal to non-mineralized collagen formed by osteoblasts) covering the mineralized bone, and multinucleated osteoclasts, not able to reach the mineralized bone. The latter will cause, together with the inability to absorb calcium and phosphorus in the intestine, a gradual decrease in plasma calcium and phosphorus levels.

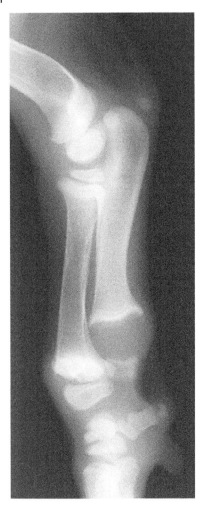

Figure 10.4 Hypophosphatemic rickets. A Great Dane of 2 months raised on food with 3.3% calcium on a dry matter basis starting at 3 weeks of age with hypophosphatemia and thus disturbed bone and cartilage mineralization. Notice the poor contrast between bone and soft tissue, the thin cortices, and the mushroom appearance of the (non-mineralized) growth plate. These radiologic signs do not differ from those of dogs with hypovitaminosis D (= rickets).

Table 10.7 Vitamin D recommendations for growing dogs.

	Vitamin D content per kg food (dry matter)
National Research Council Nutrient requirements of dogs and cats (2006)	552 IU[a] (4000 kcal ME/kg diet)
Meyer (1983)	500–1000 IU
Association of American Feed Control Officials (AAFCO) (2022)	500 IU[b] (4000 kcal ME/kg diet)

1 µg cholecalciferol = 40 IU vitamin D. ME, metabolizable energy.
[a] Recommended allowance.
[b] AAFCO minimum.

Dietary vitamin D is absorbed in the intestine by passive diffusion, transported in plasma bound to chylomicrons, lipoproteins, and vitamin D-binding proteins (DBP), and routed to the liver, where 40–60% will be absorbed and 25OHvitD$_3$ is formed. In the kidneys, further hydroxylation results in 1,25(OH)$_2$vitD$_3$ and 24,25(OH)$_2$vitD$_3$, which appear in the plasma, whereas hydroxylation at other sites (like the intestine, growth plates, and placenta) is not reflected. A variety of factors, related to breed, age, and dietary composition, influence the plasma concentrations of these main metabolites.

Since the main role of 1,25(OH)$_2$vitD$_3$ is mineralization of newly formed cartilage and osteoid, hypovitaminosis D (i.e. rickets) in young growing animals is radiologically characterized by wide growth plates (this is contrary to alimentary hyperparathyroidism), and by thin cortices with possibly curved bones and/or greenstick fractures. Histologic investigation of bone biopsies will also reveal broad (unmineralized) osteoid seams (Figure 10.3c), formed by a large amount of osteoblasts, whereas osteoclasts are seldom attached to mineralized bone. The diagnosis can be confirmed by laboratory investigation. Hypocalcemia is secondary to decreased intestinal calcium absorption and bone resorption,

and lean meat (like poultry) have low levels of vitamin D. Commercially available dog and cat food does not need any vitamin D supplementation, regardless of the season or the latitude, especially because vitamin D content is in most cases above the recommended daily requirement (Table 10.7).

which will cause hyperparathyroidism and hypophosphatemia due to the same causes as the hypocalcemia plus the hyperparathyroidism-induced hyperphosphaturia. The plasma concentrations of the vitamin D metabolites (especially 25OHvitD$_3$ and 24,25 (OH)$_2$vitD$_3$) will be very low, whereas 1,25(OH)$_2$vitD$_3$ may be in the low-normal range (Table 10.6).

Rickets is only seen under extreme circumstances, including with unsupplemented homemade foods, in dogs with an inability to absorb fat and thus also vitamins soluble in fat, and in cases of inborn errors of vitamin D3 metabolism. Treatment includes normalization of the diet. In cases where vitamin D deficiency is the only abnormality, vitamin D supplementation up to 500 IU/kg BW/d is sufficient. In most cases the daily requirements of a variety of nutrients, vitamins, and minerals will not be met, and thus a complete, balanced, commercially available dog or cat food should be advised.

In three weeks, restoration of the skeleton can be noticed, since cartilage and osteoid are waiting to become mineralized. After complete mineralization of the cortices and callus formation occur around the fractures, orthopedic correction can be performed when indicated.

Inborn errors of vitamin D metabolism are resistant to even prolonged vitamin D therapy; treatment with calcitriol (which warrants careful monitoring of plasma calcium and phosphorus levels) can be indicated until the skeleton is normally mineralized and growth is completed. Calcitriol can then be discontinued in order to avoid abnormal, soft tissue mineralization or kidney stone formation.

Deficiency of Other Trace Minerals

In an extreme situation, such as feeding a home-prepared diet based solely on potatoes, milk products, and cereals without supplementation, it is possible that there is a deficiency in one of the trace minerals; it can be anticipated that an excess of calcium might cause a deficiency in other bivalent ions like copper and zinc (Dobenecker et al. 2006; Zentek and Meyer 1991). However, Stockman et al. (2017) could not demonstrate a consistent difference in phosphorus or magnesium digestibility in adult Labradors fed a food supplemented with 7.1 times the recommended amount of calcium (NRC 2006) in comparison with a group fed 1.7 times the recommended amount. Although there are concerns about zinc absorption due to calcium supplementation (Dobenecker et al. 2006; Zentek and Meyer 1991), as revealed in studies in elderly men (Wood and Zheng 1997), no consistent influence on zinc digestibility could be demonstrated in the study of Stockman et al. (2017) in adult dogs fed a diet supplemented with calcium.

Phosphorus deficiency can be a concern in cases of calcium excess, especially when the calcium excess is started during partial weaning (Schoenmakers et al. 2000) leading to hypophosphatemic rickets (Figure 10.4), as also reported by Dobenecker et al. (2006).

Calcium Excess (Alimentary Hypercalcitoninism)

The calcium requirement will differ widely for different growing animals, depending on their growth rate. Meta-analysis revealed that the relationship between true calcium absorption (as determined with the aid of calcium tracer studies) during the first six months of life was directly proportional to the calcium content of the food (i.e. intake$^{0.82}$, with dietary calcium ranging from 0.33 to 3.3 g/100 g food dm), but independent of the breed with extremely different growth rates: that is, both miniature poodles and Great Danes (Tryfonidou et al. 2002). Evolution of terrestrial mammals has been directed to a calcium-deficient environment; young animals with a very functional paracellular, passive absorption of calcium cannot refuse an excess of dietary calcium. This is unlike mature animals, where the paracellular pathway has been sealed in such a way that calcium and other molecules cannot diffuse through the intestinal wall.

Feeding an excess of calcium to young large-breed dogs is common practice by many owners concerned about the skeletal diseases described earlier. For that reason, owners supplement dog food with minerals to prevent calcium deficiency. The addition of 2 tsp of calcium carbonate to a balanced diet of a 3-month-old fast-growing dog will almost double the daily calcium intake and thus double its calcium absorption. The source of calcium – bone meal, fresh bones, or dairy products – does not make a lot of difference; it is the amount of calcium eaten and absorbed that counts. In a study in dogs raised on food with triple the recommended amount of calcium and phosphorus, even more severe skeletal disturbances like osteochondrosis were seen than in the group with calcium excess alone (Schoenmakers et al. 2000). These abnormalities were seen also more frequently and more severe in Great Danes raised on ad libitum provided complete food, in comparison with restricted-fed littermates (Hedhammar et al. 1974).

In their efforts to produce a food for all breeds and all life stages, manufacturers enrich their foods with plenty of calcium. Feeding a 3-month-old fast-growing dog an adult maintenance diet (320 kcal/100 g; 1.6% Ca dm) instead of a puppy diet (420 kcal/100 g; 0.8% Ca cm) with a daily requirement of 2700 kcal means that it will consume 5.1 g of calcium with the puppy food and 13.5 g of calcium with the adult maintenance diet. Highly digestible food with high-quality ingredients will result in a relatively higher degree of ME (= gross energy content minus fecal plus urinary energy values; Chapter 3); the daily calcium intake of the food with the lower ME but the same calcium content will be higher than with the food with the higher ME. Since the ME values are often calculated values, this makes comparison of diets and thus dietary advice not easy. In addition, bone meal as a source of protein is used in some complete foods, thus providing both protein

and an excess of calcium (and phosphorus) at the same time. This information can be hidden behind the expression of "minimal content" instead of the actual content on the label. Calcium content above 2.5% in dry and canned mixed products is no exception (Kallfelz and Dzanis 1989).

In addition, there is a discrepancy between the energy requirements (related to the metabolic body weight, $BW^{0.67}$) and the calcium requirement for growing bones (related to body weight) (Meyer and Zentek 2005). Feeding a product that has been formulated to optimally meet the energy and calcium requirements at 10 kg to a growing dog with an adult body weight of 40 kg may create the risk of oversupplementation of calcium when fed at a younger age with a lower body weight. This makes no single calcium-to-energy ratio suitable for the entire growth period for all breeds. The lowest possible ratio for large and giant breeds will minimize the risk of oversupplementation with calcium (Nap et al. 2000). The tendency of dog owners to maximize growth velocity, rather than optimize it by lowering energy supply, will thus increase the chances of too high a calcium intake, with skeletal diseases as a possible consequence. A large-breed food for growing dogs with a level of 0.8% calcium (per 4200 ME kcal/kg) has been both calculated and proven to be safe for raising large- and giant-breed pups throughout the growth period (Nap et al. 2000).

High calcium intake will cause hyperplasia of CT-producing C cells and thus an increased response in CT secretion following calcium absorption during a meal, even months after normalization of the calcium content of such a meal (Figure 10.5) (Schoenmakers et al. 2000). The CT-depressed osteoclast activity will lead to decreased bone remodeling, with consequences for blood vessels running through the cortex of long bones. Great Dane puppies nourished by the bitch and given a high-calcium diet (3.3% calcium dm) only between the ages of 3 and 6 weeks (i.e. in the period of partial weaning) had an increased CT response and an

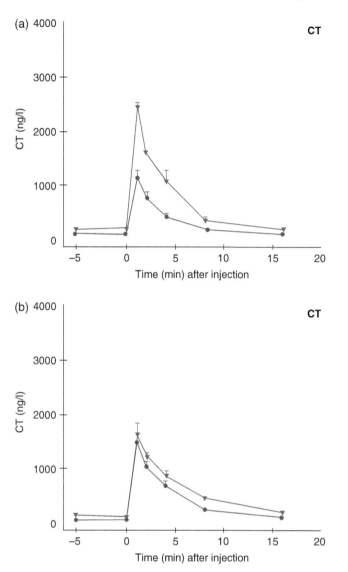

Figure 10.5 Alimentary-induced hypercalcitoninism. Two groups of Great Danes, raised on food (as a gruel from 3–6 weeks) only differing in its calcium content, i.e. 1.04 (n = 9, blue) and 3.11 (n = 5, red) g per 100 g dry matter (dm) food (both with phosphorus equal to 0.85 g and vitamin D equal to 110 IU per 100 g dm) starting at 3 weeks of age. From 6 weeks to 6 months of age, both groups received the food with a Ca content of 1.04%. At time point 0, a Ca bolus intravenous injection (2.5 mg Ca/kg body weight) was given, and the calcitonin (CT) plasma concentrations were determined at the time points indicated at the ages of (a) 13 weeks and (b) 26 weeks. Notice the increased basal level and response even seven weeks after normalization of the food, with a normalized response at 26 weeks of age. See the discussion of alimentary hypercalcitoninism for the clinical relevance. *Source:* Data from Hazewinkel et al. (2000).

increase in plasma calcium concentration until 17 weeks, and in all these dogs radiologically confirmed enostosis (panosteitis eosinophilia) (Figure 10.6) was diagnosed, but not in the (control) Great Danes raised on food containing 1.1% calcium (dm) from 3 to 17 weeks of age (Schoenmakers et al. 2000). So a high calcium intake for a short but crucial period in life, and only in addition to the bitch's milk, can have major consequences in later

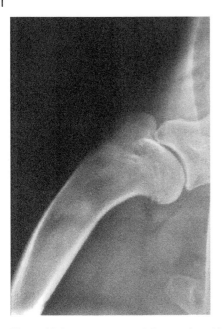

Figure 10.6 Inside the medullary cavity, white confluating spots are visible, indicating areas of mineralization as radiologic signs of panosteitis, which is clinically characterized by shifting lameness, varying in severity and location, with pain reaction upon deep palpation of the long bones.

life. Although multiple hypotheses are proposed to describe the etiopathogenesis of panosteitis, no other dietary cause has been found thus far (Hazewinkel et al. 2000).

The clinical signs (shifting lameness of differing severity, and pain upon deep bone palpation) together with the radiologic signs (white confluent areas within the medullary cavity, starting near the nutrient foramen) in young dogs of large breeds until the age of 24 months is strong evidence for this disease. The treatment is to prescribe a diet with a calcium content matching the requirement (with possibly a three-week period of calcium deficiency to induce skeletal remodeling) together with non-steroidal anti-inflammatory drugs (NSAIDs) to help the animal overcome painful periods until the age of 24 months. In order to prevent panosteitis, a diet designed for young dogs of large breeds with a calcium content no

greater than 1.1% dm should be fed during the growth period, starting at partial weaning.

Chronic calcium excess can result in a decreased widening of the foramen for blood vessels and the spinal cord. Great Danes provided free access to food (Table 10.5) (Hedhammar et al. 1974; Lavelle 1989) or limited intake of food but with a high calcium content (3.3% Ca dm) (Hazewinkel 1985) had narrowing of the cranial aperture of the cervical vertebral bodies, causing Wallerian degeneration of the spinal cord and the typical signs of wobbler syndrome: ataxia and crossed extensor reflexes. With imaging techniques, narrowing of the spinal canal without herniation of the nucleus pulposus can be detected. Surgical techniques may be indicated, although the damage to the nerve tissue may already be irreversible. Dietary corrections and medical treatment are often too late to have any impact. Differential diagnoses include vertebral or spinal cord malformations, cervical vertebral instability as seen in older dogs, discospondylitis, and meningitis.

High calcium intake will have a tendency to cause the calcium level to increase and therefore increase CT secretion and suppress PTH secretion, and 1α-hydroxylase formation lowering 1,25(OH)$_2$vitD synthesis. The increase of CT and the lowering of PTH as seen in large-breed dogs may be the cause of the high incidence and severe signs of osteochondrosis in young dogs raised on a diet with a high calcium content. Support for this comes from the finding that the influence of high calcium intake did not decrease PTH levels significantly in young dogs of small breeds (Nap et al. 1993c). In this study, Great Danes, but not miniature poodles, raised on diets with a high calcium content or with an increased calcium and phosphorus ratio had severe signs of retained cartilage cones (considered to be osteochondrosis of the growth plates) with radius curvus as a consequence; that is, elbow incongruity, bowing of the radius, and valgus deformation of the front and rear feet (Hazewinkel 1985; Schoenmakers et al. 2000) (Figure 10.7). These

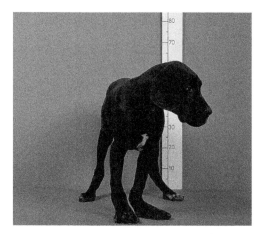

Figure 10.7 A 4-month-old Great Dane with radius curvus syndrome raised on a food with calcium excess, calcium and phosphorus excess, or vitamin D excess. *Source:* Schoenmakers et al. (2000) / Elsevier B.V. and Tryfonidou et al. (2003) / Elsevier.

Great Danes developed osteochondrosis at typical locations in joint cartilage. In some cases, where Great Danes were raised on a diet with excess calcium, it was not the distal growth plate of the ulna that was the most affected but the growth in length of the radius, resulting in incongruity of the elbow with a shortened radius (Hazewinkel 1985; Schoenmakers et al. 2000). Lavelle (1989) and Slater et al. (1992) demonstrated a correlation between calcium supplementation and the development of skeletal diseases, especially in large-breed dogs. In beagles and crossbred foxhounds, Dobenecker et al. (2006) could demonstrate a significantly higher calcium retention in the beagles on supplemented food when compared with control beagles and the foxhounds, with a >13% decreased growth in length of the antebrachium in the beagles compared with controls.

In conclusion, a variety of skeletal abnormalities can develop in dogs when raised on excess food (Hedhammar et al. 1974), excess calcium (Hazewinkel 1985), excess calcium and phosphorous (Schoenmakers et al. 2000), or excess calcium plus phosphorus, manganese, iron, zinc, and copper (Dobenecker et al.

2006). Calcium retention increases proportionally with the calcium content of the food and is in young dogs not less than 25–40% (Dobenecker et al. 2006; Hazewinkel 1985; Hedhammar et al. 1974; Nap et al. 1993a; Schoenmakers et al. 2000), and thus a disturbance of the balance in calciotropic hormones can be caused. Other dietary effects and other causes, including breed effects and genetic predisposition for disturbances in skeletal growth disturbances and development, cannot be excluded on the basis of the studies reviewed here. Especially when owners of breeds at risk are consulting the practicing veterinarian for dietary advice, this discussion will help to formulate scientifically supported advice.

Vitamin D Excess

Vitamin D is an essential vitamin in dogs and cats, since it cannot be synthesized in these species in their skin under the influence of sunlight (How et al. 1994). Since it is soluble in fat and transported to the liver for hydroxylation, the nutritional content of vitamin D is connected to the fat and liver content of the ingredients. In balanced dog foods, the raw ingredients are supplemented with vitamin D together with other essential nutrients by the manufacturer in the vitamin pre-mix. The content of the pre-mix is not declared on the label of the end product and thus the level of the separate vitamins and minerals cannot be included in the analysis. As a result, the available diets for companion animals can have a vitamin D content exceeding recommended levels (Table 10.7) (Weidner and Verbrugghe 2016).

In a study focused on the development of the medial coronoid process (MCP) of the ulna, with two groups of Labrador puppies, offspring of two Labradors with medial coronoid disease (MCD), one group was raised on a weaning diet (1.3% Ca, 1.03% P, and 130 IU vitamin D/100 g dm), the other group with 5000 IU vitamin D/100 g added, and both groups were followed during a maximum of 18 weeks with two-weekly radiologic and CT scanning of the elbow joints and histologic investigation in all dogs. Plasma calcium, phosphorus, total protein, and albumin levels did not differ between groups, whereas the 25OHvitD and 1,25(OH)$_2$vitD levels were twice as high in the supplemented group in comparison with the controls. Two dogs of the supplemented group developed MCD and one also had a shortened radius. The subchondral bone of the MCP contained retained hyaline cartilage, more in the MCD-positive dogs of the supplemented group than in the MCD-positive dogs of the dogs on the control diet. The supplemented group revealed significant more collagen-X staining than the controls, reflecting more hypertrophic chondrocyte activity as seen in delayed endochondral ossification in cases of osteochondrosis, leading to the conclusion that vitamin D supplementation does not prevent MCD and that optimal vitamin D intake in young dogs is important in breeds at risk for osteochondrosis-related developmental skeletal diseases (Corbee et al. 2015a).

Dogs raised on a diet containing a 135-fold increase in the recommended dietary vitamin D content (54 000 vs. 4560 IU cholecalciferol/kg diet, which corresponds to a mean [± standard deviation, SD] of 1615 ± 60 vs. 15 ± 1 IU vitamin D/kg/BW/d) starting at the age of 6 weeks demonstrated an adaptation mechanism through which the increased hydroxylation of excess vitamin D occurred in both 25OHvitD and 1,25(OH)$_2$vitD, without signs of increased calcium absorption or pathologic mineralization, as is commonly seen in vitamin D intoxication. This adaptation mechanism results in increased plasma concentrations of 24,25(OH)$_2$vitD and decreased levels of 1,25(OH)$_2$vitD, however with severe disturbances of endochondral ossification as a consequence resulting in retained cartilage cones at the age of 15 weeks, and eventually radius curvus syndrome (Figure 10.7). In dogs raised on an excess of vitamin D alone, the disturbed endochondral ossification cannot be explained by a direct influence of calcium on maturing chondrocytes. However, in these dogs plasma levels of PTH were significantly decreased and CT was significantly increased when compared with controls, which mimics the situation described under "calcium excess." This suggests that osteochondrosis is caused in these dogs by an imbalance in calciotropic hormones and/or adaptations in the vitamin D metabolism, generalized or locally at growth-plate level, rather than due to high calcium levels per se (Tryfonidou et al. 2002).

Chronic vitamin D intoxication due to ingestion of rat poison or due to excessive doses of vitamin D or its metabolites will be characterized by hypercalcemia, hyperphosphatemia, muscle weakness, nausea, kidney failure, and possibly death. Chronic intake of 10 000 IU/kg BW/d or a single dose of 200 000 IU/kg BW results in clinical signs including polyuria and vomiting (Spangler et al. 1979).

Vitamin A Excess

Vitamin A is essential in bone metabolism and influences chondrocyte proliferation, and osteoblast and osteoclast activity, in addition to a variety of other functions. Vitamin A (C$_{20}$H$_{29}$OH) is present in animal fat and can, in dogs but not in cats, be synthesized out of beta-carotene (C$_{40}$H$_{56}$) by cleavage with the aid of carotenase, as present in the intestinal mucosa and liver cells. Therefore, the dietary requirement of vitamin A for cats is higher than for dogs. Another difference between dogs and cats regarding vitamin A metabolism is in its inactivation: dogs, but not cats, can form retinyl esters to inactivate vitamin A, and dogs are able to excrete 15–60% of the daily intake as retinyl palmitate in the urine.

Cats absorb all the vitamin A from food ingredients that contain retinol and retinyl esters, and although this could induce vitamin A toxicity, cats can sequester larger quantities of vitamin A in the liver with no apparent adverse effect. In addition, cats form retinyl stearate out of retinol and low-density lipoproteins. No apparent deleterious effects were caused by high intakes of vitamin A alone: adult cats, even after a period of three years on 50 and 100 times the vitamin A content of the control cats (on 6 mg retinol equivalents) did not develop pathologic signs (Freytag et al. 2003). It was hypothesized that not only the high vitamin A content but also the high vitamin D content are prerequisites for the bone pathology typical of cats on a chronic raw liver diet. Subtle skeletal changes (i.e. new bone formation) and liver pathology (i.e. fibrosis) developed after 18 months of intake of food with a 100-fold increase of vitamin A and a concomitant 5- or 65-fold increase of vitamin D; the study revealed, however, that the 5-fold increase in vitamin D protected against liver fibrosis, unlike the 65-fold vitamin D intake. This suggests an optimum level of vitamin D protection (Corbee et al. 2014).

In adult cats excessive vitamin A intake will stimulate osteoclastic bone resorption as well as mineralization of newly formed osteoid by vitamin A-induced increase of 24-hydroxylase and thus of 24,25(OH)2vitD levels. Due to traction of tendons on the weakened bone, bone bridges can be formed (Figure 10.8). The most significant finding in the adult cats on excessive vitamin A was subclinical liver fibrosis due to retinol storage in the stellate cells,

transforming into myofibroblasts (Corbee et al. 2014). Adult cats fed a food with 100 times the vitamin A plus 65 times the vitamin D content of the food of control cats resulted in an increase of plasma retinol and 25OHvitD levels, osteophytosis and subtle new bone formation in the vertebrae, and signs of early subclinical liver fibrosis, the latter due to hepatic stellate cells overloaded with vitamin A (Corbee et al. 2014). The level of vitamin A (50% of vitamin A content of beef liver), the calcium content of this food (much higher than beef liver), and the short duration of the study (18 months compared with 2–5 years in clinical cases) may explain the subtlety of the pathology, compared with clinical hypervitaminosis A in adult cats (Hazewinkel 1994). In kittens, teratogenic effects of high vitamin A intake by the queen (1–2 times the safe upper limit of vitamin A as given by NRC 2006) include cleft palate, craniofacial and pelvic abnormalities, shallow ophthalmic orbits, and vascular abnormalities (Freytag et al. 2003).

Hypervitaminosis A can be caused in kittens and puppies after several weeks of oversupplementation. Such kittens and puppies will have reduced growth in length and osteoporosis of long bones together with flaring of the metaphyseal regions. Hypervitaminosis A in dogs results in anorexia, decreased weight gain,

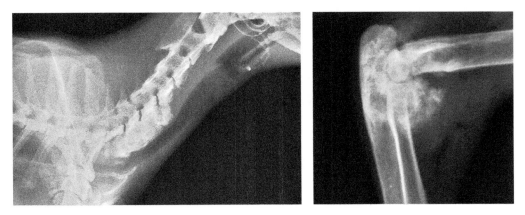

Figure 10.8 Extensive new bone formation without bone resorption throughout the spinal column and around large peripheral joints has been described in cats fed on raw fish or raw liver for a prolonged time, referred to as hypervitaminosis A. *Source:* Hazewinkel and Schoenmakers (1995).

narrowing growth plate cartilage, new bone formation, and thin cortices. Concentrations of vitamin A in plasma will exceed the normal ranges for dogs (i.e. 1800–18 000 IU/l) (Hayes 1971). Hypervitaminosis A is seen more frequently in cats than in dogs, especially in cats at an older age (3–13 years) and fed raw liver and/or fish daily. Hypervitaminosis A in cats may coincide with a stiff neck and/or enlarged joints from the front and hind legs (mainly elbow and stifle joint) (Figure 10.8) due to ankylosis, dull hair coat, change in character (probably due to hypersensitivity and/or bone pain), anorexia, and weight loss (Hazewinkel 1994).

The recommended concentration of vitamin A in dog foods is 1515 μg or 5050 IU/kg dm with a safe upper limit 10 times this amount (NRC 2006). In dogs, a history of diet supplementation with cod liver oil may help to make the diagnosis. In cats, the history can indicate a prolonged preference for raw fish, raw liver, or supplements, although this is not always the case. In a study in adult cats, a 10^6 IU vitamin A/kg diet failed to produce the classic skeletal signs of hypervitaminosis A in three years, suggesting an individual predisposition (Morris 2002a). The clinical and radiologic signs can support the diagnosis. Laboratory investigation may reveal that retinol levels in the liver are increased, contrary to plasma retinol levels, which can be normal, as shown in a study where 20% of cats with hypervitaminosis A had normal plasma levels (Morris 2002a). Corbee (2014a) designed a food for research cats with increased vitamin A and a low calcium level, thus mimicking a liver diet, and described small exostosis on vertebrae and larger joints.

In typical clinical cases of cats with hypervitaminosis A (Hazewinkel 1994; Figure 10.8), bone lesions originate from the tendon insertion areas, resulting in restricted movement and finally extra-articular new bone formation leading to ankylosis (Seawright et al. 1965). Radiographs showed deforming cervical spondylosis and formation of osteophytes and exostoses at the insertion site of tendons, ligaments, and joints. Hypervitaminosis A is therefore considered by some as a secondary form of osteoarthritis in the vertebrae and the large joints (Corbee 2014a). Therapy should be started as soon as the diagnosis is made, including analgesia and food adaptation. It may be better to have a board certified veterinary nutritionist® formulate a balanced homemade diet without vitamin A added to it (or oxidized by cooking), since all commercially available foods contain at least the required amount of vitamin A (Hazewinkel 1994).

A low dose of NSAIDs can be provided to relieve the skeletal pain and pain due to any nerve entrapment. Since cats with hypervitaminosis A may have hepatic lipidosis, the dosage of analgesia may need to be reduced. General improvement can be seen four weeks after starting treatment; although ankylosis will not disappear, the cats may remain lame, but this is not due to pain.

Nutrient Requirements for Skeletal Maintenance in Adult Animals

In the adult dog under balanced conditions, both mineralization of the skeleton and bone resorption are 4–8 mg/kg BW/d, which is almost 100 times less than in young fast-growing dogs (Hazewinkel 1989). Endogenous fecal excretion (i.e. losses of calcium via bile or mucosal cells) is approximately 10–30 mg/kg and urinary losses approximately 1–7 mg/kg BW/d. The losses can be compensated for by an intake of 50 mg Ca/kg BW/d. But even when this is not reached, the skeleton represents such a large reservoir of calcium that losses can be compensated for by an increase in bone resorption. A study in adult dogs fed a lowered calcium intake (0.5 g/1000 kcal) for six months revealed no adjusted fractional calcium excretion, leading to a negative calcium balance with increased bone resorption as a result to maintain calcium homeostasis (Schmitt 2018), this due to the fact that the endogenous fecal calcium excretion is not under hormonal (e.g. PTH) control and represents a fixed amount of calcium (Schoenmakers et al. 1999a). Pathologic fractures in adult dogs or cats do not generally occur secondary to an unbalanced diet, but rather under strenuous physiologic conditions such as gestation and lactation without adequate compensatory food intake. Two groups of nine adult Labradors fed a high-calcium diet (7.1 g/1000 kcal) or a test diet (1.7 g/1000 kcal) for 40 weeks did not reveal any difference in general or skeletal health, kidney or hormonal functions (of both PTH and calcitriol levels), or in blood biochemistry, including plasma ionized calcium concentration; only fecal calcium excretion and renal calcium excretion (the latter to a much lower extent) increased in the high-calcium group in such a way that there could be no difference registered in the calcium balance in both groups of dogs, indicating a developmental adaptation in adult dogs to regulate calcium uptake (Stockman et al. 2017). In a meta-analysis including more than 400 individual digestion trials in dogs and 156 in cats, it was revealed that true absorption for calcium in adult dogs is 13% without significant differences between groups with a calcium-to-phosphorus ratio of 1–2 or >2, respectively, and 25% for adult cats, with 26% for the same ratio of 1–2 and 19% when >2 (Mack et al. 2015).

A true safe upper limit for vitamin D intake, supported by clear scientific evidence for reproduction/growth and for adult maintenance, is not currently known in dogs (Wedner and Verbrugghe 2016). In human nutrition, the 25OHvitD plasma level is used as a reference of adequate vitamin D intake. However in dogs, a variety of different factors influence the plasma level of 25(OH)D, including breed and growth rates (Tryfonidou et al. 2003b), vitamin D intake (Hazewinkel and Tryfonidou 2002), and in cases of cancer also type of tumor (osteosarcoma, lymphoma, and mast cell tumor), as well as plasma concentration of 24,25(OH)$_2$D and ionized calcium (Weidner et al. 2017), and

thus it might be interesting to use the biologically most active, but more expensive to determine, metabolite 1,25(OH)$_2$D as an indicator for sufficient or excessive vitamin D intake (Table 10.6). Normal values for healthy adult dogs of different breeds (ranging from dachshund to German pointer) have been published for 25OHvitD (38.5 ± 14.5 ng/ml), 24,25(OH)$_2$D (40.0 ± 17.0 ng/ml), and 1,25(OH)$_2$D (76.2 ± 15.3 pg/ml) (Corbee et al. 2012). A novel C-3 epimer of 25OHvitD, ranging from 30 to 75% of the native 25OHvit D level, has been identified in cats but not in dogs (Parker et al. 2017).

Unlike postmenopausal humans, dogs do not increase bone resorption after loss of ovarian hormonal influences. Working dogs may lose extra calcium with saliva, but this is only a limited amount and hardly requires any compensation.

The major clinical problems in relation to orthopedics in adult companion animals are excessive energy intake (see later), excessive phosphorus intake together with decreased renal function, and excessive vitamin A intake, especially in cats (see earlier).

In the case of renal insufficiency, in both young and adult dogs, calcium is lost in the urine whereas phosphorus is insufficiently excreted, resulting in sequestration of calcium intracellularly as calcium phosphates and at different locations with increased pH values (lungs, stomach, and kidneys), thereby lowering the plasma calcium concentration even further. This will lead to hyperparathyroidism (i.e. renal secondary hyperparathyroidism) with increased osteoclast activity causing demineralization of the skeleton. An increase in calcitriol formation under the influence of high PTH levels helps to increase intestinal calcium absorption, but the hydroxylation of 25OHvitD in the kidney is often disturbed in a case of chronic renal insufficiency. Although PTH will lower the threshold for phosphorus in the kidneys and thus increase renal phosphorus excretion, this mechanism is also disturbed in chronic renal failure. Dietary phosphorus restriction will keep the plasma phosphorus level in the normal range until renal function becomes inadequate.

Due to the high turnover in cancellous bone, bone pathology is often initially seen clinically as severe bone loss in the jaws. Loosening of teeth and lowering of the arch can be noticed in adult dogs with chronic renal failure (i.e. hypostotic osteodystrophy), whereas hyperostotic osteodystrophy is characteristic for growing dogs with renal insufficiency (as is the case with hydronephrosis or other birth defects) (Figure 10.9). In these young dogs, their noses are much broader than normal and the gingiva seems to be thickened, all due to compensatory growth of non-mineralized fibrous tissue, and the teeth are often loose. Clinical pathology will reveal low to normal calcium; very high phosphorus, urea, and creatinine levels; and low 1,25(OH)2vitD$_3$ levels. Radiographs will show a loss of the lamina dura dentis and a loss of contrast in the skull compared to the teeth, which do not lose their mineral content. Mineral loss of the skeleton is often irreversible together with the deteriorating general health of the patient.

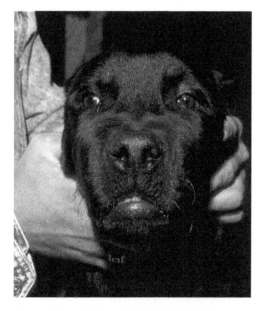

Figure 10.9 A 5-month-old Rottweiler with poor renal function and hydronephrosis and broadening of the maxilla.

Implementation of Nutrition in Clinical Orthopedics

There are numerous foods available on the commercial market, making it impossible to comment on each food. It should be recognized that the driving force of food intake in each individual, especially growing dogs, is the need for energy. Together with energy come the essential nutrients for skeletal growth, including calcium, phosphorus, and vitamin D. In addition to the requirement per kg body weight of growing dogs, the expression of these elements on an energy basis (kcal/kg diet) is also common, although more active dogs need more energy but not necessarily more minerals (i.e. calcium and phosphorus). Owners feed their dogs more often on a weight or volume basis rather than calculating the energy intake. When a diet is calculated for a growing dog of a certain body weight, the amount should be regularly adjusted when the dog becomes heavier as it matures. This can be done through consultation with a veterinary nutritionist. One must account for not only the chemical composition but also the availability and biological value of the nutrients in the diet.

It is virtually impossible to judge the quality of a diet from the label. A diet with a high grain and phytate content may need a higher calcium level to provide the required calcium for absorption and a higher phosphate content, since the phosphate in phytate is not absorbable. This may explain why a meta-analysis reported that at 2 months of age, 260–830 mg Ca/kg BW/d appears to be safe for skeletal growth; decreasing to 210–540 mg Ca/kg BW/d at 5 months of age (Figure 10.1) (Hazewinkel and Mott 2006).

To stay away from all these confusing figures, it is advised that young dogs be raised on a diet formulated for the growth and special hormonal typicalities of the breed. Small-breed dogs undergo a slow growth rate and therefore have a wide safety margin to deal with nutrient concentrations above or below the dog's requirements. Giant-breed dogs, with their balanced, but vulnerable, equilibrium of hormonal regulators, do not reveal this safety margin. Couple this with the inherited developmental diseases such as hip and elbow dysplasia with a large degree of environmental influence, including nutrition, and one can understand the importance of educating the breeder and new owner of young large-breed dogs that the dogs should be fed a diet adapted to their special needs; that is, a calcium content at the lower end of the safety spectrum. In general, in foods with a protein content of high biological value, the calcium content should be between 0.8% and 1.0% on a dry matter basis (for a food with 4200 ME kcal/kg diet) (Nap et al. 2000). This range is present in the diets of the major dog food manufacturers, but is still not seen in many smaller brands and in diets supplemented by owners themselves.

In summary, skeletal growth is limited to endochondral ossification, periosteal growth, and remodeling with a limited amount of cell types. These cells are working under the influence of different growth factors, of which they have the calciotropic hormones (PTH, vitamin D, CT) in common. Calcium as a vital mineral will be regulated in plasma as tightly as possible under all circumstances, including rapid growth and extreme calcium (and vitamin D) intakes. The adaptation mechanisms to maintain calcium homeostasis may have consequences for the maturing skeleton and thus for later life. A thorough understanding of the pathophysiologic mechanisms and thus recognition of different expressions of the same disturbance (greenstick and compression fractures, osteochondrosis, radius curvus syndrome, and wobbler syndrome) will help give guidance for the nutritional prevention (and at times treatment) of generalized skeletal diseases in dog breeds at risk. The occurrence of these dietary orthopedic diseases is increasing since the feeding of BARF and homemade diets has become more popular.

Influence of Nutrition in the Occurrence of Orthopedic Diseases

Elbow Dysplasias

Elbow dysplasias (EDs) are a serious problem for certain populations. EDs can be separated into different disease entities, including ununited anconeal process (UAP), fragmented coronoid process (FCP), osteochondritis dissecans (OCD) of the medial humeral condyle, and incongruities of the elbow joint (INC) (Figure 10.10a). EDs should be considered as different diseases, which may all cause lameness and may all cause osteoarthritis (OA) of the elbow joint (Figure 10.10b).

Depending on the specific subpopulation and the method of investigation, EDs are seen in 46–50% of Rottweilers, 36–70% of Bernese mountain dogs, 12–14% of Labrador retrievers, 15–20% of golden retrievers, 30% of Newfoundlands, and 18–21% of German shepherd dogs, and in many other breeds (Temwichitr et al. 2010). The clinical investigation starts with determination of the breed and the age at which the first signs appeared, most typically between 4 and 10 months. The elbow is often effused on palpation, the range of motion can be decreased, and subtle crepitation can be recognized. Diagnosis of EDs can be confirmed by radiographs in most cases by demonstrating the primary disease (UAP, OCD, INC, and in certain cases even FCP), or secondary changes as part of OA development, taking into account the osteophytes and sclerosis of the semilunar notch in making the diagnosis (Figure 10.10). Most instances of EDs occur bilaterally in 30–70% of cases, and therefore both elbow joints should be investigated, even in cases of unilateral lameness. In cases where there are no radiographic abnormalities in dogs with clinical lameness, and other causes of front leg lameness are excluded (including panosteitis, OCD in the shoulder joint, sesamoid fractures, and biceps tendon pain), auxiliary techniques including computed tomography, bone scintigraphy, and arthroscopy can be of value.

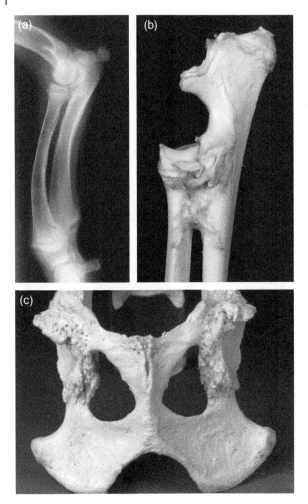

Figure 10.10 Radiograph and pathologic specimens revealing (a) incongruity (too short radius) of the joint in a Great Dane raised on food with increased calcium and phosphorus content (Schoenmakers et al. 2000); (b) osteoarthritis of the elbow joint – notice the shortened radius and the dislocated medial coronoid process; and (c) osteoarthritis of the hip joint due to hip dysplasia characterized by osteophyte formation and cartilage breakdown.

Early surgical intervention provides the best prognosis for the future status of the joint in lame dogs, although some experts advocate a more conservative approach. The UAP can be removed, or re-attached in instances of partial or acute detachment. When cartilage of the medial humeral condyle is unattached in cases of OCD, or when the apex of the coronoid process is fractured in cases of FCP, the loose bodies are removed. When fissures are present in the apex of the medial coronoid or cartilage is weakened due to chondromalacia, the apex should also be removed. INC due to a short radius is frequently seen in Bernese mountain dogs and in dogs raised on food supplemented with excess minerals (Figure 10.10b). Congruity is restored after the removal of the FCP or UAP at the same surgical intervention. The prognosis ranges from good in cases with minimal cartilage damage to poor in cases of severe OA (Innes 2009).

Role of Nutrition in Elbow Dysplasias

A combination of FCP and OCD has been described by Olsson (1993) as a disturbance of endochondral ossification and as such as expressions of the same disease. Although this may still be true in cases of chondromalacia, in the other forms of FCP (loose apex or fragmentation) primary mechanical overload of subchondral bone or joint cartilage is considered as the primary cause (Wolschrijn and

Weijs 2004). OCD and FCP are seen more frequently in certain breeds and certain subpopulations with a chi-square of less than 0.3, suggesting a considerable influence of environmental factors including nutrition. It has been demonstrated in well-controlled studies that endochondral ossification can be disturbed by high food intake (Hedhammar et al. 1974; Lavelle 1989) and excessive calcium intake (Hazewinkel 1985; Schoenmakers et al. 2000), as well as by oversupplementation of a balanced diet with vitamin D (Tryfonidou et al. 2003b).

Protein-rich rations have not been shown to have a disturbing influence on skeletal development (Nap et al. 1991). In a study in Great Danes raised on food with an increased calcium and phosphorus intake (3.3 and 3.0%, respectively, compared to controls on 1.1% and 0.9%, respectively) starting at the age of weaning (i.e. 3 weeks of age) until 17 weeks, the dogs developed disturbances in endochondral ossification in the growth plates of the distal radius and/or ulna. As a consequence, elbow incongruity developed, due either to a severe disturbance of growth in the length of the radius or to a severe radius curvus syndrome with disturbed growth in the length of the ulna (Hazewinkel 1985; Schoenmakers et al. 2000). The former may coincide with overloading and thus fracturing of the MCP, while the latter may coincide with an UAP or the painful pressure of the humeral condyle against the UAP, all leading to OA of the elbow joint. Lau et al. (2013) demonstrated in immature Labradors that FCP development was due to a disturbance of endochondral ossification, especially with delayed calcification in the calcifying zone. Since vitamin D influences skeletal development by stimulating the terminal differentiation of chondrocytes, matrix remodeling, and bone mineralization (Hazewinkel and Tryfonidou 2002), Corbee (2014a) investigated the effect of vitamin D supplementation on the development of the coronoid process. He found, however, that vitamin D supplementation did not normalize endochondral ossification in the coronoid area or prevent the development of MCD in these Labrador puppies (Corbee et al. 2014b, 2015a).

In a study in Labrador retrievers, it has been shown that OA in multiple joints (including hips, elbows, and shoulders) developed in overweight dogs and less frequently in restrictively fed, slim littermates (Huck et al. 2009; Kealy et al. 1992). The frequency and severity of the occurrence of disturbances in endochondral ossification as a common factor in EDs can be decreased in breeds at risk by dietary management, including the feeding of a diet with an appropriate calcium-to-energy ratio, a quantitative restriction of energy intake, and by not adding vitamin D to a balanced diet.

Hip Dysplasia

Although much is known about the symptoms and treatment modalities, little is known about the etiology of hip dysplasia (HD) in dogs. Symptoms include laxity of both hip joints (Bardens and Hardwick 1968), with an increased pressure load on the joint surface causing cartilage disruption of the acetabulum and femoral head, and eventually deformity of the joint and increased bone formation in the subchondral area (Figure 10.9). Pain is the dominant clinical sign during the first phase of HD with reluctance to play and walk, whereas in the advanced stages OA symptoms dominate (i.e. stiffness after rising, warming up, inability to move the joint in a normal range). Laxity of the hip joint is a constant feature in HD. The laxity can be controlled in the dog in lateral recumbency, without or with anesthesia, by moving the femur in an upward direction. Originally this was performed at 4 weeks of age with a claimed error of 5%, although no follow-up was presented (Bardens and Hardwick 1968). Noticeable laxity begins to be evident at 4 months of age, but becomes a more accurate predictor as the dog ages (Ginja et al. 2010; Smith 2004; Vezzoni et al. 2005). In mature dogs, laxity can also be evaluated clinically with the Ortolani and Bardens test, and radiologically by measuring the Norberg angle (Schawalder et al. 1998). Other radiologic techniques may include enforced lateralization of the femoral heads with the aid of a fulcrum between the thighs, as described by Smith (2004) and Vezzoni et al. (2005), or enforced craniodorsal pressure with abduction of the proximal femurs with the dog in dorsal recumbency, according to Fluckiger et al. (1999).

In different studies the genetic influence of HD has been proven, although the chi-square indicates a strong environmental influence, including nutrition, activity, and perhaps other factors.

Nutritional Influences Seen in Hip Dysplasia

The collodiaphyseal angle (the angle of inclination) is approximately 135°, but larger angles (coxa valga) are seen in conjunction with HD. In a longitudinal study in Great Danes raised on food provided ad libitum, the angle between the collum femoris and the femoral shaft was larger than in the control group raised on a calorie-restricted, but similar, diet (Hedhammar et al. 1974). The increased energy (and thus also mineral) intake may have caused hypercalcitoninism with decreased osteoclast activity and, as a consequence, hampered skeletal remodeling during maturation, with a more obtuse collodiaphyseal angle than the control dogs (Hedhammar et al. 1974).

The acetabulum is formed out of four ossification centers connected by cartilage fusions. During proportional growth of the femoral head, these ossification centers can drift away, thus remodeling during skeletal growth. Normally these ossification centers fuse at approximately 6 months of age. Asynchronous maturation of the head and acetabulum may be etiologic factors in the development of poor joint conformation as present in HD. In a colony of fast-growing Labradors, fusion of the acetabular ossification centers occurred at 5 months of age, resulting in more HD than in slower-maturing dogs (Lust et al. 1985). A

disturbed development of the os acetabulare quatrum as a form of osteochondrosis causing OA of the affected hip joint has been described by Schawalder et al. (1998). Madsen et al. (1991) registered a delayed ossification of the femoral head during the development of HD in large-breed dogs. Late fusion of secondary ossification centers, together with severe osteochondrosis, has been described in Great Danes raised on food with increased calcium content (Voorhout and Hazewinkel 1987), suggesting a disturbance in endochondral ossification of the fusion of the acetabular bones in case of HD. This, together with mechanical overloading, may explain why overnutrition and thus fast growth are etiologic factors for the development of dysplastic hips (Hedhammar et al. 1974; Kasström 1975; Kealy et al. 1992; Lust et al. 1985; Richardson et al. 2010). In addition, it may explain the involvement of multiple joints, as reported in overweight dogs (Kasström 1975; Kealy et al. 1992; Lust 1993). Interestingly, young dogs under 12 weeks of age with joint laxity did not develop HD when raised on a low-caloric intake regime during growth (Richardson et al. 2010).

The dorsal acetabular rim (DAR) is cartilaginous until 3–4 months of age, and is vulnerable to deformity in cases of joint laxity. The dorsocranial rim can develop from a separate ossification center by endochondral ossification (Morgan et al. 2000). This DAR can be visualized on radiographs with the X-ray beam parallel to the longitudinal axis of the pelvis. The line through the DAR should make an angle with the line horizontal through the pelvis (or perpendicular to the spinal processes) of <7.5° (Slocum and Devine 1990) or even –1 or –2° (Vezzoni et al. 2005). If the angle becomes larger (i.e. the angle of inclination of the roof of the acetabulum becomes larger), the femoral head will have a tendency to slip outside the acetabulum. Constant lateralization of the femoral head plus increased production of synovial fluid may stretch the joint capsule and thus elongate it, allowing for subluxation of the femoral head. The round ligament, which connects the femoral head with the acetabulum, is far too long to keep the head inside the socket. In addition, the cartilaginous rim will erode, deform, and even disappear, causing joint inflammation and irreversible malformation (Figure 10.10c). Also, acetabular filling and the presence of dorsal osteophytes can be noticed. DAR malformation can be caused by a disturbance in endochondral ossification, especially in dogs that are overweight during growth.

HD is called a biomechanical disease, representing a disparity between primary muscle mass and disproportionately rapid skeletal growth (Riser 1993). The iliopsoas muscle, with its origin at the lumbar spine and pelvis and insertion on the trochanter minor of the femur, and the pectineus muscle, originating from the os pubis with insertion on the medial femur, can both subluxate the femoral head by becoming relatively shortened during fast skeletal growth (Bowen et al. 1972). In addition to selection for muscle strength, as has been proven in livestock genetics, muscle growth can be stimulated by protein intake. Nap et al. (1993c) demonstrated that in Great Danes fed three levels of protein (31.6%, 23.1%, and 14.6% dm) in an isoenergetic, balanced dry dog food from 7 to 18 weeks of age, the group with highest protein intake had a more advanced body maturation reflected by a significant higher body weight without adiposities and without a difference in height or any skeletal abnormalities. Also Tvedten et al. (1977) could not detect an altered incidence of HD in a study with a twofold elevation of dietary protein.

Synovial fluid is partly formed by the synovial membrane (mucine) and is partly a dialysate of plasma (the watery component). In the case of OA, inflammatory mediators cause vasodilation with increased dialysis of plasma through the joint capsule and thus more and more watery synovial fluid than normal. It has been suggested by Kealy et al. (1993) that a dietary anion gap (DAG) has a direct influence on the osmolality of the joint fluid,

explaining the increased synovial fluid volume in the hip joints of dysplastic dogs. However, the anion gap in the entire diet was not calculated and the absorbed ions were not measured, nor was the osmolality of the synovial fluid determined (Kealy et al. 1993). Although the DAG may play a role, an increase in dialysate due to inflammatory mediators, including prostaglandins in cases of OA, seems to be a more likely explanation for the increase in fluid volume in a limited number of joints.

Overweightness and obesity have been proven to enhance OA development due to overloading of the joint cartilage (Marshall et al. 2009) and possibly also due to hormonal influences. Labradors fed 30% more food than controls developed more frequent and more severe signs of OA in different joints, including the hip joints. These overweight dogs had significantly higher IGF-I plasma levels and lower GH levels than controls (Hazewinkel et al. 1999a). These hormonal findings correspond to similar findings in overweight postmenopausal women with thickened subchondral bone and loss of articular cartilage, resulting in severe OA. This, together with the decreasing water-binding capacity of degraded proteoglycans in articular cartilage secondary to aging, may explain the increasing number of dogs, both overweight and lean, with OA in old age, as reported by Kealy and Smith in a longitudinal study in Labradors (Smith et al. 2006).

In cases of severe OA with constant production of a superfluous amount of synovial fluid, the intra-articular pressure will increase and thus the joint capsule will be extended. Three months of cage rest combined with maintenance of a lean body weight has been demonstrated to improve ground reaction forces by 70% in dogs suffering from HD (Hazewinkel 1991). This is likely due to a decrease in joint inflammation allowing for restoration of cartilage damage and normalization of intra-articular pressure. A reduction in body weight, increased muscle force, chondroprotective agents, and NSAIDs have been proven or are expected to have a positive influence on the clinical outcome of medically managed cases (Ginja et al. 2010; Harper 2017).

Hypertrophic Osteodystrophy (or Metaphyseal Osteopathy) in Dogs

Hypertrophic osteodystrophy (HOD) is most commonly seen in Great Danes (with an odds ratio of 40) and other large-breed dogs during their rapid growth phase (i.e. at 4–5 months of age). It is characterized by an inability to stand, fever, and malaise. Affected dogs are extremely painful at the metaphyseal areas of all long bones, especially at the distal antebrachium. The etiology is obscure, and the disease has occurred in different studies in Great Danes overfed with minerals, including excessive calcium and phosphorus. Analogous to Paget disease in humans (Hoyland et al. 2003), particles of distemper virus have been demonstrated in osteoclasts in the area of increased osteoclasia. In cases of HOD, osteoclasia can be seen just 2–3 mm away from the growth plate, in the metaphyses (Mee et al. 1993). This is represented on radiographs by a black line, parallel to the growth plates at the early stage of the disease; in more advanced stages periosteal new bone formation leads to a bony cuff surrounding the zone of excessive bone absorption (Figure 10.11). The area of excessive bone resorption is histologically characterized by acute inflammation of the osteochondral region, and thickened trabeculae of the metaphyseal bone with a thick cartilage core, necrosis, microfractures, debris, and fibrosis (Hazewinkel 1998).

A similar pathologic area of fractured metaphyseal bone and debris has been described in children with hypovitaminosis C (also known as scurvy). Vitamin C plays an important role in collagen biosynthesis; that is, the hydroxylation of proline and lysine. Due to collagen fragility, blood vessel disruptions around the belly and near joints can be seen in cases of scurvy in humans and guinea pigs. However, vitamin C is not an essential vitamin in dogs and cats, as demonstrated in a study in puppies raised for approximately five months on a diet

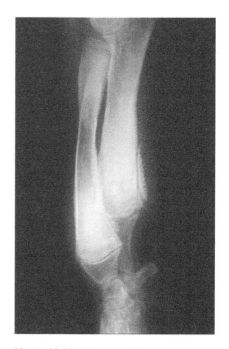

Figure 10.11 Hypertrophic osteodystrophy (HOD) is characterized by a very painful episode, lasting approximately three weeks, followed by a slow rehabilitation with periosteal new bone formation in the metaphyseal area where a discontinuity of the bony tissue (pathognomonic for HOD) has been present.

without vitamin C (NRC 2006). Due to the radiologic similarities between scurvy in children and HOD in dogs, the etiology has long been mistaken as hypovitaminosis C in dogs and is frequently mentioned as such on the internet and in the popular press. The lowered vitamin C content of the blood can be explained by the excessive oxidation of vitamin C in cases of high fever, not due to a metabolic disturbance in its formation. Contrarily, high vitamin C intake has been reported to increase calcium absorption (Teare et al. 1979) and thereby increases the chance that endochondral ossification will be disturbed (Hazewinkel et al. 1985; Hedhammar 1974), thus aggravating the disease. Therapy includes good nursing care during the period of the appearance of bony lesions in the metaphyseal areas (i.e. during a 3–4-week period), antipyretics, and analgesics. After three weeks, many dogs will start to walk. Caution should be used, as early weight bearing might aggravate the size of the bony cuffs, which will then not remodel completely.

Prevention of Nutritionally Related Orthopedic Diseases

There are three major aspects of nutritionally related orthopedic diseases that are of importance: the quality of the food, the quantity of the food, and the stage of life when the animal is vulnerable to dietary mistakes.

The quality of the food is difficult to judge based solely on the label (see Chapter 6). Although deficient foods are uncommon, the veterinarian should be aware of the differences in dietary composition between the spectrum of products as they pertain to the various life stages and the treatment of different diseases. For example, homemade or commercially available limited-antigen foods may be deficient in calcium for growth; weight-reducing diets may be rich in phytates that can bind calcium to unabsorbable complexes; diets intended solely for adult maintenance may contain dangerously high concentrations of calcium for young fast-growing dogs (see the discussion of calcium excess).

The energy requirements of healthy animals vary considerably between different stages of growth (more per kg metabolic body weight during the fast-growth period than later), between different breeds (smaller dogs require more energy based on their body weight; less energy is required in dogs with long hair), between different individual animals (there can be >50% difference between individual dogs), and between different activities (restrained young dogs eat less than active dogs, neutered dogs are less active). Furthermore, energy requirements can be impacted by husbandry practices such as the method of feeding (many dogs eat more when the food is provided ad libitum) and housing conditions (less energy is required in a warm than in a cold environment) (Gross et al. 2000). Figure 10.12 shows that the manufacturer's feeding guidelines do not take into account all of these variables; they are based on the average dog in the average household.

Since the driving force behind food intake is the animal's energy requirement, the ratio of the ingredients to the energy content of the food is of great importance; this is especially true in minerals that will be absorbed and not excreted or metabolized, like calcium (Tryfonidou et al. 2002). Calcium is >99%

Figure 10.12 Growth chart of German shepherd dogs based on information from 23 breeders for a total of 442 German shepherd puppies, revealing the heavies, the lightest, and the average weight. This illustrates the variation in body weight gain and daily requirements. *Source:* Corbee R.J. (2014) / Corbee R.J.

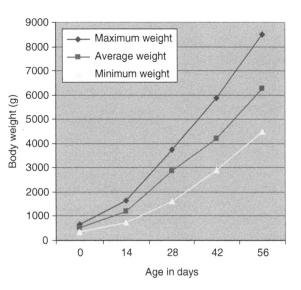

deposited in the skeleton and is related to actual body weight (Meyer and Zentek 2005), rather than the energy requirement that is related to metabolic body weight ($BW^{0.67}$) Little is known about the optimal amount of training and playing for young dogs with a developing skeleton; it should be realized that excessive activity demands extra food intake, which includes extra mineral intake. There may be a need for the former, but not necessarily the latter.

The influence of nutrition during different stages of development can be well illustrated by a summary of the results of a study performed in Great Danes fed a diet with 3.3% calcium and compared with Great Danes fed a control diet with 1.1% calcium (dm). Fed to pregnant bitches, this had no consequence for her or the skeletal development of her offspring. When fed to dogs only during partial weaning (3–6 weeks of age), it led to decreased osteoclast activity (panosteitis) three months later; when fed to pups from 3 to 17 weeks old it caused hypophosphatemic rickets; and when fed from 6 to 21 weeks it caused severe osteochondrosis. Miniature poodles on the same diet did not develop clinical signs of any skeletal disease (Hazewinkel et al. 1999b; Nap et al. 1993c). Increased calcium intake can start as early as weaning, when pups are superfluously fed with artificial milk, with possible effects at older age due to calcitonin-producing C-cell hypertrophy (Corbee et al. 2011; Schoenmakers et al. 2000).

Taken together, the author recommends the following: restricted feeding of a puppy food with a calcium and vitamin D content not to exceed the percentages demonstrated in controlled studies to result in skeletal problems (i.e. calcium ~1.0% dm, vitamin D content 12.5–25 µg/kg diet), maintaining an optimal body condition during growth, and activity adapted to the vulnerability of the skeleton. This leaves the genetic aspect of many developmental diseases in companion animals to the responsibility of breeders.

Diets to Support Treatment of Patients with Osteoarthrosis

Cartilage contains chondroblasts, proteoglycans, and collagen. Proteoglycans are built from glycosaminoglycans (GAGs) and a core protein called aggrecan. Aggrecan is an important proteoglycan in joint cartilage, with keratin sulfate and chondroitin sulfate as GAGs. About 200 aggrecan molecules are bound via a glycoprotein to a hyaluran molecule, binding a large quantity of extracellular water, determining the compressibility of cartilage. Collagen molecules in cartilage contain large amounts of hydroxyl proline and hydroxyl lysine. The molecules form a triple helix structure, bound to fibrils and these to fibers that form a labyrinth that holds proteoglycans in place. During aging, the length of the GAGs decreases, the proteoglycan content decreases, and thus the water content and the flexibility to withstand loading also decline. Moreover, reactive oxygen species (ROS), free radicals formed during different metabolic processes, trauma, infection, and irradiation, may damage GAGs.

Regeneration can occur in cases of microtrauma, by proliferation of undamaged chondrocytes, and de novo synthesis of proteoglycans and collagen. Severe cellular damage will lead to scarring, fibrotic cartilage scars without cells and a low content of proteoglycans.

Under normal circumstances proteolytic enzymes, mainly matrix metalloproteinases (MMPs), will be suppressed by "tissue inhibitors of MMPs" (i.e. TIMPs), but in cases of OA MMPs will be formed by mast cells and synovial cells under the influence of the cytokine interleukin-I (IL-I) and tumor necrosis factor (TNF)-alpha, released by synovial cells, monocytes, macrophages, and T cells. These cytokines also stimulate chondrocytes and osteoclasts to produce MMPs as soon as their surrounding cartilage has been destroyed. In addition, IL-I stimulates the release of arachidonic acid metabolites, including

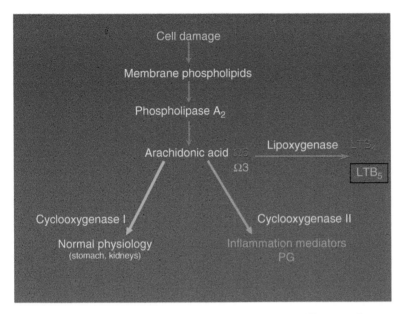

Figure 10.13 Origin of inflammatory mediators in the joint. LTB$_4$, pro-inflammatory leukotriene B$_4$; LTB$_5$, anti-inflammatory leukotriene B$_5$; PG, prostaglandin.

prostaglandin (PG) from chondrocytes and synovial membrane PGE$_2$ and leukotriene B$_4$ (LTB$_4$) (Hazewinkel and Mott 2006) (Figure 10.13).

Causative Role of Nutrition

The causes of OA can be divided into primary OA (this is without any other cause other than aging) and secondary OA (which has a primary cause such as disturbances in development, trauma, and septic or non-septic OA). The occurrence of primary OA may depend on the breed; that is, the mean age of dogs varies by breed, ranging from 3.5 years in Rottweilers to 9.3 years in miniature poodles (Patronek et al. 1997).

Many orthopedic developmental diseases have a low chi-square, as in ED (chi-square = 0.4–0.7), leaving a large influence from the environment. OCD is seen more frequently in certain breeds and subpopulations and can be aggravated by high energy intake (Alexander et al. 1988; Hedhammar et al. 1974; Kasström 1975; Kealy et al. 1992; Lavelle 1989)

and excessive calcium intake (Dobenecker et al. 2006; Hazewinkel 1985), as well as by oversupplementation of balanced foods with vitamin D (Tryfonidou et al. 2002). Rations rich in protein do not have a disturbing influence on skeletal development (Nap et al. 1993c). Great Danes raised on diets with an increased calcium and phosphorus intake (3.3% Ca and 3.0% P vs. controls on 1.1% Ca and 0.9% P, all dm) but with the same calcium-to-phosphorus ratio developed disturbances in endochondral ossification in the growth plates of the distal radius or ulna. As a consequence, elbow incongruity developed, due either to a severe disturbance of growth in the length of the radius or to a severe radius curvus syndrome with disturbed growth in the length of the ulna (Hazewinkel 1985; Schoenmakers et al. 1999b). In a study in Labradors it has been shown that OA in multiple joints (including hips, elbows, and shoulders) was seen in overweight dogs and less frequently in slim littermates (Huck et al. 2009; Kealy et al. 1992). The frequency and severity of the occurrence of osteochondrosis can thus be decreased by

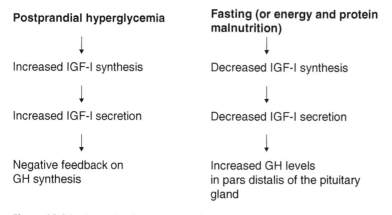

Postprandial hyperglycemia

↓

Increased IGF-I synthesis

↓

Increased IGF-I secretion

↓

Negative feedback on
GH synthesis

Fasting (or energy and protein malnutrition)

↓

Decreased IGF-I synthesis

↓

Decreased IGF-I secretion

↓

Increased GH levels
in pars distalis of the pituitary
gland

Figure 10.14 Excessive food intake or fasting may influence growth hormone (GH) and insulin-like growth factor (IGF)-I plasma levels.

dietary management, including feeding a diet with an appropriate calcium-to-energy ratio, a quantitative restriction of food intake, and not adding vitamin D to a balanced diet.

It is plausible to imagine that the specific activity of the dog may advance degeneration of joint cartilage by overuse. Overloading of the joint, either due to overuse or to over-weightness or obesity, is the main cause for increased complaints in dogs with OA. Higher energy intake (Hedhammar et al. 1974; Kasström 1975; Kealy et al. 1992; Lavelle 1989) and higher calcium intake (Hazewinkel 1985; Schoenmakers et al. 1999b) may increase the frequency and severity of OA at maturity. This is nicely illustrated by the study performed by Kealy and coworkers. In two groups of Labradors, litter mates of the same sex were pair fed; that is, one group ad libitum, the other two-thirds the amount (Kealy et al. 2000). Housing, food, and maintenance were the same, except for the amount of energy, but as a consequence the body weights were different between the groups. The average body weight was 32 kg for the dogs fed ad libitum and 23 kg for the restricted-fed dogs. At 5 years of age, 12 out of 23 ad libitum and 3 out of 23 restricted-fed dogs had OA of the hip joints; at 8 years, 12 of the 23 dogs fed ad libitum and 2 of the restricted-fed dogs had OA in multiple joints (Smith et al. 2006). The pathophysiologic

explanation for how obesity can induce OA has been reviewed (Marshall et al. 2009). It has been demonstrated that in overweight Labradors (i.e. 32 vs. 23 kg) the plasma concentration of IGF-I was significantly increased and the plasma concentration of GH was significantly decreased (Hazewinkel et al. 1999a) (Figure 10.14).

It has recently become clear that adipose tissue is not only a storage form of excess calories, but is also an important source of inflammatory adipokines, including leptin, IL-1, IL-6, and TNF-alpha. Leptin activates hypothalamic receptors and thus regulates appetite, but also has pro-inflammatory activity. In addition, IL-1 and TNF-alpha are produced by activated synoviocytes, mononuclear cells, and articular cartilage, and can upregulate matrix metalloproteinase gene expression involved in cartilage breakdown. Levels of these adipokines are elevated in joints affected by OA, and these adipokines can induce catabolic processes in chondrocytes, leading to cartilage matrix degradation (Issa and Griffin 2012).

Therapeutic Role of Nutrition

Nonsurgical therapy includes weight loss and medication (Harper 2017). A significant improvement was recorded by Impellizeri et al. (2000) in dogs with HD, following a decrease in body weight by 11–18%. This clinical finding was supported quantitatively by force-plate analysis by Burkholder et al. (2000). Adaptation to the amount and kind of activity that does the least possible harm to the joint, preferably hydrotherapy (swimming), should coincide with a weight-reduction program (Mlacnik et al. 2006). Marshall et al. (2010) demonstrated in a prospective study in 14 obese (i.e. 20% overweight) dogs that a weight-reduction program improved locomotion (measured on a visual analog scale) when weight loss was 6% or more, and resulted in better locomotion measured with force-plate analysis when weight loss was 8.8% or more. This demonstrates that dogs can reveal improvement even before they reach their optimal body weight, not only due to reduced biomechanical overloading, but possibly also due to reduction of pro-inflammatory adipokine release. Treatment of overweight varies from diminished food intake to food dilution with green beans, special commercial diets, and total starvation (Hazewinkel and Corbee 2011).

Corticosteroids suppress phospholipase activity, and consequently stabilize the blood vessel walls and the lysosomes. Joints will be less painful and less synovia is produced. Since regeneration of cartilage will be decreased under the influence of corticosteroids, long-lasting or repetitive use of corticosteroids, especially intra-articular and at higher dosages, is contraindicated. NSAIDs have actions against cyclooxygenase (COX) enzymes; COX1 stimulates the production of PGs that protect the body, whereas COX2 stimulates the production of PGE_2, which is responsible for clinical signs like pain and hyperemia. The latter results in warm joints and the overproduction of joint fluid. Selective COX2 inhibitors, with or without suppressive action on lipoxygenase, are available for dogs and claim to have fewer side effects than COX1 and COX2 inhibitors. NSAIDs, with a low incidence of side effects, should be prescribed for a prolonged period,

not to mask pain but to improve the metabolic condition of the diseased joint.

To support regeneration of joint cartilage and to shorten or lower the dosage of NSAIDs, there is a constant search for nutritional support for patients with OA. The term "nutraceutical" has been introduced, combining the terms "nutrition" and "pharmaceutical," and includes foods and dietary supplements that have a benefit in reducing the risk of developing a disease or managing it once it occurs (Bauer 2005). Nutraceuticals can be incorporated into functional foods or pharmaceutical preparations and do not fall under the legal categories of foods or drugs (see Chapter 5), but are included in the area between the two. The development of food components that provide benefits beyond their traditional nutritional value has great interest in several sectors: commercial, public, academic, and regulatory. The challenges relate to quality, safety, and efficacy. Most patients' owners who use nutraceuticals are of the opinion that natural remedies with a long history of use are safe, whereas neither clinical efficacy, quality, nor side effects are of concern. Nutraceuticals, whether for human or veterinary use, need more pre-clinical and clinical research to evaluate the mechanisms of action, safety aspects, and efficacy, thereby allowing the veterinarian to make evidence-based decisions regarding prescription or advice on their use. These supplements, or disease-modifying osteoarthritis agents (DMOAs), include chondroitin sulfate, glucosamine, polyunsaturated fatty acids, and antioxidants (Harper 2017; Hazewinkel and Mott 2006).

Chondroitin sulfate increases in vitro the production of proteoglycans and as such the regeneration of cartilage (Bassleer et al. 1998). It prevents synthesis of MMPs by IL-3 and thus cartilage damage when given prophylactically in rabbits.

Glucosamine is a precursor of GAGs that stimulates the synthesis of GAGs, prostaglandins, and collagen by chondrocytes in vitro (Bassleer et al. 1998). In cases of substitution of glucosamines in the medium of chondrocytes, the mRNA content of aggrecan is increased, MMPs decreased, and synthesis of proteoglycan increased (Henrotin et al. 2005). In rabbits with a cranial cruciate ligament (CCL) rupture, 120 mg/kg BW of prophylactic glucosamine decreased the amount of chondropathy in comparison with controls (Conrozier 1998). In a study in dogs with a CCL rupture as a model, it has been demonstrated that these dogs had less cartilage swelling, less total and active metalloproteinase, and lower pathologic scores when injected with 4 mg/kg BW glycosaminoglycan polysulfuric acid (GAGPS) twice weekly for 4–8 weeks, starting four weeks after the CCL rupture (Altman et al. 1989). It is suggested by Altman et al. (1989) that GAGPS suppresses proteoglycan breakdown by MMPs or by directly inhibiting MMPs in cartilage, rather than by increasing synthesis of proteoglycans by chondrocytes. De Haan et al. (1994) demonstrated in a clinical, double-blind, placebo-controlled trial that in dogs with HD, 4.4 mg/kg GAGPS administered intramuscularly every 3–5 days improved lameness scores, range of motion, and joint pain, and had no side effects after eight injections. The placebo group of dogs only demonstrated a small improvement.

Combinations of chondroitin sulfate and glucosamine given to dogs with OA subjectively allowed for more normal locomotion and joint movement than untreated controls (Hulse 1998). Prophylactically provided, this combination decreased inflammation in dogs with induced arthritis (Canapp et al. 1999), possibly due to a modulation in the metabolism of the articular cartilage. The latter was suggested to take place in dogs with CCL ruptures, supplemented with a mixture of chondroitin sulfate, glucosamine hydrochloride, and manganese ascorbate (Johnson et al. 2001).

Polyunsaturated free fatty acids (PUFAs) have a potentially beneficial role in immune-related disorders and OA (Bauer 1994). In vitro studies in canine cartilage indicated that only cartilage exposed to eicosapentaenoic acid

(EPA) revealed abrogation of cartilage degradation (Caterson et al. 2005). Leukotrienes are formed from arachidonic acid (AA; 20:4n-6) and EPA (20:6n-3) originating from cellular membranes, under the influence of the enzyme 5-lipoxygenase. Pro-inflammatory LTB_4 originates from AA, anti-inflammatory LTB_5 from EPA (Figure 10.13). The amount and type of these eicosanoids are determined by the availability of the PUFA precursor. A higher omega-3 intake results in decreased membrane AA levels and thus a decreased synthesis of eicosanoids from AA and an increase in eicosanoids derived from EPA. In joints with OA, the LTB_4 content is increased (Herlin et al. 1990). In 36 dogs with elbow OA due to ED, a double-blind efficacy study was performed by feeding an increased omega-3 content (omega-3 of 4% and omega-6 of 20%) versus a high omega-6 content (omega-3 of 0.8% and omega-6 of 38%). The dogs that consumed the high concentrations of omega-3 fatty acids had significant increases in plasma LTB_5 concentrations, although lameness scored by ground reaction force analysis did not differ between the groups of dogs (Hazewinkel et al. 1998).

A clinical trial including force-plate analysis performed in two groups of dogs fed either a control food or an EPA-supplemented diet for a 90-day period revealed that 31% of the controls and 82% of the EPA-supplemented group improved their weight bearing (Schoenherr 2005).

Antioxidants may decrease the damage to synovial cells by reducing ROS. For this purpose, vitamins A, C, and E and the beta-carotene content in the diet can be increased.

Combinations of chondroitin sulfate, glucosamine, and PUFAs are present in green-lipped mussels (GLMs). The flesh part of the GLM will contain saturated, monounsaturated, and polyunsaturated fatty acids. Of the latter, a large amount is omega-3 fatty acid, mainly EPA and docosahexaenoic acid (DHA), with a final ratio of omega-6 to omega-3 of 1 : 10. GLM is claimed to be a 5-lipoxygenase- pathway inhibitor. Freeze-dried GLM powder also contains a variety of nutrients that may have a beneficial effect on joint health, including amino acids (glutamine, methionine), vitamins (E, C), and minerals (zinc, copper, manganese). The combination of omega-3 PUFAs and other ingredients may have the synergistic potential to limit the progression of OA. In a double-blind, randomized controlled trial, 17 dogs were given a GLM supplement powder and 15 dogs a GLM supplement oil (both in a daily dosage of 1000 mg when BW >34 kg; 750 mg when BW between 34 and 25 kg; 450 mg when BW <25 kg) and compared with 15 controls, all with OA. A non-objective score of arthritic signs ranging from no clinical signs to severe clinical signs was given for mobility and for all major joints individually, before the start of the study and at six weeks. Joint swelling, pain, and crepitus were reported to improve in the GLM powder-supplemented group in comparison with the controls; the GLM-supplemented group was only significantly different in joint pain and crepitus scores (Bierer and Bui 2002). All three doses resulted in a similar improvement in total arthritic score and all were significantly different from controls. However, no significant effects were observed with regard to mobility and reduction in range of joint movement with the addition of GLM in any of the studies. Longer studies and more sensitive assessment methods may be helpful in detecting any possible effects in these parameters (Bierer and Bui 2002).

There is great interest in the discovery of natural products to be used as DMOAs, based on the aversion to "chemical substances" (i.e. NSAIDs) that exists among many dog owners. This interest, as well as the laxity in efficacy control, dosage, and purity, makes them easy to incorporate into dog food. There is a growing need for double-blind clinical efficacy studies with objective criteria to support the in vitro evidence that these DMOAs, nutraceuticals, and supplements may be beneficial to patients suffering from OA. Meta-analyses of the efficacy of glucosamine and chondroitin sulfate for treatment of OA in

humans led to different conclusions: the ingestion of glucosamine or chondroitin sulfate demonstrated some efficacy in some symptom-relieving parameters, but the ability to modify the structure of articular cartilage was not confirmed (Table 10.8) (McAlindon et al. 2000). At the level at which these substances are included in most pet foods there is scant research available to demonstrate a direct therapeutic effect to support their use in the treatment of OA in dogs (Schoenherr 2005). Claims for different concentrations or combinations of nutraceuticals, the period when efficacy can be expected, the use in particular breeds or sizes of dogs, and the indication for different joints or stages of OA will keep the scientific world busy until the onus of proof is laid in the hands of those who claim the efficacy.

Other supplements are under study (Curtis et al. 2004), including green tea and herbal extracts. As can be seen from the findings already discussed, preliminary information provided should be considered with care. Results should be gathered in the target species (i.e. the dog) and not in small laboratory animals, in humans, or in in vitro studies. The dosage, duration, and route of the DMOAs should be taken into account. Since most of these products are not pharmaceuticals, neither purity nor content is per se under strict control, even though the package or information material may suggest otherwise. The daily intake, together with the food, can have practical advantages; that is, client compliance is greater and the supplement will get a chance to have long-term effects. However, parenteral application has an advantage to overcome biological unavailability, used only when (still) indicated, or stopped and replaced by other prescriptions or modalities when not effective.

Double-blind studies are a necessity, and the use of objective measures (e.g. force plate, determination of relevant markers) makes multicentric trials possible to learn more about the efficacy of these and future nutraceuticals.

The varying responses in these and other trials have been suggested to be due to the lack

Table 10.8 Nutraceuticals and claimed effects on joints with osteoarthritis (OA).

Supplement	Function	Effect on joints	Oral dose in dogs
Glucosamine[a]	Precursor of GAG	Limits or delays OA in senior patients	0.02 mg/kg
Chondroitin sulfate[b]	GAG	Stimulates GAG synthesis, inhibits degradative enzyme action	25 mg/kg
Polysulfated GAG[c]		Analgesic, anti-inflammatory, chondroprotective	5 mg/kg
Omega-3 fatty acids[d]	Precursor of EPA and DHA	Anti-inflammatory	
Vitamin E[e]	Antioxidants	Minimize damage from free radicals	Vitamin E 2.5 mg/kg
Green-lipped mussel[f]	FA 3:6 = 1:10 (EPA and DHA) chondroitin, (6.9%), glutamine (0.0005%), and antioxidants	Anti-inflammatory, blocking COX and lipoxygenase pathway	Body weight >34 kg: 1000 mg; 34–25 kg: 750 mg; <25 kg: 450 mg

COX, cyclooxygenase; DHA, docosahexaenoic acid; EPA, eicosapentaenoic acid; FA, fatty acids; GAG, glycosaminoglycan.
[a] Setnikar et al. (1991).
[b] Usually given in combination with other chondroprotective agents.
[c] Setnikar et al. (1991), De Haan et al. (1994), Altman et al. (1989).
[d] Bauer (1994).
[e] Greenwald (1991); Kurz et al. (2002).
[f] Bierer and Bui (2002).

of stabilizing processes, avoidance of heat during the processing of the diets, the ratio of omega-3 to omega-6 fatty acids (i.e. the effect of the background diet), the purity and dosage of the product, and the significant placebo effect (Cobb and Ernst 2006; Curtis et al. 2004; Dobenecker et al. 2002). That there is a strong influence of the latter caused by the awareness of the owner concerning the OA of their pet and the necessity of adapting the dog's or cat's lifestyle is the experience of most veterinary surgeons who evaluate therapies (Marcillin-Little 2004), but is perhaps not as high as in human studies (~60%) (Clegg et al. 2006). Dobenecker et al. (2002) described that some symptoms improved even more in the placebo group than in supplemented groups, and concluded that studies assessing the efficacy of chondroprotective agents must therefore be carried out with placebo-controlled, double-blinded trials, and preferably with objective study measures. A caregiver placebo effect in a study with cat owners has been described by Gruen et al. with a strong placebo effect (Gruen et al. 2017). The effect of a supplement containing green-lipped mussel (*Perna canaliculus*), curcumin (*Curcuma longa*), and blackcurrant (*Ribes nigrum*) leaf extract on locomotion and behavior in client-owned dogs and cats suffering from mild to moderate osteoarthritis has been studied in a double-blind, randomised, crossover, placebo-controlled trial for 10 weeks in cats and 16 weeks in dogs. In dogs, the clinical signs improved significantly in the supplement group compared to baseline, but was not different than the placebo group. In cats, the ability to groom, activity level, playfulness, and walking up the stairs improved in the supplement group. No differences were found on objective OA scores and on force-plate analysis in dogs (Corbee 2022).

Osteoarthrosis in Cats

There is increasing interest in concern about OA in cats, the etiology and clinical signs, and the role of dietary adaptations as part of therapeutic measurements. Like in dogs, body condition plays a role in the etiology of OA in cats. Adult age in cats (>2 years), sex (male, neutered), and no outdoor confinement are all factors correlated with overweight or even obesity (19% and 7.8% of 385 cats, respectively) (Corbee 2014a). Obese cats are 4.9 times as likely to develop lameness requiring veterinary care, even more frequently than diabetes mellitus and non-allergic skin conditions. Body weight peaks in cats between 5 and 10 years of age (the middle–aged cat); a large proportion of cats older than 12 years of age are underweight compared with other age groups. In addition to an increase in maintenance energy requirements in this age group (partially due to a decrease in musculature and activity), it has been identified that older cats may experience a reduction in protein and an increase in fat-digestive capabilities, which could contribute to weight loss in aging cats (Laflamme 2005). Body condition score can therefore vary throughout a cat's life. Although overweight cats are more likely to suffer from lameness, a cross-sectional study of 100 cats >6 years revealed 61% of cats with degenerative joint disease, with the vertebrae, elbows, hips, shoulders, and tarsi as the most affected joints, but body condition score was not correlated with the presence or severity of OA (Slingerland et al. 2011), which is in accordance with the findings of Hardie et al. (2002) in 99 cats >12 years with 65% OA. The increase in body weight at young adult age and the increase in lifespan plus the increase in awareness of OA among owners make OA in cats a current topic for the practicing veterinarian.

Unlike dogs, most cats suffer from primary OA; that is, there is not a primary cause like ED or CCL rupture, but only increasing age. Solely HD is diagnosed as a primary cause of OA in 6–23% of cats, depending on the breed and the age of the investigated cat population (Lascelles 2010). It is the general opinion among authors that the sensitivity of an orthopedic investigation in cats is low, especially for the smaller joints, and the complaints of the owner are non-specific and very much related to behavior change in the cat. These changes in combination with the radiologic signs of joints support the diagnosis of OA in cats (Lascelles 2010; Slingerland et al. 2011).

Therapeutic measures include weight loss when overweight is present (Laflamme 2005), adaptation of the environment (Bennett et al. 2012), and NSAIDs such as meloxicam (Sul et al. 2014; Monteiro et al. 2016) or tramadol (Monteiro et al. 2016), as demonstrated in clinical trials. In a randomized, double-blinded, placebo-controlled cross-over design study, the efficacy of omega-3 fatty acid supplementation (fish oil: 1.53 g EPA and 0.31 g DNA, both per 1000 kcal ME) was noticed by the owners of 16 cats, and was registered by a survey before and after adding the supplement or the placebo, each during a 10-week period. Cats were more active, walking more frequently on stairs, and jumping higher during the period of supplementation with fish oil compared to the period of supplementation with placebo (Corbee et al. 2013). These findings are in conjunction with results in cats with OA provided with a special food with increased levels of omega-3 fatty acids (Lascelles 2010). Since no side effects are noticed after extended periods of fish oil supplementation in cats, this supplementation might be an aid in OA therapeutic measures, although a caregiver placebo effect in each of these measures can play a major role in cats with OA (Gruen et al. 2017).

Summary

- Nutrition plays an important role in undisturbed skeletal growth and bone remodeling.
- Both deficiency and excess of minerals (calcium, phosphorus) and vitamins (vitamin D) may be the causative factor in a variety of orthopedic diseases in dogs, including pathologic fractures, rickets, radius curvus syndrome, wobbler syndrome, panosteitis, osteochondrosis, incongruity of the elbow joint, and possibly other forms of elbow dysplasia and dysplasia of the hip joint.
- In cats minerals (calcium) and vitamins (A and D) play a role in skeletal growth. Deficiency of calcium and/or vitamin D and chronic excess of vitamin A are known to cause disturbances in skeletal integrity in cats.
- Growing dogs, of large breeds especially, should be fed according to, and not exceeding, the nutrient requirements.
- Minerals and vitamins are part of the diet that provide the energy for growth and activity. Individual variation, increased growth rate and/or level of activity, or food with a lowered level of metabolizable energy may lead to exceeding the daily requirements of minerals and vitamins, and thus to disturbance of skeletal growth as a cause of frequently diagnosed orthopedic diseases.
- Obesity in dogs is linked to lameness due to osteoarthritis.
- Osteoarthritis in cats is often without a primary cause, becomes more frequent and more severe with advancing age, and is not linked to the body condition score. Supplementation of the daily ration with fish oil might have a beneficial effect on mobility and related behavior disturbances.
- Insight into mineral and bone metabolism and into the pathophysiology of orthopedic diseases related to deficient or excessive intake of food constituents will help to understand and thus to prevent these diseases and to educate clients accordingly.

References

AAFCO (2022). *Official Publication*. Champaign, IL: Association of American Feed Control Officials.

Alexander, J.E., Moore, M.P., and Wood, L.L.H. (1988). Comparative growth studies in Labrador retrievers fed 5 commercial calorie-dense diets. *Mod. Vet. Pract.* 69: 144–148.

Altman, R.D., Dean, D.D., Muniz, O.E., and Howell, D.S. (1989). Therapeutic treatment of canine OA with glucosaminoglycan polusulfuric acid ester. *Arthritis Rheum.* 32: 179–766.

Atwal, J., Stockman, J., Gilham, M. et al. (2021). No observed adverse effects on health were detected in adult beagle dogs when fed a high-calcium diet for 40 weeks. *Animals (Basel)* 11 (6): 1799.

Bardens, J.W. and Hardwick, H. (1968). New observations on the diagnosis and cause of hip dysplasia. *Vet. Med. Small Anim. Clin.* 63: 238–245.

Bassleer, C., Rovati, L., and Franchimont, P. (1998). Stimulation of proteoglycan production by glucosamine sulfate in chondrocytes isolated from human osteoarthritic articular cartilage *in vitro*. *Osteoarthr. Cartil.* 6: 427–434.

Bauer, J.E. (1994). The potential for dietary polyunsaturated fatty acids in domestic animals. *Aust. Vet. J.* 71: 342–345.

Bauer, J.E. (2005). Nutraceuticals. In: *Textbook of Veterinary Internal Medicine, Diseases of the Dog and Cat*, 6e (ed. S.J. Ettinger and E.C. Feldman), 515–517. St. Louis, MO: Elsevier.

Bennet, D., Zainal, A.S.M., and Johnston, P. (2012). Osteoarthritis in the cat: 2. How should it be managed and treated. *Feline Med. Surg.* 14: 76–84.

Bierer, T.L. and Bui, L.M. (2002). Improvement of arthritic signs in dogs fed green-lipped mussel (Perna canaliculus). *J. Nutr.* 132 (Suppl 2): 1634S–1636S.

Bowen, J.M., Lewis, R.E., Kneller, S.K. et al. (1972). Progression of hip dysplasia in German shepherd dogs after unilateral pectineal myotomy. *J. Am. Vet. Med. Assoc.* 161: 899–904.

Burkholder, W.J., Taylor, L., and Hulse, D.A. (2000). Weight loss to optimal body condition increases ground reactive forces in dogs with osteoarthritis (abstract). Proceedings Purina Nutrition Forum 2000. *Compend. Contin. Edu. Pract. Vet.* 23: 74.

Canapp, S.O., McLaughlin, R.M., Hoskinson, J.J. et al. (1999). Scintigraphic evaluation of dogs with acute synovitis after treatment with glucosamine hydrochloride and chondroitin sulphate. *Am. J. Vet. Res.* 60: 1552–1557.

Caterson, B., Little, C.B., Cramp, J. et al. (2005). Eicosapentaenoate supplementation abrogates canine articular cartilage degeneration in *in vitro* explant culture systems. *Proceedings, Hill's European Symposium on Osteoarthritis and Joint Health*, Genoa, Italy, 14–19 April 2005 (ed. J. Debraekeleer and H. Goldberg).

Chicco, C.F., Ammerman, C.B., Feaster, J.P., and Dunavant, B.G. (1973). Nutritional interrelationship of dietary calcium, phosphorus and magnesium in sheep. *J. Anim. Sci.* 36: 986–993.

Clegg, D.O., Reda, D.J., Harris, C.L. et al. (2006). Glucosamine, chondroitin sulphate, and the two in combination for painful knee osteoarthritis. *N. Engl. J. Med.* 354: 795–808.

Cloutier, M., Rousseau, L., Gascon-Barré, M., and D'Amour, P. (1993). Immunological evidence for post-translational control of parathyroid function by ionized calcium in dogs. *Bone Miner.* 22: 197–207.

Cobb, C.S. and Ernst, E. (2006). Systematic review of a marine nutriceutical supplement in clinical trials for arthritis: the effectiveness of the New Zealand green-lipped mussel Perna canaliculus. *Clin. Rheumatol.* 25: 275–284.

Conrozier, T. (1998). Anti-arthrosis treatments, efficacy and tolerance of chondroitin sulfates. *Presse Med.* 27 (36): 1862–1865.

Corbee R.J. (2014a). Nutrition and skeletal health in dogs and cats. PhD thesis. Utrecht University.

Corbee, R.J. (2014b). Obesity in show cats. *Anim. Physiol. Anim. Nutr. (Berl).* 98 (6): 1075–1080.

Corbee, R. (2022). The efficacy of a nutritional supplement containing green-lipped mussel, curcumin and blackcurrant leaf extract in dogs and cats with osteoarthritis. *Vet. Med. Sci.* 8: 1025–1035.

Corbee, R.J., Tryfonidou, M.A., Beckers, I.P., and Hazewinkel, H.A.W. (2011). Composition and use of puppy milk replacers in German Shepherd puppies in the Netherlands. *J. Anim. Physiol. Anim. Nutr.* 96 (3): 395–402.

Corbee, R.J., Tryfonidou, M.A., Meij, B.P. et al. (2012). Vitamin D status before and after hypophysectomy in dogs with pituitary-dependent hypercortisolism. *Domest. Anim. Endocrinol.* 42: 43–49.

Corbee, R.J., Barnier, M.M., van de Lest, C.H., and Hazewinkel, H.A. (2013). The effect of dietary long-chain omega-3 fatty acid supplementation on owner's perception of behaviour and locomotion in cats with naturally occurring osteoarthritis. *J. Anim. Physiol. Anim. Nutr. (Berl.)* 97: 846–853.

Corbee, R.J., Tryfonidou, M.A., Grinwis, G.C. et al. (2014). Skeletal and hepatic changes induced by chronic vitamin A supplementation in cats. *Vet. J.* 202: 503–509.

Corbee, R.J., Tryfonidou, M.A., Grinwis, G.C.M. et al. (2015a). Dietary vitamin D supplementation during early growth is not protective for medial coronoid disease development in Labradors. *J. Vet. Med. Res.* 2 (4): 1–8.

Corbee, R.J., Vaandrager, A.B., Kik, M.J.L. et al. (2015b). Cutaneous vitamin D synthesis in carnivorous species. *J. Vet. Med. Res.* 2: 1–4.

Corbellini, C.N., Krook, L., Nathanielz, P.W., and Kallfelz, F.A. (1991). Osteochondrosis in fetuses of ewes overfed calcium. *Calcif. Tissue Int.* 48: 37–45.

Curtis, C.L., Harwood, J.L., Dent, C.M., and Caterson, B. (2004). Biological basis for the benefit of nutraceutical supplementation in arthritis. *Drug Discov. Today* 9: 165–172.

De Haan, J.L., Goring, R.L., and Beale, B.S. (1994). Evaluation of polysulfated GAGs for the treatment of hip dysplasia in dogs. *VCOT* 7: 58.

Dobenecker, B. (2004). Apparent calcium absorption in growing dogs of two different sizes. *J. Nutr.* 134: 2151S–2153S.

Dobenecker, B., Beetz, Y., and Kienzle, E. (2002). A placebo-controlled double-blind study on the effect of nutraceuticals (chondroitin sulphate and mussel extract) in dogs with joint diseases as perceived by their owners. *J. Nutr.* 132: 1690S–1691S.

Dobenecker, B., Kasbeitzer, N., Flinspach, S. et al. (2006). Calcium-excess causes subclinical changes of bone growth in Beagles but not in Foxhound-crossbred dogs, as measured in X-rays. *J. Anim. Physiol. Anim. Nutr.* 90: 394–401.

Driessen, F.C.M. (1980). Probable phase composition of the mineral in bone. *Z. Naturforsch. C Biosci.* 35: 357–362.

FEDIAF (2021). *Nutritional Guidelines for Complete and Complementary Pet Food for Cats and Dogs*. Brussels: FEDIAF.

Fluckiger, M.A., Friedrich, G.A., and Binder, H. (1999). A radiographic stress technique for evaluation of coxofemoral joint laxity in dogs. *Vet. Surg.* 28: 1–9.

Freytag, T.L., Liu, S.M., Rogers, Q.R., and Morris, J.G. (2003). Teratogenic effects of chronic ingestion of high levels of vitamin A in cats. *J. Anim. Physiol. Anim. Nutr.* 87: 42–51.

Ginja, M.M., Silvestre, A.M., Gonzalo-Orden, J.M., and Ferreira, A.J. (2010). Diagnosis, genetic control and preventive management of canine hip dysplasia: a review. *Vet. J.* 184 (3): 269–276.

Greenwald, R.A. (1991). Oxygen radicals, inflammation and arthritis: pathophysiological considerations and implications for treatment. *Semin. Arthritis Rheum.* 20 (4): 219–240.

Gross, K.L., Wedekind, K.J., Cowell, C.S. et al. (2000). Nutrients. In: *Small Animal Clinical Nutrition* (ed. M.S. Hand, C.D. Thatcher, R.L. Remillard, et al.), 21–101. Topeka: Mark Morris Institute.

Gruen, M.E., Dorman, D.C., and Lascelles, B.D.X. (2017). Caregiver placebo effect in analgesic clinical trials for cats with naturally occurring degenerative joint disease-associated pain. *Vet. Rec.* 13 (180): 473.

Hallebeek, J.M. and Hazewinkel, H.A.W. (1998). Effect of isoenergetic substitution of dietary fat (beef tallow) for carbohydrates (wheat starch) on calcium absorption in the dog. *J. Anim. Physiol. Anim. Nutr.* 78: 60–66.

Hardie, E.M., Roe, S.C., and Martin, F.R. (2002). Radiographic evidence of degenerative joint disease in geriatric cats: 100 cases (1994–1997). *J. Am. Vet. Med. Assoc.* 220: 628–632.

Harper, T.A.M. (2017). Conservative management of hip dysplasia. *Vet. Clin. North Am. Small Anim. Pract.* 47: 807–821.

Hayes, K.C. (1971). On the pathophysiology of vitamin A deficiency. *Nutr. Rev.* 29: 3–6.

Hazewinkel, H.A.W. (1985). Influences of different calcium intakes on calcium metabolism and skeletal development in young Great Danes. PhD thesis. Utrecht University, Netherlands.

Hazewinkel, H.A.W. (1989). Calcium metabolism and skeletal development. In: *Nutrition of the Dog and Cat* (ed. I.H. Burger and J.P.W. Rivers), 293–302. Cambridge: Cambridge University Press.

Hazewinkel, H.A.W. (1991). Conservative treatment in canine hip dysplasia. *Proceedings of the W.S.A.V.A. World Congress* (ed. J. Leibetseder). Vienna: Vereinigung Osterreichischer Kleintierpraktiker (11–14 October 1991).

Hazewinkel, H.A.W. (1994). Nutrition and skeletal disease. In: *The Waltham Book of Clinical Nutrition of the Dog and Cat* (ed. J.M. Wills and K.W. Simpson), 395–423. Oxford: Pergamon.

Hazewinkel, H.A.W. (1998). Bone diseases. In: *Canine Medicine and Therapeutics*, 4e (ed. N. Gorman), 796–812. Oxford: Blackwell Science.

Hazewinkel, H.A.W. and Corbee, R.J. (2011). Obesity and osteoarthritis: causes and management. Focus on obesity and obesity related diseases. *Purina Companion Animal Nutrition Summit*, Tucson, AZ (March 24–26).

Hazewinkel, H.A.W. and Mott, J. (2006). Main nutritional imbalances implicated in osteoarticular disease. In: *Encyclopedia of Canine Clinical Nutrition* (ed. P. Pibot, V. Biourge and D. Elliott), 369–405. Paris: Diffomérdia.

Hazewinkel, H.A.W. and Schoenmakers, I. (1995). Influence of protein, minerals, and vitamin D on skeletal development in dogs. *Vet. Clin. Nutr.* 2: 93–99.

Hazewinkel, H.A.W. and Tryfonidou, M.A. (2002). Vitamin D_3 metabolism in dogs. *Mol. Cell. Endocrinol.* 197: 22–33.

Hazewinkel, H.A.W., Goedegebuure, S.A., Poulos, P.W., and Wolvekamp, W.T.C. (1985). Influences of chronic calcium excess on the skeleton of growing Great Danes. *J. Am. Anim. Hosp. Assoc.* 21: 377–391.

Hazewinkel, H.A.W., van den Brom, W.E., Van 't Klooster, A.T. et al. (1991). Calcium metabolism in Great Dane dogs fed diets with various calcium and phosphorus levels. *J. Nutr.* 121: S99–S106.

Hazewinkel, H.A.W., Theyse, L.F.H., Wolvekamp, W.T. et al. (1998). The influence of dietary omega-6: omega-3 ratio on lameness in dogs with OA of the elbow joint. In: *1998 Iams Nutrition Symposium Proceedings, Recent Advances in Canine and Feline Nutrition*, vol. II (ed. G.A. Reinhart and D.P. Carey), 325–336. Wilmington, OH: Orange-Frazer Press.

Hazewinkel, H.A.W., Kealy, R.D., Mol, J.A., and Rijnberk, A. (1999a). Change in GH-IGF-1 axis in obese dogs with possible consequences for osteoarthritis. *Comp. Cont. Educ. Pract. Vet.* 21S: 51.

Hazewinkel, H.A.W., Schoenmakers, I., and Nap, R.C. (1999b). Considerations in feeding young dogs of different genetic backgrounds and life stages. *Purina Nutrition Forum Proceedings*. St. Louis, MI, 88, Nestle Purina, 21–24 October 1999.

Hazewinkel, H.A.W., Nap, R.C., Schoenmakers, I., and Voorhout, G. (2000). Dietary influence on development of enostosis in young dogs. *Vet. Surg.* 29 (3): 279.

Hedhammar, A., Wu, F., Krook, L. et al. (1974). Overnutrition and skeletal disease: an experimental study in growing Great Dane dogs. *Cornell Vet.* 64 (Suppl 5): 11–160.

Henrotin, Y., Sanchez, C., and Balligand, M. (2005). Pharmaceutical and nutraceutical management of canine osteoarthritis: present and future perspectives. *Vet. J.* 170: 113–123.

Herlin, T., Fogh, K., and Hansen, E.S. (1990). 15-HETE inhibits leukotriene B4 formation and synovial cell proliferation in experimental arthritis. *Agents Actions* 29: 52–53.

How, K.L., Hazewinkel, H.A.W., and Mol, J.A. (1994). Dietary vitamin D dependence of cat and dog due to inadequate cutaneous synthesis of vitamin D. *J. Gen. Comp. Endocrinol.* 96: 12–18.

Hoyland, J.A., Dixon, J.A., Berry, J.L. et al. (2003). A comparison of in situ hybridisation, reverse transcriptase-polymerase chain reaction (RT-PCR) and in situ-RT-PCR for the detection of canine distemper virus RNA in Paget's disease. *J. Virol. Methods* 109: 253–259.

Huck, J.L., Biery, D.N., Lawler, D.F. et al. (2009). A longitudinal study of the influence of lifetime food restriction on development of osteoarthritis in the canine elbow. *Vet. Surg.* 38 (2): 192–198.

Huis in 't Veld, M., Tryfonidou, M.A., and Hazewinkel, H.A.W. (2001). Bone mineral content and bone histomorphometry in miniature poodles and Great Danes during growth. Internal report, Department of Clinical Sciences in Companion Animals. Utrecht University.

Hulse, D. (1998). Treatment methods for pain in the osteoarthrotic patient. *Vet. Clin. North Am. Small Anim. Pract.* 28: 361–375.

Impellizeri, J.A., Tetrick, M.A., and Muir, P. (2000). Effect of weight reduction on clinical signs of lameness in dogs with hip osteoarthritis. *J. Am. Vet. Med. Assoc.* 216: 1089–1091.

Innes, J. (2009). Getting the elbow: diagnosis and management of elbow disease in dogs. *J. Small Anim. Pract.* 50: 18–20.

Issa, R.I. and Griffin, T.M. (2012). Pathobiology of obesity and osteoarthritis: integrating biomechanics and inflammation. *Pathobiol. Aging Age Relat. Dis.* 9: 2. https://doi.org/10.3402/pba.v2i0.17470.

Jee, W., Bartley, M.H., Cooper, R.R., and Dockum, N.L. (1970). Bone structure. In: *The Beagle as Experimental Dog* (ed. A.C. Anderson and L.S. Goode), 162–188. Ames, IA: Iowa University Press.

Johnson, K.A., Hulse, D.A., Hart, R.C., and Kochevar, D. (2001). Effects of an orally administered mixture of chondroitin sulphate, glucosamine hydrochloride and manganese ascorbate on synovial fluid chondroitin sulphate 3B3 and 7D4 epitope in a canine cruciate ligament transection model of OA. *Osteoarthr. Cartil.* 9: 14–21.

Kallfelz, F.A. and Dzanis, D.A. (1989). Overnutrition: An epidemic problem in pet practice? *Vet. Clin. North Am. Small Anim. Pract.* 19: 433–446.

Kasström, H. (1975). Nutrition, weight gain, and development of hip dysplasia. An experimental investigation in growing dogs with special reference to the effect of feeding intensity. *Acta Radiol. Suppl.* 344: 135–179.

Kealy, R.D., Olsson, S.E., Monti, K.L. et al. (1992). Effects of limited food consumption on the incidence of hip dysplasia in growing dogs. *J. Am. Vet. Med. Assoc.* 201: 857–863.

Kealy, R.D., Lawler, D.F., Monti, K.L. et al. (1993). Effects of dietary electrolyte balance on subluxation of the femoral head in growing dogs. *Am. J. Vet. Res.* 54 (4): 555–562.

Kealy, R.D., Lawler, D.F., Ballam, J.M. et al. (2000). Evaluation of the effect of limited food consumption on radiographic evidence of osteoarthritis in dogs. *J. Am. Vet. Med. Assoc.* 217: 1678–1680.

Kincaid, S.A. and Van Sickle, D.C. (1983). Bone morphology and postnatal osteogenesis. *Vet. Clin. North Am. Small Anim. Pract.* 13: 3–17.

Kohart, N.A., Elshafae, S.M., Breitbach, J.T., and Rosol, T.J. (2017). Animal models of cancer-associated hypercalcemia. *Vet. Sci.* 2017 (4): 21.

Kurz, B., Jost, B., and Schunke, M. (2002). Dietary vitamins and selenium diminish the development of mechanically induced osteoarthritis and increase the expression of anti-oxydant enzymes in the knee joint of mice. *Osteoarthr. Cartil.* 10: 119–126.

Laflamme, D.P. (2005). Nutrition for aging cats and dogs and the importance of body condition. *Vet. Clin. North Am. Small Anim. Pract.* 35: 713–742.

LaFond, E., Breur, E.J., and Austin, C.C. (2000). Breed susceptibility for developmental orthopedic diseases in dogs. *J. Am. Anim. Hosp. Assoc.* 38: 467–477.

Lascelles, B.D. (2010). Feline degenerative joint disease. *Vet. Surg.* 39: 2–13.

Lau, S.F., Hazewinkel, H.A.W., Grinwis, G.C. et al. (2013). Delayed endochondral ossification in early medial coronoid disease (MCD): a morphological and immunohistochemical evaluation in growing Labrador retrievers. *Vet. J.* 197: 731–738.

Lavelle, R.B. (1989). The effect of overfeeding of a balanced complete diet to a group of growing Great Danes. In: *Nutrition of the Dog and Cat. Waltham Symposium 7* (ed. I.H. Burger and J.P.W. Rivers), 303–315. Cambridge: Cambridge University Press.

Lunn, P.G. and Austin, S. (1983). Dietary manipulation of plasma albumin concentration. *J. Nutr.* 113: 1791–1802.

Lust, G. (1993). Hip dysplasia in dogs. In: *Textbook of Small Animal Surgery*, 2e (ed. D. Slatter), 1938–1944. Philadelphia, PA: WB Saunders.

Lust, G., Rendamo, V.T., and Summers, B.A. (1985). Canine hip dysplasia: concepts and diagnosis. *J. Am. Vet. Med. Assoc.* 187: 638–640.

Mack, J.K. and Kienzle, E. (2016). Inadequate nutrient supply in "BARF" feeding plans for a litter of Bernese Mountain dog-puppies. *Tierarztl. Prax.* 44: 341–347.

Mack, J.K., Alexander, L.G., Morris, P.J. et al. (2015). Demonstration of uniformity of calcium absorption in adult dogs and cat. *J. Anim. Physiol. Anim. Nutr.* 99: 801–809.

Madsen, J.S., Reimann, I., and Svalastoga, E. (1991). Delayed ossification of the femoral head in dogs with hip dysplasia. *J. Small Anim. Pract.* 32: 351–354.

Marcillin-Little, D.J. (2004). Benefits of physical therapy for osteoarthritic patients. In: *Proceedings ESVOT 2004* (ed. A. Vezzoni and M. Schramme), 100–103. Munich: European Society of Veterinary Orthopaedics and Traumatology.

Marshall, W., Bockstahler, B., Hulse, D., and Carmichael, S. (2009). A review of osteoarthritis and obesity: current understanding of the relationship and benefit of obesity treatment and prevention in the dog. *Vet. Comp. Orthop. Traumatol.* 22: 339–345.

Marshall, W.G., Hazewinkel, H.A., Mullen, D. et al. (2010). The effect of weight loss on lameness in obese dogs with osteoarthritis. *Vet. Res. Commun.* 34: 241–253.

McAlindon, T.E., LaValley, M.P., and Felson, D.T. (2000). Efficacy of glucosamine and chondroitin for treatment of osteoarthritis. *JAMA* 84: 41.

Mee, A.P., Gordon, M.T., May, C. et al. (1993). Canine distemper virus transcripts detected in the bone cells of dogs with metaphyseal osteopathy. *Bone* 14: 59–67.

Meyer, H. (1983). *Ernährung des Hundes, Grundlagen und Praxis*. Stuttgart: Eugen Verlag.

Meyer, H. and Zentek, J. (2005). *Ernähriung des Hundes*. Stuttgart: Parey Verlag.

Mlacnik, E., Bockstahler, B.A., Müller, M. et al. (2006). Effects of caloric restriction and a moderate or intense physiotherapy program for treatment of lameness in overweight dogs with osteoarthritis. *J. Am. Vet. Med. Assoc.* 229: 1756–1717.

Monteiro, B.P., Klinck, M.P., Moreau, M. et al. (2016). Analgesic efficacy of an oral transmucosal spray formulation of meloxicam alone or in combination with tramadol in cats with naturally occurring osteoarthritis. *Vet. Anesth. Analg.* 43: 643–651.

Morgan, J.P., Wind, A., and Davidson, A.P. (2000). *Hereditary Bone and Joint Diseases in the Dog*. Hanover: Schlütersche Verlag.

Morris, J.G. (1999). Ineffective vitamin D synthesis in cats is reversed by an inhibitor of 7-dehydro cholestrol-delta7reductase. *J. Nutr.* 129: 909–912.

Morris, J.G. (2002a). Idiosyncratic nutrient requirements of cats appear to be diet-induced evolutionary adaptations. *Nutr. Res. Rev.* 15: 153–168.

Morris, J.G. (2002b). Cats discriminate between cholecalciferol and ergocalciferol. *J. Anim. Physiol. Anim. Nutr.* 86 (7–8): 229–238.

Mortensen, B.M., Gautvik, K.M., and Gordeladze, J.O. (1993). Bone turnover in rats treated with 1,25-dihydroxyvitamin D3, 25-hydroxyvitamin D3 or 24,25-dihydroxyvitamin D3. *Biosci. Rep.* 13: 7–39.

Nap, R.C. and Hazewinkel, H.A.W. (1994). Growth and skeletal development in the dog in relation to nutrition: a review. *Vet. Q.* 16: 50–59.

Nap, R.C., Hazewinkel, H.A.W., Voorhout, G. et al. (1991). Growth and skeletal development in Great Dane pups fed different levels of protein intake. *J. Nutr.* 121 (Suppl. 11): 107–113.

Nap, R.C., Hazewinkel, H.A.W., and van den Brom, W.E. (1993a). ^{45}Ca Kinetics in growing miniature poodles challenged by four different dietary levels of calcium. *J. Nutr.* 123: 1826–1833.

Nap, R.C., Hazewinkel, H.A.W., and van den Brom, W.E. (1993b). Growth and skeletal development in miniature poodles fed different levels of calcium: radiographic, histologic and endocrine aspects. PhD thesis. Utrecht University.

Nap, R.C., Mol, J.A., and Hazewinkel, H.A.W. (1993c). Age-related plasma concentrations of growth hormone (GH) and insulin-like growth factor I(IGF-I) in Great Dane pups fed different dietary levels of protein. *Domest. Anim. Endocrinol.* 10: 37–47.

Nap, R.C., Hazewinkel, H.A.W., and Lepine, A.J. (2000). Clinical relevance of calcium studies and recommended feeding strategies for growing large and giant breed dogs to optimize skeletal development. In: *Recent Advances in Canine and Feline Nutrition*, vol. III (ed. G.A. Reinhart and D.P. Carey), 457–465. Wilmington, OH: Orange Fraser Press.

National Research Council (NRC) (2006). *Nutrient Requirements of Dogs*. Washington, DC: National Academies Press.

Norman, A.W., Okamura, W.H., Bishop, J.E., and Henry, H.L. (2002). Update on biological actions of 1alpha,25(OH)2-vitamin D3 (rapid effects) and 24R,25(OH)2-vitamin D3. *Mol. Cell. Endocrinol.* 197: 1–13.

Olsson, S.E. (1993). Pathophysiology, morphology, and clinical signs of osteochondrosis in the dog. In: *Disease Mechanisms in Small Animal Surgery*, 2e (ed. M.J. Bojrab), 776–796. Philadelphia, PA: Lea & Febiger.

Parker, V.J., Rudinsky, A.J., and Chew, D.J. (2017). Vitamin D metabolism in canine and feline medicine. *J. Am. Vet. Med. Assoc.* 250: 1259–1269.

Patronek, G.J., Waters, D.J., and Glickman, L.T. (1997). Comparative longevity of pet dogs and humans: implications for gerontology research. *J. Gerontol. A Biol. Sci. Med. Sci.* 52: B171–B178.

Poole, A.R., Kojima, T., Yasuda, T. et al. (2001). Composition and structure of articular cartilage: a template for tissue repair. *Clin. Orthop. Relat. Res.* 391: S26–S33.

Richardson, D.C., Zentek, J., Hazewinkel, H.A.W. et al. (2010). Developmental orthopedic disease of dogs. In: *Small Animal Clinical Nutrition* (ed. M.S. Hand, C.D. Thatcher, R.L. Remillard, et al.), 667–693. Topeka, KS: Mark Morris Institute.

Riser, W.H. (1993). Canine hip dysplasia. In: *Pathophysiology in Small Animal Surgery*, 2e (ed. M.J. Bojrab and D.D. Smeak), 797–803. Philadelphia, PA: Lea & Febiger.

Romsos, D.R., Belo, P.S., Bennink, M.R. et al. (1976). Effect of dietary carbohydrate, fat and protein on growth, body composition and blood metabolite levels in the dog. *J. Nutr.* 106: 1452–1464.

Schawalder, P., Prieur, W.D., and Koch, H. (1998). Dysplasien und Wachstumsstörungen. In: *Kleintierkrankheiten: Band 3* (ed. H. Bonath and W.D. Prieur), 356–429. Stuttgart: Verlag Eugen.

Schmitt, S.C. (2018). Untersuchung zur Anpassung des Calciumstoffwechsels adulter Hunde an längerfristige marginale Calciumversorgung [Adaptation of calcium metabolism in adult dogs under longterm low calcium intake]. PhD thesis. University of Munich, Germany.

Schoenherr, W.D. (2005). Fatty acids and evidence-based dietary management of canine osteoarthritis. *Proceedings, Hill's European Symposium on Osteoarthritis and Joint Health*, Genoa, Italy (54–59 April).

Schoenmakers, I. (1999). Modulation of calcium regulation by excessive calcium intake in dogs, doctoral thesis. Utrecht University.

Schoenmakers, I., Hazewinkel, H.A.W., and van den Brom, W.E. (1999a). Excessive Ca and P intake during early maturation in dogs alters Ca and P balance without long-term effects after dietary normalization. *J. Nutr.* 129: 1068–1074.

Schoenmakers, I., Nap, R.C., Mol, J.A., and Hazewinkel, H.A.W. (1999b). Calcium metabolism: an overview of its hormonal regulation and interrelation with skeletal integrity. *Vet. Q.* 21 (4): 147–153.

Schoenmakers, I., Hazewinkel, H.A.W., Voorhout, G. et al. (2000). Effect of diets with different calcium and phosphorus contents on the skeletal development and blood chemistry of growing great danes. *Vet. Rec.* 147: 652–660.

Schoenmakers, I., Mol, J.A., and Hazewinkel, H.A.W. (2001). Hormonal calcium regulation and calcium setpoint in offspring of bitches with different calcium intakes during pregnancy. *J. Anim. Physiol. Anim. Nutr.* 83: 1–14.

Seawright, A.A., English, P.B., and Gartner, R.J. (1965). Hypervitaminosis A and hyperostosis of the cat. *Nature* 206: 1171–1172.

Setnikar, I., Pacinic, M.A., and Revel, L. (1991). Antiarthritic effects of glucosamine sulphate studied on animal models. *Arzneimittelforschung* 41: 542–545.

Sheffy, B.E. (1979). Meeting energy-protein needs of dogs. *Comp. Cont. Educ. Pract. Vet.* 1: 345–354.

Slater, M.R., Scarlett, J.M., Donoghue, S. et al. (1992). Diet and exercise as potential risk factors for osteochondritis dissecans in dogs. *Am. J. Vet. Res.* 53 (11): 2119–2124.

Slingerland, L.I., Hazewinkel, H.A., Meij, B.P. et al. (2011). Cross-sectional study of the prevalence and clinical features of osteoarthritis in 100 cats. *Vet. J.* 187: 304–309.

Slocum, B. and Devine, T.M. (1990). Dorsal acetabular rim radiographic view for evaluation of the canine hip. *J. Am. Anim. Hosp. Assoc.* 26: 289–296.

Smith, G.K. (2004). New paradigms for hip dysplasia prevention and control performance and ethics of CHD screening as an indication for preventive strategies. In: *Proceedings ESVOT*, 125–131. Munich: European Society of Veterinary Orthopaedics and Traumatology.

Smith, G.K., Paster, E.R., Powers, M.Y. et al. (2006). Lifelong diet restriction and radiographic evidence of osteoarthritis of the hip joint in dogs. *J. Am. Vet. Med. Assoc.* 229: 690–693.

Spangler, W.L., Gribble, D.H., and Lee, T.C. (1979). Vitamin D intoxication and the pathogenesis of vitamin D nephropathy in the dog. *Am. J. Vet. Res.* 40: 73–83.

Stockman, J., Watson, P., Gilham, M. et al. (2017). Adult dogs are capable of regulating calcium balance with no adverse effects on health, when fed a high-calcium diet. *Br. J. Nutr.* 117: 1235–1243.

Stockman, J., Villaverde, C., and Corbee, R.J. (2021). Calcium, phosphorus and vitamin D in dogs and cats, beyond the bones. *Vet. Clin. Small Anim.* 51: 623–634.

Sul, R.M., Chase, D., Parkin, T., and Bennett, D. (2014). Comparison of meloxicam and a glucosamine-chondroitin supplement in management of feline osteoarthritis. A double-blind randomized, placebo-controlled, prospective trial. *Vet. Comp. Orthop. Traumatol.* 27: 20–26.

Teare, J.A., Krook, L., Kallfelz, F.A., and Hintz, H.F. (1979). Ascorbic acid deficiency and hypertrophic osteodystrophy in the dog: a rebuttal. *Cornell Vet.* 69: 384–401.

Temwichitr, J., Leegwater, P.A.J., and Hazewinkel, H.A.W. (2010). Fragmented coronoid process in the dog: a heritable disease. *Vet. J.* 185 (2): 123–129.

Tryfonidou, M.A. and Hazewinkel, H.A.W. (2004). Different effects of physiologically and pharmalogically increased growth hormone levels on cholecalciferol metabolism at prepubertal age. *J. Steroid Biochem. Mol. Biol.* 89–90: 49–54.

Tryfonidou, M.A., van den Broek, J., van den Brom, W.E., and Hazewinkel, H.A.W. (2002). Intestinal calcium absorption in growing dogs is influenced by calcium intake and age but not by growth rate. *J. Nutr.* 132: 3363–3368.

Tryfonidou, M.A., Holl, M.S., Stevenhagen, J.J. et al. (2003a). Dietary 135-fold cholecalciferol supplementation severely disturbs the endochondral ossification in growing dogs. *Domest. Anim. Endocrinol.* 24 (4): 265–285.

Tryfonidou, M.A., Holl, M.S., Vastenburg, M. et al. (2003b). Hormonal regulation of calcium homeostasis in two breeds of dogs dogs during growth at different rates. *J. Anim. Sci.* 81: 1568–1580.

Tryfonidou, M.A., Hazewinkel, H.A.W., and Kooistra, H.S. (2010). Calciotropic hormones. In: *Clinical Endocrinology of Dogs and Cats*, 2e (ed. A. Rijnberk and H.S. Kooistra), 253–289. Hanover: Schlütersche.

Tvedten, H.W., Carrig, C.B., Flo, G.L., and Romsos, D.R. (1977). Incidence of hip dysplasia in beagle dogs fed different amounts of protein and carbohydrate. *J. Am. Anim. Hosp. Assoc.* 13: 595–598.

Vezzoni, A., Dravelli, G., Corbari, A. et al. (2005). Early diagnosis of canine hip dysplasia. *Eur. J. Comp. Anim. Pract.* 15: 173–184.

Voorhout, G. and Hazewinkel, H.A.W. (1987). A radiographic study on the development of the antebrachium in Great Dane pups on different calcium intakes. *Vet. Radiol.* 28: 152–157.

Weber, M., Marescaux, L., Siliart, B. et al. (2000). Growth and skeletal development in two large breed dogs fed 2 calcium levels. *J. Vet. Intern. Med.* 14: 388.

Weidner, N. and Verbrugghe, A. (2016). Current knowledge of vitamin D in dogs. *Crit. Rev. Food Sci. Nutr.* 57: 3850–3859.

Weidner, N., Woods, J.P., Conlon, P. et al. (2017). Influence of various factors on circulating 25(OH)vitamin D concentration in dogs with cancer and healthy dogs. *J. Vet. Intern. Med.* 31: 1796–1803.

Wolschrijn, C.F. and Weijs, W.A. (2004). Development of the trabecular structure within the ulnar medial coronoid process of young dogs. *Anat. Rec. A* 278: 514–519.

Wood, R.J. and Zheng, J.J. (1997). High dietary calcium intakes reduce zinc absorption and balance in humans. *Am. J. Clin. Nutr.* 65: 1803–1909.

Wu, L.N., Genge, B.R., Ishikawa, Y. et al. (2006). Effects of 24R,25- and 1alpha, 25-dihydroxyvitamin D3 on mineralizing growth plate chondrocytes. *J. Cell. Biochem.* 98: 309–334.

Zafalon, R.V.A., Risolia, L.W., Vendramini, T.H.A. et al. (2020a). Nutritional inadequacies in commercial vegan foods for dogs and cats. *PLoS One* 15 (1): e0227046.

Zafalon, R.V.A., Ruberti, B., Rentas, M.F. et al. (2020b). The role of vitamin D in small animal bone metabolism. *Metabolites* 10: 496–517.

Zentek, J. and Meyer, H. (1991). Investigations on copper deficiency in growing dogs. *J. Nutr.* 121: S83.

11

Nutritional Management of Gastrointestinal Diseases

Nick Cave, Sean J. Delaney, and Jennifer A. Larsen

Perhaps no other organ system is so directly and immediately affected by nutrition than the gastrointestinal tract (GIT). Timing and frequency of feeding, route of feeding, and macronutrient and micronutrient compositions of the diet have profound influences on oral and intestinal health. In addition to the direct effect of diet on the body, there is a considerable indirect effect through dietary influences on the intestinal microbiota. However, there are few controlled clinical trials that have evaluated specific dietary manipulation in either prevention or management of canine and feline gastroenteric diseases. As such, this chapter draws heavily from experimental models and from human gastroenterology. Practical recommendations have been made when possible, but as new evidence emerges, empirical, pragmatic suggestions will need to be questioned.

Key Dietary Variables

Protein

Dietary protein interacts with the GIT in several ways. It is a source of essential amino acids for the GIT, a source of dispensable amino acids for oxidation by the GIT, a source of energy and amino acids for the luminal microbiota, and a source of foreign antigens (Ames et al. 1999; Bounous and Kongshavn 1985;

Brandtzaeg 2002). The digestibility of protein affects all these interactions. Protein digestibility is an inherent characteristic of the protein, but it also varies among animals in health, and notably in disease (e.g. exocrine pancreatic insufficiency), and is modified by food processing. Food processing can variably decrease the digestibility of protein and amino acids with some forms of heating (Do et al. 2021; Oba et al. 2019), including in the presence of simple carbohydrates (Bednar et al. 2000; Dust et al. 2005; Larsen et al. 2002). The glycosylation of amino acids, forming Maillard compounds, significantly reduces the efficiency of digestive enzymes and lowers the digestibility. Alternatively, some protein sources have inherently low digestibility due to antinutritional factors (e.g. legumes) or dimensional features such as numerous cross-links (e.g. collagen). In those cases, processing methods such as heating are necessary to improve digestibility.

Proteins (and amino acids) are also a key stimulus for the release of trophic hormones such as insulin, insulin-like growth factor (IGF)-1, and glucagon-like peptide (GLP)-2 (see later). Dietary protein affects motility in two main ways. First, the presence of protein in the stomach stimulates the release of gastrin, which promotes gastric, ileal, and colonic motility at the same time as ileocolic valve relaxation, as well as stimulating gastric secretion and having a trophic effect on the gastric

Applied Veterinary Clinical Nutrition, Second Edition. Edited by Andrea J. Fascetti, Sean J. Delaney, Jennifer A. Larsen, and Cecilia Villaverde.

and intestinal mucosa (Bueno and Fioramonti 1994; Hall et al. 1989; Lloyd 1994; Rehfeld et al. 2007; Strombeck and Harrold 1985; Thomas et al. 2003). The presence of dietary protein in the duodenum is also an effective stimulus for the release of cholecystokinin (CCK) from the proximal duodenum. CCK stimulates the pancreas to release pancreatic digestive enzymes, including proteases.

Dietary proteins also represent the largest source of dietary antigens, and are recognized and responded to by the mucosal immune system.

Glutamine

Glutamine is a conditionally essential amino acid, and is utilized as a significant fuel source by mucosal leukocytes, in particular lymphocytes, and by small intestinal epithelial cells (Newsholme et al. 1987; Ziegler et al. 2003). In addition, it serves as the dominant nitrogen source for purine synthesis, the requirement for which is relatively large given the mitotic rate within the normal mucosa, and at an even greater rate during periods of mucosal repair. Many animal studies have demonstrated that enteral glutamine supplementation enhances gut mucosal growth and repair, decreases bacterial translocation and inflammation, and improves nitrogen balance in animal models of intestinal atrophy, injury, and adaptation (Boza et al. 2000a; Kaya et al. 1999; Ziegler et al. 2003). It has also been shown to decrease postoperative ileus in dogs (Ohno et al. 2009). Surprisingly perhaps, glutamine may be a more effective nutrient when incorporated into highly digestible proteins or small polypeptides than when administered as a free amino acid in solution (Boza et al. 2000a, b; Preiser et al. 2003). This could be due to differences in utilization of glutamine by enterocytes or leukocytes, or to differences in the intestinal hormone–dependent trophic response to whole proteins rather than elemental diets. The difference between purified amino acid diets and whole foods was demonstrated in methotrexate-induced enteritis in cats, where a glutamine-enriched purified diet was less effective than a complex diet in preventing bacterial translocation and villous atrophy (Marks et al. 1997). Indeed, most studies found no benefit to supplemental glutamine over that provided by intact dietary proteins (Velasco et al. 2001).

Fat

Dietary fat is an important source of energy and is the macronutrient variable that determines the dry matter energy density of a diet. Animals with chronic intestinal disease are frequently malnourished from inappetence, maldigestion, and malabsorption, and thus may benefit greatly from higher energy-density diets. In addition, the absorption of dietary fat is required for the concurrent optimal absorption of the fat-soluble vitamins A, D, E, and K, as well as other fat-soluble nutrients (e.g. carotenoids, flavonoids). Long-chain polyunsaturated fatty acids (PUFAs) also have functional effects as the precursors to eicosanoids (e.g. prostaglandins and leukotrienes) (Calder and Grimble 2002; Wander et al. 1997), as ligands for nuclear transcription factors (e.g. peroxisome proliferator-activated receptors) (Kliewer et al. 1997), and as competitive inhibitors of lipopolysaccharide signaling via toll-like receptors (TLRs) expressed by leukocytes (Lee et al. 2003; Weatherill et al. 2005).

The absorption of fat through intestinal lymphatics increases lymphatic flow rates and pressure, and luminal bile acid fat micelles increase capillary permeability, resulting in a postprandial increase in intestinal lymphatic protein flux (Granger et al. 1982). Triacylglycerides (TAGs) are hydrolyzed in the intestinal lumen prior to uptake by the enterocytes, which absorb non-esterified fatty acids (NEFAs) and monoacylglycerides (MAGs), with the remaining fatty acid at the sn-2 position of the glycerol backbone. In rodents, the chain length of the NEFAs determines the proportion that is subsequently absorbed via lymph, versus the proportion that is absorbed directly into the portal veins bound to albumin. The percentage absorbed via lymphatics increases from less than 10% to 80% as chain length increases from capric acid (8 : 0) to lauric acid (12 : 0), while the MAG is still absorbed lymphatically (Mu and Hoy 2000). Thus, such medium-chain TAGs (aka medium-chain triglycerides, MCTs; 6–12 carbons) increase lymphatic pressures and protein flux less than conventional long-chain TAGs. A similar effect has been noted in dogs, although it is less pronounced, and significant absorption of MCTs via lymphatics still occurs (Jensen et al. 1994).

The presence of fat in the duodenum generates feedback signals to both the central nervous system (CNS) and the myenteric plexus. Mediators of these signals include cholecystokinin (CCK), GLP-1, and peptide YY (NPYY). In the intestine, CCK-secreting cells, known as "I cells," are located within the epithelium with their apical surfaces exposed to the lumen, and are concentrated in the duodenum and proximal jejunum (Liddle 1997). CCK release from I cells stimulates gallbladder contraction, pancreatic secretion, and intestinal peristalsis, and inhibits gastric emptying and gastric acid production. In the cat, like dogs and humans, secretion of CCK by I cells occurs in response to the luminal presence of long-chain triacylglycerides, proteins, and some amino acids (i.e. tryptophan, phenylalanine, leucine, and isoleucine) (Backus et al. 1995, 1997). The slowing of gastric emptying by small intestinal nutrients is associated with a reduction in proximal gastric tone, suppression of antral contractions, and stimulation of tonic and phasic pyloric contractions (Feinle et al. 2001; Heddle et al. 1989). The increase in phasic pyloric contractions is associated with cessation of transpyloric flow.

In addition to facilitating digestion in response to a meal, CCK is an important satiety signal, leading to meal cessation. Administration of CCK-receptor (CCK-1 receptor, formerly CCK-a receptor) antagonists before a meal delays satiety and prolongs feeding in rodents and humans. CCK-1 receptor-deficient rats have prolonged feeding periods and are prone to obesity (Beglinger et al. 2001; Bi and Moran 2002). Rats treated with CCK during a meal stop eating and commence other activities such as grooming and exploration before resting or sleeping (Antin et al. 1975). In order for CCK to influence behavior, there must be a direct or indirect connection between CCK and the CNS. It has been demonstrated that CCK mediates satiety in part by binding to receptors on vagal sensory afferent fibers innervating the stomach and small intestine and generating an ascending signal, rather than by the penetration of circulating CCK into the brain (Reidelberger et al. 2004). Surgical or chemical disruption of vagal transmission attenuates the satiating effects of CCK (Bi and Moran 2002).

In both dogs and cats, fat is a potent secretagogue for neuropeptides such as CCK. However, pharmacologic inhibition of pancreatic lipase attenuates the effects of duodenal fat on reducing gastric emptying, on appetite, and on CCK and GLP-1 secretion (Feinle et al. 2003). Thus, fat maldigestion such as occurs in exocrine pancreatic insufficiency may contribute to maldigestion of other nutrients, independent of pancreatic function.

In humans with functional dyspepsia, dietary fat is frequently incriminated as an exacerbating and potentially causative factor that leads to an exaggerated sense of fullness, nausea, and vomiting (Feinle et al. 2003). This is supported by studies that demonstrate symptoms after duodenal lipid infusions, but not after isoenergetic infusions of glucose (Feinle-Bisset et al. 2004).

Fiber and Prebiosis

Dietary fiber has been defined as the edible portion of plants or analogous carbohydrates that are resistant to digestion and absorption in the small intestine, which are then available to be completely or partially fermented by resident microbiota in the distal small intestine and large intestine (DeVries 2003). Crude fiber is the specific measure that is displayed on pet food labels in the United States, according to Association of American Feed Control Officials guidelines (AAFCO 2022). Currently there is no recommendation for fiber declaration from the European Pet Food Industry Federation (FEDIAF 2019). Crude fiber measures some although not all of the insoluble fiber but none of the soluble fiber; the latter tend to be the fermentable types of fiber. Total dietary fiber is a better measure of overall fiber including both insoluble and soluble, and this value is often available for veterinary therapeutic diets.

While not considered an essential nutrient for dogs or cats, fiber is undeniably an important component of the diet in both health and disease. The absence of plant-derived fiber has been shown to alter the microbiota in cats (Butowski et al. 2019; Kerr et al. 2014), although

there is also evidence for intestinal fermentation of prey components that suggests a fiber-like function (Depauw et al. 2012, 2013). Most plant-derived fibers are polysaccharides, although others, such as the polyphenolic compound lignin, are not (Table 11.1). Restriction of the definition to plant-derived compounds omits indigestible carbohydrates derived from animal sources (e.g. chitin) or synthetic sources (e.g. fructooligosaccharides, FOSs). Lastly, such a definition fails to include digestible carbohydrates that are in a form that is inaccessible to digestive enzymes (e.g. resistant starch). These compounds share many of the characteristics of fiber present in plant foods. Thus, a unifying definition of dietary fiber must be species specific and incorporate all compounds that share the biological characteristics of fiber in the intestine. Dietary fiber can be classified according to physical or chemical characteristics, its

Table 11.1 Dietary fiber types from plants.

Fiber	Chemistry	Source
Lignin	Complex phenolic	Cell walls of woody plants and seeds
Cellulose	Linear, insoluble glucose polymer with beta-1,4 glycosidic bonds	The main component of all higher plant cell walls
Hemicelluloses	Diverse group of polysaccharides containing hexoses and pentoses forming random amorphous structures	Found in almost all plant cell walls
Beta-glucans	Glucose polymers with a mixture of beta-1,4 glycosidic bonds and beta-1,3 glycosidic bonds	Oats and barley are rich sources
Pectins	Mostly a linear chain of alpha-1,4-linked D-galacturonic acid	Intercellular component of non-woody plants, especially citrus fruits, apples, and some berries
Gums	A complex of viscous polysaccharides of varying types, and some glycoproteins	Seeds
Inulin and oligofructose (fructans)	Inulin is a mixture of fructose chains, oligofructose is a mixture of shorter fructose chains that may terminate in glucose or fructose	Energy storage compound of some plants, e.g. rhizomes
Resistant starch	Starch that is sequestered in plant cell walls or highly dehydrated and therefore inaccessible to digestive enzymes	Bananas, legumes, raw potatoes. Can be formed during food processing by cooling and reheating

effects on bowel microbiota, or its effects on specific variables in the whole animal. In regard to its effects on gastrointestinal physiology and pathophysiology, which in turn impact the observable clinical effects of fiber, the most important characteristics are viscosity and fermentability.

Fiber Viscosity

Some types of soluble dietary fiber increase the viscosity of water when in solution and have the capacity to retain water within the viscous gel ("water-holding capacity"). This effect increases fecal water content and mass. Psyllium seed husk hydrocolloid has a greater water-holding effect than pea, oat, or sugar beet fiber (McBurney 1991). The formation of viscous gels slows gastric emptying, increases small intestinal transit times, slows the absorption, and reduces the digestibility of some nutrients (Ashraf et al. 1994; Bednar et al. 2001; Russell and Bass 1985). Viscosity of ileal contents increases greatly with certain soluble dietary fibers (Dikeman et al. 2007). This effect of fiber can be thought of as an antinutritive effect, and excessive dietary fiber may be counterproductive.

Although fibers that are soluble and capable of forming viscous gels are more likely to be fermentable, that is not always the case because the chemical requirements for both properties are different. The gel-forming component of psyllium seed husk, for instance, is not readily fermented by human colonic microbiota and contributes significantly to its effect on increasing fecal bulk (Marlett and Fischer 2003).

The ability to form viscous gels in the stomach may be the mechanism by which dietary fiber facilitates the gastrointestinal transit of ingested hair. Dietary fiber such as psyllium has been shown to increase hair transit and decrease retching and vomiting associated with hairballs, aka trichobezoars, in chronically affected cats (Dann et al. 2004; Hoffman and Tetrick 2003), while sugarcane fiber has been shown to reduce the number of trichobezoars in feces (Loureiro et al. 2014). This beneficial fiber effect on hairballs in cats is not consistent across all dietary fiber sources studied (e.g. cellulose, beet pulp, and Miscanthus grass are not generally beneficial) (Donadelli and Aldrich 2020; Loureiro et al. 2014, 2017).

Fiber as a Luminal Adsorbent

Fiber has long been recognized as an important luminal adsorbent of nutrients, bile acids, microbial toxins, and xenobiotics (Ebihara and Schneeman 1989; Floren and Nilsson 1982, 1987; Ryden and Robertson 1997). Binding of xenobiotics may reduce intestinal or systemic exposure to carcinogens, while bile acid binding may be important for protection of the colonic mucosa from damage from unabsorbed bile acids.

Non-fermentable dietary fiber lowers bile acid solubility in fecal water and reduces the potential for interactions with the colonic epithelium (Ebihara and Schneeman 1989; Gallaher and Schneeman 1986). Bile acids can have a direct effect on the epithelium through their detergent effect. However, bacterial metabolites of bile acids ("secondary bile acids") can have other biological effects. Deoxycholic acid (DCA) and chenodeoxycholic acid have been reported to induce dysplastic changes, be cytotoxic, or even be mutagenic to colonic epithelial cells. Luminal fiber directly protects the colonic epithelium by preventing direct interactions, by reducing concentrations, and indirectly by the production of the short-chain fatty acid butyrate, from microbiota fermentation (Bartram et al. 1995). Wheat bran fiber (13.5–25 g/day for up to 12 months) can significantly lower both total and secondary (e.g. DCA) bile acid concentrations in the solid phase of human feces (Alberts et al. 1996; Reddy et al. 1992).

Different fiber molecules can participate in both hydrophilic and hydrophobic interactions. The diversity of structure and fermentability, and the chemical and structural changes that occur within the intestine, alter binding capacities. Attempts to characterize the suitability of fibers for binding on the basis of

Table 11.2 Analysis of some common dietary fibers.

Fiber	Crude fiber % DM	Total dietary fiber % DM	Soluble fiber % DM	Insoluble fiber % DM
Apple pectin	0	85	78	7
Citrus pectin	1	82	82	0
Beet pectin	0	76	76	0
Guar gum	2	92	83	10
Carrageen refined	0	50	44	6
Cellulose (from wheat)	63	72	0	69

DM, dry matter.
Source: Data from Kienzle et al. (2001).

simple physicochemical classifications are inadequate, and the binding capacity for molecules of interest is best studied directly, given that various laboratory measurements of fiber types are unreliable predictors of in vivo performance (Table 11.2).

Fiber Fermentability

Just as the ability for mammals to digest polysaccharides is determined by the linkages between the monomeric subunits, so is the ability for intestinal microbes to hydrolyze and ferment dietary fiber. Dietary fibers undergoing bacterial degradation include polysaccharides such as resistant starch, pectin, inulin, guar gum, and oligosaccharides (e.g. FOSs) (Blaut 2002).

The extent to which fiber is utilized by microbiota and the fermentative by-products produced is influenced by the structure of the carbohydrate and also the composition of the microbiome within the individual. Complete fermentation will produce H_2, CO_2, and H_2O, while methane, acetone, propionate, and butyrate will be produced during less complete utilization. Utilization of fructans by lactobacilli, *Escherichia coli*, and *Clostridium perfringens* is low, while oligofructose and inulin are more completely utilized by bifidobacteria (Cummings et al. 2001). The effect of providing such substrate in the bowel lumen is to create a selection advantage to those species best adapted to its use. When the shift in microbiota has a positive effect on the host, the fiber is defined as a prebiotic. Proposed positive effects include reduction in mucosal adherence of pathogenic species, reduction in the numbers of pathogenic species, and immune modulation of the host (Bamba et al. 2002; Blaut 2002; Guarner et al. 2002; Schrezenmeir and de Vrese 2001).

Utilization of even the most fermentable fiber is never 100%, and most natural dietary fiber sources contain a range of carbohydrate structures. Thus, the fermentative by-products in cats and dogs will almost always contain short-chain volatile fatty acids (SCFAs) such as acetate, butyrate, and propionate (Bednar et al. 2001). In particular, FOSs, inulin, and resistant starch lead to significant increases in the fermentative production of butyrate in dogs, while in both cats and dogs SCFA production from other sources ranked from most to least is citrus pectin, citrus pulp, beet pulp, and cellulose (Sunvold et al. 1995; Vickers et al. 2001).

Effects of Short-Chain Volatile Fatty Acids on the Colon

In most domestic species studied, including dogs, butyrate is oxidized by colonocytes, and in dogs is also oxidized by enterocytes (Beaulieu et al. 2002; Marsman and McBurney 1995). It has been observed that when colonocytes are provided with butyrate, glutamine, glucose, and propionate, the most used substrate is butyrate (Beaulieu et al. 2002). In response to butyrate from fiber fermentation, colonocyte proliferation increases, intestinal mucosal weight increases, water and electrolyte absorption increases, and brush-border enzyme activities increase (Farness and Schneeman 1982; Forman and Schneeman 1982; Marsman and McBurney 1996; Poksay and Schneeman 1983). SCFAs, butyrate in particular, stimulate longitudinal but not circular colonic smooth muscle contractions via a direct effect on smooth muscle and improve the aboral passage of feces in the colon (McManus et al. 2002). Luminal butyrate also increases mucin secretion, which reduces microbial adhesion and translocation and improves secretory immunoglobulin (Ig)A function (Barcelo et al. 2000). Some effects may be concentration dependent, since at high concentrations butyrate can also inhibit colonocyte proliferation (Chapkin et al. 2000; Lupton 1995, 2004; Marsman and McBurney 1995). The effects of SCFAs are not limited to local impacts. Notably, in the domestic cat, propionate infused into the colon is used as a hepatic gluconeogenic precursor (Verbrugghe et al. 2012).

Effects of Butyrate on Intestinal Immunity

At reasonable physiologic concentrations, colonic luminal butyrate suppresses the immune response by inhibiting the formation of the nuclear transcription factor NF-κB in colonocytes, endothelial cells, and resident leukocytes (Luhrs et al. 2002; Yin et al. 2001). NF-κB regulates several cellular processes that vary according to the individual cell type and activation state, but include adaptive and innate immune responses in the intestinal tract, with several inflammatory cytokines and cell adhesion molecules under direct transcriptional control (Perkins 2007). The ability of butyrate to inhibit NF-κB activation and signaling appears to be the mechanism for the anti-inflammatory effect of butyrate in colitis (Luhrs et al. 2002; Venkatraman et al. 2003).

The non-toxic inhibition of lymphocyte proliferation may be a significant component of the immunologic tolerance to large numbers of microbiota in the colonic lumen.

However, not all the beneficial effects of fermentable fiber can be reduced to the luminal production and concentration of butyrate. In a model of acute colitis in rats, feeding dietary inulin (a highly fermentable fiber) prior to an insult reduced signs and histologic evidence of colitis, neutrophil recruitment, and eicosanoid production (i.e. prostaglandin E2 [PGE2], leukotriene B4 [LTB4], and thromboxane B2 [TXB2]) (Videla et al. 2001). The administration of fecal water from inulin-fed rats via an enema had a similar effect. However, neither butyrate administered via an enema nor fecal water from inulin-fed rats had a significant effect on colitis in that model. Again, that suggests a more complex effect of dietary fiber on the mucosa than that explained simply by the production and concentration of volatile fatty acids (VFAs).

The effect of fermentable fiber on immunity is not limited to cells resident within the intestinal mucosa. Feeding the highly fermentable fiber pectin to rats affects lymphocytes isolated from mesenteric lymph nodes. The production of the Th2-biased cytokines interleukin (IL)-4 and IL-10 by isolated lymphocytes is inhibited, consistent with a more Th1-biased response compared with lymphocytes isolated from cellulose-fed rats (Lim et al. 2003). This suggests that lymphocyte activation within the mucosa in the presence of luminal fermentative by-products of fiber affects the immunophenotype of the cells that subsequently leave the intestine and recirculate to other mucosal sites. Thus, dietary fiber may affect mucosal immunity throughout the intestinal tract, and probably at other mucosae as well.

Effect of Fiber on Intestinal Flora: Prebiosis

Certain fibers, such as the beta-2 fructans (e.g. inulin, FOSs), stimulate the growth and/or activity of intestinal bacteria such as *Lactobacillus* spp. and *Bifidobacterium* spp.

(Gibson et al. 1995; Kaplan and Hutkins 2000). It has been proposed that increasing the numbers of these non-pathogenic species may have several direct beneficial effects, including (i) competition with pathogens for substrate; (ii) interference with pathogen binding with, and competition for, epithelial binding sites; and (iii) direct interaction with the mucosal immune system.

Additionally, the SCFAs might acidify the colonic lumen, inhibiting species such as *Bacteroides* spp. and *Clostridia* spp. (Gibson and Wang 1994). Elimination of *Clostridium difficile* from the colonic flora within six days has been documented in mice by feeding a diet containing 20% fermentable fiber (Ward and Young 1997). Similar effects on the fecal microbiota have been seen in dogs given highly fermentable fiber (Grieshop et al. 2002). While colonic microbiota populations in cats and dogs may be relatively resistant to changes resulting from changes in dietary fiber intake (Simpson et al. 2002), there is one study that suggests that the combination of a prebiotic–probiotic supplement may reduce the incidence of diarrhea in dog shelters (Rose et al. 2017). The effect of prebiotics alone in similarly robust clinical trials in cats or dogs is still unreported, but it is reasonable to suggest that probiotics may be beneficially supported by dietary fermentable fiber or prebiotic intake.

Choice of Fiber

The combined effects of fiber fermentation with the absorptive effects of non-fermentable fiber make mixed fiber sources (e.g. psyllium seed husk) theoretically ideal for the management of colitis, over more completely fermentable fiber sources (e.g. hydrolyzed guar gum). In addition, the most highly fermentable fibers may also increase the production of methane, which has the capacity to disturb motility and exacerbate signs of colitis (see later). In other cases, more highly and rapidly fermentable sources that produce higher concentrations of butyrate in the more proximal colon may be more effective than less and more slowly fermentable sources of fiber. In a model of induced colitis in rats, both short-chain FOSs and a resistant starch (retrograded, high-amylomaize starch) were evaluated for their ability to improve clinical and histologic signs of colitis (Moreau et al. 2003). Only the resistant starch in that model improved the histologic colitis score, and there was a trend toward more rapid resolution of the diarrhea and less hematochezia. There is evidence that the addition of psyllium seed husk powder to the diet of dogs with large-bowel diarrhea results in positive outcomes in the majority of reported cases (Alves et al. 2021; Leib 2000). Other mixed and fermentable fiber sources are also incorporated into various veterinary therapeutic diets and have been used successfully for both acute and chronic colitis (Fritsch et al. 2022; Lappin et al. 2022; Rossi et al. 2020). There is little evidence to guide adjustments of specific types and amounts for non-responders, as well as a lack of characterization of the best types of fiber to use for small-bowel diarrhea. Clearly, the choice of fiber is important in certain disease states; however, insufficient information is available in feline and canine medicine to make any informed therapeutic recommendations beyond the initial introduction of mixed fermentable sources, and then proceeding with trial and error of both type and dosage based on response.

The addition of powdered fiber supplement products to diets can be easily achieved with moist diets, but can make dry diets unpalatable, even when mixed with water or animal stock or broth. Ideal non-purified sources of fiber would be very concentrated in fiber, yet highly palatable, and easy to use as dietary supplements. Some suggested rich food sources of mixed fermentable fiber are listed in Table 11.3 with comparison to psyllium seed husk. Caution must be taken to avoid essential nutrient dilution with their addition, and especially if overall dietary protein is reduced or restricted for fear of creating a sulfur amino acid deficiency, which in dogs can lead to dilated cardiomyopathy.

Table 11.3 Rich sources of dietary fiber.

Food source	Total dietary fiber % dry matter basis	Total dietary fiber in 100 g as fed
Psyllium seed husk	83%[a]	77.78[a]
Oat bran (raw)	16%	15.4
Red kidney beans (cooked or canned)	28%	6.4
Baked beans (canned)	18%	5.0
Chickpeas (cooked or canned)	15%	4.4
Green peas (cooked)	23%	3.1
Pumpkin (cooked or canned)	29%	2.9

[a] Based on manufacturer data.
Source: Data from the United States Department of Agriculture Nutrient Database for Standard Reference, Release 18.

Immune Response to Dietary Antigens (Oral Tolerance)

Immunologic Basis for Oral Tolerance

Foreign dietary antigens interact with the intestinal immune system in such a way as to prevent unnecessary and detrimental immune reactions to them. In so doing, systemic immunity is rendered effectively unresponsive if the same antigen reaches the systemic circulation. This absence of reactivity to orally administered antigens is termed oral tolerance. Oral tolerance is generated in an antigen-specific and active manner that involves the induction of an atypical immune response.

Peyer's patches are the primary inductive area of the intestinal immune system. The specialized M cells within the epithelium overlying the lymphoid follicles sample, non-specifically or by receptor-mediated uptake, particulate and insoluble antigens and whole microorganisms (Brandtzaeg 2001). Antigens and organisms are then transported to leukocytes that reside within basal membrane invaginations, namely B cells, macrophages, and dendritic cells. In the normal intestine, these antigen-presenting cells (APCs) lack co-stimulatory molecules such as CD80 and CD86. Antigens processed by these "unactivated" APCs are then presented to naïve B and T cells within the follicle, which then proliferate poorly. This occurs within a local microenvironment that differs from other sites in the body and results in induction of hyporesponsive Th2- or Th3-biased T cells (Kellermann and McEvoy 2001). Activated cells then leave via lymphatics and pass via the mesenteric lymph nodes into the systemic circulation. They will then exit at mucosal sites via engagement of cellular adhesion molecules (CAMs) specifically expressed by the high endothelial venules of mucosal tissues. Thus, activated or memory B and T lymphocytes enter the lamina propria to await a secondary encounter with their specific antigen.

The activated cells may secrete cytokines, but full differentiation into effector T cells or plasma cells may not occur without secondary exposure. For both cell types to be re-exposed to antigen, intact antigens must reach the lamina propria. Intestinal epithelial cells are responsible for the absorption of antigen, release to professional APCs, and limited antigen presentation to cells within the mucosa on major histocompatibility complex (MHC) class II. In the normal intestine, these secondary APCs will, like the primary presenters, lack co-stimulatory molecule expression and further add to the tolerogenic environment. The effector T-cell clones resident in the normal intestine secrete a bias toward Th2 and Th3 cytokines, in particular IL-10 and transforming growth factor (TGF)-beta, thus directing B-cell isotype switching to produce IgA-secreting plasma cells, while inhibiting the development of Th1 lymphocytes and IgG production.

It is important that the immune system reserves the ability to rapidly respond to pathogens. This ability to recognize pathogenicity is based on the engagement of receptors that recognize evolutionarily conserved molecular patterns such as TLRs that produce "danger signals." Predictably, expression of TLR-2 and TLR-4 is low to non-existent in the mucosal cells of the normal human intestine (which serves as the model for cats and dogs), but they can be rapidly expressed in response to inflammatory cytokines (Abreu et al. 2001). The absence of these "danger signals" results in relatively inefficient antigen processing by intestinal APCs, markedly reduced or absent tumor necrosis factor (TNF)-alpha/IL-1/IL-12 production, and the absence of CD80/86 co-stimulatory molecule expression. T cells activated by such an APC will divide less, with most clones undergoing early deletion by apoptosis, while the surviving memory cells will tend to secrete IL-10, TGF-beta, or no cytokines at all (Jenkins et al. 2001). This combination of apoptosis, functional defects in surviving clones, and T cells secreting the anti-inflammatory and IgA-supporting cytokines is the general basis for immunologic tolerance to luminal antigens.

Thus oral tolerance is composed of a delicate balance between induction of IgA, T-cell deletion, anergy (the absence of the normal immune response to a particular antigen), and immunosuppression; the retention of antigen-specific lymphocytes capable of rapidly responding to invasive pathogens though antibody isotype switching to IgM, IgE, or IgG; and the production of inflammatory cytokines such as interferon (IFN)-gamma, IL-12, and IL-6.

Loss of Tolerance to Dietary Antigens

Loss of tolerance to dietary antigens will produce a conventional but detrimental immune response against the dietary antigen. Such an inappropriate response may produce inflammation locally, or at another anatomic site. The response will be characterized by one or a combination of:

- Local cell-mediated inflammation. The resulting chronic stimulation may lead to lymphocytic intestinal infiltrates characteristic of inflammatory enteropathy.
- Local antibody production of isotypes other than IgA. The production of IgE will lead to mast cell priming and intestinal hypersensitivity, i.e. food allergy with gastrointestinal signs (vomiting and/or diarrhea).
- Systemic antibody production. Circulating IgE will lead to priming of mast cells at sites distal to the intestine such as dermal hypersensitivity, i.e. food allergy with pruritus as the clinical sign.

The initiating events that lead to loss of oral tolerance, or prevent it from developing, have not been described in either cats or dogs and remain poorly understood in any species. Suggested mechanisms include:

- Increased mucosal permeability, e.g. following mucosal injury, or in the neonatal intestine.
- Co-administration of a mucosal adjuvant that activates and changes the phenotype of intestinal dendritic cells, e.g. bacterial enterotoxins.
- Parasitism. Intestinal parasitism in cats leads to an exaggerated systemic humoral response that includes increased production of IgE (Gilbert and Halliwell 2005).

Currently, there is speculation as to the importance of infections that stimulate a Th1-biased immune response in preventing type 1 hypersensitivity reactions in people. This has been termed the "hygiene hypothesis," which states that a lack of maturation of the infant immune system from a Th2 to a Th1 type of immune response may be caused by less microbial stimulation in Western societies (Romagnani 2004). It is proposed that bacterial and viral infections during early life promote a net shift of the maturing immune system toward Th1-biased responses, and reduce potentially allergenic Th2-biased responses. The assumed reduction in the overall microbial burden is supposed to allow the natural Th2 bias of neonates to persist into maturity and enable an increase in allergy. A clinical trial supports this theory in atopic children (Bodemer et al. 2017).

The special role of parasites in modulating allergic responses to food and other allergens has been debated for over half a century. Several older reports suggested that, similar to cats and dogs, parasitized humans are more likely to suffer from allergic diseases (Carswell et al. 1977; Kayhan et al. 1978; Warrell et al. 1975). In contrast to that is the higher incidence of allergic disease in Western populations generally subject to less parasitism, as well as the growing incidence of allergic disease in developing nations as parasitism is also reduced. Elevations of anti-inflammatory cytokines, such as IL-10, that occur during long-term helminth infections have been shown to be inversely correlated with allergy. It has been suggested recently that the host's response to the parasite determines their predisposition to develop allergic diseases, and that the induction of a robust anti-inflammatory regulatory response (e.g. IL-10) induced by persistent immune challenge offers a unifying explanation for the observed inverse association of many infections with allergic disorders (Yazdanbakhsh et al. 2002). In either cats or dogs, the role of parasitism and other infections that would fall within the hygiene hypothesis has yet to be defined in determining the development of food hypersensitivity. Since the immunologic mechanism for the majority of food sensitivities may not be IgE mediated, the story may be even more complicated.

Food Immunogenicity

Adverse reactions to food are surprisingly common in both cats and dogs and have been reported to be present in up to 29% of all cases of chronic gastrointestinal disease in cats (Guilford et al. 2001). In addition, inflammatory enteropathy is the single most common cause of chronic gastrointestinal disease, and novel/uncommon antigen and hydrolyzed-ingredient diets are commonly reported to be effective in its management (Guilford and Matz 2003; Mandigers et al. 2010; Marks et al. 2002; Nelson et al. 1984). However, although the involvement of immunologic mechanisms in a proportion of these adverse reactions is suspected, it is unproven. Indeed, the normal immunologic response to ingested dietary antigens in cats has only been partially described (Cave and Marks 2004). Surprisingly, cats develop robust serum IgG and IgA responses to dietary proteins when fed as either aqueous suspensions or as part of canned diets, and it is likely that dogs are similar.

As obligate carnivores, felids have evolved on a low-fiber, highly digestible diet (Morris 2002). It may be assumed that since cats have relatively short intestinal tracts, they may be poorly suited to poorly digestible diets. However, it has been reported that cats have approximately six times more mucosal area per unit of serosal length compared to rats (Wood 1944). Regardless, diet digestibility remains an important and clinically relevant consideration. It is well established that heat processing, including the commercial canning process, decreases protein digestibility and that this has biologically significant effects in cats (Kim et al. 1996; Larsen et al. 2002).

In rodents and rabbits, intact particulate and insoluble antigens are preferentially absorbed across the intestine through M cells overlying the Peyer's patches (Frey et al. 1996). Classically, such antigens tend to invoke active immunity appropriate for microorganisms. In contrast, soluble antigens have been found to be associated with oral tolerance (Wikingsson and Sjoholm 2002). It has also been shown that oral tolerance can be abrogated or evaded when soluble proteins are fed in oil-in-water emulsions, resulting in robust systemic humoral responses (Kaneko et al. 2000). This effect may also have relevance to the pet food industry, where interactions between dietary proteins and lipids in canned or extruded diets during the cooking and manufacturing process could feasibly result in novel interactions not present in their native states or when cooked separately.

In stark contrast to rodents is the intestinal response in chickens, where particulate antigens induce tolerance, while soluble antigens provoke active immunity (Klipper et al. 2001). If the physical nature of the proteins within the natural diet of a species dictates how the intestinal immune system has evolved, this might have special relevance to species that are commonly fed diets different from their ancestors, like cats and dogs.

Most commercial pet foods are subjected to heating during the manufacturing process. The effect of heat treatment on proteins mostly changes the three-dimensional conformation of the protein. Although this may disrupt some antigens, it may equally uncover previously hidden antigenic determinants, or create new ones. Other reactions that occur at high temperatures include the Maillard reactions, which involve the reactions between certain amino acids, and the reduction of sugars to produce less digestible compounds called melanoidins, which give a characteristic brown color. Melanoidins tend to be less digestible, less soluble, and certain melanoidins have been shown to be more "allergenic" than the original uncooked protein (Maleki et al. 2000, 2003). Increasing antigenicity does appear to be a consistent effect across different but similar foods and processing methods (Abramovitch et al. 2017; Cuadrado et al. 2020; Mattison et al. 2016).

The effect of heating during the canning process on the immunogenicity of dietary proteins has been evaluated in cats (Cave and Marks 2004). Using soy and casein proteins, the canning or retorting process resulted in the creation of new antigens not present in the uncooked product. In addition, a product of heated casein induced a salivary IgA response that was not induced by the raw product. Thus, commercial food processing can qualitatively and quantitatively alter the immunogenicity of food proteins. Although the significance of this finding is uncertain at present, it emphasizes the need for feeding highly digestible protein sources, or perhaps even hydrolyzed proteins, when enteritis is present.

Acute Gastrointestinal Disease

Acute gastroenteritis is a common reason for presentation of cats and dogs to veterinarians. Common causes include bacterial toxin ingestion (e.g. staphylococcal enteritis), bacterial endotoxin production (e.g. *C. perfringens* enteritis), viral enteritis (e.g. rotavirus, coronavirus, parvovirus), self-limiting infections (e.g. *Cryptosporidium felis* and *parvum*, *Coccidia* spp.), and adverse reactions to food (both food allergies and food intolerances). Because of the transient and non-life-threatening nature of many cases, the cause of the majority remains undetermined. Despite ignorance of the exact cause, standard therapy is instigated, of which dietary management remains the cornerstone.

Withholding Food for Acute Non-specific Gastroenteritis

Standard dietary recommendations for dogs and cats with acute gastroenteritis have been to withhold food for 24–48 hours, followed by the introduction of small quantities of a "bland" diet fed 4–6 times per day for 3–7 days. These dietary recommendations have stood the test of time, but are based on common assumptions rather than any specific research.

Arguments frequently offered in support of withholding food are that it does the following:

1) **Provides Bowel Rest** It is presumed that the presence of ingesta and the physical and metabolic demands of digestion and absorption will delay recovery. In acute colitis, feeding can indeed increase the severity of signs. When there is significant colonic inflammation, the normal motor response to a meal is altered. When ingesta enter the colon during the late postprandial period, an excessive number of giant migrating contractions may be stimulated. These giant migrating contractions may be associated with postprandial abdominal discomfort and increased frequency of defecation (Sethi and Sarna 1991).

However, fasting in a normal animal is associated with intense migrating motor complexes ("housekeeper" contractions) extending from the pylorus to the ileum (Hall et al. 1983). These vigorous contractions, described as "hunger pains" by some humans, are inhibited by the presence of luminal nutrients (Defilippi 2003). In almost all cases of enteritis, regardless of the etiology, there is decreased motility with delayed gastric emptying and reduced segmental contractions (Hotokezaka et al. 1996; Shi and Sarna 2004). Thus, fasting does not immediately provide physical bowel "rest," and in most cases reduced motility or ileus is present. Feeding has been shown to decrease the development and duration of ileus from various intestinal insults. A meta-analysis on the recovery of human patients following a wide range of abdominal surgical procedures demonstrated that early introduction of feeding resulted in shorter time to the presence of bowel sound and a trend toward shorter hospital stays (Charoenkwan et al. 2007). One model of large-bowel resection in dogs showed that enteral feeding instituted one day post surgery hastened return to normal motility and was associated with possible improvements in nutritional status when compared to parenteral nutrition (Kawasaki et al. 2009). At worst continuing oral feeding will have no detrimental effect on motility, and at best it will promote normal motility and prevent ileus.

2) **Reduces the Risk of Vomiting** It has been suggested that vomiting is less likely to occur in the fasted state than the fed state, and that withholding food until vomiting has decreased or stopped is important to reduce the risk of aspiration. The early introduction of enteral feeding in dogs with severe hemorrhagic gastroenteritis did indeed result in increased vomiting when a hydrolyzed protein diet was initially introduced, despite being fed at below maintenance rates (Will et al. 2005). Nonetheless, vomiting decreased rapidly in the fed group and dogs were tolerant of enteral feeds within 2–3 days.

In contrast, the prokinetic effect of feeding may decrease the emetic response. In dogs with severe parvoviral enteritis, the time to cessation of vomiting following admission was significantly shorter when forced feeding was instigated within 12 hours of admission, compared with dogs that were fasted orally until 12 hours after vomiting cessation (Mohr et al. 2003). Additionally, the luminal presence of a complex diet supports mucosal integrity and decreases the magnitude of an enteric insult. Cats that were fed a complex diet did not vomit when given a toxic dose of methotrexate, while cats fed a purified diet did vomit (Marks et al. 1999).

However, foods that prolong gastric retention, especially high-fat diets and highly viscous diets (high soluble fiber; see later), or diets that contain poorly digestible starch may promote emesis (Heddle et al. 1989; Lin et al. 1992; Meyer et al. 1994). Maldigestion can lead to distension and stimulation of the gut that increases the chance of vomiting. Predictably, gastric retention times increase with increasing meal size, but also with increased dry matter content (Goggin et al. 1998).

Thus feeding can have either an emetic or antiemetic effect. Small, frequent feedings have been recommended in order to limit the duration of acid secretion at each meal and to minimize gastric distension, which can provoke nausea when the stomach is inflamed.

3) **Decreases Bacterial Proliferation** Undigested food provides nutrients for luminal bacterial fermentation and proliferation. However, fasting increases the rate of bacterial adherence and translocation in most experimental models (Bark et al. 1995; Marks et al. 1997; Tenenhaus et al. 1994). In addition, acidification of the lumen through the production of VFAs (e.g. butyrate, propionate) by microbiota capable of fermentation can make the environment less suitable for other pH-sensitive pathogenic bacteria such as *Campylobacter* and *Clostridium* spp. (Cummings et al. 2001).

4) **Decreases Osmotic Diarrhea** Unlike acute diarrhea in humans, the majority of cases of feline and canine diarrhea are not thought to involve a significant secretory component. Although this may be simplistic, it appears that the osmotic effect of unabsorbed nutrients and endogenously derived osmoles are more important as contributors to the diarrhea. With almost any mucosal insult, the absorptive capacity of the intestine is reduced and exudation may be increased. Undigested fat is susceptible to oxidation, hydroxylation, and the formation of by-products that can increase intestinal secretion, and increase vascular permeability, fluid secretion, and as a consequence the severity and duration of diarrhea (Ramakrishna et al. 1994).

5) **Decreases Presence of Food Antigens** At times, it will be suggested that feeding in the midst of generalized gastrointestinal inflammation may increase the risk of developing food allergies due to impaired digestion and increased gut permeability, leading to presentation of intact ingested polypeptides/food antigens to the gastrointestinal immune system. This theory is unproven, and as already noted enterocyte/gut health has been shown to be enhanced with intraluminal food, as will be further discussed later.

It can be seen that the arguments presented here can be rebutted, or satisfied by optimal feeding. Thus, the long-held belief in the value of bowel rest for the treatment of diarrhea has been challenged by the benefits of "feeding through" diarrhea. Recent studies of acute diarrhea in several species have shown that feeding through diarrhea maintains greater mucosal barrier integrity.

Benefits of Luminal Nutrition in Acute Gastroenteritis

Even in the absence of enteritis, fasting for even as short a period as one day in rats causes a significant decrease in villous height and/or crypt depth in the jejunum, ileum, and, to a lesser extent, colon (Kudsk 2003; Ziegler et al. 2003). In addition, fasting is associated with gut mucosal cell impairment marked by decreased concentrations of reduced glutathione (GSH), the major intracellular antioxidant, enhanced permeability to macromolecules, increased bacterial translocation from the lumen, and increased rates of enterocyte apoptosis (Jonas et al. 1999). Even with total parenteral nutrition, after 14 days of oral fasting in cats, small intestinal villous atrophy occurs, as well as fusion and infiltration of the lamina propria with lymphocytes, plasma cells, and neutrophils (Lippert et al. 1989). Thus, oral fasting alone, and in the absence of nutritional deficiency, induces an intestinal insult.

Fasting also significantly reduces the specific activity and expression of certain digestive enzymes in the small-bowel mucosa such as disaccharidases, which can lead to impaired digestion following the reintroduction of food (Holt and Yeh 1992). Transient lactase deficiency is common, particularly after rotavirus gastroenteritis (Zijlstra et al. 1997). Occasionally it persists, and lactose intolerance may be a cause of post-gastroenteritis diarrhea. Gastric and pancreatic secretions are markedly reduced following a period of undernutrition (Winter 2006).

Generalized malnutrition, protein depletion, or deficiencies of specific nutrients, including essential fatty acids, folate, zinc, vitamin A, and vitamin B12, inhibit the growth and turnover of the intestinal mucosa. It has long been recognized that small intestinal enterocytes utilize luminally derived glutamine as their main oxidative fuel (see earlier). In addition, glutamine provides the carbon skeleton and amino nitrogen required for purine synthesis and hence is critical for the normal DNA synthesis involved in enterocyte turnover.

Oral supplementation with zinc improves histologic recovery, normalizes absorption, decreases permeability, and decreases NF-κB nuclear binding in experimental models of diarrhea (Altaf et al. 2002; Sturniolo et al. 2001). Additional mechanisms for the effect of zinc treatment on the duration of diarrhea include improved absorption of water and electrolytes, increased levels of brush-border enzymes, and faster regeneration of the intestinal epithelium.

Intestinal Recovery and Adaptation

Multiple factors, including luminal nutrients, pancreatico-biliary secretions, and humoral agents, have been implicated in controlling the intestinal adaptive response after an intestinal insult. Despite the multifactorial regulation of intestinal adaptation, luminal nutrients are fundamental to the adaptive response such that recovery is minimized or prevented in the absence of luminal nutrients. This conclusion is largely based on studies that show significant adaptive intestinal regrowth in rats and dogs fed orally compared with those fed parenterally following an intestinal resection. Indeed, even in the absence of an intestinal insult, parenteral nutrition causes dramatic intestinal atrophy in dogs, cats, rats, and humans (Lippert et al. 1989; Renegar et al. 2001; Thor et al. 1977). This fasting-induced atrophy is accompanied by inflammatory cell infiltrates in the lamina propria, increased intestinal permeability, and increased bacterial translocation.

The ileum, and to a lesser extent the colon, is important in intestinal adaptation and recovery. The ileum and colon are the primary intestinal sites of synthesis and secretion of GLP-2 and IGF-1 (Dube et al. 2006). GLP-2 is a 33 amino acid peptide hormone released from the intestinal endocrine cells (L cells) following nutrient ingestion. GLP-2 exerts trophic effects on the small- and large-bowel epithelium via stimulation of cell proliferation and inhibition of apoptosis (Ljungmann et al. 2001). GLP-2 also decreases gastric acid secretion and decreases antral contractions, thus contributing to the "ileal brake" (Wojdemann et al. 1998). In experimental models of intestinal disease, GLP-2 reverses parenteral nutrition–induced mucosal atrophy and accelerates the process of endogenous intestinal adaptation following major small-bowel resection (Chance et al. 2000; Drucker et al. 1997; Ljungmann et al. 2001; Sangild et al. 2006). GLP-2 also markedly attenuates intestinal injury and weight loss in mice with chemically induced colitis, and significantly reduces mortality, bacterial infection, and intestinal mucosal damage in mice with indomethacin-induced enteritis. IGF-1 production by the ileum produces a similar increase in enterocyte proliferation, leads to an expansion of the proliferative compartment in the crypt, inhibits enterocyte apoptosis, and increases enterocyte migration (Dube et al. 2006). Thus luminal nutrients are essential for maximal and rapid mucosal recovery, which is stimulated largely by enterically derived GLP-2 and IGF-1.

Effect of Luminal Nutrients on Inflammation

It has long been known that the immunologic derangements that accompany malnutrition cannot all be prevented when nutrients are delivered parenterally (Dionigi et al. 1977). A lack of luminal nutrients results in an increased expression of proinflammatory adhesion molecules, especially intercellular adhesion molecule (ICAM)-1 (Fukatsu et al. 1999). This results in an increased number of primed neutrophils adhered to the microvasculature throughout the intestinal tract, where they are able to contribute to oxidative and enzymatic tissue damage following activation. Fasting or total parenteral nutrition results in decreases in IL-4 and IL-10 that correlate with decreases in IgA and increases in ICAM-1 (Fukatsu et al. 2001). Lack of enteral feeding impairs the coordinated system of sensitization, distribution, and interaction of T and B cells that is important in the production of IgA, in the maintenance of normal gut cytokines, and in the regulation of endothelial inflammation (Ikeda et al. 2003; Johnson et al. 2003; Kudsk 2003; Renegar et al. 2001). Thus the lack of luminal nutrients has been described as a "first hit" and increases the inflammatory response to a secondary insult in the GIT, but also the lungs, liver, and potentially other organs as well.

Glutamine

The amino acid glutamine reverses many of these defects and favorably influences the proinflammatory effects of gut starvation (Kudsk et al. 2000). The source of supplemental glutamine can influence gut mucosal glutamine concentrations, suggesting differences in its availability or utilization. Glutamine-rich intact proteins such as casein, whey, and soy appear to be more effective in increasing mucosal glutamine content than glutamine-enriched solutions (Marks et al. 1999).

Arginine

Arginine is an essential amino acid for cats because of their inability to synthesize sufficient quantities in the fasting state. However, beyond its role as an essential intermediate in the ornithine cycle, dietary arginine has long been known to enhance certain aspects of immunity. L-arginine is oxidized to L-citrulline + nitric acid (NO) by NO synthase. The inducible form within leukocytes (inducible NO synthase, or iNOS) produces much greater amounts of NO than the constitutive endothelial (eNOS) or neuronal (nNOS) forms. The production of NO after induction of iNOS in an activated phagocyte is limited mostly by the availability of free arginine. Therefore any increase in available arginine will increase the NO produced by any given inflammatory stimulus (Eiserich et al. 1998).

NO is a free radical. However, compared with other free radical species, in physiologic conditions the molecule is relatively stable, reacting only with oxygen and its radical derivatives, transition metals, and other radicals. This low reactivity, combined with its lipophilicity, allows the molecule to diffuse away from its place of synthesis, and to function as a signaling molecule on an intracellular, intercellular, and perhaps even systemic level.

NO is required for normal intestinal epithelial maturation. It may be the principal inhibitory neurotransmitter in intestinal motility and is essential for the maintenance of normal mucosal blood flow. In addition, NO inhibits the expression of CAMs, limiting unnecessary leukocyte entry, especially into the mucosal tissues. NO inhibits T-cell proliferation, decreases NF-kB activation, and induces a Th2 bias to local responses. However, in contrast to the paradigm that NO inhibits the key proinflammatory transcription factor NF-κB, some studies have suggested that iNOS inhibition can increase proinflammatory cytokine production.

As mentioned, NO is relatively unreactive with non-radical molecules. However, reaction with the free radical superoxide (O_2^-) to form peroxynitrite (NO_3^-) is diffusion limited. Peroxynitrite is not a free radical, though it is a powerful oxidant, and has been shown to elicit a wide array of toxic effects ranging from lipid peroxidation to protein oxidation and nitration, leading to inactivation of enzymes and ion channels, DNA damage, and inhibition of mitochondrial respiration (Virag et al. 2003). The cellular effect of NO_3^- oxidation is concentration dependent; for instance, very low concentrations will be handled by protein and lipid turnover and DNA repair, higher concentrations induce apoptosis, whereas very high concentrations induce necrosis. Since both NO and O_2^- are produced in sites of inflammation, it is reasonable to propose that NO_3^- might be involved in the pathogenesis of many cases.

In light of differences in the radius of effect of both NO and O_2^-, co-localization of both molecules within the same cell would be expected to lead to disease. In this context, the finding that iNOS is capable of generating O_2^- in conditions when L-arginine is unavailable is significant. This has been demonstrated recently in macrophages, where limiting L-arginine availability resulted in the simultaneous production of functionally significant amounts of NO and O_2^-, and the immediate intracellular formation of NO_3^- (Xia and Zweier 1997).

The large number of conflicting studies evaluating the role of NO in inflammatory disease has resulted in a polarization of viewpoints between those who argue that NO is protective, and those who argue that it contributes to pathogenesis. This is unfortunate since both views are probably correct. The fate of any individual molecule of NO is determined by multiple variables that determine its role in pathogenesis, including:

- Site of production.
- Timing of production of the molecule within the local disease process.
- Amount of NO produced.
- Redox status of the immediate environment.
- Chronicity of the disease.

Overall, it appears that supplemental arginine, either parenterally or orally administered, enhances the depressed immune response of individuals suffering from trauma, surgery, malnutrition, or infection. This action is presumably through its ability to augment the production of NO by iNOS in activated neutrophils and macrophages.

However, in cases of severe sepsis (i.e. infection accompanied by a systemic inflammatory response), augmentation of NO production might be detrimental because of its effect as a negative cardiac ino- and chronotrope, its ability to inhibit coagulation, and its potent venous and arterial dilator effects (Suchner et al. 2002).

Most commercial enteral nutrition formulas suitable for feeding to cats contain 1.5–2 times the minimum requirement of arginine for growth. However, supplementation of diets for intensive care nutrition has frequently been recommended and is widely used in human critical care medicine for enhancement of the immune system. Although clinical improvements in some studies have been reported, critically ill patients with systemic inflammatory response syndrome, sepsis, or organ failure may actually deteriorate as the result of arginine supplementation (Stechmiller et al. 2004). Thus there may be cases where supplementation with arginine, beyond that provided by a conventional protein source, may be beneficial, while in other cases it may be detrimental.

Intestinal Permeability

Even short periods of enteral fasting result in an increase in intestinal permeability in humans (Hernandez et al. 1999). Early refeeding of cats and dogs with acute gastroenteritis has been shown to reduce the increase in intestinal permeability that occurs in response to inflammation and apoptosis (Marks et al. 1999; Mohr et al. 2003). Some of the effects of luminal feeding may come from the luminal provision of glutamine alone, which can restore enterocyte glutathione concentrations and protein synthesis, and normalize intestinal permeability. Even in single-layer cell cultures of enterocytes, the application of glutamine to the apical (luminal) membrane normalizes permeability to a large molecular weight molecule, whereas applying glutamine to the basal membrane (simulating parenteral nutrition) does not (Le Bacquer et al. 2003).

Veterinary Evidence

The effect of early enteral nutrition has been evaluated in dogs with various naturally occurring disease states, including pancreatitis, severe parvoviral enteritis, and septic peritonitis, and in cats with severe mucosal damage from experimental methotrexate toxicity. Dogs tolerate tube feeding when instituted within 2 days of hospital admission for acute pancreatitis or within 24 hours of surgery for septic peritonitis (Hoffberg and Koenigshof 2017; Mansfield et al. 2011). Beyond its being safe and tolerated, another study demonstrated positive impacts of early enteral feeding on return to voluntary consumption in dogs with pancreatitis (Harris et al. 2017). Further, early enteral nutrition in canine parvovirus reduced the time for normalization of demeanor, appetite, vomiting, and diarrhea, increased body weight, and may have improved mucosal permeability compared with the traditional approach of fasting until resolution of vomiting (Mohr et al. 2003). In methotrexate-induced enteritis, feeding a complex diet abrogated the proximal small intestinal atrophy and bacterial translocation associated with feeding an amino acid–based purified diet and was associated with a marked attenuation of the clinical signs associated with the toxicity (Marks et al. 1999). In contrast, when dogs that presented with severe hemorrhagic gastroenteritis were fed a commercial dry hydrolyzed protein diet soon after presentation, there was an initial increase in the frequency of vomiting, despite being fed at below maintenance rates (Will et al. 2005).

Thus early reintroduction of feeding does not seem to exacerbate disease even in severely ill animals, and complex diets appear to be superior to purified diets in some models. However, clinicians must make individual decisions about the risks and benefits of feeding in patients with persistent vomiting. The risk of aspiration of vomitus is significant in patients that are moribund or unconscious, and in patients with concurrent dysphagia or laryngeal dysfunction.

Recommendations

It may be seen that not only can the traditional concerns of feeding in acute gastroenteritis be allayed, but there are considerable arguments for not delaying feeding at all. The current recommendations are for oral rehydration over a period of 3–4 hours as required, followed by immediate reintroduction of oral feeding. However, it is unlikely that attempting to feed the daily maintenance energy requirement (MER) is a sensible approach in the short-term management of cats and dogs suffering from acute diarrhea, and certainly not in cases of frequent vomiting. Therefore, if only 25% of the animal's resting energy requirement (RER) is fed as a highly digestible, low-fat diet, mucosal recovery may be optimized, and exacerbation of diarrhea or vomiting minimized. This has led to the concept of "minimal luminal nutrition."

At the current point of understanding, the ideal dietary characteristics would be:

- High digestibility. This is easier to recommend than it is to specifically practice. Most commercial high-quality dry diets would qualify, as would many home-prepared ingredients. For protein sources, cooked fresh chicken or fish, cottage cheese, or egg would qualify. Cooked white rice or potato is a suitable carbohydrate source, although rice may be superior (see later). Commercially canned or retorted diets generally have a lower digestibility than dry diets, often have a high fat or viscous fiber content, and thus cannot be recommended over a similar dry product. However, there is no evidence that the difference in digestibility has any clinically measurable consequences.
- Low fat. No fat-titration studies have been performed to guide firm recommendations. However, a pragmatic recommendation especially to promote gut motility would be to choose the lowest fat content available. An almost arbitrary cutoff of 20% of metabolizable energy (ME) could be made.
- Novel antigen content. For acute gastroenteritis, strict adherence to ingredient novelty is not prioritized over other considerations and simple avoidance of the staple or most commonly fed ingredients of the particular

patient is prudent, without being excessive. Some hydrolyzed diets are also excellent choices (Cave 2006), and an elemental diet (meaning no intact peptides) may prove useful in some cases.

- Dietary fiber content. Some fermentable fiber is almost always beneficial, while excessive contents can exacerbate delayed gastric emptying, diarrhea, flatulence, and abdominal pain. An empirical recommendation is to select diets that contain less than 8% total dietary fiber or less than 5% crude fiber.
- Initial feeding should not exceed 25% of the calculated RER, divided into three feeds per day. This amount can be rapidly increased with clinical improvement.

Examples of suitable, short-term, home-prepared recipes are presented in Table 11.4.

Therefore, these diets possess ideal macro-nutrient profiles, are highly digestible, and are highly palatable. There may be an advantage to the use of boiled white rice as the carbohydrate source in diets for acute gastroenteritis. A small molecular weight (<1.5 kDa), lipophilic, non-protein compound isolated from boiled white rice inhibits the activity of chloride-secretory channels in intestinal epithelial cells, which is increased in secretory diarrhea (Mathews et al. 1999). This so-called rice factor may be responsible for the improvement of oral rehydration solutions in humans with diarrhea when rice is incorporated (Alam et al. 1992; Gore et al. 1992). Rice is also very lean, low in fiber, usually palatable, and relatively energy dense when compared to other more voluminous carbohydrate sources such as potato, in addition to being inexpensive and easy to source and prepare.

Few commercial diets are currently available that could be considered ideal in all respects for acute non-specific gastroenteritis, and commercial formulations change often enough that firm recommendations cannot be made. Most commercial diets provide significantly more fat (>25% of ME) but are complete and

Table 11.4 Suitable home-prepared diets for the short-term management of acute gastroenteritis in dogs and cats.

Cottage cheese and rice	
Cottage cheese (1% milk fat)	1 unit
Boiled white rice	1 unit
ME density: 4.8 kJ/g or 1 kcal/g as fed	
Nutrient composition (% of ME):	
Digestible protein	33%
Fat	6%
Carbohydrate (and ash)	61%
Chicken and rice	
Boiled chicken breast (skin and visible fat removed)	1 unit
Boiled white rice	4 units
ME density: 5.5 kJ/g or 1.3 kcal/g as fed	
Nutrient composition (% of ME):	
Digestible protein	26%
Fat	6%
Carbohydrate (and ash)	68%

ME, metabolizable energy.

balanced. In addition, when feeding as little as 25% of RER, it is unlikely that the fat content will be sufficient to exacerbate vomiting or diarrhea if the diet contains less than 30% of ME from fat. Diets formulated with hydrolyzed ingredients such as Hill's Prescription Diet z/d canine/feline (Hill's Pet Nutrition, Guildford, UK), Nestlé Purina Pro Plan Veterinary Diets HA canine/feline (Nestlé Purina PetCare, St. Louis, MO, USA), Royal Canin Veterinary Health Nutrition Hydrolyzed Protein canine/feline, Royal Canin Anallergenic canine/feline (aka Ultamino in the United States; Royal Canin USA, Hackettstown, NJ, USA), Blue Natural Veterinary Diets HF Hydrolyzed canine/feline (Blue Buffalo, Wilton, CT, USA), and SquarePet Veterinarian Formulated Solutions Skin & Digestive Support canine (SquarePet, Los Angeles, CA, USA) warrant further study and evaluation, as does Nestlé Purina Pro Plan Veterinary Diets EL canine, an elemental diet. Despite the variable and sometimes greater than ideal fat content of many diets in this category, the combination of high digestibility and reduced antigenicity makes them attractive options for the management of acute gastroenteritis.

Chronic Gastrointestinal Disease

Periodontal Disease

Periodontal disease can be considered the scourge of domesticated dogs and cats because of its prevalence, the morbidity it is associated with, the expense of treatment, and the hassle of prevention. In a study in North America of 31 484 dogs and 15 226 cats of all ages, the prevalence of calculus and gingivitis was around 20%. Predictably, "dental disease" was the most commonly reported disease (Lund et al. 1999). In another study it was found that 80% of dogs older than 6 years had moderate to severe periodontitis (Hamp et al. 1984). The frequency of "marginal periodontitis" was found to be 82.3% in dogs aged 6–8 years, 82.9% in dogs aged 9–11 years, and 95.7% in dogs aged 12–14 years.

These are staggering figures and give (one-sided) support to the hypothesis that a natural diet protects against periodontitis, while commercial and soft homemade diets lead to periodontitis in almost all animals eventually. We imagine the effects of chewing skin, connective tissue, and bone – and the teeth-cleaning effects these actions have – and we assume that periodontal disease occurs with a low frequency in the wild because selective pressure over the millennia would have produced animals that were resistant to such disease when consuming their normal diet. In contrast, when we feed domestic cats and dogs dry extruded diets – or, perhaps worse, rolls, canned, wet, or retorted diets – it is intuitive that periodontal disease might be more common in those animals, whose teeth may not be naturally cleaned by a more abrasive diet.

It is clear that periodontitis will develop in almost all animals fed standard commercial diets, which do not have other regular measures to prevent the disease. Even more so, softer diets appear convincingly to be worse. Cats fed dry food develop less calculus and gingivitis than cats fed exclusively canned food (Studer and Stapley 1973). In a large survey of domestic cats in Japan, calculus was more common in cats fed canned or home-cooked meals than cats fed dry foods (41% vs. 25%) (Japan Small Animal Veterinary Association 1985). Similarly, it was shown many years ago that soaking dry food prior to feeding is a reliable method of inducing the rapid formation of plaque, calculus, gingivitis, and eventually periodontitis in dogs (Burwasser and Hill 1939). In a study of dogs in Brazil, those that were fed diets of home-prepared foods and scraps had significantly more dental disease than those fed commercial dry diets (Domingues et al. 1999).

Additionally, when commercial diets are supplemented with more abrasive, "natural" ingredients, the development of periodontitis is retarded, or even prevented. Feeding raw oxtails as a supplement to a dry food has been shown to be effective in minimizing the development of gingivitis and periodontitis in long-term (>6 years) studies in beagles (Brown and Park 1968). Once-weekly feeding of oxtails was shown to remove existing calculus to 5% of previous amounts within two weeks and to maintain them at that level for years. Further, a diet consisting of raw bovine trachea and attached tissues was much more effective in reducing plaque, calculus, and gingivitis than the same diet when fed minced (Egelberg 1965a). Another study used raw beef bones in beagles for effective calculus reduction for up to 20 days, although other measures of periodontal health were not assessed (Marx et al. 2016).

Thus, commercial diets are associated with periodontal disease, and softer diets are worse than dry diets, though perhaps there is less difference between the two types of commercial diets than one might expect. In addition, the supplementation of commercial diets with "natural" chews, such as oxtails, dramatically improves oral health.

These conclusions are consistent with the hypothesis that cats and dogs that consume commercial diets have a very high risk of eventually developing periodontal disease. So what evidence is there that a "natural" diet protects against periodontal disease in feral or wild cats and dogs?

Periodontitis in Feral and Wild Animals

The skulls of 29 African wild dogs were examined for evidence of periodontal disease, as a model for the domestic dog's "natural" diet (Steenkamp and Gorrel 1999). The diet of these dogs is almost exclusively small antelope. Wild dogs have shorter maxillae than wolves, making them tend toward brachygnathism, and the upper third premolar is often rotated to make room for the other, overlapping permanent molars. This gives a more powerful bite, but may predispose to periodontitis. Signs of teeth wearing were seen in 83% of teeth, and 48% of skulls had fractured teeth, with signs of endodontic disease in half of those. There was evidence of periodontitis in 41% of dogs, but interestingly, mild calculus deposits were

found on only two skulls. Therefore, the wild dog on a "natural" diet is affected by dental disease at similar rates to domesticated dogs, and, surprisingly, the "natural" diet does not protect against dental disease. This is despite its efficacy at preventing the formation of calculus.

In a study of feral cats on Marion Island, the skulls of 301 cats that had been trapped and killed were examined (Verstraete et al. 1996). Evidence of periodontitis was found in 61.8% of cats and in 14.8% of teeth. Again, however, calculus was found on only 9% of cats and on 0.76% of teeth – consistent with their diet, which was mostly birds (95% of diet). Therefore, the cause of periodontitis is unclear, but it is not prevented by natural diet or by inhibiting calculus formation. In contrast, odontoclastic resorptive lesions were infrequent, with 14.3% of cats affected and 1.2% of teeth.

In a study in Australia, there was significantly less calculus on the teeth of 29 feral cats that consumed a diet of rats, mice, lizards, birds, and insects than on a sample of 20 domestic cats fed dry or canned food (Clarke and Cameron 1998). However, once again, there was no difference in the prevalence of periodontal disease between the two groups.

These studies then throw considerable doubt on the central hypothesis. Although it appears that a "natural" diet protects against, or at least minimizes, the development of calculus, it does little to protect against the development of periodontitis and tooth loss, in either cats or dogs.

This then leads us to ask two questions: (i) what, if any, chewing activity protects against periodontitis; and (ii) how can there be any dissociation between the development of calculus and periodontitis? Or put another way: is protection against the formation of calculus different from protection against periodontitis?

Evidence of the Protective Effect of Chewing Activities

In a survey of 1350 client-owned dogs in North America, the association of calculus, gingival inflammation, and periodontal bone loss with chewing activity was analyzed (Harvey et al. 1996). It was found that there was progressively less accumulation of calculus, gingivitis, and periodontal bone loss in dogs given access to a variety of chewing activities. Although this study also suggested that rawhide chews were the most effective, no chewing material was consistently effective in all dogs. Access to bones was associated with protection against calculus and gingivitis, but still did not protect against periodontitis in premolars or molars in general. These disparities could be due to differences in chewing techniques, or could represent differences between dogs, unrelated to the act of chewing.

In prospective trials evaluating specific chews, the results are again consistent with the realization that plaque and calculus might be reduced, but not prevented, and that such reductions do not necessarily translate to protection against gingivitis or periodontitis. In a relatively long-term trial, 38 mixed-breed dogs were fed a dry diet plus Pedigree Denta Rask® (Pedigree PetFoods, McLean, VA, USA) for 6 out of 7 days, over 21 months. Both plaque and calculus were reduced (15–20%), but there was no reduction in gingivitis after 18 months (Gorrel and Bierer 1999).

In another study using a different "multi-ingredient" chew for four weeks, plaque was reduced by 38%, gingivitis by 39%, and calculus by 49%. The addition of a proprietary antimicrobial to the chew did not further the benefit (Brown and McGenity 2005). In an evaluation of rawhide chews, the development of plaque over seven days while feeding a dry diet was reduced by approximately 20% by daily chewing on one rawhide chew (Hennet 2001).

Using the C.E.T.® Forte chews (Virbac, Westlake, TX, USA) daily as a dietary supplement to cats for four weeks reduced plaque by 20%. There was a 40% reduction in calculus, but no significant reduction in gingivitis. Also, only 6 out of 15 dogs consumed the chews every day (Gorrel et al. 1998). In a further study of C.E.T. Forte, the chews were added in pieces, three hours after the morning meal. After four

weeks there was a 64% reduction in calculus, a 15% reduction in plaque, but a non-significant reduction in gingivitis (Ingham et al. 2002).

Feeding Hill's Prescription Diet t/d for six months reduced plaque by 39% and gingivitis by 36% in 20 mixed-breed dogs (Logan et al. 2002). In a comparison of feeding Hill's t/d with a normal dry diet plus a daily Pedigree Denta Rask, there was no difference in the efficacy of reducing plaque, calculus, or gingivitis between the two (Rawlings et al. 1997).

In none of these studies has a product or diet been shown to have 100% efficacy, and some do not demonstrate any benefit in the scores of gingivitis. In no trials have the interventions been long enough to demonstrate any efficacy in preventing the development of periodontitis.

Dental Diets

Several food companies now produce diets with claims of benefits for dental health. Such diets are either formulated to abrade the teeth (Hill's and Nestlé Purina), plus contain additives that function as inhibitors of calculus formation and as plaque retardants (Royal Canin). Some components may also function as antibacterial agents, such as green tea polyphenols, and some chew treats also include chlorhexidine, an antiseptic.

Sodium hexametaphosphate (HMP) or tripolyphosphate (TPP) forms soluble complexes with most cations and reduces the availability of calcium for incorporation into plaque to form calculus. It has been proposed that the HMP–calcium complexes are "washed away" in the saliva. The calcium then dissociates within the acid environment of the stomach, and HMP does not reduce dietary calcium bioavailability. The addition of an HMP solution to a dry diet reduced calculus formation in dogs by almost 80% when softened biscuits were fed (Stookey et al. 1995). However, no long-term studies have been performed to demonstrate that reducing calculus formation in such a manner has any effect on the long-term production of gingivitis or periodontitis in cats or dogs. From the other studies mentioned, one would not be hopeful of such an effect.

High concentrations of ascorbate inhibit the growth of several species of oral bacteria in vitro. A stable form of vitamin C (sodium ascorbyl phosphate) has been added to an experimental diet and fed to cats. After 28 days, plaque and calculus were reduced slightly, and the development of gingivitis was almost completely prevented compared with the control group (Wehr et al. 2004). Other attempts to control oral bacteria include the addition of green tea polyphenols, which have been shown to have in vitro antibacterial activity against important oral pathogens. To date, no clinical studies have been performed to confirm their in vivo efficacy.

Clearly, although most "dental therapeutic diets" have some proven efficacy, they are inadequate to prevent periodontitis in the long term, despite significantly reducing calculus. It is likely that combinations of approaches will have additive effects (e.g. a dental diet plus rawhide chew plus occasional bones), but this remains untested and is not without other risks such as dental fractures with the use of bones.

There is a trend, therefore, that reducing, or even preventing, the development of dental calculus is insufficient to prevent gingivitis and is presumably insufficient to prevent the development of periodontitis in either cats or dogs. This applies to both experimental means and the "natural" diet.

There does not seem to be a clear or simple relationship between the amount of plaque, and especially the amount of calculus on a tooth, and the severity of gingivitis associated with it. Some studies have shown a reduction in gingivitis in the absence of calculus reduction by adding dental chews (Rawlings et al. 1998), while others have demonstrated a reduction in calculus and plaque with no appreciable reduction in gingivitis (Gorrel et al. 1998).

Therefore, mechanical debridement or simply reducing plaque or calculus formation is unlikely to be the panacea for the prevention of dental disease. So do all these approaches fall short because they are unable to effectively remove plaque, or because simply removing or preventing plaque is insufficient to prevent gingivitis and periodontitis?

The Effect of Gingival Stimulation

Tooth brushing has long been held to be the gold standard of oral care in cats and dogs and is effective in the long term, even in reversing pre-existing oral disease. Daily tooth brushing can return gingivae to health in naturally occurring gingivitis, and daily brushing prevented plaque and gingivitis in a four-year study (Lindhe et al. 1975). In dogs with "perfect" oral health, brushing three times weekly is sufficient to maintain gingival health for 24 weeks, whereas once-weekly is not (Tromp et al. 1986). The same group then evaluated the effect of frequency of brushing once gingivitis was established and found that daily (but only daily) brushing would normalize the gingivae (prior to the development of calculus). Gorrel and Rawlings (1996) found that brushing every other day was insufficient to prevent plaque and gingivitis from developing within four weeks in dogs fed a dry food, but this was improved significantly if a dental chew was added. A subsequent study demonstrated that the addition of 0.2% chlorhexidine to the chew reduced plaque accumulation, but had no further benefit to preventing the development of gingivitis (Rawlings et al. 1998). This emphasizes the importance of the effect of mechanical stimulation of the gingivae to prevent gingivitis.

Mechanical stimulation of the gingivae by tooth brushing enhances proliferation of fibroblasts, collagen synthesis, and a reduction in gingivitis in dogs. When daily tooth brushing, including brushing of the gingivae, was compared with removal of plaque with a supragingival curette in dogs fed a softened diet, tooth brushing reduced inflammatory cell infiltration into the gingival tissues, and increased fibroblast proliferation and collagen synthesis after five weeks (Horiuchi et al. 2002). In addition, a greater effect of brushing was seen with twice-daily than once-daily brushing (Yamamoto et al. 2004). This difference was apparent despite the complete prevention of plaque accumulation by use of the curette. A more recent comparison study showed that daily tooth brushing was far superior to either daily dental diet or dental chew in controlling plaque accumulation in dogs, which may be due to more active and prolonged stimulation of gingivae (Allen et al. 2019).

Mechanical stimulation by tooth brushing has been found to enhance pocket oxygen tension, decrease exudation, increase microcirculation in gingivae, and increase saliva flow following the induction of gingivitis in dogs (Tanaka et al. 1998). If the rate of gingival tissue turnover and desquamation is increased, access to the gingival tissues of the sulcus may be reduced. Thus the mechanical stimulation by brushing contributes to the prevention of periodontal pocket formation and can promote epithelial reattachment.

The Influence of Diet on Saliva and the Flora

Normal saliva contains lysozyme, myeloperoxidase, lactoperoxidase, lactoferrin, and histatins, a group of small peptides that bind to hydroxyapatite and can kill *Candida albicans* and *Streptococcus mutans*, and are inhibitory for *Porphyromonas gingivalis*, *Prevotella*, and *Bacteroides* spp. Saliva also contains IgA and leukocytes, and probably has a "flushing" effect, inhibiting the attachment of bacteria to the gingival tissues. In dogs, synthetic, topically applied histatin preparations can significantly inhibit the development of experimental gingivitis (Paquette et al. 1997).

Animals maintained on liquid diets develop salivary gland atrophy within days (Scott et al. 1990). The atrophy is rapidly reversible once a hard diet is reintroduced. The saliva secreted by such animals has a 50% reduction in protein content (Johnson 1984). These findings have been observed in species ranging from rodents to humans. Therefore, food

consistency affects the synthesis of salivary proteins and the volume of saliva produced. In humans, an inverse relationship exists between the lysozyme concentration in stimulated parotid saliva and the mass of plaque that develops in 48 hours (Jalil et al. 1992).

In humans, modification of the diet to be of a firmer texture resulted in a 40% increase in the flow rate of stimulated parotid saliva, as well as an increased plaque pH, and salivary flow rates were significantly correlated with the bite force required to consume the diet (Yeh et al. 2000). The flow rate of saliva is significantly increased when human subjects chewed four sticks of sugar-free gum per day for eight weeks.

Interestingly, dogs fed a hard diet develop a different oral flora from those fed a soft diet – prior to the establishment of clinically apparent periodontitis. Fusiforms and spirochetes rapidly dominate the normal flora when a softened diet is introduced (Krasse and Brill 1960). Dogs that are fed via feeding tubes develop plaque and gingivitis as rapidly as those fed soft diets (Egelberg 1965b). Thus chewing modifies the oral environment in ways that are independent of a simple clearing or debridement activity.

Recommendations

The following conclusions can therefore be drawn:

- Periodontal disease is the most common disease (unless obesity is considered a disease) affecting domestic cats and dogs. Paradoxically, there is little evidence that the "natural" diet protects against periodontal disease.
- Although chewing activities and dietary additives may be sufficient to reduce plaque or even prevent calculus, only those activities that provide appropriate gingival stimulation will prevent gingivitis and periodontitis.
- Diet influences the oral flora and saliva and can thus influence the development of

periodontal disease independent of anti-plaque or anticalculus activities. Animals that require prolonged or permanent tube feeding are at risk of rapidly developing periodontal disease.

- Tooth brushing, recreational chewing, mouth rinsing, and the addition of a bacteriostat (note that the bacteriostat xylitol can result in severe and life-threatening hypoglycemia) to drinking water or mouth rinses should all be considered.

The data presented here clearly demonstrate that while it may be helpful, no single individual dietary intervention is sufficient to prevent a disease that is almost certain to develop. Multiple strategies are required to minimize the risk of periodontal disease if regular daily tooth brushing is not practiced. For cats, they might include proven dental diets or treats, or chicken or turkey necks or wings that have been previously frozen, then seared on the outside quickly to reduce microbial contamination. For dogs, these might include feeding diets proven to reduce plaque and gingivitis development; providing therapeutic chewing activities such as dental chews or pathogen-free bones large enough to be chewed on, but not chewed up/consumed; and dental toys. Reasonable arguments against the practice of feeding bones include dental damage, including fracture and intestinal trauma. However, in the author's practice those adverse events have not been seen when poultry necks are fed. Future research must move toward understanding the relative importance of saliva production and composition, gingival stimulation, and oral microbiota.

Esophageal Disease

Motility Disorders and Megaesophagus
Esophageal motility disorders can result from failure of sensory afferent pathways or from motor neuron or neuromuscular disease. Sensory afferent failure prevents the initiation of peristalsis when the food bolus enters the proximal esophagus, such as occurs in idiopathic megaesophagus (Tan and Diamant 1987). In those cases, primary peristalsis is profoundly reduced and secondary peristalsis is not initiated. Firm, large food boluses that stimulate the esophagus are more likely to elicit contractions than soft food or gruels. In contrast, the neuromuscular dysfunction that accompanies myasthenia gravis prevents muscular contraction despite intact sensation. The differences in sensory and motor dysfunction between patients with esophageal disease probably dictate the physical properties of the food that is best tolerated. The food that best suits a given cat or dog with megaesophagus may be a liquid gruel, meat or dog roll chunks, or even kibble (Davenport et al. 2010; Guilford and Strombeck 1996; van Geffen et al. 2006). Thus experimentation or evaluation of esophageal motility using barium admixed food and fluoroscopy is needed to identify the ideal food consistency for feeding cats and dogs with megaesophagus.

Recommendations
Elevated feeding to promote passage via gravity is usually recommended, whatever food is selected. When practical, the goal should be that the cervical and thoracic portions of the esophagus are elevated during, and immediately following, eating. Elevating a food bowl may raise the cervical portion, but may still allow accumulation of food in the thoracic portion if that remains horizontal. Hand feeding chunks of meat or "meatballs" of canned/retorted pet food while the patient remains in a seated position is laborious but very effective. Experimentation with different food consistencies is recommended, if chunks or soft meatballs are not tolerated.

Esophagitis
Esophageal pain can be debilitating and lead to pronounced anorexia. In cases where oral feeding is not possible, gastrostomy tube placement is indicated. Where oral feeding is possible, a selection of soft food or even slurries is

usually better tolerated than abrasive dry kibble. The main feeding concern for patients with esophagitis is the risk of promoting gastroesophageal reflux and exacerbating the esophagitis.

After a meal, food settles to the dependent part of the stomach body while gas bubbles coalesce and accumulate dorsally in the fundus and cardia, activating stretch receptors in the wall of the cardia (McNally et al. 1964). Afferent vagal fibers (ventral branch of the subdiaphragmatic vagus nerve) arising from the cardia of the stomach (in the dog) induce isolated (i.e. in the absence of peristalsis) transient lower esophageal relaxations (TLORs) of the gastroesophageal segment (GES) (Martin et al. 1986; Reynolds and Effer 1988; Sang and Goyal 2000). These are relatively prolonged relaxations of the GES in the absence of swallowing that have a pattern distinctly different from swallow-induced lower esophageal sphincter relaxation (Wyman et al. 1990). The TLORs are elicited by gaseous distension of the cardia and not by fluid distension, nor by distension of the fundus (Straathof et al. 2001; Strombeck et al. 1988). This reflex in response to the presence of gastric gas has been termed the "belch reflex." As gas is refluxed through the relaxed GES postprandially, leakage of gastric contents and acid may occur. Belching and acid reflux in normal human adults often occur simultaneously. In fact, the majority of transient GES relaxations are accompanied by reflux, either of liquid, gas, or both (Sifrim et al. 1999). In the dog, liquid and gas reflux occur during transient GES relaxations that are very similar to those during reflux in humans (Patrikios and Martin 1986).

Dietary fat restriction has long been the most commonly recommended dietary adjustment for patients with esophagitis (Guilford and Strombeck 1996). This recommendation has been based on studies that have shown that the ingestion of fat decreases GES tone, and the concern that it therefore increases the risk of gastroesophageal reflux. In humans, the GES tone decreases after ingestion of pure

fat and a combined protein–fat meal, whereas ingestion of pure protein and glucose increases GES tone (Nebel and Castell 1973). Indeed, the difference in fat content need not be great in some circumstances, since whole milk but not non-fat milk lowers the GES tone in humans (Babka and Castell 1973). However, it has recently been observed that there is a difference between pure fat ingestion and whole foods. In experiments where GES tone has been measured following a meal in healthy humans, it appears that meal size (volume) has the most impact; neither increasing energy from fat (up to 58% of ME) nor increasing energy density (by 50%) resulted in differences in GES tone or in proportion of time where pH < 4 (Pehl et al. 1999, 2001; Colombo et al. 2002). The differences between these and earlier studies are probably the volume and total energy content of the fluids ingested.

As discussed, distension of the gastric cardia initiates transient reductions in GES tone (TLORs) immediately postprandially. Increasing the volume of a meal enhances gastric cardia distension and increases the number of TLORs in the immediate postprandial period (Maher et al. 1977). Increasing the osmolarity of an ingested yogurt solution from 145 to 500 mOsm/l while maintaining the same volume and fat content increases the rate of TLORs and gastroesophageal reflux by 50% in human patients with reflux disease (Salvia et al. 2001). Similarly, increasing the volume by only 50% has an identical effect on the rate of TLORs.

Although the volume of the ingested meal appears to increase gastroesophageal reflux, the rate of gastric distension is more important than the end volume (Straathof et al. 2002). Slow meal ingestion reduces the effect of volume on the rate of TLORs (Wildi et al. 2004).

Gastroesophageal reflux is commonly reported during high-intensity endurance exercise in otherwise healthy asymptomatic humans, and is due to tonic reductions in GES tone (Maddison et al. 2005). Similar studies have not been conducted in cats or dogs, and in the absence of evidence it is prudent to assume that the case is similar in those species.

Recommendations

It is now clear that the most important variables that increase gastroesophageal reflux induced by a meal are volume, total energy content, osmolarity, rate of ingestion of the meal, and possibly postprandial exercise. However, gastroesophageal reflux is not affected by the fat content or energy density when the diet consumed is a complete food. On that basis it appears that the long-standing recommendations of feeding a low-fat diet may not be ideal. It is clear that frequent small meals are considerably better than single boluses and that slowing the rate of ingestion would be beneficial, if difficult or impractical. It may be that high-fat meals have the advantage that smaller volumes can be fed and reflux minimized. Until species-specific research answers this question, it is recommended that efforts be directed toward increasing the frequency of feeding, decreasing the volume of meals, elevation of the thoracic esophagus, and avoiding high-osmolarity foods such as hydrolysates, and that restriction of dietary fat not be prioritized.

Small Intestinal Disease

Chronic Intestinal Inflammation and Idiopathic Enteropathy

The inflammatory bowel diseases (IBDs) are the most common causes of chronic vomiting and diarrhea in dogs and cats and refer to a group of idiopathic, chronic GIT disorders, characterized by infiltration of the lamina propria by lymphocytes, plasma cells, eosinophils, macrophages, neutrophils, or combinations of these cells (Guilford 1996). Diagnosis requires the comprehensive exclusion of potential causes of gastrointestinal inflammation, including intestinal parasites, small intestinal bacterial overgrowth, bacterial enterocolitis, dietary intolerances, and neoplasia

(Guilford 1996). More recently, the term chronic enteropathy has also been adopted, with dogs being further subcategorized, based on clinical response to treatment, into food-responsive, antibiotic-responsive, and immunosuppressant-responsive enteropathy (Dandrieux and Mansfield 2019). In cats this subcategorization is not as commonly used, and the term chronic enteropathy may include not only food- and immunosuppressant-responsive disease but also small-cell lymphoma (Marsilio 2021). Chronic enteropathy that responds to immunosuppressants is also referred to as IBD; however, intestinal inflammation and other characteristic histopathologic findings such as villus blunting may be reported for dogs and cats with any of the disorders on this spectrum (Allenspach 2011).

The etiology of canine and feline chronic enteropathy is poorly understood, but the main hypothesis for the etiopathogenesis of human IBD is that there is dysregulation of mucosal immune responses to intestinal microbiota and/or dietary antigens (Belsheim et al. 1983; Giaffer et al. 1991; Guarner et al. 2002; Magne 1992). There is evidence from clinical observations and animal models to incriminate normal luminal bacteria or bacterial products in the initiation and perpetuation of the disease (Rutgers et al. 1995). In addition, antibiotics are often empirically administered in cases of chronic enteropathy as adjunctive or primary therapy, and there is widespread acceptance of their efficacy (Jergens 1994; Tams 1993). This practice may also help with subcategorization of a specific canine patient as antibiotic responsive, although trying other therapies first may be warranted given the important considerations for appropriate antibiotic stewardship (Cerquetella et al. 2020). Finally, genetic predispositions appear to play an important role in risk or at least in the phenotypical expression of disease, and research is ongoing (Hirokawa et al. 2021; Luckschander-Zeller et al. 2019).

Regardless of the underlying etiology for any given patient, abnormal immune responses to dietary antigens are often suspected, and the clinical response to novel- and hydrolyzed-ingredient diets supports that hypothesis (Nelson et al. 1984, 1988; Tolbert et al. 2022). Exaggerated humoral and cellular responses and clinical food intolerance have been recorded in human IBD patients (Pearson et al. 1993; Van Den et al. 2001, 2002). Serum IgG concentrations specific to dietary antigens are consistently greater in dogs with chronic gastrointestinal disease than normal dogs, and fecal IgE specific to dietary antigens is consistently found in soft-coated wheaten terriers with chronic enteropathy (Foster et al. 2003; Vaden et al. 2000). However, the frequency with which these might occur and the significance that immune responses play in the pathogenesis of canine and feline chronic enteropathy are unknown.

Also unknown in any given patient is whether any abnormal immune response to the diet is the cause or result of a mucosal infiltrate and/or any disruption to the microbiota (Wang et al. 2019). If abnormal immune response is the cause, it is expected that removal of the inciting antigen would lead to improvement. If abnormal immune response is the effect, it still may be that removing the largest single source of antigen during an elimination diet trial is sufficient to reduce the inflammatory stimulus, allowing restoration of normal intestinal immunity.

Because of the consistent partial or complete response, restriction or manipulation of individual dietary components is perhaps the single most important factor in the treatment of chronic enteropathy, and it may be sufficient in mild cases. Despite this fact, there is a paucity of information pertaining to the nutritional requirements of dogs and cats with chronic enteropathy.

Nutritional Derangements in Chronic Enteropathy

Protein-energy malnutrition. The disruptions of absorptive area, normal epithelial function, permeability, and motility that occur with chronic enteropathy result in disturbed nutrient absorption. Caloric insufficiency, intestinal protein loss, increased catabolism, and decreased absorption can result in hypoalbuminemia, panhypoproteinemia, and muscle wasting in a significant number of cases on presentation (Hart et al. 1994). Similar findings are reported in humans with IBD, with protein-energy malnutrition documented to occur in 20–85% of IBD patients (Gee et al. 1985).

Magnesium. Hypomagnesemia has been identified in approximately one-third of canine and feline admissions to intensive care facilities when intestinal disease was the primary complaint (Martin et al. 1994; Toll et al. 2002). Whether hypomagnesemia is a common feature of IBD on presentation has not been reported. However, the combination of malabsorption, anorexia, and therapy with magnesium-free fluids (e.g. lactated Ringer's solution) is predicted to lead to hypomagnesemia. The possibility of hypomagnesemia should be suspected if cachexia and hypokalemia are concurrently present and if intestinal ileus cannot easily be rectified.

Iron. Anemia is a relatively common finding upon presentation and can result from blood loss or systemic suppression of hematopoiesis. In addition, iron-deficiency anemia has been reported in conjunction with chronic enteropathy in dogs (Ristic and Stidworthy 2002) and cats (Hunt and Jugan 2021).

Vitamin B12 and folate deficiency. Low serum B12 and/or folate have been described in cats and dogs in association with a wide variety of gastrointestinal diseases including IBD (Allenspach et al. 2007; Hunt and Jugan 2021; Reed et al. 2007; Simpson et al. 2001). In one study, cats with chronic enteropathy apparently had a greatly decreased serum half-life of B12, which may have contributed to the deficiency (Simpson et al. 2001). However, not all authors have reported common B12 deficiency in cats with chronic enteropathy. In one study in the United Kingdom, B12 deficiency was extremely rare, although only five cats with chronic enteropathy were included (Ibarrola et al. 2005). In a further study of serum B12 and folate concentrations in cats with a variety of diseases in the United Kingdom, there was no association between the presence of gastrointestinal disease and serum B12 or folate concentrations (Reed et al. 2007).

Cats with low serum B12 and with low B12/folate have been reported to have a lower body condition score than non-deficient cats (Reed et al. 2007). It is likely that mucosal repair is impeded in the initial management of chronic enteropathy when B12 is deficient and its absorption impaired. There is anecdotal evidence that the correction of the deficiency may reduce the requirement for immunosuppression or that the response to therapy may be limited until it is corrected. In a study of cats severely deficient in B12 with chronic enteropathy, vitamin B12 supplementation resulted in increased weight gain, reduced vomiting, and reduced diarrhea in most cats (Ruaux et al. 2005). Unfortunately, the numbers of cats studied were small, the specific diseases were not defined, and there was no control group.

Consideration should be given to B12 assays in the initial evaluation of dogs and cats with chronic enteropathy, with supplementation as indicated. Dogs and cats are typically supplemented with B12 at a dose of 250 µg (cats) or 500 µg (dogs) per dose, subcutaneously or intramuscularly, weekly for 4–5 weeks (Simpson et al. 2001). Oral supplementation is also effective (0.25–1 mg cyanocobalamin/day/dog and 0.25 mg/day/cat) (Chang et al. 2022; Toresson et al. 2017, 2018). No study has yet evaluated the clinical response to folate supplementation in dogs or cats with chronic enteropathy.

Vitamin K. Vitamin K deficiency leading to coagulopathy and clinically recognizable hemorrhage has been reported to occur commonly in cats in association with chronic enteropathy and may also occur in dogs (Center et al. 2000). Coagulation tests normalized in all the cats reported that were treated with parenteral vitamin K1 (2.5–5 mg/cat, repeated two or three times at 12-hour intervals). All affected cats

had severe IBD, and some had concurrent cholangiohepatitis.

Antioxidants. In human patients with ulcerative colitis (UC) or Crohn's disease (CD), deficiencies in zinc and vitamins A, E, B6, thiamine, and riboflavin have also been described and may contribute to mucosal oxidative damage, anemia, increased intestinal permeability, and persistent inflammation. A recent study assessed the plasma antioxidant status and proinflammatory cytokines of 26 CD patients. Decreased selenium concentrations and erythrocyte glutathione peroxidase activity were found in these patients. In addition, glutathione peroxidase activity was inversely correlated with plasma TNF-alpha concentrations, and serum selenium was inversely correlated with plasma levels of both TNF-alpha and the soluble receptor of IL-2 (Reimund et al. 2000). It is likely that similar deficiencies occur in severely affected feline and canine patients, and consideration of parenteral fat-soluble vitamin administration is warranted in severely malnourished cases.

Zinc. The possibility that zinc deficiency might coexist in patients with chronic enteropathy bears special consideration, since zinc deficiency exacerbates diarrhea in humans and rodents. Oral supplementation improves histologic recovery, normalizes absorption, and decreases NF-κB nuclear binding in experimental models of diarrhea (Altaf et al. 2002). In a study of CD patients with increased intestinal permeability, daily oral zinc supplementation improved symptoms and normalized the permeability in 80% of cases (Sturniolo et al. 2001). Additional mechanisms for the effect of zinc treatment on the duration of diarrhea include improved absorption of water and electrolytes, increased levels of brush-border enzymes, and faster regeneration of the intestinal epithelium.

Potential Role of Dietary Antigens in the Pathogenesis of Chronic Enteropathy

As stated, exaggerated responses to dietary antigens are often suspected in canine and feline chronic enteropathy, and dietary therapy can be extremely successful even as the sole therapy in some cases (Tolbert et al. 2022). Elimination diets have proved to be effective in dogs and cats with small and large intestinal lymphocytic-plasmacytic, eosinophilic, and mixed cellular infiltrates (Guilford et al. 2001; Hirt and Iben 1998; Nelson et al. 1984, 1988). In a study of 16 feline cases of elimination challenge–proven dietary hypersensitivity with chronic gastrointestinal signs, all 16 cats had mild to severe inflammatory infiltrates in at least one region of the bowel (Guilford et al. 2001). The infiltrates were lymphocytic, lymphocytic-plasmacytic (most cases), or eosinophilic (two cases). All cases responded completely to the elimination diet alone and offending foods were identified in all cases. In a report of 13 dogs with lymphocytic-plasmacytic colitis, clinical signs resolved in all 13 with the introduction of an elimination diet, and of 11 dogs rechallenged with their original diet, 9 relapsed (Nelson et al. 1988). In a further report of 6 cats with lymphocytic-plasmacytic colitis, all 6 responded completely to an elimination diet (Nelson et al. 1984). A complete clinical response to an elimination diet has been reported in a cat with duodenal and ileal lymphocytic infiltrates so severe that a histologic diagnosis of intestinal lymphosarcoma was made (Wasmer et al. 1995).

The theoretical basis for the use of protein hydrolysate diets in chronic enteropathy is that a reduction in immunogenic epitopes being presented to the mucosal immune system while dysregulation is present will increase the potential for resolution. Thus the argument for the use of a hydrolysate diet is independent of whether a dietary-specific immunologic response is suspected to be present or not. Experience with protein hydrolysate diets is increasing, and anecdotally they appear to be very effective adjuncts to pharmacologic therapy, or even as sole therapy. Clinical resolution with histologic improvement has been reported in 4 of 6 dogs with refractory chronic enteropathy when treated with a hydrolyzed soy protein diet alone

(Marks et al. 2002). A similar study of dogs with chronic enteropathy documented equally beneficial results utilizing a different hydrolyzed soy protein diet (Mandigers et al. 2010).

It remains unknown why many cases of chronic enteropathy are food responsive, and some show improved or resolved clinical signs with appropriate diet modification alone. One case series showed that dogs with food-responsive disease had lower clinical disease severity scores and had better outcomes compared to antibiotic- and immunosuppressant-responsive disease; hydrolyzed and elimination diets were equally successful (Allenspach et al. 2016). This reflected some findings of an earlier study that reported that dogs with food-responsive disease tended to be younger, less severely ill, and have primarily large-bowel diarrhea compared to those requiring steroid therapy (Allenspach et al. 2007). Interestingly, 31 of 39 dogs showed no recurrence of clinical signs when switched back to their original diet (Allenspach et al. 2007). Taken together, this evidence could suggest that food-responsive enteropathy may represent a transient or temporary disruption in dietary tolerance that may involve the local immune system and likely also the microbiota.

It is possible that nutritional factors other than protein hydrolysis or ingredient novelty are responsible for positive responses to diet modification. These could include dietary digestibility, correction of vitamin or mineral deficiencies, and a lowered n-6 : n-3 fatty acid ratio, and the potential for an immunomodulatory effect of soy isoflavones within the diet. However, it is equally possible that eliminating the quantitatively most significant antigen source is sufficient to eliminate clinical signs, reduce inflammation, and allow restoration of normal mucosal immunity, even if dietary hypersensitivity is not the primary pathogenic process.

Nutritional Strategies for Therapy of Chronic Enteropathy

Pre- and probiotics. It is increasingly clear that dietary influences on the intestinal flora are involved in health and disease. On heating, the amino acid lysine reacts with reducing sugars to form Maillard compounds that cannot be digested or absorbed in a usable form (Larsen et al. 2002). This serves as substrate for luminal bacteria in the small intestine, leading to quantitative and/or qualitative changes in the flora. This leads to increased bile acid deconjugation and loss of the bile acid conjugate taurine, thus increasing the dietary requirement for taurine in canned compared with dry diets. This effect is reversible with antibiotics (Kim et al. 1996). Additionally, fermentable fiber has been shown to profoundly affect intestinal flora, in addition to its effect on enterocytes, by promoting the development of beneficial species (see earlier) (Bamba et al. 2002). This prebiotic effect reduces or prevents inflammation in experimental models of IBD (Guarner et al. 2002; Kanauchi et al. 2002). Therefore, a fermentable fiber source should probably be included as part of dietary therapy, although information regarding which type (e.g. resistant starch, FOSs, inulin) and how much is lacking. The addition of FOSs to feline diets at 0.75% dry matter did not affect duodenal flora, but it did increase the numbers of lactobacilli and reduce the numbers of *E. coli* in the fecal flora of healthy cats (Sparkes et al. 1998a, 1998b). Healthy German shepherd dogs believed to have bacterial overgrowth were supplemented with FOSs at 1.0% of their diet as fed (Willard et al. 1994). Changes were recognized in the duodenal bacterial flora, but these changes were of less magnitude than seen in normal dogs for these parameters. The clinical significance of these studies in cats and dogs with IBD is unknown.

A probiotic has been defined as "a preparation containing viable, defined microorganisms in sufficient numbers, which alter the established intestinal microbiota by implantation or colonization in a compartment of the host, and by that exert beneficial health effects in the host" (Schrezenmeir and de Vrese 2001). Unfortunately, most commercial veterinary probiotic preparations have not

historically been accurately represented by label claims, reflecting the poor quality control for most commercial veterinary probiotics (Weese and Arroyo 2003). Evidence of efficacy is mixed (Pilla et al. 2019; Rossi et al. 2020), and given the wide range of specific individual or mixes of probiotic species in various products, generalized guidance for management of clinical cases is not yet possible.

Much work is required to define what constitutes optimal numbers and species of intestinal microorganisms. However, it is likely that through interaction with the gut flora, certain diets may protect against or possibly predispose to chronic enteropathy. Until further data are available, it is prudent to select diets with a high digestibility in the management of chronic enteropathy, though with a source of fermentable fiber. An avoidance of canned diets in feline cases seems rational at present.

Glutamine. It has been proposed that gut mucosal turnover and barrier function are compromised during chronic enteropathy, due in part to a relative glutamine deficiency. This is supported by experimental studies that have demonstrated a reduction in mucosal inflammation and lipid peroxidation products following luminal glutamine supplementation in models of mucosal inflammation (Kaya et al. 1999). Caution should be heeded in interpreting many of the experimental studies, as disparate dietary effects are often seen. It is clear that the availability of glutamine is probably beneficial in all causes of acute and chronic enteritis. However, it is uncertain if any benefit will be provided by supplementation beyond that present in adequate amounts of intact protein. Studies of spontaneous IBD in human patients have yet to provide any evidence that "extra" glutamine provides any benefit over conventional levels (Goh and O'Morain 2003). This finding is consistent with the previously discussed finding that glutamine supplementation beyond that provided by intact dietary protein has no further benefit in acute gastrointestinal disease.

Arginine and nitric oxide. The main potential mechanism for the positive action of luminal arginine supplementation in chronic enteropathy is via modulation of NO production within the mucosa. In the past 10 years, it has become clear that NO is an important molecule in normal intestinal homeostasis and in the inflamed intestine. Numerous studies have attempted to elucidate whether NO production during intestinal inflammation is beneficial or deleterious, producing conclusions that range from bad through indifferent to essential (Perner and Rask-Madsen 1999). NO is produced in low amounts constitutively by endothelial and neuronal NO synthases (eNOS and nNOS). During inflammation, and under the transcriptional control of NF-κB, a third NO synthase enzyme is induced (iNOS) in most activated leukocytes and activated epithelial cells, which produce much greater amounts of NO than is produced constitutively (Grisham et al. 2002). Recently it has been reported that iNOS is expressed in canine IBD, and that NO-derived nitrite is increased in the colonic lumen of affected dogs (Gunawardana et al. 1997; Jergens et al. 1998).

Constitutively produced NO serves to maintain intestinal perfusion, inhibit longitudinal smooth muscle contraction, inhibit the expression of broad-spectrum endothelial adhesion molecules, coordinate epithelial cell turnover, and promote barrier integrity (Perner and Rask-Madsen 1999). In large iNOS-dependent quantities, studies have shown that NO can scavenge free radicals, preserve epithelial integrity or promote epithelial apoptosis with loss of barrier integrity and increased bacterial translocation, induce or inhibit inflammatory cytokines, and lead to irreversible host–protein nitrosylation and dysfunction (Pavlick et al. 2002). Variables that affect the role of NO include the cellular source, timing of production in relation to the insult, chronicity of the disease, quantity produced, and the presence of superoxide leading to the formation of peroxynitrite. It is not surprising then that such a heterogeneous collection of responses under different experimental and clinical settings has led to controversy about whether inhibition of iNOS in IBD might be beneficial or detrimental. Importantly, most experimental models of intestinal inflammation mimic human forms of IBD and probably do not reflect the same pathogenesis as that seen in feline and canine IBD. Further research, specific to feline and canine disease, needs to be performed before the use of iNOS inhibitors or even NO donors or precursors could be recommended therapeutically.

Antioxidants. Increased free radical production is a cardinal characteristic of almost any inflammatory disease and has been demonstrated convincingly in human IBD patients. In addition, as previously stated, deficiencies in vitamins and minerals associated with oxidant defense (vitamins A, E, C; zinc, manganese, copper) are commonly associated with IBD, and their supplementation has been shown to be effective in reducing the effects of intestinal damage following experimental insults. Although it is expected that oxidative stress is a feature of canine and feline chronic enteropathy, the absence of significant numbers of the major oxidant-producing species (neutrophils and macrophages) in the majority of intestinal infiltrates suggests it is less significant than in its human analogs. Nonetheless, supplementation of dietary antioxidants seems prudent until reasons are provided to suggest their lack of efficacy or detrimental effects. It is currently unknown what the optimal dose and combination of antioxidants are for patients with chronic enteropathy.

Dietary fat. A fat-restricted diet is important in the management of a variety of gastrointestinal diseases in dogs, even though fat is a valuable caloric source and enhances the palatability of the diet. Fat delays gastric emptying (Lin et al. 1990; Meyer et al. 1994), and fat-restricted diets appear to be better tolerated in a variety of gastrointestinal diseases. The assimilation of dietary fat is a relatively complex process, and malabsorbed fatty acids are hydroxylated by intestinal and colonic bacteria. These hydroxy fatty acids stimulate colonic water secretion and exacerbate diarrhea and fluid loss (Poley and Hofmann 1976). Fat malassimilation can also be associated with malabsorption of bile acids, resulting in deconjugation of unabsorbed bile acids and increased mucosal permeability and secretion (Cummings et al. 1978). Dietary fat restriction is particularly important in patients diagnosed with lymphangiectasia, with many patients needing restriction to less than 15% fat kJ or kcal. Unfortunately, there are few commercial veterinary diets available that contain less than 15% fat kJ or kcal. It is the author's opinion that when severe lymphangiectasia is suspected or confirmed, priority should be given to the feeding of a restricted-fat diet over antigenic novelty. Further studies are warranted to document the touted benefits of MCTs, as increasing evidence has highlighted their limitations based on high cost, low palatability, and evidence that at least in the dog, absorption still occurs via intestinal lymph (Jensen et al. 1994).

It is becoming increasingly clear that the significance of fat malabsorption is far less in cats with chronic intestinal disease than in dogs. One study evaluated 60 cats with chronic, nonspecific diarrhea of at least one month's duration (Laflamme et al. 2011). They were fed either a high-fat (23.2% dry matter [DM] basis) or a low-fat (10.5% DM basis) diet for six weeks. Improvement in fecal consistency was seen in most cats in both groups, and there was no difference in rates or degrees of improvement between groups. It is likely that affected cats either had an adverse reaction to food, or idiopathic IBD, or both, consistent with the prevalence previously described (Guilford et al. 2001). Thus this study emphasized the important role of dietary manipulation in chronic intestinal disease, and the lack of importance, at least in that study population, of dietary fat restriction in cats with chronic diarrhea.

Polyunsaturated n-3 fatty acids. Dietary PUFAs can modulate immunity via several mechanisms (Calder et al. 1990; Calder and Grimble 2002; Dooper et al. 2002; Geyeregger

et al. 2005; Kearns et al. 1999; Lee et al. 2003; Weatherill et al. 2005). For this reason, enriched diets may be of benefit to dogs with chronic enteropathy (Ontsouka et al. 2010). The dietary content of PUFAs determines the proportions of the n-6 and n-3 PUFAs incorporated into leukocyte cell membrane phospholipids. The n-3 PUFA eicosapentaenoic acid (EPA) competes with the n-6 arachidonate (AA) as a substrate for cyclooxygenase (COX) and lipoxygenase (LOX) after cleavage from the cell membrane, and the dietary proportions of n-6 and n-3 PUFAs determine if the prostaglandins, thromboxanes, leukotrienes, and platelet activating factor (eicosanoids) are produced from EPA or AA. EPA is a less efficient substrate for COX, resulting in reduced prostaglandin production. Eicosanoids produced from EPA range from antagonistic to equipotent to those derived from AA, and the overall effect on immunity is not explained simply by the reduced efficacy of EPA-derived eicosanoids. The effects and mechanisms of modulation of eicosanoids by dietary lipid are complex, although there is some value to the generalization that diets enriched in n-3 PUFAs will reduce inflammation relative to diets enriched in n-6 PUFAs.

PUFAs also directly affect gene transcription through the peroxisome proliferator-activated receptors (PPARs), a family of cytosolic proteins that, once bound to an appropriate ligand, diffuse into the nucleus and promote or inhibit gene transcription. PPARs are expressed by macrophages, lymphocytes, and dendritic and endothelial cells (Glass and Ogawa 2006). Activation of PPARs by EPA leads to reduced TNF-alpha, IL-6, and IL-1 production by macrophages, and reduced IL-2 production by lymphocytes (Glass and Ogawa 2006; Kliewer et al. 1997; Kostadinova et al. 2005).

The incorporation of EPA in place of AA in phospholipid membranes of lymphocytes affects the function of the lipid rafts within which T-cell receptors (TCRs) are localized. This decreases signal transduction through the TCR-reducing T-cell activation (Geyeregger et al. 2005). Lastly, both EPA and docosahexaenoic acid (DHA) antagonize the interaction between Gram-negative lipopolysaccharide (LPS or endotoxin) and TLRs, reducing the production of COX, TNF-alpha, IL-1, IL-6, and IL-8, and improving morbidity in severe sepsis (Lee et al. 2004; Mayer et al. 2003; Weatherill et al. 2005).

Predicting the effect of PUFAs within a diet has to take into account (i) the total fat content; (ii) the relative proportions of 18-carbon and 20-carbon n-3 and n-6 PUFAs; (iii) the absolute amounts of all individual n-3 and n-6 PUFAs; (iv) the previous dietary history of the animal; and (v) the duration of exposure to the diet in question. Describing the fat content of a diet by a simple ratio of n-6 to n-3 PUFA provides very limited and potentially misleading information. In addition, supplementation of a diet with a source of n-3 PUFAs (e.g. marine fish oil) will have varying effects depending on the diet and the patient. Most commercial diets are highly concentrated in n-6 PUFAs, and the addition of a small amount of n-3 PUFAs will achieve little.

Where information on specific dietary fatty acid concentrations is not available, a ratio of total n-6 to n-3 of less than 5 : 1 may be effective for reducing pruritis in atopic dermatitis, whereas a ratio less than 3.5 : 1 may be needed for more serious inflammatory diseases, and ratios as low as 1.3 : 1 may be optimal (Bauer 2007; LeBlanc et al. 2007, 2008; Saker et al. 1998). The exact amount of fish oil required to be added depends on the basal diet.

A class of transcription factors that may have an important role in chronic enteropathy is the PPARs. Upon binding with their ligand, PPARs dimerize with the retinoid X receptor (RXR) co-receptor, then translocate to the nucleus and bind to PPAR-response elements. Although the understanding of the range of action of PPARs and their ligands in cats and dogs is rudimentary, it is interesting to note that NF-κB-dependent gene transcription is decreased by PPAR-gamma ligands. Indeed, it has been shown that PPAR-gamma ligands can potently inhibit NF-κB-dependent cytokine production by the murine colonic epithelium,

and significantly decrease intestinal inflammation in an experimental model of IBD (Takagi et al. 2002). This is especially interesting given that certain n-3 fatty acids are known PPAR-gamma ligands (Kliewer et al. 1997).

Lastly, although as yet unproven, aberrant immunologic responses to enteric flora are considered a key component to the dysregulation of immunity in feline and canine chronic enteropathy (Burgener et al. 2008). If this is the case, the recent finding that n-3 PUFAs are capable of acting as competitive agonists of the bacterial LPS receptor complex (Toll-like receptor 4) is another potential mechanism by which these PUFAs could be beneficial in chronic enteropathy (Lee et al. 2003).

Fish oil supplementation has been reported to be beneficial in UC and CD patients, but the results are controversial. One study of 18 patients with UC demonstrated a reduction in the number of CD3-positive cells within the intestinal mucosa, reduced expression of MHC II antigens, and reduced plasma cell numbers following treatment with fish oil extract compared with placebo (Almallah et al. 1998). However, a larger, randomized, double-blind trial comprising 96 patients with UC failed to reveal any benefit in remission maintenance or treatment of relapse on 4.5g of EPA daily, despite a significant reduction in LTB4 synthesis by blood peripheral neutrophils (Hawthorne et al. 1992). The differences between the reports regarding study design, supplement composition, dose, whole diet n-6 : n-3 ratios, and assessment of clinical improvement may in part explain the conflicting results. One study compared the efficacy of fish oil to sulfasalazine in the treatment of mild to moderate active UC in humans (Dichi et al. 2000). Treatment with fish oil resulted in greater disease activity as detected by a significant increase in platelet count, erythrocyte sedimentation rate, C-reactive protein, and total fecal nitrogen excretion. Often overlooked is the increase in lipid peroxidation after fish oil supplementation is instituted (Girelli et al. 1994). Antioxidant supplementation may be able to counteract the potentially adverse effects of n-3 fatty acids. Most of the literature regarding n-3 fatty acid administration fails to address the amount of attendant antioxidant supplementation.

There are no reports in the veterinary literature demonstrating the efficacy of n-3 fatty acid supplementation in managing canine or feline IBD. Studies in healthy dogs fed a diet with an n-6 : n-3 ratio of 1.4 : 1 demonstrated a decreased production of PGE2 by stimulated peripheral blood mononuclear cells, and a decreased delayed-type hypersensitivity response, compared to dogs fed a diet with a ratio of 5.4 : 1 (Wander et al. 1997). Increases in certain long-chain n-3 fatty acids and decreases in arachidonic acid were identified in the small intestine and colonic mucosa of healthy beagles fed the same ratios (Reinhart and Vaughn 1995). There is insufficient evidence to make firm recommendations for disease modulation in cats using dietary PUFAs. Using a dietary fat content of approximately 70 g/kg DM basis, Saker and colleagues found that a total n-6 : n-3 ratio of 1.3 : 1 (using corn oil, animal fat, and menhaden fish oil) reduced platelet aggregation (Saker et al. 1998). Such a value provides a very rough estimate of the proportions required for modulating eicosanoid production, although the concentrations of EPA and AA were not specifically assayed. In addition, the dietary concentrations required for the other effects of n-3 PUFAs are unknown. However, most commercial veterinary therapeutic diets marketed for management of chronic enteropathy include EPA and DHA. Further research is necessary to determine the clinical benefits in dogs and cats with chronic enteropathy and currently no effective, established dosages exist.

Recommendations

The optimal nutritional approach for dogs and cats with chronic enteropathy remains to be determined and certainly varies from animal to animal. The available literature is reviewed elsewhere (Rudinsky et al. 2018; Tolbert et al. 2022). Although there are several mechanisms by which diet can affect the progression, maintenance, or resolution of chronic mucosal inflammation, it is undetermined how important any individual component is. Nonetheless, proper dietary management can result in decreased utilization or dosage of pharmacologic therapy and in some cases can lead to clinical resolution as a sole therapy.

The current recommended management following diagnosis is as follows:

- Assess the nutritional status of the patient. This will include physical parameters such as historical and serial body condition, lean body mass, weight trends, current appetite, hydration, presence of edema, and coat condition. Clinicopathologic indices include serum albumin concentration, serum electrolyte concentrations, erythrocyte and leukocyte indicators of malnutrition, evidence of protein-losing gastroenteritis (PLGE; panhypoproteinemia, hypocholesterolemia, lymphopenia), serum PIVKA (proteins invoked by vitamin K antagonism) measurement or coagulation panel to assess vitamin K status, serum vitamin B12 concentration, and folate.
- Address specific concerns regarding malnutrition. This may include vitamin B12, folate, or vitamin K1 supplementation.
- Address anorexia through pharmacologic means and consider supplemental or supportive nutrition in severely malnourished individuals. Indicators for the need for supportive nutrition would include persistent anorexia, recent weight loss of >10% body weight, anemia, hypoalbuminemia, and a body condition score of 3 or less on a 9-point scale with poor appetite.
- Select a highly digestible, novel- or hydrolyzed-ingredient diet and feed exclusively until immunosuppressive therapy can be discontinued.
- Consider fat restriction in severe cases, or where there is histologic evidence of lymphangiectasia.
- If dietary fat is not limiting, then consider enrichment of the diet with n-3 PUFAs using fish oil to achieve a crude n-6 : n-3 ratio of <2 : 1.

Protein-Losing Enteropathies

Increased lymphatic flow as the result of mucosal inflammation is expected, and dilation of intestinal lacteals is a common finding on histopathology (Wilcock 1992). Lymphatic obstruction from extraluminal fibroplasia and constriction, intraluminal adhesions, and debris can lead to a net loss of intestinal lymph. Panhypoproteinemia and hypocholesterolemia, with or without lymphopenia, suggest loss of intestinal lymph. A concern in managing lymphangiectasia is in prioritizing dietary therapy, since in many cases chronic intestinal inflammation accompanies the lymphatic obstruction (Kull et al. 2001). Many limited and uncommon or hydrolyzed-ingredient diets suitable for the management of chronic enteropathies in dogs and cats contain higher fat concentrations than would be ideal for severe lymphangiectasia. As already stated, when severe lymphangiectasia accompanies chronic enteropathy, priority should be given to the feeding of a restricted-fat diet over antigenic novelty, since the hypoproteinemia is often the most life-threatening derangement. Reducing dietary fat decreases lymphatic flow, reduces lacteal dilation and pressure, and hence limits lymphatic protein loss (Olson and Zimmer 1978). Practically, this means the selection of diets that provide <20% of kJ or kcal as fat, of which there are currently few commercial diets. The reduced lymphatic pressures reduce protein loss and can lead to normalization of serum protein concentrations (Olson and Zimmer 1978). Addition to the diet of MCTs cannot be recommended given their high cost, low palatability, and evidence that at least in the dog some absorption still occurs via intestinal lymph (Jensen et al. 1994).

In severe cases, there is sufficient disruption of the mucosa that marked malabsorption accompanies the enteric protein loss. In those cases, semi-elemental or even elemental diets may be required. There is currently only one veterinary elemental diet (Nestlé Purina EL for dogs), and no ideal human formulas. Commercial human formulas may be excessive in fat, of too high an osmolarity, contain lactose, be too low in amino acids, and/or be deficient in one or more vitamins or minerals. In this author's practice, a human elemental diet can be supplemented with a lactose-free whey protein isolate, multivitamins and minerals, and canola oil (as a source of linoleic and alpha-linolenic acids) for use in canine and feline patients.

Adverse Food Reactions
and Food-Responsive Enteropathy

Cases of gastrointestinal disease that respond completely to appropriate dietary management may or may not show histologic evidence of enteritis or morphologic changes (Allenspach et al. 2007; German et al. 2001). In practice, cats and dogs that present with chronic vomiting and/or diarrhea will usually be subjected to an elimination dietary trial and/or medication trials prior to the collection of intestinal biopsies. Therefore, when vomiting or diarrhea resolves with an elimination trial and no intestinal biopsies have been taken, the disease could be dietary hypersensitivity, dietary intolerance, or mild inflammatory enteropathy. In those cases, the term "food-responsive enteropathy" or "adverse food reaction" is appropriate. However, there are some circumstances that lead to procurement of intestinal biopsies prior to a dietary trial, which in some cases can produce unremarkable histologic findings. In those cases, an adverse reaction to food cannot and should not be excluded.

The ideal diagnostic and long-term diets for patients with adverse food reactions are based mostly on ingredient novelty and/or protein hydrolysis. However, other mechanisms than the immunologic responses to dietary antigens are probably more important when no inflammatory mucosal infiltrate is present. In a study of 55 cats with chronic vomiting and/or diarrhea, 16 cats were diagnosed as having food sensitivity based on elimination-challenge trials (Guilford et al. 2001). However, a further 11 cats responded completely to an elimination diet, but did not recrudesce during a challenge trial. Similar to the food-sensitive cats, the non-food-sensitive cats had a range of histopathologic changes from no to moderate lymphocytic-plasmacytic enteritis.

Recommendations

It is clear, then, that a large number of dogs and cats with chronic idiopathic gastrointestinal disease will respond completely to dietary manipulation. In the absence of a specific protein hypersensitivity, the mechanisms remain obscure. Possible mechanisms are listed in Table 11.5. However, ignorance of underlying mechanisms further increases the desire to manage such cases with highly digestible diets that contain as few ingredients as possible. The same general approach to the dietary choices for acute gastroenteritis is probably suitable for such cases.

Short Bowel Syndrome

Short bowel syndrome (SBS) is used to describe the nutritional and metabolic sequelae that accompany resection of sufficient small intestine to cause clinically significant malabsorption and malnutrition. Neoplasia,

Table 11.5 Potential mechanisms for non-immunologic adverse food reactions.

Factor	Mechanism
Digestibility	Poorly digestible nutrients leading to bacterial fermentation, osmotic diarrhea, etc.
Lactase deficiency	Undigested lactose leading to fermentation and osmotic diarrhea
Nutrient deficiency	For example, zinc, B12 leading to mucosal dysfunction
Fiber	Fiber-responsive diarrhea – promotion of water resorption, restored motility, prebiosis, increased fecal bulk, passage of hairballs
Food additives	Idiosyncratic, pharmacologic

intussusception, linear foreign bodies, trauma, infarction, and mesenteric torsion are all diseases that may require massive intestinal resection. Resection of at least 70% of the small intestine is required to induce SBS (Yanoff et al. 1992). In addition, the terminal ileum and ileocolic valves are of great physiologic value, and animals will perform much poorer even with only 50% resections if they are removed (Joy and Patterson 1978).

Pathophysiology

Following large-scale resection, postprandial motility is altered such that gastric emptying is delayed, and intestinal transit times are increased across the remaining portions (Johnson et al. 1996). The modification of motility appears to be an important part of the compensation for the loss of intestinal mass. Nonetheless, compensation through altered motility may be inadequate in the face of massive resection, such that artificially increasing intestinal transit times by inducing periods of retrograde movement of ingesta in portions of small intestine can lead to significantly increased absorption and clinical improvement (Gladen and Kelly 1980). These findings emphasize the importance of mixing and retaining ingesta in the remaining portion of the intestine, and highlight problems that accompany overfeeding at any one meal.

Loss of the absorptive area results in the inability to sustain adequate absorption of water, electrolytes, and other essential nutrients when fed conventional diets. Diarrhea, steatorrhea, water and electrolyte imbalances, nutrient deficiencies, and weight loss are likely to occur. Simple compensation through increased intake may be sufficient in mildly affected cases, but the majority require significant dietary adjustment. Dehydration, generalized protein-calorie malnutrition, and multiple nutrient deficiencies can result. Initial clinical signs include vomiting, diarrhea, and rapid weight loss (Johnson et al. 1996; Yanoff et al. 1992).

The active uptake of bile acids occurs in the ileum and is mediated by a sodium-dependent bile acid transporter in the brush-border membranes. Similarly, the enterocyte membrane receptor for the B12-intrinsic factor complex is expressed in the terminal ileum (Levine et al. 1984). Therefore, loss of the ileum leads to bile acid and vitamin B12 malabsorption. Given that both dogs and cats conjugate bile salts exclusively with taurine, ileal malabsorption can also lead to excessive losses of this amino acid.

Intestinal Adaptation

Through the mechanisms discussed (intestinal recovery and adaptation), the presence of luminal nutrients stimulates the remaining small intestine to undergo a period of hypertrophy and hyperplasia, which may continue for months. The colon also becomes an important digestive organ in patients with SBS (Jeppesen and Mortensen 1998). Sodium, water, and some amino acids are absorbed in the colon, as well as energy from absorbed short-chain fatty acids. Thus, a source of readily fermentable fiber should be included in all diets, while insoluble nonfermentable fiber should be kept to a minimum, to maximize nutrient digestibility (Roth et al. 1995).

Feeding Recommendations

Dietary management is complex and needs to be individualized for each patient on the basis of the residual intestine, nutritional state, current diet, underlying disease, and the client's lifestyle limitations. In addition to nutrient intake, management of SBS also requires appropriate oral rehydration, vitamin and mineral supplementation, and pharmacotherapy. Several medications provide a useful adjunctive function to dietary intervention, including antidiarrheal agents, H2 antagonists and proton pump inhibitors, pancreatic enzymes, and antibiotics. Future therapy will likely involve direct stimulation of intestinal adaptation through the administration of trophic factors such as GLP-2. The following list provides guidelines.

Resection of jejunum with intact duodenum, ileocolic valve, and colon. Feeding multiple small meals will improve absorption and decrease episodes of vomiting. Clinical improvements have been seen in the author's practice by increasing the frequency of feeding up to six times daily in some cases. Evenly spacing meals as much as possible will also help. As with most intestinal diseases, diets with high digestibility for fat, protein, and digestible carbohydrate should be preferred.

Fat is probably the limiting nutrient in absorption, and fat malabsorption likely exacerbates the diarrhea or vomiting in most cases. Avoidance of high-fat diets is recommended, although it is not known how restricted fat should be, and individualization is stressed. An empirical recommendation is to feed less than 25% of ME as fat, and reducing intake further if diarrhea or vomiting continues.

Dietary fiber is important to stimulate intestinal adaptation, maximize colonic absorption, and bind unabsorbed bile acids. However, excessive fiber will decrease diet digestibility, impair nutrient absorption, and exacerbate diarrhea. Psyllium and wheat bran have been shown to effectively bind bile acids, while guar gum is less effective, and cellulose is ineffective (Buhman et al. 1998; Ebihara and Schneeman 1989; Floren and Nilsson 1987; Ryden and Robertson 1997). The addition to the diet of 5% psyllium or wheat bran on a dry matter basis is reasonable, depending on the fiber content of the chosen diet, but improvements have been seen in the author's practice with the addition of up to 10% on a dry matter basis. Commercial high-fiber diets containing predominantly cellulose are not recommended. Any introduction or increase of fiber should be gradual over 3–5 days. Immediately after intestinal resection, water and electrolyte balances should be carefully monitored. Serum B12, folate, and taurine should be intermittently monitored after 2–4 weeks.

Hydrolyzed protein diets may be beneficial, although protein digestion and absorption are not thought to be limiting in most patients. In addition, currently available hydrolysate diets may not be restricted enough in their fat content for severely affected patients (Cave 2006).

Greater than 50% resection of the small intestine with partial resection of ileum. Bile salt–induced diarrhea is common and may not be adequately controlled through dietary fiber. If 5% (DM basis) psyllium or wheat bran is insufficient in controlling diarrhea, administration of cholestyramine 100–300 mg/kg orally every 12 h is recommended to bind bile salts left unabsorbed by the resected ileum. Supplemental taurine is advised in both cats and dogs with long-term cholestyramine treatment, and also may be needed if ileal reabsorption is insufficient to maintain normal status. Vitamin B12 absorption should be measured and, if low, the patient should be replenished by injecting vitamin B12, 250 μg (cats) or 500 μg (dogs) per dose, subcutaneously or intramuscularly, weekly for 4–5 weeks, then every 1–4 weeks as indicated; oral supplementation is not recommended.

Complete resection of ileum. Fat restriction is mandatory. Diets with less than 25% ME fat are indicated, and home-prepared diets formulated by a veterinary nutritionist may be required. With the larger resection, the bile acid pool can become depleted, and cholestyramine may not be beneficial. Parenteral vitamin B12 replacement and taurine (500 mg/day) supplementation are required.

Massive (>70%) resection of jejunum and ileum. Total parenteral nutrition or partial peripheral nutrition may be initially required. However, a delay in the introduction of enteral nutrition can limit the degree of intestinal adaptation. Initial oral feeding does not need to meet the nutritional requirement of the patient if parenteral nutrition is supplied, and as little as 25% of the patient's RER can be fed over several meals. After the initial period of parenteral nutrition, a concerted attempt should be made to wean patients onto an oral diet as soon as possible. An elemental diet may be required, although fiber supplementation is still likely to be beneficial, and careful attention to nutrient deficiency is still necessary (see earlier).

Large Intestinal Disease

Colitis

Acute Colitis

Ingestion and colonic passage of indigestible material form probably the most common cause of acute colitis; bone fragments, fabric, food packaging, and plant material are frequently incriminated in the author's experience. Other causes include infectious agents such as *Trichuris* spp., *Giardia* spp., and possibly bacterial pathogens such as *Campylobacter* spp., and *C. difficile* and *C. perfringens*. In many cases, the original insult has resolved or been passed by the time of presentation. As such, most cases resolve without specific diagnosis or management.

When colitis is present, there is an increase in the number of giant migrating peristaltic waves, while segmental contractions are decreased or even absent (Sethi and Sarna 1991). The absence of segmental contraction leads to frequent defecation following colonic peristalsis and produces urgency to defecate in the patient. A single colonic insult can result in prolonged disturbances of motility that can last 2–3 weeks, despite histologic resolution of inflammation (Sethi and Sarna 1991).

Normally in response to a meal there is an increase in segmental contractions along the colon, both immediately and several hours after a meal when ingesta enter the colon. Giant migrating contractions occur rarely in the first eight hours following a meal (Sarna and Lang 1989). When the colon is inflamed, that postprandial increase in segmental contractions does not occur, but instead feeding further increases the giant migrating waves that are increased by the inflammation (Sethi and Sarna 1991). The entry of ingesta into the inflamed colon during the late postprandial period stimulates an excessive number of giant migrating contractions. These peristaltic waves may be associated with postprandial abdominal discomfort and contribute to an increased frequency of defecation.

There are no published studies that have evaluated different dietary compositions for the management of acute colitis in dogs or cats. In light of the known effects of luminal ingesta on signs of colitis (e.g. diarrhea, urgency to defecate, abdominal discomfort), it seems prudent to recommend feeding a diet that results in the least possible amount of ingesta to be passed into the colon. Such a diet would be referred to as "low residue." Highly digestible diets formulated for small intestinal disease would therefore qualify. Avoiding high-fat diets may be warranted because of the effect of unabsorbed fatty acids on the colonic mucosa (see earlier). However, the caloric density and digestibility of fat allow for feeding smaller meals with lower residue. In addition, the presence of fat in the jejunum slows ileocolonic transit times in humans (Hammer et al. 1998). Lastly, in cats, dietary fat restriction has not been shown to be beneficial (Laflamme et al. 2011).

In direct contrast to the argument for highly digestible diets to be fed to patients with acute colitis is the observation that dietary fiber may be of benefit in many cases. The effect of dietary fiber in the colon has already been discussed. Fibers with differing degrees of fermentability produce different clinical effects. Variables that affect the response to dietary fiber in any patient include, but are not limited to, existing colonic microbiota, colonic motility, disease type, disease severity and heterogeneity along the colon, and background diet. At present, the interaction between differing fiber types and different diseases is not understood, nor is the disease in affected patients completely understood in most cases. For those reasons, it seems prudent when adding dietary fiber to recommend the empirical use of mixed fermentable sources such as psyllium husk, and, if the condition is poorly responsive, to try more fermentable sources such as hydrolyzed guar gum. When selecting commercial diets in cases of acute colitis, most commercial fiber sources could be considered to be mixed sources (e.g. pea hulls, soy fiber, rice bran) and would likely qualify empirically. There is still much to learn.

Chronic Colitis

Dietary requirements for chronic colitis are similar to those for acute colitis, namely the contrasting features of high digestibility to limit the passage of ingesta into the colon, and the provision of adequate dietary fiber. As for acute colitis, the ideal fiber quantity and type are not known, and likely differ between patients. Butyrate enemas have been shown to reduce inflammation and symptoms in humans suffering from CD or UC, demonstrating the need for some fermentable fiber to be present (Breuer et al. 1997; Luhrs et al. 2002; Patz et al. 1996). Additional benefits of non-fermentable fiber include adsorption of colonic bile acids and other mucosal irritants and the symptomatic improvement of fecal consistency.

In chronic colitis, the role of dietary antigens should also be considered. As in chronic small intestinal enteropathies, aberrant immune responses to luminal dietary antigens are prominent components of the disease in many patients. Many cases of canine food hypersensitivity that produce gastrointestinal signs have signs of large intestinal disease (Paterson 1995). In a study of 9 proven food-allergic dogs, 8 of the dogs had histologic evidence of mild to moderate lymphocytic-plasmacytic inflammation (Allenspach et al. 2006). In that same study, when the antigens, proven to be allergens by oral challenge, were injected into the colonic mucosa during colonoscopy, 17 of 23 allergens produced visible mucosal reactions (wheal and flare). In a report of 13 dogs with lymphocytic-plasmacytic colitis, clinical signs resolved in them all with the introduction of an elimination diet, and 9 of 11 dogs rechallenged with their original diet relapsed (Nelson et al. 1988). In a further report of 6 cats with lymphocytic-plasmacytic colitis, all responded completely to an elimination diet (Nelson et al. 1984). Thus aberrant (hypersensitive) immune responses to dietary antigens commonly affect the colon, whether or not signs of colonic disease are present. Conversely, when signs of chronic colitis are present, food hypersensitivity should be considered.

Similarly to chronic small intestinal inflammatory disease, the value of dietary enrichment with n-3 PUFAs for the management of chronic colitis has not been determined in dogs and cats. In the absence of evidence either way, it is reasonable to consider it as an intervention that may help. In mild cases of colonic IBD, a long-term clinical effect might occur as part of the general dietary manipulation, and in more severe cases, it may reduce the dependence on or dose of immunosuppressive therapy.

Previous reports of dogs with large-bowel signs and characterized as food responsive demonstrated that successful treatment included both hydrolyzed- and uncommon-ingredient diets (Allenspach et al. 2007, 2016). Overall recommendations are to select a diet that has highly digestible protein, fat, and carbohydrate components. Most high-quality veterinary therapeutic commercial diets would satisfy this requirement. If an initial response to dietary manipulation is not successful, adjust the dietary fiber content. It is currently impossible to know which animal will respond to what type and amount of dietary fiber, and empirical recommendations are misleading. Additionally, unless total dietary fiber values are provided by the manufacturer, diet comparisons are not possible, since the ingredient list and crude fiber measurements are of limited value. Mixed fermentable sources such as psyllium can be slowly introduced up to 10% of dry matter, while highly fermentable sources such as guar gum can be slowly introduced up to 5% of dry matter. It is unlikely that a clinical response will be seen with greater amounts. Lastly, enrichment of the diet with long-chain n-3 PUFAs may be tried (for suggested amounts, see earlier).

Idiopathic Large-Bowel Diarrhea

Idiopathic large-bowel diarrhea is diagnosed when chronic large-bowel diarrhea is present, when there is an absence of histologic evidence of colitis, and when inciting causes have been eliminated (Leib 2000). Several diagnostic terms would fall under this definition, including irritable bowel syndrome (IBS), colonic dysmotility, fiber-responsive diarrhea, stress-induced colitis, and non-specific dietary sensitivity. By definition, these cases have not responded to a strict, limited, novel-, or hydrolyzed-ingredient diet trial, but they may have idiosyncratic improvements when switched from one diet to another. In one study of 37 cases of idiopathic large-bowel diarrhea, 63% responded excellently to the addition of psyllium husk powder to a highly digestible fat-restricted diet (Leib 2000). Only one case had a very poor response. The dosage used was approximately 1 g/kg/day, with a range of 0.3–4.9 g psyllium/kg/day.

Dogs with intermittently poorly formed feces that respond to a change in diet for which no mechanism is clear are referred to as being affected with non-specific dietary sensitivity. In the majority of these cases, a clear hypersensitivity is not demonstrated. Additionally, affected dogs appear to more consistently suffer from colonic dysfunction than small intestinal dysfunction (Zentek et al. 2002). Common histologic findings in the colon include reduced mucosal crypt depth, crypt widening, and increased numbers of intraepithelial T lymphocytes (Rolfe et al. 2002; Zentek et al. 2002). Water absorption may be reduced, which is associated with reduced sodium and chloride absorption (Rolfe et al. 2002). This problem appears more common in large- rather than small-breed dogs. Fecal water content is likely to be decreased if dry extruded food is fed in preference to high-moisture canned diets, although overall fecal consistency is not necessarily improved in affected dogs by simply changing to a dry extruded diet (Zentek et al. 2004). In addition, the fecal quality of some dogs may not improve with increased soluble and insoluble dietary fiber.

Thus idiopathic large-bowel diarrhea may respond to increased dietary fiber, or it may be responsive to other dietary manipulations for reasons that are not clear. Failure to respond to one empirical dietary manipulation (e.g. the addition of fiber) should not sway the clinician away from further empirical dietary choices.

Constipation and Megacolon

Constipation can be defined as incomplete or infrequent defecation of hardened feces, often with a decreased water content, and is usually associated with tenesmus. Constipation can occur as the result of excessive dehydration of the luminal contents and/or impaired motility. Dietary variables that lead to constipation have not been well defined in dogs or cats. However, in cats, risk factors may include obesity, increased age, chronic kidney disease, and previous episodes of constipation (Benjamin and Drobatz 2020). Ingestion of large amounts of indigestible material such as bone or wool is commonly incriminated (Nemeth et al. 2008). In normal humans, colonic transit time is decreased as insoluble fiber is increased, while in patients with chronic constipation, increased insoluble fiber does not speed fecal transit (Muller-Lissner 1988). Whether that reflects a cause or effect is uncertain, as is the significance to canine and feline patients. It is likely that colonic transit time partly determines the response to dietary manipulation, as it does in people (Hagiwara and Tomita 2008). However, there are no established diagnostic protocols for clearly determining colonic motility in dogs or cats and no evidence for recommending one intervention over another.

Insoluble non-fermentable fiber increases fecal bulk and the frequency of defecation in a normal individual. Increasing fecal bulk may exacerbate constipation in an individual with impaired colonic motility. Perhaps the poorest choice of dietary fiber in constipation is a non-fermentable, insoluble fiber that increases

fecal dry matter but not fecal water content, such as cellulose (Wichert et al. 2002). Fiber that produces viscous gels (e.g. psyllium husk) will increase the fecal water content, in addition to increasing fecal dry matter. Some evidence supports the successful use of a moderate amount of mixed fiber sources, including psyllium seed husk, as a long-term treatment for constipation in cats (Freiche et al. 2011; Wernimont et al. 2020).

Short-chain fatty acids from colonic fermentation have been shown to stimulate longitudinal colonic smooth muscle contractions in kittens and adult cats in vitro (Rondeau et al. 2003). However, highly fermentable fiber may also result in the production of methane. Methane production varies greatly between individuals, and in humans it appears to be dependent on the presence of specific organisms and is produced in about half of normal individuals (McKay et al. 1985). Recently, it has been shown that physiologic concentrations of methane slow small intestinal transit by augmenting ileal circular muscle contractions (Pimentel et al. 2006). In addition, when methane is the bacterial fermentation product in human patients with IBS, those patients almost universally suffer from constipation, and small intestinal contractile activity and discomfort are increased in IBS patients who produce methane (Pimentel et al. 2003, 2006). Thus the induction of non-propulsive segmental contractions by methane may be a cause of motility dysfunction in dogs and cats. Consequently, the supplementation of diets with rapidly fermentable purified fiber sources such as hydrolyzed guar gum may exacerbate some cases of constipation, IBS, and other diseases that involve disturbances of motility.

Thus, individualization is key to successful dietary modification in patients with chronic constipation. When colonic motility is known or suspected to be impaired (e.g. megacolon), diets with moderate (<10% dm basis) contents of total dietary fiber are recommended in order to reduce fecal volume. When colonic motility is still suspected to be reasonable, increasing non-fermentable, gel-forming fiber is likely to be beneficial. A total dietary fiber content of 10–20% on a dry matter basis is reasonable.

Intestinal Gas and Flatulence

Intestinal Gas Transit and Borborygmus

Gas that is present in the small and large intestine can originate from aerophagia or be endogenously formed. Intestinal CO_2 is mostly formed from the reaction between bicarbonate and gastric acid producing water and CO_2 in the upper small intestine. For each mol of H^+ neutralized by pancreatic HCO_3^-, 1 mol of CO_2 is produced. In the three hours following a meal, a dog may produce 6 mEq H^+, which will result in the production of 134 ml CO_2 (Thor et al. 1977). Most of the CO_2 diffuses into the circulation, but some remains within the luminal contents. The remaining gases are produced from microbial fermentation, predominantly in the distal small intestine and colon.

Gas is moved along the intestine independently of solids and liquids, and in humans gas transit is more effective in the erect than supine position, illustrating the active propulsion of gas (Dainese et al. 2003). The rate of gas passage is influenced by dietary fat, but not by the moisture content of the diet (Gonlachanvit et al. 2006). Intestinal gas can be rapidly propelled aborally in normal dogs such that the infusion of air at 2 ml/min does not produce apparent abdominal discomfort (Pimentel et al. 2006). In humans, up to 30 ml/min can be infused jejunally without discomfort. Gas is actively propelled by a sustained contraction proximal to the gas, but it is still not known if intestinal gas induces classical peristaltic waves responsible for the movement of liquid and solid ingesta (Tremolaterra et al. 2006). Following a meal, the presence of lipid within the duodenum induces intestinal relaxation and leads to an increase in the intraluminal pool (Hernando-Harder et al. 2004). In humans, drinking water does not influence gas transit, while food increases the rate of transit and volume of gas that reaches the anus

(Gonlachanvit et al. 2006). The presence of duodenal lipid has the most profound inhibitory effect on gas transit times, while fiber (psyllium husk) also slows intestinal gas transit, as well as increasing the volume of gas produced from fermentation (Gonlachanvit et al. 2004; Harder et al. 2006; Hernando-Harder et al. 2004). In contrast, the intestinal transit of gas is not influenced by the moisture content of the diet (Gonlachanvit et al. 2006).

In humans, the retention of infused gas can be halved and the retardant effect of duodenal lipid can be reversed by gentle physical exercise (peddling on an adapted bicycle ergometer not sufficient to raise heart rate or blood pressure) (Villoria et al. 2006). Although not directly studied in dogs, flatulence is reported less frequently by owners of dogs that exercise frequently than by owners of sedentary dogs (Jones et al. 1998).

Borborygmus can result from excessive intestinal gas or altered motility. Humans with IBS who have bloating and borborygmus as symptoms have impaired gas transit and develop intestinal gas retention, intestinal distension, and pain in response to gas loads that are well tolerated by normal individuals (Passos et al. 2005). In those patients, proximal intestinal gas rather than large intestinal gas is responsible for their symptoms (Salvioli et al. 2005).

Flatulence

The dominance of atmospheric gases in flatus illustrates that ingested gas forms the largest component. However, odiferous compounds are the result of microbial fermentation of luminal contents. In dogs, flatulence is more likely to occur within two hours of feeding, although the presence of sulfur gases is not temporally related to feeding (Collins et al. 2001; Yamka et al. 2006). Thus ingested air is likely rapidly transported and passed after a meal, while fermentative by-products may accumulate at other times. Malodor is strongly correlated with the presence of hydrogen sulfide, and the production of hydrogen sulfide is highly variable among animals fed the same diet (Collins et al. 2001). Sulfur gases are produced by sulfate-reducing bacteria such as the genera *Desulfotomaculum*, *Desulfobacter*, *Desulfomonas*, and *Desulfobulbus*, and differences in sulfur gas production between animals likely represent differences in microbiota (Gibson et al. 1988). Sources of sulfur compounds for fermentation include endogenously derived amino acids from mucin, sulfate in cruciferous vegetables and nuts, and poorly digestible sulfated polysaccharides such as the gelling agent carrageenan.

As noted earlier, fiber slows intestinal gas transport, but fermentable fiber is also a substrate for the luminal production of intestinal gas, and in normal humans fiber intake is positively associated with the number of daily flatus emissions (Bolin and Stanton 1998; Gonlachanvit et al. 2004; Marthinsen and Fleming 1982; Tomlin et al. 1991). Thus, high-fiber diets can increase gas production by colonic flora and inhibit gas transit, leading to gas retention, notable borborygmus, abdominal pain, and flatulence (Gonlachanvit et al. 2004). Ingestion of a "fiber-free" diet for 48 hours significantly reduces the total volume of flatus (Tomlin et al. 1991). Highly purified, highly fermentable fibers will increase flatus volumes more than non-fermentable fiber and will also alter the composition of the flatus. For instance, xylan and pectin cause higher flatus volume, hydrogen, CO_2, and methane levels than cellulose or corn bran (Marthinsen and Fleming 1982). In addition, intestinal and/or microbial adaptation to changes in fiber content has been demonstrated, such that flatus volumes do not stabilize until 2–5 days of feeding have accrued (Marthinsen and Fleming 1982).

The exact nature of flatus then is affected by the composition and quantity of diet fed, its digestibility, and the type and abundance of bacterial flora. Any disease causing maldigestion or malabsorption will increase and alter the substrate available for fermentation and will thus alter the volume and odor of flatus produced.

In the absence of a primary diagnosis, the symptomatic management of borborygmus and flatulence should begin with a change to a highly digestible, low-fat diet. As with any dietary variable, there is no absolute value that constitutes "high" or "low," and they remain relative and subjective terms. Importantly, an attempt should be made to introduce a diet that has a greater digestibility and a lower fat content than the current diet. Empirical choices would be select protein diets with less than 20% ME as fat. Hydrolyzed-ingredient diets have high protein digestibility, and most contain highly digestible carbohydrate sources as well; however, the fat content may be greater than ideal. Diets with fermentable fiber sources (e.g. gums, carrageenan, pectins, resistant starches) in greater concentrations than the current diet should be avoided (Tomlin et al. 1991). Empirically, crude fiber contents of less than 3% would probably suffice.

Another option is a homemade diet comprising highly digestible protein and carbohydrate sources appropriately balanced with vitamins and minerals. Suitable home-prepared diets for managing acute gastroenteritis or dietary indiscretion in dogs and cats include cottage cheese (see Table 11.4). Therefore, it has an ideal macronutrient profile, with an easy energy density to calculate the amount to feed. For diagnostic and short-term purposes, nutrient balancing of the diet is unnecessary, and these diets can be fed safely to a previously well-nourished animal for at least seven days without concern.

The possibility of food hypersensitivity should also be considered in any patient with chronic flatulence or borborygmus, and novel- or hydrolyzed-ingredient diets should be introduced. It is recommended that a short-term switch to a highly digestible, low-fat diet be considered prior to concerns of novelty. If the initial dietary change is unsuccessful, a home-prepared or commercial novel or hydrolyzed protein should be tried. Of course, an ideal initial management of both acute and chronic borborygmus and flatulence is to feed a diet that is limited, novel or hydrolyzed, highly digestible, very low in fat, and very low in fermentable fiber. Appropriately balanced home-prepared recipes are probably the only diets that achieve all the stated goals.

As mentioned before, flatulence is reported less frequently by owners of dogs that exercise frequently than by owners of sedentary dogs (Jones et al. 1998). The effect of exercise would be consistent with findings in humans. It is not known, however, if the timing of exercise relative to meals is important, nor what amount of exercise is required. Experiments in humans suggest that very little activity is necessary to promote gas movement. On that basis, it is prudent to recommend an increase in daily exercise for dogs, and to encourage physical activity in cats for whom flatulence is problematic.

Increasing the frequency of feeding is often suggested as a potential therapy for flatulence, ostensibly to slow the delivery of nutrients to the small intestine and allow greater digestion or absorption. In normal pigs, increasing the feeding frequency from once to twice daily increased protein digestibility in one study, but not in another (Holt et al. 2006; Mroz et al. 1994). In pigs with ligated pancreatic ducts there was no effect of the frequency of feeding on digestibility (Kammlott et al. 2005). There is no evidence that changing the frequency of feeding has any effect on digestibility in dogs or cats. A study of flatulence in dogs revealed a decrease in the frequency of flatus in dogs fed twice (9.9 flatuses/day) compared with once (13.5 flatuses/day) a day (Yamka et al. 2006). Owners of dogs fed more than once a day did not report flatulence in their dogs more frequently than owners that fed only once daily (Jones et al. 1998). Thus, increasing the frequency of feeding may, in some dogs or cats, decrease flatulence, but at best the effect is mild.

Symptomatic therapy for eructation centers on attempts to reduce aerophagia. However, there are no studies that have evaluated the efficacy of methods for reducing aerophagia.

Avoiding situations that provoke nervousness and discouraging greedy eating (for instance, by ensuring that a dog does not have to compete for its food) may be helpful. Feeding multiple small meals may reduce the gastric distension secondary to aerophagia by allowing sufficient time between a series of mouthfuls for eructation to occur. Head elevation may reduce aerophagia in some dogs, but could also increase it in others.

In the rare event that dietary manipulation and regular exercise are not successful in eliminating signs, the patient should be evaluated for the presence of organic or functional intestinal disease such as described for small intestinal diarrhea. Alternatively, symptomatic pharmacologic management can be tried.

Summary

- Timing and frequency of feeding, route of feeding, and macronutrient and micronutrient compositions of the diet have profound influences on oral and intestinal health. There is also a considerable indirect effect through dietary influences on the intestinal microbiota.
- Periodontal disease is the most common disease affecting domestic dogs and cats. Although chewing activities and dietary additives may be sufficient to reduce plaque or even prevent calculus, only those activities that provide appropriate gingival stimulation will prevent gingivitis and periodontitis.
- Elevated feeding to promote passage via gravity is usually recommended in patients with megaesophagus, whatever food is selected. Hand feeding chunks of meat or meatballs while the patient remains in a seated position is very effective.
- The main feeding concern for patients with esophagitis is the risk of promoting gastroesophageal reflux. The most important variables that increase gastroesophageal reflux induced by a meal are volume, total energy

content, osmolarity, rate of ingestion of the meal, and possibly postprandial exercise.

- In cases where oral feeding is not possible in patients with esophageal disease, gastrostomy tube placement is indicated.
- The optimal nutritional approach for dogs and cats with chronic enteropathy remains to be determined and certainly varies from animal to animal. Regardless of the underlying etiology for any given patient, abnormal immune responses to dietary antigens are often suspected, and the clinical response to novel-protein diets supports that hypothesis.
- When severe lymphangiectasia accompanies chronic enteropathy, priority should be given to the feeding of a restricted-fat diet over antigenic novelty, since the hypoproteinemia is often the most life-threatening derangement.
- The ideal diagnostic and long-term diets for patients with adverse food reactions are based mostly on a limited number of ingredients that are novel, hydrolyzed, or elemental.
- Dehydration, generalized protein-calorie malnutrition, and multiple nutrient deficiencies can result in animals with short bowel syndrome. Simple compensation through increased intake may be sufficient

in mildly affected cases, but the majority require significant dietary adjustment.

- Overall recommendations for the management of chronic colitis are first to change to a limited-, novel-, hydrolyzed-, or elemental-ingredient diet. If an initial response to dietary manipulation is not successful, adjust the dietary fiber content.
- Idiopathic large-bowel diarrhea may respond to increased dietary fiber or may be responsive to other dietary manipulations for reasons that are not clear. Failure to respond to one empirical dietary manipulation (e.g. the addition of fiber) should not sway the clinician away from further empirical dietary choices.
- When colonic motility is known or suspected to be impaired (e.g. megacolon), low-residue diets with moderate (<10% dry matter basis) contents of total dietary fiber are recommended. When colonic motility is still suspected to be reasonable, increasing non-fermentable, gel-forming fiber is likely to be beneficial.
- In the absence of a primary diagnosis, the symptomatic management of borborygmus and flatulence should begin with a change to a highly digestible, low-fat diet. Feeding small, multiple meals and increasing activity may also help manage these conditions.

References

AAFCO (2022). *Official Publication*. Oxford, IN: Association of American Feed Control Officials.

Abramovitch, J.B., Lopata, A.L., O'Hehir, R. et al. (2017). Effect of thermal processing on T cell reactivity of shellfish allergens – discordance with IgE reactivity. *PLoS One* 12 (3): e0173549.

Abreu, M.T., Vora, P., Faure, E. et al. (2001). Decreased expression of Toll-like receptor-4 and MD-2 correlates with intestinal epithelial cell protection against dysregulated proinflammatory gene expression in response

to bacterial lipopolysaccharide. *J. Immunol.* 167 (3): 1609–1616.

Alam, N.H., Ahmed, T., Khatun, M. et al. (1992). Effects of food with two oral rehydration therapies: a randomised controlled clinical trial. *Gut* 33 (4): 560–562.

Alberts, D.S., Ritenbaugh, C., Story, J.A. et al. (1996). Randomized, double-blinded, placebo-controlled study of effect of wheat bran fiber and calcium on fecal bile acids in patients with resected adenomatous colon polyps. *J. Natl. Cancer Inst.* 88 (2): 81–92.

Allen, R.M., Adams, V.J., and Johnston, N.W. (2019). Prospective randomized blinded clinical trial assessing effectiveness of three dental plaque control methods in dogs. *J. Small Anim. Pract.* 60: 212–217.

Allenspach, K. (2011). Clinical immunology and immunopathology of the canine and feline intestine. *Vet. Clin. North Am. Small Anim. Pract.* 41: 345–360.

Allenspach, K., Vaden, S.L., Harris, T. et al. (2006). Evaluation of colonoscopic allergen provocation as a diagnostic tool in dogs with proven food hypersensitivity reactions. *J. Small Anim. Pract.* 47 (1): 21–26.

Allenspach, K., Wieland, B., Gröne, A., and Gaschen, F. (2007). Chronic enteropathies in dogs: evaluation of risk factors for negative outcome. *J. Vet. Intern. Med.* 21 (4): 700–708.

Allenspach, K., Culverwell, C., and Chan, D.L. (2016). Long-term outcome in dogs with chronic enteropathies: 203 cases. *Vet. Rec.* 178 (15): 368–368.

Almallah, Y.Z., Richardson, S., O'Hanrahan, T. et al. (1998). Distal procto-colitis, natural cytotoxicity, and essential fatty acids. *Am. J. Gastroenterol.* 93 (5): 804–809.

Altaf, W., Perveen, S., Rehman, K.U. et al. (2002). Zinc supplementation in oral rehydration solutions: experimental assessment and mechanisms of action. *J. Am. Coll. Nutr.* 21 (1): 26–32.

Alves, J.C., Santos, A., Jorge, P., and Pitaes, A. (2021). The use of soluble fibre for the management of chronic idiopathic large-bowel diarrhoea in police working dogs. *BMC Vet. Res.* 17 (1): 100.

Ames, J.M., Wynne, A., Hofmann, A. et al. (1999). The effect of a model melanoidin mixture on faecal bacterial populations *in vitro*. *Br. J. Nutr.* 82 (6): 489–495.

Antin, J., Gibbs, J., Holt, J. et al. (1975). Cholecystokinin elicits the complete behavioral sequence of satiety in rats. *J. Comp. Physiol. Psychol.* 89 (7): 784–790.

Ashraf, W., Lof, J., Jin, G. et al. (1994). Comparative effects of intraduodenal psyllium and senna on canine small bowel motility. *Aliment. Pharmacol. Ther.* 8 (3): 329–336.

Babka, J.C. and Castell, D.O. (1973). On the genesis of heartburn. The effects of specific foods on the lower esophageal sphincter. *Am. J. Dig. Dis.* 18 (5): 391–397.

Backus, R.C., Rosenquist, G.L., Rogers, Q.R. et al. (1995). Elevation of plasma cholecystokinin (CCK) immunoreactivity by fat, protein, and amino acids in the cat, a carnivore. *Regul. Pept.* 57 (2): 123–131.

Backus, R.C., Howard, K.A., and Rogers, Q.R. (1997). The potency of dietary amino acids in elevating plasma cholecystokinin immunoreactivity in cats is related to amino acid hydrophobicity. *Regul. Pept.* 72 (1): 31–40.

Bamba, T., Kanauchi, O., Andoh, A. et al. (2002). A new prebiotic from germinated barley for nutraceutical treatment of ulcerative colitis. *J. Gastroenterol. Hepatol.* 17 (8): 818–824.

Barcelo, A., Claustre, J., Moro, F. et al. (2000). Mucin secretion is modulated by luminal factors in the isolated vascularly perfused rat colon. *Gut* 46 (2): 218–224.

Bark, T., Katouli, M., Svenberg, T. et al. (1995). Food deprivation increases bacterial translocation after non-lethal haemorrhage in rats. *Eur. J. Surg.* 161 (2): 67–71.

Bartram, H.P., Scheppach, W., Englert, S. et al. (1995). Effects of deoxycholic acid and butyrate on mucosal prostaglandin E2 release and cell proliferation in the human sigmoid colon. *JPEN J. Parent Enter. Nutr.* 19 (3): 182–186.

Bauer, J.E. (2007). Responses of dogs to dietary omega-3 fatty acids. *J. Am. Vet. Med. Assoc.* 231 (11): 1657–1661.

Beaulieu, A.D., Drackley, J.K., Overton, T.R. et al. (2002). Isolated canine and murine intestinal cells exhibit a different pattern of fuel utilization for oxidative metabolism. *J. Anim. Sci.* 80 (5): 1223–1232.

Bednar, G.E., Murray, S.M., Patil, A.R. et al. (2000). Selected animal and plant protein sources affect nutrient digestibility and fecal characteristics of ileally cannulated dogs. *Arch. Tierernahr.* 53 (2): 127–140.

Bednar, G.E., Patil, A.R., Murray, S.M. et al. (2001). Starch and fiber fractions in selected food and feed ingredients affect their small intestinal digestibility and fermentability and their large bowel fermentability *in vitro* in a canine model. *J. Nutr.* 131 (2): 276–286.

Beglinger, C., Degen, L., Matzinger, D. et al. (2001). Loxiglumide, a CCK-A receptor antagonist, stimulates calorie intake and hunger feelings in humans. *Am. J. Physiol. Regul. Integr. Comp. Physiol.* 280 (4): R1149–R1154.

Belsheim, M.R., Darwish, R.Z., Watson, W.C. et al. (1983). Bacterial L-form isolation from inflammatory bowel disease patients. *Gastroenterology* 85 (2): 364–369.

Benjamin, S.E. and Drobatz, K.J. (2020). Retrospective evaluation of risk factors and treatment outcome predictors in cats presenting to the emergency room for constipation. *J. Feline Med. Surg.* 22 (2): 153–160.

Bi, S. and Moran, T.H. (2002). Actions of CCK in the controls of food intake and body weight: lessons from the CCK-A receptor deficient OLETF rat. *Neuropeptides* 36 (2–3): 171–181.

Blaut, M. (2002). Relationship of prebiotics and food to intestinal microflora. *Eur. J. Nutr.* 41 (Suppl 1): 111–116.

Bodemer, C., Guillet, G., Cambazard, F. et al. (2017). Adjuvant treatment with the bacterial lysate (OM-85) improves management of atopic dermatitis: a randomized study. *PLoS One* 12 (3): e0161555.

Bolin, T.D. and Stanton, R.A. (1998). Flatus emission patterns and fiber intake. *Eur. J. Surg. Suppl.* 582: 115–118.

Bounous, G. and Kongshavn, P.A. (1985). Differential effect of dietary protein type on the B-cell and T-cell immune responses in mice. *J. Nutr.* 115: 1403–1408.

Boza, J.J., Maire, J.-C., Bovetto, L. et al. (2000a). Plasma glutamine response to enteral administration of glutamine in human volunteers (free glutamine versus protein-bound glutamine). *Nutrition* 16 (11–12): 1037–1042.

Boza, J.J., Moennoz, D., Vuichoud, J. et al. (2000b). Protein hydrolysate vs free amino acid-based diets on the nutritional recovery of the starved rat. *Eur. J. Nutr.* 39 (6): 237–243.

Brandtzaeg, P. (2001). Nature and function of gastrointestinal antigen-presenting cells. *Allergy Suppl* s67: 16–20.

Brandtzaeg, P. (2002). Current understanding of gastrointestinal immunoregulation and its relation to food allergy. *Ann. N. Y. Acad. Sci.* 964: 13–45.

Breuer, R.I., Soergel, K.H., Lashner, B.A. et al. (1997). Short chain fatty acid rectal irrigation for left-sided ulcerative colitis: a randomised, placebo controlled trial. *Gut* 40 (4): 485–491.

Brown, W.Y. and McGenity, P. (2005). Effective periodontal disease control using dental hygiene chews. *J. Vet. Dent.* 22 (1): 16–19.

Brown, M.G. and Park, J.F. (1968). Control of dental calculus in experimental beagles. *Lab. Anim. Care* 18 (5): 527–535.

Bueno, L. and Fioramonti, J. (1994). Neurohormonal control of intestinal transit. *Reprod. Nutr. Dev.* 34 (6): 513–525.

Buhman, K.K., Furumoto, E.J., Donkin, S.S. et al. (1998). Dietary psyllium increases fecal bile acid excretion, total steroid excretion and bile acid biosynthesis in rats. *J. Nutr.* 128 (7): 1199–1203.

Burgener, I.A., Konig, A., Allenspach, K. et al. (2008). Upregulation of toll-like receptors in chronic enteropathies in dogs. *J. Vet. Intern. Med.* 22 (3): 553–560.

Burwasser, P. and Hill, T.J. (1939). The effect of hard and soft diets on the gingival tissues of dogs. *J. Dental Res.* 18: 389–393.

Butowski, C.F., Thomas, D.G., Young, W. et al. (2019). Addition of plant dietary fibre to a raw red meat high protein, high fat diet, alters the faecal bacteriome and organic acid profiles of the domestic cat (*Felis catus*). *PLoS One* 14 (5): e0216072.

Calder, P.C. and Grimble, R.F. (2002). Polyunsaturated fatty acids, inflammation and immunity. *Eur. J. Clin. Nutr.* 56 (Suppl 3): S14–S19.

Calder, P.C., Bond, J.A., Harvey, D.J. et al. (1990). Uptake and incorporation of saturated and unsaturated fatty acids into macrophage lipids and their effect upon macrophage adhesion and phagocytosis. *Biochem J.* 269 (3): 807–814.

Carswell, F., Merrett, J., Merrett, T.G. et al. (1977). IgE, parasites and asthma in Tanzanian children. *Clin. Allergy* 7 (5): 445–453.

Cave, N.J. (2006). Hydrolyzed protein diets for dogs and cats. *Vet. Clin. North Am. Small Anim. Pract.* 36 (6): 1251–1268.

Cave, N.J. and Marks, S.L. (2004). Evaluation of the immunogenicity of dietary proteins in cats and the influence of the canning process. *Am. J. Vet. Res.* 65 (10): 1427–1433.

Center, S.A., Warner, K., Corbett, J. et al. (2000). Proteins invoked by vitamin K absence and clotting times in clinically ill cats. *J. Vet. Intern. Med.* 14: 292–297.

Cerquetella, M., Rossi, G., Suchodolski, J.S. et al. (2020). Proposal for rational antibacterial use in the diagnosis and treatment of dogs with chronic diarrhoea. *J. Small Anim. Pract.* 61 (4): 211–215.

Chance, W.T., Sheriff, S., Foley-Nelson, T. et al. (2000). Maintaining gut integrity during parenteral nutrition of tumorbearing rats: effects of glucagon-like peptide 2. *Nutr. Cancer* 37 (2): 215–222.

Chang, C.-H., Lidbury, J.A., Suchadolski, J.S. et al. (2022). Effect of oral or injectable supplementation with cobalamin in dogs with hypocobalaminemia caused by chronic enteropathy or exocrine pancreatic insufficiency. *J. Vet. Intern. Med.* 36 (5): 1607–1621.

Chapkin, R.S., Fan, Y., and Lupton, J.R. (2000). Effect of diet on colonic-programmed cell death: molecular mechanism of action. *Toxicol. Lett.* 112–113: 411–414.

Charoenkwan, K., Phillipson, G., and Vutyavanich, T. (2007). Early versus delayed (traditional) oral fluids and food for reducing complications after major abdominal gynaecologic surgery. *Cochrane Database Syst. Rev.* (4): CD004508.

Clarke, D.E. and Cameron, A. (1998). Relationship between diet, dental calculus and periodontal disease in domestic and feral cats in Australia. *Aust. Vet. J.* 76 (10): 690–693.

Collins, S.B., Perez-Camargo, G., Gettinby, G. et al. (2001). Development of a technique for the *in vivo* assessment of flatulence in dogs. *Am. J. Vet. Res.* 62 (7): 1014–1019.

Colombo, P., Mangano, M., Bianchi, P.A. et al. (2002). Effect of calories and fat on postprandial gastro-oesophageal reflux. *Scand. J. Gastroenterol.* 37 (1): 3–5.

Cuadrado, C., Sanchiz, A., Vicente, F. et al. (2020). Changes induced by pressure processing on immunoreactive proteins of tree nuts. *Molecules* 25 (4): 954.

Cummings, J.H., Wiggins, H.S., Jenkins, D.J. et al. (1978). Influence of diets high and low in animal fat on bowel habit, gastrointestinal transit time, fecal microflora, bile acid, and fat excretion. *J. Clin. Invest.* 61 (4): 953–963.

Cummings, J.H., Macfarlane, G.T., and Englyst, H.N. (2001). Prebiotic digestion and fermentation. *Am. J. Clin. Nutr.* 73 (2 Suppl): 415S–420S.

Dainese, R., Serra, J., Azpiroz, F. et al. (2003). Influence of body posture on intestinal transit of gas. *Gut* 52 (7): 971–974.

Dandrieux, J.D.S. and Mansfield, C.S. (2019). Chronic enteropathy in canines: prevalence, impact, and management strategies. *Vet. Med. (Auckl.)* 10: 203–214.

Dann, J.R., Adler, M.A., Duffy, K.L. et al. (2004). A potential nutritional prophylactic for the reduction of feline hairball symptoms. *J. Nutr.* 134 (8 Suppl): 2124S–2125S.

Davenport, D.J., Leib, M.S., and Remillard, R.L. (2010). Pharyngeal and esophageal disorders. In: *Small Animal Clinical Nutrition*, 5the (ed. M.S. Hand, C.D. Thatcher, R.L. Remillard, et al.), 1014–1022. Topeka, KS: Mark Morris Institute.

Defilippi, C. (2003). Canine small bowel motor activity in response to intraduodenal infusion of nutrient mixtures of increasing caloric load in dogs. *Dig. Dis. Sci.* 48 (8): 1482–1486.

Depauw, S., Bosch, G., Hesta, M. et al. (2012). Fermentation of animal components in strict carnivores: a comparative study with cheetah fecal inoculum. *J. Anim. Sci.* 90 (8): 2540–2548.

Depauw, S., Hesta, M., Whitehouse-Tedd, K. et al. (2013). Animal fibre: the forgotten nutrient in strict carnivores? First insights in the cheetah. *J. Anim. Physiol. Anim. Nutr. (Berl.)* 97 (1): 146–154.

DeVries, J.W. (2003). On defining dietary fiber. *Proc. Nutr. Soc.* 62 (1): 37–43.

Dichi, I., Frenhane, P., Dichi, J.B. et al. (2000). Comparison of omega-3 fatty acids and sulfasalazine in ulcerative colitis. *Nutrition* 16 (2): 87–90.

Dikeman, C.L., Murphy, M.R., and Fahey, G.C. Jr. (2007). Diet type affects viscosity of ileal digesta of dogs and simulated gastric and small intestinal digesta. *J. Anim. Physiol. Anim. Nutr. (Berl.)* 91 (3–4): 139–147.

Dionigi, R., Ariszonta, L.D. et al. (1977). The effects of total parenteral nutrition on immunodepression due to malnutrition. *Ann. Surg.* 185 (4): 467–474.

Do, S., Phungviwatnikul, T., de Godoy, M.R.C. et al. (2021). Nutrient digestibility and fecal characteristics, microbiota, and metabolites in dogs fed human-grade foods. *J. Anim. Sci.* 99 (2): skab028.

Domingues, L.M., Alessi, A.C., Canola, J.C. et al. (1999). Type and frequency of dental diseases and disorders in dogs in the region of Jaboticabal, Sp. *Arq Bras. Med. Vet. Zootec* 51 (4): 323–328.

Donadelli, R.A. and Aldrich, C.G. (2020). The effects of diets varying in fibre sources on nutrient utilization, stool quality and hairball management in cats. *J. Anim. Physiol. Anim. Nutr. (Berl.)* 104 (2): 715–724.

Dooper, M.M., Wassink, L., M'Rabet, L. et al. (2002). The modulatory effects of prostaglandin-E on cytokine production by human peripheral blood mononuclear cells are independent of the prostaglandin subtype. *Immunology* 107 (1): 152–159.

Drucker, D.J., DeForest, L., and Brubaker, P.L. (1997). Intestinal response to growth factors administered alone or in combination with human [Gly2]glucagon-like peptide 2. *Am. J. Physiol.* 273 (6 Pt 1): G1252–G1262.

Dube, P.E., Forse, C.L., Bahrami, J. et al. (2006). The essential role of insulin-like growth factor-1 in the intestinal tropic effects of glucagon-like peptide-2 in mice. *Gastroenterology* 131 (2): 589–605.

Dust, J.M., Grieshop, C.M., Parsons, C.M. et al. (2005). Chemical composition, protein quality, palatability, and digestibility of alternative protein sources for dogs. *J. Anim. Sci.* 83 (10): 2414–2422.

Ebihara, K. and Schneeman, B.O. (1989). Interaction of bile acids, phospholipids, cholesterol and triglyceride with dietary fibers in the small intestine of rats. *J. Nutr.* 119 (8): 1100–1106.

Egelberg, J. (1965a). Local effect of diet on plaque formation and development of gingivitis in dogs. I. Effect of hard and soft diets. *Odontol. Revy* 16: 31–41.

Egelberg, J. (1965b). Local effect of diet on plaque formation and development of gingivitis in dogs. 3. Effect of frequency of meals and tube feeding. *Odontol. Revy* 16: 50–60.

Eiserich, J.P., Patel, R.P., and O'Donnell, V.B. (1998). Pathophysiology of nitric oxide and related species: free radical reactions and modification of biomolecules. *Mol. Aspects Med.* 19 (4–5): 221–357.

Farness, P.L. and Schneeman, B.O. (1982). Effects of dietary cellulose, pectin and oat bran on the small intestine in the rat. *J. Nutr.* 112 (7): 1315–1319.

FEDIAF (European Pet Food Industry Federation) (2019). Code of good labelling practice for pet food. https://europeanpetfood. org/wp-content/uploads/2022/02/FEDIAF_labeling_code_2019_onlineOctober2019.pdf (accessed 12 December 2022).

Feinle, C., Rades, T., Otto, B. et al. (2001). Fat digestion modulates gastrointestinal sensations induced by gastric distention and duodenal lipid in humans. *Gastroenterology* 120 (5): 1100–1107.

Feinle, C., O'Donovan, D., Doran, S. et al. (2003). Effects of fat digestion on appetite, APD motility, and gut hormones in response to duodenal fat infusion in humans. *Am. J. Physiol. Gastrointest. Liver Physiol.* 284: G798–G807.

Feinle-Bisset, C., Vozzo, R., Horowitz, M. et al. (2004). Diet, food intake, and disturbed physiology in the pathogenesis of symptoms in functional dyspepsia. *Am. J. Gastroenterol.* 99 (1): 170–181.

Floren, C.H. and Nilsson, A. (1982). Binding of bile salts to fiber-enriched wheat bran. *Hum. Nutr. Clin. Nutr.* 36 (5): 381–390.

Floren, C.H. and Nilsson, A. (1987). Binding of bile salts to fiber-enriched wheat fiber. *Scand. J. Gastroenterol. Suppl.* 129: 192–199.

Forman, L.P. and Schneeman, B.O. (1982). Dietary pectin's effect on starch utilization in rats. *J. Nutr.* 112 (3): 528–533.

Foster, A.P., Knowles, T.G., Moore, A.H. et al. (2003). Serum IgE and IgG responses to food antigens in normal and atopic dogs, and dogs with gastrointestinal disease. *Vet. Immunol. Immunopathol.* 92 (3–4): 113–124.

Freiche, V., Houston, D., Weese, H. et al. (2011). Uncontrolled study assessing the impact of a psyllium-enriched extruded dry diet on faecal consistency in cats with constipation. *J. Feline Med. Surg.* 13 (12): 903–911.

Frey, A., Giannasca, K.T., Weltzin, R. et al. (1996). Role of the glycocalyx in regulating access of microparticles to apical plasma membranes of intestinal epithelial cells: implications for microbial attachment and oral vaccine targeting. *J. Exp. Med.* 184 (3): 1045–1059.

Fritsch, D.A., Jackson, M.I., Wernimont, S.M. et al. (2022). Microbiome function underpins the efficacy of a fiber-supplemented dietary intervention in dogs with chronic large bowel diarrhea. *BMC Vet. Res.* 18 (1): 244.

Fukatsu, K., Lundberg, A.H., Hanna, M.K. et al. (1999). Route of nutrition influences intercellular adhesion molecule-1 expression and neutrophil accumulation in intestine. *Arch. Surg.* 134 (10): 1055–1060.

Fukatsu, K., Kudsk, K.A., Zarzaur, B.L. et al. (2001). TPN decreases IL-4 and IL-10 mRNA expression in lipopolysaccharide stimulated intestinal lamina propria cells but glutamine supplementation preserves the expression. *Shock* 15 (4): 318–322.

Gallaher, D. and Schneeman, B.O. (1986). Intestinal interaction of bile acids, phospholipids, dietary fibers, and cholestyramine. *Am. J. Physiol.* 250 (4 Pt 1): G420–G426.

Gee, M.I., Grace, M.G., Wensel, R.H. et al. (1985). Protein-energy malnutrition in gastroenterology outpatients: increased risk in Crohn's disease. *J. Am. Diet. Assoc.* 85 (11): 1466–1474.

German, A.J., Hall, E.J., and Day, M.J. (2001). Immune cell populations within the duodenal mucosa of dogs with enteropathies. *J. Vet. Intern. Med.* 15 (1): 14–25.

Geyeregger, R., Zeyda, M., Zlabinger, G.J. et al. (2005). Poly-unsaturated fatty acids interfere with formation of the immunological synapse. *J. Leukocyte Biol.* 77 (5): 680–688.

Giaffer, M.H., Cann, P., and Holdsworth, C.D. (1991). Long-term effects of elemental and exclusion diets for Crohn's disease. *Aliment. Pharmacol. Ther.* 5 (2): 115–125.

Gibson, G.R. and Wang, X. (1994). Enrichment of bifidobacteria from human gut contents by oligofructose using continuous culture. *FEMS Microbiol. Lett.* 118 (1–2): 121–127.

Gibson, G.R., Macfarlane, G.T., and Cummings, J.H. (1988). Occurrence of sulphate-reducing bacteria in human faeces and the relationship of dissimilatory sulphate reduction to methanogenesis in the large gut. *J. Appl. Bacteriol.* 65 (2): 103–111.

Gibson, G.R., Beatty, E.R., Wang, X. et al. (1995). Selective stimulation of bifidobacteria in the human colon by oligofructose and inulin. *Gastroenterology* 108 (4): 975–982.

Gilbert, S. and Halliwell, R.E. (2005). The effects of endoparasitism on the immune response to orally administered antigen in cats. *Vet. Immunol. Immunopathy* 106 (1–2): 113–120.

Girelli, D., Olivieri, O., Stanzial, A.M. et al. (1994). Factors affecting the thiobarbituric acid test as index of red blood cell susceptibility to lipid peroxidation: a multivariate analysis. *Clin. Chim. Acta* 227 (1–2): 45–57.

Gladen, H.E. and Kelly, K.A. (1980). Enhancing absorption in the canine short bowel syndrome by intestinal pacing. *Surgery* 88 (2): 281–286.

Glass, C.K. and Ogawa, S. (2006). Combinatorial roles of nuclear receptors in inflammation and immunity. *Nat. Rev. Immunol.* 6 (1): 44–55.

Goggin, J.M., Hoskinson, J.J., Butine, M.D. et al. (1998). Scintigraphic assessment of gastric emptying of canned and dry diets in healthy cats. *Am. J. Vet. Res.* 59 (4): 388–392.

Goh, J. and O'Morain, C.A. (2003). Review article: nutrition and adult inflammatory bowel disease. *Aliment. Pharmacol. Ther.* 17 (3): 307–320.

Gonlachanvit, S., Coleski, R., Owyang, C. et al. (2004). Inhibitory actions of a high fiber diet on intestinal gas transit in healthy volunteers. *Gut* 53 (11): 1577–1582.

Gonlachanvit, S., Coleski, R., Owyang, C. et al. (2006). Nutrient modulation of intestinal gas dynamics in healthy humans: dependence on caloric content and meal consistency. *Am. J. Physiol. Gastrointest. Liver Physiol.* 291 (3): G389–G395.

Gore, S.M., Fontaine, O., and Pierce, N.F. (1992). Impact of rice-based oral rehydration solution on stool output and duration of diarrhea: meta-analysis of 13 clinical trials. *BMJ* 304 (6822): 287–291.

Gorrel, C. and Bierer, T.L. (1999). Long-term effects of a dental hygiene chew on the periodontal health of dogs. *J. Vet. Dent.* 16 (3): 109–113.

Gorrel, C. and Rawlings, J.M. (1996). The role of toothbrushing and diet in the maintenance of periodontal health in dogs. *J. Vet. Dent.* 13 (4): 139–143.

Gorrel, C., Inskeep, G., and Inskeep, T. (1998). Benefits of a "dental hygiene chew" on the periodontal health of cats. *J. Vet. Dent.* 15 (3): 135–138.

Granger, D.N., Perry, M.A., Kvietys, P.R. et al. (1982). Permeability of intestinal capillaries: effects of fat absorption and gastrointestinal hormones. *Am. J. Physiol.* 242 (3): G194–G201.

Grieshop, C.M., Flickinger, E.A., and Fahey, G.C. Jr. (2002). Oral administration of arabinogalactan affects immune status and fecal microbial populations in dogs. *J. Nutr.* 132 (3): 478–482.

Grisham, M.B., Pavlick, K.P., Laroux, F.S. et al. (2002). Nitric oxide and chronic gut inflammation: controversies in inflammatory bowel disease. *J. Invest. Med.* 50: 272–283.

Guarner, F., Casellas, F., Borruel, N. et al. (2002). Role of microecology in chronic inflammatory bowel diseases. *Eur. J. Clin. Nutr.* 56 (Supplement 4): S34–S38.

Guilford, W.G. (1996). Idiopathic inflammatory bowel diseases. In: *Strombeck's Small Animal Gastroenterology* (ed. W.G. Guilford, S.A. Center, D.R. Strombeck, et al.), 211–239. Philadelphia, PA: WB Saunders.

Guilford, W.G. and Matz, M.E. (2003). The nutritional management of gastrointestinal tract disorders in companion animals. *N. Z. Vet. J.* 51 (6): 284–291.

Guilford, W.G. and Strombeck, D.R. (1996). Diseases of swallowing. In: *Strombeck's Small Animal Gastroenterology* (ed. W.G. Guilford, S.A. Center, D.R. Strombeck, et al.), 451–487. Philadelphia, PA: WB Saunders.

Guilford, W.G., Jones, B.R., Markwell, P.J. et al. (2001). Food sensitivity in cats with chronic idiopathic gastrointestinal problems. *J. Vet. Intern. Med.* 15 (1): 7–13.

Gunawardana, S.C., Jergens, A.E., Ahrens, F.A. et al. (1997). Colonic nitrite and immunoglobulin G concentrations in dogs with inflammatory bowel disease. *J. Am. Anim. Hosp. Assoc.* 211: 318–321.

Hagiwara, N. and Tomita, R. (2008). Pathophysiology of chronic constipation of the slow transit type from the aspect of the type of rectal movements. *Hepatogastroenterology* 55 (85): 1298–1303.

Hall, K.E., Diamant, N.E., El-Sharkawy, T.Y. et al. (1983). Effect of pancreatic polypeptide on canine migrating motor complex and plasma motilin. *Am. J. Physiol.* 245 (2): G178–G185.

Hall, J.A., Twedt, D.C., and Curtis, C.R. (1989). Relationship of plasma gastrin immunoreactivity and gastroesophageal sphincter pressure in clinically normal dogs and in dogs with previous gastric dilatation-volvulus. *Am. J. Vet. Res.* 50 (8): 1228–1232.

Hammer, J., Hammer, K., and Kletter, K. (1998). Lipids infused into the jejunum accelerate small intestinal transit but delay ileocolonic transit of solids and liquids. *Gut* 43 (1): 111–116.

Hamp, S.E., Olsson, S.E., Farso-Madsen, K. et al. (1984). A macroscopic and radiologic investigation of dental disease of the dog. *Vet. Radiol.* 25 (2): 86–92.

Harder, H., Hernando-Harder, A.C., Franke, A. et al. (2006). Effect of high- and low-caloric mixed liquid meals on intestinal gas dynamics. *Dig. Dis. Sci.* 51 (1): 140–146.

Harris, J.P., Parnell, N.K., Griffith, E.H. et al. (2017). Retrospective evaluation of the impact of early enteral nutrition on clinical outcomes in dogs with pancreatitis: 34 cases (2010–2013). *J. Vet. Emerg. Crit. Care* 27 (4): 425–433.

Hart, J.R., Shaker, E., Patnaik, A.K. et al. (1994). Lymphocytic-plasmacytic enterocolitis in cats: 60 cases (1988–1990). *J. Am. Anim. Hosp. Assoc.* 30: 505–514.

Harvey, C.E., Shofer, F.S., and Laster, L. (1996). Correlation of diet, other chewing activities and periodontal disease in North American client-owned dogs. *J. Vet. Dent.* 13 (3): 101–105.

Hawthorne, A.B., Daneshmend, T.K., Hawkey, C.J. et al. (1992). Treatment of ulcerative colitis with fish oil supplementation: a prospective 12 month randomised controlled trial. *Gut* 33 (7): 922–928.

Heddle, R., Collins, P.J., Dent, J. et al. (1989). Motor mechanisms associated with slowing of the gastric emptying of a solid meal by an intraduodenal lipid infusion. *J. Gastroenterol. Hepatol.* 4 (5): 437–447.

Hennet, P. (2001). Effectiveness of an enzymatic rawhide dental chew to reduce plaque in beagle dogs. *J. Vet. Dent.* 18 (2): 61–64.

Hernandez, G., Velasco, N., Wainstein, C. et al. (1999). Gut mucosal atrophy after a short enteral fasting period in critically ill patients. *J. Crit. Care* 14 (2): 73–77.

Hernando-Harder, A.C., Serra, J., Azpiroz, F. et al. (2004). Sites of symptomatic gas retention during intestinal lipid perfusion in healthy subjects. *Gut* 53 (5): 661–665.

Hirokawa, M., Takahashi, K., Miyajima, M. et al. (2021). Expression of genes encoding inflammasome sensor subunits in the duodenal and colonic mucosae of dogs with chronic enteropathy. *J. Vet. Med. Sci.* 20–0519.

Hirt, R. and Iben, C. (1998). Possible food allergy in a colony of cats. *J. Nutr.* 128 (12): 2792S–2794S.

Hoffberg, J.E. and Koenigshof, A. (2017). Evaluation of the safety of early compared to late enteral nutrition in canine septic peritonitis. *J. Am. Anim. Hosp. Assoc.* 53: 90–95.

Hoffman, L.A. and Tetrick, M.A. (2003). Added dietary fiber reduces feline hairball frequency. *J. Vet. Intern. Med.* 17 (3): 431.

Holt, P.R. and Yeh, K.Y. (1992). Effects of starvation and refeeding on jejunal disaccharidase activity. *Dig. Dis. Sci.* 37 (6): 827–832.

Holt, J.P., Johnston, L.J., Baidoo, S.K. et al. (2006). Effects of a high-fiber diet and frequent feeding on behavior, reproductive performance, and nutrient digestibility in gestating sows. *J. Anim. Sci.* 84: 946–955.

Horiuchi, M., Yamamoto, T., Tomofuji, T. et al. (2002). Tooth-brushing promotes gingival fibroblast proliferation more effectively than removal of dental plaque. *J. Clin. Periodontol.* 29 (9): 791–795.

Hotokezaka, M., Combs, M.J., Mentis, E.P. et al. (1996). Recovery of fasted and fed gastrointestinal motility after open versus laparoscopic cholecystectomy in dogs. *Ann. Surg.* 223 (4): 413–419.

Hunt, A. and Jugan, M.C. (2021). Anemia, iron deficiency, and cobalamin deficiency in cats with chronic gastrointestinal disease. *J. Vet. Intern. Med.* 35 (1): 172–178.

Ibarrola, P., Blackwood, L., Graham, P.A. et al. (2005). Hypocobalaminaemia is uncommon in cats in the United Kingdom. *J. Feline Med. Surg.* 7 (6): 341–348.

Ikeda, S., Kudsk, K.A., Fukatsu, K. et al. (2003). Enteral feeding preserves mucosal immunity despite *in vivo* MAdCAM-1 blockade of lymphocyte homing. *Ann. Surg.* 237 (5): 677–685.

Ingham, K.E., Gorrel, C., and Bierer, T.L. (2002). Effect of a dental chew on dental substrates and gingivitis in cats. *J. Vet. Dent.* 19 (4): 201–204.

Jalil, R.A., Ashley, F.P., and Wilson, R.F. (1992). The relationship between 48-h dental plaque accumulation in young human adults and the concentrations of hypothiocyanite, 'free' and 'total' lysozyme, lactoferrin and secretory immunoglobulin A in saliva. *Arch. Oral Biol.* 37 (1): 23–28.

Japan Small Animal Veterinary Association (1985). *Survey on the Health of Pet Animals, 2nd Report*. Tokyo: Japan Small Animal Veterinary Association.

Jenkins, M.K., Khoruts, A., Ingulli, E. et al. (2001). *In vivo* activation of antigen-specific CD4 T cells. *Annu. Rev. Immunol.* 19: 23–45.

Jensen, G.L., McGarvey, N., Taraszewski, R. et al. (1994). Lymphatic absorption of enterally fed structured triacylglycerol vs physical mix in a canine model. *Am. J. Clin. Nutr.* 60 (4): 518–524.

Jeppesen, P.B. and Mortensen, P.B. (1998). The influence of a preserved colon on the absorption of medium-chain fat in patients with small bowel resection. *Gut* 43 (4): 478–483.

Jergens, A.E. (1994). Rational use of antimicrobials for gastrointestinal disease in small animals. *J. Am. Anim. Hosp. Assoc.* 30 (2): 123–131.

Jergens, A.E., Carpenter, S.L., and Wannemuehler, Y. (1998). Molecular detection of inducible nitric oxide synthase in canine inflammatory bowel disease. *J. Vet. Intern. Med.* 12: 205.

Johnson, D.A. (1984). Changes in rat parotid salivary proteins associated with liquid diet-induced gland atrophy and isoproterenol-induced gland enlargement. *Arch. Oral Biol.* 29 (3): 215–221.

Johnson, C.P., Sama, S.K., Zhu, Y.-r. et al. (1996). Delayed gastroduodenal emptying is an important mechanism for control of intestinal transit in short-gut syndrome. *Am. J. Surg.* 171 (1): 90–96.

Johnson, C.D., Kudsk, K.A., Fukatsu, K. et al. (2003). Route of nutrition influences generation of antibody-forming cells and initial defense to an active viral infection in the upper respiratory tract. *Ann. Surg.* 237 (4): 565–573.

Jonas, C.R., Estivariz, C.F., Jones, D.P. et al. (1999). Keratinocyte growth factor enhances glutathione redox state in rat intestinal mucosa during nutritional repletion. *J. Nutr.* 129 (7): 1278–1284.

Jones, B.R., Jones, K.S., Turner, K. et al. (1998). Flatulence in pet dogs. *N. Z. Vet. J.* 46 (5): 191–193.

Joy, C.L. and Patterson, J.M. (1978). Short bowel syndrome following surgical correction of a double intussusception in a dog. *Can. Vet. J.* 19 (9): 254–259.

Kammlott, E., Karthoff, J., Stemme, K. et al. (2005). Experiments to optimize enzyme substitution therapy in pancreatic duct-ligated pigs. *J. Anim. Physiol. Anim. Nutr. (Berl.)* 89 (3–6): 105–108.

Kanauchi, O., Suga, T., Tochihara, M. et al. (2002). Treatment of ulcerative colitis by feeding with germinated barley foodstuff: first report of a multicenter open control trial. *J. Gastroenterol.* 37 (Suppl 14): 67–72.

Kaneko, T., Terasawa, Y., Senoo, Y. et al. (2000). Enhancing effect of dietary oil emulsions on immune responses to protein antigens fed to mice. *Int. Arch. Allergy Immunol.* 121 (4): 317–323.

Kaplan, H. and Hutkins, R.W. (2000). Fermentation of fructooligosaccharides by lactic acid bacteria and bifidobacteria. *Appl. Environ. Microbiol.* 66 (6): 2682–2684.

Kawasaki, N., Suzuki, Y., Nakayoshi, T. et al. (2009). Early postoperative enteral nutrition is useful for recovering gastrointestinal motility and maintaining the nutritional status. *Surg. Today* 39: 225–230.

Kaya, E., Gur, E.S., Ozguc, H. et al. (1999). L-glutamine enemas attenuate mucosal injury in experimental colitis. *Dis. Colon Rectum* 42 (9): 1209–1215.

Kayhan, B., Telatar, H., and Karacadag, S. (1978). Bronchial asthma associated with intestinal parasites. *Am. J. Gastroenterol.* 69 (5): 605–606.

Kearns, R.J., Hayek, M.G., Turek, J.J. et al. (1999). Effect of age, breed and dietary omega-6 (n-6): omega-3 (n-3) fatty acid ratio on immune function, eicosanoid production, and lipid peroxidation in young and aged dogs. *Vet. Immunol. Immunopathol.* 69 (2–4): 165–183.

Kellermann, S.A. and McEvoy, L.M. (2001). The Peyer's patch microenvironment suppresses T cell responses to chemokines and other stimuli. *J. Immunol.* 167 (2): 682–690.

Kerr, K.R., Dowd, S.E., and Swanson, K.S. (2014). Faecal microbiota of domestic cats fed raw whole chicks v. an extruded chicken-based diet. *J. Nutr. Sci.* 25 (3): e22.

Kienzle, E., Schrag, I., Butterwick, R. et al. (2001). Calculation of gross energy in pet foods: new data on heat combustion and fiber analysis in a selection of foods for dogs and cats. *J. Anim. Physiol. Anim. Nutr. (Berl.)* 85 (5–6): 148–157.

Kim, S.W., Rogers, Q.R., and Morris, J.G. (1996). Maillard reaction products in purified diets induce taurine depletion in cats which is reversed by antibiotics. *J. Nutr.* 126 (1): 195–201.

Kliewer, S.A., Sundseth, S.S., Jones, S.A. et al. (1997). Fatty acids and eicosanoids regulate gene expression through direct interactions with peroxisome proliferator-activated receptors alpha and gamma. *Proc. Natl. Acad. Sci. U. S. A.* 94 (9): 4318–4323.

Klipper, E., Sklan, D., and Friedman, A. (2001). Response, tolerance and ignorance following oral exposure to a single dietary protein antigen in *Gallus domesticus. Vaccine* 19 (20–22): 2890–2897.

Kostadinova, R., Wahli, W., and Michalik, L. (2005). PPARs in diseases: control mechanisms of inflammation. *Curr. Med. Chem.* 12 (25): 2995–3009.

Krasse, B. and Brill, N. (1960). Effect of consistency of diet on bacteria in the gingival pocket in dogs. *Odontol. Revy* 11: 152.

Kudsk, K.A. (2003). Effect of route and type of nutrition on intestine-derived inflammatory responses. *Am. J. Surg.* 185 (1): 16–21.

Kudsk, K.A., Wu, Y., Fukatsu, K. et al. (2000). Glutamine enriched total parenteral nutrition maintains intestinal interleukin-4 and mucosal immunoglobulin A levels. *JPEN. J. Parenter. Enteral Nutr.* 24 (5): 270–274.

Kull, P.A., Hess, R.S., Craig, L.E. et al. (2001). Clinical, clinicopathologic, radiographic, and ultrasonographic characteristics of intestinal lymphangiectasia in dogs: 17 cases (1996–1998). *J. Am. Vet. Med. Assoc.* 219: 197–202.

Laflamme, D.P., Xu, H., and Long, G.L. (2011). Effect of diets differing in fat content on chronic diarrhea in cats. *J. Vet. Intern. Med.* 25 (2): 230–235.

Lappin, M.R., Zug, A., Hovenga, C. et al. (2022). Efficacy of feeding a diet containing a high concentration of mixed fiber sources for management of acute large bowel diarrhea in dogs in shelters. *J. Vet. Intern. Med.* 36 (2): 488–492.

Larsen, J.A., Calvert, C.C., and Rogers, Q.R. (2002). Processing of dietary casein decreases bioavailability of lysine in growing kittens. *J. Nutr.* 132 (6): 1748S–1750S.

Le Bacquer, O., Laboisse, C., and Darmaun, D. (2003). Glutamine preserves protein synthesis and paracellular permeability in Caco-2 cells submitted to 'luminal fasting'.

Am. J. Physiol. Gastrointest. Liver Physiol. 285 (1): G128–G136.

LeBlanc, C.J., Dietrich, M.A., Horohov, D.W. et al. (2007). Effects of dietary fish oil and vitamin E supplementation on canine lymphocyte proliferation evaluated using a flow cytometric technique. *Vet. Immunol. Immunopathol.* 119 (3–4): 180–188.

LeBlanc, C.J., Horohov, D.W., Bauer, J.E. et al. (2008). Effects of dietary supplementation with fish oil on *in vivo* production of inflammatory mediators in clinically normal dogs. *Am. J. Vet. Res.* 69 (4): 486–493.

Lee, J.Y., Plakidas, A., Lee, W.H. et al. (2003). Differential modulation of Toll-like receptors by fatty acids: preferential inhibition by n-3 polyunsaturated fatty acids. *J. Lipid Res.* 44 (3): 479–486.

Lee, J.Y., Zhao, L., Youn, H.S. et al. (2004). Saturated fatty acid activates but polyunsaturated fatty acid inhibits Toll-like receptor 2 dimerized with Toll-like receptor 6 or 1. *J. Biol. Chem.* 279 (17): 16971–16979.

Leib, M. (2000). Treatment of chronic idiopathic large-bowel diarrhea in dogs with a highly digestible diet and soluble fiber: a retrospective review of 37 cases. *J. Vet. Intern. Med.* 14: 27–32.

Levine, J.S., Allen, R.H., Alpers, D.H. et al. (1984). Immuno-cytochemical localization of the intrinsic factor-cobalamin receptor in dog-ileum: distribution of intracellular receptor during cell maturation. *J. Cell. Biochem.* 98 (3): 1111–1118.

Liddle, R.A. (1997). Cholecystokinin cells. *Ann. Rev. Physiol.* 59: 221–242.

Lim, B.O., Lee, S.H., Park, D.K. et al. (2003). Effect of dietary pectin on the production of immunoglobulins and cytokines by mesenteric lymph node lymphocytes in mouse colitis induced with dextran sulfate sodium. *Biosci. Biotechnol. Biochem.* 67 (8): 1706–1712.

Lin, H.C., Doty, J.E., Reedy, T.J. et al. (1990). Inhibition of gastric emptying by sodium oleate depends on length of intestine exposed to nutrient. *Am. J. Physiol.* 259 (6 Pt 1): G1031–G1036.

Lin, H.C., Kim, B.H., Elashoff, J.D. et al. (1992). Gastric emptying of solid food is most potently inhibited by carbohydrate in the canine distal ileum. *Gastroenterology* 102 (3): 793–801.

Lindhe, J., Hamp, S.E., and Loe, H. (1975). Plaque induced periodontal disease in beagle dogs. A 4-year clinical, roentgenographical and histometrical study. *J. Periodontal Res.* 10 (5): 243–255.

Lippert, A.C., Faulkner, J.E., Evans, A.T. et al. (1989). Total parenteral nutrition in clinically normal cats. *J. Am. Vet. Med. Assoc.* 194 (5): 669–676.

Ljungmann, K., Hartmann, B., Kissmeyer-Nielsen, P. et al. (2001). Time-dependent intestinal adaptation and GLP-2 alterations after small bowel resection in rats. *Am. J. Physiol. Gastrointest. Liver Physiol.* 281 (3): G779–G785.

Lloyd, K.C. (1994). Gut hormones in gastric function. *Baillieres Clin. Endocrinol. Metab.* 8 (1): 111–136.

Logan, E.I., Finney, O., and Hefferren, J.J. (2002). Effects of a dental food on plaque accumulation and gingival health in dogs. *J. Vet. Dent.* 19 (1): 15–18.

Loureiro, B.A., Sembenelli, G., Maria, A.P.J. et al. (2014). Sugarcane fibre may prevent hairball formation in cats. *J. Nutr. Sci.* 3: e20.

Loureiro, B.A., Monti, M., Pedreira, R.S. et al. (2017). Beet pulp intake and hairball faecal excretion in mixed-breed shorthaired cats. *J. Anim. Physiol. Anim. Nutr. (Berl.)* 101 (Suppl 1): 31–36.

Luckschander-Zeller, N., Hammer, S.E., Ruetgen, B.C. et al. (2019). Clonality testing as complementary tool in the assessment of different patient groups with canine chronic enteropathy. *Vet. Immunol. Immunopathol.* 214: 109893.

Luhrs, H., Gerke, T., Muller, J.G. et al. (2002). Butyrate inhibits NF-κB activation in lamina propria macrophages of patients with ulcerative colitis. *Scand. J. Gastroenterol.* 37 (4): 458–466.

Lund, E.M., Armstrong, P.J., Kirk, C.A. et al. (1999). Health status and population characteristics of dogs and cats examined at private veterinary practices in the United States. *J. Am. Vet. Med. Assoc.* 214 (9): 1336–1341.

Lupton, J.R. (1995). Butyrate and colonic cytokinetics: differences between *in vitro* and *in vivo* studies. *Eur. J. Cancer Prev.* 4 (5): 373–378.

Lupton, J.R. (2004). Microbial degradation products influence colon cancer risk: the butyrate controversy. *J. Nutr.* 134 (2): 479–482.

Maddison, K.J., Shepherd, K.L., Hillman, D.R. et al. (2005). Function of the lower esophageal sphincter during and after high-intensity exercise. *Med. Sci. Sports Exerc.* 37 (10): 1728–1733.

Magne, M.L. (1992). Pathophysiology of inflammatory bowel disease. *Semin. Vet. Med. Surg. (Small Anim.)* 7 (2): 112–116.

Maher, J.W., Crandall, V., and Woodward, E.R. (1977). Effects of meal size on postprandial lower esophageal sphincter pressure (LESP). *Surg. Forum* 28: 342–344.

Maleki, S.J., Chung, S.Y., Champagne, E.T. et al. (2000). The effects of roasting on the allergenic properties of peanut proteins. *J. Allergy Clin. Immunol.* 106 (4): 763–768.

Maleki, S.J., Viquez, O., Jacks, T. et al. (2003). The major peanut allergen, Ara h 2, functions as a trypsin inhibitor, and roasting enhances this function. *J. Allergy Clin. Immunol.* 112 (1): 190–195.

Mandigers, P.J., Biourge, V., van den Ingh, T.S.G.A.M. et al. (2010). A randomized, open-label, positively-controlled field trial of a hydrolyzed protein diet in dogs with chronic small bowel enteropathy. *J. Vet. Intern. Med.* 24 (6): 1350–1357.

Mansfield, C.S., James, F.E., Steiner, J.M. et al. (2011). A pilot study to assess tolerability of early enteral nutrition via esophagostomy tube feeding in dogs with severe acute pancreatitis. *J. Vet. Intern. Med.* 25: 419–425.

Marks, S.L., Cook, A.K., Griffey, S. et al. (1997). Dietary modulation of methotrexate-induced enteritis in cats. *Am. J. Vet. Res.* 58 (9): 989–996.

Marks, S.L., Cook, A.K., Reader, R. et al. (1999). Effects of glutamine supplementation of an amino acid-based purified diet on intestinal mucosal integrity in cats with methotrexate-induced enteritis. *Am. J. Vet. Res.* 60 (6): 755–763.

Marks, S.L., Laflamme, D.P., and McCandlish, A.P. (2002). Dietary trial using a commercial hypoallergenic diet containing hydrolyzed protein for dogs with inflammatory bowel disease. *Vet. Ther.* 3 (2): 109–118.

Marlett, J.A. and Fischer, M.H. (2003). The active fraction of psyllium seed husk. *Proc. Nutr. Soc.* 62 (1): 207–209.

Marsilio, S. (2021). Feline chronic enteropathy. *J. Small Anim. Pract.* 62: 409–419.

Marsman, K.E. and McBurney, M.I. (1995). Dietary fiber increases oxidative metabolism in colonocytes but not in distal small intestinal enterocytes isolated from rats. *J. Nutr.* 125 (2): 273–282.

Marsman, K.E. and McBurney, M.I. (1996). Dietary fiber and short-chain fatty acids affect cell proliferation and protein synthesis in isolated rat colonocytes. *J. Nutr.* 126 (5): 1429–1437.

Marthinsen, D. and Fleming, S.E. (1982). Excretion of breath and flatus gases by humans consuming high-fiber diets. *J. Nutr.* 112 (6): 1133–1143.

Martin, C.J., Patrikios, J., and Dent, J. (1986). Abolition of gas reflux and transient lower esophageal sphincter relaxation by vagal blockade in the dog. *Gastroenterology* 91 (4): 890–896.

Martin, L., Matteson, V., and Wingfield, W. (1994). Abnormalities of serum magnesium in critically ill dogs: incidence and implications. *J. Vet. Emerg. Crit. Care* 4: 15–20.

Marx, F.R., Machado, G.S., Pezzali, J.G. et al. (2016). Raw beef bones as chewing items to reduce dental calculus in Beagle dogs. *Aust. Vet. J.* 94: 18–23.

Mathews, C.J., MacLeod, R.J., Zheng, S.X. et al. (1999). Characterization of the inhibitory effect of boiled rice on intestinal chloride secretion in Guinea pig crypt cells. *Gastroenterology* 116 (6): 1342–1347.

Mattison, C.P., Bren-Mattison, Y., Vant-Hull, B. et al. (2016). Heat-induced alterations in cashew allergen solubility and IgE binding. *Toxicol. Rep.* 3: 244–251.

Mayer, K., Meyer, S., Reinholz-Muhly, M. et al. (2003). Shorttime infusion of fish oil-based lipid emulsions, approved for parenteral nutrition, reduces monocyte proinflammatory cytokine generation and adhesive interaction with endothelium in humans. *J. Immunol.* 171 (9): 4837–4843.

McBurney, M.I. (1991). Potential water-holding capacity and short-chain fatty acid production from purified fiber sources in a fecal incubation system. *Nutrition* 7 (6): 421–424.

McKay, L.F., Eastwood, M.A., and Brydon, W.G. (1985). Methane excretion in man—a study of breath, flatus, and faeces. *Gut* 26 (1): 69–74.

McManus, C.M., Michel, K.E., Simon, D.M. et al. (2002). Effect of short-chain fatty acids on contraction of smooth muscle in the canine colon. *Am. J. Vet. Res.* 63 (2): 295–300.

McNally, E.F., Kelly, J.E. Jr., and Ingelfinger, F.J. (1964). Mechanism of belching: effects of gastric distension with air. *Gastroenterology* 46: 254–259.

Meyer, J.H., Elashoff, J.D., Domeck, M. et al. (1994). Control of canine gastric emptying of fat by lipolytic products. *Am. J. Physiol.* 266 (6 Pt 1): G1017–G1035.

Mohr, A.J., Leisewitz, A.L., Jacobson, L.S. et al. (2003). Effect of early enteral nutrition on intestinal permeability, intestinal protein loss, and outcome in dogs with severe parvoviral enteritis. *J. Vet. Intern. Med.* 17 (6): 791–798.

Moreau, N.M., Martin, L.J., Toquet, C.S. et al. (2003). Restoration of the integrity of rat caeco-colonic mucosa by resistant starch, but not by fructo-oligosaccharides, in dextran sulfate sodium-induced experimental colitis. *Br. J. Nutr.* 90 (1): 75–85.

Morris, J.G. (2002). Idiosyncratic nutrient requirements of cats appear to be diet-induced evolutionary adaptations. *Nutr. Res. Rev.* 15 (1): 153–168.

Mroz, Z., Jongbloed, A.W., and Kemme, P.A. (1994). Apparent digestibility and retention of nutrients bound to phytate complexes as influenced by microbial phytase and feeding regimen in pigs. *J. Anim. Sci.* 72 (1): 126–132.

Mu, H. and Hoy, C.E. (2000). Effects of different medium-chain fatty acids on intestinal absorption of structured triacylglycerols. *Lipids* 35 (1): 83–89.

Muller-Lissner, S.A. (1988). Effect of wheat bran on weight of stool and gastrointestinal transit time: a meta analysis. *Br. Med. J. (Clin. Res. Ed.)* 296 (6622): 615–617.

Nebel, O.T. and Castell, D.O. (1973). Inhibition of the lower oesophageal sphincter by fat – a mechanism for fatty food intolerance. *Gut* 14 (4): 270–274.

Nelson, R.W., Dimperio, M.E., and Long, G.G. (1984). Lymphocytic-plasmacytic colitis in the cat. *J. Am. Vet. Med. Assoc.* 184 (9): 1133–1135.

Nelson, R.W., Stookey, L.J., and Kazacos, E. (1988). Nutritional management of idiopathic chronic colitis in the dog. *J. Vet. Intern. Med.* 2 (3): 133–137.

Nemeth, T., Solymosi, N., and Balka, G. (2008). Long-term results of subtotal colectomy for acquired hypertrophic megacolon in eight dogs. *J. Small Anim. Pract.* 12: 618–624.

Newsholme, P., Gordon, S., and Newsholme, E.A. (1987). Rates of utilization and fates of glucose, glutamine, pyruvate, fatty acids and ketone bodies by mouse macrophages. *Biochem. J.* 242 (3): 631–636.

Oba, P.M., Utterback, P.L., Parsons, C.M. et al. (2019). Chemical composition, true nutrient digestibility, and true metabolizable energy of chicken-based ingredients differing by processing method using the precision-fed cecectomized rooster assay. *J. Anim. Sci.* 97 (3): 998–1009.

Ohno, T., Mochiki, E., Ando, H. et al. (2009). Glutamine decreases the duration of postoperative ileus after abdominal surgery: an experimental study of conscious dogs. *Dig. Dis. Sci.* 54 (6): 1208–1213.

Olson, N.C. and Zimmer, J.F. (1978). Protein-losing enteropathy secondary to intestinal lymphangiectasia in a dog. *J. Am. Vet. Med. Assoc.* 173 (3): 271–274.

Ontsouka, C.E., Burgener, I.A., Mani, O., and Albrecht, C. (2010). Polyunsaturated fatty acid-enriched diets used for the treatment of canine chronic enteropathies decrease the abundance of selected genes of cholesterol homeostasis. *Domest. Anim. Endocrinol.* 38 (1): 32–37.

Paquette, D.W., Waters, G.S., Stefanidou, V.L. et al. (1997). Inhibition of experimental gingivitis in beagle dogs with topical salivary histatins. *J. Clin. Periodontol.* 24 (4): 216–222.

Passos, M.C., Serra, J., Azpiroz, F. et al. (2005). Impaired reflex control of intestinal gas transit in patients with abdominal bloating. *Gut* 54 (3): 344–348.

Paterson, S. (1995). Food hypersensitivity in 20 dogs with skin and gastrointestinal signs. *J. Small Anim. Pract.* 36 (12): 529–534.

Patrikios, J., Martin, C.J., and Dent, J. (1986). Relationship of transient lower esophageal sphincter relaxation to postprandial gastroesophageal reflux and belching in dogs. *Gastroenterology* 90 (3): 545–551.

Patz, J., Jacobsohn, W.Z., Gottschalk-Sabag, S. et al. (1996). Treatment of refractory distal ulcerative colitis with short chain fatty acid enemas. *Am. J. Gastroenterol.* 91 (4): 731–734.

Pavlick, K.P., Laroux, F.S., Fuseler, J. et al. (2002). Role of reactive metabolites of oxygen and nitrogen in inflammatory bowel disease. *Free Radic. Biol. Med.* 33 (3): 311–322.

Pearson, M., Teahon, K., Levi, A.J. et al. (1993). Food intolerance and Crohn's disease. *Gut* 34 (6): 783–787.

Pehl, C., Waizenhoefer, A., Wendl, B. et al. (1999). Effect of low and high fat meals on lower esophageal sphincter motility and gastroesophageal reflux in healthy subjects. *Am. J. Gastroenterol.* 94 (5): 1192–1196.

Pehl, C., Pfeiffer, A., Waizenhoefer, A. et al. (2001). Effect of caloric density of a meal on lower oesophageal sphincter motility and gastro-oesophageal reflux in healthy subjects. *Aliment. Pharmacol. Ther.* 15 (2): 233–239.

Perkins, N.D. (2007). Integrating cell-signalling pathways with NF-kappaB and IKK function. *Nat. Rev. Mol. Cell Biol.* 8 (1): 49–62.

Perner, A. and Rask-Madsen, J. (1999). Review article: the potential role of nitric oxide in chronic inflammatory bowel disorders. *Aliment. Pharmacol. Ther.* 13 (2): 135–144.

Pilla, R., Guard, B.C., Steiner, J.M. et al. (2019). Administration of a synbiotic containing enterococcus faecium does not significantly alter fecal microbiota richness or diversity in dogs with and without food-responsive chronic enteropathy. *Front. Vet. Sci.* 6: 277.

Pimentel, M., Mayer, A.G., Park, S. et al. (2003). Methane production during lactulose breath test is associated with gastrointestinal disease presentation. *Dig. Dis. Sci.* 48 (1): 86–92.

Pimentel, M., Lin, H.C., Enayati, P. et al. (2006). Methane, a gas produced by enteric bacteria, slows intestinal transit and augments small intestinal contractile activity. *Am. J. Physiol. Gastrointest. Liver Physiol.* 290 (6): G1089–G1095.

Poksay, K.S. and Schneeman, B.O. (1983). Pancreatic and intestinal response to dietary guar gum in rats. *J. Nutr.* 113 (8): 1544–1549.

Poley, J.R. and Hofmann, A.F. (1976). Role of fat maldigestion in pathogenesis of steatorrhea in ileal resection. Fat digestion after two sequential test meals with and without cholestyramine. *Gastroenterology* 71 (1): 38–44.

Preiser, J.C., Peres-Bota, D., Eisendrath, P. et al. (2003). Gut mucosal and plasma concentrations of glutamine: a comparison between two enriched enteral feeding solutions in critically ill patients. *Nutr. J.* 2: 13.

Ramakrishna, B.S., Mathan, M., and Mathan, V.I. (1994). Alteration of colonic absorption by long-chain unsaturated fatty acids. Influence of hydroxylation and degree of unsaturation. *Scand. J. Gastroenterol.* 29 (1): 54–58.

Rawlings, J.M., Gorrel, C., and Markwell, P.J. (1997). Effect of two dietary regimens on gingivitis in the dog. *J. Small Anim. Pract.* 38 (4): 147–151.

Rawlings, J.M., Gorrel, C., and Markwell, P.J. (1998). Effect on canine oral health of adding chlorhexidine to a dental hygiene chew. *J. Vet. Dent.* 15 (3): 129–134.

Reddy, B.S., Engle, A., Simi, B. et al. (1992). Effect of dietary fiber on colonic bacterial enzymes and bile acids in relation to colon cancer. *Gastroenterology* 102 (5): 1475–1482.

Reed, N., Gunn-Moore, D., and Simpson, K. (2007). Cobalamin, folate and inorganic phosphate abnormalities in ill cats. *J. Feline Med. Surg.* 9 (4): 278–288.

Rehfeld, J.F., Friis-Hansen, L., Goetze, J.P. et al. (2007). The biology of cholecystokinin and gastrin peptides. *Curr. Top. Med. Chem.* 7 (12): 1154–1165.

Reidelberger, R.D., Hernandez, J., Fritzsch, B. et al. (2004). Abdominal vagal mediation of the satiety effects of CCK in rats. *Am. J. Physiol. Regul. Integr. Comp. Physiol.* 286 (6): R1005–R1012.

Reimund, J.M., Hirth, C., Koehl, C. et al. (2000). Antioxidant and immune status in active Crohn's disease. A possible relationship. *Clin. Nutr.* 19 (1): 43–48.

Reinhart, G.A. and Vaughn, D.M. (1995). *Dietary Fatty Acid Ratios and Tissue Fatty Acid Content*. Lake Buena Vista, FL: InnoPet.

Renegar, K.B., Johnson, C.D., Dewitt, R.C. et al. (2001). Impairment of mucosal immunity by total parenteral nutrition: requirement for IgA in murine nasotracheal antiinfluenza immunity. *J. Immunol.* 166 (2): 819–825.

Reynolds, R.P. and Effer, G.W. (1988). The effect of differential vagal nerve cooling on feline esophageal function. *Clin. Invest. Med.* 11 (6): 452–456.

Ristic, J.M. and Stidworthy, M.R. (2002). Two cases of severe iron-deficiency anaemia due to inflammatory bowel disease in the dog. *J. Small Anim. Pract.* 43: 80–83.

Rolfe, V.E., Adams, C.A., Butterwick, R.E. et al. (2002). Relationships between fecal consistency and colonic microstructure and absorptive function in dogs with and without

nonspecific dietary sensitivity. *Am. J. Vet. Res.* 63 (4): 617–622.

Romagnani, S. (2004). The increased prevalence of allergy and the hygiene hypothesis: missing immune deviation, reduced immune suppression, or both? *Immunology* 112 (3): 352–363.

Rondeau, M.P., Meltzer, K., Michel, K.E. et al. (2003). Short chain fatty acids stimulate feline colonic smooth muscle contraction. *J. Feline Med. Surg.* 5 (3): 167–173.

Rose, L., Rose, J., Gosling, S. et al. (2017). Efficacy of a probiotic-prebiotic supplement on incidence of diarrhea in a dog shelter: a randomized, double-blind, Placebo controlled trial. *J. Vet. Intern. Med.* 31 (2): 377–382.

Rossi, G., Cerquetella, M., Gavazza, A. et al. (2020). Rapid resolution of large bowel diarrhea after the administration of a combination of a high-fiber diet and a probiotic mixture in dogs. *Vet. Sci.* 7 (1): 21.

Roth, J.A., Frankel, W.L., Zhang, W. et al. (1995). Pectin improves colonic function in rat short bowel syndrome. *J. Surg. Res.* 58 (2): 240–246.

Ruaux, C.G., Steiner, J.M., and Williams, D.A. (2005). Early biochemical and clinical responses to cobalamin supplementation in cats with signs of gastrointestinal disease and severe hypocobalaminemia. *J. Vet. Intern. Med.* 19 (2): 155–160.

Rudinsky, A.J., Rowe, J.C., and Parker, V.J. (2018). Nutritional management of chronic enteropathies in dogs and cats. *J. Am. Vet. Med. Assoc.* 253 (5): 570–578.

Russell, J. and Bass, P. (1985). Canine gastric emptying of fiber meals: influence of meal viscosity and antroduodenal motility. *Am. J. Physiol.* 249 (6 Pt 1): G662–G667.

Rutgers, H.C., Batt, R.M., Elwood, C.M. et al. (1995). Small intestinal bacterial overgrowth in dogs with chronic intestinal disease. *J. Am. Vet. Med. Assoc.* 206 (2): 187–193.

Ryden, P. and Robertson, J.A. (1997). Characterisation of the binding capacities and affinities of wheat bran, fruit and vegetable fibers for MeIQx, before and after fermentation. *Cancer Lett.* 114 (1–2): 47–49.

Saker, K.E., Eddy, A.L., Thatcher, C.D. et al. (1998). Manipulation of dietary (n-6) and (n-3) fatty acids alters platelet function in cats. *J. Nutr.* 128 (12 Suppl): 2645S–2647S.

Salvia, G., Vizia, B., Manguso, F. et al. (2001). Effect of intragastric volume and osmolality on mechanisms of gastroesophageal reflux in children with gastroesophageal reflux disease. *Am. J. Gastroenterol.* 96: 1725–1732.

Salvioli, B., Serra, J., Azpiroz, F. et al. (2005). Origin of gas retention and symptoms in patients with bloating. *Gastroenterology* 128 (3): 574–579.

Sang, Q. and Goyal, R.K. (2000). Lower esophageal sphincter relaxation and activation of medullary neurons by subdiaphragmatic vagal stimulation in the mouse. *Gastroenterology* 119 (6): 1600–1609.

Sangild, P.T., Tappenden, K.A., Malo, C. et al. (2006). Glucagon-like peptide 2 stimulates intestinal nutrient absorption in parenterally fed newborn pigs. *J. Pediatr. Gastroenterol. Nutr.* 43 (2): 160–167.

Sarna, S.K. and Lang, I.M. (1989). Colonic motor response to a meal in dogs. *Am. J. Physiol.* 257 (5 Pt 1): G830–G835.

Schrezenmeir, J. and de Vrese, M. (2001). Probiotics, prebiotics, and synbiotics – approaching a definition. *Am. J. Clin. Nutr.* 73 (2 Suppl): 361S–364S.

Scott, J., Berry, M.R., Gunn, D.L. et al. (1990). The effects of a liquid diet on initial and sustained, stimulated parotid salivary secretion and on parotid structure in the rat. *Arch. Oral Biol.* 35 (7): 509–514.

Sethi, A.K. and Sarna, S.K. (1991). Colonic motor response to a meal in acute colitis. *Gastroenterology* 101: 1537–1546.

Shi, X.Z. and Sarna, S.K. (2004). G protein-mediated dysfunction of excitation-contraction coupling in ileal inflammation. *Am. J. Physiol. Gastrointest. Liver Physiol.* 286 (6): G899–G905.

Sifrim, D., Silny, J., Holloway, R.H. et al. (1999). Patterns of gas and liquid reflux during transient lower oesophageal sphincter relaxation: a study using intraluminal electrical impedance. *Gut* 44 (1): 47–54.

Simpson, K.W., Fyfe, J., Cornetta, A. et al. (2001). Subnormal concentrations of serum cobalamin (vitamin B12) in cats with gastrointestinal disease. *J. Vet. Intern. Med.* 15: 26–32.

Simpson, J.M., Martineau, B., Jones, W.E. et al. (2002). Characterization of fecal bacterial populations in canines: effects of age, breed and dietary fiber. *Microb. Ecol.* 44 (2): 186–197.

Sparkes, A.H., Papasouliotis, K., Sunvold, G. et al. (1998a). Bacterial flora in the duodenum of healthy cats, and effect of dietary supplementation with fructo-oligosaccharides. *Am. J. Vet. Res.* 59 (4): 431–435.

Sparkes, A.H., Papasouliotis, K., Sunvold, G. et al. (1998b). Effect of dietary supplementation with fructooligosaccharides on fecal flora of healthy cats. *Am. J. Vet. Res.* 59 (4): 436–440.

Stechmiller, J.K., Childress, B., and Porter, T. (2004). Arginine immunonutrition in critically ill patients: a clinical dilemma. *Am. J. Crit. Care* 13 (1): 17–23.

Steenkamp, G. and Gorrel, C. (1999). Oral and dental conditions in adult African wild dog skulls: Apreliminary report. *J. Vet. Dent.* 16 (2): 65–68.

Stookey, G.K., Warrick, J.M., and Miller, L.L. (1995). Effect of sodium hexametaphosphate on dental calculus formation in dogs. *Am. J. Vet. Res.* 56 (7): 913–918.

Straathof, J.W., Ringers, J., Lamers, C.B. et al. (2001). Provocation of transient lower esophageal sphincter relaxations by gastric distension with air. *Am. J. Vet. Gastroenterol.* 96 (8): 2317–2323.

Straathof, J.W., van Veen, M.M., and Masclee, A.A. (2002). Provocation of transient lower esophageal sphincter relaxations during continuous gastric distension. *Scand. J. Gastroenterol.* 37 (10): 1140–1143.

Strombeck, D.R. and Harrold, D. (1985). Effect of gastrin, histamine, serotonin, and adrenergic amines on gastroesophageal sphincter pressure in the dog. *Am. J. Vet. Res.* 46 (8): 1684–1690.

Strombeck, D.R., Turner, W.D., and Harrold, D. (1988). Eructation of gas through the gastroesophageal sphincter before and after gastric fundectomy in dogs. *Am. J. Vet. Res.* 49 (1): 87–89.

Studer, E. and Stapley, R.B. (1973). The role of dry foods in maintaining healthy teeth and gums in the cat. *Vet. Med. Small Anim. Clin.* 68 (10): 1124–1126.

Sturniolo, G.C., Di, L., Ferronato, A. et al. (2001). Zinc supplementation tightens "leaky gut" in Crohn's disease. *Inflamm. Bowel Dis.* 7 (2): 94–98.

Suchner, U., Heyland, D.K., and Peter, K. (2002). Immune-modulatory actions of arginine in the critically ill. *Br. J. Nutr.* 87 (Suppl 1): S121–S132.

Sunvold, G.D., Hussein, H.S., Fahey, G.C. Jr. et al. (1995). *in vitro* fermentation of cellulose, beet pulp, citrus pulp, and citrus pectin using fecal inoculum from cats, dogs, horses, humans, and pigs and ruminal fluid from cattle. *J. Anim. Sci.* 73 (12): 3639–3648.

Takagi, T., Naito, Y., Tomatsuri, N. et al. (2002). Pioglitazone, a PPAR-gamma ligand, provides protection from dextran sulfate sodium-induced colitis in mice in association with inhibition of the NF-kappaB-cytokine cascade. *Redox Rep.* 7 (5): 283–289.

Tams, T.R. (1993). Feline inflammatory bowel disease. *Vet. Clin. North Am. Small Anim. Pract.* 23 (3): 569–586.

Tan, B.J. and Diamant, N.E. (1987). Assessment of the neural defect in a dog with idiopathic megaesophagus. *Dig. Dis. Sci.* 32 (1): 76–85.

Tanaka, M., Hanioka, T., Kishimoto, M. et al. (1998). Effect of mechanical toothbrush stimulation on gingival microcirculatory functions in inflamed gingiva of dogs. *J. Clin. Periodontol.* 25 (7): 561–565.

Tenenhaus, M., Hansbrough, J.R., Zapata-Sirvent, R.L. et al. (1994). Supplementation of an elemental enteral diet with alanyl-glutamine decreases bacterial translocation in burned mice. *Burns* 20 (3): 220–225.

Thomas, R.P., Hellmich, M.R., Townsend, C.M. Jr. et al. (2003). Role of gastrointestinal hormones in the proliferation of normal and neoplastic tissues. *Endocr. Rev.* 24 (5): 571–599.

Thor, P.J., Copeland, E.M., Dudrick, S.J. et al. (1977). Effect of long-term parenteral feeding on gastric secretion in dogs. *Am. J. Physiol.* 232 (1): E39–E43.

Tolbert, M.K., Murphy, M., Gaylord, L., and Witzel-Rollins, A. (2022). Dietary management of chronic enteropathy in dogs. *J. Small Anim. Pract.* 63: 425–434.

Toll, J., Erb, H., Birnbaum, N. et al. (2002). Prevalence and incidence of serum magnesium abnormalities in hospitalized cats. *J. Vet. Intern. Med.* 16 (3): 217–221.

Tomlin, J., Lowis, C., and Read, N.W. (1991). Investigation of normal flatus production in healthy volunteers. *Gut* 32 (6): 665–669.

Toresson, L., Steiner, J.M., Olmedal, G. et al. (2017). Oral cobalamin supplementation in cats with hypocobalaminaemia: a retrospective study. *J. Feline Med. Surg.* 19 (12): 1302–1306.

Toresson, L., Steiner, J.M., Razdan, P. et al. (2018). Comparison of efficacy of oral and parenteral cobalamin supplementation in normalising low cobalamin concentrations in dogs: a randomised controlled study. *Vet. J.* 232: 27–32.

Tremolaterra, F., Villoria, A., Serra, J. et al. (2006). Intestinal tone and gas motion. *Neurogastroenterol. Motil.* 18 (10): 905–910.

Tromp, J.A., Jansen, J., and Pilot, T. (1986). Gingival health and frequency of tooth brushing in the beagle dog model. Clinical findings. *J. Clin. Periodontol.* 13 (2): 164–168.

Vaden, S.L., Hammerberg, B., Davenport, D.J. et al. (2000). Food hypersensitivity reactions in soft coated wheaten terriers with protein-losing enteropathy or protein-losing nephropathy or both: gastroscopic food sensitivity testing, dietary provocation, and fecal immunoglobulin E. *J. Vet. Intern. Med.* 2000 (14): 60–67.

Van Den, B.J., Kamm, M.A., and Knight, S.C. (2001). Immune sensitization to food, yeast and bacteria in Crohn's disease. *Aliment. Pharmacol. Ther.* 15 (10): 1647–1653.

Van Den, B.J., Cahill, J., Emmanuel, A.V. et al. (2002). Gut mucosal response to food antigens in Crohn's disease. *Aliment. Pharmacol. Ther.* 16 (11): 1903–1915.

Van Geffen, C., Saunders, J.H., Vandevelde, B. et al. (2006). Idiopathic megaoesophagus and intermittent gastrooesophageal intussusception in a cat. *J. Small Anim. Pract.* 47: 471–475.

Velasco, N., Hernandez, G., Wainstein, C. et al. (2001). Influence of polymeric enteral nutrition supplemented with different doses of glutamine on gut permeability in critically ill patients. *Nutrition* 17 (11–12): 907–911.

Venkatraman, A., Ramakrishna, B.S., Shaji, R.V. et al. (2003). Amelioration of dextran sulfate colitis by butyrate: role of heat shock protein 70 and NF-κB. *Am. J. Physiol. Gastrointest. Liver Physiol.* 285 (1): G177–G184.

Verbrugghe, A., Hesta, M., Daminet, S. et al. (2012). Propionate absorbed from the colon acts as gluconeogenic substrate in a strict carnivore, the domestic cat (*Felis catus*). *J. Anim. Physiol. Anim. Nutr. (Berl.)* 96 (6): 1054–1064.

Verstraete, F.J., van Aarde, R.J., Nieuwoudt, B.A. et al. (1996). The dental pathology of feral cats on Marion Island, part II: periodontitis, external odontoclastic resorption lesions and mandibular thickening. *J. Comp. Pathol.* 115 (3): 283–297.

Vickers, R.J., Sunvold, G.D., Kelley, R.L. et al. (2001). Comparison of fermentation of selected fructooligosaccharides and other fiber substrates by canine colonic microflora. *Am. J. Vet. Res.* 62 (4): 609–615.

Videla, S., Vilaseca, J., Antolin, M. et al. (2001). Dietary inulin improves distal colitis induced by dextran sodium sulfate in the rat. *Am. J. Gastroenterol.* 96 (5): 1486–1493.

Villoria, A., Serra, J., Azpiroz, F. et al. (2006). Physical activity and intestinal gas clearance in patients with bloating. *Am. J. Gastroenterol.* 101 (11): 2552–2557.

Virag, L., Szabo, E., Gergely, P. et al. (2003). Peroxynitrite-induced cytotoxicity: mechanism and opportunities for intervention. *Toxicol. Lett.* 140–141: 113–124.

Wander, R.C., Hall, J.A., Gradin, J.L. et al. (1997). The ratio of dietary (n-6) to (n-3) fatty acids influences immune system function, eicosanoid metabolism, lipid peroxidation and vitamin E status in aged dogs. *J. Nutr.* 127 (6): 1198–1205.

Wang, S., Martins, R., Sullivan, M.C. et al. (2019). Diet-induced remission in chronic enteropathy is associated with altered microbial community structure and synthesis of secondary bile acids. *Microbiome* 7: 126.

Ward, P.B. and Young, G.P. (1997). Dynamics of *Clostridium difficile* infection. Control using diet. *Adv. Exp. Med. Biol.* 412: 63–75.

Warrell, D.A., Fawcett, I.W., Harrison, B.D. et al. (1975). Bronchial asthma in the Nigerian savanna region. A clinical and laboratory study of 106 patients with a review of the literature on asthma in the tropics. *Quar. J. Med.* 44 (174): 325–347.

Wasmer, M.L., Willard, M.D., Helman, R.G. et al. (1995). Food intolerance mimicking alimentary lymphosarcoma. *J. Am. Anim. Hosp. Assoc.* 31 (6): 463–466.

Weatherill, A.R., Lee, J.Y., Zhao, L. et al. (2005). Saturated and polyunsaturated fatty acids reciprocally modulate dendritic cell functions mediated through TLR4. *J. Immunol.* 174 (9): 5390–5397.

Weese, J.S. and Arroyo, L. (2003). Bacteriological evaluation of dog and cat diets that claim to contain probiotics. *Can. Vet. J.* 44 (3): 212–216.

Wehr, U., Elsbett, K., and Krammer, S. (2005). Effects of stable vitamin C (STAY-C 50) on oral health in cats. *2004 Nestle Purina Nutrition Forum Proceedings: A Supplement to Compendium for Continuing Education for Veterinarians* 27 (3A): 76.

Wernimont, S.M., Fritsch, D.A., Schiefelbein, H.M. et al. (2020). Food with specialized dietary fiber sources improves clinical outcomes in adult cats with constipation or diarrhea. *FASEB J.* 34 (S1): 1–1.

Wichert, B., Schuster, S., Hofmann, M. et al. (2002). Influence of different cellulose types on feces quality of dogs. *J. Nutr.* 132 (6 Suppl 2): 1728S–1729S.

Wikingsson, L. and Sjoholm, I. (2002). Polyacryl starch microparticles as adjuvant in oral immunisation, inducing mucosal and systemic immune responses in mice. *Vaccine* 20 (27–28): 3355–3363.

Wilcock, B. (1992). Endoscopic biopsy interpretation in canine or feline enterocolitis. *Semin. Vet. Med. Surg. (Small Anim.)* 7 (2): 162–171.

Wildi, S.M., Tutuian, R., and Castell, D.O. (2004). The influence of rapid food intake on postprandial reflux: studies in healthy volunteers. *Am. J. Gastroenterol.* 99 (9): 1645–1651.

Will, K., Nolte, I., and Zentek, J. (2005). Early enteral nutrition in young dogs suffering from hemorrhagic gastroenteritis. *J. Vet. Med. A Physiol. Pathol. Clin. Med.* 52 (7): 371–376.

Willard, M.D., Simpson, R.B., Delles, E.K. et al. (1994). Effects of dietary supplementation of fructo-oligosaccharides on small intestinal bacterial overgrowth in dogs. *Am. J. Vet. Res.* 55 (5): 654–659.

Winter, T.A. (2006). The effects of undernutrition and refeeding on metabolism and digestive function. *Curr. Opin. Clin. Nutr. Metab. Care* 9 (5): 596–602.

Wojdemann, M., Wettergren, A., Hartmann, B. et al. (1998). Glucagon-like peptide-2 inhibits centrally induced antral motility in pigs. *Scand. J. Gastroenterol.* 33 (8): 828–832.

Wood, H.O. (1944). The surface area of the intestinal mucosa oin the rat and in the cat. *J. Anat.* 78: 103–105.

Wyman, J.B., Dent, J., Heddle, R. et al. (1990). Control of belching by the lower oesophageal sphincter. *Gut* 31 (6): 639–646.

Xia, Y. and Zweier, J.L. (1997). Superoxide and peroxynitrite generation from inducible nitric oxide synthase in macrophages. *Proc. Natl. Acad. Sci.* 94 (13): 6954.

Yamamoto, T., Tomofuji, T., Ekuni, D. et al. (2004). Effects of toothbrushing frequency on proliferation of gingival cells and collagen synthesis. *J. Clin. Periodontol.* 31 (1): 40–44.

Yamka, R.M., Harmon, D.L., Schoenherr, W.D. et al. (2006). in vivo measurement of flatulence and nutrient digestibility in dogs fed poultry by-product meal, conventional soybean meal, and low-oligosaccharide low-phytate soybean meal. *Am. J. Vet. Res.* 67 (1): 88–94.

Yanoff, S.R., Willard, M.D., Boothe, H.W. et al. (1992). Short-bowel syndrome in four dogs. *Vet. Surg.* 21 (3): 217–222.

Yazdanbakhsh, M., Kremsner, P.G., and van Ree, R. (2002). Allergy, parasites, and the hygiene hypothesis. *Science* 296 (5567): 490–494.

Yeh, C.K., Johnson, D.A., Dodds, M.W. et al. (2000). Association of salivary flow rates with maximal bite force. *J. Dent. Res.* 79 (8): 1560–1565.

Yin, L., Laevsky, G., and Giardina, C. (2001). Butyrate suppression of colonocyte NF-κB activation and cellular proteasome activity. *J. Biol. Chem.* 276 (48): 44641–44646.

Zentek, J., Hall, E.J., German, A. et al. (2002). Morphology and immunopathology of the small and large intestine in dogs with nonspecific dietary sensitivity. *J. Nutr.* 132 (6): 1652S–1654S.

Zentek, J., Fricke, S., Hewicker-Trautwein, M. et al. (2004). Dietary protein source and manufacturing processes affect macronutrient digestibility, fecal consistency, and presence of fecal *Clostridium perfringens* in adult dogs. *J. Nutr.* 134: 2158S–2161S.

Ziegler, T.R., Evans, M.E., Fernandez-Estivariz, C. et al. (2003). Trophic and cytoprotective nutrition for intestinal adaptation, mucosal repair, and barrier function. *Annu. Rev. Nutr.* 23: 229–261.

Zijlstra, R.T., Donovan, S.M., Odle, J. et al. (1997). Protein-energy malnutrition delays small-intestinal recovery in neonatal pigs infected with rotavirus. *J. Nutr.* 127 (6): 1118–1127.

12

Nutritional Management of Exocrine Pancreatic Diseases

Cecilia Villaverde and Marta Hervera

The main function of the exocrine pancreas is to synthesize and secrete substances to allow for the proper digestion and absorption of food. The pancreas synthesizes and secretes digestive enzymes that break down protein, fat, and carbohydrates into their smaller, absorbable components. These enzymes are secreted as inactive zymogens, which are kept separate from lysosomes in the pancreatic tissue to avoid premature activation. Other protection mechanisms include pancreatic trypsin inhibitors present in pancreatic juice (which can inactivate free trypsin) and antiproteases present in plasma (such as alpha-macroglobulin) that capture proteases that escape into circulation (Mansfield and Jones 2001).

The pancreas also secretes bicarbonate, to reach optimal pH in the small intestine for enzyme activity; intrinsic factor, to allow absorption of vitamin B12; and bacteriostatic substances, to prevent bacterial proliferation in the small intestine.

Diet plays an important role in regulating pancreatic secretion (Strombeck 1996). A complex system involving the nervous and endocrine systems is responsible for pancreatic secretion regulation. The cephalic phase is mediated by the autonomous nervous system. The gastric phase is mediated by gastrin, a hormone released in response to gastric distention and the presence of nutrients (such as protein). The intestinal phase is mediated by cholecystokinin (CCK) and secretin (also gastrin and vasoactive intestinal peptide), which are hormones synthesized by the intestinal mucosa. Secretin release is stimulated by the presence of acid in the intestine and intraluminal fatty acids (Watanabe et al. 1986). CCK secretion is stimulated by amino acids, acidic pH, and long-chain fatty acids (Figure 12.1). CCK not only stimulates pancreatic secretion, it also results in delayed gastric emptying and voiding of the gall bladder.

The relative potency of different nutrients to stimulate CCK secretion seems to be species specific. In humans, amino acids, protein, and long-chain triglycerides are more effective than carbohydrates (Karhunen et al. 2008). In dogs, fatty acids (Sun et al. 1992), amino acids, and peptides stimulate CCK release, but intact proteins do not (Meyer and Kelly 1976). Cats secrete CCK in response to long-chain triglycerides and proteins (Backus et al. 1995). Although amino acids also stimulate CCK release in the cat, intact protein is more potent (Backus et al. 1997).

Applied Veterinary Clinical Nutrition, Second Edition. Edited by Andrea J. Fascetti, Sean J. Delaney, Jennifer A. Larsen, and Cecilia Villaverde.

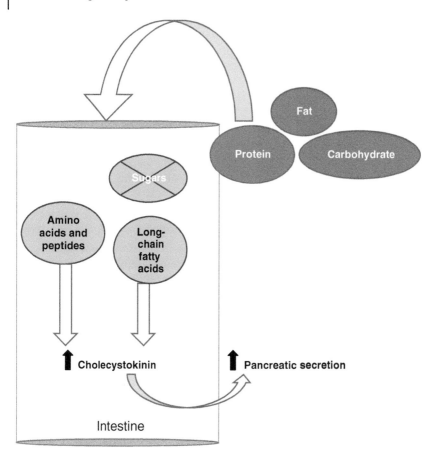

Figure 12.1 Response of cholecystokinin secretion by intestinal mucosal cells to different macronutrients in the small intestinal lumen.

Pancreatitis

Pancreatitis is defined as inflammation of the pancreas, but also includes disorders that involve necrosis or fibrosis (Xenoulis 2015). Currently there is no standardized classification of the disease in veterinary medicine. One way of classification is to extrapolate from human medicine as acute or chronic (Steiner and Williams 1999; Williams and Steiner 2005). Acute pancreatitis refers to inflammation that completely resolves with removal of the inciting cause, whereas chronic pancreatitis is characterized by irreversible histopathologic changes in the pancreas (such as fibrosis and atrophy).

The differentiation is based on histopathology and not on clinical signs, although in veterinary medicine pancreatic biopsies are not commonly collected. Canine acute pancreatitis does not just tend to have sudden onset, but also is accompanied by severe clinical signs and is often associated with systemic complications. Canine chronic pancreatitis has milder clinical signs and a more insidious course. This is less true in cats, where a study has shown that there is poor correlation between clinical signs and histopathology findings (Ferreri et al. 2003). Histopathologically, chronic pancreatitis is the most common form of the disease in cats (De Cock et al. 2007).

The main clinical signs in dogs include vomiting and abdominal pain, and also depression, anorexia, fever, and diarrhea (Williams and Steiner 2005). In cats, signs are highly variable and can be quite vague; most commonly lethargy and anorexia are reported (Hill and Van Winkle 1993; Ferreri et al. 2003). Chronic cases can be subclinical or result in hyporexia and weight loss. Clinical signs can be associated with co-morbidities, which are very common in cats (Armstrong and Williams 2012). In cats, pancreatitis can be associated with hepatic and/or gastrointestinal disease (Weiss et al. 1996), and it is also a co-morbidity found in dogs and cats with diabetes mellitus (Hess et al. 2000; Forcada et al. 2008).

Diagnosis of pancreatitis can be difficult, especially in cats (Forman et al. 2021). Clinical examination findings and standard blood analysis (complete blood cell count, serum biochemistry) show nonspecific alterations (Steiner 2003; Armstrong and Williams 2012; Xenoulis 2015). Serum lipase and amylase increases, which have been traditionally used to diagnose pancreatitis, are neither sensitive nor specific enough to be reliable tests (particularly in cats) (Steiner 2003; Xenoulis and Steiner 2008). Ultrasound can be an effective diagnostic tool (Hess et al. 1999), and can help rule out other diseases with a similar clinical presentation. One study in cats found that abdominal ultrasound had a sensitivity of 80% and specificity of 88% (Forman et al. 2004), but it has been suggested that these values might change depending on the operator (Xenoulis and Steiner 2008) and might actually be higher now with the advances in equipment and training (Xenoulis 2015). Specific tests measuring pancreatic lipase have been developed (canine and feline pancreatic lipase immunoreactivity, cPLI and fPLI, respectively). The cPLI test is specific and sensitive for the disease (Steiner 2003). One multicenter clinical study with 84 dogs with or without acute pancreatitis reported a sensitivity of different cPLI methods of 75–93% and a specificity of 72–78% (McCord et al. 2012). Another study found that

fPLI had a sensitivity and specificity of close to 100% in cats with moderate to severe disease (Forman et al. 2004). The less severe the disease, the less sensitive is this test (Xenoulis and Steiner 2008; Lee et al. 2020; Forman et al. 2021). Definitive diagnosis is made by histopathology. Even so, the diagnosis can be missed in a biopsy due to irregular distribution of the inflammation (Steiner 2003; Forman et al. 2021).

Pathophysiology

It is widely thought that pancreatitis develops as a consequence of pancreas autodigestion resulting from premature activation of the zymogens within the acinar cells (Steiner and Williams 2005; Williams and Steiner 2005). How the protective mechanisms of the pancreas are overwhelmed and autodigestion is initiated, though, is unclear and an underlying cause is rarely identified.

Experimental pancreatitis can be initiated by hyperstimulation with CCK analogs (Morita et al. 1998; Saluja et al. 2007), but the importance of these mechanisms in spontaneous disease is unknown.

Risk factors in dogs include heredity, hyperlipidemia, drugs (such as phenobarbital and potassium bromide; Gaskill and Cribb 2000; Steiner et al. 2008), trauma, and ischemia. Nutrition-related risk factors include obesity and high-fat/low-protein diets (Hess et al. 1999; Williams and Steiner 2005; Lem et al. 2008). In one retrospective study, 26% of dogs with fatal acute pancreatitis were hyperlipidemic (Hess et al. 1998), but hyperlipidemia is not present in all natural cases of pancreatitis (Whitney et al. 1987). Hyperlipidemia can be the cause or result of pancreatitis. The proposed etiologic mechanisms include the formation of toxic fatty acid products within the pancreas due to high triglycerides in pancreatic capillaries, formation of microthrombi by fatty acids, and formation of damaging calcium soaps (Petersen et al. 2009; Tsuang et al. 2009). Some breeds are considered at higher risk for pancreatitis due to their predisposition to hyperlipidemia (such as miniature schnauzers, Shetland sheepdogs, and Siamese cats).

A retrospective paper (Lem et al. 2008) noted that ingestion of unusual food items, intake of table scraps, and garbage eating were associated with a higher risk of pancreatitis in dogs. Its authors also found a positive association of canine obesity with pancreatitis. One study (Akol et al. 1993) found that 43% of dogs with acute pancreatitis were overweight or obese. Another study also reported an association between being overweight and acute fatal pancreatitis in dogs (Hess et al. 1999).

In cats, there is much less information regarding etiology and pathophysiology, and most cases are called "idiopathic" (Mansfield and Jones 2001; Steiner and Williams 2005; Armstrong and Williams 2012; Forman et al. 2021). Less commonly, pancreatitis in cats has been associated with trauma and feline infectious peritonitis (FIP). Potential causes include hyperlipidemia, toxins, ischemia, and ascending infections. Increased age and gastrointestinal and liver diseases have been positively associated with chronic pancreatitis (Akol et al. 1993; Weiss et al. 1996; De Cock et al. 2007). The link between fatty foods, table scraps, medications, and obesity with pancreatitis in cats has not been proven.

Nutritional Management

Controversies Regarding Nutritional Management

The nutritional management of the pancreatitic patient (especially cats) is quite controversial and more research in this area is needed. Some of the more conflicting points are presented in this section.

When to Start Feeding in Acute Pancreatitis?
Traditional approaches to the patient with pancreatitis, especially if vomiting, consisted of "resting the pancreas" by withholding food and water for 24–48 hours or as long as vomiting persists. The goal was to minimize pancreatic stimulation by nutrients and minimize enzyme secretion as well as reduce vomiting. A secondary goal was to prevent aspiration pneumonia. Moreover, some of these patients have severe abdominal pain, which might be further compounded by feeding.

This approach has been challenged. There is one study in dogs with parvovirosis (Mohr et al. 2003), in which the dogs that underwent early enteral nutrition despite vomiting (within 12 hours of admission) recovered earlier and gained more weight than the dogs that were not fed until vomiting stopped for at least 12 hours (an average of 50 hours after admission). The authors hypothesize that early nutrition might have prevented malnutrition and improved the barrier function of the gut, thus improving outcome. A couple of other studies have tried to elucidate if a similar positive effect would be seen in pancreatitis, which has a very different pathophysiology from a viral enteritis. A small pilot study (Mansfield et al. 2011) with 10 dogs diagnosed with severe acute pancreatitis compared feeding enterally via an esophagostomy tube (using a low-fat diet) versus using parenteral nutrition within 24 hours of admission. There was a lower incidence of vomiting and regurgitation in the enteral nutrition group, with no detectable postprandial pain. A second study (Harris et al. 2017), with a larger sample size (34 cases) but retrospective, evaluated the effect of early enteral nutritional support in dogs with acute pancreatitis. This study compared early enteral feeding (within 48 hours of admission) with delayed feeding and found that dogs fed earlier showed a faster return to voluntary feed intake and met their energy requirements earlier; moreover, dogs fed earlier showed fewer incidences of gastrointestinal intolerance, independent of the severity of the disease. There were no differences noted in hospitalization length.

In a study with dogs with experimentally induced disease (Qin et al. 2003), early intrajejunal feeding did increase the plasma concentrations of CCK and other enteral hormones compared to parenteral nutrition; however, this did not result in an increase in pancreatic enzyme secretion. This suggests that the inflamed pancreas may not respond to nutrients in the same way as the healthy pancreas. In addition, the animals fed enterally were not clinically worse, and results suggested that their intestinal barrier function was improved, and that bacterial translocation was lower compared to the dogs fed parenterally (Qin et al. 2002). However, information on enteral nutrition in naturally occurring disease is still lacking.

There is a lack of studies in cats on the effect of nutrition on pancreatitis. One retrospective study (Klaus et al. 2009) with 55 cases assessed the use of nasogastric feeding in cats with suspected acute pancreatitis. The mean start of enteral feeding was 33.5 hours ($\pm$ 15.0) from admission. Overall, cats tolerated feedings well and there was a low incidence of complications (diarrhea, vomiting, and mechanical problems). Due to the risk of hepatic lipidosis in fasting cats (Armstrong and Blanchard 2009), nutritional support should be instituted as soon as possible, especially since vomiting is not a common clinical feature of pancreatitis in cats (Ferreri et al. 2003; Forman et al. 2021). In addition, therapy in the acute phase should ideally include fluid support, pain control, and medications to control nausea. Some authors recommend starting nutrition when the cat has been anorexic for 3–5 days (Zoran 2006; Chan 2009) or earlier, within 48 hours of admission or immediately if previous anorexia was longer than 5 days (Jensen and Chan 2014). In some cases this might require the placement of a feeding tube. In cats, the most common type is an esophageal feeding tube (Figure 12.2).

In humans with acute pancreatitis, one meta-analysis from 2010, including eight randomized clinical trials (Al-Omran et al. 2010) comparing enteral versus parenteral nutrition support, showed that enteral nutrition resulted in lower mortality, less systemic infection, and less multiorgan dysfunction. The current

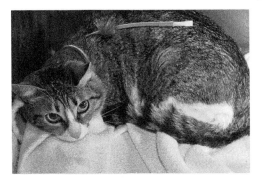

Figure 12.2 Cat with pancreatitis and concurrent hepatic lipidosis with an esophageal feeding tube in place.

recommendation in human medicine is to start enteral feeding as soon as possible in acute pancreatitis (Anand et al. 2017).

How Low Is a "Low-Fat" Diet?

The use of generalized terms like "low-fat" or "high-fat" is confusing because there is no established definition of what a "standard" or "typical" dietary fat concentration is. This problem is further compounded by the different ways in which it is possible to express dietary fat concentrations. The most common are percentage as is or as fed (which is how pet food labels report fat), percentage of dry matter, and percentage of metabolizable energy (ME; e.g. the proportion of calories provided by fat). Ideally, percentage of ME is the ideal way to compare different foods, since it allows for comparison between foods with varying amounts of moisture, fiber, and ash. The fat content of commercial canine and feline diets ranges from 20% to levels as high as 70% on an ME basis. As a rule (but not always), feline diets are higher in fat than canine diets, and canned diets are higher in fat than dry diets. For most of the population eating commercial diets, a diet that has less than 20% fat on an ME basis will be considered low fat, but the term "low fat" is relative to the patient's usual diet. This is especially important in animals with hyperlipidemia, where the degree of fat restriction should be relative to the current diet that is associated with problems.

It is important to note that diets marketed for the management of gastrointestinal disorders vary greatly in fat content, and the diet chosen may or may not be lower fat depending on the diet history of the patient.

Does Fat Have to Be Restricted in Canine Acute Pancreatitis?

Low fat diets have classically been recommended for the management of acute pancreatitis in dogs (Mansfield 2012); however, there is a lack of studies comparing different diets. Some authors have recommended using highly digestible diets not restricted in fat (34–51% ME) unless there is evidence of hyperlipidemia (Jensen and Chan 2014). One study of 10 healthy dogs fed four diets differing in fat (16% vs. 38% ME, with or without digestive enzyme supplementation) in a crossover design for one week per period, did not find any differences in blood PLI, TLI, or gastrin concentrations (James et al. 2009). However, these tests might not be sensitive enough to conclude that enzyme secretion is unaffected by dietary fat, and dogs with pancreatitis might respond differently than healthy ones.

A retrospective study of 34 dogs with acute pancreatitis found a trend toward fewer episodes of gastrointestinal intolerance in dogs fed low-fat diets, but this did not reach significance, which suggests that the sample size was too small to draw any conclusions (Harris et al. 2017).

The main drawback of feeding low-fat diets is their comparatively decreased energy density, which would require a higher volume to feed in order to meet energy needs. In the authors' experience, it is in many cases possible to meet energy requirements using highly digestible low-fat diets (<20% ME) in dogs via voluntary feed intake or tube feeding. There is one liquid diet available (Royal Canin Veterinary Health Nutrition Canine Gastrointestinal Low Fat Liquid, Royal Canin, Saint Charles, MO, USA) that is low in fat and with similar energy density to standard fat solutions (1 and 0.9 kcal/ml for the European and US

versions, respectively). If energy needs can be met, the use of a low-fat diet has no drawbacks and is recommended until more information is available.

How Important Is Fat Restriction in Feline Pancreatitis?

There is a paucity of data regarding pancreatitis in cats in general, and more so regarding the effect of diet on pancreatitis management in this species. As previously mentioned, intact protein and triglycerides both stimulate CCK, whereas carbohydrates have only a weak effect (Backus et al. 1995), so protein and fat moderation may be indicated. Dietary fat also decreases gastric emptying and slows down gastrointestinal transit time (Strombeck 1996), which may be undesired in patients with gastrointestinal disease.

However, as opposed to dogs, consumption of food items high in fat has not been associated with naturally occurring pancreatitis in cats. In the retrospective study cited earlier (Klaus et al. 2009), where 55 cats were fed via nasogastric feeding tubes, the diet used provided approximately 45% fat ME. The cats seemed to tolerate the feedings well, but there is no control diet to compare the results. There are currently no data to recommend for or against moderate or severe fat restriction in these patients. Fat restriction in cats can be challenging, since many commercial diets moderate in fat for cats are also high in fiber, and thus are not the first choice for patients with gastrointestinal signs. In these authors' experience, it is reasonable to try a moderate-fat diet in cats with hyperlipidemia and when other approaches are not giving the desired results.

Dietary Management

The main goals to manage the patient with pancreatitis are to provide enough calories and nutrients to support recovery while decreasing pancreatic stimulation. This can be accomplished in a variety of ways and will vary

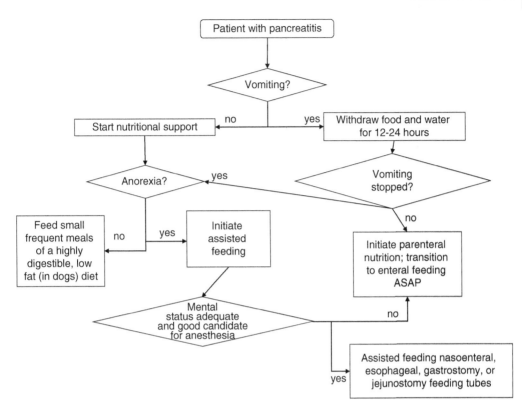

Figure 12.3 When and how to start nutritional support. ASAP, as soon as possible

depending on the clinicians' personal experience. The flowchart presented in Figure 12.3 can be used as a guide to decide if, when, and how to initiate nutritional support for each individual patient.

When to Feed

As a general rule, nutritional support should be instituted as soon as feasible, especially in severe acute pancreatitis (Mansfield and Beths 2015). As previously discussed, it is likely not indicated to withhold food until clinical signs abate in order to "rest the pancreas." Before offering any food, water should be offered first. If water is well tolerated, feeding the animal a low-fat (particularly in dogs), highly digestible diet is indicated.

Cats that have been anorectic for more than three days should be fed as soon as possible despite the presence or absence of clinical signs in order to avoid hepatic lipidosis.

Route of Feeding

Enteral feeding is preferred over parenteral, if possible, in order to avoid enterocyte atrophy and bacterial translocation and to keep costs down. If the patient is anorectic, nutritional support is indicated. Esophagostomy and gastrostomy tubes are indicated if the risk for aspiration pneumonia is minimal. If there is risk of aspiration, jejunostomy feeding tubes will bypass the duodenum to avoid prompting CCK release and can be used to feed enterally while minimizing pancreatic stimulation (Ragins et al. 1973). The main challenge with jejunostomy tubes is the need for anesthesia and surgery for placement. There is one report (Jennings et al. 2001) where a feeding tube was placed in the jejunum of a cat with pancreatitis via a percutaneous endoscopic gastrostomy (PEG) tube. This technique, while still uncommon, may prove a viable alternative in the future to surgically placed jejunostomy tubes.

In human medicine nasojejunal feeding tubes are commonplace; however, studies comparing nasogastric versus nasojejunal in acute pancreatitis in humans have not shown a particular advantage of feeding directly into the jejunum (Zhu et al. 2016).

Nasoesophageal or nasogastric feeding tubes are also an option, especially if the patient is not a good candidate for anesthesia. Due to their small lumen size, they can only be used with liquid diets, thus limiting diet choices and making it more difficult to provide a patient's full caloric requirements. There are few liquid veterinary enteral formulas, but one canine formula controlled in fat is available in the United States and in Europe. Some human enteral formulations are adequately low in fat, but are only adequate for short-term management due to cost and nutritional inadequacy for dogs and especially cats.

Parenteral nutrition is indicated in cases of intractable vomiting, when the patient is obtunded or cannot protect its airway for any other reason, and when feeding tubes cannot be placed due to instability for anesthesia. Gut atrophy has been proposed as a possible complication of parenteral nutrition in animal models (Frost and Bihari 1997; MacFie et al. 2006); thus, trickle feeding with a nasogastric/nasoesophageal tube if at all possible (e.g. provide 10% of the total daily calories) with a low-fat (in dogs) liquid diet could help maintain gut integrity.

Lipid emulsions can be included in parenteral nutrition solutions, since intravenously administered fat has not been associated with worsening the disease or stimulating the pancreas (Meier et al. 2006). However, if the patient is hyperlipidemic, fat in the solution should be minimized to keep serum triglycerides as low as possible (Chan and Freeman 2006).

In cats with mild to moderate pancreatitis, appetite stimulants might help ensure voluntary food intake (Forman et al. 2021). Mirtazapine and capromorelin are the most common drugs used in feline inappetence, although studies are lacking evaluating their efficacy in patients with pancreatitis. Mirtazapine transdermal ointment can be used in cats and generally is well tolerated and efficacious (Poole et al. 2019) and in addition has antiemetic activity (Quimby and Lunn 2013). Nevertheless, adverse effects have been reported (e.g. vocalization, agitation, vomiting, abnormal gait or ataxia, tremors, hypersalivation, tachypnea, tachycardia, lethargy) in a dose-dependent fashion (Ferguson et al. 2016). Oral capromorelin efficacy has been reported in healthy cats (Wofford et al. 2018).

Diet Selection

An ideal diet for the dog with acute pancreatitis is highly digestible, low in fat, and palatable. A good starting point is a mixture of cottage cheese (2% milk fat) and cooked white rice (in a volume ratio of 1 : 1), which provides ~220 kcal per 8 fl oz cup (237 ml) and 10% fat on an ME basis. This mixture can also be pureed in a blender or food processor and fed through an esophagostomy or gastrostomy feeding tube if the patient is anorectic. After 2–3 days, if this is well tolerated, the animal can be transitioned to a balanced, commercial, highly digestible, low-fat diet.

In cats, diets marketed for the management of intestinal disease can be used orally or via a feeding tube. If a low-fat diet is desired, the mixture of cottage cheese and white rice described can be used. If it is not palatable, other options include tuna (canned in water) plus baby rice cereal, or chicken breast plus baby rice cereal. For example, three-eighths of a cup of cooked roasted chicken breast (skinless and boneless) plus three-quarters of a cup of baby rice cereal (measured dry before reconstitution) provides ~200 kcal and 14% fat on an ME basis. Mixing 2 oz (56 g) of tuna in water (drained solids only) with seven-eighths of a cup of baby rice cereal (measured dry before reconstitution) also provides ~200 kcal and only 9% fat on an ME basis.

If a jejunostomy tube is placed, low-fat diets continue to be preferred for dogs, since there is still some pancreatic stimulation, as suggested by one study with experimentally induced disease in dogs (Qin et al. 2003). Due to the size of the tube and the lack of elasticity of the jejunum, liquid diets have to be used, ideally delivering via constant-rate infusion to avoid overloading the gut.

It has been proposed that the diet fed through a jejunostomy tube should also be "elemental" to mimic what would normally be absorbed by the jejunum (proteins should be supplied in the form of free amino acids and short peptides, while carbohydrates should be supplied as simple starches and sugars), but this is controversial even in human medicine (Niv et al. 2009). There is a meta-analysis in human pancreatitis patients that did not find any difference in outcome comparing "intact" versus "elemental" diets (Petrov et al. 2009). There are no studies in veterinary medicine assessing the need for elemental formulations, so there are no data to support or reject the use of "intact" liquid diets. However, if there is persistent diarrhea, an elemental human diet formula can be attempted. See Chapters 20 and 21 for more details on enteral and parenteral nutrition support.

Energy Requirements

During hospitalization, the goal is to provide the resting energy requirement (RER) initially (Chan and Freeman 2006). Once RER is achieved, body weight and body condition should be monitored to adjust the calories provided as necessary. A very slow increase in the calories provided is preferred to prevent metabolic derangements (critically ill animals in a catabolic state can often have significant electrolyte abnormalities) and to avoid overwhelming the gut. These patients are generally inactive during the hospital stay, and a conservative approach is necessary to avoid complications of overfeeding. Sadly, our knowledge of energy requirements in critically ill animals is very limited.

Long-Term Management

After acute, one-time episodes of nonhyperlipidemic canine pancreatitis, it is frequently possible to go back to the dog's original maintenance diet, especially if the trigger has been identified (such as dietary indiscretion, "garbage gut," surgery, or drugs). A slow transition back to the original complete and balanced diet over several days is indicated.

However, in cases of chronic pancreatitis, hyperlipidemic animals, or recurrent acute pancreatitis, a diet considerably lower in fat than the usual diet is indicated. The goal is to select a diet low enough in fat to maintain fasting triglycerides within acceptable ranges (see Chapter 17), to control chronic pancreatitis, and to prevent further episodes of recurrent acute pancreatitis. One empiric approach used by the authors is to approximately halve the fat concentration on a ME basis from the diet at the time of diagnostics.

Diet selection in these cases will depend on assessment of the diet history. If the original diet is higher in fat (i.e. >35–40% fat on an ME basis), commercial options that provide approximately 50% of that dietary fat are available. However, if that is not the case, sometimes a balanced, home-cooked diet is the best option for the patient. Commercially available, highly digestible, low-fat diets formulated for gastrointestinal disease include Royal Canin Veterinary Health Nutrition Canine Gastrointestinal Low Fat Canine canned and dry, Hill's Prescription Diet i/d Low Fat Canine canned, stew, and dry (Hill's Pet Nutrition, Topeka, KS, USA), and Purina Pro Plan Veterinary Diets Canine EN Low Fat canned and dry (Nestlé Purina PetCare, St. Louis, MO, USA), among others. These range from 16% to 22% fat on an ME basis, and an accurate diet history will need to be obtained to decide if any of these is adequate for the particular case.

Currently for cats, the lowest-fat dry veterinary diets are Hill's Prescription Diet r/d Feline dry (24% on an ME basis in the United States, 26% ME in Europe) and Purina Pro Plan Veterinary Diets OM Overweight Management Feline dry (23.4% on an ME basis in the United States, 22% ME in Europe). As is common, canned varieties are higher in fat (at least 31% on a ME basis). Both dry options listed are weight-loss diets that are very high in fiber (so less digestible) and are not energy dense. Thus, they are not typically the first choice in severe feline pancreatitis. In general, finding moderate-fat diets in cats is very challenging, since they tend to be lower in carbohydrate than canine diets and protein is an expensive ingredient. In general, therapeutic diets formulated for intestinal disease are used for these patients; however, they can vary greatly in their fat content and their effect on the patient should be carefully monitored via control of any hypertriglyceridemia, clinical signs, ultrasound, and pancreatic lipase measurements. Presence of other co-morbidities (common in cats) will also affect diet choice, and the use of highly digestible diets suitable for elimination trials (based on hydrolyzed protein or uncommon ingredients) can be considered if chronic enteropathy is suspected or confirmed.

It is important always to assess the fat concentrations of diets and compare them to the previous diet. Some commercial foods marketed as lower or reduced fat are still too high in fat for pancreatitic patients. In some cases, the difference in fat content between the canned and the dry formula of the same product is drastic.

In obese dogs, due to the epidemiologic link between obesity and pancreatitis (Lem et al. 2008), a plan using a low-fat, therapeutic, weight-loss diet that is lower in fat than the previous diet is indicated until an ideal body condition score is reached (see Chapter 9 on weight management).

Pancreatitis is a very challenging disease, both to diagnose and to treat, and there is no agreement upon the best way to manage it nutritionally. In the authors' experience, using low-fat diets (especially in acute canine cases) that are highly digestible and feeding enterally as soon as vomiting is controlled are appropriate and prudent. Provision of adequate energy is not sacrificed with this approach. If enteral nutrition is not possible, the parenteral route may be considered. Long-term management will depend greatly on the previous diet

history, concurrent diseases, and response to treatment. There are hundreds of diets available that might be successful for individual patients, and in some cases a complete and balanced home-cooked diet may be the best option to control clinical signs.

Foods to Avoid in Chronic Pancreatitis

A thorough diet history is crucial to determine the level of dietary fat that is tolerated by the individual patient, especially in canine acute pancreatitis. If the pancreatitis episode was associated with the ingestion of a particular food item, efforts should be made to determine the concentration of fat of that particular food and avoid feeding close to or above that fat concentration in the future.

In any case, a patient diagnosed with chronic pancreatitis should be fed complete and balanced diets, treats, and human foods that are low or moderate in fat, to avoid recurrence of disease. Protein is the second most important nutrient in stimulating CCK, so very high-protein diets should also be avoided, especially in the feline patient.

Some commercial therapeutic diets are very high in fat. These include energy-dense diets that use fat as a concentrated energy source (such as therapeutic diets formulated for critical care), low-carbohydrate diets that use fat as the main energy source (such as feline diabetes management diets), and protein-restricted diets that are high in fat to promote palatability (such as diets formulated for kidney disease, liver disease, and even urolithiasis). In patients with pancreatitis and co-morbidities such as kidney disease, a home-cooked diet to accommodate the nutritional needs of each disease might be indicated if fat moderation is required.

There is a variety of over-the-counter diets that can also be very high in fat and sometimes in protein. Some examples include the carnivorous-type diets that do not use grains in their formulation, some raw-meat diets and canned diets, and some very palatable sausage-like diets. It is important to consider that the

Table 12.1 Common foods to avoid in chronic canine/feline pancreatitis.

Fatty animal products	Fatty fish	Dairy	Commercial treats	Other
Beef	Salmon	Cheese (non low fat), including spreadable cream cheese	Meaty treats (sausage-like)	Tofu
Lamb	Sardines	Full-fat yogurt	Dry meat treats (jerky)	Peanut butter
Rabbit				Oils and butter
Goat		Meaty treats (sausage-like)		
Cured meats		Dry meat treats (jerky)		
Sausage				

fat content of all these diets can vary greatly between the dry and the canned formulations.

Some commercial treats can also be very high in fat and protein, especially the meaty ones, and should be avoided. Carbohydrate-based biscuits are generally acceptable.

Regarding food usually used for human consumption and table scraps, fruits and vegetables are excellent treats for dogs and event some cats with chronic pancreatitis, since they are mostly carbohydrate and are also low in energy density, which helps prevent undesired weight gain. Some common human foods to avoid are listed in Table 12.1.

Exocrine Pancreatic Insufficiency

Pathophysiology

Exocrine pancreatic insufficiency (EPI) results from a severe loss of exocrine pancreatic function. It has been reported that 90% of acinar cells must be lost before clinical signs arise (Westermarck et al. 2005).

There are several mechanisms by which pancreatic mass can be lost. In young dogs, the most common cause of EPI (Westermarck et al. 2005) is pancreatic acinar atrophy (PAA), which has been described in German shepherd dogs and other breeds such as rough-coated collies. The mechanisms of PAA are not completely understood. It is believed to have an important genetic component, and the published research supports that PAA is preceded by a lymphocytic infiltration of the pancreas (Wiberg et al. 1999), which has led to the hypothesis that PAA is an autoimmune disease. There is a case series, which suggests that chronic pancreatitis can also be a cause of EPI in dogs (Watson 2003), but its relative importance is unknown. Other less common possible causes of EPI in dogs include pancreatic hypoplasia and pancreatic neoplasia.

In cats, it is believed that the most common cause of EPI is chronic pancreatitis that ends up destroying the acini (Steiner and Williams 1999; Steiner 2012). This process has also been demonstrated in humans (Gupta et al. 2009). PAA has not been described in the cat.

When the pancreas is unable to provide enough digestive enzymes, bicarbonate, and other substances for proper digestion and absorption, signs of fat, protein, and carbohydrate malassimilation occur, mainly weight loss, poor body condition, diarrhea (with steatorrhea), and polyphagia (Westermarck and Wiberg 2003; Thompson et al. 2009). Figure 12.4 shows a dog with a dull coat and very poor body condition, secondary to the

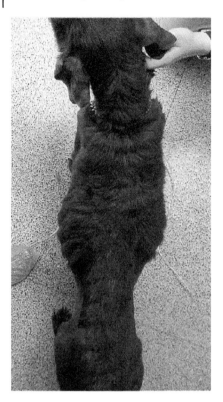

Figure 12.4   Dog with exocrine pancreatic insufficiency.

maldigestion and malabsorption classic for this disease.

Due to fat malabsorption, fat-soluble vitamins (which need fat for proper absorption) might be deficient. One study found that serum vitamin A was lower in dogs with experimental EPI compared to control dogs (Adamama-Moraitou et al. 2002). Low serum concentrations of retinol, α-tocopherol (Barko and Williams 2018), and taurine (Tayler et al. 2020) have been reported in some dogs with EPI. Additional research is needed to determine the clinical relevance of these findings, to determine whether EPI was the primary cause of this low concentration and the therapeutic potential of its supplementation, although those findings highlight the importance of ensuring that nutrient requirements are sufficiently met in patients with EPI.

There is no information on macro- and trace minerals absorption in patients with EPI. In one study in dogs with experimental EPI, the investigators found lower serum and tissue concentrations of copper and zinc compared to control dogs, but the significance of these findings is unknown (Adamama-Moraitou et al. 2001).

The pancreas secretes intrinsic factor, essential for vitamin B12 (cobalamin) absorption. In dogs the stomach also secretes intrinsic factor, but it is less important than the pancreas (Vaillant et al. 1990), and in the cat it seems the pancreas is the only significant source. Hypocobalaminemia has been reported in most dogs (Simpson et al. 1989) and cats (Thompson et al. 2009) with EPI. In dogs, this can be partly due to dysbiosis, which has been described in dogs (but not in cats) with EPI (Williams et al. 1987; Westermarck et al. 1993).

Nutritional Management

Controversies Regarding Nutritional Management

Is a Low-Fat Diet Important for Management?

Enzyme supplementation is the mainstay for the therapy of patients with EPI. The activity of lipase, however, never reaches concentrations comparable to healthy animals due to destruction by acid (DiMagno et al. 1977) and proteases (Thiruvengadam and DiMagno 1988) in the stomach, and many treated patients still have some degree of steatorrhea. For this reason, feeding a moderate- to low-fat diet has been proposed as a strategy to limit fat malabsorption. A possible downside of severe fat restriction is reduction of the energy density of the diet, which is not ideal in very underweight animals.

One study (Simpson et al. 1994) found that a group of dogs with EPI gained weight after being treated with pancreatic enzymes and a low-fat diet. However, there was no control group, and the dogs continued to do well after they were switched to a variety of different diets.

Two studies from Westermarck and collaborators (Westermarck et al. 1995; Westermarck and Wiberg 2006) investigated the importance of fat restriction and diet change in managing dogs with EPI. In the first study, the effect of a low-fat diet (13% on an ME basis) was compared to the dogs' original diet (which varied in fat content from 14% to 30% on an ME basis, approximately). In the latter study, three diets were used: a high-fat diet (51% on an ME basis), a high-fiber, low-fat diet (22% fat on an ME basis), and a moderate-fat, highly digestible diet (30% fat on an ME basis). The most important finding of these studies was that response to fat restriction varied greatly from dog to dog: some animals responded favorably, others were not affected, others were negatively affected. There are studies in experimentally induced EPI in dogs that suggest that fat restriction actually worsens lipase activity (Suzuki et al. 1997, 1999), since fat and protein protect lipase during aboral intestinal transit. Biourge and Fontaine (2004) published a case series where three German shepherd dogs with EPI and concurrent skin disease attributed to an adverse reaction to food were treated with a hydrolyzed diet (soy based) and pancreatic enzyme supplementation. The three dogs did well with the diet and the supplementation, even though the fat content of this diet was high (40.8% on an ME basis). A retrospective study looking at dogs with EPI did not find a positive (or negative) effect of changing to a low-fat diet (Batchelor et al. 2007).

Thus, current information indicates that a low-fat diet is not necessary unless steatorrhea is uncontrollable, at least initially. There is no information published regarding the specific effect of dietary fat on feline EPI. One retrospective study with 150 cases of feline EPI did not find any association of diet change with a positive response (Xenoulis et al. 2016).

Are Medium-Chain Triglycerides Preferred over Long-Chain Triglycerides?

Medium-chain triglycerides (MCTs) have medium- chain fatty acids (6–12 carbons) esterified to the glycerol moiety. They have been used in human medicine to manage malabsorption diseases, since it is believed that they are absorbed via the portal circulation instead of being transported in chylomicrons via lymphatic vessels. Research in cats and dogs is lacking.

Rutz et al. (2004) studied the effect of three diets (containing 0%, 16%, or 35% of the total fat content as MCTs) in a randomized controlled double-blind crossover trial. They found increased blood concentration of cholesterol and some fat-soluble vitamins, but there was no difference between the groups regarding appetite, attitude, drinking behavior, volume of feces, defecation frequency, color of feces, consistency of feces, flatulence, or borborygmus, as subjectively assessed by the clients.

High concentrations of MCTs have been associated with palatability problems in dogs (Matulka et al. 2009), although not all studies have reported this (for example, Berk et al. 2022), and even low to moderate levels of MCTs seem to be unpalatable to cats (MacDonald et al. 1985). Currently, there is not enough positive evidence to support the use of MCTs in dogs and cats with EPI.

Dietary Management

The main treatment of EPI is lifelong enzyme replacement therapy (Westermarck et al. 2005). There are several commercial sources of these enzymes, although raw pancreas can also be used; however, it still carries the same risks associated with feeding any raw animal product, including the potential for zoonotic diseases. Supplemental enzymes are given with every meal (with no need to preincubate them with food).

The main nutritional goals in patients with EPI are to provide enough energy and nutrients to maintain ideal body condition, avoid nutrient deficiencies, and minimize diarrhea. In light of the published data, it appears that there is not one single diet characteristic that can successfully achieve these goals. In the study from Westermarck and Wiberg (2006), some dogs responded to diet change, but to different types of diet depending on the patient. An individual choice of diet should be made for each patient, and in many cases this process will be one characterized by trial and error. Initially, a diet change might not be necessary (unless there is a concurrent disease that requires it, such as with adverse food reactions). Once enzyme supplementation has been in place for 3–4 weeks, the diet can be changed if the clinical response is not ideal. For example, since some enzymes can be affected by fiber, some authors recommend low-fiber (i.e. highly digestible) diets (Steiner and Williams 1999). Some preliminary data presented as research abstracts suggest that digestibility is an important dietary factor. Dogs with EPI and on enzyme replacement therapy, even with no clinical signs and good body condition, can have lower digestibility of macronutrients compared to healthy controls (Oliveira et al. 2021), and a highly digestible diet improves macronutrient digestibility (Oliveira et al. 2022). In addition, the studied EPI dogs had a higher dysbiosis index than the healthy dogs, which the diet did not correct in the time frame of two months. These reports have practical implications, not just for diet choice, but also for the need to consider that patients might require more food than average in order to compensate for this digestibility deficit. Examples of highly digestible foods are the veterinary therapeutic diets formulated for gastrointestinal diseases. In dogs with poor body condition, a high-fat, more energy-dense diet to promote weight gain might be attempted.

Regarding individual deficiencies, animals with low cobalamin should be supplemented with this vitamin until normalization. Parenteral supplementation is the classic recommendation, although recent studies have suggested that oral supplementation can be adequate in dogs (Toresson et al. 2016, 2021; Chang et al. 2022) and cats (Toresson et al. 2017) with chronic enteropathy. In a

retrospective study with 18 dogs with EPI and cobalamin deficiency, oral supplementation with 0.25–1.0 mg/d cobalamin resulted in significantly increased serum cobalamin concentrations (Toresson et al. 2021). A recent prospective clinical trial including 46 dogs with hypocobalaminemia caused by chronic enteropathy or EPI found that both oral (250 µg in <10 kg dogs; 500 µg in 10–19 kg dogs; 1000 µg in ≥20 kg dogs) and injectable supplementation succeeded in normalizing serum cobalamin. However, in dogs with EPI only, oral supplementation showed a significant decrease of methylmalonic acid (Chang et al. 2022). A study in Brazil (abstract only) noted that a highly digestible diet enriched in prebiotic fibers and in B12 (1.5 vs. 0.17 ppm) also resulted in higher serum cobalamin in EPI dogs. In both dogs and cats, hypocobalaminemia has been identified as a poor prognostic indicator (Batchelor et al. 2007; Thompson et al. 2009; Soetart et al. 2019) and can be a reason for treatment failure. One retrospective study by Xenoulis et al. (2016) noted that 77% of cats presented with hypocobalaminemia, and that vitamin B12 supplementation was significantly correlated with clinical improvement.

As for fat-soluble vitamins, they can be supplemented orally if there are signs of clinical deficiency (e.g. skin disease or coagulopathy). In many cases, feeding a complete and balanced diet and controlling the disease via enzyme supplementation seems to be sufficient.

Both retrospective studies on feline EPI (Thompson et al. 2009, 16 cases; and Xenoulis et al. 2016, 150 cases) have shown that concurrent diseases are common (63% and 58%, respectively), which might affect the dietary choice of these patients.

Regarding feed management, ad libitum feeding is not an option in these patients, since pancreatic enzymes must be given with every meal. Also, it is important to avoid or at least minimize treats and to make sure that the patient does not have access to unmonitored food sources.

Summary

- Voluntary or assisted feeding should be instituted as soon as feasible in animals with acute pancreatitis. The main nutritional goal is to provide energy and nutrients while minimizing pancreatic secretion.
- Fat is the most potent stimulator for pancreatic secretion, and its oral intake must be restricted during an episode of acute pancreatitis, especially in dogs. In chronic pancreatitis, lifelong fat restriction or moderation might be needed. Very high concentrations of dietary protein should also be avoided.
- Long-term nutritional management of acute canine pancreatitis should address any predisposing factors for the disease such as obesity, hyperlipidemia, and consumption of fatty foods.
- The existence of concurrent disease (such as intestinal or liver diseases) should be considered accordingly when deciding on the nutritional management of the cat with pancreatitis.
- Nutritional goals for the management of exocrine pancreatic insufficiency (EPI) are to provide energy for a healthy body condition, provide nutrients to avoid deficiencies, and minimize steatorrhea. A highly digestible diet can be useful in cases where regular maintenance diets fail to achieve these goals.
- Hypocobalaminemia is a cause for treatment failure of EPI and a poor prognostic indicator in dogs and cats; supplementation is indicated if present.
- Moderate- to high-fat diets can be useful in patients with EPI with very poor body condition.
- The presence of concurrent diseases in dogs and especially cats will affect the diet choice in these patients with EPI.

References

Adamama-Moraitou, K., Rallis, T., Papasteriadis, A. et al. (2001). Iron, zinc, and copper concentration in serum, various organs, and hair of dogs with experimentally induced exocrine pancreatic insufficiency. *Dig. Dis. Sci.* 46: 1444–1457.

Adamama-Moraitou, K.K., Rallis, T.S., Prassinos, N.N. et al. (2002). Serum vitamin a concentration in dogs with experimentally induced exocrine pancreatic insufficiency. *Int. J. Vitam. Nutr. Res.* 72: 177–182.

Akol, K.G., Washabau, R.J., Saunders, H.M. et al. (1993). Acute pancreatitis in cats with hepatic lipidosis. *J. Vet. Intern. Med.* 7: 205–209.

Al-Omran, M., Albalawi, Z.H., Tashkandi, M.F. et al. (2010). Enteral vs parenteral nutrition for acute pancreatitis. *Cochrane Database Syst. Rev.* 20: CD002837. https://doi.org/10.1002/14651858.CD002837.pub2.

Anand, N., Park, J.H., and Wu, B.U. (2017). Modern management of acute pancreatitis. *Gastroenterol. Clin. N. Am.* 41: 1–8.

Armstrong, P.J. and Blanchard, G. (2009). Hepatic lipidosis in cats. *Vet. Clin. N. Am.: Small Anim. Pract.* 39: 599–616.

Armstrong, P.J. and Williams, D.A. (2012). Pancreatitis in cats. *Top. Compan. Anim. Med.* 27: 140–147.

Backus, R.C., Rosenquist, G.L., Rogers, Q.R. et al. (1995). Elevation of plasma cholecystokinin (CCK) immunoreactivity by fat, protein, and amino acids in the cat, a carnivore. *Regul. Pept.* 57: 123–131.

Backus, R.C., Howard, K.A., and Rogers, Q.R. (1997). The potency of dietary amino acids in elevating plasma cholecystokinin immunoreactivity in cats is related to amino acid hydrophobicity. *Regul. Pept.* 72: 31–40.

Barko, P.C. and Williams, D.A. (2018). Serum concentrations of lipid-soluble vitamins in dogs with exocrine pancreatic insufficiency treated with pancreatic enzymes. *J. Vet. Intern. Med.* 32 (5): 1600–1608.

Batchelor, D.J., Noble, P.J., Taylor, R.H. et al. (2007). Prognostic factors in canine exocrine pancreatic insufficiency: prolonged survival is likely if clinical remission is achieved. *J. Vet. Intern. Med.* 21: 54–60.

Berk, B.A., Packer, R.M., Fritz, J. et al. (2022). Oral palatability testing of a medium-chain triglyceride oil supplement (MCT) in a cohort of healthy dogs in a non-clinical setting. *Animals* 12 (13): 1639.

Biourge, V.C. and Fontaine, J. (2004). Exocrine pancreatic insufficiency and adverse reaction to food in dogs: a positive response to a high-fat, soy isolate hydrolysate-based diet. *J. Nutr.* 134 (Suppl. 8): 2166–2168.

Chan, D.L. (2009). The inappetent hospitalised cat: clinical approach to maximising nutritional support. *J. Feline Med. Surg.* 11: 925–933.

Chan, D.L. and Freeman, L.M. (2006). Nutrition in critical illness. *Vet. Clin. N. Am.: Small Anim. Pract.* 36: 1225–1241.

Chang, C.H., Lidbury, J.A., Suchodolski, J.S. et al. (2022). Effect of oral or injectable supplementation with cobalamin in dogs with hypocobalaminemia caused by chronic enteropathy or exocrine pancreatic insufficiency. *J. Vet. Intern. Med.* 36 (5): 1607–1621.

De Cock, H.E., Forman, M.A., Farver, T.B. et al. (2007). Prevalence and histopathologic characteristics of pancreatitis in cats. *Vet. Pathol.* 44: 39–49.

DiMagno, E.P., Malagelada, J.R., Go, V.L. et al. (1977). Fate of orally ingested enzymes in pancreatic insufficiency. Comparison of two dosage schedules. *N. Engl. J. Med.* 296: 1318–1322.

Ferguson, L.E., McLean, M.K., Bates, J.A. et al. (2016). Mirtazapine toxicity in cats: retrospective study of 84 cases (2006–2011). *J. Feline Med. Surg.* 18 (11): 868–874.

Ferreri, J.A., Hardam, E., Kimmel, S.E. et al. (2003). Clinical differentiation of acute necrotizing from chronic nonsuppurative pancreatitis in cats: 63 cases (1996–2001). *J. Am. Vet. Med. Assoc.* 223: 469–474.

Forcada, Y., German, A.J., Noble, P.J. et al. (2008). Determination of serum fPLI concentrations in cats with diabetes mellitus. *J. Feline Med. Surg.* 10: 480–487.

Forman, M.A., Marks, S.L., De Cock, H.E. et al. (2004). Evaluation of serum feline pancreatic lipase immunoreactivity and helical computed tomography versus conventional testing for the diagnosis of feline pancreatitis. *J. Vet. Intern. Med.* 18: 807–815.

Forman, M.A., Steiner, J.M., Armstrong, P.J. et al. (2021). ACVIM consensus statement on pancreatitis in cats. *J. Vet. Intern. Med.* 35 (2): 703–723.

Frost, P. and Bihari, D. (1997). The route of nutritional support in the critically ill: physiological and economical considerations. *Nutrition* 13 (Suppl. 9): 58–63.

Gaskill, C.L. and Cribb, A.E. (2000). Pancreatitis associated with potassium bromide/ phenobarbital combination therapy in epileptic dogs. *Can. Vet. J.* 41: 555–558.

Gupta, R., Wig, J.D., Bhasin, D.K. et al. (2009). Severe acute pancreatitis: the life after. *J. Gastrointest. Surg.* 13: 1328–1336.

Harris, J.P., Parnell, N.K., Griffith, E.H. et al. (2017). Retrospective evaluation of the impact of early enteral nutrition on clinical outcomes in dogs with pancreatitis: 34 cases (2010–2013). *J. Vet. Emerg. Crit. Care* 27: 425–433.

Hess, R.S., Saunders, H.M., Van Winkle, T.J. et al. (1998). Clinical, clinicopathologic, radiographic, and ultrasonographic abnormalities in dogs with fatal acute pancreatitis: 70 cases (1986–1995). *J. Am. Vet. Med. Assoc.* 213: 665–670.

Hess, R.S., Kass, P.H., Shofer, F.S. et al. (1999). Evaluation of risk factors for fatal acute pancreatitis in dogs. *J. Am. Vet. Med. Assoc.* 214: 46–51.

Hess, R.S., Saunders, H.M., Van Winkle, T.J. et al. (2000). Concurrent disorders in dogs with diabetes mellitus: 221 cases (1993–1998). *J. Am. Vet. Med. Assoc.* 217: 1166–1173.

Hill, R.C. and Van Winkle, T.J. (1993). Acute necrotizing pancreatitis and acute suppurative pancreatitis in the cat. A retrospective study of

40 cases (1976–1989). *J. Vet. Intern. Med.* 7: 25–33.

James, F.E., Mansfield, C.S., Steiner, J.M. et al. (2009). Pancreatic response in healthy dogs fed diets of various fat compositions. *Am. J. Vet. Res.* 70: 614–618.

Jennings, M., Center, S.A., Barr, S.C. et al. (2001). Successful treatment of feline pancreatitis using an endoscopically placed gastrojejunostomy tube. *J. Am. Anim. Hosp. Assoc.* 37: 145–152.

Jensen, K.B. and Chan, D.L. (2014). Nutritional management of acute pancreatitis in dogs and cats. *J. Vet. Emerg. Crit. Care* 24: 240–250.

Karhunen, L.J., Juvonen, K.R., Huotari, A. et al. (2008). Effect of protein, fat, carbohydrate and fibre on gastrointestinal peptide release in humans. *Regul. Pept.* 149: 70–78.

Klaus, J.A., Rudloff, E., and Kirby, R. (2009). Nasogastric tube feeding in cats with suspected acute pancreatitis: 55 cases (2001–2006). *J. Vet. Emerg. Crit. Care* 19: 337–346.

Lee, C., Kathrani, A., and Maddison, J. (2020). Retrospective study of the diagnostic utility of spec fPL in the assessment of 274 sick cats. *J. Vet. Intern. Med.* 34 (4): 1406–1412.

Lem, K.Y., Fosgate, G.T., Norby, B. et al. (2008). Associations between dietary factors and pancreatitis in dogs. *J. Am. Vet. Med. Assoc.* 233: 1425–1431.

MacDonald, M.L., Rogers, Q.R., and Morris, J.G. (1985). Aversion of the cat to dietary medium-chain triglycerides and caprylic acid. *Physiol. Behav.* 35: 371–375.

MacFie, J., Reddy, B.S., Gatt, M. et al. (2006). Bacterial translocation studied in 927 patients over 13 years. *Br. J. Surg.* 93: 87–93.

Mansfield, C.S. (2012). Acute pancreatitis in dogs: advances in understanding, diagnostics, and treatment. *Top. Compan. Anim. Med.* 27: 123–132.

Mansfield, C.S. and Beths, T. (2015). Management of acute pancreatitis in dogs: a critical appraisal with focus on feeding and analgesia. *J. Small Anim. Pract.* 56: 27–39.

Mansfield, C.S. and Jones, B.R. (2001). Review of feline pancreatitis part one: the normal feline pancreas, the pathophysiology, classification, prevalence and aetiologies of pancreatitis. *J. Feline Med. Surg.* 3: 117–124.

Mansfield, C.S., James, F.E., Steiner, J.M. et al. (2011). A pilot study to assess tolerability of early enteral nutrition via esophagostomy tube feeding in dogs with severe acute pancreatitis. *J. Vet. Intern. Med.* 25: 419–425.

Matulka, R.A., Thompson, D.V., and Burdock, G.A. (2009). Lack of toxicity by medium chain triglycerides (MCT) in canines during a 90-day feeding study. *Food Chem. Toxicol.* 47: 35–39.

McCord, K., Morley, P.S., Armstrong, J. et al. (2012). A multi-institutional study evaluating the diagnostic utility of the Spec cPL™ and SNAP® cPL™ in clinical acute pancreatitis in 84 dogs. *J. Vet. Intern. Med.* 26: 888–896.

Meier, R., Ockenga, J., Pertkiewicz, M. et al. (2006). ESPEN guidelines on enteral nutrition: pancreas. *Clin. Nutr.* 25: 275–284.

Meyer, J.H. and Kelly, G.A. (1976). Canine pancreatic responses to intestinally perfused proteins and protein digests. *Am. J. Physiol.* 231: 682–691.

Mohr, A.J., Leisewitz, A.L., Jacobson, L.S. et al. (2003). Effect of early enteral nutrition on intestinal permeability, intestinal protein loss, and outcome in dogs with severe parvoviral enteritis. *J. Vet. Intern. Med.* 17: 791–798.

Morita, Y., Takiguchi, M., Yasuda, J. et al. (1998). Endoscopic and transcutaneous ultrasonographic findings and greyscale histogram analysis in dogs with caerulein-induced pancreatitis. *Vet. Q.* 20: 89–92.

Niv, E., Fireman, Z., and Vaisman, N. (2009). Post-pyloric feeding. *World J. Gastroenterol.* 15: 1281–1288.

Oliveira, V.V., Henriquez, L.B.F., Rentas, M.F. et al. (2021). Comparison of macronutrient digestibility of client-owned dogs with exocrine pancreatic insufficiency given pancreatic enzymes and healthy dogs. In: *25th ESVCN Congress Proceedings*, 136. Vienna: ESVCN.

Oliveira, V.V., Teixeira, F.A., Ishii, P.E. et al. (2022). High digestible diet with higher cobalamin and prebiotic content improves serum cobalamin and digestibility of dogs with exocrine pancreatic insufficiency but did not improve dysbiosis and gut permeability. In: *26th ESVCN Congress Proceedings*, 81. Vienna: ESVCN.

Petersen, O.H., Tepikin, A.V., Gerasimenko, J.V. et al. (2009). Fatty acids, alcohol and fatty acid ethyl esters: toxic Ca^{2+} signal generation and pancreatitis. *Cell Calcium* 45: 634–642.

Petrov, M.S., Loveday, B.P., Pylypchuk, R.D. et al. (2009). Systematic review and meta-analysis of enteral nutrition formulations in acute pancreatitis. *Br. J. Surg.* 96: 1243–1252.

Poole, M., Quimby, J.M., Hu, T. et al. (2019). A double-blind, placebo-controlled, randomized study to evaluate the weight gain drug, mirtazapine transdermal ointment, in cats with unintended weight loss. *J. Vet. Pharmacol. Ther.* 42 (2): 179–188.

Qin, H.L., Su, Z.D., Hu, L.G. et al. (2002). Effect of early intrajejunal nutrition on pancreatic pathological features and gut barrier function in dogs with acute pancreatitis. *Clin. Nutr.* 21: 469–473.

Qin, H.L., Su, Z.D., Hu, L.G. et al. (2003). Parenteral versus early intrajejunal nutrition: effect on pancreatitic natural course, entero-hormones release and its efficacy on dogs with acute pancreatitis. *World J. Gastroenterol.* 9: 2270–2273.

Quimby, J.M. and Lunn, K.F. (2013). Mirtazapine as an appetite stimulant and anti-emetic in cats with chronic kidney disease: a masked placebo-controlled crossover clinical trial. *Vet. J. (London, England: 1997)* 197 (3): 651–655.

Ragins, H., Levenson, S.M., Signer, R. et al. (1973). Intrajejunal administration of an elemental diet at neutral pH avoids pancreatic stimulation. Studies in dog and man. *Am. J. Surg.* 126: 606–614.

Rutz, G.M., Steiner, J.M., Bauer, J.E. et al. (2004). Effects of exchange of dietary medium chain triglycerides for longchain triglycerides on serum biochemical variables and subjectively assessed well-being of dogs with exocrine pancreatic insufficiency. *Am. J. Vet. Res.* 65: 1293–1302.

Saluja, A.K., Lerch, M.M., Phillips, P.A. et al. (2007). Why does pancreatic overstimulation cause pancreatitis? *Annu. Rev. Physiol.* 69: 249–269.

Simpson, K.W., Morton, D.B., and Batt, R.M. (1989). Effect of exocrine pancreatic insufficiency on cobalamin absorption in dogs. *Am. J. Vet. Res.* 50: 1233–1236.

Simpson, J.W., Maskell, I.E., Quigg, J. et al. (1994). Long term management of canine exocrine pancreatic insufficiency. *J. Small Anim. Pract.* 35: 133–138.

Soetart, N., Rochel, D., Drutand, A. et al. (2019). Serum cobalamin and folate as prognostic factors in canine exocrine pancreatic insufficiency: an observational cohort study of 299 dogs. *Vet. J. (London, England: 1997)* 243: 15–20.

Steiner, J.M. (2003). Diagnosis of pancreatitis. *Vet. Clin. N. Am.: Small Anim. Pract.* 33: 1181–1195.

Steiner, J.M. (2012). Exocrine pancreatic insufficiency in the cat. *Top. Compan. Anim. Med.* 27: 113–116.

Steiner, J.M. and Williams, D.A. (1999). Feline exocrine pancreatic disorders. *Vet. Clin. N. Am.: Small Anim. Pract.* 29: 551–575.

Steiner, J. and Williams, D. (2005). Feline exocrine pancreatic disease. In: *Textbook of Veterinary Internal Medicine*, 6e, 1489. St. Louis, MO: Elsevier Saunders.

Steiner, J.M., Xenoulis, P.G., Anderson, J.A. et al. (2008). Serum pancreatic lipase immunoreactivity concentrations in dogs treated with potassium bromide and/or phenobarbital. *Vet. Ther.* 9: 37–44.

Strombeck, D.R. (1996). Small and large intestine: normal structure and function. In: *Strombeck's Small Animal Gastroenterology*, 3e (ed. W.G. Guilford, S.A. Center, D.R. Strombeck, et al.), 318–350. Philadelphia, PA: W.B. Saunders.

Sun, G., Chang, T.M., Xue, W.J. et al. (1992). Release of cholecystokinin and secretin by sodium oleate in dogs: molecular form and bioactivity. *Am. J. Physiol.* 262: 35–43.

Suzuki, A., Mizumoto, A., Sarr, M.G. et al. (1997). Bacterial lipase and high-fat diets in canine exocrine pancreatic insufficiency: a new therapy of steatorrhea? *Gastroenterology* 112: 2048–2055.

Suzuki, A., Mizumoto, A., Rerknimitr, R. et al. (1999). Effect of bacterial or porcine lipase with low- or high-fat diets on nutrient absorption in pancreatic-insufficient dogs. *Gastroenterology* 116: 431–437.

Tayler, S., Seo, J., Connolly, D.J. et al. (2020). Blood taurine concentrations in dogs with exocrine pancreatic insufficiency. *Am. J. Vet. Res.* 81 (12): 958–963.

Thiruvengadam, R. and DiMagno, E.P. (1988). Inactivation of human lipase by proteases. *Am. J. Physiol.* 255: 476–481.

Thompson, K.A., Parnell, N.K., Hohenhaus, A.E. et al. (2009). Feline exocrine pancreatic insufficiency: 16 cases (1992–2007). *J. Feline Med. Surg.* 11: 935–940.

Toresson, L., Steiner, J.M., Suchodolski, J.S. et al. (2016). Oral cobalamin supplementation in dogs with chronic enteropathies and hypocobalaminemia. *J. Vet. Intern. Med.* 30: 101–107.

Toresson, L., Steiner, J.M., Olmedal, G. et al. (2017). Oral cobalamin supplementation in cats with hypocobalaminemia: a retrospective study. *J. Feline Med. Surg.* 19: 1302–1306.

Toresson, L., Steiner, J.M., Spodsberg, E. et al. (2021). Effects of oral cobalamin supplementation on serum cobalamin concentrations in dogs with exocrine pancreatic insufficiency: a pilot study. *Vet. J. (London, England: 1997)* 269: 105619.

Tsuang, W., Navaneethan, U., Ruiz, L. et al. (2009). Hypertri-glyceridemic pancreatitis: presentation and management. *Am. J. Gastroenterol.* 104: 984–991.

Vaillant, C., Horadagoda, N.U., and Batt, R.M. (1990). Cellular localization of intrinsic factor in pancreas and stomach of the dog. *Cell Tissue Res.* 260: 117–122.

Watanabe, S., Chey, W.Y., Lee, K.Y. et al. (1986). Secretin is released by digestive products of fat in dogs. *Gastroenterology* 90: 1008–1017.

Watson, P.J. (2003). Exocrine pancreatic insufficiency as an end stage of pancreatitis in four dogs. *J. Small Anim. Pract.* 44: 306–312.

Weiss, D.J., Gagne, J.M., and Armstrong, P.J. (1996). Relationship between inflammatory hepatic disease and inflammatory bowel disease, pancreatitis, and nephritis in cats. *J. Am. Vet. Med. Assoc.* 209: 1114–1116.

Westermarck, E. and Wiberg, M. (2003). Exocrine pancreatic insufficiency in dogs. *Vet. Clin. N. Am.: Small Anim. Pract.* 33: 1165–1179.

Westermarck, E. and Wiberg, M.E. (2006). Effects of diet on clinical signs of exocrine pancreatic insufficiency in dogs. *J. Am. Vet. Med. Assoc.* 228: 225–229.

Westermarck, E., Myllys, V., and Aho, M. (1993). Effect of treatment on the jejunal and colonic bacterial flora of dogs with exocrine pancreatic insufficiency. *Pancreas* 8: 559–562.

Westermarck, E., Junttila, J.T., and Wiberg, M.E. (1995). Role of low dietary fat in the treatment of dogs with exocrine pancreatic insufficiency. *Am. J. Vet. Res.* 56: 600–605.

Westermarck, E., Wiberg, M., Steiner, J. et al. (2005). Exocrine pancreatic insufficiency in dogs and cats. In: *Textbook of Veterinary Internal Medicine*, 6e, vol. 2 (ed. S.J. Ettinger and E.C. Feldman), 1492–1495. St. Louis, MO: Elsevier Saunders.

Whitney, M.S., Boon, G.D., Rebar, A.H. et al. (1987). Effects of acute pancreatitis on circulating lipids in dogs. *Am. J. Vet. Res.* 48: 1492–1497.

Wiberg, M.E., Saari, S.A., and Westermarck, E. (1999). Exocrine pancreatic atrophy in German shepherd dogs and rough-coated collies: an end result of lymphocytic pancreatitis. *Vet. Pathol.* 36: 530–541.

Williams, D. and Steiner, J. (2005). Canine exocrine pancreatic disease. In: *Textbook of Veterinary Internal Medicine*, 6e, vol. 2 (ed. S.J. Ettinger and E.C. Feldman), 1482–1488. St. Louis, MO: Elsevier Saunders.

Williams, D.A., Batt, R.M., and McLean, L. (1987). Bacterial overgrowth in the duodenum of dogs with exocrine pancreatic insufficiency. *J. Am. Vet. Med. Assoc.* 191: 201–206.

Wofford, J.A., Zollers, B., Rhodes, L. et al. (2018). Evaluation of the safety of daily administration of capromorelin in cats. *J. Vet. Pharmacol. Ther.* 41 (2): 324–333.

Xenoulis, P.G. (2015). Diagnosis of pancreatitis in dogs and cats. *J. Small Anim. Pract.* 56: 13–26.

Xenoulis, P.G. and Steiner, J.M. (2008). Current concepts in feline pancreatitis. *Top. Compan. Anim. Med.* 23: 185–192.

Xenoulis, P.G., Zoran, D.L., Fosgate, G.T. et al. (2016). Feline exocrine pancreatic insufficiency: a retrospective study of 150 cases. *J. Vet. Intern. Med.* 30: 1790–1797.

Zhu, Y., Yin, H., Zhang, R. et al. (2016). Nasogastric nutrition versus nasojejunal nutrition in patients with severe acute pancreatitis: a meta-analysis of randomized controlled trials. *Gastroenterol. Res. Pract.* 2016: 6430632.

Zoran, D.L. (2006). Pancreatitis in cats: diagnosis and management of a challenging disease. *J. Am. Anim. Hosp. Assoc.* 42: 1–9.

13

Nutritional Management of Hepatobiliary Diseases

Stanley L. Marks and Aarti Kathrani

The liver is a crucial metabolic organ, playing a pivotal role in integrating numerous biochemical pathways of protein, lipid, carbohydrate, mineral, and vitamin metabolism, all of which are essential for a well-nourished state. Consequently, malnutrition is a significant co-morbidity in patients with advanced liver disease, being documented in almost 40% of humans (Gheorghe et al. 2013). Malnutrition has also been shown to be a predictor of morbidity and mortality, as well as poor health-related quality of life in humans with cirrhosis (Maharshi et al. 2015; Rojas-Loureiro et al. 2017).

The unique position of the liver between the intestinally derived portal venous circulation and the systemic venous circulation makes it susceptible to a myriad of inflammatory and degenerative conditions. The liver is also unique because it derives most of its own nutrient supply from a vein rather than an artery. Hepatotropic factors in portal venous blood modulate the functional and structural integrity of the liver (Diehl 1991). Several hormones increase after hepatic injury or resection and may affect the ensuing hepatic regenerative growth (Bucher and Malt 1971). Therefore, optimal nutrition is important not only to correct malnutrition associated with advanced liver disease, but also to help regulate the hormonal milieu after hepatic injury. However, the specific nutritional requirements of dogs and cats with liver disease have not been well defined to date.

Unlike most terminally differentiated cells, hepatocytes in adult liver retain the capacity to proliferate. After partial (70%) hepatectomy, compensatory hyperplasia begins within minutes of resection and is typically completed within two weeks in rats and in less than one month in humans (Higgins and Anderson 1931; Francavilla et al. 1990). The management of dogs and cats with liver disease should thus be predicated on using this capacity to the maximum advantage.

Metabolic Alterations in Liver Failure

Hepatocellular dysfunction is responsible for a number of metabolic disturbances that alter the utilization of various nutrients by the body. Changes in protein, carbohydrate, and lipid metabolism (Table 13.1) are particularly prominent in the fasting state (McCullough and Tavill 1991). Attempts to correct these alterations by manipulating nutrient supply represent an important strategy in the nutritional management of patients with advanced liver disease. In addition, impaired hepatic metabolism and storage may result in vitamin and mineral deficiencies. A combination of these alterations usually exists in patients with hepatic disease, and each must be given

Applied Veterinary Clinical Nutrition, Second Edition. Edited by Andrea J. Fascetti, Sean J. Delaney, Jennifer A. Larsen, and Cecilia Villaverde.
© 2024 John Wiley & Sons, Inc. Published 2024 by John Wiley & Sons, Inc.

Table 13.1 Metabolic alterations in hepatic failure.

Alteration	Mechanism
Hyperglucagonemia	Portosystemic shunting
	Impaired hepatic degradation
	Increased plasma aromatic amino acids
	Hyperammonemia
Hyperinsulinemia	Increased peripheral insulin resistance
	Decreased insulin-to-glucagon ratio
	Impaired hepatic degradation
Increased plasma epinephrine and cortisol	Impaired hepatic degradation
Decreased liver and muscle carbohydrate stores	Accelerated glycogenolysis
	Impaired glycogenesis
Increased gluconeogenesis	Hyperglucagonemia
Hyperglycemia (fasting and postprandial)	Portosystemic shunting
	Increased gluconeogenesis
	Decreased insulin-dependent glucose uptake
	Decreased insulin-hepatic glycolysis
Increased plasma aromatic amino acids[a]	Decreased hepatic clearance and incorporation into proteins
	Increased release into the circulation
Decreased plasma branched-chain amino acids[a]	Hyperinsulinemia and excessive uptake
	Increased utilization as an energy source
Increased plasma methionine, glutamine, asparagine, and histidine[a]	Decreased hepatic clearance

[a] Tietge et al. (2003).

consideration before appropriate dietary therapy can be instituted.

Carbohydrate Metabolic Alterations

In healthy individuals, the liver accounts for approximately 90% of endogenous glucose production (Ekberg et al. 1999). The liver is able to maintain euglycemia for obligate glucose-consuming cell types, such as neurons, red blood cells, and renal medullary cells, by utilizing gluconeogenesis, glycogenolysis, glycogen synthesis, glycolysis, and other pathways (Rizza 2010). Consequently, advanced hepatic disease can be associated with a decrease in glycogen storage and glucose synthesis,

contributing to fasting hypoglycemia. Hepatic glycogen can usually meet glucose needs for obligate cells for 24–36 h. In humans with hepatic cirrhosis, glycogen stores are more rapidly depleted (10–12 h) due to diminished stores, which results in premature protein catabolism to supply amino acids for gluconeogenesis (Owen et al. 1981). Fasting hypoglycemia is uncommon in patients with liver disease as euglycemia can be maintained with as little as one-fourth to one-third of normal liver parenchymal mass (Zakim 1982). In addition, fasting hypoglycemia is prevented by a compensatory drop in peripheral glucose oxidation.

However, hepatogenic hypoglycemia can occur and is most common in dogs with cirrhosis, congenital portosystemic vascular anomalies, fulminant hepatic failure, septicemia, and extensive hepatic neoplasia (Center 1996a, b). Normally one-third of an enteral glucose load is taken up by the liver; however, this may be impaired in liver disease due to reduced parenchymal mass or the presence of portosystemic shunting (Kruszynska et al. 1993) and therefore may be a contributory mechanism causing hypoglycemia. Nevertheless, glucose intolerance is more common than hypoglycemia in humans with severe liver dysfunction and approximately 15–30% of patients have overt diabetes mellitus (Bianchi et al. 1994).

Hyperglycemia is suspected to occur due to insulin resistance from chronic inflammation in the liver (Hotamisligil 2006) and concurrent increase in glucagon (Marco et al. 1973). In addition, hepatic inflammation also increases the ability of glucagon to stimulate hepatic glucose production (Chen et al. 2012). Interestingly, hyperglucagonemia has been suggested to occur in dogs with cirrhosis that develop an uncommon necrotizing dermatopathy (i.e. superficial necrolytic dermatitis [SND], hepatocutaneous syndrome). This disorder is characterized by skin erosions and ulcerations with alopecia, exudation, and crusting on the footpads and mucocutaneous junctions (Outerbridge et al. 2002). The mean plasma amino acid concentrations for dogs with SND were significantly lower than for dogs with acute and chronic hepatitis. A metabolic hepatopathy in which there is increased hepatic catabolism of amino acids is hypothesized to explain the hypoaminoacidemia seen in SND (Outerbridge et al. 2002) (For further discussion on SND, see Chapter 11.)

Protein and Amino Acid Metabolic Alterations

The liver is responsible for four main functions in the metabolism of proteins (Charlton 1996). The first is the synthesis of proteins. The liver synthesizes the majority of circulating plasma proteins. The most abundant is albumin, which represents 55–60% of the total plasma protein pool (Center 1996c). The other proteins synthesized and secreted by the liver are usually glycosylated proteins (i.e. glycoproteins) that function in hemostasis, protease inhibition, transport, and ligand binding.

The second function of the liver in protein metabolism is amino acid interconversion; this is particularly important for de novo protein synthesis and gluconeogenesis (Charlton 1996).

The third function is amino acid deamination or breakdown to produce energy (Charlton 1996). Therefore, alterations in amino acids are one of the most important metabolic changes in chronic liver failure. Increased muscle breakdown and liver insufficiency induce an increase in the concentrations of the aromatic amino acids (AAAs; i.e. tyrosine, phenylalanine, tryptophan) and a reduction in those of the branched-chain amino acids (BCAAs; i.e. leucine, isoleucine, valine) (Strombeck and Rogers 1978; Dejong et al. 2007). In addition, it is believed that changes in protein metabolism that occur in chronic liver disease play a role in the complications seen in this condition, such as hepatic encephalopathy (HE), ascites, and protein-calorie malnutrition. Consistent alterations in the plasma amino acid profiles may suggest a potential role for amino acids in the pathogenesis of HE. It has been hypothesized that as AAAs are able to cross the blood–brain barrier and act as false neurotransmitters, they may play a role in HE (Fischer and Baldessarini 1971). This characteristic profile of amino acid changes formed the basis for the initial formulation of solutions enriched in BCAAs as a potentially effective nutritional modality for the treatment of chronic liver disease and HE (Khanna and Gopalan 2007). However, subsequent studies have not supported this approach and although supplementation with BCAAs decreased plasma concentrations of AAAs, they did not consistently improve signs of encephalopathy (Johnson et al. 2013). Alterations in protein metabolism, seen with chronic hepatic disease, can result in protein-calorie malnutrition, which is associated with higher in-hospital mortality in humans with cirrhosis and portal hypertension (Sam and Nguyen 2009). Therefore, protein restriction is discouraged in human patients with cirrhosis, firstly as there are advantages of adequate protein intake for overall nutritional status and faster improvement in encephalopathy scores. Secondly, there are no scientific data in humans to support the use of dietary protein restriction in patients with cirrhosis (Cordoba et al. 2004; Gheorghe et al. 2005).

The fourth function of the liver in protein metabolism is in the conversion of ammonia to urea in the urea cycle (Charlton 1996). Alterations in nitrogen metabolism manifested by hyperammonemia are a common finding and probably result from a combination of factors, including active amino acid deamination and gluconeogenesis, bacterial degradation of protein in the intestine, impaired ureagenesis, and inadequate delivery of ammonia to the liver because of portosystemic vascular shunting (Dimski 1994; Center 1996c). Studies in human patients with liver failure have shown that nitrogen balance can be improved if the diet is divided into small frequent meals, including a snack at bedtime (Swart et al. 1989).

Lipid Metabolic Alterations

The liver plays an important role in lipid metabolism and is involved in lipoprotein uptake, formation, and export into the circulation. After hepatic glycogen stores are depleted, fatty acids are mobilized from adipose tissue, and their rate of hepatic oxidation increases. The release of free fatty acids from adipocytes is greatly accelerated by epinephrine, which stimulates the activation of hormone-sensitive triacylglycerol lipase. Since insulin counterbalances this effect of epinephrine, reduced insulin activity will result in activation of triacylglycerol lipase with consequent hydrolysis of triacylglycerols. The end result is increased release of free fatty acids from adipose tissue into the circulation.

Lipoprotein lipase activity is also decreased in liver failure, resulting in a reduced clearance capacity for exogenous triglycerides. Patients with liver failure can thus be intolerant of large amounts of dietary fat (Barber and Teasley 1984).

The liver is also a major site of cholesterol synthesis from acetyl-CoA. Hypocholesterolemia has been recognized in animals with portosystemic vascular anomalies and acquired hepatic insufficiency (Center 1996c), whereas hypercholesterolemia has been seen in animals with obstruction to bile flow. The changes in lipoprotein metabolism associated with cirrhosis generally reflect the degree of impairment of hepatic function, with serum total, low-density lipoprotein (LDL), and high-density lipoprotein (HDL) cholesterol being inversely correlated with severity of cirrhosis in human patients (Ghadir et al. 2010).

Vitamin and Mineral Abnormalities

Vitamin deficiencies are commonly found in patients with chronic liver disease. Deficient dietary intake and malabsorption are the principal causes of vitamin deficiency, although decreased storage, metabolism defects, and increased requirements also play a role (Mezey 1978). In human patients with cirrhosis, the hepatic concentrations of folate, riboflavin, nicotinamide (from dietary niacin), pantothenic acid, vitamin B6 (pyridoxine), vitamin B12 (cyanocobalamin), and vitamin A have been found to be decreased (Leevy et al. 1970). The requirements for water-soluble vitamins are determined by the caloric intake. With complete anorexia there is a low requirement (Strombeck et al. 1983b), but with resumption of caloric intake, water-soluble vitamins are necessary to replenish co-enzymes involved in metabolic processes in the liver and other tissues (Strombeck et al. 1983b). Due to the variety of vitamin deficiencies that may develop and the inability to quantitatively appraise these changes, water-soluble vitamins are often empirically supplemented at a doubled daily dose. Subnormal concentrations of vitamin B12 have been demonstrated in some cats with cholangitis and hepatic lipidosis associated with chronic inflammatory bowel disease (IBD). Vitamin B12 can be supplemented parenterally at a dose of 250 µg per cat subcutaneously (SQ) once weekly for six consecutive weeks, followed by administration every [q]2–3 weeks for an indefinite period. Alternatively, one retrospective study showed that oral cobalamin supplementation was effective in increasing serum cobalamin to supranormal concentrations in cats with hypocobalaminemia (Toresson et al. 2017).

Vitamin C is produced by the canine and feline liver and lower plasma concentrations of ascorbate are present in dogs and cats with hepatic disease (Strombeck et al. 1983a). Vitamin C should thus be supplemented, and dogs will tolerate doses of 25 mg/kg body weight orally (PO) per day. However, vitamin C status has been shown not to be impaired in dogs with a portosystemic shunt (PSS) (Hishiyama et al. 2006).

Malabsorption of fat-soluble vitamins is typically seen in patients with chronic bile-duct occlusion, biliary cirrhosis, end-stage cholangitis, or liver disorders occurring concurrent with pancreatic or intestinal disease, causing steatorrhea. It has been shown that as the severity of liver disease progresses in humans, the fat-soluble vitamins tend to become more deficient (Abbott-Johnson et al. 2011). Caution should be exercised with the administration of vitamin A, as this vitamin can interact synergistically with chemicals and endotoxins to injure the liver, despite the use of vitamin A concentrations that are not normally hepatotoxic (Strombeck et al. 1983b).

Suboptimal stores of vitamin D can be associated with both cholestatic and non-cholestatic liver disease and may be attributed to lower vitamin D intake, fat malabsorption, bile acid deficiency, and impaired hepatic function (Pappa et al. 2008). Although 90% of human patients with advanced liver disease are deficient in vitamin D (Arteh et al. 2010), the status in dogs and cats with liver disease is unknown. Therefore, additional studies are needed in dogs and cats before supplementation with vitamin D can be recommended for those with liver disease.

Vitamin E may be beneficial for the management of patients with copper-associated liver damage because of its antioxidant effects that protect against lipid peroxidation. Vitamin E should be supplemented at doses of 10–15 IU/kg/day.

Vitamin K stores in the liver are limited and can be rapidly depleted when dietary sources are inadequate or lipid malabsorption is severe (Strombeck et al. 1983b). One study showed that 25% of human patients with primary biliary cirrhosis had subnormal plasma vitamin K1 (phylloquinone) concentrations (Kowdley et al. 1997). Endogenous production of vitamin K by intestinal bacteria can maintain requirements for one month following the lack of dietary supplementation. With bleeding due to hepatic disease, the function for synthesis of the prothrombin-complex clotting factors is always lost before the storage of vitamin K is depleted (Center 1996b, c). Vitamin K deficiency can be diagnosed with a PIVKA (proteins induced by vitamin K antagonism or absence) assay clotting time. Normalization of prolonged clotting times after parenteral administration of vitamin K1 (0.5–1.0 mg/kg SQ) documents vitamin K deficiency.

There is considerable evidence that zinc deficiency is prevalent in liver disease (Riggio et al. 1991). Urea synthetic capacity is reduced in zinc-deficient canine patients due to reduced hepatic ornithine transcarbamylase (OTC) activity and increased muscle glutamine synthetase activity Cats are dependent on dietary arginine and not ornithine conversion to citrulline and then citrulline conversion to arginine like dogs, so this reduced enzyme activity is likely insignificant for them (Morris 2002). Zinc deficiency could thus adversely influence multiple aspects of ammonia metabolism (Mullen and Weber 1991), whereas excess zinc inhibits the intestinal absorption of copper and its deposition in the liver (Fisher et al. 1983). Zinc deficiency in human cirrhotic patients may lead to anorexia due to altered taste and smell (Allis and Leopold 2012). Zinc should be orally supplemented as zinc gluconate or zinc citrate (5 mg/kg body weight/day). Improved zinc status has been associated with improvement in liver function in human patients with cirrhosis (Rahelic et al. 2006).

Hypokalemia is common in human cirrhotic patients, in whom it may be associated with glucose intolerance. Potassium depletion may occur secondary to inadequate dietary intake, vomiting, diarrhea, secondary hyperaldosteronism, and use of non-potassium-sparing diuretic drugs. Potassium repletion in these patients is associated with a reversal of subnormal insulin and growth hormone concentrations (Podolsky et al. 1973).

Copper hepatotoxicity is a well-documented cause of liver disease in genetically predisposed dogs and can also occur secondary to cholestatic disorders. Secondary copper accumulation rarely exceeds 2000 ppm (µg/g) dry weight (dw) in liver tissue; normal <400 ppm (µg/g) dw (Thornburg 2000; Hoffmann et al. 2006; Spee et al. 2006).

Malnutrition in Liver Disease

Malnutrition is a common finding in humans with advanced liver disease, and in human cirrhotic patients has been associated with increased morbidity and mortality, compromised immune function, delayed wound healing, and decreased muscle mass (Johnson et al. 2013). It is important to recognize that weight loss commonly occurs in the face of normal dietary intake, suggesting that factors other than caloric intake are involved in the malnutrition of these patients. Protein-calorie malnutrition occurs in almost 40% of human patients with cirrhosis and progresses as liver function declines (Cheung et al. 2012; Gheorghe et al. 2013). Potential causes of malnutrition in animals with liver disease include (i) anorexia, nausea, and vomiting; (ii) impaired nutrient digestion, absorption, and metabolism; (iii) increased energy requirements; and (iv) accelerated protein catabolism with impaired protein synthesis. Additional causes of malnutrition in human patients with cirrhosis include imposed protein and sodium restriction,

modified taste perception due to zinc deficiency, early satiety, delayed gastric emptying, impaired gut motility, and small intestinal bacterial overgrowth (Kalaitzakis 2014; Thandassery and Montano-Loza 2016). Also, hypermetabolism from increased beta-adrenergic activation along with other metabolic aberrations, such as increased lipid utilization and insulin resistance, has also been shown to contribute to malnutrition in humans with cirrhosis (Greco et al. 1998).

Prolonged fasting in cirrhosis leads to a rapid consumption of fat stores, and increased gluconeogenesis results in depletion of structural and functional proteins (Munoz 1991). Approximately 80% of humans with cirrhosis have depletion of visceral protein (Caregaro et al. 1996). In addition, the chronic administration of lactulose and/or neomycin for HE may lead to nutrient malabsorption, secondary to decreased intestinal transit time and suppressed activity of microbiota. Cholestatic liver disorders are associated with decreased intraluminal concentration of bile salts, resulting in lipid malabsorption and depletion of body fat stores (Kowdley 1998). The steatorrhea that occurs in approximately 40% of human patients with hepatic cirrhosis is related to decreased delivery of bile salts into the intestinal lumen, impaired intestinal capacity for absorption of long-chain fatty acids (Malagelada et al. 1974), interference with lipid absorption by neomycin, and in some cases concurrent exocrine pancreatic insufficiency (Lee and Lai 1976).

Nutritional Management of Common Hepatobiliary Disorders

The early identification and resolution of the factors causing hepatic insult are integral to the successful repair and regeneration of the hepatocyte. Nutritional management is frequently delayed in small animal patients with liver disease owing to the insidious onset and lack of understanding of pathophysiologic mechanisms. In addition, therapeutic diets may need to be modified depending on the patient's nutritional status and underlying liver disorder. Sufficient carbohydrate and fat must be provided in the diet to prevent protein catabolism for energy needs and consequent ammonia formation. Although nutritional therapy only plays a supportive role in the management of most hepatic diseases, it is the primary treatment for feline idiopathic hepatic lipidosis (HL) and HE, and is an important component of the treatment of copper-associated hepatotoxicity in dogs.

Feline Idiopathic Hepatic Lipidosis

Feline HL is a well-recognized syndrome characterized by the accumulation of excess triglycerides in hepatocytes (see Figures 13.1 and 13.2) with resulting cholestasis and hepatic dysfunction (Biourge et al. 1990). The prognosis for this life-threatening disorder has improved dramatically over the past two decades as a consequence of the increased utilization of long-term (3–8 weeks or longer) enteral feeding devices (Biourge et al. 1990, 1993; Center 2005). Despite this progress, the underlying pathophysiology of this syndrome remains incompletely understood. Potential

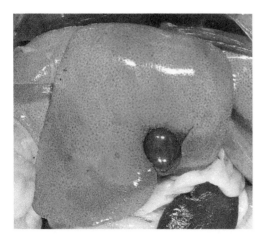

Figure 13.1 Fatty liver from a cat diagnosed with hepatic lipidosis showing the pale-colored surface, swollen parenchyma, and rounded borders. Courtesy of Dr. Eunju (April) Choi, Department of Pathology, Microbiology, and Immunology, University of California, Davis, School of Veterinary Medicine.

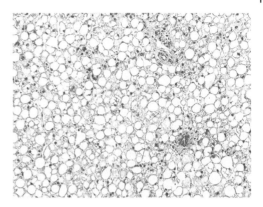

Figure 13.2 Hepatic biopsy from a cat's liver showing a diffuse vacuolar hepatopathy consistent with hepatic lipidosis. Magnification 20X. Courtesy of Dr. Eunju (April) Choi, Department of Pathology, Microbiology, and Immunology, University of California, Davis, School of Veterinary Medicine.

causes include protein deficiency, excessive peripheral lipolysis, excessive lipogenesis, inhibition of lipid oxidation for gluconeogenesis, and inhibition of the synthesis of very low-density lipoproteins (Center 2005).

Most cats with this disorder are obese and usually present with a history of anorexia and weight loss following a stressful event (Biourge et al. 1990, 1993; Center 2005). Initial management should be directed toward correcting cardiovascular, fluid, and electrolyte abnormalities, HE, and any infection. Resolution of HL associated with pancreatitis, infections, and drugs is dependent on the success in treating the underlying disorder (Center 2005). Early tube feeding via esophagostomy or gastrostomy tubes remains the cornerstone of therapy. If the cat cannot be safely anesthetized for placement of an enteral feeding tube, a nasoesophageal tube should be placed, and a liquid, enteral formula should be administered until the cat is stabilized for placement of a longer-lasting esophagostomy or gastrostomy tube (see Chapter 20 for further discussion on enteral feeding).

Energy

Provision of adequate daily energy intake is pivotal for the successful management of cats with HL; however, there are no guidelines for estimated energy needs in cats with HL other than clinical experience. Most cats tolerate feeding to meet their resting energy requirement (RER). This can be increased slightly to 1.1–1.2 times RER when the cat is managed at home. Force-feeding is contraindicated because it may be associated with a conditioned food aversion, is stressful for the cat, may result in human caretaker injury, and is unlikely to provide adequate nutrition. The use of appetite stimulants such as diazepam, oxazepam, cyproheptadine, capromorelin, and mirtazapine can be attempted, but usually results in failure to meet the cat's caloric requirement and frustration for the human companion. Caution should be heeded with the use of diazepam in cats with hepatic disease because of the associated fulminant hepatic failure that can ensue (Center et al. 1996).

Esophagostomy and gastrostomy tubes are well tolerated by cats and help ensure the administration of adequate calories. Nasoesophageal tubes have the advantages of relatively low cost and the lack of chemical restraint needed for their placement. Nasoesophageal tubes are a simple and efficient choice for the short-term (under 10 days) nutritional support of most anorectic hospitalized animals that have a normal mentation, nasal cavity, pharynx, esophagus, and stomach (Crowe 1986). Nasoesophageal tube feeding is contraindicated in animals that are vomiting, comatose, or lack a gag reflex. Polyvinylchloride (infant feeding tube, Argyle Division of Sherwood Medical, St. Louis, MO, USA) or red rubber tubes (Robinson catheter, Sherwood Medical) are the least expensive tubes for cats, although the polyvinylchloride tubes may harden within two weeks of insertion and cause irritation or ulceration of the pharynx or esophagus. Tubes made of polyurethane (MILA International, Erlanger, KY, USA) or silicon (Global Veterinary Products, New Buffalo, MI, USA) are more expensive; however, they are less irritating and more resistant to gastric acid, allowing prolonged usage. A 5- to 8-French tube is more comfortable for cats and smaller dogs.

The tube should terminate in the distal esophagus to decrease the likelihood of reflux esophagitis (Balkany et al. 1977), and this is facilitated by ensuring that the length of the tube approximates the distance from the tip of the nose to the seventh or eighth intercostal space. However, one study did not identify a difference in complication rate between nasoesophageal and nasogastric feeding tubes in dogs (Yu et al. 2013), and therefore further studies are needed in cats to determine the optimal terminal location of nasoenteral feeding tubes. The small diameter of the tube (i.e. 5- to 8-French) necessitates the feeding of a liquid enteral formula, and clogging can be a significant problem. Commercially available canned pâté or loaf-style pet foods that are diluted with water will invariably clog the feeding tube. The caloric density of most human and veterinary liquid enteral formulas varies from 1.0 to 2.0 kcal/ml. These liquid diets are fed full strength on continuous (pump infusion) or bolus feeding schedules.

The most common complications associated with the use of nasoesophageal tubes include epistaxis, rhinitis, dacryocystitis, tracheal intubation with secondary pneumonia, vomiting, diarrhea, early removal or displacement, and clogged tubes (Crowe 1986; Abood and Buffington 1992; Klaus et al. 2009; Campbell et al. 2010; Holahan et al. 2010). Vomiting associated with delayed gastric emptying can often be controlled with metoclopramide (0.2–0.4 mg/kg SQ) 15 min before each meal. Mild hypokalemia can be treated with oral potassium chloride or potassium gluconate supplementation (5–10 mEq/day with meals; i.e. 375 mg potassium chloride to 750 mg potassium chloride per day).

Protein

Dietary protein should not be restricted in cats with HL unless the cat is showing signs of encephalopathy. Protein restriction for cats with HE should not fall below minimum protein requirements. Commercial veterinary diets containing between 25% and 30% protein on a metabolizable energy (ME) basis and 60–68% fat on an ME basis have been well tolerated in most cats with HL that are not encephalopathic (Biourge et al. 1993). Caution should be heeded in the feeding of human liquid enteral formulas, which are typically deficient in the essential amino acids arginine and taurine and contain inadequate concentrations of protein. Arginine is an important urea cycle substrate and arginine deficiency has been associated with the development of hyperammonemia in cats fed a single meal of a complete amino acid diet without arginine (Morris and Rogers 1978). Taurine deficiency has been shown to increase lipolysis in peripheral tissues and increasing dietary taurine decreased total liver lipid content in cats (Cantafora et al. 1991).

There are a variety of veterinary liquid enteral diets that are marketed for small animal use. These formulas should be fed at room temperature and kept refrigerated between meals. Tube feedings should be started at three to four times daily with a gradual increase in the volume administered. Feeding should be initiated at 25% of the calculated RER and then slowly increased by 25% increments daily, depending on the animal's tolerance to the diet until full RER is reached on at least day 4. Gradually increasing to full RER over at least four days may also help to prevent refeeding syndrome (i.e. sudden intracellular shifts in potassium, phosphorus, and magnesium causing potentially life-threatening hypokalemia, hypophosphatemia, and hypomagnesemia), which has been reported in a cat with HL (Brenner et al. 2011). Commercial canned diets should be blended with water to provide a gruel for gastrostomy or esophagostomy tube feeding. The advantage of using a balanced commercial diet is that additional protein, minerals, and vitamins do not need to be added. For further guidance on enteral or tube feeding, see Chapter 20.

Food aversion appears to be an important component of the anorexia of cats with HL (Biourge 1997). Cats that refuse to eat a diet that they associate with nausea may continue to avoid that diet even after full recovery, due to their association with the unpleasant sensation. One should therefore tube-feed these cats as soon as the diagnosis of HL has been made, rather than offer several commercial diets to which the cat can develop an aversion. Cats with HL should not be offered any food by mouth for approximately 10 days following placement of a feeding tube. Cats that express an interest in eating can then be presented with a novel diet that they have not been fed before. The prognosis for HL is influenced to a large degree by the ability of the clinician or human caretaker to aggressively meet the cat's caloric requirements via enteral feeding. In addition, a decrease in serum beta-hydroxybutyrate, a ketone body, which likely reflects an improvement in catabolic state, during hospitalization in cats with HL was associated with survival (Kuzi et al. 2017).

Potassium

Hypokalemia is a relatively common finding in cats with HL and may develop due to inadequate potassium intake, vomiting, magnesium depletion, and concurrent renal failure. In one study, hypokalemia was present in 19 of 66 cats (29%) with severe HL and was significantly related to non-survival in this group of cats (Center et al. 1993). However, a recent study documented hypokalemia in 16% of survivors and 38% of non-survivors at the time of presentation to the hospital in cats with HL, and this difference was not statistically significant (Kuzi et al. 2017). Hypokalemia is deleterious because it can exacerbate HE and anorexia, and cause muscle weakness and ileus. Diets for cats with HL should be potassium replete (0.8–1% potassium on a dry matter basis, or 1.5 g/Mcal), or potassium can be orally supplemented at 2–6 mEq potassium gluconate per day (or 465 mg–1.395 g potassium gluconate per day).

l-Carnitine

Food and biosynthesis by the liver are the primary sources of carnitine for animals. Carnitine is an essential co-factor for transport of long-chain fatty acids across the inner mito-chondrial membrane into the mitochondrial matrix for beta-oxidation. Carnitine also removes potentially toxic acyl groups from cells and equilibrates ratios of free co-enzyme A (CoA)/acetyl-CoA between the mitochondria and cytoplasm. Thus, carnitine plays a very important role in utilizing lipid as a cellular energy source.

Several studies have investigated the relationship between carnitine, weight loss in obese cats, and feline HL. Jacobs et al. (1990) found that mean concentrations of carnitine in plasma, the liver, and skeletal muscle were significantly greater in cats with HL than in control cats. In contrast, other studies have shown that feline diets supplemented with L-carnitine benefit obese cats undergoing rapid weight loss (Center et al. 2000; Blanchard et al. 2002). In addition, dietary L-carnitine supplementation protected obese cats from hepatic lipid accumulation during caloric restriction and rapid weight loss (Ibrahim et al. 2003). Center and colleagues have also previously shown that food supplemented with L-carnitine can safely facilitate rapid weight loss in privately owned obese cats (Center et al. 2000). Supportively, dietary L-carnitine supplementation appeared to facilitate fatty acid oxidation in overweight colony-housed cats undergoing rapid weight loss (Center et al. 2012).

Based on these findings, L-carnitine has been recommended for the management of cats with HL at an oral dose of 250–500 mg L-carnitine/cat/day. Although there have not been any rigorous placebo-controlled clinical trials evaluating the benefits of L-carnitine in these patients, the clinical impression is one of faster recovery and increased survival rates.

Cyanocobalamin/Vitamin B12

Cats with HL frequently have concurrent IBD or intestinal lymphoma and pancreatitis. Serum concentrations of vitamin B12 are commonly decreased in cats with HL in association with concurrent IBD (Simpson et al. 2001).

Other Nutrient Considerations

Additional dietary supplements that are inconsistently used by some clinicians in cats with severe HL include taurine (250–500 mg/day PO), subcutaneous vitamin K1 (0.5–1.0 mg/kg at 12 h intervals for three doses), thiamine (100–200 mg/day PO), and antioxidants such as vitamin E (d-α-tocopherol acetate; 10–15 IU/kg/day PO) and S-adenosylmethionine (SAMe; 20 mg/kg/day PO). See later in the chapter for a detailed description of antioxidants for liver disease.

Copper-Associated Hepatotoxicity in Dogs

There are three causes of hepatic copper accumulation. One cause is a hereditary defect that inhibits biliary excretion of copper, resulting in hepatocellular lysosomal copper accumulation, which is the primary form of copper storage disease in humans (Wilson's disease) and Bedlington terrier dogs (Su et al. 1982; Brewer 1998; Thornburg 2000; see Figure 13.3). A second cause is altered biliary excretion of copper due to hepatic inflammation, fibrosis, and/or cholestasis, although this has not been proven definitively in the dog (Hoffmann et al. 2006; Spee et al. 2006). A third known and suggested cause of hepatic copper accumulation is from excessive dietary intake (van den Ingh et al. 2007; Center et al. 2021). Absorption of copper is also enhanced by amino acids and

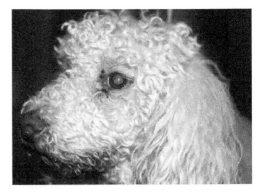

Figure 13.3 Bedlington terrier diagnosed with primary copper-associated hepatotoxicity.

high dietary protein, and reduced by zinc, ascorbate, and fiber.

In non-hereditary, secondary copper storage disease, copper accumulation is mainly restricted to periportal areas and hepatic copper concentrations are usually less than 2000 ppm (µg/g) dw (Thornburg 2000; Hoffmann et al. 2006). In contrast, copper accumulation with primary hereditary copper storage disorders is always centrilobular, and hepatic copper concentrations are usually greater than 2000 ppm (µg/g) dw (Hultgren et al. 1986; Hoffmann et al. 2006). Normal hepatic copper concentrations are considered to be less than 400 ppm (µg/g) dw (Hoffmann et al. 2006; Spee et al. 2006).

Breed-associated hepatic copper accumulation with reports of greater than 2000 ppm (µg/g) dw has been identified in Bedlington terriers, West Highland white terriers, Skye terriers, Dalmatians, Doberman pinschers, and Labrador retrievers (see Figure 13.4; Rolfe and Twedt 1995; Cooper et al. 1997; Haywood et al. 1988; Hoffmann et al. 2006; Mandigers et al. 2007). Recently, it has also been reported in a Pembroke Welsh corgi (Rifkin and Miller 2014). In Bedlington terriers, copper-associated hepatitis has been identified as an autosomal recessive

Figure 13.4 Hepatic biopsy from a Labrador retriever with copper associated hepatitis showing diffuse copper staining (brown pigment) using a Rhodanine stain. Magnification 20X. Courtesy of Dr. Eunju (April) Choi, Department of Pathology, Microbiology, and Immunology, University of California, Davis, School of Veterinary Medicine.

disease (Johnson et al. 1980). A deletion in the *COMMD1* gene (formerly *MURR1*) results in reduced biliary excretion of copper and marked accumulation of copper within hepatocytes (Forman et al. 2005). Recently, two missense mutations in the copper transporters *ATP7B* (Wilson's disease gene) and *ATP7A* (Menkes disease gene) were positively and negatively associated with hepatic copper concentrations, respectively, in Labrador retrievers (Fieten et al. 2016). In addition to genetic susceptibility, hepatic copper concentrations in Labrador retrievers are also influenced by dietary copper intake (Fieten et al. 2012). Copper is highly toxic when not bound to protein. In the presence of superoxide ions, copper catalyzes the formation of hydroxyl radicals causing oxidative damage to lipids and proteins, resulting in chronic hepatitis (Forman et al. 2005).

Energy

There are no guidelines for estimated energy needs in dogs with vacuolar, inflammatory, or toxic hepatopathies. Provision of adequate daily energy intake to allow for protein synthesis and prevent tissue catabolism with subsequent ammoniagenesis is important. Most hospitalized patients are fed at their RER.

Dietary Copper Restriction

The goal of treatment in dogs with copper-associated hepatotoxicity is to create a negative copper balance by restricting copper intake and increasing urinary copper excretion via the use of chelators. Studies have shown that a low-copper and high-zinc diet may be beneficial in preventing or postponing reaccumulation of copper in Labrador retrievers that were initially treated with a copper chelator (Hoffmann et al. 2009; Fieten et al. 2014). In addition, hepatic copper concentrations could be normalized in one study with dietary intervention alone in 15 out of 28 subclinical Labrador retrievers with increased hepatic copper (Fieten et al. 2015). However, some study individuals continued to accumulate copper despite being fed a low-copper and high-zinc diet. Therefore, response to dietary treatment should be evaluated with repeat liver biopsy of multiple locations/lobes and copper staining and quantification due to individual variation in dietary response, which is likely the result of differences in genetic background.

Commercially available therapeutic diets are available for dogs and cats with liver disease. These formulations differ from those pre-scribed for patients with renal disease in that the hepatic formulas are generally less protein restricted (14–15.5% protein on an ME basis) than most renal diets. In addition, the hepatic diets are restricted in dietary copper, have increased concentrations of dietary zinc and B vitamins, are controlled in sodium, and are fortified with antioxidants.

An alternative option for anorectic dogs that refuse to eat commercial diets or that have concurrent disorders warranting a com-plex dietary formulation that is not commer-cially available is to feed a complete and balanced homemade diet that has been for-mulated by a board certified veterinary nutri-tionist® or a Diplomate of the European College of Veterinary and Comparative Nutrition. Care should be taken to fortify any copper-restricted, canine homemade diet with a supplement that does not contain added copper (Balance IT® Canine -Cu, DVM Consulting, Davis, CA, USA) or a multivita-min that uses cupric oxide with low to no bio-availability such as Centrum Kids Chewable (https://www.centrum.com/products/multivitamins/centrum-kids). Homemade diets should exclude liver, nuts, shellfish, mushrooms, and organ meats that are all high in copper content (Center 1996b). Supplementation of vitamin C is controver-sial in small animals, with some clinicians preferring to avoid its use because of *in vitro* studies documenting increased transition metal oxidation. In contrast, others advocate a lower dose of vitamin C supplementation (25 mg/kg body weight/day) because plasma ascorbic acid concentrations can be decreased in dogs with hepatic failure (Strombeck et al. 1983b).

Pharmacologic Reduction of Copper

Copper chelators or zinc therapy are warranted if the liver biopsy of a dog with chronic hepati-tis or copper hepatotoxicity shows significant hepatic copper accumulation. Hepatic copper concentrations >1000 ppm (μg/g) dw liver require therapy to be reduced. Animals with >2000 ppm (μg/g) dw copper content should all have chelator therapy for at least three months.

Zinc

Zinc salts are effective in preventing copper accumulation in the livers of humans with Wilson's disease (Jaffe et al. 1964). In addition, zinc has antifibrotic and hepatoprotective properties. Zinc ions induce the synthesis of metallothionein, which binds copper tightly, rendering it unabsorbable from the intestine and possibly also detoxifying it in the liver (Center et al. 2002). Copper bound to metal-lothionein in the intestinal cell is then lost in the feces when the intestinal cell is sloughed. Zinc acetate or zinc gluconate is the recom-mended source, since the sulfate form may be associated with gastric irritation and vomiting in people. The zinc should be administered on an empty stomach and regardless of form still has the common side effect of vomiting. An initial induction dose of 15 mg/kg body weight of elemental zinc given twice daily 1 h before meals is recommended. The dose can be halved after 1–3 months of therapy. The goal is to maintain serum zinc concentrations between 200 and 500 μg/dl. Excess zinc may interfere with the absorption and utilization of iron and copper and can cause hemolytic ane-mia (Center 1996b). Plasma zinc concentra-tions exceeding 1000 μg/dl may result in hemolysis, and therefore plasma zinc concen-trations should be monitored during treatment.

Copper Chelators

Copper chelators bind copper either in the blood or the tissues and promote its urinary excretion. D-penicillamine (Cuprimine®, 250 mg capsules, Bausch Health, Bridgewater, NJ, USA), the most frequent copper chelator recommended for use in dogs, should be given at a dose of 10–15 mg/kg PO twice a day on an empty stomach (Center 1996b; Langlois et al. 2013). Anorexia and vomiting are the most common side effects in dogs and can be alleviated by reducing the dose or giving a long-acting antiemetic 1 h prior to administration (Langlois et al. 2013).

In addition to its chelating properties, D-penicillamine may have other beneficial effects such as immunomodulation and antifibrotic activities (Lipsky and Ziff 1978; Siegel 1977). D-penicillamine therapy has also been associated with a pyridoxine (vitamin B6) deficiency in human patients (Jaffe et al. 1964). Although this problem has not been recognized to occur in dogs, the diet should be high in this B vitamin, or supplemental amounts should be given daily. It is thought that penicillamine induces the production of a hepatic copper-binding protein, metallothionein, thus binding and sequestering copper in a non-toxic form in the liver.

Continuous life-long D-penicillamine treatment is not recommended in Labrador retrievers due to the risk of hepatic copper and zinc deficiency (Fieten et al. 2013). However, a model has recently been published that can be used as a guideline for the duration of D-penicillamine treatment based on hepatic copper concentrations in this breed (Fieten et al. 2013). Periodic liver biopsies are recommended with the use of copper chelators to monitor hepatic copper concentrations and need for ongoing therapy.

A second copper chelator is trientine (Syprine®, Bausch Health), which has been manufactured for patients that are intolerant to penicillamine. The drug is administered at a dose of 15 mg/kg PO twice daily on an empty stomach and is better tolerated than D-penicillamine. Anti-inflammatory agents such as prednisone also may be of benefit in the management of chronic hepatitis in Bedlington terriers and West Highland white terriers.

Antioxidants

Considerable evidence shows that free radicals are generated in chronic hepatitis and participate in the pathogenesis of oxidative liver injury in dogs and cats. Decreased hepatic glutathione concentrations have been documented in dogs and cats with naturally occurring liver disease (Center et al. 2002). Normally there is an extensive system of cytosolic and membrane-bound enzymatic and non-enzymatic antioxidants that function to prevent oxidative damage by scavenging or quenching free radicals that are formed.

Vitamin E

Vitamin E (d-α tocopherol) functions as a major membrane-bound intracellular antioxidant, protecting membrane phospholipids from peroxidative damage when free radicals are formed. Vitamin E protects against the effects of copper, bile acids, and other hepatotoxins, and is administered at 10–15 IU/kg/day. Because bile acids are required for fat-soluble vitamin E absorption and may be reduced in cholestatic liver disease, a water-soluble formulation (e.g. forms with acetate, succinate, or phosphate esters) is recommended.

S-adenosylmethionine

SAMe is a precursor of glutathione, an important component of the liver antioxidant system. In a placebo-controlled feline model of oxidant injury from acetaminophen, SAMe-treated cats had reduced Heinz body formation and erythrocyte destruction compared with cats that received acetaminophen alone. Hepatic and blood glutathione concentrations increased with SAMe administration (Webb et al. 2003). There was also evidence of protection in hepatic glutathione (GSH)-treated cats. SAMe and silybin (aka silibinin, see more below under milk thistle) in combination have been shown to decrease cytokine-induced prostaglandin E2 (PGE2), interleukin (IL)-8, and monocyte chemoattractant protein-1 (MCP1) production and to increase glutathione in canine hepatocytes *in vitro* (Au et al. 2013). In addition, a combination of SAMe and silybin was shown to minimize increased liver enzyme activity in dogs receiving CCNU chemotherapy (Skorupski et al. 2011).

It is important to recognize that there are two well-characterized stereoisomers of the SAMe molecule, denoted as "−" SAMe (S,S-SAMe) and "+" SAMe (R,S-SAMe) isomers. This nomenclature refers to the orientation at the sulfonium chiral center. The S,S-SAMe isomer is the predominant form synthesized in cells and is biologically active, whereas <4% of the R,S-SAMe is found in tissues. Both *in vitro* and *in vivo* studies indicate that only the S,S-SAMe isomer has preferential high reactivity with most methyltransferases that have been studied (Beaudouin et al. 1993). SAMe is administered at a dose of 20 mg/kg body weight once daily on an empty stomach (given 1–2 hours before feeding). While the stereoisomeric composition of SAMe products is important in determining their biological effects, this information typically is not disclosed for marketed products or may not be known. Analysis of Denosyl® (Nutramax Laboratories Veterinary Sciences, Lancaster, SC, USA), a SAMe product proven to produce biological responses in healthy dogs and cats and in a canine and feline model of acetaminophen toxicity (Wallace et al. 2002; Webb et al. 2003), demonstrated a 74% content of the biologically active S,S-SAMe stereoisomer, while analysis of another veterinary brand disclosed a 57% S,S-SAMe isomer content.

Milk Thistle

The active extract of milk thistle is silymarin, which contains four flavonoid stereoisomers; the most biologically potent is silybin. Important functions showing the hepatoprotective properties of silymarin include its role as an antioxidant and free-radical scavenger in the liver. There is also evidence that silymarin has effects in inhibiting hepatotoxin binding, increasing glutathione concentrations and iron chelation, and promoting choleresis (Crocenzi et al. 2003). Silybin and the more bioavailable silybin-phosphatidylcholine complex were shown to inhibit canine hepatocyte activation by the pro-inflammatory cytokine IL-1beta *in vitro* (Au et al. 2011). In cats, oral supplementation with silibinin-phosphatidylcholine complex increased granulocyte glutathione content

and phagocytic function (Webb et al. 2009). The oral uptake and bioavailability of silybin are low, but significantly increase when complexed with phosphatidylcholine (Filburn et al. 2007).

Milk thistle as silybin or silymarin extract is dosed at 5–15 mg/kg body weight/day PO. To date, limited clinical studies have evaluated the efficacy of silymarin in liver disease in dogs and cats. In one placebo-controlled experimental study of dogs poisoned with the *Amanita phalloides* mushroom, silybin had a significant positive effect on liver damage and survival outcome (Vogel et al. 1984). Also, one study showed that silymarin was able to protect liver tissue against oxidative stress in cats that had received a single oral administration of toxic amounts of acetaminophen (Avizeh et al. 2010).

Portosystemic Shunts and Hepatic Encephalopathy

Hepatic encephalopathy is currently defined as "a brain dysfunction caused by liver insufficiency and/or portosystemic shunt; it manifests as a wide spectrum of neurological or psychiatric abnormalities ranging from subclinical alterations to coma" (Vilstrup et al. 2014). The syndrome is most often recognized in dogs or cats with congenital anomalies of the portal vascular system (Figures 13.5–13.7); however,

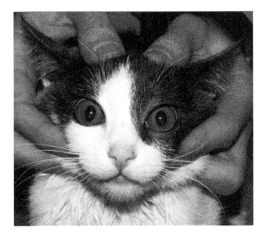

Figure 13.5 Copper-colored irises in an encephalopathic kitten diagnosed with a portosystemic shunt.

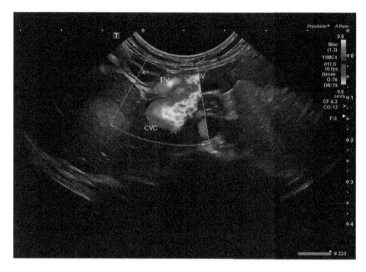

Figure 13.6   Abdominal ultrasound using color flow doppler interrogation in a 6-month female toy-poodle with a single extrahepatic portosystemic shunt. CVC, caudal vena cava; PV, portal vein; SV, shunt vessel. Courtesy of Dr. Eric G. Johnson, Department of Surgical and Radiological Sciences, University of California, Davis, School of Veterinary Medicine.

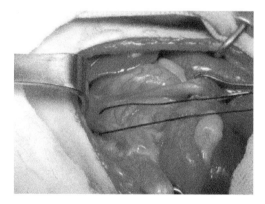

Figure 13.7   Exploratory laparotomy in a cat with a single extrahepatic shunt showing the ligature around the aberrant vessel.

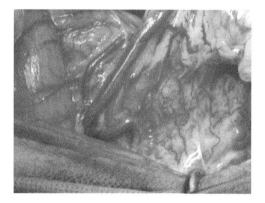

Figure 13.8   Exploratory laparotomy in a dog showing a plexus of multiple extrahepatic shunt vessels secondary to portal hypertension from hepatic cirrhosis.

it may occur in association with chronic progressive hepatic disorders that lead to end-stage liver failure (Figure 13.8). An understanding of the pathogenesis and precipitating factors for the development of HE is integral to successful patient management.

The goals of therapy in patients with HE are threefold: (i) early recognition and correction of precipitating causes of encephalopathy (e.g. gastrointestinal bleeding, constipation, hypokalemia); (ii) reduction of the intestinal production and absorption of toxins; and (iii) provision of

supportive and symptomatic care. Clinicians should refrain from the use of sedatives, narcotics, and anesthetic agents in patients with HE. Non-potassium-sparing diuretics, in particular furosemide, should be judiciously utilized, because overzealous use may cause hypokalemic alkalosis and hypovolemia. Treatments based on the mechanism of intestinal production and absorption of toxins (i.e. ammonia, mercaptans, short-chain fatty acids, indoles and skatoles, and biogenic amines) include decreasing or modifying dietary protein, altering intestinal flora, and decreasing intestinal transit time (Center 1996b). Supportive care includes correction of hypovolemia, electrolyte, and acid–base abnormalities (Center 1996b).

Animals with PSSs and an absence of HE should not be unduly protein restricted. Instead, efforts should be made to provide normal dietary intake in patients with chronic stable liver disease. Likewise, not all animals with surgically repaired PSSs require protein restriction, and these animals are typically slowly weaned onto normal maintenance diets within 4–6 weeks following surgery. Any evidence of dietary protein intolerance on a maintenance diet is usually managed with a moderately protein-restricted diet in the form of a commercially manufactured hepatic diet. Alternatively, higher dietary protein concentrations can be fed in the form of vegetable or milk-based proteins to these animals, with every effort made to avoid the feeding of animal proteins.

Dietary Protein

Protein supplementation remains an enigma of great concern for clinicians caring for patients with HE secondary to hepatic cirrhosis, because these patients may have significantly increased protein requirements due to their liver disease and possible catabolism from a reduced insulin/glucagon ratio (Soeters et al. 1977; Swart et al. 1988). However, dietary protein should not be restricted in animals with PSSs that are not encephalopathic, and these animals should be fed as much protein as they will tolerate without becoming clinically encephalopathic. A study showed that 2.1 g of crude protein/kg body weight/day with 80% or greater bioavailability was adequate at maintaining body protein stores in dogs with PSSs, without causing HE (Laflamme et al. 1993).

Renal diets are best avoided in animals with liver disease due to the source of dietary protein (often animal/organ meats), and efforts should be made to feed vegetable or dairy proteins if higher concentrations of dietary protein are associated with encephalopathy. Decreased portal venous perfusion or markedly reduced hepatic mass permits encephalogenic material derived from the gut, diet, or endogenous metabolism to enter the systemic circulation. Subsequent exposure to the blood–brain barrier allows access to the central nervous system. Nitrogen is normally metabolized to ammonia and detoxified in the hepatic urea cycle. Ingestion of a meat-based high-protein diet, gastrointestinal bleeding, and azotemia are the most common causes of HE in animals with severe liver disease or PSSs (Center 1996b). The source of protein is critically important in the management of animals with HE. Dogs with experimentally created PSSs had significantly prolonged survival and fewer signs of encephalopathy when fed a milk-based diet as opposed to a meat-based diet (Condon 1971). It is possible that heme, RNA, and other nitrogenous bases in the meat-based diet contributed to the exacerbation of HE and shortened survival. The presence of diarrhea and soft stools in the dogs receiving the milk-based diet was a possible cause for decreased nitrogen absorption secondary to shortened intestinal transit time and lowering of colonic pH. The latter hypothesis is supported by the finding that encephalopathy is worse in Eck fistula dogs with constipation, and clinical signs are reduced following administration of enemas. The benefits of feeding milk proteins are unlikely to be the result of a favorable amino acid composition of the protein's amino acids, because the ratio between BCAAs and AAAs is similar for proteins in cottage cheese, meat, and fish. The benefits of cottage cheese are thus likely to be associated with its optimal digestibility and lack of porphyrins such as heme and other nitrogenous bases.

The feeding of vegetable-based diets (e.g. soybeans) is also preferred over the feeding of meat-based diets in patients with cirrhosis (Weber et al. 1985). The effect of vegetable-based diets on nitrogen metabolism can be mainly accounted for by the increased intake of dietary fiber and increased incorporation and elimination of nitrogen in fecal bacteria (Weber et al. 1985). The benefits of feeding a protein-restricted soy-based diet versus a protein-restricted poultry-based diet to dogs with congenital PSSs were documented when the dogs on the soy-based diet had significantly lower plasma ammonia concentrations compared to the dogs ingesting the poultry-based diet (Proot et al. 2009). Casein-based diets have been fed to both dogs and cats with liver disease; however, these diets have the potential for low arginine concentrations, warranting supplementation of this essential amino acid if administered to cats. Dietary arginine deficiency in otherwise healthy cats can cause hyperammonemia and encephalopathy signs within 30 min of consumption of a high-protein, arginine-deficient diet (Morris 1985).

Parenteral or enteral supplemental formulas containing increased BCAAs and reduced AAAs designed to normalize circulating amino acids have been evaluated in a number of clinical trials of HE. Despite the large number of investigations, it is difficult to analyze the data because of marked differences in the study designs, lack of randomization, and the varying formulas utilized (Wahren et al. 1983; Cerra et al. 1985; Michel et al. 1985). A recent review, including 16 randomized clinical trials, found that BCAAs had a beneficial effect on symptoms and signs of HE in humans but no effect on mortality (Gluud et al. 2017). Additional beneficial effects demonstrated for BCAAs in humans include overall improvement in nutrition status and energy metabolism, decreased frequency of hospitalization, and improved overall quality of life (Marchesini et al. 2003; Muto et al. 2005). Unfortunately, BCAA supplementation is extremely expensive (Morgan 1990) and may have reduced palatability.

Protein-restricted renal and hepatic diets are often recommended for cats and dogs with HE, although there are as yet no published studies demonstrating the benefits of these diets for liver disease. Renal diets are not optimal for the management of HE due to the large quantities of organ meats in some of these diets. Homemade diets formulated by a board certified veterinary nutritionist®, which avoid the use of meat-based protein sources, can be used as effective alternatives to commercial diets. Fat- and water-soluble vitamins should be supplemented in the diet. Zinc should also be supplemented, since depletion of this mineral has been suggested as a precipitant of HE in people with liver failure (van Der Rijt et al. 1991). In addition, the administration of zinc has induced psychomotor improvements in human cirrhotic patients with mild HE (Reding et al. 1984) and together with oral supplementation of antioxidants has been shown to improve minimal HE in human patients with cirrhosis (Mousa et al. 2016).

Management of animals with urate stones in the urinary bladder secondary to PSSs remains a challenge for clinicians, as these stones are not amenable to dissolution with dietary intervention. Such stones are typically removed surgically via cystotomy or with lithotripsy (see Chapter 16).

Nonabsorbable Disaccharides

Lactulose administration is considered to be one of the treatments of choice in HE. It is a synthetic disaccharide that is hydrolyzed by colonic bacteria, principally to lactic and acetic acids (Lieberthal 1988). Lactulose appears to exert its beneficial effects by (i) lowering colonic pH with subsequent trapping of ammonium ions; (ii) inhibiting ammonia generation by colonic bacteria through a process known as catabolite repression; (iii) decreasing intestinal transit time due to its cathartic properties; and (iv) suppressing bacterial and intestinal ammonia generation by providing a carbohydrate source. The dose to achieve these goals is somewhat variable, although most dogs and cats can be managed with lactulose at 0.25–0.5 ml/kg body weight PO q8–12 h. The dose should be reduced if liquid diarrhea develops. One recent retrospective study did not find a significant effect on estimated median survival times for dogs with PSSs with the addition of lactulose compared to dietary change alone (Favier et al. 2020).

Lactulose is also highly effective when added to enema fluid (a ratio of 30% lactulose to 70% water) and given as a retention enema. Approximately 20–30 ml/kg body weight of this lactulose enema solution is infused and retained in the colon for 20–30 min before evacuation. Lactulose requires intestinal bacteria to be activated; however, neomycin and other antibiotics inhibit bacterial growth. Despite this antagonism, the two agents have successfully been used simultaneously with additive or synergistic effects (Weber et al. 1982).

Antimicrobials

A number of antimicrobials have been advocated for use in patients with HE. Most drugs effective in this capacity are inhibitory to the urease-producing bacteria that frequently comprise Gram-negative anaerobic bacteria. Administration of ampicillin or neomycin appears to provide short-term clinical benefit in both dogs and cats with acute HE associated with portosystemic vascular anomalies. Cats demonstrating ptyalism as a sign of HE appear particularly responsive to ampicillin, fluid therapy, and temporary withdrawal of food. Although metronidazole has broad-spectrum activity against enteric anaerobes such as *Bacteroides* spp. that are believed to metabolize nitrogenous dietary substances, it should be avoided in patients with HE due to its adverse effects (i.e. ataxia, seizures, anorexia) that can mimic manifestations of HE.

Chronic Hepatitis

Chronic hepatitis is a poorly defined clinico-pathologic entity characterized by parenchymal necrosis, particularly piecemeal necrosis, with associated lymphocytic inflammation (Thornburg 1982). The disease can have an insidious onset, contributing to the poor understanding of its etiopathogenesis and advanced stage when recognized. Nutritional management is, thus, frequently delayed and is directed at arresting inflammation, correcting nutritional derangements, and resolving fibrosis. Specific therapy involves the use of immunomodulatory drugs such as corticosteroids (with or without cyclosporine or azathioprine), choleretics such as ursodeoxycholic acid (Meyer et al. 1997), copper chelators (if warranted based on copper quantitation of liver biopsies), zinc, and antioxidants such as SAMe and vitamin E. Protein intake should not be restricted unless the patient shows signs of protein intolerance. The principles of nutritional support are similar to those for the patient with copper-associated hepatotoxicity, although copper does not need to be restricted unless warranted based on copper quantification of liver biopsies.

Parenteral nutrition offers the possibility of increasing or ensuring nutrient intake in patients in whom sufficient nutrition by the oral or enteral route alone is insufficient or impossible. Parenteral nutrition should be considered in patients with acute hepatotoxicity with subsequent HE in which enteral feeding is either contraindicated or not tolerated by the patient. Central parenteral administration to dogs and cats with chronic hepatitis and cholangitis was associated with a mortality rate of approximately 50% (Reuter et al. 1998; Pyle et al. 2004). The relatively high mortality rate was more likely a reflection of the increased selection of critically ill patients unable to tolerate enteral nutritional support, and not those whose prognosis was unaltered or worsened with the advent of central parenteral nutrition support.

Ascites should be managed by avoiding excess dietary sodium and judicious use of diuretics. Commercially available hepatic diets are controlled in sodium and are recommended. Sodium-controlled homemade diets can also be prepared. Spironolactone, administered at 1–2 mg/kg PO twice daily, is the diuretic of choice since it blocks the action of aldosterone at the distal renal tubules and collecting ducts

(Boyer and Warnock 1983). Diuretics must be dosed cautiously to prevent dehydration and hypovolemia, with secondary exacerbation of HE. In addition, corticosteroids are catabolic to body proteins and could precipitate a worsening of clinical signs caused by the associated increase in ammonia production.

Summary

- The specific nutritional requirements of dogs and cats with liver disease are currently not defined.
- The underlying cause of liver disease should be identified and treated whenever feasible.
- Malnutrition is a significant co-morbidity in patients with advanced liver disease and therefore nutrition is important in the management of these cases.
- Anorexia is a common manifestation of liver disease and adequate energy and nutrient intake can easily be facilitated with the use of enteral feeding devices.
- Early nutritional support with nasoesophageal, esophagostomy, or gastrostomy tubes remains the cornerstone of therapy for cats with hepatic lipidosis.
- A copper-restricted diet is an important component for the treatment of copper-associated hepatotoxicity in dogs.
- Dietary protein should not be restricted in non-encephalopathic animals with liver disease, including those with portosystemic shunts.
- In animals with hepatic encephalopathy, highly digestible vegetable and dairy proteins are better tolerated than animal proteins.
- There is increasing evidence that liver support in the form of supplementation with antioxidants (e.g. vitamin E, SAMe, milk thistle) has a hepatoprotective role, particularly in inflammatory hepatopathies.

References

Abbott-Johnson, W., Kerlin, P., Clague, A. et al. (2011). Relationships between blood levels of fat soluble vitamins and disease etiology and severity in adults awaiting liver transplantation. *J. Gastroenterol. Hepatol.* 26: 1402–1410.

Abood, S.K. and Buffington, C.A. (1992). Enteral feeding of dogs and cats: 51 cases (1989–1991). *J. Am. Vet. Med. Assoc.* 201: 619–622.

Allis, T.J. and Leopold, D.A. (2012). Smell and taste disorders. *Facial Plast. Surg. Clin. North Am.* 20: 93–111.

Arteh, J., Narra, S., and Nair, S. (2010). Prevalence of vitamin D deficiency in chronic liver disease. *Dig. Dis. Sci.* 55: 2624–2628.

Au, A.Y., Hasenwinkel, J.M., and Frondoza, C.G. (2011). Silybin inhibits interleukin-1beta-induced production of pro-inflammatory mediators in canine hepatocyte cultures. *J. Vet. Pharmacol. Ther.* 34: 120–129.

Au, A.Y., Hasenwinkel, J.M., and Frondoza, C.G. (2013). Hepatoprotective effects of S-adenosylmethionine and silybin on canine hepatocytes in vitro. *J. Anim. Physiol. Anim. Nutr. (Berl)* 97: 331–341.

Avizeh, R., Najafzadeh, H., Razijalali, M., and Shirali, S. (2010). Evaluation of prophylactic and therapeutic effects of silymarin and N-acetylcysteine in acetaminophen-induced hepatotoxicity in cats. *J. Vet. Pharmacol. Ther.* 33: 95–99.

Balkany, T.J., Baker, B.B., Bloustein, P.A. et al. (1977). Cervical esophagostomy in dogs. Endoscopic, radiographic and histopathologic evaluation of esophagitis induced by feeding tubes. *Ann. Otol. Rhinol. Laryngol.* 86: 588–593.

Barber, J.R. and Teasley, K.M. (1984). Nutritional support of patients with severe hepatic failure. *Clin. Pharm.* 3: 245–253.

Beaudouin, C., Haurat, G., Laffitte, J.A. et al. (1993). The presence of (+)-S-adenosyl-L-methionine in the rat brain and its lack of effect on phenylethanolamine N-methyltransferase activity. *J. Neurochem.* 61: 928–935.

Bianchi, G., Marchesini, G., Zoli, M. et al. (1994). Prognostic significance of diabetes in patients with cirrhosis. *Hepatology* 20: 119–125.

Biourge, V. (1997). Nutrition and liver disease. *Semin. Vet. Med. Surg.* 12: 34–44.

Biourge, V., MacDonald, M.J., and King, L. (1990). Feline hepatic lipidosis: pathogenesis and nutritional management. *Comp. Cont. Educ. Pract. Vet.* 12: 1244–1258.

Biourge, V., Pion, P., Lewis, J. et al. (1993). Spontaneous occurrence of hepatic lipidosis in a group of laboratory cats. *J. Vet. Intern. Med.* 7: 194–197.

Blanchard, G., Paragon, B.M., Milliat, F., and Lutton, C. (2002). Dietary L-carnitine supplementation in obese cats alters carnitine metabolism and decreases ketosis during fasting and induced hepatic lipidosis. *J. Nutr.* 132: 204–210.

Boyer, T.D. and Warnock, D.G. (1983). Use of diuretics in the treatment of cirrhotic ascites. *Gastroenterology* 84: 1051–1055.

Brenner, K., Kukanich, K.S., and Smee, N.M. (2011). Refeeding syndrome in a cat with hepatic lipidosis. *J. Feline Med. Surg.* 13: 614–617.

Brewer, G.J. (1998). Wilson disease and canine copper toxicosis. *Am. J. Clin. Nutr.* 67: 1087S–1090S.

Bucher, N.L.R. and Malt, R.A. (1971). *Regeneration of Liver and Kidney*, 143–176. Boston, MA: Little, Brown.

Campbell, J.A., Jutkowitz, L.A., Santoro, K.A. et al. (2010). Continuous versus intermittent delivery of nutrition via nasoenteric feeding tubes in hospitalized canine and feline patients: 91 patients (2002–2007). *J. Vet. Emerg. Crit. Care* 20: 232–236.

Cantafora, A., Blotta, I., Rossi, S.S. et al. (1991). Dietary taurine content changes liver lipids in cats. *J. Nutr.* 121: 1522–1528.

Caregaro, L., Alberino, F., Amodio, P. et al. (1996). Malnutrition in alcoholic and virus-related cirrhosis. *Am. J. Clin. Nutr.* 63: 602–609.

Center, S.A. (1996a). Acute hepatic injury: hepatic necrosis and fulminant hepatic failure. In: *Strombeck's Small Animal Gastroenterology*, 3e (ed. W.G. Guilford, S.A. Center, D.R. Strombeck, et al.), 654–704. Philadelphia, PA: W.B. Saunders.

Center, S.A. (1996b). Chronic hepatitis, cirrhosis, breed-specific hepatopathies, copper storage hepatopathy, suppurative hepatitis, granulomatous hepatitis and idiopathic hepatic fibrosis. In: *Strombeck's Small Animal Gastroenterology*, 3e (ed. W.G. Guilford, S.A. Center, D.R. Strombeck, et al.), 705–765. Philadelphia, PA: W.B. Saunders.

Center, S.A. (1996c). Pathophysiology of liver disease: normal and abnormal function. In: *Strombeck's Small Animal Gastroenterology*, 3e (ed. W.G. Guilford, S.A. Center, D.R. Strombeck, et al.), 553–632. Philadelphia, PA: W.B. Saunders.

Center, S.A. (2005). Feline hepatic lipidosis. *Vet. Clin. North Am. Small Anim. Pract.* 35: 225–269.

Center, S.A., Crawford, M.A., Guida, L. et al. (1993). A retrospective study of 77 cats with severe hepatic lipidosis: 1975–1990. *J. Vet. Intern. Med.* 7: 349–359.

Center, S.A., Elston, T.H., Rowland, P.H. et al. (1996). Fulminant hepatic failure associated with oral administration of diazepam in 11 cats. *J. Am. Vet. Med. Assoc.* 209: 618–625.

Center, S.A., Harte, J., Watrous, D. et al. (2000). The clinical and metabolic effects of rapid weight loss in obese pet cats and the influence of supplemental oral L-carnitine. *J. Vet. Intern. Med.* 14: 598–608.

Center, S.A., Richter, K.P., Twedt, D.C. et al. (2021). Is it time to reconsider current guidelines for copper content in commercial dog foods? *J. Am. Vet. Med. Assoc.* 258: 357–364.

Center, S.A., Warner, K.L., and Erb, H.N. (2002). Liver glutathione concentrations in dogs and cats with naturally occurring liver disease. *Am. J. Vet. Res.* 63: 1187–1197.

Center, S.A., Warner, K.L., Randolph, J.F. et al. (2012). Influence of dietary supplementation with (L)-carnitine on metabolic rate, fatty acid oxidation, body condition, and weight loss in overweight cats. *Am. J. Vet. Res.* 73: 1002–1015.

Cerra, F.B., Cheung, N.K., Fischer, J.E. et al. (1985). Disease specific amino acid infusion (F080) in hepatic encephalopathy: a prospective, randomized, double-blind, controlled trial. *J. Parenter. Enteral Nutr.* 9: 288–295.

Charlton, M.R. (1996). Protein metabolism and liver disease. *Baillière's Clin. Endocrinol. Metab.* 10: 617–635.

Chen, Z., Sheng, L., Shen, H. et al. (2012). Hepatic TRAF2 regulates glucose metabolism through enhancing glucagon responses. *Diabetes* 61: 566–573.

Cheung, K., Lee, S.S., and Raman, M. (2012). Prevalence and mechanisms of malnutrition in patients with advanced liver disease, and nutrition management strategies. *Clin. Gastroenterol. Hepatol.* 10: 117–125.

Condon, R.E. (1971). Effect of dietary protein on symptoms and survival in dogs with an Eck fistula. *Am. J. Surg.* 121: 107–114.

Cooper, V.L., Carlson, M.P., Jacobson, J. et al. (1997). Hepatitis and increased copper levels in a Dalmatian. *J. Vet. Diagn. Invest.* 9: 201–203.

Cordoba, J., Lopez-Hellin, J., Planas, M. et al. (2004). Normal protein diet for episodic hepatic encephalopathy: results of a randomized study. *J. Hepatol.* 41: 38–43.

Crocenzi, F.A., Sanchez Pozzi, E.J., Pellegrino, J.M. et al. (2003). Preventive effect of silymarin against taurolithocholate-induced cholestasis in the rat. *Biochem. Pharmacol.* 66: 355–364.

Crowe, D.T. (1986). Clinical use of an indwelling nasogastric tube for enteral nutrition and fluid therapy in the dog and cat. *J. Am. Anim. Hosp. Assoc.* 22: 675–682.

Dejong, C.H., van de Poll, M.C., Soeters, P.B. et al. (2007). Aromatic amino acid metabolism during liver failure. *J. Nutr.* 137: 1579S–1585S.

Diehl, A.M. (1991). Nutrition, hormones, metabolism, and liver regeneration. *Semin. Liver Dis.* 11 (4): 315–320.

Dimski, D.S. (1994). Ammonia metabolism and the urea cycle: function and clinical implications. *J. Vet. Intern. Med.* 8: 73–78.

Ekberg, K., Landau, B.R., Wajngot, A. et al. (1999). Contributions by kidney and liver to glucose production in the postabsorptive state and after 60 h of fasting. *Diabetes* 48: 292–298.

Favier, R.P., De Graaf, E., Corbee, R.J., and Kummeling, A. (2020). Outcome of non-surgical dietary treatment with or without lactulose in dogs with congenital portosystemic shunts. *Vet. Q.* 40: 108–114.

Fieten, H., Biourge, V.C., Watson, A.L. et al. (2014). Nutritional management of inherited copper-associated hepatitis in the Labrador retriever. *Vet. J.* 199: 429–433.

Fieten, H., Biourge, V.C., Watson, A.L. et al. (2015). Dietary management of Labrador retrievers with subclinical hepatic copper accumulation. *J. Vet. Intern. Med.* 29: 822–827.

Fieten, H., Dirksen, K., Van Den Ingh, T.S. et al. (2013). D-penicillamine treatment of copper-associated hepatitis in Labrador retrievers. *Vet. J.* 196: 522–527.

Fieten, H., Gill, Y., Martin, A.J. et al. (2016). The Menkes and Wilson disease genes counteract in copper toxicosis in Labrador retrievers: a new canine model for copper-metabolism disorders. *Dis. Model. Mech.* 9: 25–38.

Fieten, H., Hooijer-Nouwens, B.D., Biourge, V.C. et al. (2012). Association of dietary copper and zinc levels with hepatic copper and zinc concentration in Labrador Retrievers. *J. Vet. Intern. Med.* 26: 1274–1280.

Filburn, C.R., Kettenacker, R., and Griffin, D.W. (2007). Bioavailability of a silybin-phosphatidylcholine complex in dogs. *J. Vet. Pharmacol. Ther.* 30: 132–138.

Fischer, J.E. and Baldessarini, R.J. (1971). False neurotransmitters and hepatic failure. *Lancet* 2: 75–80.

Fisher, P.W.F., Giroux, A., and L'Abbe, M.R. (1983). Effects of zinc on mucosal copper binding and on kinetics of copper absorption. *J. Nutr.* 113: 462–469.

Forman, O.P., Boursnell, M.E.G., Dunmore, B.J. et al. (2005). Characterization of the COMMD1 (MURR1) mutation causing copper toxicosis in Bedlington terriers. *Anim. Genet.* 36: 497–501.

Francavilla, A., Panella, C., Polimeno, L. et al. (1990). Hormonal and enzymatic parameters of hepatic regeneration in patients undergoing major liver resections. *Hepatology* 12: 1134–1138.

Ghadir, M.R., Riahin, A.A., Havaspour, A. et al. (2010). The relationship between lipid profile and severity of liver damage in cirrhotic patients. *Hepat. Mon.* 10: 285–288.

Gheorghe, L., Iacob, R., Vadan, R. et al. (2005). Improvement of hepatic encephalopathy using a modified high-calorie high-protein diet. *Rom. J. Gastroenterol.* 14: 231–238.

Gheorghe, C., Pascu, O., Iacob, R. et al. (2013). Nutritional risk screening and prevalence of malnutrition on admission to gastroenterology departments: a multicentric study. *Chirurgia (Bucur)* 108: 535–541.

Gluud, L.L., Dam, G., Les, I. et al. (2017). Branched-chain amino acids for people with hepatic encephalopathy. *Cochrane Database Syst. Rev.* (5): CD001939. https://doi.org/10.1002/14651858.CD001939.pub2.

Greco, A.V., Mingrone, G., Benedetti, G. et al. (1998). Daily energy and substrate metabolism in patients with cirrhosis. *Hepatology* 27: 346–350.

Haywood, S., Rutgers, H.C., and Christian, M.K. (1988). Hepatitis and copper accumulation in Skye terriers. *Vet. Pathol.* 25: 408–414.

Higgins, G.M. and Anderson, R.M. (1931). Experimental pathology of the liver: restoration of the liver by the white rat following partial surgical removal. *Arch. Pathol.* 12: 186–202.

Hishiyama, N., Kayanuma, H., Matsui, T. et al. (2006). Plasma concentration of vitamin C in dogs with a portosystemic shunt. *Can. J. Vet. Res.* 70: 305–307.

Hoffmann, G., Jones, P.G., Biourge, V. et al. (2009). Dietary management of hepatic copper accumulation in Labrador Retrievers. *J. Vet. Intern. Med.* 23: 957–963.

Hoffmann, G., van den Ingh, T.S., Bode, P., and Rothuizen, J. (2006). Copper-associated chronic hepatitis in Labrador retrievers. *J. Vet. Intern. Med.* 20: 856–861.

Holahan, M., Abood, S., Hauptman, J. et al. (2010). Intermittent and continuous enteral nutrition in critically ill dogs: a prospective randomized trial. *J. Vet. Intern. Med.* 24: 520–526.

Hotamisligil, G.S. (2006). Inflammation and metabolic disorders. *Nature* 444: 860–867.

Hultgren, B.D., Stevens, J.B., and Hardy, R.M. (1986). Inherited, chronic progressive hepatic degeneration in Bedlington terriers with increased liver copper concentrations: clinical and pathologic observations and comparison with other copper-associated liver diseases. *Am. J. Vet. Res.* 47: 365–377.

Ibrahim, W.H., Bailey, N., Sunvold, G.D., and Bruckner, G.G. (2003). Effects of carnitine and taurine on fatty acid metabolism and lipid accumulation in the liver of cats during weight gain and weight loss. *Am. J. Vet. Res.* 64: 1265–1277.

Jacobs, G., Cornelius, L., Keene, B. et al. (1990). Comparison of plasma, liver, and skeletal muscle carnitine concentrations in cats with idiopathic hepatic lipidosis and in healthy cats. *Am. J. Vet. Res.* 51: 1349–1351.

Jaffe, I., Altman, K., and Merryman, P. (1964). The antipyridoxine effects of penicillamine in man. *J. Clin. Investig.* 43: 1869–1873.

Johnson, G.F., Sternlieb, I., Twedt, D.C. et al. (1980). Inheritance of copper toxicosis in Bedlington terriers. *Am. J. Vet. Res.* 41: 1865–1866.

Johnson, T.M., Overgard, E.B., Cohen, A.E., and Dibaise, J.K. (2013). Nutrition assessment and management in advanced liver disease. *Nutr. Clin. Pract.* 28: 15–29.

Kalaitzakis, E. (2014). Gastrointestinal dysfunction in liver cirrhosis. *World J. Gastroenterol.* 20: 14686–14695.

Khanna, S. and Gopalan, S. (2007). Role of branched-chain amino acids in liver disease: the evidence for and against. *Curr. Opin. Clin. Nutr. Metab. Care* 10: 297–303.

Klaus, J.A., Rudloff, E., and Kirby, R. (2009). Nasogastric tube feeding in cats with suspected acute pancreatitis: 55 cases (2001–2006). *J. Vet. Emerg. Crit. Care* 19: 337–346.

Kowdley, K.V. (1998). Lipids and lipid-activated vitamins in chronic cholestatic diseases. *Clin. Liver Dis.* 2: 373–389.

Kowdley, K.V., Emond, M.J., Sadowski, J.A., and Kaplan, M.M. (1997). Plasma vitamin K1 level is decreased in primary biliary cirrhosis. *Am. J. Gastroenterol.* 92: 2059–2061.

Kruszynska, Y.T., Meyer-Alber, A., Darakhshan, F. et al. (1993). Metabolic handling of orally administered glucose in cirrhosis. *J. Clin. Investig.* 91: 1057–1066.

Kuzi, S., Segev, G., Kedar, S. et al. (2017). Prognostic markers in feline hepatic lipidosis: a retrospective study of 71 cats. *Vet. Rec.* 181: 512.

Laflamme, D.P., Allen, S.W., and Huber, T.L. (1993). Apparent dietary protein requirement of dogs with portosystemic shunt. *Am. J. Vet. Res.* 54: 719–723.

Langlois, D.K., Lehner, A.F., Buchweitz, J.P. et al. (2013). Pharmacokinetics and relative bioavailability of D-penicillamine in fasted and nonfasted dogs. *J. Vet. Intern. Med.* 27: 1071–1076.

Lee, S.P. and Lai, K.W. (1976). Exocrine pancreatic function in hepatic cirrhosis. *Am. J. Gastroenterol.* 65: 244–248.

Leevy, C.M., Thompson, A., and Baker, H. (1970). Vitamins and liver injury. *Am. J. Clin. Nutr.* 23: 493–498.

Lieberthal, M.M. (1988). The pharmacology of lactulose. In: *Hepatic Encephalopathy: Management with Lactulose and Related Carbohydrates* (ed. H.O. Conn and J. Bircher), 146–175. East Lansing, MI: Medi-Ed Press.

Lipsky, P.E. and Ziff, M. (1978). The effect of D-penicillamine on mitogen-induced human lymphocyte proliferation: synergistic inhibition by D-penicillamine and copper salts. *J. Immunol.* 120: 1006–1013.

Maharshi, S., Sharma, B.C., and Srivastava, S. (2015). Malnutrition in cirrhosis increases morbidity and mortality. *J. Gastroenterol. Hepatol.* 30: 1507–1513.

Malagelada, J.R., Pihl, O., and Linscher, W.G. (1974). Impaired absorption of micellar long chain fatty acid in patients with alcoholic cirrhosis. *Am. J. Dig. Dis.* 19: 1016–1020.

Mandigers, P.J., Bode, P., van Wees, A.M. et al. (2007). Hepatic ^{64}Cu excretion in Dobermans with subclinical hepatitis. *Res. Vet. Sci.* 83: 204–209.

Marchesini, G., Bianchi, G., Merli, M. et al. (2003). Nutritional supplementation with branched-chain amino acids in advanced cirrhosis: a double-blind, randomized trial. *Gastroenterology* 124: 1792–1801.

Marco, J., Diego, J., Villanueva, M.L. et al. (1973). Elevated plasma glucagon levels in cirrhosis of the liver. *N. Engl. J. Med.* 289: 1107–1111.

McCullough, A.J. and Tavill, A.S. (1991). Disordered energy and protein metabolism in liver disease. *Semin. Liver Dis.* 11: 265–277.

Meyer, D.J., Thompson, M.B., and Senior, D.F. (1997). Use of ursodeoxycholic acids in a dog with chronic hepatitis: effects on serum hepatic tests and endogenous bile acid composition. *J. Vet. Intern. Med.* 11: 195–197.

Mezey, E. (1978). Liver disease and nutrition. *Gastroenterology* 74: 770–783.

Michel, H., Bories, P., Aubin, J.P. et al. (1985). Treatment of acute hepatic encephalopathy in cirrhotics with a branched chain amino acids enriched versus a conventional amino acid mixture: a controlled study of 70 patients. *Liver* 5: 282–289.

Morgan, M.Y. (1990). Branched chain amino acids in the management of chronic liver disease: facts and fantasies. *J. Hepatol.* 11: 133–141.

Morris, J.G. (1985). Nutritional and metabolic responses to arginine deficiency in carnivores. *J. Nutr.* 115: 524–531.

Morris, J.G. (2002). Idiosyncratic nutrient requirements of cats appear to be diet-induced evolutionary adaptations. *Nutr. Res. Rev.* 15: 153–168.

Morris, J.G. and Rogers, Q.R. (1978). Ammonia intoxication in the near-adult cat as a result of a dietary deficiency of arginine. *Science* 199: 431–432.

Mousa, N., Abdel-Razik, A., Zaher, A. et al. (2016). The role of antioxidants and zinc in minimal hepatic encephalopathy: a randomized trial. *Therap. Adv. Gastroenterol.* 9: 684–691.

Mullen, K.D. and Weber, F.L. (1991). Role of nutrition in hepatic encephalopathy. *Semin. Liver Dis.* 11: 292–304.

Munoz, S.J. (1991). Nutritional therapies in liver disease. *Semin. Liver Dis.* 11: 278–291.

Muto, Y., Sato, S., Watanabe, A. et al. (2005). Effects of oral branched-chain amino acid granules on event-free survival in patients with liver cirrhosis. *Clin. Gastroenterol. Hepatol.* 3: 705–713.

Outerbridge, C.A., Marks, S.L., and Rogers, Q.R. (2002). Plasma amino acid concentrations in 36 dogs with histologically confirmed superficial necrolytis dermatitis. *Vet. Dermatol.* 13: 177–186.

Owen, O.E., Reichle, F.A., Mozzoli, M.A. et al. (1981). Hepatic, gut, and renal substrate flux rates in patients with hepatic cirrhosis. *J. Clin. Investig.* 68: 240–252.

Pappa, H.M., Bern, E., Kamin, D., and Grand, R.J. (2008). Vitamin D status in gastrointestinal and liver disease. *Curr. Opin. Gastroenterol.* 24: 176–183.

Podolsky, S., Zimmerman, H.J., Burrows, B.A. et al. (1973). Potassium depletion in hepatic cirrhosis: a reversible cause of impaired growth hormone and insulin response to stimulation. *N. Engl. J. Med.* 13: 644–648.

Proot, S., Biourge, V., Teske, E., and Rothuizen, J. (2009). Soy protein isolate versus meat-based low-protein diet for dogs with congenital portosystemic shunts. *J. Vet. Intern. Med.* 23: 794–800.

Pyle, S.C., Marks, S.L., and Kass, P.H. (2004). Evaluation of complications and prognostic factors associated with administration of total parenteral nutrition in cats: 75 cases (1994–2001). *J. Am. Vet. Med. Assoc.* 225: 242–250.

Rahelic, D., Kujundzic, M., Romic, Z. et al. (2006). Serum concentration of zinc, copper, manganese and magnesium in patients with liver cirrhosis. *Coll. Antropol.* 30: 523–528.

Reding, P., Duchateau, J., and Bataille, C. (1984). Oral zinc supplementation improves hepatic encephalopathy: results of a randomised controlled trial. *Lancet* 2: 493–495.

Reuter, J.D., Marks, S.L., Rogers, Q.R., and Farver, T.B. (1998). Use of total parenteral nutrition in dogs: 209 cases (1988–1995). *J. Vet. Emerg. Crit. Care* 8: 201–213.

Rifkin, J. and Miller, M.D. (2014). Copper-associated hepatitis in a Pembroke welsh corgi. *Can. Vet. J.* 55: 573–576.

Riggio, O., Merli, M., and Capocaccia, L. (1991). The role of zinc in the management of hepatic encephalopathy. In: *Progress in Hepatic Encephalopathy* (ed. F. Bengtsson and B. Jeppsson), 303–312. Boca Raton, FL: CRC Press.

Rizza, R.A. (2010). Pathogenesis of fasting and postprandial hyperglycemia in type 2 diabetes: implications for therapy. *Diabetes* 59: 2697–2707.

Rojas-Loureiro, G., Servin-Caamano, A., Perez-Reyes, E. et al. (2017). Malnutrition negatively impacts the quality of life of patients with cirrhosis: an observational study. *World J. Hepatol.* 9: 263–269.

Rolfe, D.S. and Twedt, D.C. (1995). Copper-associated hepatopathies in dogs. *Vet. Clin. North Am. Small Anim. Pract.* 25: 399–417.

Sam, J. and Nguyen, G.C. (2009). Protein-calorie malnutrition as a prognostic indicator of mortality among patients hospitalized with cirrhosis and portal hypertension. *Liver Int.* 29: 1396–1402.

Siegel, R.C. (1977). Collagen cross-linking. Effect of D-penicillamine on cross-linking in vitro. *J. Biol. Chem.* 252: 254–259.

Simpson, K.W., Fyfe, J., Cornetta, A. et al. (2001). Subnormal concentrations of serum cobalamin (vitamin B12) in cats with gastrointestinal disease. *J. Vet. Intern. Med.* 15: 26–32.

Skorupski, K.A., Hammond, G.M., Irish, A.M. et al. (2011). Prospective randomized clinical trial assessing the efficacy of Denamarin for prevention of CCNU-induced hepatopathy in tumor-bearing dogs. *J. Vet. Intern. Med.* 25: 838–845.

Soeters, P.B., Weir, G., Ebeid, A.M., and Fischer, J.E. (1977). Insulin, glucagon, portal systemic shunting, and hepatic failure in the dog. *J. Surg. Res.* 23: 183–188.

Spee, B., Arends, B., van den Ingh, T.S. et al. (2006). Copper metabolism and oxidative stress in chronic inflammatory and cholestatic liver diseases in dogs. *J. Vet. Intern. Med.* 20: 1085–1092.

Strombeck, D.R., Harrold, D., Rogers, Q.R., and Wheeldon, E. (1983a). Plasma amino acids, glucagon, and insulin concentrations in dogs with nitrosamine-induced hepatic disease. *Am. J. Vet. Res.* 44: 2028–2036.

Strombeck, D.R. and Rogers, Q.R. (1978). Plasma amino acid concentrations in dogs with hepatic disease. *J. Am. Vet. Med. Assoc.* 173: 93–96.

Strombeck, D.R., Schaeffer, M.C., and Rogers, Q.R. (1983b). Dietary therapy for dogs with chronic hepatic insufficiency. In: *Current Veterinary Therapy VIII* (ed. R.W. Kirk), 817–821. Philadelphia, PA: W.B. Saunders.

Su, L.C., Owen, C.A. Jr., McCall, J.T. et al. (1982). A defect of biliary excretion of copper in copper-laden Bedlington terriers. *Am. J. Physiol.* 243: G231–G236.

Swart, G.R., van den Berg, J.W.O., Wattimena, J.L.D. et al. (1988). Elevated protein requirements in cirrhosis of the liver investigated by whole body protein turnover studies. *Clin. Sci.* 75: 101–107.

Swart, G.R., Zillikens, M.C., van Vuure, J.K., and van den Berg, J.W. (1989). Effect of a late evening meal on nitrogen balance in patients with cirrhosis of the liver. *Br. Med. J.* 299: 1202–1203.

Thandassery, R.B. and Montano-Loza, A.J. (2016). Role of nutrition and muscle in cirrhosis. *Curr. Treat. Options Gastroenterol.* 14: 257–273.

Thornburg, L.P. (1982). Chronic active hepatitis: what is it and does it occur in dogs? *J. Am. Anim. Hosp. Assoc.* 18: 21–22.

Thornburg, L.P. (2000). A prospective on copper and liver disease in the dog. *J. Vet. Diagn. Invest.* 12: 101–110.

Tietge, U.J.F., Bahr, M.J., Manns, M.P., and Boker, K.H.W. (2003). Hepatic amino acid metabolism in liver cirrhosis and in the long-term course after liver transplantation. *Transpl. Int.* 16: 1–8.

Toresson, L., Steiner, J.M., Olmedal, G. et al. (2017). Oral cobalamin supplementation in cats with hypocobalaminaemia: a retrospective study. *J. Feline Med. Surg.* 19: 1302–1306.

Van den Ingh, T.S., Punte, P.M., Hoogendijk, E.N. et al. (2007). Possible nutritionally induced copper-associated chronic hepatitis in two dogs. *Vet. Rec.* 161: 728.

Van Der Rijt, C.C.D., Schalm, S.W., Schat, H. et al. (1991). Overt hepatic encephalopathy precipitated by zinc deficiency. *Gastroenterology* 100: 1114–1118.

Vilstrup, H., Amodio, P., Bajaj, J. et al. (2014). Hepatic encephalopathy in chronic liver disease: 2014 practice guideline by the American Association for the Study of Liver Diseases and the European Association for the Study of the liver. *Hepatology* 60: 715–735.

Vogel, G., Tuchweber, B., Trost, W., and Mengs, U. (1984). Protection by silibin against *Amanita phalloides* intoxication in beagles. *Toxicol. Appl. Pharmacol.* 73: 355–362.

Wahren, J., Denis, J., Desurmont, P. et al. (1983). Is intravenous administration of branched chain amino acids effective in the treatment of hepatic encephalopathy? A multicenter study. *Hepatology* 3: 475–480.

Wallace, K.P., Center, S.A., Hickford, F.H. et al. (2002). S-adenosyl-L-methionine (SAMe) in the treatment of acetaminophen toxicity in a dog. *J. Am. Anim. Hosp. Assoc.* 38: 246–254.

Webb, C.B., Mccord, K.W., and Twedt, D.C. (2009). Assessment of oxidative stress in leukocytes and granulocyte function following oral administration of a silibinin-phosphatidylcholine complex in cats. *Am. J. Vet. Res.* 70: 57–62.

Webb, C.B., Twedt, D.C., Fettman, M.H., and Mason, G. (2003). S-adenosylmethionine (SAMe) in a feline acetaminophen model of oxidative injury. *J. Feline Med. Surg.* 5: 69–75.

Weber, F.L. Jr., Fresard, K.M., and Lally, B.R. (1982). Effects of lactulose and neomycin on urea metabolism in cirrhotic subjects. *Gastroenterology* 82: 213–217.

Weber, F.L. Jr., Minco, D., Fresard, K.M., and
Banwell, J.G. (1985). Effects of vegetable diets
on nitrogen metabolism in cirrhotic subjects.
Gastroenterology 89: 538–544.

Yu, M.K., Freeman, L.M., Heinze, C.R. et al.
(2013). Comparison of complication rates in
dogs with nasoesophageal versus nasogastric
feeding tubes. *J. Vet. Emerg. Crit. Care* 23:
300–304.

Zakim, D. (1982). Metabolism of glucose and
fatty acids by the liver. In: *Hepatology: A
Textbook of Liver Disease*, 2e (ed. D. Zakim and
T.D. Boyer), 65–96. Philadelphia, PA:
W.B. Saunders.

14

Nutritional Management of Skin Diseases

Catherine A. Outerbridge and Tammy J. Owens

The skin and hair coat can provide cues and clues to underlying systemic health, with their appearance influenced by the nutritional intake of the animal. The skin can also develop lesions secondary to nutritional deficiencies or certain excesses. Additionally, certain skin diseases are managed by alterations to the diet, such as changes to ingredients fed or the addition of supraphysiologic supplementation of specific nutrients or dietary elements. This chapter will discuss dermatologic diseases or conditions that result from nutritional deficiencies and those managed by changes in diet or nutritional supplementation.

Evaluation of Diet in the Context of Dermatologic Disease

Dermatologic disease is often multifactorial; however, diet or specific nutrients may play a role in either the development and/or resolution of clinical signs. Additionally, specific dietary supplementation may be utilized to improve clinical manifestations of specific dermatologic conditions, even when there is no (known) direct role of diet in the disease process. For these reasons, it is imperative to collect diet histories, as they may provide relevant information treatment.

Several resources are available to help in the collection of diet histories. It is important to emphasize that all items consumed by a veterinary patient (including the main diet, treats, table scraps, supplements, flavored medications, or via frequent hunting or scavenging behavior, etc.) will be important in the context of certain dermatologic conditions. Thus, it is worthwhile to collect a written diet history and/or have the pet's owner keep a journal or log. In addition, the pet owner should also be asked to describe the pet's diet using an open-ended statement or question such as "Tell me about everything your pet eats throughout the day, starting from first thing in the morning until the end of the day." Using open-ended questions or similar statements is often more efficient at eliciting the desired scope of information (MacMartin et al. 2015). Similar to diet surveys, they will also elicit disclosure of more diet-related items than the common "What kind of food is he/she on?" (Coe et al. 2020). Also, in these authors' experience, it is most helpful if the client can provide pictures of food packaging to ensure correct information and avoid miscommunication or false assumptions.

The provided information needs to be evaluated to determine if the pet is consuming an appropriate, complete and balanced diet, or if there is reasonable concern for a nutritional deficiency or imbalance. A good place to start

Applied Veterinary Clinical Nutrition, Second Edition. Edited by Andrea J. Fascetti, Sean J. Delaney, Jennifer A. Larsen, and Cecilia Villaverde.
© 2024 John Wiley & Sons, Inc. Published 2024 by John Wiley & Sons, Inc.

is by assessing whether the main diet(s) provides a nutritional adequacy statement to indicate it is intended to be adequate for the species and life stage of interest, as well as how this was determined (e.g. by formulation or feeding trial). It is also very important to remember that these diets balance the concentration of individual nutrients to the energy density of the food, such that a sufficient intake of that food is still required in order to ensure appropriate total intake of individual nutrients for the day. For example, if greater than 90% of total daily calories are provided by complete and balanced diets and the pet consumes at least resting energy requirements, the overall diet is typically sufficient. However, deficiencies can still occur due to formulation or manufacturing errors or in animals requiring very few calories relative to their size (such as those with below average energy needs or "easy keepers") or those who consume too many of their calories from foods that are nutritionally incomplete (e.g. too many treats or table foods). Specific nutrients of concern will be addressed individually throughout the chapter.

Nutritional Deficiencies and Excesses

Some cutaneous manifestations of nutritional deficiencies have been linked to inadequate or unbalanced diets. In the case of improper diets, multiple nutritional deficiencies and imbalances may occur (rather than single, isolated deficiencies), which could affect the constellation of presenting clinical signs. Nutritional deficiencies and excesses should not typically occur in healthy animals without a genetic or metabolic abnormality if they are consuming adequate amounts of complete and balanced diets appropriate for their life stage. They could be noted, however, in pets fed unbalanced or defective diets, if too many of the daily calories are provisioned by foods other than the "complete and balanced diet,"

Table 14.1 Dermatologic signs associated with nutritional deficiencies.

Dietary deficiency	Skin lesions
Protein	Scaling, patchy alopecia, thin brittle hair shafts, loss of hair pigment, decreased wound healing
Essential fatty acids	Mild scaling, lack of luster to coat, with chronicity skin thickens and becomes greasy
Zinc	In dogs: erythema, scaling, adherent scaling and crusts develop around mucocutaneous junctions and pressure points
Copper	Hair depigmentation and rough, dull hair coat
Vitamin A	Scaling, follicular hyperkeratosis, dull hair coat
Vitamin E	In cats: steatitis – firm, nodular, painful subcutaneous swellings
Vitamin B complex	Dry hair coat with scaling; cheilosis with riboflavin deficiency

or if the pet has an abnormality affecting their ability to utilize nutrients. Some deficiencies are recognized in particular breeds, suggesting a possible alteration in absorption or metabolism within those individuals. Nutrient deficiencies that can result in cutaneous manifestations include total protein, specific amino acids, essential fatty acids (EFAs), zinc, copper, vitamin A, vitamin B complex, and vitamin E (Table 14.1).

Protein

Protein deficiency can occur when animals consume diets deficient in protein, inadequate amounts of lower-protein diets, diets in which the protein is poorly digestible, when a severe catabolic process or illness leads to excessive protein use or loss, or with starvation. These situations affect the skin in particular due to its high requirements for protein and energy: hair is 95% protein and hair growth can utilize up to 30% of the daily protein intake (Watson 1998; Scott et al. 2001). Longer-haired breeds may also have relatively increased protein needs. Lesions tend to be most prominent in young, growing animals whose total protein requirements are higher than adults. Certain amino acids, particularly cysteine and tyrosine, are also particularly important for the production, growth, and color of normal hair and skin. Hair contains large amounts of the sulfur-containing amino acids methionine and cysteine. Cysteine can form disulfide bonds to make cystine, a major constituent of hair, with several of the keratin-associated proteins in hair fibers containing large amounts (Shimomura et al. 2003). Tyrosine, which can be synthesized from phenylalanine, is an important precursor of melanin and is required for normal production of the eumelanin and pheomelanin found in hair (Yu et al. 2001).

Thin, inelastic, hyperpigmented skin, scaling, brittle hair, loss of hair pigment, and/or patchy alopecia (easily shed hair that is slow to regrow) can be seen in animals related to dermatologic lesions connected to protein deficiency. Hair shafts become thinner and the overall hair coat quality is poor, with dry, dull, brittle hair shafts. In humans, a mean hair root diameter of less than 0.06 mm suggests protein deficiency, but no similar specifications are available for animals (Scott et al. 2001). These hair shaft lesions, together with scales and/or crusts, may appear symmetrically on the head, back, thorax, abdomen, and/or the feet and legs. If total protein intake is adequate, but there are deficiencies in certain specific amino acids, a change in hair color may be noted. For example, black cats or dogs may start turning brown or orange when phenylalanine deficiency results in inadequate tyrosine synthesis.

Ill or metabolically stressed animals may suffer from anagen or telogen defluxion. In some cases this could result from inadequate protein and energy intake during these periods (e.g. sick animals may become hypo- or anorexic). Anagen (growth-phase) defluxion or effluvium (thinning or shedding of hair) results in alopecia when hairs that are in the anagen stage are lost or damaged. This can also occur with certain metabolic disorders, endocrinopathies, or administration of antimitotic drugs. Telogen (resting-phase) defluxion or effluvium occurs when there is a sudden growth arrest of numerous anagen follicles and then synchronization of these follicles into telogen. Causes of telogen defluxion also include severe illness, high fever, physiologic shock, surgery or anesthesia, or pregnancy. Typically, over a 1–3-month period after the insult, the majority of hairs from these follicles are shed as a new hair follicle cycle begins.

Wound healing will be delayed due to impaired collagen synthesis; consequently, wound dehiscence and decubital ulcers are possible cutaneous lesions resulting from protein deficiency (Rhoads et al. 1942). Wound healing can also be negatively impacted by certain micronutrient deficiencies (e.g. zinc), so a poor diet may influence this through multiple routes. Increasing consumption of high-quality protein should resolve many cutaneous signs, providing there is not a complicating disease process or other nutritional deficiencies. Insufficient intake resulting from illness may require placement of an assisted feeding device to support healing.

Most protein or amino acid deficiencies result from consumption of diets that are not complete and balanced (e.g. an unbalanced homemade diet or being fed too many table scraps/treats) or from inadequate consumption of a low-protein diet. The protein and amino acid needs of dogs and cats can be estimated and compared to their intake to gauge the likelihood of protein deficiency in an individual. One way to evaluate this is to compare the estimated daily intake of protein (g/day) to the daily recommended allowance outlined by the National Research Council (NRC) for nutrient requirements of dogs and cats (NRC 2006); see Table 14.2. There are several caveats to this, however. These recommended allowances (and the even lower minimum requirements) were determined in a limited population of healthy, adult laboratory dogs and cats, and the general

Table 14.2   Daily recommended allowances for protein in adult animals.

	Minimum requirement (assumes complete bioavailability)	Recommended allowance (RA) (daily intake should typically be ≥ RA)
Adult cat	$3.97\,g$ protein $\times$ (body weight$_{kg}$)$^{0.67}$	$4.96\,g$ protein $\times$ (body weight$_{kg}$)$^{0.67}$
Adult dog	$2.62\,g$ protein $\times$ (body weight$_{kg}$)$^{0.75}$	$3.28\,g$ protein $\times$ (body weight$_{kg}$)$^{0.75}$

Note: Growing animals have higher daily needs depending on stage of growth, and needs may be overestimated in overweight animals.
Source: Data from NRC (2006).

applicability to all individuals, all breeds, or those with varying disease or aging states is not entirely clear. They are determined in animals with ideal body condition, and this can sometimes introduce uncertainty when utilizing for under- or overweight animals. Consideration must also be given to other factors that could influence the actual utilization, including the digestive and absorptive capacity of the animal and the protein quality (a combination of essential amino acid profile and protein digestibility). Still, if an individual has clinical signs consistent with possible protein deficiency and intake is questionable, this information is clinically useful. Ultimately, protein and/or amino acid deficiencies can potentially be confirmed by testing plasma and whole blood amino acid profiles, available at specialized diagnostic facilities.

Essential Fatty Acids

Animals have an essential requirement for fats, which provide a concentrated source of energy, serve as the carrier for fat-soluble vitamins, and must provide sufficient amounts of EFAs. These EFAs in dogs and cats are polyunsaturated fatty acids (PUFA) omega 6 (n-6) and omega 3 (n-3), which must be acquired from the diet, as the animal cannot synthesize them. These lipids serve structural and functional roles in the body. Specifically, EFAs are needed to maintain normal structure and function of the skin. Additionally, different types of fat impart varying fluid properties to cell membranes (depending on the degree of

unsaturation), and several key PUFAs are precursors for various eicosanoids (metabolites that include prostaglandins, leukotrienes, and thromboxanes).

The essential n-6 fatty acid for all mammals is linoleic acid (LA). This fatty acid is found in certain vegetable and seed oils (e.g. safflower, sunflower, corn, walnut) or certain animal fats (e.g. chicken fat and egg yolk). Other common oils such as olive or coconut oil are very poor sources of LA. Arachidonic acid (AA), another n-6 PUFA, is found only in terrestrial animals and is semi-essential in cats. Unlike dogs, cats do not have the ability to efficiently biotransform LA to AA, instead relying on consumption of prey to supply larger amounts of this fatty acid. Although strict essentiality for adult maintenance is debated (e.g. there are no overt signs of health defects in non-reproducing adults), AA is certainly conditionally essential for growth and reproduction and it is generally prudent to include AA in all feline diets. Gamma linolenic acid (GLA), another n-6 fatty acid, derived from seed oils of evening primrose, borage seed, or blackcurrant, can be used to substitute for animal-derived AA if needed, because it bypasses the rate-limiting step in conversion of LA to AA.

The n-3 PUFA alpha-linolenic acid (ALA) is also an EFA. Although signs of deficiency are more subtle, several long-chain derivatives (EPA, DPA, DHA) are metabolically important and themselves conditionally essential (especially in growth). The first step in the pathway converting ALA to eicosapentaenoic acid (EPA) relies on the same enzyme (delta-6 desaturase) used in conversion of LA to its derivatives and is rate limiting in cats. In both cats and dogs, ALA conversion may be affected by the concentration of LA in the diet and vice versa. Conversion of ALA to EPA and docosapentaenoic acid (DPA) is relatively low overall and is somewhat further suppressed by the presence of large amounts of LA (NRC 2006). Additionally, dogs cannot effectively convert EPA/DPA to docosahexaenoic acid (DHA) (Dunbar et al. 2010). These inefficiencies in converting ALA to other n-3 PUFAs is why marine-sourced oils (e.g. algae, krill, or fish oils) are often preferred, since they contain higher concentrations of preformed EPA and DHA. This is in contrast to terrestrially sourced grain and seed oils, which only really provide ALA (Bauer et al. 2006). Dietary sources used to provide ALA include seed and grain oils (e.g. canola or flaxseed, aka linseed). If providing ALA alone, the ratio of LA to ALA should be controlled due to the competitive interactions for enzymes between LA and ALA. However, if more LA is present in the diet, then it may be prudent to include more ALA for metabolic balance and effects on downstream eicosanoid production. A ratio of 2.6 : 26 of LA : ALA (2.6 : 16 in gestation/lactation) is considered safe in dogs, along with a safe upper limit for LA and EPA + DHA of 16.3 and 2.8 g/1000 kcal, respectively (NRC 2006).

EFAs, especially n-6, have multiple functions in the skin and are important in the maintenance of dermatologic health and integrity. Skin is both the largest organ of the body and easily visualized; therefore, it is an important indicator for signs of EFA deficiency. In growing dogs and cats, deficiency in the skin leads to hypotrichosis, alopecia, scaling, sebaceous gland hypertrophy, and increased transepidermal water loss (TEWL). In cats without sufficient intake of EFA (even with LA and ALA provided), coats can be dry and lusterless with dandruff (NRC 2006).

Linoleic acid in particular is an important component of ceramides, which are necessary in maintaining the cornified lipid envelope or skin barrier. In fact, epidermal water barrier function depends on the LA content of ceramides extruded by epidermal keratinocytes to enhance cohesion between lipid sheets of intercellular lamellae. This is why many dogs with dull, dry coats or scaling, non-pruritic skin disease may temporarily improve with fat or oil supplementation that contains LA or LA + ALA, but adaptation may eventually occur if this EFA deficiency is not the only issue.

Arachidonic acid is a fundamental component of skin, comprising 20–25% of its total cell membrane fatty acids. Since skin lacks the enzymes to convert LA to AA, it is typically circulated to the skin after either being ingested pre-formed or made from LA in the liver. Availability of AA in the skin can alter physiologic response, and the release of AA in skin tissue cells (keratinocytes, neutrophils, platelets, macrophages, endothelial cells, etc.) is a rate-limiting step in eicosanoid production. This can influence epidermal proliferation via the production of prostaglandin E2 (PGE2), which is generally vasodilatory and can be pro-inflammatory in the skin. Provision of alternative substrates (such as EPA) for cyclooxygenase and lipoxygenase, the enzymes responsible for eicosanoid production, may allow competitive substitution for AA. This modulates eicosanoid production and the overall physiologic response, including inflammation. This will be further discussed later in the chapter.

If LA and AA are deficient in the diet, cutaneous signs of EFA deficiency can occur (Codner and Thatcher 1993; Watson 1998; Scott et al. 2001). This might occur if the diet is too low in fat and/or EFA (e.g. unbalanced home-prepared diet) or if the diet has been poorly preserved (e.g. exposure to high heat, use of rancid raw material during production, or inadequate inclusion of protective antioxidants). In rare cases, intestinal malabsorptive disease, exocrine pancreatic disease, or chronic hepatic disease can affect the absorption of EFAs or the production and distribution of other physiologically important fatty acids, leading to cutaneous signs of deficiency.

EFA deficiency in dogs and cats is characterized biochemically in the skin by the absence of LA and AA, and by the accumulation of the monounsaturated fatty acids oleic acid and mead acid. When these fatty acids replace AA in cell membranes membrane integrity is compromised, and when oleic acid replaces LA in ceramides there is increased TEWL. Decrease in AA may also result in decreases in PGE2 and lead to epidermal proliferation. Signs of deficiency may take 2–3 months to appear (Watson 1998). Clinically, in early EFA deficiency a fine scaling is observed, with a loss of hair coat luster and sheen due to decreased surface lipid production. Chronic EFA deficiency results in increasing seborrhea, skin thickening with greasiness (particularly in the ears and intertriginous zones), alopecia, and eventual skin infections and pruritus (Watson 1998; Scott et al. 2001).

The diagnosis is confirmed by response to EFA supplementation, either by feeding a better-quality diet with higher fatty acid content or administration of a veterinary fatty acid supplement. A better-quality dog food is preferred, as EFA deficiency may indicate other potential issues (such as overall poor quality or other nutrient deficiencies), and it will then be better suited to also meet all nutritional needs for vitamins and minerals. For example, when PUFA intake increases, requirements for vitamin E and other nutrients involved in fatty acid metabolism and utilization (such as zinc, vitamin A, B vitamins) will also increase (Miller 1989). Response to dietary change or supplementation is typically rapid, with improvement seen within 4–8 weeks, although severe cases may take up to 6 months (Hensel 2010).

Zinc

Zinc is an important dietary element. It is present in most tissues, helps stabilize biological membranes, and serves as a cofactor in numerous transcription factors and more than 300 enzyme systems involved in all important metabolic pathways, as well as RNA and DNA polymerases. It is therefore very important in any tissues or systems that frequently undergo cell renewal, such as the skin and immune system. Specifically, zinc is important for the biosynthesis of fatty acids, vitamin A metabolism, and normal epithelialization (Watson 1998). Zinc-dependent matrix metalloproteinases are involved in keratinocyte migration and wound healing. The skin contains approximately 20% of the total body zinc stores, and the highest concentrations are found in the keratinized tissue of the nasal planum, tongue, and foot pad in dogs (Lansdown and Sampson 1997). There are several recognized syndromes associated with either disturbances in zinc assimilation or zinc deficiency that present with cutaneous signs. There are two naturally occurring syndromes of zinc-responsive dermatosis seen clinically in dogs. Syndrome I can be seen in dogs with abnormal zinc metabolism whose needs cannot be met by ingestion of standard zinc concentrations. Syndrome II can be seen in dogs fed poor-quality ("generic") diets. Additionally, zinc is associated with an unresponsive lethal process in young bull terriers.

In experimentally induced cases of zinc deficiency in dogs, clinical signs can occur as early as two weeks later; however, it is important to note that severity of signs can vary between dogs, even from the same litter.

Zinc-Responsive Dermatoses

Syndrome I has been identified in Siberian huskies, Alaskan Malamutes, and Samoyeds; occasionally other breeds have also been reported. Age of onset can vary, but patients often present as younger adult dogs (mean age reported is 3.4 years; White et al. 2001). It is speculated that these dogs have a genetic defect in the intestinal absorption or the metabolism of zinc. For example, it was shown that Malamutes affected with chondrodysplasia have a decreased capability for intestinal zinc absorption (Brown et al. 1978). Skin lesions develop despite adequate consumption of diets with sufficient bioavailable zinc. Affected syndrome I dogs typically present with crusting, scaling, and alopecia of the facial mucocutaneous junctions, particularly the periocular region, perioral, and pinnal margins, but elbows, pressure points, and foot-pad margins can also be affected. Lesions progress from erythema, followed by variable alopecia with fine silver scaling that becomes adherent, or develops into crusting with underlying suppuration, most commonly around the mouth, chin, eyes, and ears. Lesions are often well demarcated and can initially be unilateral, but become symmetric as the disease progresses (see Figures 14.1 and 14.2). Lesions develop early in adulthood (1–3 years of age) and progress at a variable rate. Lesions may be pruritic in about half of affected dogs (Colombini and Dunstan 1997).

Syndrome II occurs most often in rapidly growing puppies, or juvenile larger-breed dogs. In these cases, zinc deficiency is likely caused by a combination of low zinc intake and/or the effects of excessive calcium or phytate intake interfering with zinc absorption. This absolute or relative dietary deficiency has often been associated with the use of poor-quality ("generic") dog food where either there is a deficiency in bioavailable zinc, the zinc in the diet has been chelated (such as high cereal or soy diets with high concentrations of phytates), or the diet has been oversupplemented with calcium, iron, and/or copper (Watson 1998). It can also occur in dogs given excessive calcium or other supplementation. Although phytates can bind to various dietary minerals, they bind more strongly to zinc compared to copper or manganese, and this effect can be further exacerbated by high concentrations of calcium or magnesium (NRC 2006). The required amount of dietary zinc is therefore dependent on both the form of zinc (which affects absorption) and on the effect of other dietary elements on overall bioavailability and absorption.

Affected syndrome II dogs have marked crusting lesions, often over pressure points or on the muzzle. Foot pads can be very

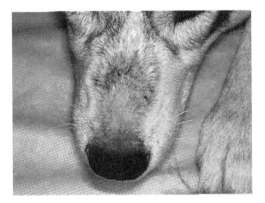

Figure 14.1 Type 1 zinc deficiency in a husky dog. Adherent scale, crusts, and erythema with alopecia are present over the dorsal muzzle. Courtesy of UC Davis Dermatology Service.

Figure 14.2 Type 1 zinc deficiency in a non-arctic breed dog. There is a well-demarcated area of alopecia with thick adherent silver-colored scale in the periocular region. Courtesy of UC Davis Dermatology Service.

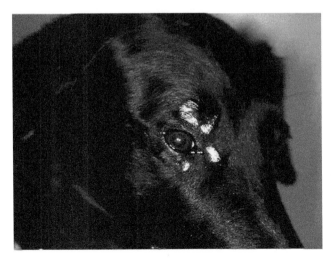

hyperkeratotic with fissuring. Another interesting feature of zinc deficiency is possible hypogeusia (diminished sense of taste) and/or an altered sense of smell, both of which can contribute to a depressed appetite (Miller 1989; Watson 1998). Since immunocompetency can be affected by zinc deficiency, there have also been reports of recurrent bacterial folliculitis in dogs with depressed appetites, in which clinical signs resolved with zinc supplementation (Miller 1989). With longer-term deficiency, weight loss and impaired wound healing can also be noted, potentially along with generalized lymphadenopathy (Watson 1998).

Diagnosis of syndrome I zinc-responsive dermatosis is based on appropriate signalment, diet history, typical cutaneous lesions, and histopathology of skin biopsies. Marked follicular and epidermal parakeratotic hyperkeratosis is evident histologically. Diagnosis of syndrome II zinc dermatosis is based on compatible signalment, diet history, and clinical signs, with histopathology similar to that seen in syndrome I. Diagnosis is further confirmed by response to zinc supplementation. Unfortunately, quantification of zinc levels in serum, plasma, leukocytes, and hair does not appear to be a reliable indicator of zinc status in dogs (van den Broek and Stafford 1988; Logas et al. 1993). There is too much overlap in values of healthy and zinc-deficient dogs. Values can be affected by other disease states such as hepatic disease, hypothyroidism, and infections, as well as influenced by age, sex, and other factors (Miller 1989). Biomarkers of zinc status in general are also often inconsistent in any cases of mild to moderate zinc deficiency (Knez et al. 2017). Additionally, oral zinc tolerance tests vary too widely and are reportedly unhelpful (White et al. 2001).

Therapy requires zinc supplementation with a recommended dosage of 2–3 mg/kg/body weight (BW) of elemental zinc in the form of zinc sulfate, zinc gluconate, or zinc methionine (White et al. 2001). Zinc oxide should not be used as it is not very bioavailable. When fed as a zinc–amino acid chelate (such as zinc

methionine), the zinc is thought to be more bioavailable; however, that may be most important when there are dietary or physiologic conditions that limit zinc availability or increase the need for it (Roudebush and Wedekind 2002). To date there do not appear to be differences in clinical response associated with the use of the different listed forms or salts used for zinc supplementation in dogs with syndrome I zinc-responsive dermatosis (White et al. 2001). Clinical signs are typically improved within 2–6 weeks (Hensel 2010). Affected female dogs often respond to lower dosages of zinc after being spayed, suggesting that zinc needs are greater during estrus or that zinc and estrogen compete for carrier proteins (White et al. 2001). Syndrome I dogs will require zinc supplementation for life and female dogs may need to be spayed, whereas syndrome II dogs may initially need supplementation, but then should respond to maintenance on a higher-quality diet with adequate zinc (especially after they have finished growing). Dietary mineral supplements that could interfere with zinc absorption should be avoided.

In dogs with either syndrome of zinc-responsive dermatosis, fat absorption may be lower, with fasting and postprandial concentrations of serum triglycerides significantly lower in successfully treated dogs compared with normal dogs (van den Broek and Simpson 1992). EFA deficiency impairs zinc absorption, and supplementation with EFAs appears to enhance zinc absorption (Huang et al. 1982; White et al. 2001). Zinc and EFA metabolism in rodents are closely linked; zinc deficiency accelerates the development of clinical signs of EFA deficiency and the clinical signs of zinc deficiency can be partially reversed by supplementing with EFA (Cunnane and Horrobin 1980). Several manifestations of zinc deficiency are mediated by a relative state of EFA deficiency, attributed in part to reduced delta-6-desaturase enzyme activity, which requires zinc as a cofactor and is a critical enzyme in fatty acid metabolism (particularly with conversion of LA or ALA to downstream

PUFAs). Therefore, additional supplementation with oils providing higher amounts of LA and ALA, or even GLA as well as other key PUFAs (AA, EPA, DHA), may help. Low-dose corticosteroids may be indicated in some dogs that do not respond to zinc (± EFA supplementation) alone. Corticosteroids are known to increase metallothionein, a zinc carrier protein, and they may also have some direct anti-inflammatory effects on the skin.

There has been a report of zinc-responsive dermatitis in related pharaoh hound puppies (Campbell and Crow 2006). Dogs developed cutaneous lesions in the first months of life that histologically were suggestive of an underlying zinc deficiency. Affected puppies also had systemic signs of lethargy, poor growth, and mental dullness. Dogs did not respond to oral supplementation; intravenous supplementation with zinc sulfate was required to produce amelioration of clinical signs.

Kittens with zinc deficiency have been studied experimentally, although naturally occurring deficiency in cats has not been recognized. These kittens primarily displayed poor growth followed by weight loss and/or parakeratotic skin lesions, especially around mucocutaneous junctions (NRC 2006). Parakeratosis associated with zinc deficiency is thought to be related to an increase in epidermal cell turnover time and/or a decrease in function of lytic enzymes requiring zinc (White et al. 2001).

Zinc-Unresponsive Lethal Acrodermatitis in White Bull Terriers

Lethal acrodermatitis (LAD) is an autosomal recessive disease seen in white bull terriers. The homozygous-affected puppies show clinical signs in the first few weeks of life and have a median survival of seven months, typically succumbing to bronchopneumonia and sepsis. Bull terriers that are heterozygous affected may exhibit increased risk for the development of pyoderma. A disease in humans called acrodermatitis enteropathica occurs as both a heritable disease and an acquired form, and has some similarities to both the clinical and histopathologic features of acrodermatitis in white bull terriers. The heritable disease in humans has been shown to be an autosomal recessive genetic defect in a zinc transporter protein (Wang et al. 2002). A similar disturbance in zinc transport has not yet been proven in the bull terrier breed.

Skin lesions in LAD-affected dogs are characterized by a progressive crusting dermatitis of the distal extremities and mucocutaneous junctions. Abnormal keratinization of paw pads can result in splaying of the feet. Claw dystrophy and paronychia may be present. Secondary infections of the skin with bacteria and yeast are common. Dogs with LAD also often have an abnormally arched hard palate, retarded skeletal growth, abnormal mentation, diarrhea, and bronchopneumonia. In a report of 28 affected dogs, all had difficulty eating, stunted growth, and splayed digits, and they had developed skin lesions by 12 weeks of age (McEwan et al. 2003b). The cutaneous signs are suggestive of severe zinc deficiency. Serum zinc and copper concentrations were lower (P < 0.05) in dogs with LAD, compared with values for control dogs (Uchida et al. 1997); however, other studies have not found serum zinc concentrations to be a useful diagnostic tool for LAD (McEwan et al. 2003b). Dogs with LAD have been shown to have significantly lower immunoglobulin (Ig)A levels than a control group of dogs (McEwan et al. 2003a).

A diagnosis of LAD can be strongly suspected in any bull terrier or mini bull terrier showing a combination of the aforementioned signs from an early age. Skin biopsy reveals a marked parakeratotic hyperkeratosis. Although many of the clinical signs and the pathology of this condition suggest zinc deficiency, zinc supplementation is of little benefit and there is no effective therapy. A variant in the *MKLN1* gene that codes for the protein muskelin 1 has been identified in affected dogs (Bauer et al. 2018). A genetic test is available through PennGen (https://www.vet.upenn.edu/research/academic-departments/clinical-sciences-advanced-medicine/research-labs-centers/

penngen/penngen-tests/genetic-tests), Antagene (https://antagene.com/chien/bull-terrier-standard), and Genoscoper Laboratories (now part of Mars Petcare) to allow breeders to screen dogs for being carriers.

Copper

Copper is essential in the function of many important enzymes, including lysyl oxidase (connective tissue formation), tyrosinase (melanin pigment formation and normal hair color), and superoxide dismutase (defense against oxidative damage). It is therefore required for melanin production and keratin synthesis. Cutaneous lesions seen with copper deficiency include hypopigmentation and dull, rough hair coat (Scott et al. 2001). Hypopigmentation may also present as "fading coat color." In growing puppies with copper deficiency, loss of hair pigmentation as well as hyperextension of distal joints (e.g. phalanges) would be expected (NRC 2006).

White bull terriers with LAD have been shown to be copper deficient in their sera (Uchida et al. 1997). Copper deficiency is otherwise uncommon with the use of commercial diets, as they generally contain more than adequate copper; however, oversupplementation with other minerals such as zinc, iron, or calcium could cause imbalances by negatively affecting the bioavailability/absorption of copper in the intestines. For example, zinc stimulates production of metallothionein in enterocytes, which then preferentially binds copper and is lost when enterocytes slough. Zinc-induced dietary copper deficiency has been reported in kittens (Hendriks et al. 2001). Additionally, if supplementation with cupric oxide is relied upon to provide sufficient copper in home-cooked diets or in lower-quality commercial diets, this could be problematic due to its lower bioavailability.

Therapeutic diets formulated to address copper-associated hepatopathy in dogs may contain lower concentrations of copper compared to typical daily recommended allowances according to AAFCO; however, a minimum requirement has not been defined in dogs (NRC 2006). Although these diets appear generally well tolerated, if a dog consuming one of these diets were to develop signs consistent with copper deficiency (e.g. loss of hair color and/or poor hair coat), it should be considered (especially if the dog is also concurrently receiving supplements that could impair copper absorption, such as zinc, calcium, or iron, and/or long-term treatment with D-penicillamine).

Vitamin A

Vitamin A is a group of related compounds with biological actions equivalent to retinol, which by conversion to retinoic acid has an important role in the health of the skin. These retinoids mainly work via regulation of gene expression to influence cellular proliferation and differentiation of keratinizing epithelium. Vitamin A is also important in immune function and reduced or delayed response to antigens. Both vitamin A deficiency and hypervitaminosis A (chronic oversupplementation) can manifest with scaling, poor hair coat, alopecia, seborrhea, poor wound healing, and an increased tendency for pyoderma (Watson 1998; Scott et al. 2001; Hensel 2010). Sebaceous gland hyperkeratosis can also lead to duct occlusion with firm, papular eruptions. Acute toxicosis with vitamin A can cause skin peeling, as well as general malaise and more serious signs such as muscle convulsions, pain, paralysis, and death (Miller 1989; Hensel 2010). Chronic hypervitaminosis is probably more common in cats, with associated classic skeletal changes, when liver is a main component of the daily diet, or when cod liver oil or other vitamin A–containing substances are oversupplemented. There is only one report of true vitamin A deficiency in a dog, which had severe seborrheic skin lesions, hyperpigmentation, and alopecia (Scott et al. 2001).

There are important species differences in the absorption, transport, uptake, and potential conversion of certain pro-vitamin A carotenoids (e.g. beta-carotene) within tissues. Cats cannot synthesize vitamin A from precursor carotenoids and ferrets are very inefficient with conversion; therefore, they must consume pre-formed retinol in their diet. Even in dogs, which can convert pro-vitamin A carotenoids to retinol, quantitative conversion efficiency has not been estimated. Interestingly, there are also species differences in the ability to accumulate beta-carotene in the blood (felids and ferrets do, canids do not) and to store it in tissues (ferrets do, cats and dogs do not).

There are also a variety of factors that may influence the bioavailability of these carotenoids, even within species that can potentially utilize them as vitamin A precursors. These compounds can also be more safely ingested at very high intakes without the apparent toxic effects that would occur with ingestion of retinol. Interestingly, animals such as birds (e.g. flamingos) and fish may have their coloration affected via dietary ingestion and absorption of certain carotenoids.

As fat-soluble vitamins, both carotenoids and retinol require dietary fat and bile salts for efficient absorption. It appears that there are species differences in the amount of fat required for optimal absorption, as well as influences on conversion and uptake by type of dietary fat (Green and Fascetti 2016). Other factors that influence absorption or excretion of fat and fat-soluble compounds could potentially also influence vitamin A. Retinol is highly susceptible to oxidation and therefore must be in an esterified (palmitate or acetate) form in pet food to protect it. It is thus conceivable that dietary deficiencies could occur in dogs and cats with fat malabsorptive disease or other digestive issues, with unbalanced diets (such as home-prepared diets too low in fat or without sufficient retinol and/or carotenoids, depending on species), or with commercial foods using inappropriate sources of vitamin A. However, clinical signs may take a while to present depending on the animal's pre-existing vitamin A status (there can be substantial body storage of this vitamin, especially in the stellate cells of the liver and particularly in carnivores). In dogs and cats, circulating retinyl esters (but not retinol) may be affected by vitamin A status; therefore, serum or plasma retinol concentrations are not necessarily good indicators of total vitamin A status (Green and Fascetti 2016).

Vitamin A deficiency can be seen in captive reptiles and birds (particularly parrots) when nutritional needs are not met (e.g. feeding a seed-based diet). Birds develop hyperkeratotic skin, blepharitis, rhinitis, and white plaques of the oral mucosa. In reptiles, they may also develop hyperkeratosis of the skin and mouth, squamous metaplasia, aural abscesses, periocular edema, and conjunctivitis. Therapy should consist of supplementation (intramuscular injections: 2000 IU/kg in reptiles and 5000–20 000 IU/kg in birds), as well as a long-term diet change to include vitamin A and/or pro-vitamin A carotenoid–containing foods (Hensel 2010).

Vitamin E

Vitamin E is the major fat-soluble antioxidant, but also has more minor non-oxidant roles. Its deficiency can lead to seborrhea, immunosuppression, and/or pansteatitis. Different tocopherols and tocotrienes (members of the vitamin E family) exert varying levels of activity, with RRR-alpha-tocopherol having the greatest biological activity. Due to its fat-soluble nature, its major route of excretion is via bile and any factors that may influence fat digestion, emulsification, or absorption (e.g. fat malabsorptive diseases) could contribute to a vitamin E deficiency.

Vitamin E partitions into cell membrane bilayers, where there is the highest concentration of PUFA. By scavenging free radicals and single oxygens it exerts its protective effect and it is important in maintaining the stability of cell membranes. Working with other antioxidants, vitamin E can protect cells against the adverse effects of reactive oxygen and other free radicals that initiate the oxidation of membrane phospholipids. Lipid metabolism is a major source of toxic oxygen radicals and, therefore, vitamin E requirements are linked directly to dietary intake of PUFA. Additionally, glutathione peroxidase (which also requires selenium), ascorbic acid, and ubiquinone are other antioxidants needed to regenerate vitamin E after it has been reversibly oxidized. Even though supplementation with other antioxidants can help rescue or prevent signs of vitamin E deficiency, oversupplementation with vitamin C should be avoided, as it appeared to actually increase the vitamin E requirement in rats (NRC 2006).

Fat can also oxidize during processing or storage and a relative deficiency can then occur with diets excessive in PUFAs, or in fatty diets that are poorly prepared and/or stored. It is difficult, consequently, to define a single minimum requirement for intake. The necessary concentration of vitamin E in the diet will depend on the total concentration of fat in the diet and the proportion of PUFAs, the degree of peroxidation of those fatty acids, the presence or absence of other antioxidants, and the concentration of selenium. Additionally, vitamin E alcohols are not very stable and/or are quickly depleted in commercially extruded dog and cat food. It is therefore necessary to use vitamin E esters (e.g. tocopherol acetate) to improve recovery and reduce storage losses. When diets contain higher concentrations of PUFAs, a ratio of at least 0.6 mg alpha-tocopherol : 1 g PUFA must be maintained.

Pansteatitis is associated with diets that are relatively low in vitamin E and high in PUFAs. Cats have historically been more susceptible to developing this condition because their typical diet is higher in fat and/or contains more fish-based PUFAs compared to most dog diets. A diet composed entirely of raw oily fish is a classic example. Cats with pansteatitis develop firm, painful, nodular swellings, often associated with the inguinal and abdominal fat pads. The swellings result from the inflammation and necrosis associated with the peroxidative damage of adipose tissue causing ceroid accumulation. Cats may be painful and reluctant to move, anorexic, or febrile. It is important to differentiate this disease from panniculitis caused by infectious agents such as the opportunistic mycobacteria that can often cause nodular lesions on the ventral abdomen. Diagnosis is made based on a diet history and histologic evidence of steatitis on biopsy. Biopsy reveals lobular panniculitis with macrophages and giant cells, and there is ceroid within lipocytes. Correcting the dietary deficiency with vitamin E supplementation (10 mg/kg/day, 1 mg = 1 IU) will improve clinical signs (Watson 1998).

Experimentally induced vitamin E deficiency has been reported in dogs to cause a cornification disturbance: initially a dry scaling that becomes more inflamed with erythema, skin thickening, and increased greasiness (Scott and Sheffy 1987). Cutaneous signs resolved within 10 weeks of feeding a diet with adequate vitamin E supplementation. Deficiency in dogs has also been linked to subcutaneous edema (as well as skeletal muscle degeneration, retinal degeneration, and several other signs).

It is important to avoid oversupplementation of vitamin E due to toxicity concerns.

Vitamin B Complex

The B vitamins are water soluble and very important coenzymes in numerous metabolic pathways. Deficiencies could occur if animals have prolonged anorexia, impaired absorption (e.g. chronic enteropathies), decreased production by gut microbiota (e.g. receiving prolonged courses of antibiotics), or increased excretion (e.g. polyuria). The most common clinical skin change seen with deficiencies of the B vitamin complex is a dry scaling with alopecia. Clinical signs associated with individual B vitamin deficiencies have been described, but are rare. Since thiamin has the most limited body storage of the B vitamins, and is not associated with dermatologic manifestations, conditions or diets with multiple B vitamin deficiencies may generally be expected to be associated with other signs before skin changes. However, if deficiencies of B vitamins exclusive of thiamin do occur, skin lesions could be expected. There is a large margin of safety with the ingestion of B vitamins, however, so pre-emptive supplementation is recommended if there is concern.

Biotin is an essential coenzyme in four very important carboxylase enzymes involved in energy metabolism (pyruvate, proprionyl-coenzyme A [CoA], methyl-crotonyl-CoA, and acetyl-CoA carboxylases). Deficiency can result in facial and periocular alopecia in dogs, which can progress to more generalized crusting lesions (Watson 1998; Scott et al. 2001) with hyperkeratotis of superficial and follicular epithelia. In the cat, generalized dermatitis with crusted papules has been described (Scott et al. 2001). Deficiency in cats has been associated with accumulation first of salivary, nasal, and lacrimal secretions, with progressive alopecia that starts at the extremities and progresses to the entire body, as well as achromotrichia and scaly dermatitis. As the deficiency progresses, loss of body weight and diarrhea in the terminal stages can be seen (NRC 2006). Biotin is generally well distributed in foods stuffs and liberated by digestive enzymes, but there is also some synthesized by the gut microbial population. Biotin deficiency can occur when prolonged courses of certain antibiotics are used or if the diet includes large amounts of raw egg whites, which contain avidin. Avidin binds biotin and prevents its absorption.

Chronic riboflavin deficiency in dogs can cause a dry, scaling, or flaking dermatitis around the eyes (typically bilateral) and the ventrum, and a marked cheilosis (Lewis et al. 1987). This may be seen with corneal opacities, watery purulent eye discharge, and muscular weakness as well. In cats, an acute deficiency causes periauricular alopecia with epidermal atrophy, along with anorexia and decreasing body weight (chronic deficiency is associated with cataracts and fatty liver).

Riboflavin deficiency also impacts the body status of other vitamins because of its role in the flavin coenzymes important in the metabolism of folic acid, pyridoxine, niacin, vitamin K, and vitamin D. However, riboflavin deficiency is unlikely if the diet contains any meat or dairy products or is a complete commercial food. Most riboflavin in food is in the form of flavin coenzymes flavin adenine dinucleotide (FAD) or flavin mononucleotide (FMN) or is bound to proteins; however, it is mostly in the free form in milk. Most food sources that contain high concentrations of riboflavin will also contain other B vitamins. It is worth noting that riboflavin is sensitive to acidic and alkaline conditions, as well as to ultraviolet (UV) light (so certain processes could degrade it in foods).

Niacin (vitamers with nicotinamide bioactivity) deficiency results in pellagra, which is well known for causing the 4 "Ds" in humans (diarrhea, dermatitis, dementia, death). Known as "black tongue" in dogs, it is characterized by a reddened inside upper lip that progresses to inflamed and ulcerated mucous membrane, especially of the buccal and pharyngeal areas. Severely affected dogs may develop profuse salivation with ropy blood-stained drool, foul or fetid breath, diarrhea with changes to gastrointestinal mucosa, emaciation, and (in some dogs) pruritic dermatitis of the ventral abdomen and hind legs (Scott et al. 2001; NRC 2006). In cats, deficiency is associated with a fiery red tongue with ulceration, as well as anorexia, increased body temperature, congestion, and decreased weight associated with respiratory disease.

Niacin is endogenously synthesized in most animals from L-tryptophan, but deficiency is possible if a diet is low in animal protein and high in cereals, in which the limiting amino acid is tryptophan and the majority of the niacin is in a bound form that cannot be used. Unprocessed corn, for example, can be particularly problematic, as it is both poor in tryptophan and its niacin is only released after exposure to high pH. Animal tissue, however, contains niacin in the form of nicotinamide adenine dinucleotide (NAD), nicotinamide adenine dinucleotide phosphate (NADP), and some free nicotinamide. Cats, as obligate carnivores, must consume niacin in their diet preformed, as they are unable to perform the conversion from tryptophan. Although B vitamin supplementation has a large margin of safety, hypervitaminosis can occur with excessive supplementation (e.g. 133–145 mg/kg/day in dogs or ~2 g/day; or >350 mg/kg/day in most animals) and has been associated with toxicity, such as bloody feces followed by convulsions and death in dogs.

Vitamin B6 (pyridoxine, pyridoxamine, pyridoxal) is available from both animal and plant sources. In cats, it appears that requirements increase with increasing protein in the diet. Deficiency signs in dogs and cats affect a multitude of systems; however, deficiency relating to dermatologic manifestations has only been effectively demonstrated in an experimental setting in cats. The cats developed a dull, waxy, "unkempt" hair coat with generalized fine scaling and focal alopecia involving the face and extremities (Norton 1987; Scott et al. 2001). It is noteworthy that the active form of the vitamin (pyridoxal-5′-phosphate or PLP) is a coenzyme for more than 100 reactions involved in a multiplicity of processes, including synthesis of niacin and several neurotransmitters (from tryptophan). PLP is also a modulator of steroid actions. In rats with B6 deficiency, conversion of LA to AA is impaired. Additionally, the circulating level of PLP is decreased when riboflavin status is low. This demonstrates how inter-related metabolic actions of various B vitamins may be and that deficiencies in certain B vitamins may impact the action or function of others.

Cobalamin (vitamin B12) deficiency is not typically related to dermatologic signs; however, in young kittens with induced cobalamin deficiency, their hair coat was reported to have a "wet" appearance. It is overall relatively rare to see dermatologic manifestations of deficiencies in only one B vitamin, especially if it is related to an issue of dietary intake (more likely that multiple vitamins are affected). If a deficiency is suspected, it may be recommended to supplement B complex vitamins orally or parentally, and to look for other non-dermatologic signs related to these possible deficiencies.

Vitamin C

Famous as the deficiency causing scurvy in people, vitamin C (L-ascorbic acid) is not an essential nutrient in most mammalian species, including dogs and cats, as they produce it endogenously from glucose. Guinea pigs and humans, however, are unable to perform this conversion and, without the appropriate dietary intake of the pre-formed vitamin, clinical deficiency can occur. Guinea pigs require 10 mg/kg daily (30 mg/kg for gestating females). Typical signs of deficiency can include poor coat quality, seborrhea, and ulcerations, as well as hematomas, petechiations, and ecchymoses. Vitamin C deficiency is relatively rarer in reptiles, but has been associated with spontaneous skin rupture in snakes (particularly boas and pythons), as well as gingival bleeding.

Correction of the diet is paramount to long-term health and some guinea pigs may also benefit from additional daily oral supplementation. If clinical manifestations are present, subcutaneous injections (50–100 mg/guinea pig/day or 10–20 mg/kg in snakes) should be used until signs resolve (Hensel 2010) or until sufficient oral supplementation is instituted to correct. Oversupplementation with excessively high doses of vitamin C should be avoided due to potential side effects or undesired interactions with other nutrients (e.g. effect on vitamin E requirement, increased urinary excretion of oxalic acid, etc.).

Generic Dog Food Dermatosis

A dermatosis associated with the exclusive feeding of a poor-quality dog food was reported in the 1980s (Sousa et al. 1988). This disease is seen less commonly in North America since

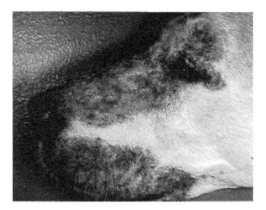

Figure 14.3 Generic dog food disease in a young Labrador. There are areas of well-demarcated crusted plaques with erythematous borders periorally and periocularly. Courtesy of UC Davis Dermatology Service.

the adoption of additional pet food regulations. Many of the affected dogs were typically less than 1 year of age and were undergoing a period of rapid growth.

The dermatosis is characterized by the presence of well-demarcated, thick, crusted plaques with fissures and erosions (see Figure 14.3). These lesions are typically located on the muzzle, at mucocutaneous junctions, over pressure points, and on distal extremities. Affected dogs can also have concurrent pyrexia, malaise, dependent edema, and lymphadenopathy. A deficiency of multiple trace minerals, vitamins, EFAs, and amino acids was likely the cause of the cutaneous lesions. Diagnosis is based on a compatible diet history and histopathologic evaluation of skin biopsies. Histopathology of representative skin lesions reveals a markedly acanthotic epidermis with parakeratosis, crusting, and spongiosis. Lesions resolve when the dog is fed a better-quality diet.

Skin Diseases That Benefit from Nutritional or Dietary Management

The next section will discuss dermatologic diseases for which dietary modifications are paramount for the management of skin disease.

Cutaneous Adverse Food Reactions

"Food allergy" is a term often incorrectly utilized in veterinary medicine to describe all adverse reactions following food intake. Cutaneous adverse food reactions (CAFR) can occur as the result of either an immunologic or non-immunologic response to a dietary ingredient. Non-immunologic cutaneous reactions to food include intolerances or idiosyncratic reactions to foods or other ingredients (e.g. preservatives or dyes), but also include dose-related toxic reactions (e.g. histamine in scombroid fish poisoning), occur in any individual, and are associated with histamine, tyramine (old cheese), or bacterial toxins (Scott et al. 2001). CAFR is perhaps a better term than food allergy, as a positive response to diet changes may not be due to avoidance of an adverse immunologic response. When CAFR occurs in dogs with atopic dermatitis, it can also be referred to as food-induced atopic dermatitis.

In human medicine, IgE-mediated type 1 hypersensitivity appears to play a role in the pathogenesis of food allergy in young children and is the best-defined immunologic mechanism causing food allergy (Sampson and Burks 2009). In humans, food allergens are often glycoproteins with a molecular weight of 10–70 kDa; however, the exact molecular size of food allergens is not actually known for dogs and cats. The pathogenesis of CAFR in small animals is not well understood and the immunologic mechanisms occurring are not known in the majority of cases. In the literature, type 1, 3, and 4 hypersensitivity reactions are stated to possibly be involved in causing CAFR in small animals (Gross et al. 2005; Verlinden et al. 2006).

There are numerous potential food allergens and, because of the large number of ingredients in a typical commercial pet food, it is nearly impossible to implicate which one might be a causative allergen for each animal suspected of having a CAFR. "Common" allergens tend to be common because of their abundance in many pet foods, exposing the greatest number of pets over prolonged periods of time, but theoretically an animal could develop an intolerance to any dietary ingredient fed consistently enough. A recent review and analysis of evidence in published studies reports that the most commonly reported food allergens contributing to CAFR in dogs are beef (34%), dairy products (17%), chicken (15%), wheat, (13%), and lamb (14.5%). Less commonly reported items included soy (6%), corn (4%), pork (2%), fish (2%), and rice (2%), as well as a few items reported for single dogs only (barley, rabbit, chocolate, kidney beans, and tomato). In the same review, the most common food allergens reported for cats were beef (18%), fish (17%), and chicken (5%). Less common (at 4% each) were wheat, corn, dairy, and lamb. Egg, barley, and rabbit were reported in single cats (Mueller et al. 2016). A previous review of the literature also revealed that at the time the most commonly implicated food allergens included beef, dairy, wheat, lamb, egg, chicken, and soy in dogs and beef, dairy, fish, chicken, and lamb in cats (Verlinden et al. 2006). It is noteworthy that the authors of this chapter have also had cases in which one of the offending foods has not made an appearance in these reports. Thus, even though it may not be a commonly reported allergen, a food should not be excluded from the list of possible offenders.

Some studies have shown that a significant number of dogs and cats (35–50%) had adverse reactions to more than one food ingredient (Harvey 1993; Patterson 1995; Jeffers et al. 1996). In humans with food allergies, some foods can exhibit cross-reactivity between proteins from similar sources (e.g. seafood, cereals, nuts). There is conflicting evidence as to whether this is clinically relevant in small animals. Some studies have shown that there was not cross-reactivity between milk and beef proteins (Jeffers et al. 1996), while another study showed that bovine IgG in milk may confer cross-reactivity to beef and possibly to proteins from other ruminants that may have shared immunoglobulin homology, such as lamb (Martin et al. 2004).

CAFR is considered to be the third most common allergic skin disease in dogs after flea allergy dermatitis and atopic dermatitis. CAFR in the cat is reported to be second in frequency to flea allergy dermatitis. The exact incidence of CAFR in all small animals is unknown. One study reported that 17.45% of dogs completing an elimination diet trial had CAFR (Chesney 2001), and another that CAFR was the cause of pruritus in 23% of non-seasonal pruritic dogs (Reedy et al. 1997).

CAFR appears to affect 1–2% of dogs and <1% of cats presented to veterinarians. For those pets presented for skin disease, CAFR was responsible for 0–24% of these cases in dogs and 3–6% of cats (Olivry and Mueller 2017). In a previous report, CAFR was reported as 1% of all skin disease and 10% of all allergic skin disease (Scott et al. 2001). However, the prevalence does appear to be increased in dogs (9–40%) and cats (12–21%) with pruritus (Olivry and Mueller 2017). CAFR is also seen more commonly in individuals with other allergies. Since pruritus is a threshold phenomenon, reported information about incidence may be influenced by the type and prioritization of diagnostic evaluations utilized in reporting studies.

Clinical Signs

CAFR affects any age, breed, or sex. Food reactions have been reported in pets from less than 1 year of age up to 13 years (Olivry and Mueller 2019a). In contrast to other allergies that typically take years to develop, anywhere from 22 to 50% of reported dogs diagnosed with CAFR developed clinical signs before 1 year of age (Scott et al. 2001; Olivry and Mueller 2019a). In addition, while an increased risk in certain breeds has been reported, there is no statistical evidence of breed predilections.

In the dog, urticaria is possible; however, CAFR most commonly results in non-seasonal pruritus with localized or generalized secondary self-trauma. It is important to remember, however, that periodic signs could occur (and reoccur) if the pet only has intermittent access to the offending food (e.g. table scraps, hunting, scavenging, etc.). The clinical signs of CAFR can also be very pleomorphic and mimic or be complicated by other dermatologic diseases, including atopic dermatitis, flea allergy dermatitis, ectoparasitism, *Malassezia* dermatitis, and pyoderma. Primary skin lesions seen with CAFR include erythema and papules. Secondary skin lesions then result from the self-trauma associated with pruritus or the development of secondary infections, and can include alopecia, pustules and collarettes, erosions, excoriations, lichenification, and hyperpigmentation. This can involve any area, but the face, ears, paws, and ventrum are the most commonly involved sites in dogs, with the perineum less commonly targeted (Olivry and Mueller 2019a). Pruritus in these areas may be demonstrated by foot licking or face rubbing in addition to scratching or chewing pruritic sites. Secondary pyoderma and *Malassezia* are also common in dogs with CAFR. Otitis externa is a common manifestation of CAFR and in some animals is the only clinical sign.

CAFR in cats has no age or sex predilections, although cats generally appear to develop signs later than dogs (Olivry and Mueller 2019a). Siamese cats are reported to be at increased risk (Gross et al. 2005). Cats with CAFR may present with a number of reaction patterns. Pruritus is often very severe and centered on the face, neck, and pinnae (Figure 14.4). Miliary dermatitis, eosinophilic plaques or eosinophilic granulomas, and feline lip ulcers may also occur in CAFR cats. Pruritus causing self-traumatic alopecia might also involve the limbs, ventral abdomen, and/or inguinal area and is often symmetric. Otitis externa can be a feature of CAFR in cats as it is in dogs.

Concurrent gastrointestinal signs may accompany pruritic skin disease caused by CAFR in small animals, but the reported incidence varies in the literature. It is estimated in most publications that fewer than 20% of animals with CAFR have concurrent gastrointestinal signs (White 1998). Adverse food reactions should also be considered in dogs and cats suffering from symmetric lupoid onychitis, concurrent conjunctivitis, or sneezing (Olivry and Mueller 2018).

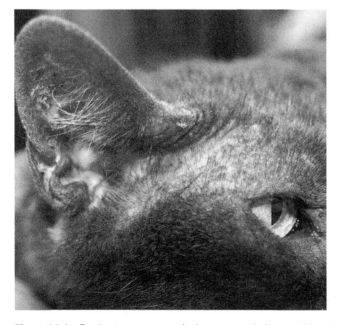

Figure 14.4 Erythematous pre-auricular areas and pinnae with evidence of self-trauma in a cat with confirmed cutaneous adverse food reaction. Courtesy of UC Davis Dermatology Service.

Diagnosis and Treatment

An elimination diet trial is the most important and only reliable diagnostic test to evaluate and diagnose CAFR in a dog or cat (Jeffers et al. 1991). This involves exclusively feeding a diet that avoids ingredients previously fed, for an accepted period of time. If the clinical signs resolve, then the patient should be challenged with the original diet to confirm a food reaction. If clinical signs return upon challenge and abate again on the elimination diet, a diagnosis of CAFR is made. The timing of utilizing a diet trial may also be important: any pre-existing infections or other sources of pruritus should be addressed. If the pet is flea allergic or atopic, choosing a season when these factors may be minimized (e.g. winter) may provide an advantage in limiting confounding variables. Prior to starting a diet trial, the animal should be evaluated for any concurrent secondary infections with bacteria and/or yeast and treated appropriately. Depending on the geographic location of the animal, it is also important to be sure that flea control is being used appropriately. A large commitment is required by the owner to successfully complete an elimination-and-rechallenge diet trial, but it is the only way to conclusively identify patients with adverse reactions to food.

Neither serology with food-specific IgE or IgG, intradermal testing, fecal IgE, or other diagnostic methods such as endoscopic testing or hair and saliva tests provide clinically reliable information about the food proteins to which an animal is allergic (Mueller and Olivry 2017). Despite its frequent use, a number of studies have shown that serologic evaluation for IgE levels to dietary proteins has little to no clinical utility in predicting which dietary protein is actually acting as an allergen (Jeffers et al. 1991; Mueller and Tsohalis 1998; Scott et al. 2001) and its use should be discouraged as it is misleading. However, negative patch test reactions may have high negative predictability in dogs for choosing ingredients used in elimination diets, and lymphocyte proliferation tests may have increased accuracy with

CAFR but are currently impractical (Mueller and Olivry 2017).

There is no such thing as a "hypoallergenic diet." A diet might be non-allergenic or non-stimulatory to an individual if it contains ingredients that the animal has never eaten before and there is no cross-reactivity (although this phenomenon is uncertain in dogs and cats). In order to ascertain appropriate elimination diet options for an individual, a complete diet history is necessary. This should include all diets (current and prior), treats, table foods, supplements and medications with flavoring, or capsules containing any possible glycoprotein sources, as well as consideration of any other possible antigen sources that could occur from scavenging (consideration of home environment is therefore important).

During an elimination diet trial all previous food items are removed, including treats or any supplements containing natural protein-based flavorings, and a new trial diet that meets certain criteria is chosen. The trial diet should contain a limited number of ingredients. The protein source should be novel if possible (i.e. the patient has never been exposed to it before) or hydrolyzed. If this is not possible, a protein that the pet is not currently exposed to from any source, including treats and table foods, and has had relatively little exposure to in the past could be tried if necessary. It should be noted that anything cellular will contain proteins; therefore, carbohydrates and fats (if not a purified starch or oil verified to be DNA free) will also contain glycoproteins, which can be sources of potential antigenic stimulation. Therefore, purified fats and carbohydrates should be used or the ingredients providing them should also be novel or of limited previous exposure. Many preferred carbohydrate sources are also relatively low in protein as an additional precaution (e.g. potato). The diet should avoid vasoactive amines and meet the nutritional needs for that animal at its current life stage (e.g. a growth diet is still needed for a puppy or kitten).

There are a number of options for trial diets to be used during an elimination diet trial. These include home-cooked diets with a single, novel protein and a novel carbohydrate component (see Chapter 8 on home-prepared diets), commercial uncommon protein diets that are novel for the individual animal, or commercial hydrolyzed protein diets. Which diet is chosen depends on the thoroughness and accuracy of the past diet history, other possible special nutritional needs of the animal, palatability, and practicality for the owner. If pets have other medical conditions, in addition to CAFR, that benefit from dietary management, they will likely benefit from commercial veterinary therapeutic multifunction diets or customized home-cooked diets formulated by a board-certified veterinary nutritionist®.

Home-cooked diet trials have the advantage that there is more control as to what ingredients are fed, they are less processed, and there are no additives or preservatives. However, they are very labor intensive and can be quite expensive, especially for large-breed dogs or when using certain protein sources, and not all animals will willingly or consistently eat home-cooked diets. Home-cooked diets are very often not nutritionally complete and balanced, which is a concern when used for any length of time, particularly in certain life stages such as growth. There are reputable commercial resources and various veterinary nutrition services that can offer formulation of appropriate complete and balanced home-cooked diets. This is generally recommended, as most elimination diet trials will take a minimum of 8–12 weeks to complete, and sometimes more than one diet trial is needed. Although some supplements may not be needed during the beginning of an elimination diet trial in adult dogs and cats, B vitamins (especially thiamin) can be very quickly depleted and should be supplemented even in the short term. Additionally, taurine should be added at 125–250 mg/kg BW for cats. Fatty acid and total protein or specific amino acid deficiencies could then also contribute to lack of improvement or development of new signs. For these reasons, it is generally recommended to work with a veterinary nutritionist to provide appropriate dietary recommendations, even in the short term. Despite these issues, there are reports of patients who will respond better to a home-cooked diet compared to its commercial equivalent, so it is worth considering, especially in pets failing multiple diet trials with commercial products (White 1986; White and Sequoia 1989; Jeffers et al. 1991; Leistra and Willemse 2002). If chosen for long-term management of CAFR, the home-cooked diet must be balanced by a veterinary nutritionist or with commercially available software with appropriate nutritional supplements to provide all essential dietary needs for that individual (see Chapter 8).

Commercial uncommon protein diets are typically, but not always, nutritionally balanced and are more practical for most owners. However, additives are present, and the antigenic properties of dietary ingredients may be altered during the processing of the diet. Although this is not problematic for the majority of pets, it is a consideration, especially if multiple commercial diets fail to be tolerated. It has also been shown in several studies that unexpected additional proteins other than those stated on the label can be found within diets used for elimination diet trials, particularly any over-the-counter diet. It is suspected that this more commonly reflects contamination during the manufacturing process, rather than intentional addition or mislabeling (Raditic et al. 2011; Willis-Mahn et al. 2014). Confidence in the reliability of the diet might be increased if the manufacturer utilizes polymerase chain reaction (PCR) testing or mass spectroscopy to screen for contaminant proteins post production.

Hydrolyzed diets are made utilizing proteins that have been enzymatically hydrolyzed to smaller peptides and amino acids, or even using purified amino acids. This decreases the molecular size of the proteins and hopefully the antigenicity and allergenicity of the protein are then diminished. This approach is based on research indicating that IgE-mediated CAFR in humans involves allergenic proteins cross-linking IgE antibodies on the surface of mast cells to trigger inflammation, and that these proteins are typically larger than 10 kDa (Bizikova and Olivry 2016). Similar information is not known for dogs or cats and the various veterinary hydrolyzed diets are hydrolyzed to varying extents.

Despite larger proteins being typically implicated in human IgE-mediated reactions, 3–5 kDa peptides could theoretically also act as haptens to elicit an immune response, or even smaller peptides (0.5 kDa or larger) might be involved in non-IgE-mediated CAFR by activating lymphocytes (Bizikova and Olivry 2016). Most of the commercially available hydrolyzed protein diets utilize common proteins (e.g. poultry products and soy) and the proteins within the diet are hydrolyzed to different extents. The individual diets currently available provide proteins anywhere from 0 to 88% as single amino acids, 78–95% below 1 kDa, and 1–7% exceeding 5–6 kDa (Bizikova 2016). Additionally, the diets may differ from one another in other ingredients as well (e.g. carbohydrates), which may themselves either be purified of proteins or utilized as whole ingredients. This is why comparing ingredient lists between products is important, as even the dry and canned products from the same line may have differences that could prove important for the individual.

It is therefore also possible for a hydrolyzed diet to fail to identify or manage CAFR. However, for the majority of animals with confirmed CAFR, there is good evidence that hydrolyzed diets can control their clinical signs. Studies have shown that a majority of soy-sensitized dogs did not respond to oral administration of hydrolyzed soy protein (Jackson et al. 2003; Puigdemont et al. 2006). However, in one of these studies using a hydrolyzed soy and cornstarch diet, 3/14 dogs (all 3 had been demonstrated to react to both soy and corn and 1 to cornstarch) reacted with CAFR to the diet (Jackson et al. 2003). In one

report, a hydrolyzed chicken liver diet led to flares in 4/10 confirmed chicken-induced CAFR, whereas a hydrolyzed poultry feather diet did not cause flares in any of those same 10 dogs (Bizikova and Olivry 2016). Further studies, especially in cats, are warranted.

Overall, the veterinary therapeutic hydrolyzed diets have a reported efficacy of anywhere from 60 to 75% (Hensel 2010). Additionally, it has been previously noted that, in some cases, partially hydrolyzed diets may actually worsen clinical signs, with 20–50% of dogs worsening when they ingested partial hydrolysates of foods to which they were hypersensitive (Olivry and Bizikova 2010). Therefore, although hydrolyzed diets may be highly effective for many patients, there is variability in percent efficacy between individual hydrolyzed diets and they cannot completely eliminate allergenicity for all.

A recent survey of dog owners highlights the importance of the veterinary healthcare team providing appropriate owner education and specific diet recommendations. If the veterinarian is involved in changing the diet in dogs with suspected CAFR, a much larger percentage of pet owners will utilize a veterinary diet with a decrease in the use of alternate over-the-counter diets and raw or home-made diets (Tiffany et al. 2019).

Once the diet has been chosen, it is vital that the owner fully understands that the animal cannot have access to any other food items. This includes all treats, human food items, foods given to hide oral medications, flavored toothpaste, and flavored medications or supplements, including heartworm preventives. For example, it has been shown that food-allergic dogs will react to the flavored heartworm preventive Interceptor® (milbemycin with pork liver and soy; Novartis, Basel Switzerland) with increased pruritus and increased serum IgE within days of getting the medication (Jackson and Hammerberg 2002). Some of the current flea and tick preventives also have hydrolyzed soy as a base, while others contain intact soy or pork protein.

It is possible that despite changing the diet of the pet, a large percentage (up to 75% in one survey) of dogs will still have instances of food indiscretions during a trial, including provision of treats by the pet owner (e.g. dental chews, rawhides, jerky, etc.) or access to unmonitored food sources (including garbage, litter boxes or other sources of feces, and prey; Tiffany et al. 2019). Since ingestion of even small quantities of other foods could impair success of an elimination diet trial, it is important to discuss with owners what strategies will be used to prevent access to these foods. Other considerations must include food handling and possible cross-contamination (utensils, bowls, counters, storage, etc.) and, if there are any other animals in the household, whether the pet to be evaluated may be exposed to potential oral allergens by contact with the other animal (e.g. grooming, licking the other's food bowl, flavored toys or treats, coprophagia, etc.). Sometimes it is necessary to place all animals in a house on the same diet to ensure an effective trial.

Another important consideration is food storage and handling, as the presence of contaminants, such as various microbial agents including mold, or cross-contamination from other foods could confound a food trial. An example of this is the presence of storage mites in stored food, which have been shown to exacerbate clinical signs in dogs with atopic dermatitis already sensitized to the house dust mite, despite them being different species. Therefore, these atopic dogs could flare and be erroneously diagnosed with CAFR (Olivry and Mueller 2019b). Storage mites are typically undetectable in new bags of pet food, provided that the seal is intact and they have been stored in temperate indoor conditions; however, mites will proliferate more on crushed kibble, in bags with broken seals, or even in those with intact seals stored in higher temperatures or humid conditions. Smaller (more quickly consumed and therefore fresher) bags of food may be preferred for diet trials. Storage mites can also affect other dry feed stuffs, including grains and flours. Therefore, utilizing fresh, appropriately stored feeds is important, especially during a diet trial or rechallenge, as food contaminants could lead to false-positive results. This is also worthwhile considering even when utilizing home-prepared diets, and bulk-purchased items may need to be avoided in the testing stages (or if there are recurrent problems).

A review indicates that in order to diagnose CAFR in more than 90% of dogs and cats, an elimination diet trial should last for a minimum of 8 weeks (Olivry et al. 2015), but 10–12 weeks (or more) may be required for others or to achieve further amelioration, especially if concurrent pruritic diseases/triggers are still being managed. The patient should be reevaluated after four weeks to ascertain if all infections have been adequately eliminated and to reassess the intensity and distribution of pruritus. Although maximum improvement may take longer, significant improvement can often be seen within the first six weeks, provided that all other concurrent diseases contributing to pruritus are also addressed (e.g. pyoderma, *Malassezia* dermatitis, or flea allergy dermatitis). There is recent evidence that the needed length of a diet trial can be shortened if, at initiation, any visible inflammation of the skin is treated with a tapering course of corticosteroids (Favrot et al. 2019).

Up to 75% of dogs with CAFR will concurrently have other allergic triggers (Scott et al. 2001). Consequently, only a partial improvement may be seen during the food trial. To prove if any decrease in the animal's pruritus is due to CAFR, a rechallenge needs to be done with the original diet. Animals with CAFR will have a recurrence or exacerbation of their pruritus within hours to days, with most having a recurrence within 3–7 days. If after two weeks there is no change in the degree of pruritus, the animal does not have CAFR, but the diagnosis of food allergy or CAFR is confirmed if the animal's pruritus returns or worsens, and the degree of pruritus again improves when the animal is placed on the novel protein diet. It is important to continue therapy for any concurrent dermatologic diseases during the rechallenge portion of the trial. If infections recur, this could exacerbate pruritus and lead to erroneous interpretations of the rechallenge.

In order to determine the specific offending allergen, provocation tests with single ingredients from the diet are required. If the animal is allergic to a particular food ingredient, pruritus will increase after introduction of that ingredient. Typically, clinical signs will occur within minutes to hours of rechallenge; however, they can take up to 14 days to manifest (Jeffers et al. 1996), so only one new item should be offered every 2 weeks at most. CAFR is managed long term by avoidance of any offending dietary allergens, confirmed with provocative testing or by strictly feeding a diet that is known not to induce CAFR.

Although the prognosis for controlling CAFR with dietary management is generally good (with patient compliance), recurrence can sometimes occur and a new dietary sensitivity can develop to other proteins, necessitating another diet change if this occurs. It is unclear if extended avoidance of the originally offending allergens can eventually result in future tolerance to them, although this phenomenon has been reported in people (Hensel 2010).

Figure 14.5 presents an algorithm for evaluating CAFR with an elimination diet trial.

Cutaneous Xanthomatosis

The formation of cutaneous xanthomas is rare and often reflects underlying dyslipoproteinemia secondary to diabetes mellitus, therapy with megestrol acetate, or hereditary defects in lipid metabolism. Cutaneous xanthomas in cats have been reported with hereditary hyperchylomicronemia (i.e. lipoprotein lipase deficiency), megestrol acetate–induced diabetes mellitus, or naturally occurring diabetes mellitus. Cutaneous xanthomas have been reported in dogs with diabetes mellitus.

Affected animals may be consuming a diet rich in fats. Cutaneous xanthomas typically appear as multiple pale yellow to white plaques, papules, or nodules with erythematous borders. They are often located on the face, ventral trunk, and over bony prominences. Larger masses may ulcerate and exude inspissated necrotic material. Cats with inherited hyperchylomicronemia may also demonstrate peripheral neurologic signs due to nerve compression from subcutaneous xanthoma formation. Histologic evaluation of skin biopsies reveals large foamy macrophages and giant cells. Serum biochemistry evaluations for diabetes mellitus, hypercholesterolemia, and hypertriglyceridemia should be obtained. The feeding of a low-fat diet, as well as identification and correction of the underlying disturbance in lipid metabolism, is recommended for patients that have had cutaneous xanthomas identified.

Superficial Necrolytic Dermatitis

Hepatocutaneous syndrome (HCS) is an uncommon skin disorder associated with systemic metabolic disease. It has also been called superficial necrolytic dermatitis (SND), metabolic epidermal necrosis (MEN), diabetic dermatopathy, and necrolytic migratory erythema (NME). More recently the term aminoaciduric canine hypoaminoacidemic hepatopathy (ACHES) has been proposed to reflect recognized metabolic derangement (Loftus 2022). The first English-language reference comparing it to the histologically similar human disease NME was in 1986, when SND was described in four dogs with diabetes mellitus and was therefore called diabetic dermatopathy (Walton et al. 1986). As different disease processes appear to cause similar histologic skin lesions, it might be more accurate to refer to the skin disease as either SND or MEN. The disease has been most commonly described in older dogs, although there are reports of a histologically equivalent disease

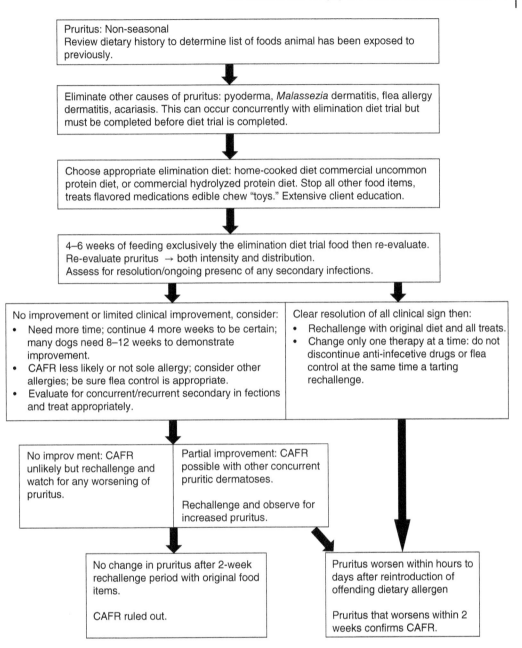

Figure 14.5 Algorithm evaluating for cutaneous adverse food reaction (CAFR) with elimination diet trial.

in cats and the black rhinoceros (Patel et al. 1996; Day 1997; Munson et al. 1998; Asakawa et al. 2013). The etiopathogenesis of this disease is unclear, but it is likely multifactorial.

Most often, human NME occurs in association with a glucagon-secreting tumor. Unlike people with NME, association with glucagonoma has not been consistently demonstrated in the majority of dogs with the skin lesions of SND. The term canine glucagonoma-associated necrolytic migratory erythema (canine NME) has been used to describe the disease in a dog with confirmed glucagonoma (Oberkirchner et al. 2009) The vast majority of dogs afflicted with SND have a characteristic concurrent hepatopathy, thus the use of the term HCS. The hepatic pathology seen in dogs with HCS has not been reported to occur in those dogs with confirmed glucagonoma-associated SND. In addition to the association with hepatic pathology, dogs with the skin lesions of SND that have a history of phenobarbital administration have been reported (Bloom et al. 1992; Byrne 1999; March et al. 2004), and some with gastrointestinal signs and malabsorption (Florant et al. 2000).

The severe vacuolar liver disease seen in the majority of dogs with the skin lesions of SND and the association in some dogs with concurrent diabetes mellitus suggests that an underlying hormonal or metabolic disturbance is occurring in dogs with HCS. Diabetes mellitus has been reported to occur in 25–40% of dogs with HCS (Byrne 1999; Outerbridge et al. 2002). Hypoaminoacidemia has been documented to occur in all reported dogs with SND skin lesions that have, thus far, had concentrations of plasma amino acids measured. Most dogs had non-glucagonoma-associated disease or HCS, and only three dogs for which plasma amino acids were measured were confirmed to have a pancreatic tumor (Bond et al. 1995; Torres et al. 1997; Allenspach et al. 2000). The pattern of the plasma amino acid panels in dogs with SND appears to be significantly different from that seen in dogs with acute or chronic hepatitis.

The liver plays a critical role in amino acid balance. In both chronic and acute hepatitis, the compromised hepatic metabolism results in increased concentrations of many plasma amino acids. However, this is not seen in dogs with SND, as the majority of individual plasma amino acid concentrations are less than 60% of normal (see Figure 14.6). Total amino acid concentrations documented in dogs with SND are approximately 30% of the concentrations documented in healthy dogs or dogs with acute or chronic hepatitis (Outerbridge et al. 2002). These differences suggest that the hypoaminoacidemia in dogs with SND cannot be explained by compromised hepatic metabolism. The ratio of branch-chain amino acids (BCAA) to aromatic amino acids (AAA) has

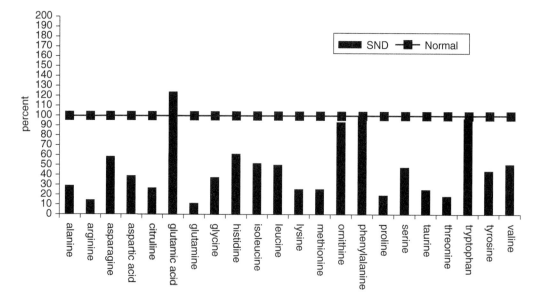

Figure 14.6 Plasma amino acids in 36 dogs with histologically confirmed superficial necrolytic dermatitis (SND) as a percentage of normal. The majority of individual plasma amino acid concentrations in dogs with SND are less than 60% of normal. *Source:* Data from Outerbridge et al. (2002).

been recognized as an indicator of hepatic insufficiency, and this ratio decreases with the severity of hepatic dysfunction or portal-systemic shunting. The mean BCAA : AAA ratio in dogs with SND in one study was 2.6 : 1.0, which is not indicative of severe hepatic dysfunction (Outerbridge et al. 2002). It seems probable that an as yet unexplained increase in hepatic catabolism of amino acids might account for the severity of the hypoaminoacidemia documented in dogs with SND. Intravenous administration of amino acids initially bypasses the portal circulation, resulting in the delivery of amino acids to peripheral tissues before hepatic uptake and catabolism can occur. The fact that some dogs respond better to therapy with intravenous amino acid infusions rather than oral protein hyperalimentation supports the hypothesis that there is increased hepatic catabolism of amino acids in dogs with SND.

The etiopathogenesis of the hepatic pathology seen in the majority of dogs with SND remains unknown, and it is unclear what metabolic pathways may link liver or pancreatic disease with the skin lesions seen in SND. Hyperglucagonemia, if it were present, could explain the risk for the development of diabetes mellitus and hypoaminoacidemia seen in dogs with SND. Glucagon is not a hormone routinely measured in dogs and assays may not detect all biologically active metabolites of glucagon. The catabolism of almost all amino acids, except tryptophan, is influenced by glucagon (Shepartz 1973). Tryptophan concentrations are not significantly decreased in dogs with SND (Outerbridge et al. 2002). It is possible that a disturbance in glucagon metabolism may have a role in the HCS form of SND. Adding to the confusion about the pathogenesis of this disease is the fact that dogs with histologically confirmed glucagonomas do not seem to have the same hepatic pathology as seen in dogs with HCS. Yet the clinical skin lesions, histologic skin pathology, and amino acid levels measured are similar to those dogs with the hepatic pathology-associated form of SND.

The actual etiopathogenesis for the skin lesions seen in dogs with SND or in humans with NME is not known, although a number of mechanisms have been proposed (Sohier et al. 1980; Peterson et al. 1984; Mullans and Cohen 1998; Marinkovich et al. 1995; Almdal et al. 1990). EFA and zinc deficiencies have both been proposed to contribute to the development of NME, because the histologic appearance of skin lesions in patients with zinc deficiency (acrodermatitis enteropathica) or EFA deficiency share some similarities, and skin lesions improved in some patients after zinc or EFA supplementation, although it was not helpful for long-term resolution (Kasper 1992). In dogs with SND associated with glucagonoma, pancreatic tumor excision or treatment with somatostatin has resolved skin lesions (Torres et al. 1997; Oberkirchner et al. 2009). As different disease processes appear to be able to produce the same characteristic histologic skin lesions, this suggests that perhaps they may all be due to a common metabolic disturbance. The fact that severe hypoaminoacidemia is documented to occur in all cases of SND in which plasma amino acids have been measured, regardless of associated disease, makes it likely that this metabolic derangement is directly contributing to the cutaneous lesions seen in affected dogs.

Clinical Presentation

The disease is typically diagnosed in older dogs. Upon review of the literature, the mean age of all reported cases is 10 years, with a range of 4–16 years. Male dogs comprise 64% of reported cases. Shetland Sheepdogs, West Highland White Terriers, Cocker Spaniels, and Scottish Terriers may have a predisposition to develop HCS as they appear to be overrepresented (Outerbridge et al. 2002). There is a report of a group of Shih Tzus, some of which were related, that all developed SND (Hall-Fonte et al. 2016). It is unknown how genetic influences may predispose to the development of SND.

The most common clinical sign is the development of visually distinctive skin lesions with a characteristic distribution. In a review of all published cases, 94% of dogs had affected footpads with marked crusting, fissuring, and ulcerations (Outerbridge 2010). These footpad lesions are highly suggestive of SND (Figures 14.7 and 14.8). Erythema, crusting, exudation, ulceration, and alopecia can also involve the periocular or perioral regions, anal–genital regions, and pressure points on the trunk and limbs. The skin lesions in dogs with HCS may precede any other clinical signs. Secondary cutaneous infections with bacteria, yeast (i.e. *Malassezia, Candida*) or dermatophytes, particularly involving the feet, are often present in dogs with SND. Lameness secondary to footpad lesions, inappetence, and weight loss can also be associated with SND. Polydipsia and polyuria may be present when there is concurrent diabetes mellitus or if significant liver dysfunction is present.

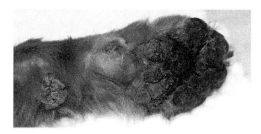

Figure 14.7 Foot-pad lesions in a dog with superficial necrolytic dermatitis.

Histopathologic findings of representative skin biopsies are unique and confirm the diagnosis. These findings include a marked parakeratotic epidermis with striking inter- and intracellular edema, keratinocyte degeneration in the upper epidermis, and hyperplastic basal cells that create the characteristic "red, white, and blue" histologic lesion. Evaluation of serum biochemistry panels often demonstrates an increase in liver enzyme activities and a decrease in serum albumin concentration. Serum bile acid evaluations are abnormal in about half of affected dogs. A past review of all reported cases at that time found hypoaminoacidemia in all dogs, elevated glucagon in 4 out of 4 dogs that had a glucagonoma, and increased serum insulin concentrations in 8 out of 11 dogs (Outerbridge 2010).

Abdominal ultrasound may demonstrate a unique "honeycomb" pattern to the liver consisting of variably sized hypoechoic regions surrounded by hyperechoic borders. Hepatic histopathology often documents a distinctive vacuolar hepatopathy with parenchymal collapse. Grossly, the liver may appear irregular, have multiple nodules, and be mistaken for being cirrhotic. There exists some contradiction as to whether the hepatic lesions in SND reflect true cirrhosis. Despite some histologic descriptions of micronodular cirrhosis, one study, using special stains, confirmed only a minimal increase in collagen within portal areas (Gross et al. 1993). Extensive fibrosis and

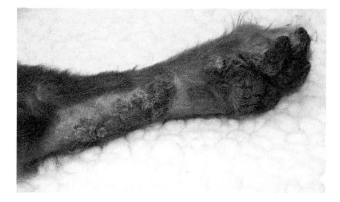

Figure 14.8 Adherent crusting over pressure point on the tarsus and severe hyperkeratosis of the foot pads with fissures in a dog with superficial necrolytic dermatitis (SND). Courtesy of UC Davis Dermatology Service.

reduced liver size characteristic of chronic cirrhosis are not seen in livers that only have the hepatic lesion associated with SND.

Diagnosis and Treatment

Diagnosis of SND is based on obtaining skin biopsies with the typical histopathologic changes. The characteristic dermatohistopathology can be focal within a given lesion. Whenever possible, multiple representative samples should be obtained and submitted. Biopsies should be chosen, if possible, from easily accessible sites with attempts to avoid general anesthesia. The documented occurrence of abnormal laboratory findings, which can include elevated liver enzymes (serum alkaline phosphatase, alanine transferase) or hyperglycemia if concurrent diabetes mellitus is present, should increase the clinical suspicion of SND in dogs with compatible cutaneous lesions. If abdominal ultrasound is available, it can provide further support for the diagnosis if the characteristic honeycomb pattern is documented. If this ultrasonographic pattern to the liver is not visualized in a dog with a confirmed histologic diagnosis of SND, evaluation for a possible pancreatic tumor is necessary. Pancreatic tumors may not be readily visible with an abdominal ultrasound examination, so measurement of plasma glucagon is also recommended. If plasma glucagon concentrations are abnormally increased or a pancreatic mass is visible on ultrasound, the option for exploratory laparotomy and tumor excision can be considered. However, postoperative morbidity and mortality have been high. Plasma amino acids, if measured, should document a characteristic severe hypoaminoacidemia.

The most effective symptomatic or palliative therapy for dogs with SND appears to be the administration of intravenous amino acids. There are a number of crystalline amino acid solutions for parenteral administration on the market that vary in their concentration and the inclusion of electrolytes. Although there are minor differences in the amounts of essential and non-essential amino acids between manufacturers, there are no data to suggest that one product is more efficacious than another. Solutions without additional electrolytes are preferred. The following have all been used for intravenous infusions in treating dogs with SND: 10% Aminosyn® intravenous solution (Abbott Labs, NC, USA); Travasol 8.5% without electrolytes (Baxter Healthcare, Clintec Nutrition, Deerfield, IL, USA); and ProcalAmine® (3% amino acids with 3% glycerin and electrolytes; B. Braun Medical, Irvine, CA, USA). Administration of 10% Aminosyn at 25 ml/kg over 6–8 hours that is repeated at 7–10-day intervals has been suggested (Byrne 1999). However, there is a case report describing long-term management of a dog with SND that was given both amino acid and lipid infusions (Bach and Glasser 2013). These hypertonic amino acid solutions should be administered via a central vein to diminish the chance of thrombophlebitis. Inducing a hyperosmolar state is possible if administration is too aggressive. Dogs should be watched for neurologic signs and the infusion discontinued if these occur. If compromised hepatic or renal function is present, the administration of intravenous amino acids may exacerbate hepatic encephalopathy or augment increases in blood urea nitrogen (BUN). Such dogs warrant close monitoring with serial measurements of ammonia, BUN, and osmolality during intravenous amino acid administration. Some dogs show dramatic improvement in attitude with resolution of skin lesions after receiving amino acid infusions. There are no rigorously studied protocols for the administration of amino acid infusions in these dogs, and repeat infusions are performed weekly, bimonthly, monthly, or when clinical signs return.

Oral nutritional support should include a high-quality, higher protein diet (or the amount of protein tolerated without signs of hepatic encephalopathy) that can be additionally supplemented with amino acids.

The best oral nutritional approach is not known, but hyperalimentation with protein is indicated unless the dog is known to have hepatic insufficiency as documented by an abnormal liver functions test and clinical signs. The dog with SND does not require the protein moderation that is necessary for dogs suffering from hepatic insufficiency and hepatic encephalopathy. Zinc and EFA supplementation are often recommended, in part because of the reported initial improvement in some humans with NME (Kasper 1992). Feeding egg yolks (3–6 per day) has been anecdotally reported to result in clinical improvement in some dogs (Gross et al. 1993). This provides some additional protein, but also possibly micronutrients that may have an unknown role in this disease.

Secondary infections should be treated with appropriate antibiotic and antifungal therapy, with careful consideration of those drugs that may be hepatotoxic or require hepatic metabolism. Topical therapy with antibacterial and antifungal (yeast) shampoos can also be of benefit in some dogs in helping to manage secondary infections.

Therapy with glucocorticoids is not recommended. Although anti-inflammatory therapy for the skin lesions may be of some benefit, the risk of precipitating or exacerbating diabetes mellitus in these dogs makes the use of glucocorticoids contraindicated.

The prognosis for dogs with SND is generally poor and the majority have survival times of less than 6 months. However, 20% of the dogs in a study were maintained for 12 months or more with oral protein hyperalimentation and periodic parenteral intravenous amino acid infusions (Outerbridge et al. 2002). There are reports of dogs that have been maintained over two years with intravenous amino acid infusions and protein hyperalimentation (Bach and Glasser 2013; Nam et al. 2017). Cooked egg white provides high-quality protein, but requires supplementation to keep the diet complete and balanced.

Nutritional Supplementation for Management of Skin Disease

Many diets or nutritional supplements make claims to treat skin diseases and improve coat quality. The following section will review indications for the use of nutritional supplements in skin diseases and also which nutrients may impact skin health and coat quality. Some supplements contain multiple nutrients; however, specific supplements cannot be reviewed, as formulations may change. The best rule of thumb is to use supplements judiciously, review them for constituents with mechanisms of action relevant to the issue of interest and/or clinical trials to substantiate the benefit of their use, avoid supplements containing potentially harmful or unknown components, and look for evidence of quality control for that supplement. Be aware that there are concerns within the supplement industry regarding the actual presence of desired ingredients in concentrations reported and sufficient for desired effect, and absence of any undesired or undeclared substances (see Chapter 5 for further discussion on supplements).

Fatty Acid Supplementation

Fatty acid supplementation, commonly used in veterinary dermatology, may have some efficacy in ameliorating pruritic skin conditions via a number of mechanisms. Specific fatty acids or combinations have been reported to be beneficial in managing pruritus, particularly in atopic dermatitis, feline eosinophilic reaction patterns (i.e. eosinophilic plaques or granulomas), cornification disturbances, improving coat quality, and "idiopathic" seborrhea. EFA combinations have also been used to treat canine symmetric lupoid onychodystrophy (Bergvall 1998; Mueller et al. 2003), either as sole therapy or in conjunction with other therapeutics. Since various combination products were utilized in these cases, a single recommendation is not currently possible (refer to Mueller et al. 2003 for specifics).

Overall, there are many open, uncontrolled studies and comparatively few published placebo-controlled or double-blinded crossover studies regarding the efficacy of fatty acids in veterinary dermatology. Only trials with a crossover design would minimize the lack of dietary standardization between different trials. Most of these earlier trials investigated the supplementation of n-6 EFAs (e.g. LA or AA) for managing pruritus in atopic dermatitis. In dogs, the results of those crossover trials reported variable efficacy between 17% and 56% (Olivry et al. 2001). More recent studies, however, demonstrated stronger evidence for the supplementation of n-3 PUFAs (e.g. ALA, EPA, DHA) in cases of pruritus related to atopy or flea allergy dermatitis. The doses were relatively high compared to maintenance dose and therefore more supraphysiologic or 'nutraceutical' to achieve therapeutic benefit.

It appears that supplementation with n-6 LA can cause a significant decrease in TEWL (Marsh et al. 2000). This suggests that the supplementation leads to more incorporation into the intercellular lipids of the epidermis. By decreasing cutaneous permeability and via the ability of AA to influence epidermal proliferation, EFA supplementation can positively affect conditions related to defects in keratinization. Coat quality is positively affected by supplementation with these EFAs, as assessed by increased coat gloss and decreased scale (Marsh et al. 2000; Rees et al. 2001).

Certain PUFAs are thought to modulate eicosanoid production in the skin by competing with AA for incorporation into cellular membranes, eventually providing an alternative substrate for cyclooxygenase and lipoxygenase enzymes to produce less inflammatory eicosanoids than those derived from AA. The latter produces 2-series prostaglandins (e.g. PGE2) and 4-series leukotrienes (e.g. LBT4) when degraded; whereas, the n-6 fatty acid dihomogammalinolenic acid (DGLA) produces 1-series prostaglandins, while the n-3 fatty acid EPA produces 3-series prostaglandins (e.g. PGE3) and 5-series leukotrienes

(e.g. LTB5). LTB5 is 30–100 times less stimulatory than LTB4 (Waldron et al. 2012).

In dogs, it has been found that both fatty acid type and chain length affect the structure and function of neutrophil membranes independent of the n-6 : n-3 fatty acid ratio. Although both menhaden fish oil (EPA + DHA) and linseed oil (ALA) increased plasma and neutrophil membrane EPA concentrations (compared to safflower oil or beef tallow), only the fish oil increased DHA and resulted in the greatest increase in LTB5 with decreased LTB4 production (linseed oil produces this relative change to a lesser extent). Both fish oil and linseed oil also resulted in an approximately 20% decrease in production of superoxide (presumably by limiting the AA available for NADPH oxidase; Waldron et al. 2012). In addition to modulating eicosanoid production, the inflammatory response may also be influenced by production of different resolvins and protectins from EPA, alterations in cellular signaling, and inhibiting cytokine secretion. Additionally, although n-3 fatty acids are mostly utilized for their "anti-inflammatory" effect, they may also have potential antitumor effects, improve receptor and ion channel function, and positively alter blood lipid concentrations (Bauer 2011).

Some studies over the past few decades have demonstrated a benefit to adding various n-3 PUFAs when compared to placebos; however, the dose of flaxseed or canola oil (ALA sources) needed to be substantially higher than the dose of marine-sourced n-3 oils (EPA + DHA sources) in order to achieve similar results. The benefits of high doses of ALA may be due to the sparing effect exerted on conversion of LA to AA (leading to greater accumulation of LA vs. AA in the phospholipid fractions), as well as the conversion of ALA to small amounts of EPA. When directly comparing the dosing of EPA + DHA to ALA in a crossover study in pruritic dogs, greater improvement was seen in pruritus, self-trauma, and coat character in dogs receiving the fish oil (180 mg EPA + 120 mg DHA/4.55 kg BW) compared to the ALA (Logas and Kunkle 1994). It is important to note that studies prior to this were often using much lower doses and reporting variable results. A more recent study (Abba et al. 2005) also showed a greater effect of supplementing n-3 PUFAs in cases of early compared to chronic atopy. It is worthwhile noting, however, that the doses used in that study (17 mg EPA + 5 mg DHA + 35 mg ALA/kg BW) resulted in much lower intakes of EPA + DHA than the prior study. It is therefore important to realize that sufficient dosing, sufficient time of administration, and disease type or duration may all interact to determine whether fatty acid supplementation is successful in reducing clinical signs.

Based on a cumulative review of the better-designed studies supporting use of fish oil supplementation in dogs for inflammatory and immunologic conditions (e.g. atopy), the apparent median effective dose of EPA + DHA is $125\,mg \times BW(kg)^{0.75}$ or 700 mg/10 kg BW (Bauer 2011). Therefore, this dose should likely be used as a starting guideline in dogs with dermatologic disease; however, higher doses may be needed in certain individuals to see an effect. Whether addition of ALA may also have a further or synergistic effect (by affecting LA to AA conversion) is less clear, but possible. A balanced intake of n-6 : n-3 fatty acids is recommended, with supplementation of n-3 PUFAs (especially EPA + DHA) in dermatologic cases.

Although vegetable oil supplementation may be safe in dogs, it is not recommended in cats. The addition of these oils (high in LA, which cats cannot convert) dilutes the AA provided by the base diet such that, when consumed to meet energy needs, a relative deficiency of AA may be created. AA deficiency has been previously linked to dry, lusterless coats and dandruff (among other signs) and should be avoided. However, supplementation with menhaden fish oil was demonstrated to maintain baseline AA, while also providing EPA and DHA (Angell et al. 2012). Therefore, supplementation with n-3 fatty acid products is preferred. Although clinical studies using fish oil for skin disorders in cats are more sparse and harder to interpret compared to those for dogs, it does appear that (similar to other species) feline plasma and tissue do respond to dosing with n-3 PUFAs in a dose-dependent manner, with possible saturation after 600–700 mg/day (Bauer 2011). Caution with dosing EPA + DHA should be used in cats, as no safe upper limit has been determined yet, due to equivocal data (Bauer 2011).

N-3 PUFAs from marine sources (EPA and DHA) are more efficiently incorporated into membranes when compared to terrestrially sourced n-3 PUFAs such as flaxseed (primarily ALA), regardless of the ratio of n-3 : n-6 (Waldron et al. 2012). In dogs, the conversion of ALA to EPA is low (even lower conversion to DHA) because of the competitive interaction with the same enzyme system that converts LA to AA (so cats are also less efficient at converting ALA to EPA). However, even the somewhat low conversion to EPA will lead to less inflammation due to its subsequent incorporation and use (Dunbar et al. 2010). So, even though pre-formed EPA is more potent, the incorporation of some ALA may still be beneficial to balance the concentration of LA in a diet. By competing with the same enzyme as LA, less AA will accumulate in canine membranes.

It has been fairly well demonstrated that n-3 fatty acid dosing, independent of the n-3 : n-6 ratio, affects fatty acid profiles and subsequent actions in dogs (Hall et al. 2006). More controlled studies that account for total amounts and doses of the relevant n-6 and n-3 fatty acids (rather than just ratios of total n-6 : n-3) are needed to fully understand their potential impact. This applies to not only the understanding of their positive therapeutic benefits, but also to any possible unintended adverse effects. For example, there is a limited ability to interpret most of the past studies exploring potential adverse effects on platelet function in dogs and cats, due to the reporting of only n-6 : n-3 ratios, rather than total amounts and specific fatty acids (Lenox and Bauer 2013).

It is important to note that supplementation with fatty acids may have a time lag to effect of several weeks to months (Watson 1998) depending on lipid turnover in membranes, although some research has shown that a steady state is reached in four weeks (Bauer 2011). Additionally, effects may not be apparent if sufficient dosing is not utilized. Since there can be a wide variation in the fatty acid profile of base diets consumed, it is recommended first to evaluate the daily intake of key fatty acids from the base diet. Evaluating only total n-6 or n-3 is insufficient. The appropriate level of additional supplementation will then be tailored to provide at least the desired total daily intake, without exceeding the safe upper limit. For example, certain diets intended for joint, renal, or dermatologic support may already have high concentrations of EPA and DHA. These diets may or may not have sufficient concentrations to provide the desired total daily dose to the individual, depending on their food intake (Lenox and Bauer 2013). Conversely, if intake is already sufficient, blindly adding more fish oil to the diet could result in overconsumption of calories, other undesired side effects (e.g. diarrhea, or wasted money or effort for the client), or consumption of total EPA + DHA that exceeds the safe upper limit before toxicity concerns occur. From a nutritional perspective, it is also important to note what other nutrients may be added in excessive amounts via the use of these supplements. Some oils, such as cod liver or salmon oils, will naturally contain the fat-soluble vitamins A and D. Dosing needs either to consider the addition of these other nutrients to avoid toxicity concerns, or a product that has removed them via molecular distillation should be used. It is not possible to assume absence if they are not listed on the label, and the manufacturer must be contacted for confirmation.

Supplemental oils are not created equal, and recent studies in commercial human (and limited veterinary) fish oil supplements showed that a large proportion did not contain the stated concentrations of EPA or DHA. This could be due to mislabeling and lack of quality control during production; however, it may also be linked to oxidation of the PUFA into lipid peroxides, aldehydes, and ketones. This not only reduces the efficacy of the supplement, but may also result in undesired effects related to consuming oxidation products. When choosing a product, quality control by the manufacturer as well as postproduction handling should be considered. Anything with high concentrations of PUFAs is more prone to spoiling (via oxidation) and should be stored in a way to minimize contact with oxygen or UV light, at an appropriate temperature (refrigerated after opening), and with appropriate levels of antioxidants, particularly vitamin E. Unfortunately, a recent survey indicated that a large percentage of both veterinarians and pet owners are unaware of the potential for EFAs to oxidize (Martinez et al. 2020).

In conclusion, supplementation with fatty acids may be useful to improve clinical signs in some cases of dermatologic disease. Supplementation with n-6 fatty acids, specifically LA, may have a positive effect in cases of keratinization disorders in dogs, but LA supplementation is not recommended in cats, although GLA supplementation should be safe in both species and may help. N-3 fatty acid supplementation with fish oil to provide EPA + DHA, with or without additional ALA, appears useful in several types of inflammatory and pruritic skin disease, especially in dogs. Supplementation of EFA may also help improve the efficacy of antihistamines or have a dose-sparing effect on glucocorticoid administration (DeBoer 2016). Absorption of supplemental oils is best when administered with food/meals and when dosing is split (rather than one large daily dose). These steps also help minimize negative side effects (diarrhea, etc.). When dosing marine oils, it is important to ensure that administration is for a sufficient time period to allow effect (four weeks or longer) and that a sufficient total daily intake of EPA + DHA, at a dose expected to result in a therapeutic benefit, is provided. In dogs, the median dosing required for EPA + DHA appears to be $125\,mg \times BW(kg)^{0.75}$ (or ~700 mg/ 10 kg), meaning that more or less may be required for an individual, but the safe upper limit for dosing in dogs is $< 370\,mg \times BW(kg)^{0.75}$ and should not be exceeded. Less is known in cats and more cautious supplementation is recommended. Since a safe upper limit is unknown in cats, initial doses should be limited to $< 75\,mg \times BW(kg)^{0.67}$. Higher doses may be tried; however, close monitoring is recommended, and particular caution should be used in any cats with other conditions that could negatively affect platelet function (Bauer 2011).

Zinc Supplementation for Skin Disease

The zinc-responsive dermatoses have been discussed earlier. Zinc has also been used in conjunction with EFAs in a study in dogs to evaluate changes in skin and hair coat quality, assessed by measuring coat gloss, presence of scale, and TEWL (Marsh et al. 2000). The combination of zinc (100 mg/1000 kcal) and linoleic acid (15 g/1000 kcal) produced statistically significant improvements in coat gloss and decreased TEWL over a nine-week period in dogs (NRC 2006).

B Vitamin Supplementation

Pantothenic acid (B5) and nicotinamide (B3) in combination with choline and inositol, and the amino acid histidine, were shown to reduce TEWL (Watson et al. 2006). Biotin supplementation has also been advocated to improve coat quality in dogs (Frigg et al. 1989). Based on their important role in skin health, supplementation of B complex vitamins may be found in many combination veterinary dermatology supplements for skin and coat health. This supplementation may either address a relative deficiency or may enhance the effects of other supplements via synergistic mechanisms.

Vitamin A–Responsive Skin Diseases

Vitamin A–responsive dermatosis is a rare skin disease seen predominantly in Cocker Spaniels (Ihrke and Goldschmidt 1983), but also Labrador Retrievers and Miniature Schnauzers. It is an adult-onset cornification disorder in which dogs present with multifocal, well-demarcated, erythematous, alopecia plaques with thick adherent scale, most often located on the ventral abdomen and thorax. Hair shafts are often entrapped and clumped by keratinaceous debris. Overall, the hair coat is dull. Histologically, severe follicular hyperkeratosis is evident, which is highly suggestive for the diagnosis (Gross et al. 2005). Despite being fed a nutritionally balanced diet, these dogs require supraphysiologic supplementation with oral vitamin A at 600–800 IU (2000–2667 retinol equivalents or all trans-retinol)/kg BW/ day). Clinical improvement is typically seen in 6–8 weeks. Some degree of lifelong supplementation with vitamin A is often needed. High doses of vitamin A are likely to have some degree of a suppressive effect on cornification in these dogs and slow the epidermal turnover time.

There are numerous synthetic retinoids that have been developed and used for treating skin disease in humans and some have been used in small animals. The synthetic retinoids, either isotretinoin or etretinate, have been reported to be of benefit for treating primary idiopathic seborrhea, ichthyosis, solar or actinic dermatitis, sebaceous adenitis, infundibular keratinizing acanthomas, epitheliotropic T-cell lymphoma, and squamous cell carcinoma (Kwochka 1993). Due to the expense of these agents, vitamin A is often tried in the management of some of these diseases.

Anti-inflammatory corticosteroids can impair wound healing. Vitamin A and retinoids also significantly, but not completely, reverse some of the impaired wound healing seen with anti-inflammatory corticosteroids (Wicke et al. 2000).

Vitamin E–Responsive Skin Diseases

Vitamin E at supraphysiologic doses (200–400 IU/dog twice daily) has been used to treat canine discoid lupus erythematosus, dermatomyositis, and primary acanthosis nigricans with variable success (and a lag time of 30–60 days for maximum effect may be needed), even though these are not the result of a dietary deficiency (Werner and Harvey 1995; Watson 1998). It did not appear to be effective in dogs without significant epidermal changes (e.g. dogs with atopy).

It is important to be cautious about extreme oversupplementation of vitamin E. Although it has a higher margin of safety than other fat-soluble vitamins, there are reports of high doses of vitamin E interfering with the absorption and metabolic action of vitamin D and vitamin K in other species. There are limited data on toxicity in dogs and cats. No safe upper limit has been established in cats; however, cats given a salmon- and tuna-based diet overly fortified with vitamin E developed prolonged clotting times (e.g. increased prothrombin time), which were then restored by vitamin K therapy (NRC 2006). Mortality in kittens was also dose related to vitamin E, with death in all at doses of 1000 mg/kg/day and significant mortality at doses of 100–200 mg/kg/day. In dogs, a tentative upper limit of 75 IU/kg/day (or 1000–2000 IU/kg diet) has been suggested (NRC 2006).

Therapeutic Diets for Skin Health

A number of diets designed and marketed to benefit or support skin health are available. Some of these diets are targeted to address CAFRs or other food intolerances by utilizing uncommon and limited ingredients or hydrolyzed proteins ± purified starch. The diets might also contain additional modifications aimed at decreasing inflammation, supporting immune system health, and/or improving skin barrier function. Other diets may be intended for use in pets with environmental atopy or other causes of pruritus. The nutritional modifications will target similar strategies to those already discussed, but may exclude use of uncommon or hydrolyzed ingredients. Many contain additional EPA and DHA; however, not all do and it is important to look for EPA/DHA concentrations in the product guides (or call the manufacturers). Preliminarily, the ingredient list can be evaluated for sources of whole fish (fish meal has fat removed during rendering) or fish and other marine oils; flaxseed will predominantly provide ALA, so only evaluating total n-3 concentration can be misleading. Other nutrients that may be highlighted include n-6 PUFA, vitamin A, biotin and/or B complex, and zinc. These nutrients, as outlined previously, play a role in maintenance of skin health and even in specific functions such as improving TEWL. The intention is that by utilizing nutrition to improve barrier function, clinical signs of dermatitis may be improved, particularly in atopy. Manipulation of the lipid composition of the stratum corneum via altering the fatty acid composition of the diet is promising. The use of micronutrients that could stimulate barrier components, such as Vitamin A and zinc, are hoped to further enhance barrier function.

When comparing these diets, there are variations in the total concentration of each of these nutrients, ingredients, and caloric distribution (amount of protein, fat, and carbohydrate). Some diets have been utilized in clinical trials to assess efficacy for such things as coat quality, pruritus scores, potential sparing effects or delays in medication use. Their use is worth consideration but, ultimately, individual response or usefulness will vary. Regardless, the utilization of these diets may, in some cases, be superior to adding supplements/nutraceuticals to a different diet. Due to the complexity of nutrient–nutrient interactions, including possible synergism or antagonism, the presence of other bioactive food components, and/or other unknown variables, it is sometimes more useful to evaluate the effect of entire diets more holistically. Although this is different from more reductionist nutritional studies, and may obscure specifics about the effect (or lack of effect) of individual nutrients, it does offer insight into the utility of the diet as a whole. At the least, they should provide a complete and balanced diet appropriate for the species and life stage of the pet, while also including additional recommended nutritional strategies. This may be better than trying to alter a different diet with limited information or risking the creation of imbalances or oversupplementation.

Summary

- Dermatologic conditions associated with nutritional deficiencies are uncommon when the animal is fed >90% of daily kilocalorie intake from diets that meet all nutritional needs for that individual and there is no issue of malabsorption. Generic dog food disease and feline pansteatitis (associated with a diet low in vitamin E and high polyunsaturated fatty acids) are two examples of how an unbalanced diet can cause cutaneous lesions.
- The skin has relatively high demand for protein and energy.
- Essential fatty acids (EFAs) have multiple functions in the skin and are an important component of ceramides, which are necessary in maintaining the cornified lipid envelope or skin barrier.
- Zinc is an important dietary element for the development of normal epithelialization.

- There are two syndromes of zinc-responsive dermatosis seen clinically in the dog. Syndrome I most commonly affects Arctic breeds, and syndrome II affects rapidly growing puppies, often fed poor-quality dog food. Both syndromes present with clinical lesions of adherent scaling around the mouth, chin, eyes, pinnae, and foot pads. Syndrome I dogs require oral zinc supplementation on top of a good diet, while syndrome II dogs require a better diet.
- Superficial necrolytic dermatitis (SND) and cutaneous adverse food reaction (CAFR) are two skin diseases that benefit from nutritional or dietary management.
- SND is a disease seen in older dogs and in association with a number of systemic metabolic disturbances, including hypoaminoacidemia and diabetes mellitus. In most cases a characteristic histologic and ultrasonographic hepatic pathology are found. Characteristic skin changes include hyperkeratotic foot pads and adherent crusting lesions over pressure points. Intravenous amino acid infusions may provide palliative management for some dogs.
- CAFR is a cause of nonseasonal pruritus in dogs and cats. It requires an elimination-and-rechallenge diet trial to diagnose. Neither serology nor intradermal testing provides clinically relevant information regarding the specific food proteins or substances an animal does not tolerate.
- Nutritional supplementation with various EFAs, vitamin A, and zinc may be beneficial in the management of certain skin diseases.

References

Abba, C., Mussa, P.P., Vercelli, A., and Raviri, G. (2005). Essential fatty acids supplementation in different-stage atopic dogs fed on a controlled diet. *J. Anim. Physiol. Anim. Nutr (Berl).* 89: 203–207.

Allenspach, K., Arnold, P., Glaus, T. et al. (2000). Glucagon-producing neuroendocrine tumour associated with hypoaminoacidaemia and skin lesions. *J. Small Anim. Pract.* 41: 402–406.

Almdal, T.P., Heindorff, H., Bardram, L., and Vilstrup, H. (1990). Increased amino acid clearance and urea synthesis in a patient with glucagonoma. *Gut* 8: 956–948.

Angell, R.J., McClure, M.K., Bigley, K.E., and Bauer, J.E. (2012). Fish oil supplementation maintains adequate plasma arachidonate in cats, but similar amounts of vegetable oils lead to dietary arachidonate deficiency from nutrient dilution. *Nutr. Res.* 32: 381–389.

Asakawa, M.G., Cullen, J.M., and Linder, K.E. (2013). Necrolytic migratory erythema associated with a glucagon-producing primary hepatic neuroendocrine carcinoma in a cat. *Vet. Dermatol.* 24: 466–469.

Bach, J.F. and Glasser, S.A. (2013). A case of necrolytic migratory erythema managed for 24 months with intravenous amino acid and lipid infusions. *Can. Vet. J.* 54: 873–875.

Bauer, J.E. (2011). Therapeutic use of fish oils in companion animals. *JAVMA* 239 (11): 1441–1451.

Bauer, J.E., Heinnemann, K.M., Lees, G.E., and Waldron, M.K. (2006). Docosahexaenoic acid accumulates in plasma of canine puppies raised on alpha-linolenic acid-rich milk during suckling but not when fed alpha-linolenic acid-rich diets after weaning. *J. Nutr.* 136 (7 Suppl): 2087S–2089S.

Bauer, A., Jagannathan, V., Högler, S. et al. (2018). MKLN1 splicing defect in dogs with lethal acrodermatitis. *PLoS Genet.* 14 (3): e1007264.

Bergvall, K. (1998). Treatment of symmetrical onychomadesis and onychodystrophy in five dogs with n-3 and n-6 fatty acids. *Vet. Dermatol.* 9: 263–268.

Bizikova, P. and Olivry, T. (2016). A randomized, double-blinded crossover trial testing the benefit of two hydrolysed poultry-based commercial diets for dogs with spontaneous pruritic chicken allergy. *Vet. Dertmatol.* 27: 289–e70.

Bloom, P., Rosser, E.J., and Dunstan, R. (1992). Anti-convulsant hepatitis-induced necrolytic migratory erythema. *Proceedings of the Second World Congress of Veterinary Dermatology*, Montreal, Quebec, 56 (May 13–16 1992).

Bond, R., McNeil, P.E., Evans, H., and Srebernik, N. (1995). Metabolic epidermal necrosis in two dogs with different underlying diseases. *Vet. Rec.* 136: 466–471.

Brown, R.G., Hoag, G.N., Smart, M.E., and Mitchell, L.H. (1978). Alaskan malamute chondrodysplasia. V. Decreased gut zinc absorption. *Growth* 42: 1–6.

Byrne, K.P. (1999). Metabolic epidermal necrosis-hepatocutaneous syndrome. *Vet. Clin. North Am. Small Anim. Pract.* 29: 1337–1355.

Campbell, G.A. and Crow, D. (2006). Zinc responsive dermatosis in a litter of pharaoh hounds: selected abstracts from the North American veterinary dermatology forum (NAVDF), 5–9 April, Wyndham Palm Springs, Palm Springs, California, USA. *Vet. Dermatol.* 17: 207–220.

Chesney, C.J. (2001). Systematic review of evidence for the prevalence of food sensitivity in dogs. *Vet. Rec.* 148: 445–448.

Codner, E.C. and Thatcher, C.D. (1993). Nutritional management of skin disease. *Compendium* 15: 411–424.

Coe, J.B., O'Connor, R.E., MacMartin, C. et al. (2020). Effects of three diet history questions on the amount of information gained from a sample of pet owners in Ontario. *Canada. J. Am. Vet. Med. Assoc.* 256: 469–478.

Colombini, S. and Dunstan, R.W. (1997). Zinc-responsive dermatosis in northern-breed dogs: 17 cases (1990–1996). *J. Am. Vet. Med. Assoc.* 211: 451–453.

Cunnane, S.C. and Horrobin, D.F. (1980). Parenteral linoleic and gamma-linolenic acids ameliorate the gross effects of zinc deficiency. *Proc. Soc. Exp. Biol. Med.* 164: 583–588.

Day, M.J. (1997). Review of thymic pathology in 30 cats and 36 dogs. *J. Small Anim. Pract.* 38: 393–403.

DeBoer, D. (2016). 10 things you need to know about allergic skin disease. *Proceedings, OVMA Conference*, Toronto, Ontario (January 28-30, 2016).

Dunbar, B.L., Bigley, K.E., and Bauer, J.E. (2010). Early and sustained enrichment of serum n-3 long chain polyunsaturated fatty acids in dogs fed a flaxseed supplemented diet. *Lipids* 45: 1–10.

Favrot, C., Bisikova, P., Fisher, N. et al. (2019). The usefulness of short-course prednisolone during the initial phase of an elimination diet trial in dogs with food-induced atopic dermatitis. *Vet. Dermatol.* 30: 498–e149.

Florant, E., Guillot, J., Degorce-Rubiales, F., and Mailot, M. (2000). Four cases of canine metabolic epidermal necrosis. *Vet. Dermatol.* 11 (Suppl): 18.

Frigg, M., Schulze, J., and Völker, L. (1989). Clinical study on the effects of biotin on skin conditions in dogs. *Schweiz. Arch. Tierheilkd.* 131: 621–625.

Green, A.S. and Fascetti, A.J. (2016). Meeting the vitamin A requirement: the efficacy and importance of β-carotene in animal species. *Scientific World Journal* 2016: 7393620.

Gross, T.L., Song, M.D., Havel, P.J. et al. (1993). Superficial necrolytic dermatitis (necrolytic migratory erythema) in dogs. *Vet. Pathol.* 30: 75–81.

Gross, T.L., Ihrke, P.J., Walder, E.J., and Affolter, V.K. (2005). *Skin Diseases of the Dog and Cat: Clinical and Histopathologic Diagnosis*, 2e. Oxford: Blackwell Science.

Hall, J.A., Picton, R.A., Skinner, M.M. et al. (2006). The (n-3) fatty acid dose, independent of the (n-6) to (n-3) fatty acid ratio, affects the plasma fatty acid profile of normal dogs. *J. Nutr.* 136: 2338–2344.

Hall-Fonte, D.L., Center, S.A., McDonough, S.P. et al. (2016). Hepatocutaneous syndrome in Shih Tzus: 31 cases (1996–2014). *J. Am. Vet. Med. Assoc.* 248: 802–813.

Harvey, R.G. (1993). Food allergy and dietary intolerance in dogs: a report of 25 cases. *J. Small Anim. Pract.* 34: 175–179.

Hendriks, W.H., Allan, F.J., Tarttelin, M.F. et al. (2001). Suspected zinc-induced copper deficiency in growing kittens exposed to galvanised iron. *N. Z. Vet. J.* 49: 68–72.

Hensel, P. (2010). Nutrition and skin diseases in veterinary medicine. *Clin. Dermatol.* 28: 696–693.

Huang, Y.S., Cunnane, S.C., Horrobin, D.F., and Davignon, J. (1982). Most biological effects of zinc deficiency corrected by gamma-linolenic acid (18: 3 omega 6) but not by linoleic acid (18: 2 omega 6). *Art Ther.* 41: 193–207.

Ihrke, P.J. and Goldschmidt, M.H. (1983). Vitamin A-responsive dermatosis in the dog. *J. Am. Vet. Med. Assoc.* 182: 687–690.

Jackson, H.A. and Hammerberg, B. (2002). The clinical and immunological reaction to a flavored monthly oral heartworm prophylactic in 12 dogs with spontaneous food allergy. *Vet. Dermatol.* 13: 211–229.

Jackson, H.A., Jackson, M.W., Coblentz, L., and Hammerberg, B. (2003). Evaluation of the clinical and allergen specific serum immunoglobulin E responses to oral challenge with cornstarch, corn, soy and a soy hydrolysate diet in dogs with spontaneous food allergy. *Vet. Dermatol.* 14: 181–187.

Jeffers, J.G., Shanley, K.J., Meyer, E.K. et al. (1991). Diagnostic testing of dogs for food hypersensitivity. *J. Am. Vet. Med. Assoc.* 198: 245–250.

Jeffers, J.G., Meyer, E.K., and Sosis, E.J. (1996). Responses of dogs with food allergies to single-ingredient dietary provocation. *J. Am. Vet. Med. Assoc.* 209: 608–611.

Kasper, C.S. (1992). Necrolytic migratory erythema. Unresolved problems in diagnosis and pathogenesis. A case report and literature review. *Cutis* 49: 120–128.

Knez, M., Stangoulis, J.C.R., Glibetic, M. et al. (2017). The linoleic acid: Dihomo-γ-linolenic acid ratio (LA:DGLA) – an emerging biomarker of Zn status. *Nutrients* 9: 825.

Kwochka, K.W. (1993). Retinoids and vitamin A therapy. In: *Current Veterinary Dermatology* (ed. C.E. Griffin, J.M. MacDonald and K.W. Kwochka), 203. St. Louis, MO: Mosby Year Book.

Lansdown, A.B. and Sampson, B. (1997). Trace metals in keratinizing epithelia in beagle dogs. *Vet. Rec.* 141: 571–572.

Leistra, M.H.G. and Willemse, T. (2002). Double-blind evaluation of two commercial hypoallergenic diets in cats with adverse food reactions. *J. Feline Med. Surg.* 4: 185–188.

Lenox, C.E. and Bauer, J.E. (2013). Potential adverse effects of N-3 fatty acids in dogs and cats. *JVIM* 27: 217–226.

Lewis, L.D., Morris, M.L., and Hand, M.S. (1987). *Small Animal Clinical Nutrition*, 3e. Topeka, KS: Mark Morris Institute.

Loftus, J.P., Center, S.A., AStor, M. et al. (2022). Clinical features and amino acid profiles of dogs with hepatocutaneous syndrome or hepatocutaneous hepatopathy. *JVIM* 36: 97–105.

Logas, D. and Kunkle, G.A. (1994). Double-blinded cross-over study with marine oil supplementation containing high-dose icosapentanoic acid for the treatment of canine pruritic skin disease. *Vet. Dermatol.* 5 (3): 99–104.

Logas, D., Kunkle, G.A., and McDowell, L. (1993). Comparison of serum zinc levels in healthy, systemically ill and dermatologically diseased dogs. *Vet. Dermatol.* 4: 61–64.

MacMartin, C., Wheat, H.C., Coe, J.B., and Adams, C.L. (2015). Effect of question design on dietary information solicited during veterinary-client interactions in companion animal practice in Ontario, Canada. *J. Am. Vet. Med. Soc.* 246: 1203–1214.

March, P.A., Hillier, A., Weisbrode, S.E. et al. (2004). Superficial necrolytic dermatitis in 11 dogs with a history of phenobarbital administration (1995–2002). *J. Vet. Intern. Med.* 18: 65–74.

Marinkovich, M.P., Botella, R., and Sangueza, O.P. (1995). Necrolytic migratory erythema without glucagonoma in patients with liver disease. *J. Am. Acad. Dermatol.* 32: 625–629.

Marsh, K.A., Ruediueli, F.L., Coe, S.L., and Watson, T.G.D. (2000). Effects of zinc and linoleic acid supplementation on the skin and coat quality of dogs receiving a complete and balanced diet. *Vet. Dermatol.* 11: 277–284.

Martin, A., Sierra, M.P., Gonzalez, J.L., and Arevalo, M.A. (2004). Identification of allergens responsible for canine cutaneous adverse food reactions to lamb, beef and cow's milk. *Vet. Dermatol.* 15: 349–356.

Martinez, N., McDonald, B., and Martínez-Taboada, F. (2020). Exploring the use of essential fatty acids in veterinary dermatology. *Vet. Rec.* 187 (5): 190.

McEwan, N.A., Huang, H.P., and Mellon, D.J. (2003a). Immunoglobulin levels in bull terriers suffering from lethal acrodermatitis. *Vet. Immunol. Immunopathol.* 96: 235–238.

McEwan, N.A., McNeil, P.E., Thompson, H., and McCandlish, I.A.P. (2003b). Diagnostic features, confirmation and disease progression in 28 cases of lethal acrodermatitis of bull terriers. *J. Small Anim. Pract.* 41: 501–507.

Miller, W.H. Jr. (1989). Nutritional considerations in small animal dermatology. *Clin. Nutr.* 19: 497–511.

Mueller, R.S. and Olivry, T. (2017). Critically appraised topic on adverse food reactions of companion animals (4): can we diagnose adverse food reactions in dogs and cats with in vivo or in vitro tests? *BMC Vet. Res.* 13: 275–281.

Mueller, R. and Tsohalis, J. (1998). Evaluation of serum allergen-specific IgE for the diagnosis of food adverse reactions in the dog. *Vet. Dermatol.* 9: 167–171.

Mueller, R.S., Rosychuk, R.A., and Jonas, L.D. (2003). A retrospective study regarding the treatment of lupoid onychodystrophy in 30 dogs and literature review. *J. Am. Anim. Hosp. Assoc.* 39: 139–150.

Mueller, R.S., Olivry, T., and Prélaud, P. (2016). Critically appraised topic on adverse food reactions of companion animals (2): common food allergen sources in dogs and cats. *BMC Vet. Res.* 12: 9.

Mullans, E.A. and Cohen, P.R. (1998). Iatrogenic necrolytic migratory erythema: A case report and review of non-glucagonoma-associated necrolytic migratory erythema. *J. Am. Acad. Dermatol.* 38: 866–873.

Munson, L., Koehler, J.W., Wilkinson, J.E., and Miller, R.E. (1998). Vesicular and ulcerative dermatopathy resembling superficial necrolytic dermatitis in captive black rhinoceroses (*Diceros bicornis*). *Vet. Pathol.* 35: 31–42.

Nam, A., Han, S.M., and Go, D.M. (2017). Long-term management with adipose tissue-derived mesenchymal stem cells and conventional treatment in a dog with hepatocutaneous syndrome. *J. Vet. Intern. Med.* 31 (5): 1514–1519.

National Research Council (NRC) Ad Hoc Committee on Dog and Cat Nutrition (2006). *Nutrient Requirements of Dogs and Cats.* Washington, DC: National Academies Press.

Norton, A. (1987). Skin lesions in cats with vitamin B (pyridoxine) deficiency. *Proc. Annu. Members Meet. Am. Acad. Vet. Dermatol. Am. Coll. Vet. Dermatol.* 3: 24.

Oberkirchner, U., Linder, K., Zadrozny, L., and Olivry, T. (2009). Resolution of clinical signs of canine glucagonoma associated necrolytic migratory erythema with subcutaneous octreotide. *NAVDF 2009 Abstr. Vet. Dermatol.* 20: 215.

Olivry, T. and Bizikova, P. (2010). A systematic review of the evidence of reduced allergenicity and clinical benefit of food hydrolysates in dogs with cutaneous adverse food reactions. *Vet. Dermatol.* 21: 32–41.

Olivry, T. and Mueller, R.S. (2017). Critically appraised topic on adverse food reactions of companion animals (3): prevalence of cutaneous adverse food reactions in dogs and cats. *BMC Vet. Res.* 13: 51–54.

Olivry, T. and Mueller, R.S. (2018). Critically appraised topic on adverse food reactions of companion animals (5): discrepancies between ingredients and labeling in commercial pet foods. *BMC Vet. Res.* 14: 24–28.

Olivry, T. and Mueller, R.S. (2019a). Critically appraised topic on adverse food reactions of companion animals (7): signalment and cutaneous manifestations of dogs and cats with adverse food reactions. *BMC Vet. Res.* 15: 140–145.

Olivry, T. and Mueller, R.S. (2019b). Critically appraised topic on adverse food reactions of companion animals (8): storage mites in commercial pet foods. *BMC Vet. Res.* 15: 385–389.

Olivry, T., Marsella, R., and Hillier, A. (2001). The ACVD task force on canine atopic dermatitis (XXIII): are essential fatty acids effective? *Vet. Immunol. Immunopathol.* 81: 347–362.

Olivry, T., Mueller, R.S., and Prélaud, P. (2015). Critically appraised topic on adverse food

reactions of companion animals (1): duration of elimination diets. *BMC Vet. Res.* 11: 225–227.

Outerbridge, C.A. (2010). Hepatocutaneous syndrome. In: *Textbook of Veterinary Internal Medicine Diseases of the Dog and Cat*, 7e (ed. S.J. Ettinger and E.C. Feldman), 112–116. St. Louis, MO: Elsevier Saunders.

Outerbridge, C.A., Marks, S., and Rogers, Q. (2002). Plasma amino acid concentrations in 36 dogs with histologically confirmed superficial necrolytic dermatitis (SND). *Vet. Dermatol.* 13: 177–187.

Patel, A., Whitbread, T.J., and McNeil, P.E. (1996). A case of metabolic epidermal necrosis in a cat. *Vet. Dermatol.* 7: 221–226.

Patterson, S. (1995). Food hypersensitivity in 20 dogs with skin and gastrointestinal signs. *J. Small Anim. Pract.* 36 (12): 529–534.

Peterson, L.L., Shaw, J.C., Acott, K.M. et al. (1984). Glucagonoma syndrome: *in vitro* evidence that glucagon increases epidermal arachidonic acid. *J. Am. Acad. Dermatol.* 11: 468–473.

Puigdemont, A., Brazis, P., Serra, M., and Fondati, A. (2006). Immunologic responses against hydrolyzed soy protein in dogs with experimentally induced soy hypersensitivity. *Am. J. Vet. Res.* 67: 484–488.

Raditic, D.M., Remillard, R.L., and Tater, K.C. (2011). ELISA testing for common food antigens in four dry dog foods used in dietary elimination trials. *J. Anim. Physiol. Anim. Nutr. (Berl.)* 95: 90–97.

Reedy, L.M., Miller, W.H., and Willemse, T. (1997). *Allergic Skin Diseases of Dogs and Cats.* Philadelphia, PA: WB Saunders.

Rees, C.A., Bauer, J.E., Burkholder, W.J. et al. (2001). Effects of dietary flax seed and sunflower seed supplementation on normal canine serum polyunsaturated fatty acids and skin and hair coat condition scores. *Vet. Dermatol.* 12: 111–117.

Rhoads, J.D., Fliegelman, M.T., and Panzer, L.M. (1942). The mechanism of delayed wound healing in the presence of hypoproteinemia. *J. Am. Med. Assoc.* 118 (1): 21–25.

Roudebush, P. and Wedekind, K.J. (2002). Zinc responsive dermatosis in dogs: letter to the editor. *Vet. Dermatol.* 13: 61.

Sampson, H.A. and Burks, A.W. (2009). Adverse reactions to foods. In: *Middleton's Allergy: Principles and Practice*, 6e (ed. E. Middleton), 1139–1167. St. Louis, MO: Mosby.

Scott, D.W. and Sheffy, B.E. (1987). Dermatosis in dogs caused by vitamin E deficiency. *Companion Anim. Pract.* 41: 42.

Scott, D.W., Miller, W.H., and Griffin, C.E. (2001). *Muller & Kirk's Small Animal Dermatology*, 6e. Philadelphia, PA: WB Saunders.

Shepartz, B. (1973). *Regulation of Amino Acid Metabolism in Mammals*. Philadelphia, PA: WB Saunders.

Shimomura, Y., Aoki, N., Rogers, M.A. et al. (2003). Characterization of human keratin-associated protein 1 family members. *J. Investig. Dermatol. Symp. Proc.* 8: 96–99.

Sohier, J., Jeanmougin, M., Lombrail, P., and Passa, P. (1980). Rapid improvement of skin lesions in glucagonoma with intravenous somatostatin infusion. *Lancet* 1: 40.

Sousa, C.A., Stannard, A.A., Ihrke, P.J., and Reinke, S.I. (1988). Dermatosis associated with feeding generic dog food: 13 cases (1981–1982). *J. Am. Vet. Med. Assoc.* 192: 676–680.

Tiffany, S., Parr, J.M., Templeman, J. et al. (2019). Assessment of dog owners' knowledge relating to the diagnosis and treatment of canine food allergies. *Can. Vet. J.* 60: 268–274.

Torres, S.M.F., Caywood, D.D., O'Brien, T.D. et al. (1997). Resolution of superficial necrolytic dermatitis following excision of a glucagon-secreting pancreatic neoplasm in a dog. *J. Am. Anim. Hosp. Assoc.* 33: 313–319.

Uchida, Y., Moon-Fanelli, A.A., Dodman, N.H. et al. (1997). Serum concentrations of zinc and copper in Bull Terriers with lethal acrodermatitis and tail-chasing behavior. *Am. J. Vet. Res.* 58: 808–810.

Van den Broek, A.H.M. and Simpson, J.W. (1992). Fat absorption in dogs with demodicosis or zinc responsive dermatosis. *Res. Vet. Sci.* 52: 117–119.

Van den Broek, A.H. and Stafford, W.L. (1988). Diagnostic value of zinc concentrations in serum, leucocytes and hair of dogs with zinc-responsive dermatosis. *Res. Vet. Sci.* 44: 41–44.

Verlinden, A., Hesta, M., and Millet, S. (2006). Food allergy in dogs and cats: A review. *Crit. Rev. Food Sci. Nutr.* 46: 259–273.

Waldron, M.K., Hannah, S.S., and Bauer, J.E. (2012). Plasma phospholipid fatty acid and ex vivo neutrophil responses are differentially altered in dogs fed fish- and linseed-oil containing diets at the same n-6:n-3 fatty acid ratio. *Lipids* 47 (4): 425–434.

Walton, D.K., Center, S.A., Scott, D.W., and Collins, K. (1986). Ulcerative dermatosis associated with diabetes mellitus in the dog. *J. Am. Vet. Med. Assoc.* 22: 79–88.

Wang, K., Zhou, B., Kuo, Y.M. et al. (2002). A novel number of zinc transporter family is defective in acrodermatitis enteropathica. *Am. J. Hum. Genet.* 71: 66.

Watson, T.D. (1998). Diet and skin disease in dogs and cats. *J. Nutr.* 128: 2783S–2789S.

Watson, A.L., Fray, T.R., Bailey, J. et al. (2006). Dietary constituents are able to play a beneficial role in canine epidermal barrier function. *Exp. Dermatol.* 15: 74–81.

Werner, A. and Harvey, R.G. (1995). Diet and veterinary dermatology. *WALTHAM Focus* 5: 11–19.

White, S.D. (1986). Food hypersensitivity in 30 dogs. *J. Am. Vet. Med. Assoc.* 188: 695–698.

White, S.D. (1998). Food allergy in dogs. *Compend. Contin. Educ. Pract. Vet.* 20: 261–269.

White, S.D. and Sequoia, D. (1989). Food hypersensitivity in cats: 14 cases (1982–1987). *J. Am. Vet. Med. Assoc.* 194 (5): 692–695.

White, S.D., Bourdeau, P., Rosychuk, R.A.W. et al. (2001). Zinc responsive dermatosis in dogs: 41 cases and literature review. *Vet. Dermatol.* 12: 101–109.

Wicke, C., Halliday, B., Allen, D. et al. (2000). Effects of steroids and retinoids on wound healing. *Arch. Surg.* 135: 1265–1270.

Willis-Mahn, C., Remillard, R., and Tater, K. (2014). ELISA testing for soy antigens in dry dog foods used in dietary elimination trials. *J. Am. Anim. Hosp. Assoc.* 50: 383–389.

Yu, S., Rogers, Q.S., and Morris, J.G. (2001). Effects of low levels of tyrosine on the hair coat of cats. *J. Small Anim. Pract.* 42: 176–180.

15

Nutritional Management of Kidney Disease
Yann Queau and Denise A. Elliott

Chronic Kidney Disease

Dietary therapy has remained at the forefront of the management of chronic kidney disease (CKD) for decades. There are two fundamental applications of nutrition in CKD: the first is the key role that certain nutrients have in altering disease progression, and the second is the role of nutrition in maintaining body weight, controlling uremic symptoms, and improving the quality of life.

Water

Compensatory polydipsia balances excessive fluid loss associated with osmotically driven polyuria; however, some patients will fail to consume sufficient water to prevent volume depletion. Therefore, methods should be employed that encourage the patient to drink and maintain fluid balance. An increase in water turnover can be achieved by feeding diets that contain ≥70% moisture (retorted can/pouch/tray, commercially frozen ± added water, extruded kibble soaked in sufficient water, or balanced home-cooked diets ± added water) or by increasing feeding frequency (increasing number of meals per day) (Anderson 1982; Kirschvink et al. 2005). The patient should have easy access to fresh and

clean water at all times. Providing water at several locations in the house may facilitate water intake. Cats have very sensitive whiskers and many seem to prefer a large bowl in which the whiskers do not touch the sides of the bowl. A variety of water types (home filtered, distilled, bottled, warm tap water, cold tap water) can be offered. Some pets prefer running water, and water fountains are now commercially available to encourage water intake. It is important to keep the food and water bowls away from the litter box area.

When fluid balance cannot be maintained with these techniques, cautious fluid supplementation should be used to prevent dehydration and attendant vascular depletion. Maintenance fluids (e.g. Plasma-Lyte® 56 [Baxter Healthcare, Deerfield, IL, USA], 40 mEq/l; Plasma-Lyte M, 40 mEq Na/l; Normosol™ M [ICU Medical, San Clemente, CA, USA], 40 mEq/l) can be administered subcutaneously daily by the pet's caretaker. Chronic administration of lactated Ringer's solution (LRS; 130 mEq/l) or normal saline (154 mEq/l) can cause hypernatremia if sufficient free water is not provided or consumed. Conversely, 5% dextrose in water can cause cellulitis and abscess formation and should not be administered subcutaneously.

Applied Veterinary Clinical Nutrition, Second Edition. Edited by Andrea J. Fascetti, Sean J. Delaney, Jennifer A. Larsen, and Cecilia Villaverde.

Energy

Sufficient energy needs to be provided to prevent endogenous protein catabolism to support gluconeogenesis that will result in malnutrition and exacerbation of azotemia. Prevention of malnutrition by ensuring adequate energy and nutrient intake is crucial in the management of kidney disease, and lower body condition scores (BCS) in dogs and body weights in cats have been associated with shorter survival (Parker and Freeman 2011; Freeman et al. 2016; Rudinsky et al. 2018). Often, weight loss has already occurred at the time of diagnosis (Greene et al. 2014; Freeman et al. 2016). The maintenance energy requirements are a good starting point to determine the amount of calories required each day. A commonly used equation indicates that adult cats require 1.2–1.4 × RER (where RER = resting energy requirement = 70 × (BW [Kg]$^{0.75}$)), and dogs require 1.6–1.8 × RER (see Chapter 3). This starting point should be adjusted based on serial determinations of body weight and BCS. Carbohydrate and fat provide the non-protein sources of energy in the diet. Fat provides approximately twice the energy per gram compared to carbohydrate. Therefore, fat increases the energy density of the diet, which allows the patient to obtain its nutritional requirements from a smaller volume of food. A smaller volume of food minimizes gastric distension, which can reduce the likelihood of nausea and vomiting unless gastric emptying is delayed too greatly.

Protein

Dietary protein modification has been a mainstay for the management of CKD for decades. However, over the years dietary protein restriction has also been the subject of much controversy. It is clearly helpful to consider dietary protein intake within two different contexts: implementation in stage I/II disease (IRIS 2023) with the primary aim of altering disease progression and implementation in stage III/ IV disease to control uremic symptoms.

Stage I/II: Progression

The intact nephron hypothesis is the prevailing theory of the progression of renal disease (Hostetter et al. 1981; Spencer et al. 2021). In this model, once a critical threshold of functioning nephrons is reached, the remaining surviving nephrons hypertrophy and undergo an increase in glomerular plasma flow and glomerular filtration rate (GFR). The capillary blood flow and pressure gradient across the capillary wall increase, and the chemical and electrical selective glomerular barriers are impaired as a result. These changes increase the amounts of protein entering the glomerular filtrate. Ultimately the tubular resorptive processes for protein are overwhelmed. The tubular cells are stimulated to secrete cytokines and inflammatory mediators, including endothelin-1, monocyte chemoattractant protein-1 (MCP-1), and RANTES (regulated on activation, normal T-cell expressed and secreted; also known as CCL5, chemokine ligand 5), which stimulate interstitial fibrosis and inflammation, contributing to progressive renal damage (Remuzzi and Bertani 1998). Accordingly, protein restriction has been demonstrated to slow the rate of progression of renal disease in rats and people by reducing renal blood flow, GFR, and proteinuria.

It is less certain if dietary protein restriction alters the progression of renal disease in cats or dogs, as most studies do not support it (Finco et al. 1985, 1992a, b, 1994, 1998, 1999; Robertson et al. 1986; Polzin et al. 1988; Brown et al. 1991b; Adams et al. 1993). However, these studies have been performed using the remnant kidney model, which does not necessarily reflect naturally occurring disease. In addition, some of the studies have been confounded by alterations in energy and/or phosphate intake in addition to protein restriction (Brown et al. 1990, 1991b; Finco et al. 1994).

Recent research suggests that the urine protein-to-creatinine ratio (UPC) is an independent risk factor for all-cause mortality of cats with naturally occurring CKD, cats with systemic hypertension, and uremic crisis

(King et al. 2006, 2007; Kuwahara et al. 2006; Syme et al. 2006; Jepson et al. 2007, 2009; Chakrabarti et al. 2012). Furthermore, studies in dogs with naturally occurring CKD have reported that a UPC value greater than 0.5 or 1 at initial evaluation is associated with an increased risk of uremic morbidity and mortality (Jacob et al. 2005; Wehner et al. 2008; Rudinsky et al. 2018), and the risk of adverse outcomes increases as the magnitude of proteinuria increases (Jacob et al. 2005). Therefore, therapeutic strategies should be employed to minimize proteinuria (Lees et al. 2005). Angiotensin-converting enzyme (ACE) inhibitor therapy has been shown to reduce glomerular capillary pressure and to lower the UPC, and angiotensin receptor blockers (ARB) may also be used alone or in combination with an ACE inhibitor for that purpose (Vaden and Elliott 2016).

The effect of dietary protein restriction on proteinuria in cats and dogs with CKD is not clear. Initial studies in feline remnant kidney models suggested a beneficial effect of protein restriction (28% vs. 52% dry matter [dm]) on the development of glomerular lesions (Adams et al. 1993, 1994). However, the effect of protein in this study was confounded with that of calorie intake, as the low-protein diet was consumed in lesser quantities, probably as a result of lower palatability. A subsequent study in cats to evaluate the role of protein versus calorie restriction showed that calorie – and not protein – restriction was responsible for the protective effect on renal morphology and proteinuria (Finco et al. 1998). There have not been any reports on the effect of dietary protein restriction and proteinuria in dogs with naturally occurring tubulointerstitial kidney disease. However, in studies using the remnant kidney model, there was no detrimental effect of feeding higher-protein diets (31–54% dm) compared to lower-protein diets (8–19% dm) on renal lesions, disease progression, or proteinuria (Robertson et al. 1986; Polzin et al. 1988; Bovee 1991; White et al. 1991; Finco et al. 1992a, 1994), except in one study where

dietary protein intake increased the magnitude of proteinuria (Polzin et al. 1988). Dietary protein restriction may be most beneficial to limit proteinuria in glomerular disease (see later), but for cats and dogs with naturally occurring tubulointerstitial CKD, further studies are required.

Nonetheless, the current recommendation of the International Renal Interest Society (IRIS) is to implement a restricted-protein diet in conjunction with an ACE inhibitor and/or an ARB for dogs with a UPC > 0.5 and for cats with a UPC > 0.4, regardless of the IRIS stage (IRIS 2023).

Stage III/IV: Uremia

Azotemia and uremia are due to the accumulation of protein metabolites derived from excessive dietary protein and degradation of endogenous protein. High protein intake exacerbates the azotemia and morbidity of CKD, while protein malnutrition is strongly correlated with morbidity and mortality (Polzin et al. 1983).

The rationale for formulating a diet that contains a reduced quantity of high-quality protein is based on the premise that controlled reduction of non-essential amino acids results in decreased production of nitrogenous wastes, with consequent amelioration or elimination of clinical signs, even though renal function remains essentially unchanged. Indeed, the various nitrogen waste products (blood urea nitrogen [BUN] is a routinely used surrogate marker), also called "uremic toxins," have a myriad of negative effects, such as nausea, cardiovascular effects, decreased red blood cell survival, blood loss by gastrointestinal ulcerations, or impaired platelet function (Vanholder et al. 2003, 2018).

Studies have clearly shown that modifying dietary protein intake can reduce BUN and provide clinical benefits to cats and dogs with CKD (Polzin et al. 1983; Finco et al. 1985; Polzin and Osborne 1988; Leibetseder and Neufeld 1991; Hansen et al. 1992; Adams et al. 1993; Elliott et al. 2000b; Jacob et al. 2002;

Ross et al. 2006). Therefore, every patient symptomatic for stage III/IV CKD should benefit from a protein-restricted diet, while simultaneously avoiding excessive restriction to prevent the risk of protein malnutrition (i.e. hypoalbuminemia, anemia, weight loss, and/or loss of muscle mass).

The minimal dietary protein requirements of cats and dogs with CKD are not known, but have been presumed to be similar to the minimal protein requirements of healthy animals: for cats, 3.97 g/kg $BW^{0.67}$ or 40 g/Mcal; and for dogs, 2.62 g/kg $BW^{0.75}$ or 20 g/Mcal (NRC 2006). However, in recent years the degree of protein restriction adequate for animals with kidney disease has caused some controversy, especially in cats (Larsen 2016; Polzin and Churchill 2016; Scherk and Laflamme 2016). Indeed, it has been suggested that the true protein requirement of cats to maintain lean body mass is higher than previously determined, which might in part be due to the lack of sensitivity of classic assessment methods such as nitrogen balance (Laflamme and Hannah 2013). Nevertheless, there is to date no published evidence that cats fed protein concentrations close to the published recommended allowance develop protein malnutrition. In the study by Laflamme and Hannah evaluating body composition by dual X-ray absorptiometry (DEXA), there was no statistical difference in lean body mass change between the cats fed the lowest- or the highest-protein diets for two months (Laflamme and Hannah 2013). Likewise, lean body mass assessed by DEXA was maintained in older cats with early CKD (IRIS I/II) fed their maintenance energy needs with a diet containing 67 g protein/Mcal (~24% ME) over six months (Hall et al. 2019). In cats with naturally occurring CKD, there was also no apparent negative effect of feeding a protein-restricted diet (23% ME) on body weight and BCS over two years, although lean body mass could not be evaluated in this clinical setting (Ross et al. 2006).

The complexity of this controversy is that dietary protein concentration is not the only factor to consider for maintenance of lean body mass. Overall caloric intake (which ultimately affects the amount of protein ingested), protein quality (i.e. digestibility and essential amino acid profile), the role of other nutrients (such as carbohydrate) in protein turnover, and acid–base status can all contribute to changes in lean body mass and may in fact dictate the optimal protein concentration to be fed to an individual animal with kidney disease. Finally, it should be remembered that dietary protein is also a main source of phosphorus, a nutrient of great importance in the management of CKD, and that careless dietary supplementation with protein may therefore have deleterious consequences.

Based on current evidence, the consensus is to implement a restricted-protein diet to decrease azotemia in cats and dogs with stage III/IV disease and also to consider it from stage II as part of a "renal diet," especially if it enables dietary phosphorus restriction (IRIS 2023; Sparkes et al. 2016).

Phosphate

Phosphate retention is one of the most common regulatory derangements of CKD that arises secondary to reduced glomerular filtration of phosphorus. It occurs early in CKD and plays a key role in the genesis and progression of fibroblast growth factor (FGF)-23 increase, renal secondary hyperparathyroidism, hypocalcemia, relative or absolute deficiency of 1,25-dihydroxyvitamin D (calcitriol), and renal osteodystrophy (Nagode and Chew 1992; Barber and Elliott 1998; Tang et al. 2021b). CKD–mineral and bone disorder (CKD-MBD) is the term used to describe these clinical, biochemical, hormonal, and imaging abnormalities. Clinical consequences described in small animals include bone resorption (Shipov et al. 2014, 2017) and soft tissue mineralization, such as gastric or renal tubular mineralization (Chakrabarti et al. 2013; McLeland et al. 2014) when the calcium–phosphate product exceeds 70 mg^2/dl^2. Renal mineralization will promote interstitial inflammation and fibrosis, and may contribute to progressive renal damage (Nagode and Chew 1992). Dogs with higher serum phosphate and Ca-PO$_4$ product have a poorer prognosis (Lippi et al. 2014; Rudinsky et al. 2018), and in cats high serum phosphate is associated with poorer outcome (King et al. 2007; Boyd et al. 2008; Geddes et al. 2015).

In the traditional "trade-off" hypothesis, the initial increase in both intracellular and plasma phosphate concentration triggers parathyroid hormone (PTH) synthesis and secretion. PTH works at the level of the proximal tubule to decrease phosphate reabsorption and so increases the excretion of phosphate, which compensates for the reduced glomerular filtration of phosphorus. However, the trade-off for maintaining normophosphatemia is that increased PTH concentrations also trigger the release of calcium and phosphate from bone via the stimulation of calcitriol synthesis by the kidneys. As renal mass further decreases, calcitriol production becomes insufficient to limit hyperparathyroidism. Nevertheless, this hypothesis does not explain all the metabolic changes observed in renal secondary hyperparathyroidism, especially calcitriol concentrations that are below what would be expected from decreased renal mass only (de Brito Galvao et al. 2013). FGF-23 is a phosphatonin produced by osteocytes and osteoblasts, which acts with its co-factor Klotho to decrease serum phosphate. This is achieved by decreasing phosphate renal tubular reabsorption and inhibiting 1α hydroxylase activity in the kidney, thus lowering calcitriol synthesis and subsequently intestinal phosphorus absorption. In addition, FGF-23 decreases PTH production, although this might be impaired in CKD due to lower Klotho expression in parathyroid glands (de Brito Galvao et al. 2013; Geddes et al. 2013a). FGF-23 rises early in CKD, and its concentration increases with the stage of disease in both cats and dogs (Finch et al. 2013; Geddes et al. 2013a; Harjes et al. 2017; Miyakawa et al. 2020, 2022) as a result of decreased glomerular filtration and phosphate

retention. In addition, FGF-23 is an independent predictor of the development of azotemia (Finch et al. 2013), CKD progression, and mortality (Geddes et al. 2015) in both dogs and cats.

Studies have clearly shown that by minimizing hyperphosphatemia, secondary hyperparathyroidism and its sequelae can be prevented (Ross et al. 1982; Brown et al. 1991a; Finco et al. 1992a, b; Nagode and Chew 1992; Barber et al. 1999). In one study of dogs with surgically induced reduced renal function, dogs fed a low-phosphorus diet (0.44% dm) for 24 months had a 75% survival versus a 33% survival in dogs fed a high-phosphorus diet (1.44% dm) (Finco et al. 1992b). Renal function also deteriorated more rapidly in the high-phosphorus group. Ross et al. reported that cats with laboratory-induced reduced renal mass that were fed a phosphorus-restricted diet (0.24% dm) showed little or no histologic change compared with cats fed a "typical" diet containing 1.56% dm phosphorus. The cats in the "typical" dietary phosphate group had evidence of mineralization, fibrosis, and mononuclear cell infiltration in the renal tissue (Ross et al. 1982). The efficacy of dietary phosphate restriction in cats with naturally occurring CKD has also been published. Dietary phosphate restriction alone or as part of a modified diet for the management of CKD is clearly associated with a reduction in both plasma phosphate, PTH concentration, and FGF-23 (Barber et al. 1999; Elliott et al. 2000b; Geddes et al. 2013b). Furthermore, control of phosphate concentrations has been associated with a reduction in all-cause mortality in cats with naturally occurring CKD (Elliott et al. 2000b). The mechanism of how phosphate restriction slows progression of renal disease is not fully understood. It may be related to decreased phosphate retention, decreased soft tissue mineralization, prevention of secondary hyperparathyroidism, or, most likely, a combination of these factors (Boyd et al. 2008).

IRIS recommends that the phosphate concentration should be maintained at 2.7–4.5 mg/dl for stage II; <5 mg/dl for stage III, and

<6 mg/dl for stage IV disease. The first step to control plasma phosphate concentration is to limit the dietary intake of phosphate. The plasma phosphate concentration should be reassessed within two weeks of implementing dietary restriction. Commercial or homemade renal diets have different degrees of phosphorus restriction; if the first attempt is not effective in controlling the plasma phosphate concentration, a diet with lower phosphorus content can be selected. Plasma total and ionized calcium should be monitored, as hypercalcemia has been reported in cats with CKD (van den Broek et al. 2017), and may develop when feeding phosphorus-restricted diets (Geddes et al. 2021; Schauf et al. 2021; Tang et al. 2021a; van den Broek et al. 2022). It has been resolved by feeding diets with less severe phosphorus restriction (e.g. selected "senior" diets) (Geddes et al. 2021; Schauf et al. 2021); feeding renal diets with a lower calcium content and Ca : P ratio may also be attempted.

If dietary restriction alone does not allow plasma phosphate maintenance within the recommended ranges, intestinal phosphate binders should be added to the treatment plan (Table 15.1). Intestinal phosphate binding agents combine with phosphate contained in dietary and digestive secretions to form insoluble complexes that are excreted in the feces. They should be mixed with the food prior to feeding to ensure maximal phosphate binding

Table 15.1 List of intestinal phosphorus binding agents and typical doses recommended.

Aluminum hydroxide	60–90 mg/kg/day
Calcium acetate	60–90 mg/kg/day
Calcium carbonate	60–90 mg/kg/day
Calcium carbonate + chitosan	200 mg/kg twice daily
Sevelamer hydrochloride	50–160 mg/kg twice daily
Lanthanum carbonate	12.5–25 mg/kg/day
Lanthanum carbonate octahydrate	400 mg once or twice daily

effectiveness. The plasma phosphate concentration should continue to be monitored every 2–4 weeks, and dosage adjustments made accordingly until the target plasma phosphate concentration is achieved. Side effects of phosphate binders can include hyporexia/gastrointestinal signs (e.g. aluminum hydroxide, sevelamer hydroxide, lanthanum carbonate), aluminum toxicity that causes neurologic signs (i.e. aluminum hydroxide), and effects on vitamin (especially vitamin K) and possibly taurine status (e.g. sevelamer hydrochloride).

Given these side effects, dietary phosphate restriction remains the preferred means to reduce dietary intake. There are no indications for phosphate binders to be used alone and in the absence of concurrent dietary phosphate restriction.

Calcitriol replacement therapy has been advocated by some authors to help limit renal secondary hyperparathyroidism and additional renoprotective effects (Nagode et al. 1996; de Brito Galvao et al. 2013). The serum phosphate and ionized calcium concentrations should be within the reference range/interval prior to beginning therapy, and hyperparathyroidism should be confirmed by PTH concentration measurement. Calcitriol should not be given with meals because it enhances intestinal calcium and phosphate absorption. Serum calcium and phosphate concentrations need to be continuously monitored to avoid hypercalcemia and soft tissue mineralization. The risk of hypercalcemia is heightened by the concurrent administration of calcium-based intestinal phosphate binding agents (i.e. calcium acetate and calcium carbonate). The serum PTH concentration should return to normal or almost normal within several weeks of initiating therapy.

Electrolytes

Sodium

Sodium restriction has historically been recommended for patients with CKD. The rationale for this restriction was based on the reduced ability of the remaining nephrons to excrete sodium, and the concern that whole-body sodium accumulation would contribute to the development of hypertension. Hypertension is indeed more common in cats with CKD, its risk increases with time and IRIS stage (Bijsmans et al. 2015; Hori et al. 2018), and it has been implicated as a factor that contributes to the progression of CKD. Approximately 20–32% of cats with naturally occurring CKD have arterial blood pressures >175 mmHg (23.3 kPa), which places them at severe risk of target organ (i.e. kidney, eye, brain, heart) damage secondary to hypertension (Syme et al. 2002; Hori et al. 2018). Jacob et al. (2003) reported that 31% of dogs with naturally occurring CKD had systolic blood pressure >160 mmHg (21.3 kPa). Dogs with naturally occurring CKD and a systolic blood pressure >180 mmHg (24 kPa) were more likely to develop a uremic crisis and to die compared with dogs that had a normal systolic blood pressure (Jacob et al. 2003). Furthermore, the risk of developing a uremic crisis and of dying increased significantly as systolic blood pressure increased.

There have not been any published studies to demonstrate that dietary sodium restriction will alleviate hypertension or slow disease progression. In healthy cats and dogs, dietary sodium intake up to 3.1 g/Mcal in cats and 4.1 g/Mcal in dogs does not affect blood pressure or renal or cardiac functions (Xu et al. 2009, 2016; Reynolds et al. 2013; Chetboul et al. 2014; Nguyen et al. 2017). Altering sodium intake from 0.5 to 3.25 g Na/Mcal did not influence the development of hypertension nor affect GFR in dogs with surgically induced renal reduction (Greco et al. 1994a, b). A study in cats with surgically induced kidney disease reported that sodium restriction (0.6–0.7 g/Mcal) activated the renin-angiotensin-aldosterone system (RAAS), significantly lowered plasma potassium concentration, and had no effect on arterial blood pressure (Buranakarl et al. 2004). Hansen et al. (1992) reported that changes in dietary sodium intake did not affect blood pressure in nine dogs with naturally

occurring CKD. Syme (2003) reported that systolic blood pressure did not change following the introduction of a sodium-restricted "renal care" diet to cats with naturally occurring CKD. Plasma aldosterone concentration and plasma renin activity were higher when cats were consuming a sodium-restricted renal diet. Consistent with IRIS recommendations and the American College of Veterinary Internal Medicine (ACVIM) consensus statement on hypertension (Brown et al. 2007), there is currently no evidence to suggest that lowering dietary sodium will reduce blood pressure in cats or dogs with CKD. At the same time, moderately sodium-restricted therapeutic diets for the nutritional management of renal disease remain common and recommended (Pouchelon et al. 2015). Antihypertensive therapy is clearly and universally recommended to maintain the systolic blood pressure <160 mmHg (21.3 kPa) in cats and dogs with CKD (IRIS 2023; Brown et al. 2007). Note that ACE inhibitors can lead to hyperkalemia, as summarized later.

Potassium

Hypokalemia has been well recognized for decades as a complication of CKD. The mechanism of action is unclear and includes inadequate potassium intake, acidifying diets, and/or increased urinary losses. Hypokalemia occurs in about 20% of cats with CKD, although this number may underestimate the true prevalence of whole-body potassium depletion (DiBartola et al. 1987; Theisen et al. 1997). Hypokalemia can occur at any stage of disease. Elliott and Syme (2003) reported hypokalemia in 14.3% of cats with stage II, 25% of cats with stage III, and 30% of cats in stage IV disease. Segev et al. (2010) reported that hypokalemia occurred in 14% of dogs with naturally occurring CKD.

Questions have also been raised regarding hypokalemia as a cause or a consequence of feline CKD (Dow and Fettman 1992). An association between CKD and hypokalemia has been reported in cats (Dow et al. 1989). Furthermore, feeding an acidifying or potassium-depleted diet has been associated with naturally occurring CKD and a decline in GFR (Dow et al. 1987, 1990; DiBartola et al. 1993). Dow and Fettman hypothesized that potassium depletion may lead to a self-perpetuating cycle of renal damage and further potassium loss (Dow and Fettman 1992). However, the causal relationship between whole-body potassium deficit and progressive renal injury remains to be proven.

Clinically, hypokalemia is generally mild, without overt clinical signs. Hypokalemia causes generalized muscle weakness and pain that may present as cervical ventroflexion and a stiff, stilted gait (Dow et al. 1987). Hypokalemia impairs protein synthesis, promotes weight loss, and contributes to polyuria by decreasing the renal responsiveness to ADH (antidiuretic hormone). Hypokalemia also appears to be associated with an increased risk of systemic hypertension in cats with CKD (Syme et al. 2002).

Potassium supplementation is indicated when the serum potassium concentration is less than 4 mEq/l (4 mmol/l) (Sparkes et al. 2016). This may be achieved by oral potassium gluconate or potassium citrate supplementation (1–4 mEq per cat every [q]12 h) (Sieberg and Quimby 2020). Potassium chloride can be acidifying and therefore counterproductive for supplementation in CKD. Clinical improvement in appetite and activity level has been noted following potassium supplementation, although palatability of the supplement may be a concern in some cats. Muscle weakness typically resolves within five days of institution of therapy. However, a randomized controlled clinical trial failed to identify any beneficial effect of potassium gluconate supplementation on blood pressure or kidney function in cats with naturally occurring CKD (Elliott and Syme 2003). Side effects of potassium supplementation include gastrointestinal irritation, ulceration, nausea, and vomiting. The potassium dosage should be adjusted by monitoring the serum potassium concentration and response to supplementation.

It is important to note that not all cats with CKD are hypokalemic. Indeed, hyperkalemia was reported in 13% of cats with CKD in one study (Dow et al. 1989), and in 22% of cats with end-stage renal disease in another study (Elliott and Barber 1998). Segev et al. (2010) reported that 71 of 152 (41%) of dogs with naturally occurring CKD had at least one reported episode of hyperkalemia, defined as a serum potassium concentration above the reference range/interval of 5.3 mmol/l. Furthermore, 16% of dogs had at least one episode in which the serum potassium concentration was >6.5 mmol/l. Postulated contributors to hyperkalemia include advanced kidney disease, dietary potassium intake, and the concurrent use of medications such as ACE inhibitors.

Management of hyperkalemia includes ruling out contributory factors such as thrombocytosis and medications. A complete dietary history, including treats and nutritional supplements, should be obtained to ascertain the patient's daily potassium intake. This information is used to identify and implement a dietary regime that would provide less dietary potassium. It is important to note that hyperkalemia can occur in dogs with naturally occurring CKD that receive therapeutic renal diets (Segev et al. 2010). In this situation, a potassium-reduced, commercial renal diet or a home-prepared diet specifically formulated for the patient by a board certified veterinary nutritionist® or a Diplomate of the European College of Veterinary and Comparative Nutrition should be prescribed.

Acid–Base Balance

The kidneys are essential in the regulation of acid–base balance. One of their key roles is to excrete metabolically derived non-volatile acid (e.g. sulfates, hydrogen ions). As renal function declines, the capacity to excrete hydrogen ions and reabsorb bicarbonate ions is lost and metabolic acidosis ensues. Metabolic acidosis results in increased renal ammoniagenesis, which has been associated with activation of complement and may contribute to the progression of kidney disease. Metabolic acidosis increases the catabolism and degradation of skeletal muscle protein, disrupts intracellular metabolism, and promotes dissolution of bone mineral. These cellular disruptions exacerbate azotemia, contribute to the loss of lean body mass, and promote renal osteodystrophy. Metabolic acidosis also increases the likelihood that hypokalemia will occur or exacerbates pre-existing hypokalemia as potassium moves out of the cells in response to metabolic acidosis and is lost in urine.

Metabolic acidosis is typically evident in stage III–IV disease (Elliott et al. 2003a, b; Slawuta et al. 2020). Dibartola et al. (1987) reported that 62.7% of cats with CKD had a bicarbonate concentration <15 mmol/l. Another study of 59 cats with naturally occurring CKD reported that 15% of cats with late-stage III and 52.6% of cats with stage IV CKD had evidence of acidosis (Elliott et al. 2003b).

The blood bicarbonate concentration should be maintained in the range of 18–24 mmol/l. Therefore, alkalinization therapy (e.g. potassium citrate, sodium bicarbonate, calcium carbonate) should be implemented when the bicarbonate concentration is <18 mmol/l. Dietary protein restriction results in the consumption of reduced quantities of protein-derived acid precursors; however, this alone is rarely adequate to prevent metabolic acidosis. The choice and dose of alkalinization therapy will need to be individualized for each patient. Factors to consider include the effect on palatability when added to the diet, the presence of hypokalemia (where potassium salts will be chosen), the presence of hyperkalemia (where potassium salts will be avoided), the presence of hyperphosphatemia (where calcium salts may be best because of their phosphate binding capabilities provided hypercalcemia does not occur), and the concurrent presence of congestive heart failure (where sodium salts may contribute to fluid overload).

Alkalinization therapy will improve the clinical signs of anorexia, lethargy, nausea, vomiting, muscle weakness, and weight loss, in addition to limiting the catabolic effects of metabolic acidosis on protein metabolism. It remains to be determined if there is any beneficial effect to provide alkali supplementation prior to the detection of metabolic acidosis.

Long-Chain Omega-3 Fatty Acids

Long-chain omega-3 fatty acids (eicosapentaenoic acid [EPA] and docosahexaenoic acid [DHA]) compete with the long-chain omega-6 fatty acid arachidonic acid (AA), and alter eicosanoid, thromboxane, and leukotriene production (Bauer et al. 1999). Studies in laboratory-induced renal disease in dogs have reported that supplementation with menhaden fish oil (rich in long-chain omega-3 polyunsaturated fatty acids) was considered to be reno-protective compared with safflower oil (varietal rich in omega-6 polyunsaturated fatty acids; and notably not rich in the omega-9 monounsaturated fatty acid oleic acid, like the common variety available now) and beef tallow (rich in saturated fatty acids) (Brown et al. 1998). Supplementation with menhaden fish oil lowered glomerular capillary pressure, reduced proteinuria, and slowed progressive decline in the GFR (Brown et al. 1998).

Omega-6 fatty acids appeared to be detrimental to renal disease (Brown et al. 2000). Brown et al. reported that supplementation with omega-6 polyunsaturated fatty acids (using an omega-6 rich variety of safflower oil) to dogs with laboratory-induced CKD was associated with increased glomerular capillary pressure, glomerular enlargement, and increased eicosanoid excretion rates.

Similar studies have not been reported in cats. Lipid metabolism is complex in cats as they lack the enzyme delta-6-desaturase, suggesting that providing EPA and DHA may be particularly important in this species. However, one study suggests that the provision of dietary long-chain omega-3 fatty acids from marine sources versus dietary shorter-chain omega-3 fatty acids from plant sources is also important in the dog (Waldron et al. 2012). One retrospective study of 175 cats with CKD suggested that survival time was longer for cats fed diets with high concentrations of EPA (Plantinga et al. 2005). It is clear that further research is needed to evaluate the efficacy of long-chain omega-3 fatty acid supplementation in cats and dogs with CKD.

Fiber

Fiber is a simple term for a complex family of plant components that cannot be digested by the digestive tract of the dog or cat. Fiber can be broadly classified as soluble, insoluble, fermentable, non-fermentable, or mucilage. Fiber can have multiple beneficial effects on gastrointestinal health and function, from supporting the microbiota to regulating gastrointestinal motility. Alterations in gastrointestinal motility (alterations in duodenojejunal motility and decreased colonic transit time) have been reported in a study of dogs with laboratory-induced renal disease (Lefebvre et al. 2001). Cats with CKD have been found to be at higher risk of constipation (Benjamin and Drobatz 2020), with fewer bowel movements than healthy cats on average (Jones et al. 2022). The causes are numerous and include dehydration, reduced gastrointestinal motility, and as a side effect of therapeutic agents, including phosphate binders and calcium channel blockers. Therefore, dietary fiber may have a beneficial role to help promote gastrointestinal health in patients with CKD.

Fermentable fiber promotes colonic bacterial multiplication; however, a source of ammonia nitrogen is required for bacterial growth. Nitrogen sources include dietary protein that escapes small intestinal digestion, endogenous proteins (pancreatic, intestinal secretions), sloughed intestinal mucosal cells, and blood urea that diffuses across the intestines with water movement. In dogs with CKD, extrarenal pathways of urea excretion (i.e. mostly enteric) become predominant with more advanced stages of the disease (Steinbach et al. 2010). It has been hypothesized that supplementing the diet with fermentable fiber as a source of carbohydrate nutrition for gastrointestinal bacteria will result in the subsequent utilization of blood urea as a source of nitrogen for growth. Therefore, fecal nitrogen excretion in the form of the bacterial cell mass will be increased, urinary nitrogen excretion will be decreased, and the need for protein restriction will be alleviated. Studies with dietary fermentable carbohydrate in partially nephrectomized rats have documented a decrease in blood urea concentration; however, there was no net change in total nitrogen excretion, just a shift from urinary to fecal excretion (Younes et al. 1997, 1998). There have not been any studies published to date to validate this hypothesis in cats or dogs. Furthermore, the clinical relevance of a reduction in blood urea concentration is unknown, as urea is a nitrogen biomarker and not considered a uremic toxin. The traditional uremic toxins are classified as middle molecules and hence are too large to move freely with water across the intestinal barrier. More research is needed in this area before widespread recommendations can be made.

Antioxidants

Oxidation is the loss of an electron from a chemical species. Removal or loss of an electron from a chemical compound produces a free radical. Free radicals are highly reactive as they search for an electron from surrounding molecules to stabilize their structure. Free radicals are able to attack numerous compounds in the body, including lipids, proteins, and nucleic acids. Oxidative damage to these core biological components has been hypothesized to be involved in the etiology or progression of a number of diseases or conditions, including cancer, atherosclerosis, arthritis, aging, cardiovascular disease, and diabetes mellitus. Free radical damage has also been implicated as a contributing factor in the progression of

CKD in humans (Cochrane and Ricardo 2003; Locatelli et al. 2003).

Humans with CKD have been shown to have oxidative stress by evidence of lower concentrations of vitamin E and vitamin C, and high concentrations of markers of lipid peroxidation (Cochrane and Ricardo 2003; Locatelli et al. 2003). It has been hypothesized that cats and dogs with CKD may also have oxidative stress (Brown 2008). Silva et al. found that oxidative stress was greater in dogs with naturally occurring renal disease than in control dogs (Silva et al. 2013). Two studies, in a limited number of cats with naturally occurring kidney disease, have shown contradictory results regarding antioxidant capacity, but both studies suggest that antioxidant defense mechanisms are activated (Keegan and Webb 2010; Krofic Zel et al. 2014). This is supported by two other studies, reporting higher concentrations of lipid peroxidation products – markers of oxidative stress – in limited numbers of cats with various stages of naturally occurring CKD compared to healthy controls (Valle et al. 2019; Granick et al. 2021). However, in those studies, diet was not controlled among groups, and differences in dietary antioxidant supply may have affected the results.

The body contains a number of compounds and systems designed to protect against oxidative stress. This protective system includes enzymes such as superoxide dismutase and GSH reductase, peptides such as glutathione, and some vitamins, such as tocopherols, vitamin A and associated retinoids, and vitamin C. Various minerals are also required for the activity of many antioxidant enzymes. Nutritional interventions in which exogenous antioxidants such as vitamin E, vitamin C, taurine, carotenoids, and flavanols are added to the diet are also an effective way to promote a more favorable redox status in the body so that less oxidative damage can occur (Brown 2008). Together, the antioxidant systems collectively function to scavenge and neutralize free radicals and minimize oxidative stress.

Studies in rats and humans have suggested that vitamin E supplementation may slow the progression of CKD by modulating tubulointerstitial injury, proteinuria, and glomerulosclerosis (Hahn et al. 1998, 1999; Tahzib et al. 1999; Tain et al. 2007). Yu and Paetau-Robinson (2006) reported that supplementation with vitamin E, beta-carotene, and vitamin C in cats with naturally occurring stage II CKD reduced markers of DNA damage. Brown reported that vitamin E, carotenoids, and lutein supplementation to dogs with surgically induced renal mass reduction slowed the rate of reduction of the GFR, compared to dogs that did not receive antioxidant supplementation (Brown 2008). Therefore, it is clear that dietary antioxidants can be beneficial to cats and dogs with CKD. What remains to be determined, by further studies, is the actual dose and synergistic combination of dietary antioxidants that are most effective.

Nutrients That Target the Endothelium

Endothelial cells have a key role in maintaining vascular homeostasis by the generation of nitric oxide via the endothelial enzyme nitric oxide synthase. Nitric oxide has a critical role in renal hemodynamics and urine production by dilating both the afferent and efferent arterioles, augmenting estimated GFR (GFRe), and influencing the renal handling of sodium along the tubule segments. Accordingly, endothelial dysfunction is characterized by alterations in vasodilation and vasoconstriction, increased oxidative stress and inflammation, deregulation of thrombosis and fibrinolysis, and abnormal smooth muscle cell proliferation. Endothelial dysfunction is thought to contribute to systemic hypertension, glomerular pathology, progressive proteinuria, and tubulointerstitial inflammation and fibrosis in human and animal models of disease.

Endothelial dysfunction arises by decreased bioavailability of nitric oxide at the vascular level. There are several proposed mechanisms of action by which endothelial cell dysfunction arises in renal disease. These include a reduction in the renal synthesis of L-arginine, the precursor of nitric oxide; oxidative stress, which reduces nitric oxide release from the endothelium and stimulates the production of profibrotic mediators from the endothelium; and the accumulation of asymmetric dimethylarginine (ADMA), an inhibitor of endothelial nitric oxide synthase. Increasing attention is currently focused on ADMA, which is an endogenous amino acid that is structurally similar to L-arginine. ADMA competes with L-arginine as a substrate for endogenous nitric oxide synthase. Jepson et al. (2008) reported that ADMA accumulates in cats with naturally occurring stage II, III, and IV CKD, and the plasma concentration of ADMA correlated with the creatinine concentration.

There have not been any studies to date to evaluate the effect of nutrients on endothelial cell dysfunction in cats or dogs with CKD. However, there are several approaches that can be considered, including supplementation with L-arginine, flavanols, and antioxidants such as vitamin E, vitamin C, taurine, lutein, lycopene, or beta-carotene. L-arginine may increase the production of nitric oxide and counteract the inhibition induced by ADMA. However, the effect of L-arginine supplementation on human and rodent models of CKD is controversial, and further studies are clearly warranted before widespread supplementation can be recommended (Cherla and Jaimes 2004). Flavanols, a subclass of flavonoids, are polyphenolic antioxidants that are found in a variety of plants. Flavanols increase the endothelial production of nitric oxide. They are effective antioxidants that trap free radicals generated by circulatory disorders within the glomeruli that occur in CKD and have an antihypertensive action.

Clinical Efficacy

Several studies have been published evaluating the effect of dietary therapy in patients with naturally occurring, azotemic CKD (Leibetseder and Neufeld 1991; Elliott et al. 2000b; Jacob et al. 2002; Ross et al. 2006). To date, these studies have used "renal" diets that included a combination of nutrient alterations compared to maintenance diets. Therefore, it is not possible to speculate which of the nutrient alterations is responsible for differences in outcome between groups. Nevertheless, the evidence from these clinical studies indicates that nutritional intervention is clearly warranted for pets with naturally occurring CKD.

The effect of a modified-protein, low-phosphate diet on the outcome of 50 cats with stable, naturally occurring stage II/III CKD has been reported by Elliott et al. (2000b). In the study, 29 of 50 cats received a modified-protein, low-phosphate diet, and the remaining 21 of 50 cats remained on their normal diets. The median survival time of the cats fed the modified-protein, low-phosphate diet was significantly greater than the cats fed their normal maintenance diet (633 vs. 264 days, P < 0.0036). The results of this study suggest that feeding a renal diet to cats with chronic renal failure will double their life expectancy.

Ross et al. (2006), using a randomized controlled masked clinical trial, evaluated the effect of a renal diet on time to uremic crisis or renal death in 45 cats with naturally occurring stage II/III CKD. The renal diet was associated with a significantly lower number of uremic crises and renal-related deaths compared to a maintenance diet.

Jacob et al. (2002) evaluated the effect of a modified-protein, low-phosphate diet on the outcome of 28 dogs with stable, naturally occurring stage III CKD. Dogs that were fed a renal diet had a 70% reduction in the relative risk of developing a uremic crisis, remained free of uremic signs almost two and a half times longer, and had a median survival that was three times longer than dogs with CKD that were fed a maintenance diet.

With the advent of the early renal disease biomarker symmetric dimethylarginine (SDMA), which may detect CKD before the onset of azotemia (IRIS stage I) (Hall et al. 2014, 2016c), the question of earlier dietary intervention is raised. There is to date no controlled study evaluating the effect of single or combined diet modifications on the progression of renal disease to later stages or on survival. Some studies in non-azotemic geriatric cats and dogs evaluating a diet supplemented with fish oil, antioxidants (i.e. lipoic acid, vitamins E and C), and L-carnitine reported a steadier SDMA over six months compared to other diets of the human companion's choice, the composition of which was not reported (Hall et al. 2016a, b). However, the biological relevance of this is unknown, and interpretation of the results is made difficult by the variability of diet composition across the population and the small number of animals evaluated. Additional studies are therefore warranted to be able to make evidence-based recommendations on dietary intervention in stage I CKD. Better understanding of calcium phosphorus metabolism at this early stage of the disease is also needed.

Administration

The efficacy of nutritional therapy depends on the diet being fed consistently and exclusively. Humans afflicted with kidney disease, and presumably cats and dogs with CKD, have altered senses of smell and taste. In one owner survey, 52% of affected cats had poor appetite, requiring some coaxing of their diet (Markovich et al. 2015). Cats in particular also have a strong likelihood of developing food aversion, which arises when adverse events such as nausea, hospitalization, and blood sampling are associated with feeding. In this regard, it is advisable not to institute dietary changes when patients are undergoing intravenous fluid therapy to induce diuresis and/or are hospitalized. Rather, the renal support diet should be instituted in the home environment. In addition, the diet must be palatable enough to help overcome a potentially reduced sense of smell and taste.

Practical measures to improve food intake include the use of highly odorous foods, warming the food prior to feeding (Eyre et al. 2022),

and stimulating eating by positive reinforcement with petting and stroking behavior. Appetite stimulants may be judiciously administered. Mirtazapine administered orally or as a transdermal ointment on the inner pinna every other day was shown to be effective to increase appetite scores and body weight of cats with stages II–III CKD over a three-week period (Quimby and Lunn 2013; Quimby et al. 2020). Capromorelin, an orally administered ghrelin receptor agonist, is approved by the US Food and Drug Administration (FDA) for the management of weight loss in cats with CKD. However, in cases where adequate daily energy intake cannot be achieved, more aggressive therapy employing enteral feeding tubes is clinically indicated (Elliott et al. 2000c; Ross 2016). Feeding tubes (see Chapter 20) should be instituted for nutritional support upon documentation of a 10–15% loss of body weight in conjunction with a declining body condition score and a history of poor dietary intake. Feeding tubes are also advantageous, as they circumvent the need for subcutaneous fluid therapy (since water intake can be controlled by the caretaker) and ease the administration of oral medications.

Concurrent Diseases

CKD is typically a disease of middle-aged to older pets, and it is not unusual for them to have two or more chronic disease conditions. In one survey, 40% of cats with CKD also had concurrent ailments, with hyperthyroidism, heart disease, and inflammatory bowel disease being the most common (Markovich et al. 2015). In some situations, the nutritional management of these diseases can be diametrically opposed. An example is the management of a dog with CKD and a history of recurrent pancreatitis or hyperlipidemia, where one might wish to increase dietary fat to increase palatability and energy density for the CKD, but also need to decrease dietary fat given the fat intolerance. Or a cat with diabetes mellitus might benefit from a reduction in dietary carbohydrate, but CKD dietary management inherently results in a higher dietary carbohydrate concentration as protein-rich foods that are often a main source of phosphorus and fat are reduced. Clearly, for many of these disease combinations the ideal commercial therapeutic diet may not initially appear to be available. In some situations, a solution can be found in the plethora of commercial diets specifically designed for renal disease by careful analysis of the true needs of the patient, coupled with a detailed review of the nutritional features of the diets, which differ in both ingredients and concentrations of nutrients. Furthermore, some diets specifically designed for mature or senior pets may have controlled levels of phosphate and/or fat concentrations that are adequate to control the serum phosphate concentrations for pets with early-stage disease or chronic pancreatitis. In situations where a commercial diet cannot be identified, a compromise can be made to select a diet that meets the needs of the most life-threatening disease. Alternatively, a home-prepared diet can be formulated for the patient.

Home-Prepared Diets

Unfortunately, home-prepared diets are not convenient or as economical compared to commercial extruded food for the client. Unlike commercially available foods, home-prepared diets have also not been adequately tested with animal feeding trials or laboratory analysis to confirm nutrient content and nutrient availability. Home-prepared diets are often crudely balanced and may not achieve satisfactory palatability, digestibility, or safety. Furthermore, owners are likely to substitute or delete some ingredients or supplements, unbalancing the diet in a process referred to as "diet drift." In one survey, only 13% of dog owners that were provided a homemade diet recommendation at a veterinary teaching hospital were strictly adhering to the recipe a few years later (Johnson et al. 2016).

Formulating a home-prepared diet requires a complete understanding of the nutrient requirements of the pet and the effect of the disease process on the nutritional requirements. Detailed nutrient analyses of the ingredients selected and a thorough knowledge of dietary interactions and effect of preparation and storage on nutrient availability are needed. Caution should be applied when retrieving recipes from the internet or lay publications (see Chapter 8). In one report evaluating 28 and 39 recipes advocated for cats and dogs with kidney disease, respectively, assumptions on ingredient and/or supplement type were required for every recipe, and their analysis with computer software revealed that no recipe met all National Research Council nutrient recommended allowances for adult animals (Larsen et al. 2012). Deficiencies were common for essential amino acids, trace minerals, or some vitamins. There was also great variability in nutrient content, making some recipes potentially contraindicated for the management of CKD. Another study confirmed the important variability in the nutrient content of rations prepared according to recipes, and reported deviations from the projected nutrient content, which could be detrimental to the management of kidney disease such as excess protein (Davies 2014). Therefore, all recipes should be obtained from a board certified veterinary nutritionist® or Diplomate of the European College of Veterinary and Comparative Nutrition, to ensure that it is appropriate and specifically designed for the pet taking into account its current clinical condition.

Monitoring

CKD is a dynamic condition that can have multiple and variable effects on all body systems. No two patients are alike in presentation, complications, or response to therapy. Therefore, regular monitoring is crucial to ensure that dietary and medical management remains optimal for the needs of the patient. Human caretaker compliance may also be improved by frequent patient evaluation. Patients should be reevaluated within two weeks of initiating therapy and then at minimum three to four times per year. Re-evaluations should always be made two weeks following medication or dietary change. Certain medical therapies such as erythropoietin and antihypertensive therapy will initially require weekly evaluation until the appropriate maintenance dosage is achieved.

A complete history is typically indicated, including diet history, physical examination, body weight, BCS, muscle condition assessment, and laboratory evaluation, including complete blood count, biochemical panel, urinalysis, urine protein-to-creatinine ratio, urine culture, and blood pressure evaluation. Urine culture should be a routine procedure in follow-up examinations, as patients with CKD are predisposed to urinary tract infections. These patients are typically asymptomatic, or clinically "silent," and yet chronic urinary tract infections may progress to pyelonephritis, acute kidney disease, or CKD, or contribute to progression of the kidney disease.

A complete list of all medications and doses that the client is currently administering to the pet should be obtained to verify compliance. In addition, some owners will self-adjust medications or simply may be confused by previous instructions. The diet history should include the type of diet (dry/extruded, wet/retorted, home-prepared, frozen, etc.), the amount eaten each day (amount eaten is more important than amount offered), the method of feeding, and information regarding all treats, snacks, and supplements, to be able to assess if dietary management and caloric intake are appropriate.

Acute Kidney Injury

Protein-calorie malnutrition has been implicated as a possible factor influencing outcome in human patients with acute kidney injury (AKI) (Leonard et al. 1975; Acchiardo et al. 1983; Combe et al. 2001). Although there have been no reported studies evaluating the effect of nutritional status on the duration,

outcome, or recovery of renal function in canine and feline AKI patients, protein-calorie malnutrition appears to be common and is a major factor contributing to morbidity and mortality. Factors contributing to malnutrition include inadequate intake of nutrients as dietary intake is compromised by the uremia-induced consequences of anorexia, nausea, and vomiting, and coexisting catabolic illnesses. In addition, recovery from AKI may require prolonged convalescence during which animals are hypercatabolic, azotemic, hyperkalemic, acidotic, and hyperphosphatemic. Malnutrition and wasting may contribute to many aspects of uremic syndrome, including impaired immune function, increased susceptibility to infection, delayed wound healing, decreased strength and vigor, and poor quality of life. Therefore, early nutritional assessment and institution of nutritional support are crucial in the management of patients with AKI. Furthermore, nutritional supplementation should be individually tailored to compensate for the specific abnormalities in protein, lipid, and carbohydrate metabolism, and the marked alterations in fluid, electrolyte, and acid–base balance characteristic of AKI. Oliguria and anuria are complications that significantly influence the nutritional management of the patient with acute renal failure.

Metabolic status among patients with AKI varies; however, most patients have some degree of protein catabolism and negative nitrogen balance (Mitch 1998). Patients are more likely to be catabolic when the acute renal failure is caused by or associated with shock, sepsis, or rhabdomyolysis (Feinstein et al. 1981). Catabolism and marked protein breakdown in turn contribute to uremic syndrome by exacerbating azotemia, hyperkalemia, acidosis, and hyperphosphatemia.

The optimum nutritional regime for controlling accelerated catabolism and the precise nutritional requirements for cats and dogs with AKI are unknown, but a high-energy, moderate-protein, potassium- and phosphate-restricted diet comparable to those for CKD is a logical choice. AKI is a dynamic disease; hence serial clinical and laboratory assessment of the patient and modification of dietary therapy in response to changes in the patient's condition are integral to successful therapy.

Sufficient energy needs to be provided to prevent endogenous protein catabolism, which results in malnutrition and exacerbation of azotemia. Oxygen consumption has shown to be reduced in rats with experimental AKI; however, humans with AKI have increased oxygen consumption (Schneeweiss et al. 1990). This may be due to the presence of coexisting complications, including sepsis and multiple organ failure. Therefore, energy metabolism in AKI varies and depends on the presence of underlying disease. It is generally considered that there is a decrease rather than an increase in energy expenditure. The energy expenditure of an individual patient may be assessed by indirect calorimetry; however, this technique is not widely available in veterinary hospitals. The energy intake of the patient can be calculated as the RER, $70 \times (Wt_{kg})^{0.75}$. This should be used as a starting point and re-evaluated based on body weight and condition changes. Excessive energy intake should be avoided, particularly in animals with compromised respiratory function, as the increased carbohydrate and fat metabolism generate CO_2.

The dietary protein requirements for cats and dogs with acute renal failure are not known and may be influenced by the extent of protein catabolism and coexistent illnesses. Peritoneal dialysis and hemodialysis may also increase protein requirements to compensate for substrate loss during therapy (Elliott et al. 2000a). Ideally, protein intake should be matched with catabolism to promote a positive nitrogen balance. However, measurement of total nitrogen output to determine nitrogen balance is too laborious and expensive to be widely applied for clinical use.

Potassium and phosphorus intake should be restricted to prevent accumulation of these minerals; however, intakes must be modified according to the clinical status of the patient (see the section on potassium). Patients with AKI are often anorexic, have reduced appetites, and may have gastrointestinal ulceration secondary to uremia. In addition, an altered sense of taste and smell has been reported in people (Atkin-Thor et al. 1978). These factors in combination contribute to reduced caloric intake and refusal of diet. Effective dietary management can be facilitated by the placement and use of enteral feeding devices (see Chapter 20). Enteral feeding can be achieved by the administration of blended commercial extruded or retorted therapeutic diets or veterinary therapeutic liquid diets. The feeding solution can be administered intermittently or continuously using a syringe pump. Typically, feeding begins with one-quarter to one-third of the calculated daily energy allowance. The amount and concentration of the solution should be gradually increased over several days if tolerated until the nutritional requirements are met. Several enteral formulations have been specifically developed for use in renal disease in humans; however, these products may contain inadequate amounts of protein and amino acids such as arginine and taurine, and hence should be used cautiously in cats and dogs. Concentrated protein supplements and purified arginine may be utilized to supplement human enteral products to the desired protein concentration in some cases with the assistance of a board certified veterinary nutritionist® or Diplomate of the European College of Veterinary and Comparative Nutrition.

Peripheral parenteral nutrition (PPN) or central parenteral nutrition (CPN) (Chapter 21) is indicated if the nutrient requirements cannot be met by the enteral route and the patient can tolerate the additional fluid load. This additional fluid load is often the limiting factor in the nutritional management of the oliguric or anuric AKI patient. PPN involves the administration of isotonic nutritional solutions through a peripheral vein, thereby avoiding the requirement of a central vein necessary for the administration of a hyperosmolar parenteral nutrition solution. CPN refers to the provision of most of the essential nutrients and, because of the hyperosmolality of the solution, requires administration into a central vein such as the cranial vena cava. PN is indicated to allow time for vomiting to cease and gastrointestinal recovery to occur, at which time a commercial renal failure diet can be substituted enterally.

It is difficult to overcome the catabolic state in uremia and achieve a positive nitrogen balance with nutritional support alone. Therefore, recent interest has focused on evaluating pharmacologic strategies to promote anabolism in patients with AKI. Metabolic interventions including the administration of insulin, anabolic steroids, growth hormone, thyroid hormone, anti-glucocorticoids, insulin-like growth factor-1, beta-2 adrenergic agonists, intracellular proteolytic pathway inhibitors, adenine nucleotides, glutamine, arginine, ribonucleic acid, or omega-3 fatty acids to facilitate the anabolic process, reduce protein degradation, or enhance the immune system are currently being evaluated as nutritional adjunctives in human medicine. The efficacy of these interventions in patients with AKI remains to be seen.

Glomerular Disease

The term "glomerular disease" represents a diverse array of disorders of different pathogenic mechanisms, morphologic expressions, clinical courses, and response to therapy in which the glomerulus is the sole or principal tissue involved. The hallmark, and indeed one of the earliest functional defects in glomerular disease, is the loss of plasma protein in the urine (proteinuria) with inactive urinary sediment. The consequences of proteinuria include sodium retention, edema and/or ascites, hypercholesterolemia, hypertension, hypercoagulability, muscle wasting, and weight loss.

The management of glomerular disease encompasses reversing or eliminating the underlying antigenic stimulation in order to halt progression of the disease, and partnering dietary therapy with appropriate pharmacologic management (Lees et al. 2005; Brown et al. 2013). In most cases, specific antigens or antigenic sources cannot be identified. Indeed, in a study of 106 dogs with glomerular disease, an underlying cause could not be found in 43% of cases (Cook and Cowgill 1996).

The appropriate diet for glomerular disease appears to be a protein-restricted, controlled-sodium, and long-chain omega-3 fatty acid–enhanced diet. This may seem counterintuitive as the seemingly logical approach to protein-losing disease may be to increase the protein intake of the patient. However, Burkholder et al. (2004) reported that the magnitude of proteinuria increased when dogs with X-linked hereditary nephropathy were placed on a higher-protein (36.4% dry matter [DM]) versus a lower-protein (14.1% DM) diet. Studies in rats suggest that high-protein diets are actually detrimental to glomerular disease, as the additional protein load increases glomerular capillary pressure, exacerbates proteinuria, and increases progression of renal disease. Restricting the dietary protein intake of nephrotic subjects actually reduces proteinuria and increases total body albumin mass and serum albumin concentrations. In models of canine kidney disease, supplementation with long-chain omega-3 fatty acids from fish oil (i.e. EPA and DHA) was shown to decrease glomerular pressure compared to omega-6 fatty acids (Brown et al. 2000). While this strategy has not been evaluated in animals with glomerular disease, some studies in humans and the mechanism of action provide a rationale for supplementation with EPA and DHA (Brown et al. 2013).

Uncontrolled (Zatelli et al. 2016) or controlled (Valli et al. 1991; Cortadellas et al. 2014) studies evaluating the effect of renal therapeutic diet as a whole (protein restriction in association with other nutrient modifications, such as phosphorus restriction and/or omega-3 fatty acid supplementation) suggest that in dogs with glomerular disease, such dietary modifications can decrease proteinuria and glomerular damage and delay the onset and progression of renal failure. The current consensus is therefore to prescribe such diets in association with appropriate medical therapy to inhibit the RAAS (Brown et al. 2013). There have been no studies that the authors are aware of in cats, although there is renewed interest in the importance of proteinuria in CKD (see the section on protein).

Humans with protein-losing nephropathies have been reported to have additional nutritional deficiencies, primarily associated with the loss of protein-bound vitamins and minerals. However, studies of nutrient deficiencies associated with protein-losing nephropathies have not been reported in cats or dogs. It would seem rational that minimizing proteinuria, maintaining lean body mass, and ensuring appropriate daily caloric intake of a complete and balanced diet would help to minimize vitamin and mineral deficiencies.

Fanconi Syndrome

Fanconi syndrome is a disease that affects the proximal renal tubule, resulting in defective transport of water, glucose, phosphate, sodium, potassium, amino acids, and bicarbonate (Yearley et al. 2004). The disease has been reported to be inherited in basenjis and Norwegian elkhounds, with sporadic occurrences in other breeds and cats. Fanconi syndrome can also be an acquired disease secondary to drugs such as gentamicin therapy and toxins like heavy metals. A recent outbreak of Fanconi-like disease has also been reported in Australia in association with the consumption of chicken jerky treats (Thompson et al. 2013).

Glycosuria, phosphaturia, amino aciduria, bicarbonaturia, and uricosuria can have several metabolic consequences, including hypophosphatemia, hyponatremia, hypokalemia, hyperchloremic metabolic acidosis, and hypocalcemia. Most dogs do not have renal disease at the time of diagnosis; however, the development of acute renal disease due to severe metabolic acidosis and papillary necrosis is a realistic clinical concern. Indeed, renal failure has been reported to be the most common reason for death or euthanasia of affected dogs (Yearley et al. 2004).

Management needs to be customized to the individual patient and revolves primarily around management of the clinical and metabolic signs: polyuria, azotemia, acidosis, and hypokalemia. Hypokalemia is common and is due to the resorptive defect of bicarbonate: bicarbonaturia enhances renal potassium excretion. Treatment should be targeted at both the impairment in bicarbonate reabsorption by providing sodium bicarbonate therapy and by providing oral potassium supplementation to manage the hypokalemia.

Hydration should be ensured by providing adequate fresh water at all times. For dogs with no evidence of renal disease, the most appropriate diet would be a good-quality, highly digestible diet for adult dogs. The "Gonto protocol" has been designed by basenji enthusiasts and enjoys widespread anecdotal success (Gonto 2003). However, studies have not been reported that compare the efficacy of this therapy to alternative approaches. Once the patient has evidence of renal disease, dietary alterations as discussed earlier for CKD would be appropriate; however, protein intake should be carefully monitored to ensure maintenance of lean body mass and to minimize the adverse consequence of protein deficiency.

Conclusion

Diet plays an important role in the management of patients with kidney disease. Nutritional therapy introduced in stages II and III of CKD is aimed at factors that delay

Table 15.2 Summary of key nutritional factors.

	Stage I	Stage II	Stage III	Stage IV
Hydration	Fresh water at all times			
Protein modification	Dogs: UPC >2 Cats: UPC >0.4	Dogs: UPC >0.5 Cats: UPC >0.4	Appropriate dietary protein reduction to control uremia and hyperphosphatemia	
Control phosphate		2.7–4.5 mg/dl	<5 mg/dl	<6 mg/dl
Control acidosis	Maintain bicarbonate 18–24 mmol/l			
Control potassium	Control at all stages within species – specific reference intervals			
Prevent protein calorie malnutrition	Feeding tube intervention when not eating MER or 10–15% loss of body weight			

MER, maintenance energy requirements; UPC, urine protein-to-creatinine ratio.

progression, whereas once late-stage III/IV disease has been reached, clinical signs of uremia are evident, and dietary treatment is designed increasingly to improve the quality of life of the patient rather than to slow disease progression (Table 15.2). Regular monitoring to ensure that dietary and medical management remains optimal for the needs of the patient is crucial for the long-term successful treatment of the patient with kidney disease. Regardless of the disease, the diet must be tailored to the individual needs of the patient, and adjustments are to be expected throughout the course of treatment. Clinical studies have clearly proven that nutrition can improve the life expectancy and significantly minimize the risk of uremic crises in patients with CKD.

Summary

- Dietary therapy in kidney disease is only effective if it is administered appropriately.
- Kidney disease is dynamic, hence the nutritional requirements need to be tailored to the individual and altered according to the metabolic status of the patient.
- Nutritional alterations in stage II and early stage III disease are focused on slowing the progression of kidney disease.
- Management of later stage III and stage IV disease is designed to alleviate the clinical manifestations of the uremic syndrome.
- Studies have clearly shown that feeding a renal diet to cats and dogs with kidney disease will ameliorate the clinical signs and slow disease progression.

References

Acchiardo, S.R., Moore, L.W., and Latour, P.A. (1983). Malnutrition as the main factor in morbidity and mortality of hemodialysis patients. *Kidney Int. Suppl.* 16: S199–S203.

Adams, L.G., Polzin, D.J., Osborne, C.A., and O'Brien, T.D. (1993). Effects of dietary protein and calorie restriction in clinically normal cats and in cats with surgically induced chronic renal failure. *Am. J. Vet. Res.* 54 (10): 1653–1662.

Adams, L.G., Polzin, D.J., Osborne, C.A. et al. (1994). Influence of dietary protein/calorie intake on renal morphology and function in cats with 5/6 nephrectomy. *Lab. Invest.* 70 (3): 347–357.

Anderson, R.S. (1982). Water balance in the dog and cat. *J. Small Anim. Pract.* 23 (9): 588–598.

Atkin-Thor, E., Goddard, B.W., O'Nion, J. et al. (1978). Hypogeusia and zinc depletion in chronic dialysis patients. *Am. J. Clin. Nutr.* 31 (10): 1948–1951.

Barber, P.J. and Elliott, J. (1998). Feline chronic renal failure: calcium homeostasis in 80 cases diagnosed between 1992 and 1995. *J. Small Anim. Pract.* 39 (3): 108–116.

Barber, P.J., Rawlings, J.M., Markwell, P.J., and Elliott, J. (1999). Effect of dietary phosphate restriction on renal secondary hyperparathyroidism in the cat. *J. Small Anim. Pract.* 40 (2): 62–70.

Bauer, J.E., Markwell, P.J., Rawlings, J.M., and Senior, D.E. (1999). Effects of dietary fat and polyunsaturated fatty acids in dogs with naturally developing chronic renal failure. *J. Am. Vet. Med. Assoc.* 215 (11): 1588–1591.

Benjamin, S.E. and Drobatz, K.J. (2020). Retrospective evaluation of risk factors and treatment outcome predictors in cats presenting to the emergency room for constipation. *J. Feline Med. Surg.* 22 (2): 153–160.

Bijsmans, E.S., Jepson, R.E., Chang, Y.M. et al. (2015). Changes in systolic blood pressure over time in healthy cats and cats with chronic kidney disease. *J. Vet. Intern. Med.* 29 (3): 855–861.

Bovee, K.C. (1991). Influence of dietary protein on renal function in dogs. *J. Nutr.* 121 (Suppl 11): S128–S139.

Boyd, L.M., Langston, C., Thompson, K. et al. (2008). Survival in cats with naturally occurring chronic kidney disease (2000–2002). *J. Vet. Intern. Med.* 22 (5): 1111–1117.

de Brito Galvao, J.F., Nagode, L.A., Schenck, P.A., and Chew, D.J. (2013). Calcitriol, calcidiol, parathyroid hormone, and fibroblast growth factor-23 interactions in chronic kidney disease. *J. Vet. Emerg. Crit. Care* 23 (2): 134–162.

van den Broek, D.H., Chang, Y.M., Elliott, J. et al. (2017). Chronic kidney disease in cats and the risk of total hypercalcemia. *J. Vet. Intern. Med.* 31 (2): 465–475.

van den Broek, D.H.N., Geddes, R.F., Lotter, N.S. et al. (2022). Ionized hypercalcemia in cats with azotemic chronic kidney disease (2012–2018). *J. Vet. Intern. Med.* 36 (4): 1312–1321.

Brown, S.A. (2008). Oxidative stress and chronic kidney disease. *Vet. Clin. North Am. Small Anim. Pract.* 38 (1): 157–166, vi.

Brown, S.A., Finco, D.R., Crowell, W.A. et al. (1990). Single-nephron adaptations to partial renal ablation in the dog. *Am. J. Physiol.* 258 (3 Pt 2): F495–F503.

Brown, S.A., Crowell, W.A., Barsanti, J.A. et al. (1991a). Beneficial effects of dietary mineral restriction in dogs with marked reduction of functional renal mass. *J. Am. Soc. Nephrol.* 1 (10): 1169–1179.

Brown, S.A., Finco, D.R., Crowell, W.A., and Navar, L.G. (1991b). Dietary protein intake and the glomerular adaptations to partial nephrectomy in dogs. *J. Nutr.* 121 (Suppl 11): S125–S127.

Brown, S.A., Brown, C.A., Crowell, W.A. et al. (1998). Beneficial effects of chronic administration of dietary omega-3 polyunsaturated fatty acids in dogs with renal insufficiency. *J. Lab. Clin. Med.* 131 (5): 447–455.

Brown, S.A., Brown, C.A., Crowell, W.A. et al. (2000). Effects of dietary polyunsaturated fatty acid supplementation in early renal insufficiency in dogs. *J. Lab. Clin. Med.* 135 (3): 275–286.

Brown, S., Atkins, C., Bagley, R. et al. (2007). Guidelines for the identification, evaluation, and management of systemic hypertension in dogs and cats. *J. Vet. Intern. Med.* 21 (3): 542–558.

Brown, S., Elliott, J., Francey, T. et al.; IRIS Canine GN Study Group Standard Therapy Subgroup(2013). Consensus recommendations for standard therapy of glomerular disease in dogs. *J. Vet. Intern. Med.* 27 (Suppl 1): S27–S43.

Buranakarl, C., Mathur, S., and Brown, S.A. (2004). Effects of dietary sodium chloride intake on renal function and blood pressure in cats with normal and reduced renal function. *Am. J. Vet. Res.* 65 (5): 620–627.

Burkholder, W.J., Lees, G.E., LeBlanc, A.K. et al. (2004). Diet modulates proteinuria in heterozygous female dogs with X-linked hereditary nephropathy. *J. Vet. Intern. Med.* 18 (2): 165–175.

Chakrabarti, S., Syme, H.M., and Elliott, J. (2012). Clinicopathological variables predicting progression of azotemia in cats with chronic kidney disease. *J. Vet. Intern. Med.* 26 (2): 275–281.

Chakrabarti, S., Syme, H.M., Brown, C.A., and Elliott, J. (2013). Histomorphometry of feline chronic kidney disease and correlation with markers of renal dysfunction. *Vet. Pathol.* 50 (1): 147–155.

Cherla, G. and Jaimes, E.A. (2004). Role of L-arginine in the pathogenesis and treatment of renal disease. *J. Nutr.* 134 (Suppl 10): 2801S–2806S; discussion 2818S–2819S.

Chetboul, V., Reynolds, B.S., Trehiou-Sechi, E. et al. (2014). Cardiovascular effects of dietary salt intake in aged healthy cats: a 2-year prospective randomized, blinded, and controlled study. *PLoS One* 9 (6): e97862.

Cochrane, A.L. and Ricardo, S.D. (2003). Oxidant stress and regulation of chemokines in the development of renal interstitial fibrosis. *Contrib. Nephrol.* 139: 102–119.

Combe, C., Chauveau, P., Laville, M. et al. (2001). Influence of nutritional factors and hemodialysis adequacy on the survival of 1,610 French patients. *Am. J. Kidney Dis.* 37 (1 Suppl 2): S81–S88.

Cook, A.K. and Cowgill, L.D. (1996). Clinical and pathological features of protein-losing glomerular disease in the dog: a review of 137 cases (1985–1992). *J. Am. Anim. Hosp. Assoc.* 32 (4): 313–322.

Cortadellas, O., Talavera, J., and Fernández del Palacio, M.J. (2014). Evaluation of the effects of a therapeutic renal diet to control proteinuria in proteinuric non-azotemic dogs treated with benazepril. *J. Vet. Intern. Med.* 28 (1): 30–37.

Davies, M. (2014). Variability in content of homemade diets for canine chronic kidney disease. *Vet. Rec.* 174 (14): 352.

DiBartola, S.P., Rutgers, H.C., Zack, P.M., and Tarr, M.J. (1987). Clinicopathologic findings associated with chronic renal disease in cats: 74 cases (1973–1984). *J. Am. Vet. Med. Assoc.* 190 (9): 1196–1202.

DiBartola, S.P., Buffington, C.A., Chew, D.J. et al. (1993). Development of chronic renal disease in cats fed a commercial diet. *J. Am. Vet. Med. Assoc.* 202 (5): 744–751.

Dow, S.W. and Fettman, M.J. (1992). Chronic renal disease and potassium depletion in cats. *Semin. Vet. Med. Surg. (Small Anim.)* 7 (3): 198–201.

Dow, S.W., Fettman, M.J., LeCouteur, R.A., and Hamar, D.W. (1987). Potassium depletion in cats: renal and dietary influences. *J. Am. Vet. Med. Assoc.* 191 (12): 1569–1575.

Dow, S.W., Fettman, M.J., Curtis, C.R., and LeCouteur, R.A. (1989). Hypokalemia in cats: 186 cases (1984–1987). *J. Am. Vet. Med. Assoc.* 194 (11): 1604–1608.

Dow, S.W., Fettman, M.J., Smith, K.R. et al. (1990). Effects of dietary acidification and potassium depletion on acid-base balance, mineral metabolism and renal function in adult cats. *J. Nutr.* 120 (6): 569–578.

Elliott, J. and Barber, P.J. (1998). Feline chronic renal failure: clinical findings in 80 cases diagnosed between 1992 and 1995. *J. Small Anim. Pract.* 39 (2): 78–85.

Elliott, J. and Syme, H.M. (2003). Response of cats with chronic renal failure to dietary potassium supplementation (abstract). *J. Vet. Intern. Med.* 17 (3): 418.

Elliott, D.A., Marks, S.L., Cowgill, L.D. et al. (2000a). Effect of hemodialysis on plasma amino acid concentrations in healthy dogs. *Am. J. Vet. Res.* 61 (8): 869–873.

Elliott, J., Rawlings, J.M., Markwell, P.J., and Barber, P.J. (2000b). Survival of cats with naturally occurring chronic renal failure: effect of dietary management. *J. Small Anim. Pract.* 41 (6): 235–242.

Elliott, D.A., Riel, D.L., and Rogers, Q.R. (2000c). Complications and outcomes associated with use of gastrostomy tubes for nutritional management of dogs with renal failure: 56 cases

(1994–1999). *J. Am. Vet. Med. Assoc.* 217 (9): 1337–1342.

Elliott, J., Syme, H.M., and Markwell, P.J. (2003a). Acid-base balance of cats with chronic renal failure: effect of deterioration in renal function. *J. Small Anim. Pract.* 44 (6): 261–268.

Elliott, J., Syme, H.M., Reubens, E., and Markwell, P.J. (2003b). Assessment of acid-base status of cats with naturally occurring chronic renal failure. *J. Small Anim. Pract.* 44 (2): 65–70.

Eyre, R., Trehiou, M., Marshall, E. et al. (2022). Aging cats prefer warm food. *J. Vet. Behav.* 47: 86–92.

Feinstein, E.I., Blumenkrantz, M.J., Healy, M. et al. (1981). Clinical and metabolic responses to parenteral nutrition in acute renal failure. A controlled double-blind study. *Medicine (Baltimore)* 60 (2): 124–137.

Finch, N.C., Geddes, R.F., Syme, H.M., and Elliott, J. (2013). Fibroblast growth factor 23 (FGF-23) concentrations in cats with early nonazotemic chronic kidney disease (CKD) and in healthy geriatric cats. *J. Vet. Intern. Med.* 27 (2): 227–233.

Finco, D.R., Crowell, W.A., and Barsanti, J.A. (1985). Effects of three diets on dogs with induced chronic renal failure. *Am. J. Vet. Res.* 46 (3): 646–653.

Finco, D.R., Brown, S.A., Crowell, W.A. et al. (1992a). Effects of dietary phosphorus and protein in dogs with chronic renal failure. *Am. J. Vet. Res.* 53 (12): 2264–2271.

Finco, D.R., Brown, S.A., Crowell, W.A. et al. (1992b). Effects of phosphorus/calcium-restricted and phosphorus/calcium-replete 32% protein diets in dogs with chronic renal failure. *Am. J. Vet. Res.* 53 (1): 157–163.

Finco, D.R., Brown, S.A., Crowell, W.A. et al. (1994). Effects of aging and dietary protein intake on uninephrectomized geriatric dogs. *Am. J. Vet. Res.* 55 (9): 1282–1290.

Finco, D.R., Brown, S.A., Brown, C.A. et al. (1998). Protein and calorie effects on progression of induced chronic renal failure in cats. *Am. J. Vet. Res.* 59 (5): 575–582.

Finco, D.R., Brown, S.A., Brown, C.A. et al. (1999). Progression of chronic renal disease in the dog. *J. Vet. Intern. Med.* 13 (6): 516–528.

Freeman, L.M., Lachaud, M.P., Matthews, S. et al. (2016). Evaluation of weight loss over time in cats with chronic kidney disease. *J. Vet. Intern. Med.* 30 (5): 1661–1666.

Geddes, R.F., Finch, N.C., Elliott, J., and Syme, H.M. (2013a). Fibroblast growth factor 23 in feline chronic kidney disease. *J. Vet. Intern. Med.* 27 (2): 234–241.

Geddes, R.F., Elliott, J., and Syme, H.M. (2013b). The effect of feeding a renal diet on plasma fibroblast growth factor 23 concentrations in cats with stable azotemic chronic kidney disease. *J. Vet. Intern. Med.* 27 (6): 1354–1361.

Geddes, R.F., Elliott, J., and Syme, H.M. (2015). Relationship between plasma fibroblast growth factor-23 concentration and survival time in cats with chronic kidney disease. *J. Vet. Intern. Med.* 29 (6): 1494–1501.

Geddes, R.F., van den Broek, D.H.N., Chang, Y.M. et al. (2021). The effect of attenuating dietary phosphate restriction on blood ionized calcium concentrations in cats with chronic kidney disease and ionized hypercalcemia. *J. Vet. Intern. Med.* 35 (2): 997–1007.

Gonto, S. (2003). Fanconi disease management protocol for veterinarians. Basenji Club of America, Wilmington, IL. http://www.basenji.org/ClubDocs/fanconiprotocol2003.pdf (accessed August 9, 2022).

Granick, M., Leuin, A.S., and Trepanier, L.A. (2021). Plasma and urinary F2-isoprostane markers of oxidative stress are increased in cats with early (stage 1) chronic kidney disease. *J. Feline Med. Surg.* 23 (8): 692–699.

Greco, D.S., Lees, G.E., Dzendzel, G., and Carter, A.B. (1994a). Effects of dietary sodium intake on blood pressure measurements in partially nephrectomized dogs. *Am. J. Vet. Res.* 55 (1): 160–165.

Greco, D.S., Lees, G.E., Dzendzel, G. et al. (1994b). Effect of dietary sodium intake on glomerular filtration rate in partially nephrectomized dogs. *Am. J. Vet. Res.* 55 (1): 152–159.

Greene, J.P., Lefebvre, S.L., Wang, M. et al. (2014). Risk factors associated with the development of chronic kidney disease in cats evaluated at primary care veterinary hospitals. *J. Am. Vet. Med. Assoc.* 244 (3): 320–327.

Hahn, S., Kuemmerle, N.B., Chan, W. et al. (1998). Glomerulosclerosis in the remnant kidney rat is modulated by dietary alpha-tocopherol. *J. Am. Soc. Nephrol.* 9 (11): 2089–2095.

Hahn, S., Krieg, R.J. Jr., Hisano, S. et al. (1999). Vitamin E suppresses oxidative stress and glomerulosclerosis in rat remnant kidney. *Pediatr. Nephrol.* 13 (3): 195–198.

Hall, J.A., Yerramilli, M., Obare, E. et al. (2014). Comparison of serum concentrations of symmetric dimethylarginine and creatinine as kidney function biomarkers in cats with chronic kidney disease. *J. Vet. Intern. Med.* 28 (6): 1676–1683.

Hall, J.A., MacLeay, J., Yerramilli, M. et al. (2016a). Positive impact of nutritional interventions on serum symmetric dimethylarginine and creatinine concentrations in client-owned geriatric cats. *PLoS One* 11 (4): e0153654.

Hall, J.A., MacLeay, J., Yerramilli, M. et al. (2016b). Positive impact of nutritional interventions on serum symmetric dimethylarginine and creatinine concentrations in client-owned geriatric dogs. *PLoS One* 11 (4): e0153653.

Hall, J.A., Yerramilli, M., Obare, E. et al. (2016c). Serum concentrations of symmetric dimethylarginine and creatinine in dogs with naturally occurring chronic kidney disease. *J. Vet. Intern. Med.* 30 (3): 794–802.

Hall, J.A., Fritsch, D.A., Jewell, D.E. et al. (2019). Cats with IRIS stage 1 and 2 chronic kidney disease maintain body weight and lean muscle mass when fed food having increased caloric density, and enhanced concentrations of carnitine and essential amino acids. *Vet. Rec.* 184: 190.

Hansen, B., DiBartola, S.P., Chew, D.J. et al. (1992). Clinical and metabolic findings in dogs with chronic renal failure fed two diets. *Am. J. Vet. Res.* 53 (3): 326–334.

Harjes, L.M., Parker, V.J., Dembek, K. et al. (2017). Fibroblast growth factor-23 concentration in dogs with chronic kidney disease. *J. Vet. Intern. Med.* 31 (3): 784–790.

Hori, Y., Heishima, Y., Yamashita, Y. et al. (2018). Relationship between indirect blood pressure and various stages of chronic kidney disease in cats. *J. Vet. Med. Sci.* 80 (3): 447–452.

Hostetter, T.H., Olson, J.L., Rennke, H.G. et al. (1981). Hyperfiltration in remnant nephrons: a potentially adverse response to renal ablation. *Am. J. Physiol.* 241 (1): F85–F93.

IRIS, International Renal Interest Society (2023). http://iris-kidney.com/guidelines/index.html (accessed March 24, 2023).

Jacob, F., Polzin, D.J., Osborne, C.A. et al. (2002). Clinical evaluation of dietary modification for treatment of spontaneous chronic renal failure in dogs. *J. Am. Vet. Med. Assoc.* 220 (8): 1163–1170.

Jacob, F., Polzin, D.J., Osborne, C.A. et al. (2003). Association between initial systolic blood pressure and risk of developing a uremic crisis or of dying in dogs with chronic renal failure. *J. Am. Vet. Med. Assoc.* 222 (3): 322–329.

Jacob, F., Polzin, D.J., Osborne, C.A. et al. (2005). Evaluation of the association between initial proteinuria and morbidity rate or death in dogs with naturally occurring chronic renal failure. *J. Am. Vet. Med. Assoc.* 226 (3): 393–400.

Jepson, R.E., Elliott, J., Brodbelt, D., and Syme, H.M. (2007). Effect of control of systolic blood pressure on survival in cats with systemic hypertension. *J. Vet. Intern. Med.* 21 (3): 402–409.

Jepson, R.E., Syme, H.M., Vallance, C., and Elliott, J. (2008). Plasma asymmetric dimethylarginine, symmetric dimethylarginine, l-arginine, and nitrite/nitrate concentrations in cats with chronic kidney disease and hypertension. *J. Vet. Intern. Med.* 22 (2): 317–324.

Jepson, R.E., Brodbelt, D., Vallance, C. et al. (2009). Evaluation of predictors of the development of azotemia in cats. *J. Vet. Intern. Med.* 23 (4): 806–813.

Johnson, L.N., Linder, D.E., Heinze, C.R. et al. (2016). Evaluation of owner experiences and adherence to home-cooked diet recipes for dogs. *J. Small Anim. Pract.* 57 (1): 23–27.

Jones, S.E., Quimby, J.M., Summers, S.C. et al. (2022). Survey of defecation habits in apparently healthy and chronic kidney disease cats. *J. Feline Med. Surg.* 24 (2): 131–141.

Keegan, R.F. and Webb, C.B. (2010). Oxidative stress and neutrophil function in cats with chronic renal failure. *J. Vet. Intern. Med.* 24 (3): 514–519.

King, J.N., Gunn-Moore, D.A., Tasker, S. et al. (2006). Tolerability and efficacy of benazepril in cats with chronic kidney disease. *J. Vet. Intern. Med.* 20 (5): 1054–1064.

King, J.N., Tasker, S., Gunn-Moore, D.A., and Strehlau, G., and BENRIC (renal insufficiency in cats) Study Group(2007). Prognostic factors in cats with chronic kidney disease. *J. Vet. Intern. Med.* 21 (5): 906–916.

Kirschvink, N., Lhoest, E., Leemans, J. et al. (2005). Effects of feeding frequency on water intake in cats (abstract). *J. Vet. Intern. Med.* 19: 476.

Krofic Zel, M., Tozon, N., and Nemec Svete, A. (2014). Plasma and erythrocyte glutathione peroxidase activity, serum selenium concentration, and plasma total antioxidant capacity in cats with IRIS stages I-IV chronic kidney disease. *J. Vet. Intern. Med.* 28 (1): 130–136.

Kuwahara, Y., Ohba, Y., Kitoh, K. et al. (2006). Association of laboratory data and death within one month in cats with chronic renal failure. *J. Small Anim. Pract.* 47 (8): 446–450.

Laflamme, D.P. and Hannah, S.S. (2013). Discrepancy between use of lean body mass or nitrogen balance to determine protein requirements for adult cats. *J. Feline Med. Surg.* 15 (8): 691–697.

Larsen, J.A. (2016). Controversies in veterinary nephrology: differing viewpoints: role of dietary protein in the management of feline chronic kidney disease. *Vet. Clin. North Am. Small Anim. Pract.* 46 (6): 1095–1098.

Larsen, J.A., Parks, E.M., Heinze, C.R., and Fascetti, A.J. (2012). Evaluation of recipes for home-prepared diets for dogs and cats with chronic kidney disease. *J. Am. Vet. Med. Assoc.* 240 (5): 532–538.

Lees, G.E., Brown, S.A., Elliott, J. et al., and American College of Veterinary Internal Medicine(2005). Assessment and management of proteinuria in dogs and cats: 2004 ACVIM forum consensus statement (small animal). *J. Vet. Intern. Med.* 19 (3): 377–385.

Lefebvre, H.P., Ferre, J.P., Watson, A.D. et al. (2001). Small bowel motility and colonic transit are altered in dogs with moderate renal failure. *Am. J. Physiol. Regul. Integr. Comp. Physiol.* 281 (1): R230–R238.

Leibetseder, J.L. and Neufeld, K.W. (1991). Effects of medium protein diets in dogs with chronic renal failure. *J. Nutr.* 121 (Suppl 11): S145–S149.

Leonard, C.D., Luke, R.G., and Siegel, R.R. (1975). Parenteral essential amino acids in acute renal failure. *Urology* 6 (2): 154–157.

Lippi, I., Guidi, G., Marchetti, V. et al. (2014). Prognostic role of the product of serum calcium and phosphorus concentrations in dogs with chronic kidney disease: 31 cases (2008–2010). *J. Am. Vet. Med. Assoc.* 245 (10): 1135–1140.

Locatelli, F., Canaud, B., Eckhardt, K.-U. et al. (2003). Oxidative stress in end-stage renal disease: an emerging threat to patient outcome. *Nephrol. Dial. Transplant.* 18 (7): 1272–1280.

Markovich, J.E., Freeman, L.M., Labatao, M.A., and Heinze, C.R. (2015). Survey of dietary and medication practices of owners of cats with chronic kidney disease. *J. Feline Med. Surg.* 17 (12): 979–983.

McLeland, S.M., Lunn, K.F., Duncan, C.G. et al. (2014). Relationship among serum creatinine, serum gastrin, calcium-phosphorus product, and uremic gastropathy in cats with chronic kidney disease. *J. Vet. Intern. Med.* 28 (3): 827–837.

Mitch, W.E. (1998). Robert H Herman memorial award in clinical nutrition lecture, 1997. Mechanisms causing loss of lean body mass in kidney disease. *Am. J. Clin. Nutr.* 67 (3): 359–366.

Miyakawa, H., Nagatani, Y., Ogawa, M. et al. (2020). Fibroblast growth factor-23 as an early marker of CKD-mineral bone disorder in dogs: preliminary investigation. *J. Small Anim. Pract.* 61 (12): 744–751.

Miyakawa, H., Hsu, H.H., Ogawa, M. et al. (2022). Serum fibroblast growth factor-23 concentrations in young and mature adult cats with chronic kidney disease. *J. Feline Med. Surg.* 24: 815–820.

Nagode, L.A. and Chew, D.J. (1992). Nephrocalcinosis caused by hyperpara-thyroidism in progression of renal failure: treatment with calcitriol. *Semin. Vet. Med. Surg. (Small Anim.)* 7 (3): 202–220.

Nagode, L.A., Chew, D.J., and Podell, M. (1996). Benefits of calcitriol therapy and serum phosphorus control in dogs and cats with chronic renal failure. Both are essential to prevent of suppress toxic hyperparathyroidism. *Vet. Clin. North Am. Small Anim. Pract.* 26 (6): 1293–1330.

National Research Council (2006). *Nutrient Requirements of Dogs and Cats*. Washington, DC: National Academies Press https://nap. nationalacademies.org/catalog/10668/nutrient-requirements-of-dogs-and-cats.

Nguyen, P., Reynolds, B., Zentek, J. et al. (2017). Sodium in feline nutrition. *J. Anim. Physiol. Anim. Nutr. (Berl.)* 101 (3): 403–420.

Parker, V.J. and Freeman, L.M. (2011). Association between body condition and survival in dogs with acquired chronic kidney disease. *J. Vet. Intern. Med.* 25 (6): 1306–1311.

Plantinga, E.A., Everts, H., Kastelein, A.M.C., and Beynen, A.C. (2005). Retrospective study of the survival of cats with acquired chronic renal insufficiency offered different commercial diets. *Vet. Rec.* 157 (7): 185–187.

Polzin, D.J. and Churchill, J.A. (2016). Controversies in veterinary nephrology: renal diets are indicated for cats with international renal interest society chronic kidney disease stages 2 to 4: the pro view. *Vet. Clin. North Am. Small Anim. Pract.* 46 (6): 1049–1065.

Polzin, D.J. and Osborne, C.A. (1988). The importance of egg protein in reduced protein diets designed for dogs with renal failure. *J. Vet. Intern. Med.* 2 (1): 15–21.

Polzin, D.J., Osborne, C.A., Hayden, D.W., and Stevens, J.B. (1983). Influence of reduced protein diets on morbidity, mortality, and renal function in dogs with induced chronic renal failure. *Am. J. Vet. Res.* 45 (3): 506–517.

Polzin, D.J., Leininger, J.R., Osborne, C.A., and Jeraj, K. (1988). Development of renal lesions in dogs after 11/12 reduction of renal mass. Influences of dietary protein intake. *Lab. Invest.* 58 (2): 172–183.

Pouchelon, J.L., Atkins, C.E., Bussadori, C. et al. (2015). Cardiovascular–renal axis disorders in the domestic dog and cat: a veterinary consensus statement. *J. Small Anim. Pract.* 56 (9): 537–552.

Quimby, J.M. and Lunn, K.F. (2013). Mirtazapine as an appetite stimulant and anti-emetic in cats with chronic kidney disease: a masked placebo-controlled crossover clinical trial. *Vet. J.* 197 (3): 651–655.

Quimby, J.M., Benson, K.K., Summers, S.C. et al. (2020). Assessment of compounded transdermal mirtazapine as an appetite stimulant in cats with chronic kidney disease. *J. Feline Med. Surg.* 22 (4): 376–383.

Remuzzi, G. and Bertani, T. (1998). Pathophysiology of progressive nephropathies. *N. Engl. J. Med.* 339 (20): 1448–1456.

Reynolds, B.S., Chetboul, V., Nguyen, P. et al. (2013). Effects of dietary salt intake on renal function: a 2-year study in healthy aged cats. *J. Vet. Intern. Med.* 27 (3): 507–515.

Robertson, J.L., Goldschmidt, M., Kronfeld, D.S. et al. (1986). Long-term renal responses to high dietary protein in dogs with 75% nephrectomy. *Kidney Int.* 29 (2): 511–519.

Ross, S. (2016). Utilization of feeding tubes in the management of feline chronic kidney disease. *Vet. Clin. North Am. Small Anim. Pract.* 46 (6): 1099–1114.

Ross, L.A., Finco, D.R., and Crowell, W.A. (1982). Effect of dietary phosphorus restriction on the kidneys of cats with reduced renal mass. *Am. J. Vet. Res.* 43 (6): 1023–1026.

Ross, S.J., Osborne, C.A., Kirk, C.A. et al. (2006). Clinical evaluation of dietary modification for treatment of spontaneous chronic kidney disease in cats. *J. Am. Vet. Med. Assoc.* 229 (6): 949–957.

Rudinsky, A.J., Harjes, L.M., Byron, J. et al. (2018). Factors associated with survival in dogs with chronic kidney disease. *J. Vet. Intern. Med.* 32: 1977–1982.

Schauf, S., Coltherd, J.C., Atwal, J. et al. (2021). Clinical progression of cats with early-stage chronic kidney disease fed diets with varying protein and phosphorus contents and calcium to phosphorus ratios. *J. Vet. Intern. Med.* 35: 2797–2811.

Scherk, M.A. and Laflamme, D.P. (2016). Controversies in veterinary nephrology: renal diets are indicated for cats with International Renal Interest Society chronic kidney disease stages 2 to 4: the con view. *Vet. Clin. North Am. Small Anim. Pract.* 46 (6): 1067–1094.

Schneeweiss, B., Graninger, W., Stockenhuber, F. et al. (1990). Energy metabolism in acute and chronic renal failure. *Am. J. Clin. Nutr.* 52 (4): 596–601.

Segev, G., Fascetti, A.J., Weeth, L.P., and Cowgill, L.D. (2010). Correction of hyperkalemia in dogs with chronic kidney disease consuming commercial renal therapeutic diets by a potassium-reduced home-prepared diet. *J. Vet. Intern. Med.* 24 (3): 546–550.

Shipov, A., Segev, G., Meltzer, H. et al. (2014). The effect of naturally occurring chronic kidney disease on the micro-structural and mechanical properties of bone. *PLoS One* 9 (10): e110057.

Shipov, A., Shahar, R., Sugar, N., and Segev, G. (2017). The influence of chronic kidney disease on the structural and mechanical properties of canine bone. *J. Vet. Intern. Med.* 32 (1): 280–287.

Sieberg, L.G. and Quimby, J.M. (2020). Retrospective study of the efficacy of oral potassium supplementation in cats with kidney disease. *J. Feline Med. Surg.* 22: 539–543.

Silva, A.C., de Almeida, B.F., Soeiro, C.S. et al. (2013). Oxidative stress, superoxide production, and apoptosis of neutrophils in dogs with chronic kidney disease. *Can. J. Vet. Res.* 77 (2): 136–141.

Slawuta, P., Sikorska-Kopylowicz, A., and Sapikowski, G. (2020). Diagnostic utility of different models used to assess the acid-base balance in cats with chronic kidney disease. *Acta Vet. Hung.* 68 (2): 169–176.

Sparkes, A.H., Caney, S., Chalhoub, S. et al. (2016). ISFM consensus guidelines on the diagnosis and management of feline chronic kidney disease. *J. Feline Med. Surg.* 18 (3): 219–239.

Spencer, S., Wheeler-Jones, C., and Elliott, J. (2021). Hypoxia and chronic kidney disease: possible mechanisms, therapeutic targets, and relevance to cats. *Vet. J.* 274: 105714.

Steinbach, S., Binkert, B., Schweighauser, A. et al. (2010). Quantitative assessment of urea generation and elimination in healthy dogs and in dogs with chronic kidney disease. *J. Vet. Intern. Med.* 24 (6): 1283–1289.

Syme, H.M. (2003). *Studies of the Epidemiology and Aetiology of Hypertension in the Cat.* London: University of London.

Syme, H.M., Barber, P.J., Markwell, P.J., and Elliott, J. (2002). Prevalence of systolic hypertension in cats with chronic renal failure at initial evaluation. *J. Am. Vet. Med. Assoc.* 220 (12): 1799–1804.

Syme, H.M., Markwell, P.J., Pfeiffer, D., and Elliott, J. (2006). Survival of cats with naturally occurring chronic renal failure is related to severity of proteinuria. *J. Vet. Intern. Med.* 20 (3): 528–535.

Tahzib, M., Frank, R., Gauthier, B. et al. (1999). Vitamin E treatment of focal segmental glomerulosclerosis: results of an open-label study. *Pediatr. Nephrol.* 13 (8): 649–652.

Tain, Y.L., Freshour, G., Dikalova, A. et al. (2007). Vitamin E reduces glomerulosclerosis, restores renal neuronal NOS, and suppresses oxidative stress in the 5/6 nephrectomized rat. *Am. J. Physiol. Renal Physiol.* 292 (5): F1404–F1410.

Tang, P.K., Geddes, R.F., Chang, Y.M. et al. (2021a). Risk factors associated with disturbances of calcium homeostasis after initiation of a phosphate-restricted diet in cats with chronic kidney disease. *J. Vet. Intern. Med.* 35: 321–332.

Tang, P.K., Geddes, R.F., Jepson, R.E. et al. (2021b). A feline-focused review of chronic kidney disease-mineral and bone disorders – part 2: pathophysiology of calcium disorder and extraosseous calcification. *Vet. J.* 275: 105718.

Theisen, S.K., DiBartola, S.P., Radin, M.J. et al. (1997). Muscle potassium content and potassium gluconate supplementation in normokalemic cats with naturally occurring chronic renal failure. *J. Vet. Intern. Med.* 11 (4): 212–217.

Thompson, M.F., Fleeman, L.M., Kessell, A.E. et al. (2013). Acquired proximal renal tubulopathy in dogs exposed to a common dried chicken treat: retrospective study of 108 cases (2007–2009). *Aust. Vet. J.* 91 (9): 368–373.

Vaden, S.L. and Elliott, J. (2016). Management of proteinuria in dogs and cats with chronic kidney disease. *Vet. Clin. North Am. Small Anim. Pract.* 46 (6): 1115–1130.

Valle, E., Prola, L., Vergnano, D. et al. (2019). Investigation of hallmarks of carbonyl stress and formation of end products in feline chronic kidney disease as markers of uraemic toxins. *J. Feline Med. Surg.* 21 (6): 465–474.

Valli, V.E., Baumal, R., Thorner, P. et al. (1991). Dietary modification reduces splitting of glomerular basement membranes and delays death due to renal failure in canine X-linked hereditary nephritis. *Lab. Invest.* 65 (1): 67–73.

Vanholder, R., Glorieux, G., De Smet, R., and Lameire, N., and European Uremic Toxin Work Group(2003). New insights in uremic toxins. *Kidney Int. Suppl.* (84): S6–S10.

Vanholder, R., Pletinck, A., Schepers, E., and Glorieux, G. (2018). Biochemical and clinical impact of organic uremic retention solutes: a comprehensive update. *Toxins (Basel)* 10 (1): 33.

Waldron, M.K., Hannah, S.S., and Bauer, J.E. (2012). Plasma phospholipid fatty acid and ex vivo neutrophil responses are differentially altered in dogs fed fish- and linseed-oil containing diets at the same n-6:n-3 fatty acid ratio. *Lipids* 47 (4): 425–434.

Wehner, A., Hartmann, K., and Hirschberger, J. (2008). Associations between proteinuria, systemic hypertension and glomerular filtration rate in dogs with renal and non-renal diseases. *Vet. Rec.* 162 (5): 141–147.

White, J.V., Finco, D.R., Crowell, W.A. et al. (1991). Effect of dietary protein on functional, morphologic, and histologic changes of the kidney during compensatory renal growth in dogs. *Am. J. Vet. Res.* 52 (8): 1357–1365.

Xu, H., Laflamme, D.P., and Long, G.L. (2009). Effects of dietary sodium chloride on health parameters in mature cats. *J. Feline Med. Surg.* 11 (6): 435–441.

Xu, H., Laflamme, D., Bathnagar, S. et al. (2016). Effect of high sodium diet on blood pressure and cardiac function in healthy adult dogs (abstract). *J. Vet. Intern. Med.* 30 (4): 1485–1485.

Yearley, J.H., Hancock, D.D., and Mealey, K.L. (2004). Survival time, lifespan, and quality of life in dogs with idiopathic Fanconi syndrome. *J. Am. Vet. Med. Assoc.* 225 (3): 377–383.

Younes, H., Rémésy, C., Behr, S., and Demigné, C. (1997). Fermentable carbohydrate exerts a urea-lowering effect in normal and nephrectomized rats. *Am. J. Physiol.* 272 (3 Pt 1): G515–G521.

Younes, H., Garleb, K.A., Behr, S.R., and Rémésy, C. (1998). Dietary fiber stimulates the extra-renal route of nitrogen excretion in partially nephrectomized rats. *J. Nutr. Biochem.* 9 (11): 613–620.

Yu, S. and Paetau-Robinson, I. (2006). Dietary supplements of vitamins E and C and beta-carotene reduce oxidative stress in cats with renal insufficiency. *Vet. Res. Commun.* 30 (4): 403–413.

Zatelli, A., Roura, X., D'Ippolito, P. et al. (2016). The effect of renal diet in association with enalapril or benazepril on proteinuria in dogs with proteinuric chronic kidney disease. *Open Vet. J.* 6 (2): 121–127.

16

Nutritional Management of Lower Urinary Tract Disease
Joe Bartges and Ronald J. Corbee

Lower urinary tract disease occurs commonly in cats and dogs. Previous estimates of the incidence in cats in the United States and United Kingdom were 0.85–1.0% per year (Willeberg 1984; Lawler et al. 1985), while in dogs the incidence is 2.0–3.0% per year (Thomsen et al. 1986). These estimates are based on the presence of clinical signs only and did not consider actual diagnoses. Any disorder of the lower urinary tract may cause signs of lower urinary tract disease. In cats younger than approximately 10 years of age, idiopathic cystitis and urolithiasis occur most commonly (Kruger et al. 1991; Buffington et al. 1997), while in cats older than 10 years of age, bacterial urinary tract infection and urolithiasis occur most commonly (Bartges 1996). In dogs, the incidence of lower urinary tract disease increases with advancing age; bacterial urinary tract infections and urolithiasis occur most commonly (Bartges 2000; Lulich et al. 2000). Urinary tract infections are seen more often in female dogs compared to male dogs and in medium- and large-breed dogs compared to small-breed dogs (Adamama-Moraitou et al. 2017).

Crystal-Related Lower Urinary Tract Disease

Of the various causes of lower urinary tract disease, crystal-related disease accounts for 15–45% of cases. There are many minerals that may precipitate in the urinary tract to form crystals and uroliths (aka stones); however, more than 85% of uroliths from cats and more than 70% of uroliths from dogs are composed of either struvite (magnesium ammonium phosphate hexahydrate) or calcium oxalate monohydrate or dihydrate (Lulich et al. 2013b; Burggraaf et al. 2021; Kpercny et al. 2021a, b). Struvite is the most common mineral observed to occur in matrix-crystalline urethral plugs (Osborne et al. 2009).

Urolith and matrix-crystalline plug formation involves complex physiochemical processes. Major factors include (i) urine supersaturation resulting in crystal formation (nucleation); (ii) effect of inhibitors of mineral nucleation, crystal aggregation, and crystal growth; (iii) crystalloid complexors; (iv) effects of promoters of crystal aggregation and growth; (v) effects of non-crystalline matrix; and (vi) urine retention or slowed transit for the processes to occur (Brown and Purich 1992; Coe et al. 1992). Urethral matrix-crystalline plugs have only been identified in male cats and may represent an intermediate phase between lower urinary tract inflammation without crystals and urolith formation (Osborne et al. 1996b). The most important driving force behind urolith formation is urinary supersaturation with calculogenic substances (Bartges et al. 1999b); however, as mentioned before, other factors are important.

Applied Veterinary Clinical Nutrition, Second Edition. Edited by Andrea J. Fascetti, Sean J. Delaney, Jennifer A. Larsen, and Cecilia Villaverde.
© 2024 John Wiley & Sons, Inc. Published 2024 by John Wiley & Sons, Inc.

The goal of urinary crystal-related disease is to promote a reduced state of urinary saturation.

Urolithiasis

Urolithiasis refers to the formation of and consequences of mineral precipitation within the urinary system. It is not a single disease with a single cause, but the sequelae of multiple underlying abnormalities. Therefore, it can be viewed as a syndrome defined as the combination of pathophysiologic factors (i.e. familial, congenital, and/or acquired) that increase the risk of precipitation of minerals in the urinary system forming uroliths.

Calcium Oxalate

Figures 16.1–16.3 show a calcium oxalate dehydrate urocystolith in a dog.

Calcium oxalate uroliths form when urine is oversaturated with calcium and oxalate (Bartges et al. 1999b). In addition to these alterations in activities of ions, large molecular weight proteins that occur in urine, such as nephrocalcin, uropontin, and Tamm–Horsfall mucoprotein, influence calcium oxalate formation (Balaji and Menon 1997). Hydroxyproline induces oxalate excretion in cats, and therefore preventive diets for calcium oxalate should contain less than 1 g per megajoule (MJ) metabolizable energy (ME) (<4.4 g per Mcal ME) of hydroxyproline (Dijcker

et al. 2014). Hydroxyproline is mostly found in bone and collagenous tissues. We have a limited understanding of the role of these macromolecular and ionic inhibitors of calcium oxalate formation in cats and dogs. Certain metabolic factors are known to increase the risk of calcium oxalate urolith formation in several species. Medical and nutritional strategies for stone prevention have focused on amelioration of these factors.

Hypercalcemia is associated with increased risk of calcium oxalate urolith formation. In cats with calcium oxalate uroliths, hypercalcemia was observed in 35% of cases (Bartges 2001). Conversely, uroliths developed in 35% of cats with idiopathic hypercalcemia (Midkiff et al. 2000). In dogs with calcium oxalate uroliths, hypercalcemia has been observed to occur in approximately 5%; usually these dogs have primary hyperparathyroidism (Lulich et al. 1999b). Hypercalcemia results in increased calcium fractional excretion and hypercalciuria when severe.

Hypercalciuria is a significant risk factor, but not necessarily the cause of calcium oxalate urolith formation in human beings, dogs, and cats (Bartges et al. 2004a). In two studies involving calcium oxalate urolith-forming miniature schnauzers, bichon frisés, and shih tzus, and breed-matched controls, hypercalciuria was defined as a urine calcium-to-urine creatinine ratio of greater than 0.6 in fasting or

Figure 16.1 Lateral abdominal radiograph of an 8-year-old, castrated male miniature schnauzer with an urocystolith composed of calcium oxalate dihydrate (arrow).

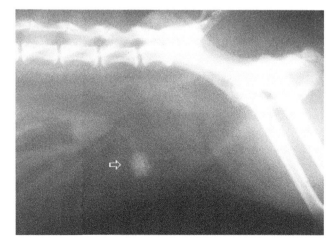

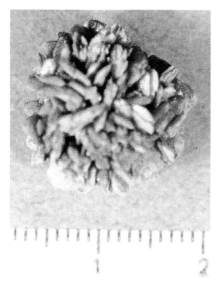

Figure 16.2 Calcium oxalate dihydrate urocystolith removed from the dog in Figure 16.1.

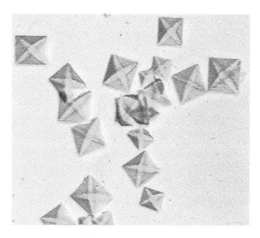

Figure 16.3 Calcium oxalate dihydrate crystals from the dog in Figure 16.1.

postprandial urine samples up to eight hours after food consumption (Furrow et al. 2015; Carr et al. 2019). Hypercalciuria can result from excessive intestinal absorption of calcium (gastrointestinal [GI] hyperabsorption), impaired renal reabsorption of calcium (renal leak), and/or excessive skeletal mobilization of calcium (resorptive) (Coe et al. 1992). In miniature schnauzers, GI hyperabsorption appears to occur most commonly, although renal leak hypercalciuria has also been observed (Lulich et al. 1991). Bone resorption was not found to be present in miniature schnauzers, bichon frisés, or shih tzus with calcium oxalate uroliths utilizing analysis of a canine-specific enzyme-linked immunosorbent assay (ELISA) for Beta-CrossLaps in serum, suggesting that bone resorption is not a primary cause of idiopathic hypercalcemia (Luskin et al. 2019).

Genetic factors may play a role in calcium oxalate urolith formation, at least in dogs. A positive correlation between the 25-hydroxyvitamin D (25(OH)D)-to-24,25-dihydroxyvitamin D ratio and the urinary calcium-to-creatinine ratio in a subset of dogs with calcium oxalate urolithiasis has been reported, suggesting that a decreased conversion of 25(OH)D might contribute to urolith risk in some dogs (Groth et al. 2019). In another study of dogs with calcium oxalate uroliths and healthy matched controls, including Pomeranians, shih tzus, Chihuahuas, miniature schnauzers, Yorkshire terriers, and Maltese, urine calcium-to-creatinine ratios were greater in urolith-forming dogs and were correlated with homozygous mutant or heterozygous genotype involving the rs852900542 single-nucleotide polymorphism of the vitamin D receptor (Chamsuwan et al. 2021).

Hypercalciuria has not been well defined in normocalcemic cats with calcium oxalate uroliths, but is thought to occur.

Hyperadrenocorticism and glucocorticoid administration are associated with increased risk of calcium oxalate urolith formation in dogs (Hess et al. 1998). The mechanisms for the increased risk are unknown; however, one author has observed hypercalciuria and increased urinary saturation for calcium oxalate in dogs with hyperadrenocorticism and calcium oxalate uroliths (Kraje et al. 2000). The degree of hypercalciuria was decreased with medical management of hyperadrenocorticism.

Metabolic acidosis promotes hypercalciuria by promoting bone turnover (release of calcium with buffers from bone), increasing serum ionized calcium concentration, resulting in increased urinary calcium excretion and decreased renal tubular reabsorption of calcium. Consumption by cats of diets supplemented with the urinary acidifier ammonium chloride has been associated with increased urinary calcium excretion (Ching et al. 1989). Aciduria (urine pH <6.2) may represent a risk factor for calcium oxalate formation because of acidemia and hypercalciuria. In addition, acidic urine alters the function and concentration of crystal inhibitors. Low urine pH decreases urinary citrate concentration by increasing renal proximal tubular citrate reabsorption. Acidic urine is known to impair function of macromolecular protein inhibitors. In a study of healthy cats, urinary saturation for calcium oxalate was less at a urine pH of 7.2 compared with 6.8 or 6.2, when the only variable was the acidification or alkalinization potential of the diet (Bartges et al. 2004b). Another study showed no difference in relative supersaturation for calcium oxalate in a pH range of 5.9–6.4 in cats (Bijsmans et al. 2021).

Inhibitors, such as citrate, magnesium, and pyrophosphate, form soluble salts with calcium or oxalic acid and reduce availability of calcium or oxalic acid for precipitation. Other inhibitors, such as Tamm–Horsfall glycoprotein and nephrocalcin, interfere with the ability of calcium and oxalic acid to combine, minimizing crystal formation, aggregation, and growth.

Oxalic acid is a metabolic end product of ascorbic acid (vitamin C) and several amino acids, such as glycine and serine, derived from dietary sources. Oxalic acid forms soluble salts with sodium and potassium ions, but a relatively insoluble salt with calcium ions. Therefore, any increased urinary concentration of oxalic acid may promote calcium oxalate formation. Dietary increases of oxalate and vitamin B6 (otherwise known as pyridoxine) deficiency are known factors increasing urinary oxalate. Hyperoxaluria has been observed experimentally in kittens consuming vitamin B6-deficient diets, but has not been associated

with naturally occurring calcium oxalate urolith formation. Genetic anomalies may also increase urine oxalic acid concentration. Hyperoxaluria has been recognized in a group of related cats with reduced quantities of hepatic D-glycerate dehydrogenase, an enzyme involved in metabolism of oxalic acid precursors (primary hyperoxaluria type II) (McKerrell et al. 1989). Hyperoxaluria has also been associated with defective peroxisomal alanine/glyoxylate aminotransferase activity (primary hyperoxaluria type I) and intestinal disease in human beings (enteric hyperoxaluria). These have not been evaluated in cats or dogs.

Decreased urine volume results in increased calcium and oxalic acid saturation and an increased risk for urolith formation. Cats can achieve urine specific gravities in excess of 1.065, indicating a marked ability to produce concentrated urine. Many cats and dogs affected with calcium oxalate uroliths have a urine specific gravity >1.040, unless there is some impairment of renal function or concentrating ability (Bartges et al. 2004a).

The detection of calcium oxalate crystals indicates that urine is supersaturated with calcium oxalate and, if persistent, this supersaturation represents an increased risk for calcium oxalate urolith formation. However, calcium oxalate crystalluria is present in fewer than 50% of feline and canine cases at time of diagnosis of urolithiasis (Bartges et al. 2004a).

Medical protocols that promote dissolution of calcium oxalate uroliths are not currently available; therefore, uroliths must be removed physically: either surgically, by cystoscopy and laser lithotripsy, or by voiding urohydropropulsion (Lulich et al. 1999a, 2009; Adams et al. 2008).

Nutritional and/or medical protocols should be considered to minimize urolith recurrence or prevent further growth of uroliths that remain in the urinary tract. A significant number of cats and dogs will develop recurrent uroliths within two years of their initial episode if prevention protocols are not initiated (Lulich et al. 2004). If possible, metabolic factors known to increase calcium oxalate risk should be corrected or minimized. The goals of dietary prevention include (i) reducing urine calcium and oxalate concentration; (ii) promoting high concentrations and activity of urolith inhibitors; (iii) reducing urine acidity; and (iv) promoting dilute urine.

Increasing urine volume is a mainstay of preventive therapy for calcium oxalate urolithiasis in humans. By increasing water intake, urinary concentrations of calculogenic minerals are reduced. In addition, larger urine volumes typically increase urine transit time and voiding frequency, thereby reducing retention time for crystal formation and growth. Feeding a canned/retorted food is the most practical means of increasing water intake and lowering calcium oxalate urine saturation. The goal is to dilute urine to a specific gravity of at least ≤1.025 or 1.030 (Kirk et al. 2003; Palm and Westropp 2011; Bartges and Callens 2015; Lulich et al. 2016). Flavoring water, enhancing water access, and adding water to dry/extruded foods may be used in dogs and cats that refuse to eat canned foods. Many nutritionists use the following equation to calculate the amount of water in g or ml to add to food of a known moisture percentage to achieve a specific overall dietary moisture. The example demonstrates how much water is needed to achieve an overall desired moisture of 85%:

Current Food Moisture % or "C" = 10% or 0.1 (see label for actual value)

Food Total Mass or "F" = 250 g (specific to each patient)

Desired Overall Moisture % or "D" = 85% or 0.85 (generally 75–85%)

Answer or "X" = g or ml Water to Add

$X = ((D \times F) - (C \times F))/(1 - D)$

OR

$X = ((0.85 \times 250) - (0.1 \times 250)) / (1 - 0.85)$

Solving for X = 1250 g or 1250 ml (as 1 g water = 1 ml water)

Using this equation can be helpful as the amount of added water is often underestimated, including when fresh or canned/

retorted food is fed (~65–75% moisture) and the desired overall moisture is high at 85%.

Consumption of high concentrations of sodium may augment renal calcium excretion in human. Epidemiologic evidence suggests that the low dietary sodium concentrations in cat and dog foods increase the risk for calcium oxalate urolithiasis and that diets that contain high dietary sodium concentrations decrease the risk (Lekcharoensuk et al. 2000a, b, 2001). Studies in healthy cats and dogs did not find increased urine calcium excretion in response to high dietary salt intake (minimal 1.2% sodium dry matter basis) (Kirk et al. 2003; Stevenson et al. 2003; Lulich et al. 2005). A study has shown that high dietary sodium chloride promotes urine dilution in cats and dogs, and while calcium excretion increased in dogs in this study, the overall urinary calcium concentration decreased, as did relative supersaturation for calcium oxalate (Queau et al. 2020). In humans with hypocitraturia, sodium supplementation has also been shown to increase urine volume and decrease urinary saturation for calcium oxalate (Stoller et al. 2009). In one study, when fed a food lower in sodium, cats with naturally occurring calcium oxalate uroliths excreted less urine calcium (Lulich et al. 2004). In healthy cats or those with marginal renal function and hypercalciuria, increased dietary sodium exacerbated calcium excretion with (Kirk et al. 2006) and without (Hughes et al. 2002; Buranakarl et al. 2004; Luckschander et al. 2004; Cowgill et al. 2007; Xu et al. 2009) increasing azotemia. Furthermore, in another study, restricting dietary sodium was associated with kaliuresis, an increased risk of hypokalemia, and a decrease in glomerular filtration rate in cats with induced chronic renal failure (Buranakarl et al. 2004). Until further data are available, orally administered sodium chloride or loop diuretics, which promote renal sodium excretion, for diuresis should be used cautiously and with careful monitoring, as they may increase one risk factor for calcium oxalate urolith formation (i.e. increased calcium excretion but not urinary calcium concentration) or worsening azotemia in some patients. As a result, recommended concentrations of sodium in foods for cats and dogs predisposed to calcium oxalate formation is debated, as diets containing as low as 0.4 g/Mcal sodium and as high as 3.5 g/Mcal sodium are available commercially. If high dietary sodium is of concern or proves to not be tolerated, the use of a high-moisture diet is generally recommended.

The solubility of calcium oxalate in urine is influenced by pH, and epidemiologic studies consistently identify acidifying diets among the most prominent risk factors for calcium oxalate urolithiasis (Kirk et al. 1995; Thumchai et al. 1996; Lekcharoensuk et al. 2000a, b; Okafor et al. 2014). In prospective studies, however, the influence of pH directly on calcium oxalate solubility is less clear, with one study showing no influence (Stevenson 2002) and another showing an increase in calcium oxalate solubility at an alkaline pH of 7.2 (Bartges et al. 2004b). In a case series of five cats with idiopathic hypercalcemia and calcium oxalate uroliths, discontinuation of acidifying diets or urinary acidifiers was associated with normalization of serum calcium concentration (McClain et al. 1999). In another study of healthy cats, urinary saturation for calcium oxalate linearly decreased with increasing urine pH (Bartges et al. 2004b). Although conclusions from one study were that urinary pH and potassium citrate had limited effects on urinary saturation for calcium oxalate in dogs, three miniature schnauzers, a breed with a higher risk for calcium oxalate formation, had lower urinary saturation for calcium oxalate with potassium citrate supplementation and alkaluria (Stevenson et al. 2000). Aciduria promotes hypocitraturia and functional impairment of endogenous urolith inhibitors. Thus, feeding an acidifying diet or administering urinary acidifiers to cats and dogs at risk for calcium oxalate is contraindicated. A target urine pH of approximately 7.5 has been suggested in cats and dogs at risk for the recurrence of calcium oxalate uroliths (Kirk et al. 2003; Bartges

et al. 2004b), despite conflicting and debated evidence (Stevenson 2002).

Although reduction of urine calcium and oxalic acid concentrations by restriction of dietary calcium and oxalic acid appears logical, it is not without risk. Reducing consumption of only one of these constituents may increase availability and intestinal absorption of the other, resulting in increased urinary excretion. Conversely, increasing dietary calcium concentrations contributes directly to increased urine calcium concentration. Because epidemiologic data suggest that marked dietary calcium restriction increases urolith risk, moderate concentrations of dietary calcium are advised in non-hypercalcemic cats (Lekcharoensuk et al. 2000a, 2002; Kirk et al. 2003). Thiazide diuretics may be administered to decrease urinary calcium excretion. A 55% decrease in urinary calcium concentration was reported in urolith-forming dogs that were treated with hydrochlorothiazide at a dose of 2 mg/kg every (q) 12 h (Lulich et al. 2000). A 65% decrease in urinary calcium oxalate-relative supersaturation was reported in clinically normal cats receiving hydrochlorothiazide at a dose of 1 mg/kg q 12 h (Hezel et al. 2007). Thiazide diuretics may induce hypercalcemia by increasing renal calcium reabsorption; therefore, monitoring of plasma calcium or ionized calcium concentrations is advised. Hypercalcemia and renal failure are contraindications for the use of thiazide diuretics.

Urinary oxalate is derived from endogenous metabolism of oxalate precursors (i.e. glycine and ascorbic acid) and dietary oxalic acid. Most pet food ingredients are low in oxalic acid, with the exception of vegetables, legumes, and several vegetable-based fermentable fibers (e.g. beet pulp and soybean fiber). Dietary oxalic acid concentrations should be reduced to the lowest possible concentration in cases of calcium oxalate urolithiasis. Suggested dietary concentration is <20 mg oxalic acid/100 g of food (dry matter basis) or about <40–45 mg oxalic acid/Mcal.

Excess intake of vitamin C, a metabolic oxalate precursor, should similarly be avoided (Kirk et al. 2003). While normal dietary vitamin C concentrations are not considered a risk in human beings, very small increases in urinary oxalate are a concern in urolith formers. Because cats and dogs do not have a dietary vitamin C requirement, supplementation should be avoided. Cranberry concentrate tablets are also contraindicated. They provide mild acidification and are high in oxalate, as well as vitamin C (Terris et al. 2001); however, in one study of human beings, cranberry juice ingestion resulted in increased citrate and decreased oxalic acid in urine (McHarg et al. 2003).

Potassium citrate is often included in diets designed for calcium oxalate prevention. In urine, citric acid combines with calcium to form soluble complexes, thereby reducing urinary ionic calcium concentration and directly inhibiting nucleation of calcium and oxalate crystals (Tiselius et al. 1993; Caudarella and Vescini 2009). Administration has also been associated with decreased urinary oxalate excretion (Ito 1991), decreased intestinal calcium absorption resulting in decreased urinary calcium excretion (Rumenapf and Schwille 1987), and increased excretion and activity of urinary inhibitory macromolecules (Caudarella and Vescini 2009). When oxidized within the tricarboxylic acid cycle, supplemental citrate results in urine alkalinization due, in part, to the production of bicarbonate (Hamm and Simon 1987; Rodman 1991), although short-term administration of citrate does not have this effect (Sakhaee et al. 1992; Stevenson et al. 2000). The metabolic alkalinization increases endogenous renal citrate excretion and reduces calcium absorption and urinary excretion (Pak et al. 1985; Kirk et al. 2003). Commercial products that add citrate but continue to acidify the urine (pH <6.5) reduce the benefit of citrate therapy. Potassium citrate may be supplemented at an initial dosage of 75 mg/kg by mouth q 12 h, with adjustment of dosage to achieve a urine pH of approximately

7.5. Potassium citrate at this dose may lower urinary relative calcium oxalate supersaturation without a significant increase in urinary pH (Stevenson et al. 2000).

Dietary phosphorus should not be restricted with calcium oxalate urolithiasis. Low dietary phosphorus is a risk factor for calcium oxalate urolith formation in cats and dogs (Lekcharoensuk et al. 2000a,b, 2001, 2002). Reduction in dietary phosphorus may be associated with activation of vitamin D, which in turn promotes intestinal calcium absorption and hypercalciuria. Additionally, phosphate status determines pyrophosphate urinary concentrations, an inhibitor of calcium oxalate urolith formation in human beings and rodents. If calcium oxalate urolithiasis is associated with hypophosphatemia and normal calcium concentration, oral phosphorus supplementation may be considered. Caution should be used, however, because excessive dietary phosphorus may predispose to formation of calcium phosphate uroliths. Whether this occurs in cats is unknown. Phosphorus concentrations in the foods for cats predisposed to calcium oxalate formation should not be excessive. Diets formulated for oxalate prevention in cats and dogs contain phosphorus from 0.3 to 2.1 g/Mcal. Concentrations from approximately 1.5 to 2.0 g/Mcal have been recommended (Kirk et al. 2003). In cats that have developed hypercalcemia due to chronic kidney disease and are on a phosphorus-restricted renal diet (e.g. <1.0 g/Mcal), feeding a diet with a moderate phosphorus concentration (e.g. 1.5 g/Mcal) can result in normalization of the plasma calcium concentration and thus reduce the risk of calcium oxalate urolithiasis (Geddes et al. 2021).

Urinary magnesium forms complexes with oxalic acid, reducing the amount of oxalic acid available to form calcium oxalate. Studies in cats associate low dietary magnesium with calcium oxalate risk (Robertson 1993; Thumchai et al. 1996; Smith et al. 1997; Lulich et al. 1999b; Lekcharoensuk et al. 2000a, 2001). In human beings, supplemental magnesium has been used to minimize recurrence of calcium oxalate uroliths; however, supplemental magnesium may increase the risk of struvite formation in cats. At this time, the risks and benefits of magnesium supplementation to cats and dogs with calcium oxalate urolithiasis have not been evaluated, and supplementation is not advised. However, it appears logical that magnesium should not be highly restricted in diets that are consumed by cats with calcium oxalate urolithiasis. Many diets that claim to benefit feline "urinary tract health" are reduced in magnesium and promote urinary acidification. These foods are designed for struvite prevention and may not be appropriate for cats at risk for calcium oxalate urolithiasis, unless data to support their use for both urolith types are available. Prudent concentrations of dietary magnesium have been suggested from 0.08 to 0.10% dry matter or approximately 200 mg magnesium/Mcal (Lekcharoensuk et al. 2001; Kirk et al. 2003).

Consumption of high amounts of animal protein by humans is associated with an increased risk of calcium oxalate formation. Dietary protein of animal origin may increase urinary calcium and oxalic acid excretion, decrease urinary citrate excretion, and promote bone mobilization in order to buffer the acid intake from the metabolism of animal proteins (Aparicio et al. 2013; Prezioso et al. 2015). In contrast, a case-controlled, retrospective study showed that higher protein concentration in cat and dog foods appeared protective against calcium oxalate uroliths (Lekcharoensuk et al. 2000a,b, 2001, 2002). Protein concentrations between 80 and 90 g protein/Mcal appeared most protective in cats. In another study of healthy cats, consumption of a diet containing 35% crude protein (dry matter) from a high-quality protein was associated with lower urine saturation for calcium oxalate and higher urinary citrate excretion when compared with diets containing either 44% or 57% crude protein (dry matter) from a high-quality protein (Paßlack et al. 2014).

Excessive concentrations of vitamin D (which promotes intestinal absorption of calcium) and vitamin C (which is a precursor of oxalic acid) should be avoided. Diets with vitamin D between 250 and 350 IU/Mcal kcal should suffice. As discussed earlier, vitamin C is an oxalate precursor, as well as a weak urinary acidifier. Both features may increase likelihood of urolith recurrence, so its addition should be avoided or minimized.

The diet should be adequately fortified with vitamin B6, because vitamin B6 deficiency promotes endogenous production and subsequent urinary excretion of oxalic acid (Bai et al. 1989). There is no evidence that increased vitamin B6 beyond that needed to meet the nutritional requirements in cats provides a benefit. Because most commercial diets designed for cats and dogs are well fortified with vitamin B6, it is unlikely that additional supplementation will be beneficial except in deficient homemade diets. Regardless, vitamin B6 is reasonably safe and sometimes provided to cats with persistent calcium oxalate crystalluria or frequent recurrences.

Increased dietary fiber intake is associated with decreasing risk of calcium oxalate recurrence in some human beings. Certain types of fiber (soy or rice bran) decrease calcium absorption from the gastrointestinal tract, which may decrease urinary calcium excretion. Also, higher-fiber diets tend to be less acidifying. In five cats with idiopathic hypercalcemia and calcium oxalate uroliths, feeding a high-fiber diet with supplemental potassium citrate resulted in normalization of serum calcium concentrations (McClain et al. 1999). It is unclear whether a reduction in dietary calcium alone would have had a similar impact, as has been suggested by editors of this text.

While the relationship of obesity to urolith formation is not understood, it remains a consistent risk factor in all studies to date; suggested effects of obesity in cats that might contribute to urolith formation, as stated by one of the authors (RJC) are less activity, less water intake, postponed use of the litter box, and therefore prolonged presence of more concentrated urine in the bladder. Also excessive caloric intake may result in excessive mineral/calcium intake. Restricting food intake to obtain an ideal weight and body condition is encouraged.

Cats and dogs that are meal fed on average have a more alkaline urinary pH, controlled food intake for obesity prevention, and a lower risk of calcium oxalate urolith formation (Kirk et al. 1995; Lekcharoensuk et al. 2000a,b). This method of feeding is also the preferred choice for canned foods, as they desiccate over time when left out. This is a relatively simple step that owners can take to improve preventive measures.

Although there are several commercially available therapeutic diets for managing calcium oxalate uroliths in cats and dogs, none has been through clinical trials with the end point of urolith recurrence, although there are some data in healthy animals and in pets that have formed calcium oxalate uroliths (Smith et al. 1998; Stevenson et al. 2002; Lulich et al. 2004). Calcium oxalate uroliths are recurrent, with an approximate 36% recurrence rate within one year if preventive measures are not undertaken (Lulich et al. 1992). Even with preventive measures, first recurrence occurs (7.1%) within 25 months (Albasan et al. 2009).

Recommendations for monitoring cats and dogs that have formed calcium oxalate uroliths include complete urinalysis and abdominal radiography every 4–6 months. Maintaining a urine pH of 7.0–7.5 and dilute urine is desired. In two studies, urine saturation for calcium oxalate was significantly lower when urine specific gravity was 1.040–1.044 (Hawthorne and Markwell 2004) and 1.034–1.040 (Buckley et al. 2011). The recommendation is to dilute urine to a specific gravity of ≤1.045, although others recommend ≤1.025 (Kirk et al. 2003; Palm and Westropp 2011; Bartges and Callens 2015; Lulich et al. 2016). In cats with hypercalcemia-associated calcium oxalate urolithiasis, maintain normocalcemia; if an underlying disease process is identified then manage appropriately, which may mean a calcium-restricted homemade diet.

Struvite

Figures 16.4–16.6 show a struvite urolith in a dog.

Struvite is another name for crystals or uroliths composed of magnesium ammonium phosphate hexahydrate. The chemical composition of struvite is $Mg^{2+}NH_4^+PO_4^{3-}*6H_2O$. In order for uroliths to form, urine must be oversaturated with respect to the minerals that precipitate to form that type of urolith. In order for struvite uroliths to form, urine must be

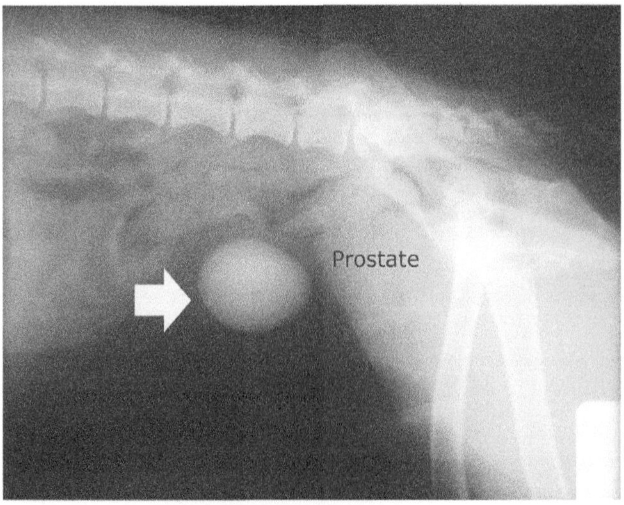

Figure 16.4 Lateral abdominal radiograph of a 10-year-old mixed-breed intact male dog with an infection-induced struvite urocystolith (arrow) and prostatomegaly.

Prostate

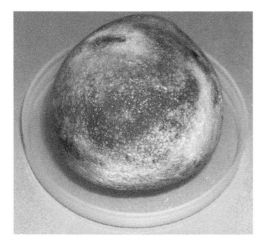

Figure 16.5 Infection-induced struvite urocystoliths removed from the dog in Figure 16.4.

oversaturated with magnesium, ammonium, and phosphate ions. Urinary oversaturation with struvite may occur as a consequence of a urinary tract infection with a urease-producing microbe (infection-induced struvite) or without the presence of a urinary tract infection (sterile struvite) (Osborne et al. 1990; Bartges et al. 1992b).

Sterile Struvite

Sterile struvite uroliths form typically in cats between 1 and 10 years of age, although they have been reported in related English cocker spaniels (Bartges et al. 1992b). Risk for struvite urolith formation decreases after approximately 6–8 years of age in cats (Smith et al. 1997). They occur with equal frequency in male and female cats. Sterile struvite uroliths form because of dietary composition as well as innate risks for urolith formation. Experimentally, magnesium phosphate and struvite uroliths formed in healthy cats that consumed calculogenic diets containing 0.15–1.0% magnesium (dry matter basis) (Finco et al. 1985; Osborne et al. 1985; Buffington 1989). These data are difficult to interpret, however, because the amount of magnesium consumption by cats in these studies may be different than the amount consumed by cats that spontaneously form sterile struvite uroliths because of the differences in commercial diets with regard to caloric density, palatability, and digestibility (Osborne et al. 1999a). The influence of magnesium on struvite formation depends on urine pH (Buffington et al. 1990) and the influence of ions, minerals, and other components in urine (Buffington et al. 1994). Alkaluria is associated with increased risk for struvite formation (Tarttelin 1987a; Bartges et al. 1998). In a clinical study including 20 cats with naturally occurring struvite urocystoliths and no detectable bacterial urinary tract infection, the mean

Figure 16.6 Struvite crystals, sperm, and blood cells from the dog in Figure 16.4.

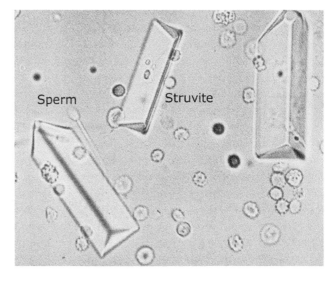

urinary pH at the time of diagnosis was 6.9 ± 0.4 (Osborne et al. 1990). An additional factor is water intake and urine volume. Consumption of increased quantities of water may result in lower concentrations of calculogenic substances in urine, thus decreasing the risk of urolith formation (Smith et al. 1998). Frequent consumption of small quantities of food rather than one or two large meals per day is associated with production of more acidic urine and a lower degree of struvite crystalluria in cats (Tarttelin 1987b; Finke and Litzenberger 1992).

Sterile struvite uroliths can be dissolved by feeding a diet that is magnesium, phosphorus, and protein restricted, and that induces aciduria relative to maintenance adult cat foods (Osborne et al. 1990). In a clinical study including 22 cats with sterile struvite urocystoliths, urocystoliths dissolved in 20 cats in a mean of 36.2 ± 26.6 days (range 14–141 days) (Osborne et al. 1990). The cats were fed a high-moisture (canned/retorted), calorically dense diet containing 0.058% magnesium (dry matter basis) and increased sodium chloride (0.79% dry matter basis). The diet induced a urine pH of approximately 6.0. Sterile struvite uroliths dissolve on average in 2–4 weeks (Osborne et al. 1990). A urinalysis and lateral abdominal survey radiograph should be performed every 4 weeks until urolith dissolution. The diet should be continued for 2 weeks past radiographic evidence of dissolution. If uroliths do not dissolve, uroliths may contain other minerals (Tefft et al. 2021) or not be composed of struvite, and surgery or a minimally invasive technique should be performed to remove them. Other considerations for attempting dietary versus surgical intervention can include whether other concurrent disease(s) prevent the use of a dissolution diet (e.g. fat intolerance, as some commercial options are higher in fat, >45% fat calories).

Prevention of sterile struvite uroliths involves inducing a urine pH less than approximately 6.8, increasing urine volume, and decreasing the excretion of magnesium, ammonium, and phosphorus. There are many diets available that are formulated to be "struvite preventive," although none has published information concerning recurrence rates. The goals for prevention of sterile struvite urolithiasis include maintaining a urine pH of <6.5 and a lack of struvite crystalluria (Tarttelin 1987a; Houston et al. 2011; Bartges et al. 2013; Lulich et al. 2013a). Whether inducing dilute urine is beneficial is unknown; however, a target urine specific gravity of <1.040 may be an appropriate goal.

Infection-Induced Struvite

Infection-induced struvite uroliths occur more commonly in dogs, but are reported to occur in cats less than 1 year and greater than 10 years of age. They are more likely to occur in female dogs, but no sex predilection has been identified in cats. Infection-induced struvite uroliths form because of an infection with a urease-producing microbe in a fashion similar to human beings (Osborne et al. 1985). In this situation, dietary composition is not important, as the production of the enzyme urease by the microbial organism is the driving force behind struvite urolith formation.

Infection-induced struvite uroliths can be dissolved by feeding a therapeutic "struvite dissolution" diet and administering an appropriate antimicrobial agent based on bacteriologic culture and sensitivity. Average dissolution time for infection-induced struvite uroliths is approximately 70 days (Osborne et al. 1990; Osborne 1999). It is important that the patient receive an appropriate antimicrobial agent during the entire time of medical dissolution, because bacteria become trapped in the matrix of the urolith and as the urolith dissolves, bacteria contained in the matrix of the urolith are released into urine. If therapeutic concentrations of an appropriate antimicrobial agent are not present in urine, then an infection will recur, and dissolution will cease. A urinalysis and lateral survey abdominal radiograph should be performed every

4 weeks until urolith dissolution. When successful, uroliths decrease in size and number by approximately 50% every 4 weeks until disappearance. The struvite dissolution diet and antimicrobial therapy should be continued for 2–4 weeks past radiographic evidence of urolith dissolution. If uroliths do not dissolve, then surgery or a minimally invasive technique should be performed to remove them.

Prevention of infection-induced struvite does not require feeding a special diet, as it is the infection that causes these struvite uroliths to form. It involves preventing a bacterial urinary tract infection from recurring and treating bacterial infections as they arise. Dietary manipulation will not prevent infection-induced struvite uroliths from recurring, because diet will not prevent recurrence of a bacterial urinary tract infection. A therapeutic diet designed for weight loss may be used in patients that are overweight or obese, as this may be a predisposing risk factor due to anatomic alterations especially around the vulva increasing the risk for an ascending urinary tract infection, as reported in people.

Purines

Uric acid is one of several biodegradation products of purine nucleotide metabolism (Bartges et al. 1999c). In most cats and dogs, allantoin is the major metabolic end product; it is the most soluble of the purine metabolic products excreted in urine. Purine accounted for 7.6% from 1999 to 2000 and 5.1% from 2002 to 2009 of feline and canine uroliths submitted to the Minnesota Urolith Center (Lulich et al. 2013b); most are composed of urate salts, with <0.2% composed of xanthine. Ammonium urate is the monobasic ammonium salt of uric acid, and it is the most common form of naturally occurring purine uroliths observed to occur in cats and dogs (Osborne et al. 2000). Other naturally occurring purine uroliths include sodium urate, sodium calcium urate, potassium urate, uric acid dihydrate, and xanthine.

Urate

Figures 16.7–16.9 show urate uroliths in a Dalmatian, and Figures 16.10–16.12 show urate uroliths in a Pomeranian with a portosystemic shunt. Figure 16.13 shows xanthine crystals in a cat.

Urate uroliths occur when urinary concentration of uric acid, and usually ammonium ion, is increased. This may occur secondary to portovascular anomalies (particularly in young animals) (Bartges et al. 1999a), but may occur in certain types of cats (e.g. domestic shorthair) or breeds of dogs (e.g. Dalmatians and English bulldogs) (Bartges et al. 1994b); in dogs without portovascular anomalies, males appear to be affected more frequently than females, but in cats, as well as in animals with portovascular anomalies, males and females appear equally likely to be affected. Dalmatians, English bulldogs, and black Russian terriers have been shown to have a mutation in the *SLC2A9* gene that encodes for a transporter for uric acid (Bannasch et al. 2008). Most urate uroliths occur before 4 years of age. Urate

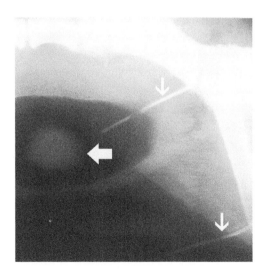

Figure 16.7 Lateral double-contrast cystogram of a 4-year-old castrated male Dalmatian with ammonium urate urocystoliths. The urocystoliths collect in the dependent portion of the contrast (large arrow). Small arrows point to an 8-French red rubber urinary catheter containing contrast inserted transurethrally.

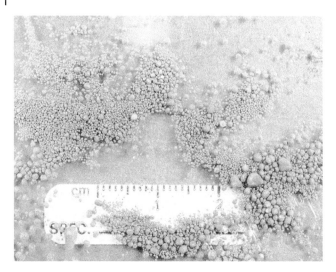

Figure 16.8 Ammonium urate urocystoliths removed from the dog in Figure 16.7.

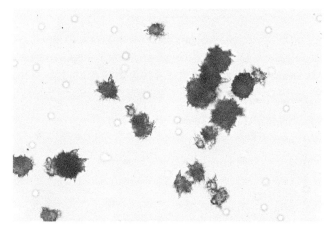

Figure 16.9 Ammonium urate crystals from the dog in Figure 16.7.

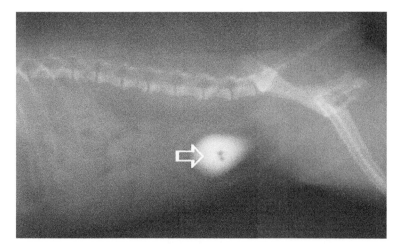

Figure 16.10 Lateral double-contrast cystogram of a 3-year-old castrated male Pomeranian with ammonium urate urocystoliths (arrow).

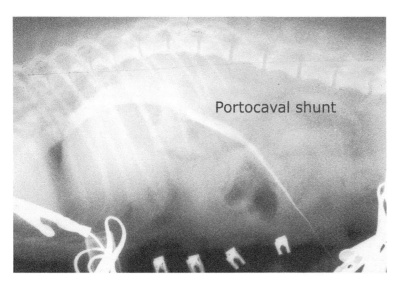

Figure 16.11 Contrast portal radiography from the dog in Figure 16.10 demonstrating a portocaval vascular shunt.

Figure 16.12 Ammonium urate urocystoliths removed from the dog in Figure 16.10.

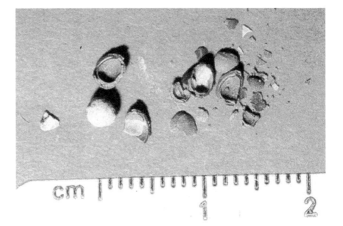

Figure 16.13 Xanthine crystals from a 3-year-old castrated male domestic shorthair cat.

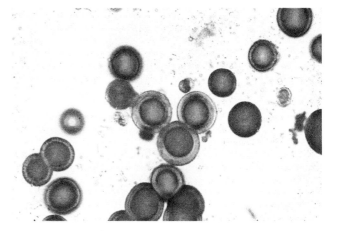

uroliths that occur in association with porto-vascular anomalies are most commonly composed of ammonium urate and are often diagnosed before 1 year of age.

Apparently there have been few studies of the biological behavior of ammonium urate uroliths in dogs with portal vascular anomalies (Marretta et al. 1981; Hardy and Klausner 1983; Johnson et al. 1987; Brain 1988) and none in cats. It is logical to hypothesize that elimination of hyperuricuria and reduction of urine ammonium concentration following surgical correction of anomalous shunts would result in spontaneous dissolution of uroliths composed primarily of ammonium urate. Appropriate clinical studies are needed to prove or disprove this hypothesis. The authors have occasionally been successful in medically dissolving urate uroliths in dogs with portal vascular anomalies by decreasing dietary purine intake and administering a low dose of allopurinol (5–10 mg/kg orally [PO] q 12 h), but have not attempted dissolution in cats with ammonium urate uroliths and portal vascular anomalies.

Medical dissolution of ammonium urate uroliths in dogs without portovascular anomalies is possible by feeding a diet that is protein and purine restricted (approximately 35–50 g protein/Mcal) and induces a diuresis and alkaluria, and by administering allopurinol (15 mg/kg PO q 12 h) (Bartges et al. 1999c). It should be noted that getting exact purine concentration data for some commercial foods can be challenging, and often foods must be selected based on total dietary protein and the protein-rich food sources (e.g. plant- and egg-based proteins) used as indicators of purine concentration. This combination is effective in approximately one-third of dogs, with a reduction in the size and number of urate uroliths facilitating non-surgical removal (voiding urohydropropulsion or catheter-assisted retrieval) in one-third; in the remaining one-third of dogs, uroliths did not change or increased in size and number (associated with xanthine formation) (Bartges et al. 1994a). A urinalysis and either abdominal ultrasonography or a double-contrast cystogram should be performed every four weeks. Urine pH should be >7.0, and urate crystals should not be present. Uroliths should decrease in size and number by 50% every four weeks until gone. If uroliths do not dissolve, then surgery or a minimally invasive procedure should be performed to remove them.

Allopurinol is a synthetic isomer of hypoxanthine. It rapidly binds to, and inhibits the action of, xanthine oxidase, and thereby decreases production of uric acid by inhibiting the conversion of hypoxanthine to xanthine, and xanthine to uric acid. The result is a reduction in serum and urine uric acid concentration within approximately two days, and a concomitant but lower degree of increase in the serum concentrations of hypoxanthine and xanthine. One author (JWB) has given this dosage to non-azotemic urate-urolith-forming dogs for up to six months without detectable consequences; however, when clients supplemented the diet with foods containing purine precursors, a layer of xanthine formed around ammonium urate uroliths or pure xanthine uroliths formed (Bartges et al. 1992a). Therefore, to minimize xanthine formation, allopurinol should be administered only to animals consuming purine-restricted foods. There is only one report of a possible immune-mediated reaction (hemolytic anemia, trigeminal neuropathy) to allopurinol administration in a dog (Pedroia 1981). The authors observed cutaneous erythema in a Dalmatian given allopurinol and ampicillin. Apparently, this may occur in human beings that are administered this combination of medication. Discontinuation of the ampicillin, but not the allopurinol, resulted in resolution of the skin lesions. Because allopurinol and its metabolites are dependent on the kidneys for elimination from humans, the dosage is commonly reduced in patients with renal dysfunction. Allopurinol has been reported to cause life-threatening erythematous desquamative skin rash, fever, hepatitis, eosinopenia, and further decline in renal function when given to human patients with renal insufficiency. Appropriate precautions should be used when considering use of allopurinol in dogs with primary renal failure.

Although no studies have been performed that evaluate the efficacy or safety of medical dissolution of urate uroliths in cats with idiopathic urate urolithiasis, one author (JWB) has successfully dissolved urate uroliths in cats using a low-protein, "renal failure" diet (50–65 g protein/Mcal) and allopurinol (7.5 mg/kg PO q 12 h). Until further studies are performed to confirm the safety and efficacy of medical dissolution, surgical removal remains the treatment of choice for urate uroliths in cats.

Prevention of urate uroliths in cats and dogs without portovascular anomalies is aimed at reducing urinary concentrations of uric acid and ammonium ions, and inducing diuresis and alkaluria. Feeding diets formulated for "renal failure" in cats or diets that are restricted in purines to dogs are effective in >90% of cases (J.W. Bartges, personal communication, 2010), despite some of these therapeutic foods using organ meats richer in purine. Administration of an alkalinizing agent (potassium citrate at 75 mg/kg PO q 12 h) may be required to achieve a urine pH >7.0. In dogs, administration of allopurinol (7–10 mg/kg PO q 12–24 h) may also be required to prevent urate uroliths from reforming; prophylactic allopurinol therapy has not been evaluated in cats. Urinalysis and abdominal ultrasonography or double-contrast cystography should be performed every 4–6 months to monitor effectiveness of prevention. Urine pH should be >7.0 and urine specific gravity should be <1.035 (cats) or <1.025 (dogs), and urate crystalluria should not be present.

In cats and dogs with portovascular anomalies, correction of the anomaly often is all that is required to prevent urate uroliths from reforming. In some animals with congenital liver disease (e.g. microvascular dysplasia), surgical correction is not possible. Preventive therapy in these patients is aimed at decreasing urinary concentrations of uric acid and ammonium ion and at managing signs of hepatoencephalopathy (see Chapter 13).

Xanthine

Xanthine uroliths may form in cats and dogs given allopurinol, especially if dietary protein and purine content are not restricted. Discontinuing allopurinol while restricting dietary protein and purine content may result in dissolution of xanthine in these patients (Bartges et al. 1994a). In such cases of xanthine urolithiasis, allopurinol may be restarted at 25–35% of the previous dosage.

Naturally occurring xanthine uroliths have been described in cats and dogs and contain pure xanthine, although a few contain small quantities of uric acid. Of 64 cats that formed xanthine uroliths in one report (Osborne et al. 2004), none of the cats had been treated with the xanthine oxidase inhibitor allopurinol. In this study, 61 xanthine uroliths were obtained from the lower urinary tract, while xanthine uroliths from 3 cats came from the upper urinary tract. Xanthine uroliths occurred in 30 neutered and 8 non-neutered males and 25 neutered females (the sex of one cat was not specified). The mean age of the cats at the time of diagnosis of xanthine uroliths was 2.8 ± 2.3 years (range 4 months–10 years). Of the 64 cats, 8 were less than 1 year old. Urinary uric acid excretion was similar between 8 xanthine urolith-forming cats and healthy cats (2.09 ± 0.8 mg/kg/d vs. 1.46 ± 0.56 mg/kg/d); however, urinary xanthine excretion (2.46 ± 1.17 mg/kg/d) and urinary hypoxanthine excretion (0.65 ± 0.17 mg/kg/d) were higher (neither is detectable in urine from healthy cats). Cavalier King Charles spaniels have a genetic predisposition to formation of idiopathic xanthine uroliths (van Zuilen et al. 1997; Gow et al. 2011; Jacinto et al. 2013). In a study of two Manchester terriers, three Cavalier King Charles spaniels, an English cocker spaniel, a dachshund, and a mixed-breed dog affected with xanthine uroliths, multiple variants in xanthine dehydrogenase or molybdenum co-factor sulfrase genes were found in a homozygous state, suggesting an autosomal recessive mode of inheritance in these dogs with hereditary xanthinuria (Tate et al. 2021).

No medical dissolution protocol for feline xanthine uroliths exists. Prevention involves feeding a diet containing approximately 50–65 g/Mcal of protein that induces alkaluria. Without preventive measures, xanthine uroliths often recur within 3–12 months following removal. In 10 cats that consumed a protein-restricted alkalinizing diet and were followed for at least two years, only one had a recurrence.

Cystine

Figures 16.14–16.16 show cystine urocystoliths removed from an English bulldog.

Cystine accounts for less than 1% of feline and canine uroliths. They occur with equal frequency in male and female cats, but occur more frequently in male dogs. Brons et al. (2013) suggested that neutering might be effective in managing cases of mild cystinuria in intact male dogs. The mean age of diagnosis of cats and dogs with cystine uroliths is 3–4 years (Osborne et al. 1999a, c). Most cats affected with cystine uroliths are domestic shorthair; English bulldogs, Newfoundlands, and dachshunds are predisposed (Case et al. 1992; Bartges et al. 1994b). In Newfoundlands, a polymorphism in the canine *SLC3A1* gene was found and can now be used as a screening test

for cystinuria (Henthorn et al. 2000; Matos et al. 2006).

Cystine uroliths occur when urine is oversaturated with cystine (the oxidized dimer of the amino acid cysteine). Cysteine is a disulfide-containing amino acid that is normally filtered and reabsorbed by proximal renal tubular cells. Therefore, cystinuria occurs when there is a defect in proximal renal tubular absorption and must be present for cystine uroliths to form. Evaluation of urine amino acid profiles from cats and dogs with cystine uroliths often reveals increased concentrations of the amino acids cysteine, arginine, lysine, and ornithine (Clark and Cuddeford 1971; DiBartola et al. 1991; Osborne et al. 1999a).

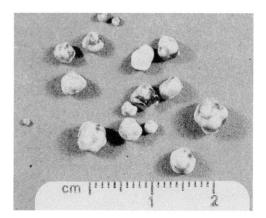

Figure 16.15 Cystine urocystoliths removed from the dog in Figure 16.14.

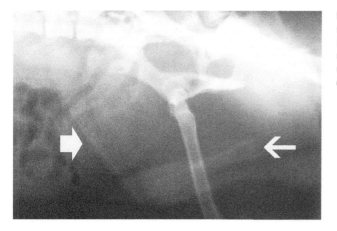

Figure 16.14 Lateral abdominal radiograph of a 3-year-old intact male English bulldog with cystine urocystoliths (large arrow) and a urethrolith at the base of the os penis (small arrow).

Figure 16.16 Cystine crystals from the dog in Figure 16.14.

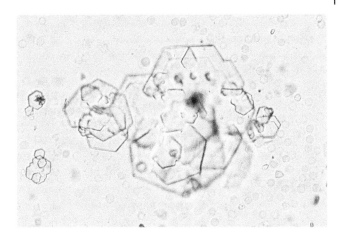

Medical protocols exist for dissolution of cystine uroliths in dogs utilizing urinary alkalinization and thiol-containing drugs, such as N-(2-mercaptopropionyl)-glycine (2-MPG); the dose for dissolution in dogs is 15 mg/kg PO q 12h with or without dietary modification (Osborne et al. 1999c). On average, cystine uroliths dissolve in 1–2 months; therefore, urinalysis and abdominal radiography should be performed monthly until urolith dissolution (Osborne et al. 1999c). Urine pH should be >7.5 and urine specific gravity <1.025. If uroliths do not dissolve, then surgery or a minimally invasive procedure should be performed to remove them.

Prevention of cystine uroliths involves feeding a protein-restricted, alkalinizing diet with or without 2-MPG. Reducing dietary protein has the potential of minimizing formation of cystine uroliths by decreasing intake and excretion of sulfur-containing amino acids and by decreasing renal medullary tonicity, resulting in larger urine volume. The solubility of cystine increases exponentially when the urine pH is greater than 7.2 (Milliner 1990). If necessary, or if dietary modification cannot be done, potassium citrate (initial dose 75 mg/kg PO q 12h; titrate to urine pH of 7.5) may be administered to induce alkaluria. For prevention, 2-MPG or d-penicillamine (15 mg/kg by mouth q 12h) may be used (Bovée 1986; Hoppe et al. 1993; Hoppe and Denneberg 2001);

however, it is often not necessary with dietary modification (Osborne et al. 1999c). Although thiol-containing drugs are used in dogs and human beings, their use has not been evaluated adequately in cats. Urinalysis and abdominal radiography should be performed every 4–6 months, and urine pH should be >7.5 and urine specific gravity <1.025 with an absence of cystine crystalluria.

Compound Uroliths

Figure 16.17 shows compound urocystoliths from a toy poodle.

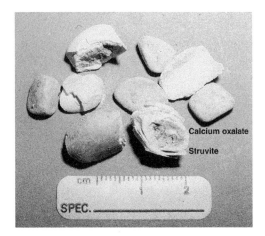

Figure 16.17 Compound urocystoliths removed from a 10-year-old castrated male toy poodle. The urocystoliths contained a nidus of calcium oxalate and outer layers of struvite, which formed because of a *Staphylococcal* urinary tract infection.

Occasionally, uroliths may be composed of more than one mineral. Most commonly, calcium phosphate apatite or ammonium urate may be mixed with struvite when induced by a urease-producing microbial urinary tract infection. These minerals become incorporated into the struvite urolith, because ammonium ions produced from the metabolism of urea by microbial urease combine with uric acid, and carbonate produced from the metabolism of urea by microbial urease combines with calcium and phosphorus in alkaluria (Osborne et al. 1999b). Medical dissolution of these uroliths is possible following protocols for dissolution of infection-induced uroliths. Direct preventive measures are toward controlling the causative bacterial urinary tract infection.

Compound uroliths also form when a urolith of one mineral forms and a different mineral precipitates around the first mineral. This occurs most commonly when a calcium oxalate urolith forms and a secondary urinary tract infection with a microbe that produces urease develops, resulting in struvite forming around the calcium oxalate urolith. Calcium oxalate uroliths must be removed physically as they cannot be dissolved, and preventive measures are directed toward prevention of calcium oxalate formation.

Surgically and Minimally Invasive Management of Uroliths

Although some uroliths, such as struvite, urate, and cystine, may be dissolved medically, others, such as calcium oxalate and compound uroliths with calcium oxalate nidus or core, are not amenable to medical dissolution. Even with uroliths composed of minerals that may be dissolved medically, sometimes it is more desirable to physically remove the uroliths. Physical removal of uroliths may be done by surgery (e.g. cystotomy, urethrotomy, and/or urethrostomy) or by minimally invasive techniques (e.g. catheter-assisted retrieval, voiding urohydropropulsion, cystoscopic removal, and/or cystoscopy with laser lithotripsy)

(Lulich and Osborne 1992; Bartges 2000; Adams et al. 2008; Lulich et al. 2009; Williams 2009).

Matrix-Crystalline Urethral Plugs

Figure 16.18 shows a matrix-crystalline urethral plug.

Urethral matrix-crystalline plugs occur in approximately 20% of male cats under 10 years of age that present with obstructive lower urinary tract disease (Kruger et al. 1991). Urethral plugs have only been observed to occur in male cats. They are composed of at least 45–50% matrix (see later for typical matrix composition) and variable amounts of mineral; they may be composed entirely of matrix (Osborne et al. 2003). Struvite is the most common mineral found in urethral plugs (84% of all minerals found in plugs) (Osborne et al. 2009). Multiple factors are thought to be associated with urethral plug formation. If a mineral is present in the urethral plug, then risk factors associated with that crystal formation, as discussed previously, are involved, at least in part. Compared with uroliths, urethral plugs contain large quantities of matrix. Components of matrix that may be important in urethral plug formation include Tamm–Horsfall mucoprotein, serum proteins, cellular debris, and

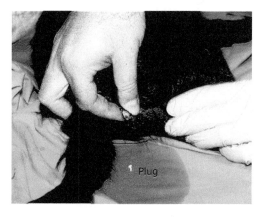

Figure 16.18 Matrix-crystalline urethral plug expressed from the distal urethra of a 6-year-old castrated male domestic shorthair cat with urethral obstruction.

virus-like particles (Kruger and Osborne 1990; Osborne et al. 1996b).

Management of urethral matrix-crystalline plugs involves relieving the obstructive uropathy (Osborne et al. 1996a). Modifying urine composition by feeding a therapeutic diet may be beneficial if minerals are present in the urethral plug. Increasing urine volume may help to decrease the concentration of minerals and matrix components in urine. Successful prevention of recurrent urethral obstruction by utilizing diets designed to reduce urine pH and urine magnesium and phosphorus concentrations has been reported (Osborne et al. 1991). Perineal urethrostomy may be considered in cats with recurrent urethral plug formation; however, it is associated with complications, including recurrent bacterial urinary tract infections, urethral stricture, and clinical signs of lower urinary tract disease (Osborne et al. 1991; Williams 2009). In one study of cats with urethral obstruction due to matrix-crystalline plugs, uroliths, or unidentified causes that were managed medically, recurrence of urethral obstruction occurred in approximately one-third; therefore, surgery may be necessary (Gerber et al. 2008).

Idiopathic Cystitis

The most common cause of lower urinary tract disease in cats less than 10 years of age is feline idiopathic cystitis (FIC) (Kruger et al. 1991; Buffington et al. 1997). Idiopathic cystitis is characterized by signs of lower urinary tract disease (i.e. hematuria, stranguria, pollakiuria, and inappropriate urination) without identifiable causes. Often the clinical signs resolve in 3–7 days; however, recurrence is variable and unpredictable. Because no specific cause has been identified, no specific treatment is available that works consistently in all cats.

The role of a canned diet in managing cats with idiopathic cystitis has been evaluated in two studies. In one non-randomized,

prospective study of cats with idiopathic cystitis, recurrence of clinical signs occurred in 11% of cats that consumed a canned/retorted food when compared with 39% of cats consuming a dry/extruded food (Markwell et al. 1999). The diets evaluated in this study were acidifying and formulated to prevent struvite crystalluria and urolithiasis. In another study, clinical improvement and decreased recurrence of clinical signs in cats with idiopathic cystitis were associated with the feeding of canned foods (Gunn-Moore and Shenoy 2004). The findings of these studies have resulted in the recommendation to feed canned food to cats with idiopathic cystitis; however, these studies were not randomized controlled trials. Furthermore, specific dietary ingredients have not been evaluated in cats with idiopathic cystitis.

Environmental modification appears to benefit many cats with idiopathic cystitis (Buffington et al. 2006). Modifications for indoor cats with idiopathic cystitis include providing a canned diet, good litter box management, climbing structures, an appropriate number of food and water dishes, and increasing water intake. Non-steroidal anti-inflammatory drugs are often described despite a lack of evidence for effectiveness. A trial with oral glucosamine (125 mg N-acetyl glucosamine per cat per day) demonstrated improvement of the owners' perceived mean health score compared to placebo, although not significantly different from the placebo group, as both groups improved due to the feeding of canned food (Gunn-Moore and Shenoy 2004).

Stress management seems to be important when managing FIC (Forrester and Towell 2015). Therapeutic urinary stress diets contain L-tryptophan and milk protein hydrolysate (also known as alpha-casozepine). L-tryptophan is a precursor for the neurotransmitter serotonin, which is important in almost all of the central nervous system integrative functions. One double-blinded, randomized placebo-controlled study evaluated the effect of short-term supplementation of L-tryptophan on behavioral responses associated with anxiety and stress-related disorder in cats. Results showed that supplementation of cats with dietary tryptophan may be a beneficial adjunct to decrease signs of stress and anxiety and improve animal welfare (Pereira et al. 2004). Furthermore, Beata et al. (2007) provided evidence for the efficacy of alpha-casozepine in the short-term management of anxiety in cats. A non-randomized short-term study has shown dietary therapy with L-tryptophan and alpha-casozepine to reduce FIC episodes that included stranguria, periuria, hematuria, dysuria, and pollakiuria (Naarden and Corbee 2020). Results from these studies suggest that supplementation of L-tryptophan and alpha-casozepine is beneficial for stress management in cats with FIC. However, evidence about the effects of supplementation of these nutrients on long-term FIC management and recurrence is not available.

Urinary Tract Infections

Management of urinary tract infections involves eradication or control of predisposing factors and antimicrobial therapy; however, several nutritional strategies may be useful in preventing recurrent bacterial urinary tract infections. Bacterial urinary tract infections occur more frequently in animals with predisposing conditions (e.g. diabetes mellitus, hyperadrenocorticism, chronic renal failure, and hyperthyroidism); therefore, management of these conditions, including diet, may help to decrease recurrent bacterial urinary tract infections (Bartges 2005). Obesity is a common nutritional disorder and the incidence of bacterial urinary tract infections is increased in obese patients.

Bacteria are able to survive in pH from 4 to 9; therefore, feeding an acidifying diet or providing a urinary acidifier is not effective in preventing recurrent bacterial urinary tract infections (Bartges 2005). Cranberry juice or extract has been recommended for preventing recurrent infections. Cranberries contain proanthocyanidins that bind to type 1 pili and P fimbriae of *Escherichia coli*, thereby preventing adhesion of *E. coli* to the uroepithelium (Howell 2007; Guirguis-Blake 2008; Jepson and Craig 2008; Wing et al. 2008; Guay 2009). Despite widespread use and availability, there are few controlled clinical trials supporting the use of cranberries as prophylaxis, although there are some. The only in vitro study with canine cells did not find benefit (Suksawat et al. 1996). Cranberries should, however, not be prescribed with concurrent calcium oxalate uroliths as they are high in oxalate (Terris et al. 2001).

Probiotics are recommended by some for prevention of recurrent infections. The theory behind probiotics is to modify enteric microbiota and, ultimately, urogenital microbiota. There is little evidence of effectiveness; however, certain strains of *Lactobacillus* have been shown to be beneficial in some women and children in controlled studies (Lee et al. 2007; Reid 2008; Abad and Safdar 2009).

There are many botanicals that have been recommended for prevention of urinary tract infections, most commonly *Uva ursi*, which contains tannins and arbutin that may be bactericidal and anti-inflammatory (Head 2008). Little evidence exists for effectiveness.

Mannose inhibits adherence of *E. coli* to the uroepithelium in vitro by binding to type 1 pili and shows promise in preliminary studies in human beings (Domenici et al. 2016; Genovese et al. 2018).

Not all feline and canine urinary tract disorders are associated with dietary factors; however, most benefit from nutritional management. It is important to understand the pathophysiology of lower urinary tract disease and the physiologic effects of foods and feeding in order to formulate the best nutritional and treatment plan for patients.

Summary

- Lower urinary tract disease occurs commonly in cats and dogs, with urolithiasis, urinary tract infections (dogs), and idiopathic cystitis (cats) occurring most frequently.

- Uroliths occur when urine is oversaturated with minerals that precipitate. Dietary modification may be useful for medically dissolving and for preventing uroliths. Calcium oxalate and struvite uroliths occur most commonly in cats and dogs.

- Dietary modification may also be useful in managing cats with idiopathic cystitis.

References

Abad, C.L. and Safdar, N. (2009). The role of lactobacillus probiotics in the treatment or prevention of urogenital infections—a systematic review. *J. Chemother.* 21 (3): 243–252.

Adamama-Moraitou, K.K., Pardali, D., Prassinos, N.N. et al. (2017). Evaluation of dogs with macroscopic haematuria: a retrospective study of 162 cases (2003–2010). *N. Z. Vet. J.* 65 (4): 204–208.

Adams, L.G., Berent, A.C., Moore, G.E., and Bagley, D.H. (2008). Use of laser lithotripsy for fragmentation of uroliths in dogs: 73 cases (2005–2006). *J. Am. Vet. Med. Assoc.* 232 (11): 1680–1687.

Albasan, H., Osborne, C.A., Lulich, J.P. et al. (2009). Rate and frequency of recurrence of uroliths after an initial ammonium urate, calcium oxalate, or struvite urolith in cats. *J. Am. Vet. Med. Assoc.* 235 (12): 1450–1455.

Aparicio, V.A., Nebot, E., Garcia-del Moral, R. et al. (2013). High protein diets and renal status in rats. *Nutr. Hosp.* 28 (1): 232–237.

Bai, S.C., Sampson, D.A., Morris, J.G., and Rogers, Q.R. (1989). Vitamin B6 requirement of growing kittens. *J. Nutr.* 119: 1020–1027.

Balaji, K.C. and Menon, M. (1997). Mechanism of stone formation. *Urol. Clin. North Am.* 24 (1): 1–11.

Bannasch, D., Safra, N., Young, A. et al. (2008). Mutations in the SLC2A9 gene cause hyperuricosuria and hyperuricemia in the dog. *PLoS Genet.* 4 (11): e1000246.

Bartges, J.W. (1996). Lower urinary tract disease in older cats: What's common, what's not? *Symposium on Health and Nutrition of Geriatric Cats and Dogs*, Orlando, FL.

Bartges, J.W. (2000). Diseases of the urinary bladder. In: *Saunders Manual of Small Animal Practice* (ed. S.J. Birchard and R.G. Sherding), 943–957. Philadelphia, PA: W.B. Saunders.

Bartges, J.W. (2001). Calcium oxalate urolithiasis. In: *Consultations in Feline Internal Medicine* (ed. J.R. August), 352–364. Philadelphia, PA: W.B. Saunders.

Bartges, J.W. (2005). Bacterial urinary tract infections. In: *Textbook of Veterinary Internal Medicine* (ed. S.J. Ettinger and E.C. Feldman), 1800–1808. Philadelphia, PA: W.B. Saunders.

Bartges, J.W. and Callens, A.J. (2015). Urolithiasis. *Vet. Clin. North Am. Small Anim. Pract.* 45: 747–768.

Bartges, J.W., Cornelius, L.M., and Osborne, C.A. (1999a). Ammonium urate uroliths in dogs with portosystemic shunts. In: *Current Veterinary Therapy XIII* (ed. J.D. Bonagura), 872–874. Philadelphia, PA: W.B. Saunders.

Bartges, J.W., Osborne, C.A., Felice, L.J. et al. (1992a). Canine xanthine uroliths: risk factor management. In: *Current Veterinary Therapy XI* (ed. R.W. Kirk and J.D. Bonagura), 900–905. Philadelphia, PA: W.B. Saunders.

Bartges, J.W., Osborne, C.A., Polzin, D.J. et al. (1992b). Recurrent sterile struviterocystolithiasiss in three related Cocker Spaniels. *J. Am. Anim. Hosp. Assoc.* 28: 459–469.

Bartges, J.W., Osborne, C.A., Koehler, L.A. et al. (1994a). An algorithmic approach to canine urate uroliths. In: *12th Annual Veterinary Medical Forum of the American College of Veterinary Internal Medicine*, 476–477. San Francisco, CA: Omnipress.

Bartges, J.W., Osborne, C.A., Lulich, J.P. et al. (1994b). Prevalence of cystine and urate uroliths in bulldogs and urate uroliths in dalmatians. *J. Am. Vet. Med. Assoc.* 204 (12): 1914–1918.

Bartges, J.W., S.L. Tarver, and Schneider, C. (1998). Comparison of struvite activity product ratios and relative supersaurations in urine collected from healthy cats consuming four struvite management diets. *Ralston Purina Nutrition Symposium*, St.Louis, MO.

Bartges, J.W., Osborne, C.A., Lulich, J.P. et al. (1999b). Methods for evaluating treatment of uroliths. *Vet. Clin. North Am. Small Anim. Pract.* 29 (1): 45–57, x.

Bartges, J.W., Osborne, C.A., Lulich, J.P. et al. (1999c). Canine urate urolithiasis. Etiopathogenesis, diagnosis, and management. *Vet. Clin. North Am. Small Anim. Pract.* 29 (1): 161–191, xii–xiii.

Bartges, J.W., Kirk, C., and Lane, I.F. (2004a). Update: management of calcium oxalate uroliths in dogs and cats. *Vet. Clin. North Am. Small Anim. Pract.* 34 (4): 969–987, vii.

Bartges, J.W., Kirk, C.A., and Moyers, T. (2004b). Influence of alkalinization and acidification on urine saturation with calcium oxalate and struvite and bone mineral density in healthy cats. *Urol. Res.* 32 (2): 172.

Bartges, J.W., Kirk, C.A., Cox, S.K. et al. (2013). Influence of acidifying or alkalinizing diets on bone mineral density and urine relative supersaturation with calcium oxalate and struvite in healthy cats. *Am. J. Vet. Res.* 10: 1347–1352.

Beata, C., Beaumont-Graff, E., Coll, V. et al. (2007). Effect of alpha-casozepine (Zylkene) on anxiety in cats. *J. Vet. Behav.: Clin. Appl. Res.* 2 (2): 40–46.

Bijsmans, E.S., Queau, Y., Feugier, A. et al. (2021). The effect of urine acidification on calcium oxalate relative supersaturation in

cats. *J. Anim. Physiol. Anim. Nutr. (Berl.)* 105 (3): 579–586.

Bovée, K.C. (1986). Canine cystine urolithiasis. *Vet. Clin. North Am. Small Anim. Pract.* 16 (2): 211–215.

Brain, P.H. (1988). Portosystemic shunts—urate calculi as a guide to diagnosis. *Aust. Vet. Pract.* 18 (1): 3–4.

Brons, A.K., Henthorn, P.S., Raj, K. et al. (2013). SLC3A1 and SLC7A9 mutations in autosomal recessive or dominant canine cystinuria: a new classification system. *J. Vet. Intern. Med.* 27: 1400–1408.

Brown, C. and Purich, D. (1992). Physical-chemical processes in kidney stone formation. In: *Disorders of Bone and Mineral Metabolism* (ed. F. Coe and M. Favus), 613–624. New York: Raven Press.

Buckley, C.M., Hawthorne, A., Colyer, A. et al. (2011). Effect of dietary water intake on urinary output, specific gravity and relative supersaturation for calcium oxalate and struvite in the cat. *Br. J. Nutr.* 106 (Suppl 1): S128–S130.

Buffington, T. (1989). Struvite urolithiasis in cats. *J. Am. Vet. Med. Assoc.* 194 (1): 7–8.

Buffington, C.A., Rogers, Q.R., and Morris, J.G. (1990). Effect of diet on struvite activity product in feline urine. *Am. J. Vet. Res.* 51 (12): 2025–2030.

Buffington, C.A., Blaisdell, J.L., and Sako, T. (1994). Effects of Tamm-Horsfall glycoprotein and albumin on struvite crystal growth in urine of cats. *Am. J. Vet. Res.* 55 (7): 965–971.

Buffington, C.A., Chew, D.J., Kendall, M.S. et al. (1997). Clinical evaluation of cats with nonobstructive urinary tract diseases. *J. Am. Vet. Med. Assoc.* 210 (1): 46–50.

Buffington, C.A., Westropp, J.L., Chew, D.J. et al. (2006). Clinical evaluation of multimodal environmental modification (MEMO) in the management of cats with idiopathic cystitis. *J. Feline Med. Surg.* 8 (4): 261–268.

Buranakarl, C., Mathur, S., and Brown, S.A. (2004). Effects of dietary sodium chloride intake on renal function and blood pressure in cats with normal and reduced renal function. *Am. J. Vet. Res.* 65 (5): 620–627.

Burggraaf, N.D., Westgeest, D.B., and Corbee, R.J. (2021). Analysis of 7866 feline and canine uroliths submitted between 2014 and 2020 in the Netherlands. *Res. Vet. Sci.* 137: 86–93.

Carr, S.V., Grant, D.C., DeMonaco, S.M., and Shepherd, M. (2019). Measurement of preprandial and postprandial urine calcium to creatinine ratios in male Miniature Schnauzers with and without urolithiasis. *J. Vet. Intern. Med.* 34: 754–760.

Case, L.C., Ling, G.V., Franti, C.E. et al. (1992). Cystine-containing urinary calculi in dogs: 102 cases (1981–1989). *J. Am. Vet. Med. Assoc.* 201 (1): 129–133.

Caudarella, R. and Vescini, F. (2009). Urinary citrate and renal stone disease: the preventive role of alkali citrate treatment. *Arch. Ital. Urol. Androl.* 81 (3): 182–187.

Chamsuwan, S., Angkanaporn, K., Dissayabutra, T. et al. (2021). The association between single nucleotide polymorphism in vitamin D receptor and calcium oxalate urolithiasis in dogs. *J. Vet. Intern. Med.* 35 (5): 2263–2270.

Ching, S.V., Fettman, M.J., Hamar, D.W. et al. (1989). The effect of chronic dietary acidification using ammonium chloride on acid-base and mineral metabolism in the adult cat. *J. Nutr.* 119 (6): 902–915.

Clark, W.T. and Cuddeford, D. (1971). A study of amino acids in urine from dogs with cystine urolithiasis. *Vet. Rec.* 88: 414–417.

Coe, F.L., Parks, J.H., and Asplin, J.R. (1992). The pathogenesis and treatment of kidney stones. *N. Engl. J. Med.* 327 (16): 1141–1152.

Cowgill, L.D., Sevgev, G., Bandt, C. et al. (2007). Effects of dietary salt intake on body fluid volume and renal function in healthy cats. *J. Vet. Intern. Med.* 21 (3): 600–601.

DiBartola, S.P., Chew, D.J., and Horton, M.L. (1991). Cystinuria in a cat. *J. Am. Vet. Med. Assoc.* 198 (1): 102–104.

Dijcker, J.C., Hagen-Plantinga, E.A., Thomas, D.G. et al. (2014). The effect of dietary hydroxyproline and dietary oxalate on urinary oxalate excretion in cats. *J. Anim. Sci.* 92 (2): 577–584.

Domenici, L., Monti, M., Bracchi, C. et al. (2016). D-mannose: a promising support for acute urinary tract infections in women. A pilot study. *Eur. Rev. Med. Pharmacol. Sci.* 20 (13): 2920–2925.

Finco, D.R., Barsanti, J.A., and Crowell, W.A. (1985). Characterization of magnesium-induced urinary disease in the cat and comparison with feline urologic syndrome. *Am. J. Vet. Res.* 46 (2): 391–400.

Finke, M.D. and Litzenberger, B.A. (1992). Effect of food intake on urine pH in cats. *J. Small Anim. Pract.* 33 (6): 261–265.

Forrester, S.D. and Towell, T.L. (2015). Feline idiopathic cystitis. *Vet. Clin. North Am. Small Anim. Pract.* 45 (4): 783–806.

Furrow, E., Patterson, E.E., Armstrong, P.J. et al. (2015). Fasting urinary calcium-to-creatinine and oxalate-to-creatinine ratios in dogs with calcium oxalate urolithiasis and breed-matched controls. *J. Vet. Intern. Med.* 29 (1): 113–119.

Geddes, R.F., van den Broek, D.H.N., Chang, Y.-M. et al. (2021). The effect of attenuating dietary phosphate restriction on blood ionized calcium concentrations in cats with chronic kidney disease and ionized hypercalcemia. *J. Vet. Intern. Med.* 35 (2): 997–1007.

Genovese, C., Davinelli, S., Mangano, K. et al. (2018). Effects of a new combination of plant extracts plus d-mannose for the management of uncomplicated recurrent urinary tract infections. *J. Chemother.* 30 (2): 107–114.

Gerber, B., Eichenberger, S., and Reusch, C.E. (2008). Guarded long-term prognosis in male cats with urethral obstruction. *J. Feline Med. Surg.* 10 (1): 16–23.

Gow, A.G., Fairbanks, L.D., Simpson, J.W. et al. (2011). Xanthine urolithiasis in a Cavalier King Charles spaniel. *Vet. Rec.* 169 (8): 209.

Groth, E.M., Lulich, J.P., Chew, D.J. et al. (2019). Vitamin D metabolism in dogs with and without hypercalciuric calcium oxalate urolithiasis. *J. Vet. Intern. Med.* 33: 758–763.

Guay, D.R. (2009). Cranberry and urinary tract infections. *Drugs* 69 (7): 775–807.

Guirguis-Blake, J. (2008). Cranberry products for treatment of urinary tract infection. *Am. Fam. Physician* 78 (3): 332–333.

Gunn-Moore, D.A. and Shenoy, C.M. (2004). Oral glucosamine and the management of feline idiopathic cystitis. *J. Feline Med. Surg.* 6 (4): 219–225.

Hamm, L.L. and Simon, E.E. (1987). Roles and mechanisms of urinary buffer excretion. *Am. J. Physiol.* 253 (4 Pt 2): F595–F605.

Hardy, R.M. and Klausner, J.S. (1983). Urate calculi associated with portal vascular anomalies. In: *Current Veterinary Therapy VIII* (ed. R.W. Kirk), 1073. Philadelphia, PA: W.B. Saunders.

Hawthorne, A.J. and Markwell, P.J. (2004). Dietary sodium promotes increased water intake and urine volume in cats. *J. Nutr.* 134 (8 Suppl): 2128S–2129S.

Head, K.A. (2008). Natural approaches to prevention and treatment of infections of the lower urinary tract. *Altern. Med. Rev.* 13 (3): 227–244.

Henthorn, P.S., Liu, J., Gidalevich, T. et al. (2000). Canine cystinuria: polymorphism in the canine SLC3A1 gene and identification of a nonsense mutation in cystinuric Newfoundland dogs. *Hum. Genet.* 107 (4): 295–303.

Hess, R.S., Kass, P.H., and Ward, C.R. (1998). Association between hyperadrenocorticism and development of calcium-containing uroliths in dogs with urolithiasis. *J. Am. Vet. Med. Assoc.* 212 (12): 1889–1891.

Hezel, A., Bartges, J.W., Kirk, C.A. et al. (2007). Influence of hydrochlorothiazide on urinary calcium oxalate relative supersaturation in healthy young adult female domestic shorthaired cats. *Vet. Ther.* 8 (4): 247–254.

Hoppe, A. and Denneberg, T. (2001). Cystinuria in the dog: clinical studies during 14 years of medical treatment. *J. Vet. Intern. Med.* 15 (4): 361–367.

Hoppe, A., Denneberg, T., Jeppson, J.-O. et al. (1993). Canine cystinuria: an extended study on the effects of 2-mercaptopropionylglycine on cystine urolithiasis and urinary cystine excretion. *Br. Vet. J.* 149 (3): 235–251.

Houston, D.M., Weese, H.E., Evason, M.D. et al. (2011). A diet with a struvite relative supersaturation less than 1 is effective in dissolving struvite stones in vivo. *Br. J. Nutr.* 106 (Suppl 1): S90–S92.

Howell, A.B. (2007). Bioactive compounds in cranberries and their role in prevention of urinary tract infections. *Mol. Nutr. Food Res.* 51 (6): 732–737.

Hughes, K.L., Slater, M.R., Geller, S. et al. (2002). Diet and lifestyle variables as risk factors for chronic renal failure in pet cats. *Prev. Vet. Med.* 55 (1): 1–15.

Ito, H. (1991). Combined administration of calcium and citrate reduces urinary oxalate excretion. *Hinyokika Kiyo* 37 (10): 1107–1110.

Jacinto, A.M., Mellanby, R.J., Chandler, M. et al. (2013). Urine concentrations of xanthine, hypoxanthine and uric acid in UK Cavalier King Charles spaniels. *J. Small Anim. Pract.* 54 (8): 395–398.

Jepson, R.G. and Craig, J.C. (2008). Cranberries for preventing urinary tract infections. *Cochrane Database Syst. Rev.* (1): CD001321. https://doi.org/10.1002/14651858.CD001321.pub5.

Johnson, C.A., Armstrong, P.J., and Hauptmann, J.G. (1987). Congenital portosystemic shunts in dogs: 46 cases (1979–1986). *J. Am. Vet. Med. Assoc.* 19 (11): 1478–1483.

Kirk, C.A., Ling, G.V., Franti, C.E. et al. (1995). Evaluation of factors associated with development of calcium oxalate urolithiasis in cats. *J. Am. Vet. Med. Assoc.* 207 (11): 1429–1434.

Kirk, C.A., Ling, G.V., Osborne, C.A. et al. (2003). Clinical guidelines for managing calcium oxalate uroliths in cats: medical therapy, hydration, and dietary therapy. In: *Managing Urolithiasis in Cats: Recent Updates and Practice Guidelines* (ed. A.C. Kraje and J.W. Bartges), 10–19. Topeka, KS: Hill's Pet Nutrition.

Kirk, C.A., Jewell, D.E., and Lowry, S.R. (2006). Effects of sodium chloride on selected parameters in cats. *Vet. Ther.* 7 (4): 333–346.

Kpercny, L., Palm, C.A., Segev, G. et al. (2021a). Urolithiasis in cats: evaluation of trends in urolith composition and risk factors (2005-2018). *J. Vet. Intern. Med.* 35 (3): 1397–1405.

Kpercny, L., Palm, C.A., Segev, G., and Westropp, J.L. (2021b). Urolithiasis in dogs: evaluation of trends in urolith composition and risk factors (2005-2018). *J. Vet. Intern. Med.* 35 (3): 1406–1415.

Kraje, A.C., Bartges, J.W., DeNovo, R.C., and Millis, D.L. (2000). Effects of op-DDD on urinary calcium excretion, parathyroid hormone concentration, and bone mineral density in dogs with spontaneously occurring pituitary dependent hyperadrenocorticism. *J. Vet. Intern. Med.* 14: 384.

Kruger, J.M. and Osborne, C.A. (1990). The role of viruses in feline lower urinary tract disease. *J. Vet. Intern. Med.* 4 (2): 71–78.

Kruger, J.M., Osborne, C.A., Goyal, S.M. et al. (1991). Clinical evaluation of cats with lower urinary tract disease. *J. Am. Vet. Med. Assoc.* 199 (2): 211–216.

Lawler, D.F., Sjolin, D.W., and Collins, J.E. (1985). Incidence rates of feline lower urinary tract disease in the United States. *Feline Pract.* 15 (5): 13–16.

Lee, S.J., Shim, Y.H., Cho, S.J., and Lee, J.W. (2007). Probiotics prophylaxis in children with persistent primary vesicoureteral reflux. *Pediatr. Nephrol.* 22 (9): 1315–1320.

Lekcharoensuk, C., Lulich, J.P., Osborne, C.A. et al. (2000a). Association between patient-related factors and risk of calcium oxalate and magnesium ammonium phosphate urolithiasis in cats. *J. Am. Vet. Med. Assoc.* 217 (4): 520–525.

Lekcharoensuk, C., Lulich, J.P., Osborne, C.A. et al. (2000b). Patient and environmental factors associated with calcium oxalate urolithiasis in dogs. *J. Am. Vet. Med. Assoc.* 217 (4): 515–519.

Lekcharoensuk, C., Osborne, C.A., Lulich, J.P. et al. (2001). Association between dietary factors and calcium oxalate and magnesium ammonium phosphate urolithiasis in cats. *J. Am. Vet. Med. Assoc.* 219 (9): 1228–1237.

Lekcharoensuk, C., Osborne, C.A., Lulich, J.P. et al. (2002). Associations between dietary factors in canned food and formation of calcium oxalate uroliths in dogs. *Am. J. Vet. Res.* 63 (2): 163–169.

Luckschander, N., Iben, C., Hosgood, G. et al. (2004). Dietary NaCl does not affect blood pressure in healthy cats. *J. Vet. Intern. Med.* 18 (4): 463–467.

Lulich, J.P. and Osborne, C.A. (1992). Catheter-assisted retrieval of urocystoliths from dogs and cats. *J. Am. Vet. Med. Assoc.* 201 (1): 111–113.

Lulich, J.P., Osborne, C.A., Nagode, L.A. et al. (1991). Evaluation of urine and serum metabolites in miniature schnauzers with calcium oxalate urolithiasis. *Am. J. Vet. Res.* 52 (10): 1583–1590.

Lulich, J.P., Perrine, L., Osborne, C.A. et al. (1992). Postsurgical recurrence of calcium oxalate uroliths in dogs. *J. Vet. Intern. Med.* 6 (2): 119.

Lulich, J.P., Osborne, C.A., Sanderson, S.L. et al. (1999a). Voiding urohydropropulsion. Lessons from 5 years of experience. *Vet. Clin. North Am. Small Anim. Pract.* 29 (1): 283–292.

Lulich, J.P., Osborne, C.A., Thumchai, R. et al. (1999b). Epidemiology of canine calcium oxalate uroliths. Identifying risk factors. *Vet. Clin. North Am. Small Anim. Pract.* 29 (1): 113–122.

Lulich, J.P., Osborne, C.A., Bartges, J.W., and Lekcharoensuk, C. (2000). Canine lower urinary tract disorders. In: *Textbook of Veterinary Internal Medicine*, vol. 2 (ed. S.J. Ettinger and E.C. Feldman), 1747–1783. Philadelphia, PA: W.B. Saunders.

Lulich, J.P., Osborne, C.A., Lekcharoensuk, C. et al. (2004). Effects of diet on urine composition of cats with calcium oxalate urolithiasis. *J. Am. Anim. Hosp. Assoc.* 40 (3): 185–191.

Lulich, J.P., Osborne, C.A., and Sanderson, S.L. (2005). Effects of dietary supplementation with sodium chloride on urinary relative supersaturation with calcium oxalate in healthy dogs. *Am. J. Vet. Res.* 66 (2): 319–324.

Lulich, J.P., Osborne, C.A., Albasan, H. et al. (2009). Efficacy and safety of laser lithotripsy in fragmentation of urocystoliths and urethroliths for removal in dogs. *J. Am. Vet. Med. Assoc.* 234 (10): 1279–1285.

Lulich, J.P., Kruger, J.M., Macleay, J.M. et al. (2013a). Efficacy of two commercially available, low-magnesium, urine-acidifying dry foods for the dissolution of struvite uroliths in cats. *J. Am. Vet. Med. Assoc.* 243 (8): 1147–1153.

Lulich, J.P., Osborne, C.A., Albasan, H. et al. (2013b). Recent shifts in the global proportions of canine uroliths. *Vet. Rec.* 172 (14): 363.

Lulich, J.P., Berent, A.C., Adams, L.G. et al. (2016). ACVIM small animal consensus recommendations on the treatment and prevention of uroliths in dogs and cats. *J. Vet. Intern. Med.* 30 (5): 1564–1574.

Luskin, A.C., Lulich, J.P., Gesch, S.C., and Furrow, E. (2019). Bone resorption in dogs with calcium oxalate urolithiasis and idiopathic hypercalciuria. *Res. Vet. Sci.* 123 (April): 129–134.

Markwell, P.J., Buffington, C.A., Chew, D.J. et al. (1999). Clinical evaluation of commercially available urinary acidification diets in the management of idiopathic cystitis in cats. *J. Am. Vet. Med. Assoc.* 214 (3): 361–365.

Marretta, S.M., Pask, A.J., Greene, R.W., and Liu, S. (1981). Urinary calculi associated with portosystemic shunts in six dogs. *J. Am. Vet. Med. Assoc.* 178 (2): 133–137.

Matos, A.J., Mascarenhas, C., Magalhães, P., and Pinto, J.P. (2006). Efficient screening of the cystinuria-related C663T Slc3a1 nonsense mutation in Newfoundland dogs by denaturing high-performance liquid chromatography. *J. Vet. Diagn. Invest.* 18 (1): 102–105.

McClain, H.M., Barsanti, J.A., and Bartges, J.W. (1999). Hypercalcemia and calcium oxalate urolithiasis in cats: a report of five cases. *J. Am. Anim. Hosp. Assoc.* 35 (4): 297–301.

McHarg, T., Rodgers, A., and Charlton, K. (2003). Influence of cranberry juice on the urinary risk factors for calcium oxalate kidney stone formation. *BJU Int.* 92 (7): 765–768.

McKerrell, R.E., Blakemore, W.F., Heath, M.F. et al. (1989). Primary hyperoxaluria (L-glyceric aciduria) in the cat: a newly recognised inherited disease. *Vet. Rec.* 125 (2): 31–34.

Midkiff, A.M., Chew, D.J., Randolph, J.F. et al. (2000). Idiopathic hypercalcemia in cats. *J. Vet. Intern. Med.* 14 (6): 619–626.

Milliner, D.S. (1990). Cystinuria. *Endocrinol. Metab. Clin. North Am.* 19 (4): 889–907.

Naarden, B. and Corbee, R.J. (2020). The effect of a therapeutic urinary stress diet on the short-term recurrence of feline idiopathic cystitis. *Vet. Med. Sci.* 6: 32–38.

Okafor, C.C., Lefebvre, S.L., Pearl, D.L. et al. (2014). Risk factors associated with calcium oxalate urolithiasis in dogs evaluated at general care veterinary hospitals in the United States. *Prev. Vet. Med.* 115: 217–228.

Osborne, C.A. (1999). Medical dissolution and prevention of canine uroliths. Seven steps from science to service. *Vet. Clin. North Am. Small Anim. Pract.* 29 (1): 1–15, ix.

Osborne, C.A., Polzin, D.J., Abdullahi, S.U. et al. (1985). Struvite urolithiasis in animals and man: formation, detection, and dissolution. *Adv. Vet. Sci. Comp. Med.* 29: 1–101.

Osborne, C.A., Lulich, J.P., Kruger, J.M. et al. (1990). Medical dissolution of feline struvite urocystoliths. *J. Am. Vet. Med. Assoc.* 196 (7): 1053–1063.

Osborne, C.A., Caywood, D.D., Johnston, G.R. et al. (1991). Perineal urethrostomy versus dietary management in prevention of recurrent lower urinary tract disease. *J. Small Anim. Pract.* 32 (6): 296–305.

Osborne, C.A., Kruger, J.M., Lulich, J.P. et al. (1996a). Medical management of feline urethral obstruction. *Vet. Clin. North Am. Small Anim. Pract.* 26 (3): 483–498.

Osborne, C.A., Lulich, J.P., Kruger, J.M. et al. (1996b). Feline urethral plugs. Etiology and pathophysiology. *Vet. Clin. North Am. Small Anim. Pract.* 26 (2): 233–253.

Osborne, C.A., Kruger, J.M., Lulich, J.P. et al. (1999a). Feline lower urinary tract diseases. In: *Textbook of Veterinary Internal Medicine*, vol. 2 (ed. S.J. Ettinger and E.C. Feldman), 1710–1746. Philadelphia, PA: W.B. Saunders.

Osborne, C.A., Lulich, J.P., Polzin, D.J. et al. (1999b). Medical dissolution and prevention of canine struvite urolithiasis. Twenty years of experience. *Vet. Clin. North Am. Small Anim. Pract.* 29 (1): 73–111, xi.

Osborne, C.A., Sanderson, S.L., and Lulich, J.P. (1999c). Canine cystine urolithiasis. Cause, detection, treatment, and prevention. *Vet. Clin. North Am. Small Anim. Pract.* 29 (1): 193–211, xiii.

Osborne, C.A., Bartges, J.W., Lulich, J.P. et al. (2000). Canine urolithiasis. In: *Small Animal Clinical Nutrition* (ed. M.S. Hand, C.D. Thatcher, R.L. Remillard and P. Roudebush), 605–688. Marceline MO: Wadsworth.

Osborne, C.A., Lulich, J.P., Albasan, H. et al. (2003). Mineral composition of feline uroliths and urethral plugs: current status. In: *Managing Urolithiasis in Cats: Recent Updates and Practice Guidelines*, vol. 26 (ed. C.A. Davis). Topeka, KS: Hill's Pet Nutrition.

Osborne, C.A., Bartges, J.W., Koehler, L.A. et al. (2004). "Feline xanthine urolithiasis: a newly recognized cause of urinary tract disease" (abstract). *Urol. Res.* 32 (2): 171.

Osborne, C.A., Lulich, J.P., Kruger, J.M. et al. (2009). Analysis of 451,891 canine uroliths, feline uroliths, and feline urethral plugs from 1981 to 2007: perspectives from the Minnesota Urolith Center. *Vet. Clin. North Am. Small Anim. Pract.* 39 (1): 183–197.

Pak, C.Y., Fuller, C., Sakhaee, K. et al. (1985). Long-term treatment of calcium nephrolithiasis with potassium citrate. *J. Urol.* 134 (1): 11–19.

Palm, C. and Westropp, J. (2011). Cats and calcium oxalate: strategies for managing lower and upper tract stone disease. *J. Feline Med. Surg.* 13 (9): 651–660.

Paßlack, N., Burmeier, H., Brenten, T. et al. (2014). Short term effects of increasing dietary salt concentrations on urine composition in healthy cats. *Vet. J.* 201 (3): 401–405.

Pedroia, V. (1981). Allopurinol-induced immune disorders. *Canine Pract.* 8 (4): 19–22.

Pereira, D.A., Aguiar, J.A.K., Hagiwara, M.K. et al. (2004). Changes in cat urinary glycosaminoglycans with age and in feline urologic syndrome. *Biochem. Biophys. Acta* 1672 (1): 1–11.

Prezioso, D., Strazzullo, P., Lotti, T. et al. (2015). Dietary treatment of urinary risk factors for renal stone formation. A review of CLU working group. *Arch. Ital. Urol. Androl.* 87 (2): 105–120.

Queau, Y., Bijsmans, E.S., Feugier, A., and Biourge, V.C. (2020). Increasing dietary sodium chloride promotes urine dilution and decreases struvite and calcium oxalate relative supersaturation in healthy dogs and cats. *J. Anim. Physiol. Anim. Nutr.* 104: 1524–1530.

Reid, G. (2008). Probiotic lactobacilli for urogenital health in women. *J. Clin. Gastroenterol.* 42 (Suppl 3 Pt 2): S234–S236.

Robertson, W.G. (1993). Urinary calculi. In: *Metabolic Bone and Stone Disease* (ed. B.E.C. Nordin, A.G. Need and H.A. Morris), 249–311. Edinburgh: Churchill Livingstone.

Rodman, J.S. (1991). Prophylaxis of uric acid stones with alternate day doses of alkaline potassium salts. *J. Urol.* 145: 97–99.

Rumenapf, G. and Schwille, P.O. (1987). The influence of oral alkali citrate on intestinal calcium absorption in healthy man. *Clin. Sci. (Lond.)* 73 (1): 117–121.

Sakhaee, K., Alpern, R., Poindexter, J., and Pak, C.Y. (1992). Citraturic response to oral citric acid load. *J. Urol.* 147 (4): 975–976.

Smith, B.H.E., Moodie, S.J., Wensley, S. et al. (1997). Differences in urinary pH and relative supersaturation values between senior and young adult cats. *J. Vet. Intern. Med.* 11 (2): 674.

Smith, B.H., Stevenson, A.E., and Markwell, P.J. (1998). Urinary relative supersaturations of calcium oxalate and struvite in cats are influenced by diet. *J. Nutr.* 128 (12 Suppl): 2763S–2764S.

Stevenson, A.E. (2002). The incidence of urolithiasis in cats and dogs and the influence of diet in formation and prevention of recurrence. PhD thesis, Institute of Urology and Nephrology, University College London.

Stevenson, A.E., Wigglesworth, D.J., Smith, B.H. et al. (2000). Effects of dietary potassium citrate supplementation on urine pH and urinary relative supersaturation of calcium oxalate and struvite in healthy dogs. *Am. J. Vet. Res.* 61: 430–435.

Stevenson, A.E., Markwell, P.J., and Blackburn, J.M. (2002). The effect of diet on calcium oxalate urinary relative supersaturation (RSS) of stone-forming (SF) and normal (N) dogs. *J. Vet. Intern. Med.* 16 (3): 377.

Stevenson, A.E., Hynds, W.K., and Markwell, P.J. (2003). Effect of dietary moisture and sodium content on urine composition and calcium oxalate relative supersaturation in healthy miniature schnauzers and labrador retrievers. *Res. Vet. Sci.* 74 (2): 145–151.

Stoller, M.L., Chi, T., Eisner, B.H. et al. (2009). Changes in urinary stone risk factors in hypocitraturic calcium oxalate stone formers treated with dietary sodium supplementation. *J. Urol.* 181 (3): 1140–1144.

Suksawat, J., Cox, H.U., O'Reilly, K.L. et al. (1996). Inhibition of bacterial adherence to canine uroepithelial cells using cranberry juice extract. *J. Vet. Intern. Med.* 10 (5): 167.

Tarttelin, M.F. (1987a). Feline struvite urolithiasis: factors affecting urine pH may be more important than magnesium levels in food. *Vet. Rec.* 121 (10): 227–230.

Tarttelin, M.F. (1987b). Feline struvite urolithiasis: fasting reduced the effectiveness of a urinary acidifier (ammonium chloride) and increased the intake of a low magnesium diet. *Vet. Rec.* 121 (11): 245–248.

Tate, N.M., Minor, K.M., Lulich, J.P. et al. (2021). Multiple variants in XDH and MOCOS underlie xanthine urolithiasis in dogs. *Mol. Genet. Metab. Rep.* 29 (September): 100792.

Tefft, K.M., Byron, J.K., Hostnik, E.T. et al. (2021). Effect of a struvite dissolution diet in cats with naturally occurring struvite urolithiasis. *J. Feline Med. Surg.* 23 (4): 269–277.

Terris, M.K., Issa, M.M., and Tacker, J.R. (2001). Dietary supplementation with cranberry concentrate tablets may increase the risk of nephrolithiasis. *Urology* 57 (1): 26–29.

Thomsen, M.K., Svane, L.C., and Poulsen, P.H. (1986). Canine urinary tract infection. Detection, prevalence and therapeutic consequences of bacteriuria. *Nord. Vet. Med.* 38 (6): 394–402.

Thumchai, R., Lulich, J., Osborne, C.A. et al. (1996). Epizootiologic evaluation of urolithiasis in cats: 3,498 cases (1982–1992). *J. Am. Vet. Med. Assoc.* 208 (4): 547–551.

Tiselius, H.G., Berg, C., Fornander, A.M., and Nilsson, M.A. (1993). Effects of citrate on the different phases of calcium oxalate crystallization. *Scanning Microsc.* 7 (1): 381–389, discussion 389–390.

Willeberg, P. (1984). Epidemiology of naturally occurring feline urologic syndrome. *Vet. Clin. North Am. Small Anim. Pract.* 14 (3): 455–469.

Williams, J. (2009). Surgical management of blocked cats. Which approach and when? *J. Feline Med. Surg.* 11 (1): 14–22.

Wing, D.A., Rumney, P.J., Preslicka, C.W., and Chung, J.H. (2008). Daily cranberry juice for the prevention of asymptomatic bacteriuria in pregnancy: a randomized, controlled pilot study. *J. Urol.* 180 (4): 1367–1372.

Xu, H., Laflamme, D.P., and Long, G.L. (2009). Effects of dietary sodium chloride on health parameters in mature cats. *J. Feline Med. Surg.* 11 (6): 435–441.

van Zuilen, C.D., Nickel, R.F., van Dijk, T.H., and Reijngoud, D.J. (1997). Xanthinuria in a family of Cavalier King Charles spaniels. *Vet. Q.* 19 (4): 172–174.

17

Nutritional Management of Endocrine Diseases

Andrea J. Fascetti and Sean J. Delaney

Metabolic regulation occurs on many levels. The diseases discussed in this chapter alter metabolic regulation and energy metabolism. The clinical signs of these diseases are manifested by alterations in subcellular homeostasis. Nutrition can be an important aspect of the management of endocrine diseases including diabetes mellitus (DM), lipid disorders, hypo- and hyperthyroidism, hyperadrenocorticism, and feline idiopathic hypercalcemia.

Diabetes Mellitus

DM is an endocrine disorder that occurs in both cats and dogs. It describes an alteration in the cellular transport and metabolism of glucose caused by insufficient insulin release from the pancreas (absolute and/or relative to sensitivity), a lack of insulin receptors, or an inability of the insulin receptors to transduce the signal. This results in elevated glucose concentrations and an inability of tissues to uptake and utilize the glucose they need. While there are various general classifications of DM described in humans, applying these classifications to dogs and cats is difficult due to the imperfect understanding of the etiopathogenesis and because familial histories and diagnostic tests used in humans are not readily available (Kirk et al. 1993; Nelson et al. 1993; Gilor et al. 2016). The terms insulin-dependent diabetes mellitus

(IDDM) and non-insulin-dependent diabetes mellitus (NIDDM) are commonly used; however, etiopathogenesis is not considered in this classification, which may impact treatment. Most dogs with diabetes are classified as IDDM. Cats can be diagnosed with either IDDM or NIDDM. To make matters more complicated, cats can have one form and then revert to the other over time. It has been hypothesized that beta-cell function in these animals can fluctuate, moving them from one category into the next (Zicker et al. 2010).

Dietary management in animals with IDDM does not eliminate the need for insulin replacement, but in some cases it may improve glycemic control. In patients with NIDDM, dietary therapy can also improve glycemic control and may (in some cases) eliminate the need for exogenous insulin therapy. Regardless of the type of diabetes, the following factors should be considered in every patient: overall health and body condition, presence of other diseases, type of diet, nutrient composition of the diet, nutritional adequacy of the diet, the animal's caloric requirement, and feeding schedule.

Nutritional Factors

Water

Often overlooked, water is one of the key nutrients for all animals and is especially important in animals with diabetes. Diabetics have

Applied Veterinary Clinical Nutrition, Second Edition. Edited by Andrea J. Fascetti, Sean J. Delaney, Jennifer A. Larsen, and Cecilia Villaverde.
© 2024 John Wiley & Sons, Inc. Published 2024 by John Wiley & Sons, Inc.

increased water losses associated with osmotic diuresis secondary to glucosuria, as well as ketonuria if diabetic ketoacidosis is present. Fresh, clean water should be available at all times.

Energy

Many cats and dogs with diabetes have the classic energy-related dichotomy of polyphagia with weight loss. In general, the clinical response of animals with DM to dietary manipulation is dependent upon the level of control of the primary disease process, and the presence or absence of secondary diseases. Weight loss may be secondary to poorly controlled diabetes or an underlying infection, and weight gain may be due to the presence of another problem such as a thyroid disorder or Cushing's disease.

In cats, like humans, the relationship between obesity and DM is well documented (Rand et al. 2004; Lund et al. 2005; Prahl et al. 2007; Laflamme 2010). Studies have shown that baseline insulin concentrations and insulin response to a glucose load increases in dogs as a function of their degree of obesity (Mattheeuws et al. 1984). In cats, the development of feline obesity was accompanied by a 52% decrease in tissue sensitivity to insulin and diminished glucose effectiveness (Appleton et al. 2001). Weight loss can reverse this and promote insulin sensitivity (Hoenig et al. 2007). The tissues of other obese species (monkeys and rodents) have decreased numbers of insulin receptors and those receptors that are present have reduced binding affinity. Over time, these changes reduce the body's ability to respond to insulin.

Fiber

Fiber is not considered nutritionally essential for dogs or cats, but is often used in diabetic dogs and cats to promote satiety, decrease energy density, and modulate gastrointestinal transit and nutrient absorption. The amount and type of dietary fiber have been the subject of extensive investigation in the management of diabetic patients. For the purposes of this discussion, dietary fiber will be classified into two broad categories: insoluble and soluble. Soluble fibers (e.g. pectins, gums, mucilages, fructooligosaccharides, and some hemicelluloses) have high water-holding capacity, delay gastric emptying, slow the rate of nutrient absorption across the intestinal surface, and are highly fermentable by intestinal bacteria. Insoluble fibers (e.g. cellulose, lignin, and most hemicelluloses) have less initial water-holding capacity, decrease gastrointestinal transit time, and are less efficiently fermented by gastrointestinal bacteria. Fiber is proposed to promote the slowed digestion and absorption of digestible dietary carbohydrate, and to reduce insulin peaks after meals. Some soluble fibers also form gels in aqueous solutions, thereby binding glucose and water and preventing their transfer to the absorptive surface of the intestine.

There have been a number of studies examining the use of dietary fiber in diabetic dogs. Most have small sample sizes and confounding factors; however, in general positive effects of fiber-enriched diets have been described. In one study, dogs with experimentally induced diabetes had significant reductions in 24-hour blood glucose fluctuations when fed a diet containing either 15% soluble or insoluble fiber on a dry matter basis (Nelson et al. 1991). Dogs consuming the high-fiber diets were consuming fewer calories than the dogs fed the control diet, and the effect may have been secondary to the fiber, a reduction in calorie intake, or both.

A second study assessed dogs with DM fed a canned diet supplemented with either 20 g of wheat bran (insoluble fiber) or 20 g of guar gum (soluble fiber) (Blaxter et al. 1990). Compared to control dogs that consumed the canned diet without added fiber, both fiber sources reduced postprandial hyperglycemia, the wheat bran to a lesser extent than the guar gum. Similar effects were observed in both diabetic and healthy control dogs.

A third study examined the long-term effects of feeding increased amounts of cellulose (insoluble fiber) to dogs with DM over two eight-month periods (Nelson et al. 1998). Dogs were fed canned diets with either 11% or 23% total dietary fiber on a dry matter basis. The composition of the diets was similar and caloric intake was controlled to maintain body weight. Nine of the eleven dogs in the study improved with respect to daily insulin requirement, fasting blood glucose, urinary glucose excretion, glycosylated hemoglobin concentrations, and serum cholesterol while eating the high-fiber food. The remaining two dogs had better glycemic control when they were eating the low-fiber diet. Overall, when dogs had better glycemic control, they were consuming fewer calories. This finding suggests that caloric intake may have partially influenced glycemic control in this study.

The effects of both insoluble and soluble dietary fiber were examined in a study in dogs with naturally occurring DM (Kimmel et al. 2000). Seven dogs were fed one of three dry diets for a one-month period. One diet was a low-fiber diet (total dietary fiber not reported), a second diet was a high-fiber diet containing only insoluble fiber (73 g/1000 kcal), and the third diet contained both soluble and insoluble fiber sources (56 g/1000 kcal). The dogs had significantly better glycemic control while consuming the high–insoluble fiber diet compared to the other two diets. Fructosamine concentrations were lower in dogs when consuming both fiber-supplemented diets, compared to the low-fiber diet. Although the calorie composition of the diets was similar and caloric intake did not differ between the groups, there were differences with respect to the soluble carbohydrate sources between the diets. It is unknown if this difference had any impact on the findings.

Another study looked at the effect of feeding a high-fiber canned diet containing a blend of insoluble and soluble fibers (Graham et al. 2002). Over the four-month study, changing to the high-fiber diet was associated with significant reductions in fructosamine concentrations, glycosylated hemoglobin concentrations, cholesterol, and 24-hour glucose concentrations. Body weight declined in the

dogs in the study by the fourth month; the authors attributed this to underfeeding the dogs. An increase in dietary fiber consumption or calorie restriction may have been responsible for the positive findings.

Finally, a study in 12 dogs with stable DM compared two commercially available diets that differed in fat content, but that both had predominantly insoluble fiber (90% insoluble; total fiber 50 g/1000 kcal) to a control diet with a mix of types (75% insoluble, 25% soluble; total fiber 35 g/1000 kcal) (Fleeman et al. 2009). Each group of four dogs was fed the diets in a different sequence in a Latin square design. When the dogs were fed the higher-fiber diet with lower energy density, lower fat, and higher protein, statistically significant weight loss occurred (although the mean was less than 2% body weight over the two-month feeding period). However, there was no difference in the insulin requirements of the dogs when they were fed the different diets.

There are very few studies specifically evaluating the effects of dietary fiber on naturally occurring DM in cats. One early study described the effects of the oral sulfonylurea drug glipizide in 20 cats fed commercial diets high or low in fiber for 12 weeks (Nelson et al. 1993). Benefits of the higher-fiber diet were reported, including one cat successfully maintained only on diet and no oral or injectable therapies for DM, but statistical analysis of response rates was not possible. A randomized crossover study in cats with DM compared the effect of the same canned diet mixed with either insoluble fiber (cellulose, 19% total dietary fiber [dry matter]) or starch (low insoluble fiber, 4.1% total dietary fiber [dry matter]) for 24 weeks (Nelson et al. 2000). Mean preprandial glucose concentrations and 12-hour mean glucose concentrations were significantly lower when cats were eating the high-fiber diet. The higher carbohydrate content in the low-fiber diet may have impacted glycemic control in the participants in this study; however, there was a greater difference in fiber content between the diets (total fiber

61 vs. 11 g/1000 kcal) than in carbohydrate content (29% vs. 37% on an energy basis).

Another study investigated the effects of a low-carbohydrate/low-fiber canned diet compared to a moderate-carbohydrate/high-fiber canned diet in 63 cats with DM (Bennett et al. 2006). While cats in both groups were able to discontinue insulin and reverted to a nondiabetic state during the 16-week trial, this was significantly more likely in the low-carbohydrate/low-fiber diet group (68% on the low-carbohydrate/low-fiber diet and 41% on the moderate-carbohydrate/high-fiber diet). It is important to note that only crude fiber was reported and was used to calculate the carbohydrate content. Since crude fiber analysis does not capture all insoluble fiber or any soluble fiber, the total fiber was undefined but certainly underestimated, and the carbohydrate concentration was therefore overestimated; the inaccuracy likely impacted the diets to a different extent based on the expected variable content of fiber types. In addition, the source of fiber, carbohydrate, and other nutrients differed between the diets. The diets were commercial products that were not controlled in energy density, in any nutrient, or in ingredient profile. The low-carbohydrate/low-fiber diet contained soybean meal and corn gluten meal, whereas the moderate-carbohydrate/high-fiber diet contained ground corn. Corn gluten meal is a high-protein product of corn with most of the soluble carbohydrates extracted and therefore will have a lower glycemic index compared to whole ground corn. Soybean meal has a low glycemic index as well. The use of carbohydrates with a lower glycemic index in the low-carbohydrate/low-fiber diet may have also influenced the overall findings of the study.

Research examining the efficacy of fiber supplementation in diabetes has raised a number of questions, perhaps more than it has answered. Most controlled studies support that increasing amounts of insoluble fiber may reduce the postprandial glycemic curve. However, is this effect from the fiber or the caloric dilution that occurs secondary to the addition of the fiber? Alternatively, is it related to the amount and type of soluble carbohydrate in the diet? Perhaps it is a combination of both. Furthermore, the ability of fiber to provide long-term health benefits, improve quality of life, or reduce or eliminate the complications associated with diabetes has not yet been determined.

Fat

Diabetic animals often have accompanying abnormalities in lipid metabolism such as hypertriglyceridemia, hypercholesterolemia, or both. Concurrent pancreatitis is common in many diabetics. Fat should be restricted in patients with these problems. The degree of fat restriction is dependent on the patient's diet history and current fat consumption at the time of diagnosis for both hyperlipidemia (see later) and pancreatitis (see Chapter 12).

Protein

Diabetic animals may have increased amino acid losses through their urine. Patients that are not well controlled will also experience muscle wasting as protein is catabolized to meet energy needs. Currently there are two basic approaches to managing diabetes in dogs and cats: high-carbohydrate/moderate-protein foods or low-carbohydrate/"high-protein" diets. It should be noted that many diets formulated to be lower in carbohydrate and higher in fat are not truly higher in protein compared to typical maintenance diets.

Digestible Carbohydrates

Glucose is one of the most important secretagogs of insulin in healthy subjects. Carbohydrates that are ingested and absorbed result in physiologic responses that are dependent upon the rate in which they enter into an animal's system (Jenkins et al. 1981). In humans, a diet that minimizes the glycemic response is desirable because this provides better control of blood glucose and its associated complications. The term "glycemic index" refers to a ranking system for food based on its effects on blood glucose concentrations. In general, because they are more slowly digested and absorbed, complex carbohydrates with more fiber (such as barley) have a lower glycemic index than starchy foods with lower fiber (such as potatoes) or simple carbohydrates with more mono- and disaccharides (such as those with fructose or sucrose). One study in healthy dogs looked at the glycemic response of five different starch sources: corn, wheat, barley, rice, and sorghum fed at 30% of the diet on a dry matter basis for two weeks (Sunvold and Bouchard 1998). Rice consumption resulted in the highest postprandial glycemic index of the five sources, sorghum the lowest. Wheat and corn generated an intermediate response, and barley had a lower response than wheat and corn. A second study in dogs examined the glucose and insulin response in healthy dogs consuming extruded diets with six different starch sources (cassava flour, brewers' rice, corn, sorghum, peas, or lentils) (Carciofi et al. 2008). This study reported greater immediate postprandial and insulin responses (area under the curve <30 minutes) for brewers' rice, corn, and cassava flour. A similar study examined the same six starch sources in extruded feline diets (de-Oliveira et al. 2008). When compared to the other five starch sources, only corn stimulated an increase in the glucose response at 4 and 10 hours following a meal. Plasma insulin concentrations increased not only when the cats were fed the diet containing corn, but also those containing sorghum, peas, and brewer's rice.

There has been a trend recently among some veterinarians, animal professionals, and pet owners to eschew carbohydrates as an unhealthful food source for dogs and cats. As an obligate carnivore, much of the focus and controversy has centered on the cat. The basis for the argument is that since starch, fiber, and sugar were not a significant part of the cat's natural diet, it is unhealthy for such products to be consumed. The simultaneous increase in the use of carbohydrate in many commercial pet foods and the increasing rates of obesity and DM in cats are frequently cited as evidence for this theory. However, the scientific evidence about to be summarized counters these claims.

Insufficient insulin secretion and impaired insulin sensitivity are the major abnormalities of feline diabetes. The "carnivore connection" paradigm hypothesizes that these abnormalities are the result of long-term feeding of dietary carbohydrate (Miller and Colaquiri 1994). While it is true that experimentally induced hyperglycemia is detrimental to feline beta-pancreatic cells, the same is true in omnivores (de-Oliveira et al. 2008; Zini et al. 2009). Furthermore, hyperglycemia has not been shown to result from either the typical starch concentrations present in commercial diets (de-Oliveira et al. 2008; Laflamme et al. 2022) or even when simple sugars are fed at high concentrations (Drochner and Muller-Schlosser 1980; Kienzle 1994).

Due to the strong association between obesity and the development of DM in cats, carbohydrate has been often blamed for both conditions. However, epidemiologic studies report that obesity is associated with high-fat foods and not high-carbohydrate foods (Scarlett and Donoghue 1998; Lund et al. 2005). In fact, there are some studies that suggest that high-carbohydrate, low-fat diets have an obesity-protective effect (Michel et al. 2005; Backus et al. 2010). Notably, prospective research has directly implicated dietary fat, not carbohydrate, as a risk factor for unwanted weight gain in neutered cats (Nguyen et al. 2004; Backus et al. 2007). Exchanging dietary carbohydrate for protein does appear to be helpful for weight loss and managing diabetes in some cats (Laflamme et al. 2022); however, a similar macronutrient exchange does not appear to prevent weight gain in ovariohysterectomized cats (Vester 2007; Laflamme et al. 2022). In addition, several studies further refute the hypothesis that either feeding dry-type extruded diets long term or dietary carbohydrate per se is the cause of obesity and diabetes in cats (Nguyen et al. 2004; Backus et al. 2007; McCann et al. 2007; Slingerland et al. 2009; Cave et al. 2012).

Recent investigations into obesity and the pathogenesis of DM in cats have led to the hypothesis that feline diabetics might have improved glycemic control, or in some cases even revert to a nondiabetic state, when dietary carbohydrate is restricted. However, there are few data investigating this theory. Of the published studies involving dietary interventions in cats with DM, only four compared two or more diets (Nelson et al. 1993, 2000; Bennett et al. 2006; Hall et al. 2009). Each study reported improvement or remission of DM for cats in every dietary group, and none of them tested the carbohydrate concentration in isolation. The two studies reporting that most cats appeared to benefit from a higher-fiber diet were described earlier (Nelson et al. 1993, 2000). In the third study, also described earlier, the diets tested differed in almost every way (macro- and micronutrient content, fiber type and amount, ingredients, digestibility, calorie density, etc.), so any conclusions related to a specific dietary difference are not possible (Bennett et al. 2006). The third published study comparing diets in cats with DM was a small clinical trial that enrolled 12 newly diagnosed or otherwise uncontrolled patients (Hall et al. 2009). Over a 10-week period, six cats were fed the dry and/or canned versions of a therapeutic diet formulated for feline DM (one each ate only dry and canned, and four ate both) and six were fed both the dry and canned versions of an over-the-counter adult cat food. The therapeutic diets were higher in protein and fiber, and lower in carbohydrate compared to the maintenance diets. One cat in each diet group achieved remission and insulin was discontinued. The cats fed the therapeutic diets had significantly lower serum fructosamine values, but other assessments did not differ between the groups. All cats had improved clinical signs and gained weight, supporting that standardized treatment and monitoring may benefit DM control. Despite the diet

comparison aspect of this study, there were four different products that varied in nutrient profile, and conclusions with regard to specific characteristics are not justified.

Of course, it is not possible in any study to accurately assess in isolation the impacts of either fiber or any macronutrient, including digestible carbohydrate, due to the resulting changes in energy density and obligatory modifications in fat and/or protein. As such, studies are not able to draw conclusions regarding positive or negative benefits of dietary starch concentration per se. There appears to be some clear evidence that supplementation with insoluble fiber helps reduce the glycemic response and may benefit diabetic patients, which may be due to the reduction in calorie density, altered gastrointestinal transit, and nutrient absorption, or any other factor. The roles of carbohydrate and protein concentrations are less clear. However, some clinicians utilize low-carbohydrate/high-protein exclusively for cats and some dogs with DM. There is no specific contraindication to this approach, although such diets are often higher in fat and calories. Assuming that it is not counter to the management of any other concurrent condition (such as pancreatitis or hyperlipidemia), and that the ideal weight can be achieved and maintained, such diets are an option for successful management of DM in dogs and cats. It seems clear that overweight or obese diabetic patients that lose weight also develop better control, or in some cases revert to a nondiabetic state. As such, weight loss to achieve an ideal body condition may be the most effective modification toward achieving better glycemic control or, in cats, reverting to a nondiabetic state.

Minerals and Vitamins

Dogs and cats with diabetes are at risk for the following vitamin and mineral abnormalities: hypophosphatemia, hypokalemia, hyponatremia, hypochloremia, hypocalcemia, hypomagnesemia, and hypovitaminosis D. Generally, adequate control of the diabetes is sufficient to avoid these problems.

Only when the primary disease is not controlled, diabetic ketoacidosis or a secondary problem develops, do these become more of a concern.

Chromium is an essential dietary trace element involved in carbohydrate and lipid metabolism. Chromium functions as a cofactor for insulin, and its presence is necessary for the cellular uptake of glucose. The effect of oral chromium supplementation on glucose tolerance in healthy dogs and cats has been evaluated with conflicting results (Spears et al. 1998; Appleton et al. 2002). The only study done to determine the effect of oral chromium supplementation on glycemic control in diabetic dogs did not support any beneficial or harmful effects in the dosage range of 20–60 μg/kg body weight (BW)/d (Schachter et al. 2001).

Food Type

Semi-moist pet foods or snacks should not be fed to diabetic pets. In dogs, postprandial blood glucose and insulin responses were highest in dogs fed semi-moist foods, compared to dry or canned foods (Holste et al. 1989). This is most likely due to the use of sucrose, fructose, and other simple carbohydrates in many semi-moist products. Despite wide tissue expression of ketohexokinase (Springer et al. 2009), cats do not appear to metabolize fructose, which may lead to intolerance and polyuria due to fructosuria (Kienzle 1994).

Feeding Recommendations and Assessment

Remembering that every patient is unique, the optimal nutritional approach to managing a diabetic patient will vary from animal to animal. It is important that the diet fed to any diabetic is readily and reliably consumed, so palatability is an important factor. In general, for most cases a dietary change is not recommended at the time of diagnosis (unless a concurrent disease is present, such as pancreatitis). The animal should remain on the normal diet while undergoing stabilization, as long as it is balanced and otherwise appropriate. However, adjustments in the feeding schedule may be needed. Particularly in dogs, consistency in the diet, amount, and timing of meals is important, so that insulin can be properly coordinated. This is likely less critical in cats, which appear to have slower gastrointestinal absorption and do not display post-meal hyperglycemia (Martin and Rand 1999; De-Oliveira et al. 2008). In patients that are difficult to regulate (and where a secondary disease process has been ruled out), a diet change, either to a high-fiber diet or in some patients, a low-carbohydrate diet may be beneficial.

If adjustments to fiber intake are desired, this may be done by changing to a fiber-enhanced food or adding fiber to the animal's current diet. Fiber can be added as a mixed fiber source such as psyllium husk powder, 1–3 tbsp per day, soluble fiber such as guar gum or wheat dextrin, 2–4 tsp per day, or insoluble fiber such as wheat bran, 1–3 tbsp per day. Fiber supplementation should be divided equally over the daily meals. Be aware that some fiber sources contain artificial sweeteners such as xylitol and should be avoided; others include sucrose and add unwanted calories and digestible carbohydrate. Using some canned food to deliver the fiber (by mixing them together) can be helpful especially in cats, but care should be taken to ensure that supplemental soluble fiber has "gelled" prior to feeding to prevent rejection of the changed texture or even a potential choking hazard. Plain canned pumpkin can be used, but due to the high moisture content it contains only about half of the fiber per unit volume of psyllium. Pumpkin pie filling should not be used due to its sugar content. Start at the lower dose and titrate up as needed (larger amounts may be needed for large- or giant-breed dogs and smaller quantities for toy or small breeds). It can take a few weeks to see an effect, so patience is warranted.

If snacks and treats are included in the animal's feeding program, it is important that they are also consistent with regard to treat type and time of day offered, as well as low in calories. Minimizing or avoiding treats high in digestible carbohydrates and fat is recommended.

Maintenance of ideal body condition is important in patients with diabetes. In overweight animals, a conservative weight loss protocol should be considered once the initial medical problems are controlled. When dogs and cats with diabetes lose weight, glucose tolerance improves. Weight loss may result in enhanced tissue sensitivity to insulin, necessitating lower daily insulin requirements. As a result, the patient should be carefully monitored and insulin doses adjusted as needed. During weight loss, frequent monitoring and caloric adjustment should be the norm, rather than the exception, in any patient with a disease process including diabetes (see Chapter 9).

Hyperlipidemia

Hyperlipidemia (also referred to as hyperlipoproteinemia) is a disturbance of lipid metabolism that results in an elevation in lipids in the blood, particularly triglycerides (triacylglycerides) and/or cholesterol (Johnson 2005). In the fasted state, hyperlipidemia is an abnormal laboratory finding and is caused by the accelerated synthesis or reduced degradation of lipoproteins. Among dogs and cats, the most clinically relevant type of hyperlipidemia is the finding of an excess blood concentration of triglycerides (hypertriglyceridemia or hypertriacylglyceridemia). Hypercholesterolemia is a state of excess cholesterol in the blood. Unlike humans, most of the cholesterol in dogs is carried on high-density lipoproteins (HDL), the smallest lipoprotein (Johnson 2005). Patients with hypercholesterolemia do not have lipemic serum (unless triglycerides are concurrently elevated), because HDL particles do not refract the light due to their small size (Whitney 1992; Johnson 2005).

Classification and Etiology

Hyperlipidemic states can be classified as postprandial, primary, or secondary. Postprandial hyperlipidemia is the most common hyperlipidemia in dogs and cats (Schenck and Elliott 2010). This is a normal physiologic phenomenon caused by increased circulating chylomicrons. In some cases (depending upon the diet and amount of fat consumed) this can persist anywhere from 7 to 12 hours after a meal (Bauer 2004). However, even when a high-fat diet is consumed, serum triglycerides are not expected to exceed 500 mg/dl in a normal animal. Circulating chylomicrons carry only a fraction of the body's cholesterol, so meal consumption has little impact on cholesterol during the 6–12-hour postprandial period.

Primary causes of hyperlipidemia are either genetic or familial. The principal forms in dogs and cats are idiopathic hyperlipidemia of miniature schnauzers and hyperchylomicronemia of cats. The disease in miniature schnauzers is characterized by excess concentrations of circulating very low-density lipoproteins (VLDL) with or without concurrent hyperchylomicronemia (Whitney et al. 1996; Jaeger et al. 2003; Xenoulis et al. 2007). Familial hyperlipidemia in cats is caused by the production of an inactive form of lipoprotein lipase (LPL), which results from a miscoding of a single amino acid; inheritance is autosomal recessive. Cats with this disease have increased fasting hyperchylomicronemia and slight elevations in VLDL (Backus et al. 2001).

Secondary hyperlipidemia is associated with endocrine disorders (i.e. DM, hypothyroidism, and hyperadrenocorticism) or pancreatitis. Hypertriglyceridemia and hypercholesterolemia can be seen with hypothyroidism (Schenck et al. 2004). In dogs with hypothyroidism, 88% had hypertriglyceridemia and 78% had hypercholesterolemia (Dixon et al. 1999). Hypertriglyceridemia is attributed to a decrease in lipid degradation, secondary to a reduction in LPL activity.

Hypercholesterolemia is believed to result from impaired low-density lipoprotein (LDL) clearance from the circulation. It is postulated that in hypothyroid dogs an absolute deficiency in T3 leads to an increase in the hepatic pool of cholesterol. Subsequently, more cholesterol is carried by LDL. In turn, LDL-receptor activity is also downregulated (Schenck 2006). Activation of hormone-sensitive lipase (HSL) by reduced insulin levels in DM causes the release of large quantities of free fatty acids into the bloodstream (Schenck and Elliott 2010). These excess free fatty acids are converted to VLDL particles by the liver and released back into the circulation. Additionally, insulin deficiency reduces the production of LPL, resulting in the reduced clearance of triglycerides from VLDL. In hyperadrenocorticism, a similar mechanism for hyperlipidemia has been proposed (Schenck and Elliott 2010). Stimulation of HSL releases free fatty acids into the bloodstream; these free fatty acids are packaged into VLDL by the liver and sent out into the circulation. Glucocorticoids inhibit LPL activity, thereby reducing the clearance of triglyceride-rich lipoproteins.

Clinical Signs and Diagnosis

Clinical signs associated with hyperlipidemia are variable and can be different in every patient. Some patients have no clinical signs and are diagnosed on routine blood work. The most common clinical presentations include vomiting (often intermittent), diarrhea, and/or abdominal discomfort. Triglyceride concentrations in excess of 1000 mg/dl have also been associated with pancreatitis, cutaneous xanthomas, lipemia retinalis, seizures, peripheral nerve paralysis, and abnormal behavior (Schenck and Elliott 2010). In addition, it is now well documented that hypertriglyceridemia is associated with glomerular injury and renal proteinuria in miniature schnauzers and likely other breeds (Smith et al. 2017). Due to these serious consequences, confirmation and therapy to control hyperlipidemia are indicated.

A blood sample to confirm hypertriglyceridemia should be obtained following a 12-hour fast. Serum should be submitted for analysis. Clear serum usually has a triglyceride concentration of less than 200 mg/dl. Serum turbidity generally begins to occur between 200 and 300 mg/dl, and lactescent serum is seen around 1000 mg/dl (Bauer 1995; Johnson 2005).

Management and Assessment

Every attempt should be made to determine the underlying cause for the hyperlipidemia. Hyperlipidemia that occurs secondary to an underlying metabolic disease often improves with correction or treatment of the problem (Whitney 1992; Johnson 2005). Dietary treatment of hyperlipidemia is a lifelong commitment, and the importance of nutritional management should be discussed and emphasized with the owner. It has been suggested that triglyceride concentrations greater than 500 mg/dl mandate treatment, even if the animal is asymptomatic, to prevent possible complications (Whitney 1992; Xenoulis and Steiner 2010). While primary hypercholesterolemia is associated with less severe complications, it is recommended that values greater than 750 mg/dl be treated (Schenck and Elliott 2010; Xenoulis and Steiner 2010).

Restriction of dietary fat is the foundation for the treatment of hypertriglyceridemia. Chylomicrons are produced from fat of dietary origin. The success of nutritional therapy is highly dependent upon the veterinarian's ability to select a product that is appropriate for the individual animal they are treating. One key piece of information that is frequently not considered or even obtained is the patient's diet history. A diet history should include not only the names and amounts of commercial food that the animal consumes, but also snacks, treats, dietary supplements, and foods used to administer medications. A diet should be selected that provides less fat than the animal is currently consuming. Most recommendations in the literature suggest feeding a diet that provides 20% of the calories or less from fat on a metabolizable energy (ME) basis (Xenoulis et al. 2020). However, in many patients more severe restriction is often indicated, sometimes as low as 10% fat ME or less. The diet history is so critical because it guides the degree of restriction that is indicated for an individual patient. For example, if the patient is currently consuming a diet that contains 25% of the calories from fat, restricting to 20% fat calories is unlikely to have a significant impact. Treats should be restricted to low-fat treats as well. Baby carrots, rice cakes, and salt-free nonfat pretzels are good human food alternatives. In addition to monitoring the fat intake, calorie intake should be carefully monitored as well. Caloric restriction is also indicated in overweight patients, as excess dietary energy increases VLDL production.

The authors have seen many animals fed fiber-enhanced or weight-loss foods based on the incorrect assumption that a high-fiber or weight-loss diet is automatically a low-fat diet. It is also important to also note that the dry and canned formulas of the same diet can be vastly different in fat content. It is important to check the fat content of the diet directly from the manufacturer's website or product guide, and provide clear guidelines to the client and support staff to ensure that the patient receives the correct product.

Diets rich in omega-3 fatty acids have been used with some success to improve hypertriglyceridemia in humans and experimental animals by reducing the production of VLDLs (Illingworth et al. 1989; Froyland et al. 1995). Fish oils are poor substrates for triglyceride-synthesizing enzymes and therefore are poor VLDL formers. In a study in healthy dogs, fish oil supplementation led to a significant reduction of serum triglyceride concentrations, suggesting that this supplement may play a role in the treatment of primary canine hypertriglyceridemia (LeBlanc et al. 2005; Xenoulis and Steiner 2010). One study reported the impact of fish oil supplementation in reducing modest fasting hyperlipidemia in 18 dogs (mean cholesterol concentrations were less than 310 mg/dl and mean triglyceride concentrations were less than 400 mg/dl) (De Albuquerque et al. 2021). Dogs were fed low- or moderate-fat diets (24 or 33 g/1000 kcal, respectively), and cholesterol and triglycerides were satisfactorily controlled in both groups after 90 days of fish oil supplementation that provided approximately 104 mg eicosapentaenoic acid (EPA) + docosahexaenoic acid (DHA)/kg BW. In the veterinary literature, menhaden fish oil has been used by some authors (220–330 mg/kg BW daily) (Bauer 1995; Schenck and Elliott 2010). It is important to remember that the administration of fish oil will increase intake of both fat and calories, which must be considered when assessing total dietary fat intake relative to meeting the goals for a particular patient.

Other measures to address hyperlipidemia in veterinary patients have also been tried, including niacin, chitosan, and high-fiber diets, as well as drugs such as HMG-CoA reductase inhibitors and fibric acid derivatives. Niacin has been used in dogs (25–100 mg/d) to reduce triglyceride concentrations (Bauer 1995). It is proposed to act by decreasing fatty acid release from adipocytes and reducing the production of VLDL particles. It has been reported to reduce serum triglyceride concentrations in dogs for several months without any negative effects (Whitney 1992; Bauer 1995; Johnson 2005). Negative side effects of using niacin include vomiting, diarrhea, erythema, pruritus, convulsions, and death (Chen et al. 1938; Bauer 1995; Xenoulis and Steiner 2010).

One study compared the efficacy of chitosan and the HMG-CoA reductase inhibitor atorvastatin in controlling cholesterol-induced hyperlipidemia in cats (Mosallanejad et al. 2016). Both strategies were successful and appeared safe, but atorvastatin was more effective. Fibric acid derivatives such as fenofibrate and bezafibrate have been used successfully in dogs with hyperlipidemia (De Marco et al. 2017; Miceli et al. 2021). Adverse effects are uncommonly reported at the doses used, and the drug is effective for both primary and secondary hypertriglyceridemia. Dietary fiber and niacin have also been used in humans to reduce cholesterol concentrations in an effort to prevent coronary artery disease. Coronary artery disease is extremely rare in dogs and cats, and the effect of fiber and niacin in reducing cholesterol levels is unknown. Dietary cholesterol comes from animal sources, so feeding a diet with reduced amounts of animal products may be helpful in reducing cholesterol concentrations. This can be accomplished in dogs using a vegetable protein–based diet and in cats by selecting animal protein sources that are lower in fat and therefore potentially lower in cholesterol (e.g. lean fish, chicken, or pork).

The patient should be reevaluated in about 4–8 weeks after starting the new, low-fat diet. If triglyceride concentrations have not decreased, several steps should be taken. A diet history should be reevaluated to ensure that the patient is getting the correct diet, not receiving additional food sources within the household, nor getting access to food outside of the house (e.g. the neighbors, outdoor cat food, etc.). The patient's medical record should be reviewed to ensure that an underlying disorder has not been overlooked. If triglyceride concentrations are not sufficiently reduced using a commercial product, a home-prepared diet can be formulated by a board certified veterinary nutritionist® to provide a ration that is lower in fat than the currently available veterinary therapeutic products (see Chapter 8). Additional treatments including drug therapy can also be considered.

Hypothyroidism and Hyperadrenocorticism in Dogs

To date, there has been no link established between nutrition and the development of either hypothyroidism or hyperadrenocorticism in dogs. Currently, nutritional management is supportive and is used to address the clinical signs of polyphagia, often leading to secondary weight gain and hyperlipidemia. The nutritional management of hyperlipidemia was discussed earlier in this chapter. Guidance on how to implement a successful weight-loss plan is covered elsewhere (see Chapter 9). However, there are potential strategies that can address polyphagia and prevent weight gain in these patients.

The first step is client education at the time of disease diagnosis. Weight gain occurs when calorie consumption exceeds energy expenditure. Dogs with both of these conditions may experience alterations on both sides of this equation. Many dogs with hypothyroidism or hyperadrenocorticism experience an increase in appetite while simultaneously reducing their energy expenditure. The result can be weight gain and constant hunger. Successfully treating the underlying disease may alleviate these signs. However, clients should be made aware of these concerns at the time the diagnosis is made and offered some advice on how to address them. In order to help abate hunger and prevent weight gain, one can recommend a diet with low calorie density so that a similar or, in some cases, greater volume of food can be fed, but still provide the same or a reduced number of calories. Diets that carry the label "lite" can be helpful in this regard due to their lower calorie density. However, calorie density should be assessed on both a weight basis (kcal/kg) and a volume basis (per cup or can, for example), in order to select a diet that is reduced relative to the currently fed product. A higher-fiber diet could also be considered. There are several studies that have reported an increase in satiety in dogs fed high-fiber diets (Jewell and Toll 1996; Jackson et al. 1997; Weber et al. 2007). In some diets, the addition of fiber also reduces the caloric density of the food. However, it is important to remember that any recommendation should be done with the dog's diet history in mind in order to ensure that the new food provides fewer kcal/g than the current diet. Whenever possible, a few specific brands should be recommended to assist the owner in this process.

Additional strategies include the use of low-calorie treats, which may include commercial snack products or human foods. Energy from treats should be included in the dog's total calorie count and should not exceed 10% of the total daily calories. It also helps if specific treats and amounts are recommended to assist the owner with this process. Feeding small, multiple meals, adding water to the food, and using food-dispensing toys or slow feeding bowls can help prolong meal consumption and may also aid with satiety.

Dietary Hyperthyroidism in Dogs

In 1987, there was a large outbreak of diet-induced hyperthyroidism involving 121 human cases associated with ground beef over a 16-month time period (Hedberg et al. 1987). Investigators identified gullet as the common exposure. In this instance the gullet was not removed at all, or not completely removed during butchering. Following this outbreak, the US Department of Agriculture (UDSA) issued a regulation (Regulation 9 CFR 310.15, www.govinfo.gov/content/pkg/CFR-1998-title9-vol2/pdf/CFR-1998-title9-vol2-sec310-15.pdf) requiring that the thyroid glands of livestock and laryngeal muscle tissue cannot be used in human food. The only permissible use is by pharmaceutical manufacturers.

Hyperthyroidism is uncommon in dogs, and dietary thyrotoxicosis likely represents a small fraction of those cases. In most cases, dogs with hyperthyroidism have differentiated autonomously functioning thyroid gland carcinomas. This was also reported in dogs secondary to the consumption of feces from a housemate that was receiving levothyroxine (Shadwick et al. 2013).

One of the earliest reports of dietary hyperthyroidism involved 12 dogs with clinical and laboratory signs of dietary hyperthyroidism based on elevated plasma thyroxine concentrations and compatible dietary history (Kohler et al. 2012). Six of the dogs displayed no clinical signs; however, thyroxine concentrations were abnormally high in those dogs. The median age of the dogs in this study was 5 years. The median plasma thyroxine concentration was 156.1 nmol/l (range 79.7–391.9 nmol/l). Thyroid-stimulating hormone was less than 0.03 ng/ml. Six of the dogs demonstrated clinical signs of aggression, weight loss, tachycardia, and panting. A diet history taken on the dogs reported that eight owners were feeding a diet containing only raw food and bones, whereas four owners were feeding a commercial diet but also adding dried gullet daily.

Another report involved two female spayed dogs living with the same owner displaying clinical and laboratory signs of hyperthyroidism (Zeugswetter et al. 2013). The dogs had polyuria and polydipsia, excessive panting, and restlessness. These two dogs were fed head meat containing thyroid gland tissue by their owner. Consultation with the slaughterhouse confirmed that thyroid tissue remained with the head meat. The authors of this study also measured iodine and hormone concentrations. Thyroxine concentrations were above reference ranges and thyroid-stimulating hormone was below the reference range.

One attribute common to most if not all cases is the consumption of a meat-based diet. Consumption of commercially available dog foods or treats containing high concentrations of thyroid hormones were implicated in 14 dogs in one report (Broome et al. 2015). Total serum thyroxine concentrations of affected dogs were high (median 8.8 μg/dl; range 4.64–17.4 μg/dl). Analysis of suspected products revealed a median thyroxine concentration of 1.52 μg/dl compared to unrelated commercial foods (0.38 μg/dl).

Investigators from the US Food and Drug Administration published a retrospective case study reporting investigations of 17 dogs with dietary thyrotoxicosis (Rotstein et al. 2021). The report included seven products comprising either jerky treats or canned food made from bison or beef. The investigations underscore the importance of a diet history in all cases, and dietary exogenous thyrotoxicosis should be considered in dogs exhibiting clinical signs compatible with hyperthyroidism, especially if consuming beef-based food.

Feline Hyperthyroidism and Idiopathic Hypercalcemia

Nutritional factors that may influence the development of both feline hyperthyroidism and idiopathic hypercalcemia have been proposed, although no definitive links have been identified. Dietary management may play a role in modulating these diseases and controlling clinical signs.

Hyperthyroidism

The etiology of feline hyperthyroidism is unknown at this time, although many nutritional risk factors have been proposed. The consumption of canned diets has been cited in numerous studies to be a risk factor for thyroid disease in cats in the United States and the United Kingdom (Scarlett et al. 1988; Kass et al. 1999; Martin et al. 2000; Edinboro et al. 2004; Wakeling et al. 2009). One group hypothesized that bisphenol A found in canned cat foods may be the causative goitrogenic substance (Edinboro et al. 2004), although research has not been published to confirm this proposal. Soybeans are another potential goitrogen used in both canine and feline diets (Court and Freeman 2002). In one study in healthy cats, short-term consumption caused an increase in serum T_4 and free T_4 concentrations (White et al. 2004). Overall, feline hyperthyroidism likely has a multifactorial etiology, and proposed dietary risk factors have not been elucidated; these are reviewed in detail elsewhere (van Hoek et al. 2015).

The trace minerals selenium and iodine also have an effect on thyroid hormone concentrations in the cat, and dietary concentrations in pet foods are highly variable. Iodine is necessary for synthesis of thyroid hormones T3 and T4.

As selenium concentrations increase in the diet, serum T3 concentrations also increase, and serum T3 has been correlated with serum selenium concentrations (Wedekind et al. 2003; Zicker et al. 2010). Selenium concentrations are also reported to be higher in canned feline diets compared to dry or canine diets (Zicker et al. 2010). Serum free thyroxine concentrations have been reported to be inversely related to dietary iodine concentrations (Tartellin et al. 1992). Although a recent study found no effect of iodine intake on total thyroxine (TT4) and total triiodothyronine (TT3) concentrations in adult cats, free thyroxine (FT4) was elevated in cats eating 8.8 mg I/kg of diet. The study suggests that the iodine requirement is lower than the current National Research Council (NRC)-recommended allowance (NRC 2006), but higher than the current Association of American Feed Control Officials (AAFCO 2022) recommendation for commercial diets formulated for adult cats (Wedekind et al. 2009). Whether any of these alterations in thyroid hormone concentrations translates into abnormalities or thyroid disease long term remains to be determined. Iodine restriction is a proposed dietary treatment for feline hyperthyroidism through reduced synthesis of thyroid hormone. There are several published reports describing the successful use of a therapeutic, iodine-restricted, feline diet in different populations of hyperthyroid cats (Fritsch et al. 2014; van der Kooij et al. 2014; Hui et al. 2015; Loftus et al. 2019). Although not all studies are prospective, masked, or even controlled, the overall evidence supports that most hyperthyroid cats fed exclusively this diet will safely achieve euthyroidism. The diet is only designed for that purpose, and is not currently recommended as a preventive diet.

In some cases, a dietary change may not be warranted (e.g. those undergoing ablation, thyroidectomy, or radioactive iodine therapy), although the clinician should review the patient's diet history to ensure that a diet appropriate for the cat's life stage is being fed. In some cases, cats will experience significant weight loss and loss of lean body mass. Successful treatment of hyperthyroidism should result in subsequent weight gain and restoration of lean body mass. In some cases cats will have been diagnosed with chronic kidney disease (CKD), or treatment of their hyperthyroidism will reveal underlying kidney disease. Patients should be monitored frequently and if CKD is diagnosed, an appropriate diet should be instituted (see Chapter 15).

Feline Idiopathic Hypercalcemia

Hypercalcemia in cats can be caused by endocrinopathy, neoplasia, hypervitaminosis D, granulomatous disease, and osteolysis. Clinical signs of hypercalcemia are nonspecific and may include polyuria/polydipsia, vomiting, lethargy, and anorexia, although in many cases the finding of hypercalcemia is incidental. Consequences can be serious and may include cardiac arrhythmia as well as renal mineralization and/or calcium oxalate urolithiasis. In many cases the underlying cause is elusive; in this case an exclusionary diagnosis of idiopathic hypercalcemia is made. Exclusive of hypervitaminosis D, no causative dietary factors are identified to date, although various nutritional links have been proposed. Hypercalcemia may be an incidental finding in many cases and can also be transient in some cats, which may complicate identification of putative nutrient associations. Medical therapy is aimed at reducing serum ionized calcium concentration and may include diuresis, steroid medications, or specific drugs targeting calcium metabolism. Positive responses to alendronate in cats with idiopathic hypercalcemia have been reported, typically in conjunction with dietary modification (de Brito Galvão et al. 2017; Kurtz et al. 2022). However, dietary therapy remains the primary and initial recommendation, although which strategies are most efficacious is unknown. Controlled studies are lacking, and most guidance comes from expert opinion and case reports. Some cats demonstrate apparently diet-responsive hypercalcemia, but the

degree and duration of response are highly variable and difficult to predict.

Based on presumptive mechanisms of action, various dietary strategies have been utilized in cats with idiopathic hypercalcemia. Some have not been described in the literature, and controlled studies to investigate any specific or general nutritional modifications are lacking. Those reported in published clinical descriptions (primarily retrospective and uncontrolled case series) and anecdotes include the following:

- Fiber supplementation, which may reduce calcium absorption (McClain et al. 1999; Fantinati and Priymenko 2020).
- Use of diets formulated to manage calcium oxalate urolithiasis with or without sodium supplementation, with the goal of controlling mineral intake and promoting a higher volume of more dilute urine (Lulich et al. 2004); high sodium intake induces calciuresis but does not increase urinary calcium concentration due to dilutional effects (Paßlack et al. 2014).
- Use of diets formulated for CKD, with the goal of controlling mineral intake and avoiding acidification (Fettman et al. 1992; Sławuta et al. 2020).
- Reducing intake of key nutrients such as vitamin D and calcium.

Although some published reports describe the use of some of these strategies to successfully manage cats with idiopathic hypercalcemia, one retrospective case series did not find a positive impact on serum ionized calcium concentrations in 11 cats fed diets formulated to be high in insoluble fiber, for CKD, or for calcium oxalate urolithiasis (Midkiff et al. 2000). Interestingly, 2/11 cats had resolution of total but not ionized hypercalcemia, which underscores the importance of accurate assessment after treatment is initiated.

Some cases of feline idiopathic hypercalcemia may respond positively to dietary calcium restriction, and ionized hypercalcemia can correct to the normal range (A.J. Fascetti and S.J. Delaney, personal communication).

Assessment of the individual diet history is crucial to determine the current total calcium intake. This will inform the degree of reduction that is necessary and may limit dietary options. A home-prepared diet is recommended if a reduction in dietary calcium below the concentrations in commercial diets is necessary. The use of a home-prepared diet also allows more precise control of the vitamin D concentration (although typical dietary concentrations of vitamin D levels have not been identified as a causative factor in feline hypercalcemia). The authors have had success in controlling hypercalcemia in cats with customized home-prepared diets containing approximately 0.6 g Ca/1000 kcal, although it is unclear if the calcium restriction or some other variable is the cause for the positive response. Oral products containing high concentrations of vitamin D, such as organ meats, some fish oils, and certain supplements, should be avoided. Patients can be monitored using ionized calcium concentrations, in addition to the other parameters normally evaluated in any patient consuming a home-prepared diet (see Chapter 8). If no response is evident after 4–6 weeks, consideration should be given to adding other dietary strategies, or instituting medical therapy such as alendronate, as the patient may not be responsive to dietary calcium restriction.

Summary

- Dietary fiber may have a role in the management of diabetes mellitus (DM). Reducing intake of carbohydrates may be beneficial in some patients.

- Current scientific evidence does not support that carbohydrates in pet foods cause an increase in the incidence of obesity and DM.
- In obese or overweight dogs and cats, weight loss to achieve an ideal body condition may be the most effective modification toward achieving improved glycemic control or, in cats, reverting to a nondiabetic state.
- Successful management of hyperlipidemia is dependent upon selecting a diet that contains less fat than the diet the animal is currently consuming.
- Endocrinopathies that cause polyphagia can be managed with foods that are lower in energy density.
- Dietary thyrotoxicosis is not common in dogs, but has been reported in dogs eating treats and diets containing the neck tissues of beef and bison. Clinical signs include polyuria, polydipsia, aggression, panting, restlessness, weight loss, and tachycardia. Thyroxine concentrations may be elevated, whereas thyroid-stimulating hormone may be below the reference range. Discontinuation of suspected diets often results in recovery.
- A dietary change may be indicated in cats with hyperthyroidism; however, if concurrent kidney disease is present or is unmasked with treatment, an appropriate therapeutic diet formulated for feline chronic kidney disease should be fed.
- Although the etiology of feline idiopathic hypercalcemia is unknown, selecting a diet that contains less calcium than the current diet is indicated. In some cases, a home-prepared, calcium-restricted diet should be considered.

References

Appleton, D.J., Rand, J.S., and Sunvold, G.D. (2001). Insulin sensitivity decreases with obesity, and lean cats with low insulin sensitivity are at greatest risk of glucose intolerance with weight gain. *J. Feline Med. Surg.* 3: 211–228.

Appleton, D.J., Rand, J.S., Sunvold, G.D. et al. (2002). Dietary chromium tripicolinate supplementation reduces glucose concentrations and improves glucose tolerance in normal-weight cats. *J. Feline Med. Surg.* 4: 13–25.

Association of American Feed Control Officials (AAFCO) (2022). Model regulations for pet food and specialty pet food. In: *Official Publication*, 113–240. Oxford, IN: Association of American Feed Control Officials.

Backus, R.C., Ginzinger, D.G., Ashbourne Excoffon, K.J.D. et al. (2001). Maternal expression of functional lipoprotein lipase and effects on body fat mass and body condition scores of mature cats with lipoprotein lipase deficiency. *Am. J. Vet. Res.* 62: 264.

Backus, R.C., Cave, N.J., and Keisler, D.H. (2007). Gonadectomy and high dietary fat but not high dietary carbohydrate induce gains in body weight and fat of domestic cats. *Br. J. Nutr.* 98 (3): 641–650.

Backus, R.C., Cave, N.J., Ganjam, V.K. et al. (2010). Age and body weight effects on glucose and insulin tolerance in colony cats maintained since weaning on high dietary carbohydrate. *J. Anim. Physiol. Anim. Nutr. (Berl.)* 94 (6): e318–e328.

Bauer, J.E. (1995). Evaluation and dietary considerations in idiopathic hyperlipidemia in dogs. *J. Am. Vet. Med. Assoc.* 206: 1684–1688.

Bauer, J.E. (2004). Lipoprotein-mediated transport of dietary and synthesized lipids and lipid abnormalities of dogs and cats. *J. Am. Vet. Med. Assoc.* 224: 668–675.

Bennett, N., Greco, D.S., Peterson, M.E. et al. (2006). Comparison of a low carbohydrate–low fiber diet and a moderate carbohydrate–high fiber diet in the management of cats with diabetes mellitus. *J. Feline Med. Surg.* 8 (2): 73–84.

Blaxter, A.C., Cripps, P.J., and Gruffydd-Jones, T.J. (1990). Dietary fibre and post prandial hyperglycemia in normal and diabetic dogs. *J. Small Anim. Pract.* 31: 229–233.

de Brito Galvão, J.F., Parker, V., Schenck, P.A. et al. (2017). Update on feline ionized hypercalcemia. *Vet. Clin. N. Am. Small Anim. Pract.* 47 (2): 273–292.

Broome, M.R., Peterson, M.E., Kemppainen, R.J. et al. (2015). Exogenous thyrotoxicosis in dogs attributable to consumption of all-meat commercial dog food or treats containing excessive thyroid hormone: 14 cases (2008–2013). *J. Am. Vet. Med. Assoc.* 246: 105–111.

Carciofi, A.C., Takakura, F.S., de-Oliveira, L.D. et al. (2008). Effects of six carbohydrate sources of dog digestibility and postprandial glucose and insulin response. *J. Anim. Physiol. Anim. Nutr.* 92: 326–336.

Cave, N.J., Allan, F.J., Schokkenbroek, S.L. et al. (2012). A cross-sectional study to compare changes in the prevalence and risk factors for feline obesity between 1993 and 2007 in New Zealand. *Prev. Vet. Med.* 107 (1–2): 121–133.

Chen, K.K., Rose, C.L., and Robbins, E.B. (1938). Toxicity of nicotinic acid. *Proc. Soc. Exp. Biol. Med.* 38: 241–245.

Court, M.H. and Freeman, L.M. (2002). Identification and concentration of soy isoflavones in commercial cat foods. *Am. J. Vet. Res.* 63: 181–185.

De Albuquerque, P., De Marco, V., Vendramini, T.H.A. et al. (2021). Supplementation of omega-3 and dietary factors can influence the cholesterolemia and triglyceridemia in hyperlipidemic Schnauzer dogs: a preliminary report. *PLoS One* 16 (10): e0258058.

De Marco, V., Noronha, K.S.M., Casado, T.C. et al. (2017). Therapy of canine hyperlipidemia with bezafibrate. *J. Vet. Intern. Med.* 31 (3): 717–722.

De-Oliveira, L.D., Carciofi, A.C., Oliveira, M.C.C. et al. (2008). Effects of six carbohydrate sources on diet digestibility and postprandial glucose and insulin responses in cats. *J. Anim. Sci.* 86: 2237–2246.

Dixon, R.M., Reid, S.W., and Mooney, C.T. (1999). Epidemiological, clinical, haematological and biochemical characteristics of canine hypothyroidism. *Vet. Rec.* 145: 481–487.

Drochner, W. and Muller-Schlosser, S. (1980). Digestibility and tolerance of various sugars in cats. In: *Nutrition of the Dog and Cat* (ed.

R.S. Anderson), 101–111. Oxford: Pergamon Press.

Edinboro, C.H., Scott-Moncrieff, C., Janovitz, E. et al. (2004). Epidemiologic study of relationships between consumption of commercial canned food and risk of hyperthyroidism in cats. *J. Am. Vet. Med. Assoc.* 224: 879–886.

Fantinati, M. and Priymenko, N. (2020). Managing feline idiopathic hypercalcemia with chia seeds (Salvia hispanica L.): a case series. *Front. Vet. Sci.* 7: 421.

Fettman, M.J., Coble, J.M., Hamar, D.W. et al. (1992). Effect of dietary phosphoric acid supplementation on acid-base balance and mineral and bone metabolism in adult cats. *Am. J. Vet. Res.* 53 (11): 2125–2135.

Fleeman, L.M., Rand, J.S., and Markwell, P.J. (2009). Lack of advantage of high-fibre, moderate-carbohydrate diets in dogs with stabilized diabetes. *J. Small Anim. Pract.* 50 (11): 604–614.

Fritsch, D.A., Allen, T.A., Dodd, C.E. et al. (2014). A restricted iodine food reduces circulating thyroxine concentrations in cats with hyperthyroidism. *Int. J. Appl. Res. Vet. Med.* 12: 24–32.

Froyland, L., Asiedu, D.K., Vaagenes, H. et al. (1995). Tetra-decylthioacetic acid incorporated into very low density lipoprotein: changes in the fatty acid composition and reduced plasma lipids in cholesterol fed hamsters. *J. Lipid Res.* 36: 2529–2540.

Gilor, C., Niessen, S.J., Furrow, E. et al. (2016). What's in a name? Classification of diabetes mellitus in veterinary medicine and why it matters. *J. Vet. Intern. Med.* 30 (4): 927–940.

Graham, P.A., Maskell, I.E., Rawlings, J.M. et al. (2002). Influence of a high fibre diet on glycaemic control and quality of life in dogs with diabetes mellitus. *J. Small Anim. Pract.* 43: 67–73.

Hall, T.D., Mahony, O., Rozanski, E.A., and Freeman, L.M. (2009). Effects of diet on glucose control in cats with diabetes mellitus treated with twice daily insulin glargine. *J. Feline Med. Surg.* 11 (2): 125–130.

Hedberg, C.W., Fishbein, D.B., Janssen, R.S. et al. (1987). An outbreak of thyrotoxicosis caused by the consumption of bovine thyroid gland in ground beef. *New Engl. J. Med.* 316: 993–998.

van Hoek, I., Hesta, M., and Biourge, V. (2015). A critical review of food-associated factors proposed in the etiology of feline hyperthyroidism. *J. Feline Med. Surg.* 17 (10): 837–847.

Hoenig, M., Thomaseth, K., Waldron, M. et al. (2007). Insulin sensitivity, fat distribution, and adipocytokine response to different diets in lean and obese cats before and after weight loss [published correction appears in Am. J. Physiol. Regul. Integr. Comp. Physiol. 2009 Apr; 296(4): R1291]. *Am. J. Physiol. Regul. Integr. Comp. Physiol.* 292 (1): R227–R234.

Holste, L.C., Nelson, R.W., Feldman, E.C. et al. (1989). Effect of dry, soft moist and canned dog foods on postprandial blood glucose and insulin concentrations in healthy dogs. *Am. J. Vet. Res.* 50 (6): 984–989.

Hui, T., Bruyette, D., Moore, G. et al. (2015). Effect of feeding an iodine-restricted diet in cats with spontaneous hyperthyroidism. *J. Vet. Intern. Med.* 29: 1063–1068.

Illingworth, D.R., Connor, W.E., Hatcher, L.F. et al. (1989). Hypolipemic effects of n-3 fatty-acids in primary hyperlipoproteinemia. *J. Intern. Med.* 225: 91–97.

Jackson, J.R., Laflamme, D.P., and Owens, D.P. (1997). Effects of dietary fiber content on satiety in dogs. *Vet. Clin. Nutr.* 4: 130–134.

Jaeger, J.Q., Johnson, S., Hinchcliff, K.W. et al. (2003). Characterization of biochemical abnormalities in idiopathic hyperlipidemia of miniature schnauzer dogs. *J. Vet. Intern. Med.* 17: 394.

Jenkins, D.J.A., Taylor, T.M.S., Barker, R.H. et al. (1981). Glycemic index of foods: a physiological basis for carbohydrate exchange. *Am. J. Clin. Nutr.* 35: 346–366.

Jewell, D.E. and Toll, P.W. (1996). Effect of fiber on food intake in dogs. *Vet. Clin. Nutr.* 3: 115–118.

Johnson, M.C. (2005). Hyperlipidemia disorders in dogs. *Compend. Contin. Educ. Pract. Vet.* 27: 361–364.

Kass, P.H., Peterson, M.E., Levy, J. et al. (1999). Evaluation of environmental, nutritional, and host factors in cats with hyperthyroidism. *J. Vet. Intern. Med.* 13: 323–329.

Kienzle, E. (1994). Blood sugar levels and renal sugar excretion after the intake of high carbohydrate diets in cats. *J. Nutr.* 124 (12 Suppl): 2563S–2567S.

Kimmel, S.E., Michel, K.E., Hess, R.S. et al. (2000). Effects of insoluble and soluble dietary fiber on glycemic control in dogs with naturally occurring insulin-dependent diabetes mellitus. *J. Am. Vet. Med. Assoc.* 216: 1076–1081.

Kirk, C.A., Feldman, E.C., and Nelson, R.W. (1993). Diagnosis of naturally acquired type-I and type-II diabetes mellitus in cats. *Am. J. Vet. Res.* 54: 463–467.

Kohler, B., Stenge, C., and Neiger, R. (2012). Dietary hyperthyroidism in dogs. *J. Small Anim. Pract.* 53: 182–184.

van der Kooij, M., Becvarova, I., Meyer, H.P. et al. (2014). Effects of an iodine-restricted food on client-owned cats with hyperthyroidism. *J. Feline Med. Surg.* 16: 491–498.

Kurtz, M., Desquilbet, L., Maire, J. et al. (2022). Alendronate treatment in cats with persistent ionized hypercalcemia: a retrospective cohort study of 20 cases. *J. Vet. Intern. Med.* https://doi.org/10.1111/jvim.16508.

Laflamme, D.P. (2010). Cats and carbohydrates: implications for health and disease. *Compend. Contin. Educ. Vet.* 32: E1–E3.

Laflamme, D.P., Backus, R.C., Forrester, S.D., and Hoenig, M. (2022). Evidence does not support the controversy regarding carbohydrates in feline diets. *J. Am. Vet. Med. Assoc.* 260 (5): 506–513.

LeBlanc, C.J., Bauer, J.E., Hosgood, G. et al. (2005). Effect of dietary fish oil and vitamin E supplementation on hematologic and serum biochemical analytes and oxidative status in young dogs. *Vet. Ther.* 6: 325–340.

Loftus, J.P., DeRosa, S., Struble, A.M. et al. (2019). One-year study evaluating efficacy of an iodine-restricted diet for the treatment of moderate-to-severe hyperthyroidism in cats. *Vet. Med. (Auckl.)* 10: 9–16.

Lulich, J.P., Osborne, C.A., Lekcharoensuk, C. et al. (2004). Effects of diet on urine composition of cats with calcium oxalate urolithiasis. *J. Am. Anim. Hosp. Assoc.* 40 (3): 185–191.

Lund, E.M., Armstrong, P.J., Kirk, C.A. et al. (2005). Prevalence and risk factors for obesity in adult cats from private US veterinary practices. *Int. J. Appl. Vet. Med. Res.* 3: 88–96.

Martin, G.J.W. and Rand, J.S. (1999). Food intake and blood glucose in normal and diabetic cats fed ad libitum. *J. Feline Med. Surg.* 1: 241–251.

Martin, K.M., Rossing, M.A., Ryland, M.L. et al. (2000). Evaluation of dietary and environmental risk factors for hyperthyroidism in cats. *J. Am. Vet. Med. Assoc.* 217: 853–856.

Mattheeuws, D., Rottiers, R., Baeyens, D. et al. (1984). Glucose tolerance and insulin response in obese dogs. *J. Am. Anim. Hosp. Assoc.* 20: 287–290.

McCann, T.M., Simpson, K.E., Shaw, D.J. et al. (2007). Feline diabetes mellitus in the UK: the prevalence within an insured cat population and a questionnaire-based putative risk factor analysis. *J. Feline Med. Surg.* 9: 289–299.

McClain, H.M., Barsanti, J.A., and Bartges, J.W. (1999). Hypercalcemia and calcium oxalate urolithiasis in cats: a report of five cases. *J. Am. Vet. Med. Assoc.* 35 (4): 297–301.

Miceli, D.D., Vidal, V.P., Blatter, M.F.C. et al. (2021). Fenofibrate treatment for severe hypertriglycertidemia in dogs. *Domest. Anim. Endocrinol.* 74: 106578.

Michel, K.E., Bader, A., Shofer, F.S. et al. (2005). Impact of time-limited feeding and dietary carbohydrate content on weight loss in group-housed cats. *J. Feline Med. Surg.* 7 (6): 349–355.

Midkiff, A.M., Chew, D.J., Randolph, J.F. et al. (2000). Idiopathic hypercalcemia in cats. *J. Vet. Intern. Med.* 14 (6): 619–626.

Miller, J. and Colaquiri, S. (1994). The carnivore connection: dietary carbohydrate in the evolution of NIDDM. *Diabetologica* 37: 1280–1286.

Mosallanejad, B., Avizeh, R., Razi Jalali, M. et al. (2016). Comparative evaluation between chitosan and atorvastatin on serum lipid profile changes in hyperlipidemic cats. *Iran. J. Vet. Res.* 17 (1): 36–40.

National Research Council (NRC) (2006). *Nutrient Requirements of Dogs and Cats.* Washington, DC: National Academies Press.

Nelson, R.W., Ihle, S.L., Lewis, L.D. et al. (1991). Effect of dietary fiber supplementation on glycemic control in dogs with alloxan-induced diabetes mellitus. *Am. J. Vet. Res.* 52: 2060–2066.

Nelson, R.W., Feldman, E.C., Ford, S.L. et al. (1993). Effect of an orally administered sulfonylurea, glipizide, for treatment of diabetes mellitus in cats. *J. Am. Vet. Med. Assoc.* 203: 821–827.

Nelson, R.W., Duesberg, C.A., Ford, S.A. et al. (1998). Effect of dietary insoluble fiber on control of glycemia in dogs with naturally acquired diabetes mellitus. *J. Am. Vet. Med. Assoc.* 212: 380–386.

Nelson, R.W., Scott-Moncrieff, C., Feldman, E.C. et al. (2000). Effect of dietary insoluble fiber on control of glycemia in cats with naturally acquired diabetes mellitus. *J. Am. Vet. Med. Assoc.* 216: 1082–1088.

Nguyen, P.G., Dumon, H.J., Siliart, B.S. et al. (2004). Effects of dietary fat and energy on body weight and composition after gonadectomy in cats. *Am. J. Vet. Res.* 65: 1708–1713.

Paßlack, N., Burmeier, H., Brenten, T. et al. (2014). Short term effects of increasing dietary salt concentrations on urine composition in healthy cats. *Vet. J.* 201 (3): 401–405.

Prahl, A., Guptill, L., Glickman, N.W. et al. (2007). Time trends and risk factors for diabetes mellitus in cats presented to veterinary teaching hospitals. *J. Feline Med. Surg.* 9 (5): 351–358.

Rand, J.S., Fleeman, L.M., Farrow, H.A. et al. (2004). Canine and feline diabetes mellitus: nature or nurture? *J. Nutr.* 134 (8 Suppl): 2072S–2080S.

Rotstein, D., Jones, J.L., Buchweitz, J. et al. (2021). Pet food-associated dietary exogenous thyrotoxicosis: retrospective study (2016–2018) and clinical considerations. *Top. Companion Anim. Med.* 43: 100521.

Scarlett, J.M. and Donoghue, S. (1998). Association between body condition and disease in cats. *J. Am. Vet. Med. Assoc.* 212: 1725–1731.

Scarlett, J.M., Moise, N.S., and Rayl, J. (1988). Feline hyperthyroidism: a descriptive and case-control study. *Prev. Vet. Med.* 6: 295–305.

Schachter, S., Nelson, R.W., and Kirk, C.A. (2001). Oral chromium picolinate and control of glycemia in insulin-treated diabetic dogs. *J. Vet. Intern. Med.* 15: 379–384.

Schenck, P.A. (2006). Canine hyperlipidemia: causes and nutritional management. In: *Encyclopedia of Canine Clinical Nutrition* (ed. P. Pibot and D.A. Elliott), 222–251. Paris: Aniwa SAS.

Schenck, P.A. and Elliott, D.A. (2010). Dietary and medical considerations in hyperlipidemia. In: *Textbook of Veterinary Internal Medicine* (ed. S.J. Ettinger and E.C. Feldman), 710–715. St. Louis, MO: Elsevier Saunders.

Schenck, P.A., Donovan, D., Refsal, K.N.R. et al. (2004). Incidence of hypothyroidism in dogs with chronic hyperlipidemia. *J. Vet. Intern. Med.* 18: 442.

Shadwick, S.R., Ridgway, M.D., and Kubier, A. (2013). Thyrotoxicosis in a dog induced by the consumption of feces from a levothyroxine-supplemented housemate. *Can. Vet. J.* 54: 987–989.

Sławuta, P., Sikorska-Kopyłowicz, A., and Sapikowski, G. (2020). Diagnostic utility of different models used to assess the acid–base balance in cats with chronic kidney disease. *Acta Vet. Hung.* 68 (2): 169–176.

Slingerland, L.I., Fazilova, V.V., Plantinga, E.A. et al. (2009). Indoor confinement and physical inactivity rather than the proportion of dry food are risk factors in the development of feline type 2 diabetes mellitus. *Vet. J.* 179 (2): 247–253.

Smith, R.E., Granick, J.L., Stauthammer, C.D. et al. (2017). Consequences of hypertriglyceridemia-associated proteinuria in miniature schnauzers. *J. Vet. Intern. Med.* 31 (6): 1740–1748.

Spears, J.W., Brown, T.T., Sunvold, G.D. et al. (1998). Influence of chromium on glucose metabolism and insulin sensitivity. In: *Recent Advances in Canine and Feline Nutrition, Proceedings from the IAMS Nutrition Symposium* (ed. G.A. Reinhart and D.P. Carey), 103–112. Wilmington, OH: Orange Frazer Press.

Springer, N., Lindbloom-Hawley, S., and Schermerhorn, T. (2009). Tissue expression of ketohexokinase in cats. *Res. Vet. Sci.* 87 (1): 115–117.

Sunvold, G.D. and Bouchard, G.F. (1998). The glycemic response to dietary starch. In: *Recent Advances in Canine and Feline Nutrition, Proceedings from the Iams Nutrition Symposium* (ed. G.A. Reinhart and D.P. Carey), 123–131. Wilmington, OH: Orange Frazer Press.

Tartellin, M.F., Johnson, L.A., Cooke, R.R. et al. (1992). Serum free thyroxine levels respond inversely to changes in levels of dietary iodine in the domestic cat. *N. Z. Vet. J.* 40: 66–68.

Vester, B.M. (2008). Effects of spaying on food intake, weight gain, body condition score, activity and body composition in cats fed high protein versus moderate protein diet. *2007 Nestle Purina Nutrition Forum Proceedings: A Supplement to Compendium for Continuing Education for Veterinarians* 30 (3A): 59.

Wakeling, J., Everard, A., Brodbelt, D. et al. (2009). Risk factors for feline hyperthyroidism in the UK. *J. Small Anim. Pract.* 50 (8): 406–414.

Weber, M., Bissot, T., Servet, E. et al. (2007). A high-protein, high-fiber diet designed for weight loss improves satiety in dogs. *J. Vet. Intern. Med.* 21 (6): 1203–1208.

Wedekind, K.J., Howard, K.A., Backus, R.C. et al. (2003). Determination of selenium requirement in kittens. *J. Anim. Physiol. Anim. Nutr.* 87: 315–323.

Wedekind, K.J., Blumer, M.E., Huntington, C.E. et al. (2009). The feline iodine requirement is lower than the 2006 NRC recommended allowance. *J. Anim. Physiol. Anim. Nutr. (Berl.)* 94: 527–539.

White, H.L., Freeman, L.M., Mahony, O. et al. (2004). Effect of dietary soy on serum thyroid hormone concentrations in healthy adult cats. *Am. J. Vet. Res.* 65: 586–591.

Whitney, M.S. (1992). Evaluation of hyperlipidemias in dogs and cats. *Semin. Vet. Med. Surg.* 7: 292–300.

Whitney, M.S., Boon, G.D., Rebar, A.H. et al. (1996). Ultra-centrifugal and electrophoretic characteristics of the plasma lipoproteins of miniature schnauzer dogs with idiopathic hyperlipoproteinemia. *J. Vet. Intern. Med.* 18: 253–260.

Xenoulis, P.G. and Steiner, J.S. (2010). Lipid metabolism and hyperlipidemia in dogs. *Vet. J.* 183 (1): 12–21.

Xenoulis, P.G., Suchodolski, J.S., Levinski, M.D. et al. (2007). Investigation of hypertriglyceridemia in healthy Miniature Schnauzers. *J. Vet. Intern. Med.* 21: 1224.

Xenoulis, P.G., Cammarate, P.J., Walzem, R.L. et al. (2020). Effect of a low-fat diet on serum triglyceride and cholesterol concentrations and lipoprotein profiles in Miniature Schnauzers with hypertriglyceridemia. *J. Vet. Intern. Med.* 34 (6): 2605–2616.

Zeugswetter, F.K., Volgelsinger, K., and Handl, S. (2013). Hyperthyroidism in dogs caused by consumption of thyroid-containing head meat. *Schweiz. Arch. Tierheilkd.* 155 (2): 149–152.

Zicker, S.C., Nelson, R.W., Kirk, C.A., and Wedekind, K.J. (2010). Endocrine Disorders. In: *Small Animal Clinical Nutrition* (ed. M.S. Hand, C.D. Thatcher, R.L. Remillard, et al.), 415–427. Topeka, KS: Mark Morris Institute.

Zini, E., Osto, M., Franchini, M. et al. (2009). Hyperglycemia but not hyperlipidaemia causes beta cell dysfunction and beta cell loss in the domestic cat. *Diabetologica* 52 (2): 336–346.

18

Nutritional Management of Cardiovascular Diseases
Lisa M. Freeman and John E. Rush

Cardiac disease is one of the most common disorders in both dogs and cats, affecting 11% of all dogs and up to 20% of some feline populations (Buchanan 1999; Cote et al. 2004; Lund et al. 1999; Paige et al. 2009; Paine et al. 2015). Although none of the common cardiac diseases in dogs and cats currently is easily corrected (although surgical replacement or repair of the mitral valve is possible where cardiopulmonary bypass is available), these diseases can be successfully managed medically. Medical therapy of cardiac disease has improved in recent years, with newer and more effective drugs, but medical therapy still is only palliative, with the goal of controlling clinical signs, slowing the progression of disease, and improving quality of life. Maintaining good quality of life is particularly important in dogs and cats, for whom owners often prefer quality of life to "quantity" of life (Oyama et al. 2008). Quality of life also is an important contributing factor to the euthanasia decision in dogs (Mallery et al. 1999).

One key component of medical therapy is nutrition. Careful attention to the diet of animals with cardiac disease is critical for the optimal treatment of these patients. In the past, the goal of nutritional management for animals with cardiac disease was purely symptomatic and focused only on sodium restriction. This was primarily due to the limited number of medications available for treatment, and in that situation, sodium restriction was beneficial for reducing fluid accumulation in animals with congestive heart failure (CHF). Now, with more effective medications available for use in dogs and cats, severe sodium restriction is not required in most animals with cardiac disease (although some sodium restriction is still important). The current emphasis in nutritional management for these patients is on maintaining optimal body composition, avoiding nutritional deficiencies and excesses, and gaining potential benefits from pharmacologic doses of certain nutrients. Optimal nutrition may improve quality of life and may slow the progression of the disease. Therefore, nutrition has an integral role in the medical management of animals with cardiac disease.

Feeding the Cat with Cardiac Disease

Hypertrophic cardiomyopathy (HCM) currently is the most common form of cardiac disease in cats, but other forms of cardiomyopathy

*Note: This chapter was written by the authors in 2017. It was reviewed by the authors in November 2022 for inaccuracies but was not updated.

Applied Veterinary Clinical Nutrition, Second Edition. Edited by Andrea J. Fascetti, Sean J. Delaney, Jennifer A. Larsen, and Cecilia Villaverde.
© 2024 John Wiley & Sons, Inc. Published 2024 by John Wiley & Sons, Inc.

(e.g. dilated, restrictive) and other diseases (e.g. heartworm disease, pericardial disease) also can occur. Cardiac disease often is perceived as a relatively uncommon disease in cats, but studies have reported a prevalence of cardiac disease in 10–18% of apparently healthy cats (Cote et al. 2004; Paige et al. 2009; Paine et al. 2015). Thus, cardiac disease appears to be a very common disease in the feline population and regardless of the cause often leads to CHF, arterial thromboembolism (ATE), syncope, or sudden death.

Hypertrophic Cardiomyopathy

Feline HCM is characterized by left ventricular hypertrophy, impaired diastolic filling, left ventricular outflow tract obstruction in some cats, and often secondary left atrial enlargement (MacDonald 2010). In cats with HCM, CHF and ATE are common clinical manifestations (Atkins et al. 1992; Fox 1999; Kittleson and Kienle 1998; Rush et al. 2002; Tilley 1975; Tilley and Weitz 1977). The most common site of ATE in cats is the terminal aorta, resulting in hindlimb paresis/paralysis, but other limbs and other sites can be affected less frequently (Fox 1999; Rush et al. 2002; Kittleson and Kienle 1998). Other clinical manifestations of HCM in cats include syncope, arrhythmias, and sudden death (Fox 1999; Rush et al. 2002; Kittleson and Kienle 1998). The majority of cats with HCM have not yet been identified to have a genetic cause for their HCM, but myosin-binding protein-C mutations have been identified in Maine Coon and Ragdoll cats (Kittleson et al. 2015). However, in both humans and cats, some patients with mutations have minimal cardiac changes, while some with the same mutation and even in the same family have severe hypertrophy with advanced clinical signs or sudden death. This variable relationship between genotype and phenotype suggests that there are other genetic or environmental modifiers of phenotype. Nutrigenomics, or nutrient–gene interactions, may play an important role in this phenotypic

variability in HCM. Studies have shown that cats with HCM are skeletally larger, more likely to be overweight, have higher concentrations of glucose and insulin-like growth factor-1, and grew more quickly in early life compared to healthy controls (Yang et al. 2008; Freeman et al. 2013, 2015). Therefore, nutrition and growth in early life may play a role in increasing or decreasing the likelihood of developing HCM in a cat that is genetically predisposed.

For cats with HCM, the dietary management depends on the stage of disease. For cats with asymptomatic HCM, much additional research is needed, but diet may play a role in the progression of disease. One randomized, single-blinded study of cats with HCM showed that diet influenced some clinical, biochemical, and echocardiographic variables (Freeman et al. 2014). A successful nutritional intervention would be especially useful considering the lack of a proven drug therapy for asymptomatic cats. Nonetheless, this is an ideal time to begin talking to the owner about the animal's overall dietary patterns (i.e. pet food, treats, table food, and medication administration) and achieving ideal body weight/body condition, as it is easier to institute dietary modifications before clinical signs have arisen. Mild sodium restriction (<100 mg/100 kcal) is recommended, although further research is needed to determine the optimal dose and timing for sodium restriction in cats with cardiac disease. Severe sodium restriction (<50 mg/100 kcal) is not recommended as this can cause early and prolonged activation of the renin-angiotensin-aldosterone (RAA) system (Pedersen 1996; Freeman et al. 2006). The authors' goal for body composition is to achieve or maintain an ideal body condition score (BCS) and normal muscle condition score (MCS) for cats with asymptomatic cardiac disease.

When cats with HCM develop mild–moderate CHF, moderate sodium restriction (i.e. <80 mg Na/100 kcal) is indicated in conjunction with medical therapy, although severe sodium restriction still is usually unnecessary.

Another important issue in cats with CHF is ideal body composition. Muscle loss (cachexia) is common in cats with CHF. Cardiac cachexia can range from mild to moderate to severe (Figure 18.1), and detecting it at an early stage is important when interventions are more likely to be successful. Although inflammation is a central mechanism in cachexia (see later), insufficient calorie and protein intake also contributes to muscle loss. Reduced food intake is a common problem in cats with CHF. Cats can develop anorexia (complete absence of food intake), hyporexia (inadequate food intake), or dysrexia (abnormal patterns of food intake) (Johnson and Freeman 2017). In one study, 38% of cats with cardiac disease had a current or past history of either anorexia or hyporexia, and cats with CHF were significantly more likely than cats without CHF to have reductions in food intake (Torin et al. 2007). Anorexia, hyporexia, and dysrexia can be caused by medication side effects (e.g. azotemia secondary to angiotensin-converting enzyme [ACE] inhibitors or excessive diuretic use), so careful monitoring of drug doses and the serum biochemistry profile for alterations in blood urea nitrogen (BUN), creatinine, and electrolytes is important. Some tips to improve food intake include switching from a dry food to a canned food or vice versa; changing to a different brand; warming the food; or adding small amounts of unsalted, cooked meat or fish (e.g. 1–2 tsp/cat/meal). Supplementation with fish oil, which is high in n-3 fatty acids, can decrease inflammatory cytokine production and improve appetite in some cats with CHF (Freeman et al. 1998; see the n-3 fatty acid section). However, more research is needed on n-3 fatty acids in cats, since one study reported that cats with HCM have *higher* plasma concentrations of docosahexaenoic acid (DHA) compared to healthy controls (compared to dogs with CHF due to dilated cardiomyopathy [DCM] that had *lower* concentrations of DHA and eicosapentaenoic acid [EPA]) (Hall et al. 2014; Freeman et al. 1998).

In addition to minimizing muscle loss, it is important to maintain optimal BCS. While a BCS of 5/9 is considered ideal in healthy cats and cats with asymptomatic cardiac disease, a higher BCS may be more desirable in cats with CHF. In contrast to the healthy cat, obesity may actually be associated with a protective effect once CHF is present – this is known as the obesity paradox. Although there are a number of hypothesized reasons for the obesity paradox, the benefit of obesity in CHF is likely due more to a *lack* of cachexia, rather than to the obesity per se, given the adverse effects associated with cachexia. However, even in cats with CHF, a BCS over 7 was still associated with shorter survival times (Finn et al. 2010). Therefore, the authors recommend maintaining a BCS of 5–6/9 for cats with CHF in addition to preventing/minimizing muscle loss.

Thiamine deficiency is known to be a cause of cardiomyopathy in people, but there has been little investigation into the role of B vitamins as a cause of or contributor to heart disease in cats (or dogs). Reduced food intake can contribute to B vitamin deficiencies, as can increased urinary losses of water-soluble vitamins due to diuretic use. One human study reported that 33% of CHF patients were thiamine deficient (Hanninen et al. 2006). Research has shown that plasma concentrations of vitamins B6, B12, and folate were significantly lower in cats with cardiomyopathy than in healthy controls, an effect that was unrelated to diet or furosemide use (Hohenhaus et al. 2000; McMichael et al. 2000). Therefore, animals with cardiac disease (at least those receiving diuretics) may have higher dietary B vitamin requirements. Although most commercial feline diets contain relatively high levels of water-soluble vitamins, B vitamin supplementation may be useful for cats with CHF, particularly those receiving large doses of diuretics. Cats eating unbalanced homemade diets or commercial diets made by companies with inadequate nutritional expertise or quality control may contain insufficient

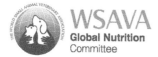

Muscle Condition Score

Muscle condition score is assessed by visualization and palpation of the spine, scapulae, skull, and wings of the ilia. Muscle loss is typically first noted in the epaxial muscles on each side of the spine; muscle loss at other sites can be more variable. Muscle condition score is graded as normal, mild loss, moderate loss, or severe loss. Note that animals can have significant muscle loss even if they are overweight (body condition score > 5/9). Conversely, animals can have a low body condition score (< 4/9) but have minimal muscle loss. Therefore, assessing both body condition score and muscle condition score on every animal at every visit is important. Palpation is especially important with mild muscle loss and in animals that are overweight. An example of each score is shown below.

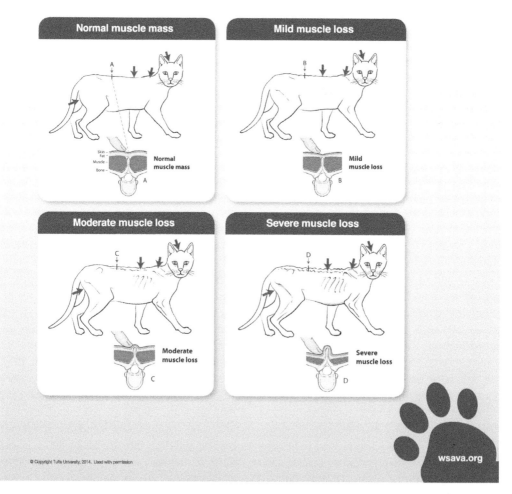

Figure 18.1   Muscle condition score chart for cats. The muscle condition score specifically assesses muscle (as opposed to the body condition score, which assesses fat stores). *Source:* Provided courtesy of the World Small Animal Veterinary Association (WSAVA). Available at the WSAVA Global Nutrition Committee Nutritional Toolkit website: https://wsava.org/global-guidelines/global-nutrition-guidelines. Accessed November, 2022. Copyright Tufts University, 2014, all rights reserved.

concentrations of B vitamins. One study found that 15.6% of 90 commercial canned cat foods were below the National Research Council recommended allowance (Markovich et al. 2014).

In severe CHF, greater restriction of dietary sodium may be beneficial, although much additional research is needed to determine optimal dose and timing of sodium restriction in cats with cardiac disease. The optimal level of dietary sodium for patients with CHF, whether human or veterinary, remains to be determined and requires much research. Of critical importance in advanced CHF is ensuring adequate food intake, since anorexia, hyporexia, and dysrexia are very common at this stage. Addressing other nutrients of concern (e.g. ensuring adequate protein intake; avoiding excessive or insufficient potassium; providing sufficient magnesium, etc.) also are critical for optimal care (see later for canine cardiac disease).

Dilated Cardiomyopathy

DCM is a disease associated with reduced myocardial contractility and dilation of all four cardiac chambers. This disease often results in CHF. DCM once was one of the most common heart diseases in cats, until the publication of a paper associating feline DCM and taurine deficiency, with reversal of cardiomyopathy following taurine supplementation (Pion et al. 1987). Since that time, the dietary taurine content of good-quality commercial cat foods has increased, and there has been a dramatic reduction in the incidence of feline DCM.

DCM is occasionally still seen in cats today, but most current cases are not taurine deficient and a taurine-independent variant of DCM is causative in most cases. Still, owners of cats with DCM should be carefully questioned about the cat's diet, as cats that have been fed unbalanced homemade, vegetarian, or other unconventional diets are at risk for taurine deficiency. In addition, commercial diets made by companies with inadequate nutritional expertise or quality control can be at risk for taurine deficiency. One study, for example, found that two commercial vegetarian diets that claimed to be complete and balanced contained only 18–24% of the Association of American Feed Control Officials (AAFCO) minimum taurine for adult cat maintenance (Gray et al. 2004). Cats with DCM should have plasma and whole blood taurine concentrations analyzed as part of the diagnostic workup and taurine should be administered (125–250 mg/cat orally [PO] every [q]12 h) until results are available. If the cat is eating a diet at risk for taurine deficiency, the owner also should be counseled to switch to a good-quality, nutritionally balanced, animal protein–based commercial cat food. Cats with taurine deficiency–induced DCM often have dramatic reversal of myocardial function after supplementation if their CHF can be successfully controlled and stabilized for at least 2–3 weeks. Cats with DCM that is unrelated to taurine deficiency have a less promising outcome unless they have been eating a nontraditional diet and the diet is changed (see Sidebar 18.1).

Sidebar 18.1   Diet-Associated Dilated Cardiomyopathy

In addition to primary DCM (the genetic form of the disease affecting dogs of certain large or giant breeds), DCM can also occur secondary to drugs, infectious agents, and nutritional causes (e.g. thiamine or taurine deficiency, diet-associated toxins). Between 2018 and 2019, the US Food and Drug Administration (FDA) published three alerts on its investigation of a potential connection between diet and DCM (FDA 2018a, 2018b, 2019). Since the initial FDA alert, there have been 15 peer-reviewed research publications on this topic (Adin et al. 2019, 2021, 2022; Bakke et al. 2022; Cavanaugh et al. 2021; Haimovitz et al. 2022; Kaplan et al. 2018; Freeman et al. 2022; Freid et al. 2021; Karp et al. 2022; Ontiveros et al. 2020; Owens et al. 2022; Quest et al. 2022; Smith et al. 2021; Walker et al. 2022). Breeds typically affected by primary DCM (e.g. Doberman pinschers) as well as breeds that do not commonly develop DCM (e.g. miniature schnauzers, pit bull–type breeds) have been affected by diet-associated DCM (Adin et al. 2019; FDA 2019; Freeman et al. 2022; Freid et al. 2021; Jones et al. 2020; Walker et al. 2022). This secondary form of DCM is unique because of the improvement in various echocardiographic variables and longer survival times after diet change, whereas dogs with primary DCM typically have limited echocardiographic improvement and shorter survival times (Adin et al. 2019; FDA 2019; Freeman et al. 2022; Freid et al. 2021; Jones et al. 2020; Kaplan et al. 2018; Walker et al. 2022). Diets fed to dogs and cats with DCM reported to the FDA and in subsequent studies (often termed "nontraditional") are typically grain-free commercial dry diets that contain pulses (e.g. peas, lentils, chickpeas) and, to a lesser extent, potatoes or sweet potatoes (Adin et al. 2019; FDA 2018, 2019; Freeman et al. 2022; Freid et al. 2021; Kaplan et al. 2018; Karp et al. 2022; Walker et al. 2022). As of July 2020, the FDA had received more than 1100 reports of dogs and more than 20 reports of cats with DCM (Jones et al. 2020).

DCM represents an advanced stage of what appears to be a spectrum of disease associated with nontraditional diets. Studies in apparently healthy dogs suggest that nontraditional diets may be associated with negative cardiac effects before the onset of overt DCM, such as larger left ventricular diameter, lower left ventricular systolic function, higher cardiac troponin I concentrations, and more arrhythmias (Adin et al. 2021; Cavanaugh et al. 2021; Freeman et al. 2022; Ontiveros et al. 2020; Owens et al. 2022).

The cause of diet-associated DCM has not yet been determined. Except in one study of golden retrievers, plasma and whole blood taurine deficiency have been uncommon in affected dogs (Adin et al. 2019; Freeman et al. 2022; Freid et al. 2021; Kaplan et al. 2018; Walker et al. 2022). Other deficiencies that can cause DCM were uncommon in evaluations of diets and small numbers of dogs with diet-associated DCM (FDA 2019; Freeman et al. 2022). A recent foodomics study compared diets associated with DCM and more traditional diets and found more than 100 biochemical compounds that differed between nontraditional and traditional diets, with most being higher in the nontraditional diets (Smith et al. 2021). This study also found that peas was one of the main ingredients that distinguished the two diet types, with this ingredient showing the greatest association with higher concentrations of biochemical compounds in the nontraditional diets (Smith et al. 2021). Grain-free and grain-inclusive pet foods containing peas and other pulses remain popular for both dogs and cats. As a result, dogs (and possibly cats) continue to be affected by diet-associated DCM, so identifying the cause and mechanism as quickly as possible is critical. The veterinary healthcare team should obtain a complete diet history on every patient at every visit, including the exact brand, product, and flavor of commercial pet food. In dogs or cats with DCM, myocardial dysfunction, subclinical cardiac abnormalities, or unexplained arrhythmias, the diet should be changed if they are eating grain-free or grain-inclusive diets containing pulses or potatoes. In the authors' experience, the presence or absence of pulses cannot be ascertained simply based on the name of the diet or if it contains/does not contain grains, so the ingredient list of the specific product should be reviewed. In addition, home-prepared diets, unless the recipe was formulated by a board-certified veterinary nutritionist and strictly followed by the owner, are likely to be nutritionally unbalanced and can put animals eating home-prepared diets at risk for a variety of deficiencies or toxicities that can result in secondary DCM.

Note: This sidebar was up to date as of November 2022.

Hypertension

Traditionally, low-sodium diets have been recommended for cats with hypertension. This has been based primarily on data from rodents or humans. Idiopathic hypertension is much less common than essential hypertension in people. In veterinary patients, high blood pressure is the result of "white coat hypertension" or is secondary to medications, renal disease, or other medical disorders in more than 80% of cases (Brown et al. 2007). In the case of secondary hypertension due to systemic diseases, medical and nutritional treatment of the underlying disease is a priority. In many cases, sodium restriction may also be a part of the recommended nutrient modifications for that disease (e.g. chronic kidney disease).

Even in people, there is much controversy over the relative role of sodium in the development of hypertension and the degree of sodium restriction that should be recommended. Reduced-sodium diets are typically recommended, although other nutrients, such as potassium and magnesium, may play as important a role in hypertension as sodium.

Despite concerns over high-sodium diets in animals with hypertension, studies in normal cats and in cats and dogs with experimentally induced kidney disease have shown no detrimental effect on blood pressure (Buranakarl et al. 2004; Cowgill et al. 2007; Greco et al. 1994; Hansen et al. 1992; Kirk et al. 2006; Xu et al. 2009; Chetboul et al. 2014; Nguyen et al. 2017). However, the effects of sodium restriction in animals with naturally occurring idiopathic hypertension are not known. Currently, medical therapy should be the primary method used to achieve control of blood pressure; however, optimal treatment of any underlying disease is important and may include modification of dietary sodium intake. Certainly, avoiding high-sodium diets seems prudent.

Feeding the Dog with Cardiac Disease

Cardiac disease is one of the most common health problems seen in dogs, with approximately 95% of affected dogs having adult-onset (acquired) cardiac disease. For dogs with adult-onset disease, the majority (75–80%) have myxomatous mitral valve disease (MMVD) or degenerative mitral valve disease (DMVD) (Buchanan 1999). Another 5–10% have DCM, and the remaining dogs with cardiac disease have pericardial disease, endocarditis, primary arrhythmias, or heartworm disease (Buchanan 1999). In dogs, small- to medium-sized breeds are predisposed to MMVD, while DCM is the most common cause of CHF in large-breed dogs. A variety of congenital heart diseases also can occur.

As in cats, the major differences for nutritional modifications are based on the severity of cardiac disease.

Asymptomatic Cardiac Disease (Myxomatous Mitral Valve Disease, Dilated Cardiomyopathy, or Other Cardiac Diseases; American College of Veterinary Internal Medicine [ACVIM] Stage B)

The sympathetic nervous system and the RAA system become increasingly activated as heart disease progresses. Thus, severe sodium restriction in animals with early heart disease could theoretically be detrimental by early and excessive activation of the RAA system (Pedersen 1996; Freeman et al. 2006). The results of one study reported that a low-sodium diet fed to dogs with asymptomatic MMVD resulted in increased aldosterone concentrations and heart rate, with no improvement in cardiac size or function (Freeman et al. 2006). Because of the potential detrimental effects and lack of documented benefits of severe sodium restriction in asymptomatic disease, the authors recommend only mild sodium restriction (<100 mg/100 kcal) in asymptomatic heart disease. However, much additional research is needed to determine the optimal dose and timing of sodium for dogs with heart disease. As in cats, this also is an opportune time to begin educating the owner about the animal's overall dietary patterns – pet food, treats, table food, dental chews, raw-hides and other chews, dietary supplements, and how medications are administered – as it is generally much easier to institute dietary modifications at this stage, before the dog develops clinical signs of CHF and food intake becomes affected to a greater degree.

In addition to mild sodium restriction in animals with asymptomatic cardiac disease, the other main goal is to achieve or maintain optimal body composition. Animals with cardiac disease may be overweight or obese, particularly those in the asymptomatic stages. At this stage, the goal should be a BCS of 4–5/9, with normal muscle condition. If dogs are overweight or obese, a carefully designed weight-reduction program should be developed for the individual, taking into account both the dog (and the owner's) preferences and key problem areas, which can be identified from a thorough diet history. In addition to careful planning, regular monitoring and adjustment are critical for a successful weight-loss program (see Chapter 9). In this stage, a lower BCS (<4/9) or muscle loss should be investigated with a thorough examination and diet history. As the cardiac disease progresses and patients get closer to developing CHF, the authors often allow the BCS to increase to 5–6/9.

Finally, there is a great deal of potential for benefit with nutritional modification in the dog with asymptomatic disease. One study compared a moderately reduced sodium cardiac diet that was enriched with n-3 fatty acids, antioxidants, arginine, taurine, and carnitine to a placebo diet in dogs with asymptomatic MMVD (Freeman et al. 2006). The cardiac diet increased circulating levels of key nutrients (e.g. antioxidants, n-3 fatty acids) and also reduced cardiac size, an effect that did not appear to be the result of sodium restriction. Future studies will help to increase our understanding of the role for nutritional modification in this early stage of disease.

Mild to Moderate Congestive Heart Failure (ACVIM Stage C)

Cardiac Cachexia

When CHF develops, additional nutritional concerns arise for the dog with cardiac disease.

Maintaining optimal body composition is of primary importance in the animal with CHF. Animals with CHF commonly begin to demonstrate muscle loss and sometimes weight loss. This muscle loss is known as cardiac cachexia and is unlike that seen in a healthy animal. A healthy animal that receives insufficient calories to meet energy requirements loses primarily fat. In an animal with CHF that receives insufficient calories, the primary tissue lost is lean body mass (Freeman 2012). This loss of lean body mass has deleterious effects on strength, immune function, and survival (Anker et al. 1997; Freeman 2012). Therefore, it is important to recognize cachexia in its earliest stages when there is the greatest opportunity to have a positive impact. Cardiac cachexia is not only the classic picture of the emaciated, end-stage patient; cachexia actually occurs on a spectrum of severity, from mild to moderate to severe (Figure 18.2).

In the early stages, cachexia can be very subtle and may even occur in obese animals (i.e. an animal may have excess fat stores but still lose lean body mass). Conversely, an animal can be thin but have a normal MCS. Loss of lean body mass is noted in the epaxial, gluteal, scapular, or temporal muscles (Figures 18.1 and 18.2), but is typically identified earliest and most readily in the epaxial muscles. Cardiac cachexia typically does not occur until CHF has developed, but can occur with any underlying cause of CHF (e.g. DCM, MMVD, congenital heart diseases). Cardiac cachexia is a common finding in dogs and cats with CHF and is a multifactorial process caused by reduced calorie and protein intake, increased energy requirement, and an increased production of inflammatory cytokines (Freeman 2012). The cytokines, tumor necrosis factor (TNF), and interleukin-1 (IL-1) are elevated in people, dogs, and cats with CHF (Freeman et al. 1998; Levine et al. 1990; Meurs et al. 2002). These cytokines cause reduced food intake, increase energy requirements, and increase the catabolism of lean body mass (Freeman 2012). In addition, TNF and IL-1 also cause cardiac myocyte hypertrophy and fibrosis and have negative inotropic effects (Mann 2002).

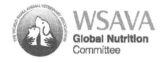

Muscle Condition Score

Muscle condition score is assessed by visualization and palpation of the spine, scapulae, skull, and wings of the ilia. Muscle loss is typically first noted in the epaxial muscles on each side of the spine; muscle loss at other sites can be more variable. Muscle condition score is graded as normal, mild loss, moderate loss, or severe loss. Note that animals can have significant muscle loss if they are overweight (body condition score > 5). Conversely, animals can have a low body condition score (< 4) but have minimal muscle loss. Therefore, assessing both body condition score and muscle condition score on every animal at every visit is important. Palpation is especially important when muscle loss is mild and in animals that are overweight. An example of each score is shown below.

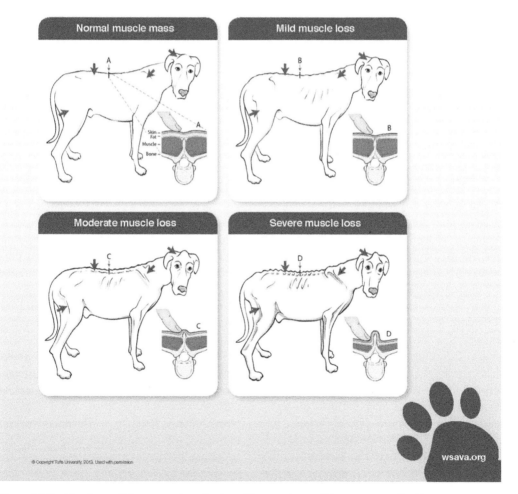

wsava.org

Figure 18.2 Muscle condition score chart for dogs. The muscle condition score specifically assesses muscle and is graded as normal muscle condition or mild, moderate, or severe muscle loss. *Source:* Provided courtesy of the World Small Animal Veterinary Association (WSAVA). Available at the WSAVA Global Nutrition Committee Nutritional Toolkit website: https://wsava.org/global-guidelines/global-nutrition-guidelines. Accessed, November 2022. Copyright Tufts University, 2014, all rights reserved.

Managing dogs with cardiac cachexia can be challenging, but is more successful when identified and addressed early in the process. Conducting a nutritional assessment on every patient at every visit can identify cachexia at its earliest stage. The nutritional assessment includes body weight, BCS, MCS, and a diet history (World Small Animal Veterinary Association 2011; https://wsava.org/global-guidelines/global-nutrition-guidelines; www.petfoodology.org). The nutritional keys to managing cachexia are ensuring adequate calorie and protein intake, modulating cytokine production, and, ideally, providing an anabolic stimulus. Anorexia, hyporexia, and dysrexia are extremely common in cardiac disease, particularly in CHF, with a prevalence of anorexia or hyporexia between 34% and 84% of dogs with cardiac disease (Freeman et al. 2003b; Mallery et al. 1999). After CHF develops, complete anorexia may not ensue, but hyporexia and dysrexia are extremely common. Dysrexia is particularly common, where owners often note changes in food preferences or "cyclical" appetite (i.e. dogs will eat one food well for several days and then refuse it, but will usually eat that specific food again days to weeks later). One of the most important issues for managing reduced food intake is to optimize medical therapy. A reduction in food intake in an animal that previously has been eating well may be an early sign of worsening CHF or a need for medication adjustment. Medication side effects, such as digoxin toxicity or azotemia secondary to ACE inhibitors or overzealous diuretic use, also can cause reduced food intake. Providing a more palatable diet can help to improve appetite (e.g. changing to a different brand or form of food, or having a balanced home-cooked diet formulated by a veterinary nutritionist). Smaller, more frequent meals also may increase food intake, as can flavor enhancers (i.e. foods added to the dog food to increase palatability), such as yogurt (check to be sure it has <100 mg of sodium/100 kcal), maple syrup, or apple sauce. Dogs with cardiac disease often appear sensitive to food temperature and may have specific preferences, so experimentation with foods at different temperatures may be helpful: some prefer the food warm, some prefer it room temperature, and some actually seem to like it best when cold. Feeding the dog on a dinner plate, rather than the usual dog food bowl, or feeding in a different place in the house also may increase food intake. Modulation of cytokine production can be beneficial for managing cardiac cachexia. Supplementation of fish oil, which is high in n-3 fatty acids, can decrease inflammatory cytokine production and improve cachexia and food intake (see the n-3 fatty acid section). A reduction of IL-1 has been correlated with survival in dogs with CHF (Freeman et al. 1998). Finally, capromorelin (Entyce®, Elanco, Greenfield, IN, USA), an appetite stimulant for dogs, is a ghrelin receptor agonist. In addition to its positive effects on food intake, ghrelin has anti-inflammatory effects and increases lean body mass through increased insulin-like growth factor-1. Whether or not capromorelin also has these effects in dogs or cats with naturally occurring disease has not been tested.

Because loss of lean body mass (i.e. cachexia) occurs in animals with CHF, it is critical to ensure adequate intake of protein in addition to calories. Protein restriction was recommended for dogs with CHF in the 1960s because of concerns over the "metabolic load" on the kidneys and liver. However, restricting protein is not currently recommended in animals with CHF because it can contribute to lean body mass loss and malnutrition. Therefore, animals with CHF should not be protein restricted, unless they have concurrent advanced renal disease (see Chapter 15). Some of the diets designed for dogs with cardiac disease are very low in protein. Similarly, renal diets, which are too protein restricted for most dogs with CHF, have previously been recommended by some authors for cardiac disease because these diets often (but not always) are moderately sodium restricted. Clinicians should also be cautious about recommending senior diets. While some senior diets have appropriate levels of protein and sodium for a patient with heart disease, others are much too low in protein or much too high in sodium. For example, one study of 37 over-the-counter senior dog foods found sodium levels ranging from 33 to 412 mg/100 kcal (Hutchinson and Freeman 2011). Unless indicated for concurrent disease, dietary protein for dogs should at least meet the AAFCO minimum of 4.5 g/100 kcal, although higher protein intake may be beneficial, particularly in animals with muscle loss.

Cardiac cachexia has many deleterious effects, but recent studies have also shown that obesity may have differential effects in otherwise healthy dogs compared to those with CHF. While obesity is a risk factor for heart disease, obesity may actually be associated with a protective effect once CHF is present – the obesity paradox. Numerous studies in people have been published showing a beneficial effect of overweight and obesity in various populations of human patients with CHF. Although there are a number of hypothesized reasons for the obesity paradox, the benefit of obesity in CHF is likely due more to a *lack* of cachexia, rather than to the obesity per se, given the adverse effects associated with cachexia. The obesity paradox also has been demonstrated in dogs and cats with CHF (Slupe et al. 2008; Finn et al. 2010).

n-3 Fatty Acids

Fat serves as a source of calories and essential fatty acids, but fatty acids also can have significant effects on immune function, inflammatory mediator production, and hemodynamics. Most pet foods contain primarily n-6 fatty acids (e.g. linoleic acid, arachidonic acid) and are low in the long-chain n-3 fatty acids, EPA, and DHA. In dogs or cats that consume a typical diet, long-chain n-3 fatty acids generally are found in low concentrations in the cell membrane compared to n-6 fatty acids; however, plasma and cell membrane concentrations can be increased by the consumption of foods or supplements high in n-3 fatty acids. There are

a number of benefits of increased dietary n-3 fatty acid intake (Freeman 2010). One is that breakdown products of the n-3 fatty acids (eicosanoids) are less potent inflammatory mediators than eicosanoids derived from n-6 fatty acids. Production of TNF and IL-1 is directly reduced by n-3 fatty acids, and n-3 fatty acid supplementation has been shown to reduce muscle loss in dogs with CHF and, in some animals, to improve appetite (Freeman et al. 1998). Another potential benefit is that n-3 fatty acids have been shown to have antiarrhythmic effects in a variety of species including boxers with ventricular arrhythmias (Smith et al. 2007). One retrospective study showed longer survival times in dogs with CHF that were receiving n-3 fatty acid supplementation (Slupe et al. 2008).

Although an optimal dose of n-3 fatty acids has not been determined, the authors currently recommend a dosage of fish oil to provide 40 mg/kg EPA and 25 mg/kg DHA for animals with CHF, especially if they have appetite issues or cachexia. Unless the diet is one of a few specially designed therapeutic diets, supplementation will be necessary to achieve this n-3 fatty acid dose. When recommending a supplement, it is important to know the exact amount of EPA and DHA in the specific brand of fish oil, since supplements vary widely. The most common formulation of fish oil, however, is 1 g capsules that contain approximately 180 mg EPA and 120 mg DHA. At this concentration, fish oil can be administered at a dose of 1 capsule/4.5 kg (10 lb) of body weight to achieve the authors' recommended EPA and DHA dosage. Fish oil supplements should always contain vitamin E as an antioxidant, but other nutrients should not be included to avoid toxicities. Cod liver oil should not be used to provide n-3 fatty acids at this dose, because it can contain high levels of vitamins A and D, which can result in toxicity. Inefficient hepatic elongation of plant-based n-3 fatty acids (i.e. α-linolenic acid) to EPA and DHA in dogs (and particularly in cats) make flax seed oil a much less effective source of n-3 fatty acids for these species (Bauer 2011). In addition, ventricular arrhythmias in dogs were not significantly reduced by flax seed oil supplementation, as they were with fish oil (Smith et al. 2007).

Sodium

Studies in the 1960s (performed at a time when few cardiac medications were available) demonstrated that low-sodium diets resulted in reduced congestion in dogs with CHF (Pensinger 1964). However, current medical therapy for dogs with CHF may make severe sodium restriction less critical for these patients. While there have been no studies documenting the benefit of sodium restriction on survival or quality of life in dogs with CHF, one study showed that a low-sodium diet (40 mg/100 kcal) reduced cardiac size in dogs with CHF compared to a diet containing 70 mg/100 kcal (Rush et al. 2000). In dogs with ACVIM Stage C, the authors recommend moderate sodium restriction (i.e. <80 mg/100 kcal).

Potassium and Magnesium

Potassium and magnesium are nutrients of concern in cardiac patients because depletion of these electrolytes can increase the risk for cardiac arrhythmias, decrease myocardial contractility, contribute to muscle weakness, and potentiate the adverse effects of certain cardiac medications. Many of the medications used in animals with CHF, such as loop diuretics (e.g. furosemide) and thiazide diuretics (e.g. hydrochlorothiazide), can predispose a patient to hypokalemia or hypomagnesemia. Inadequate dietary intake of potassium or magnesium also predisposes the animal to hypokalemia or hypomagnesemia. However, it is also important to note that hyperkalemia is just as likely as hypokalemia given the routine use of ACE inhibitors, which result in renal potassium sparing. Spironolactone, an aldosterone antagonist and potassium-sparing diuretic, is commonly used to treat CHF and this drug also can cause hyperkalemia. Finally, some commercial cardiac diets are high in potassium, which can exacerbate hyperkalemia.

Serum potassium should be routinely monitored in CHF patients, particularly in those receiving an ACE inhibitor, spironolactone, or high diuretic doses. In humans, one study suggested that the optimal potassium range for patients with CHF was narrow: between 4.1 and 4.8 mmol/l (Aldahl et al. 2017). Serum magnesium concentrations also should be measured, but clinicians should be aware that serum magnesium concentrations are a relatively poor indicator of total body stores. Nonetheless, serial evaluations in an individual patient may be useful, especially in patients with arrhythmias or in those taking high doses of diuretics. Diets vary greatly in their potassium content, so if hypo- or hyperkalemia is present, a diet with a higher or lower potassium content, respectively, should be selected. Diets high in magnesium may be beneficial in a hypomagnesemic animal. However, diet alone may not correct hypokalemia or hypomagnesemia and additional supplementation may be required.

Antioxidants

Antioxidants have received a great deal of attention in the popular press in terms of preventing and treating coronary artery disease, although enthusiasm has waned in recent years as the result of an increasing number of negative clinical trials. Nevertheless, antioxidants may play a role in canine and feline cardiac diseases. Reactive oxygen species cause cellular damage, have negative inotropic effects, and perpetuate an inflammatory response. Normally, the reactive oxygen species being produced as a result of normal oxygen metabolism are balanced by endogenously produced antioxidants. However, an imbalance can arise if there is either increased oxidant production or inadequate endogenous antioxidant protection. Some studies, but not all, have shown that in dogs with CHF there is an imbalance between oxidant production and antioxidant protection (Freeman et al. 1999, 2005; Svete et al. 2017; Reimann et al. 2017; Verk et al. 2017). Supplemental antioxidants are included in many commercial veterinary diets, including at least one cardiac diet, and can increase circulating antioxidant concentrations and reduce oxidation (Freeman et al. 2006). Even if antioxidant supplementation proves to have benefits in animals with CHF, much additional research is needed on which antioxidants, optimal doses, and appropriate timing.

Arginine

Arginine is an essential amino acid for both dogs and cats. In addition, it is a precursor for nitric oxide, an endogenous vascular smooth muscle relaxant. Nitric oxide is synthesized from L-arginine and oxygen and is catalyzed by one of the three forms of nitric oxide synthase (NOS): inducible NOS (iNOS), endothelial NOS (eNOS), or neuronal NOS (nNOS). Both eNOS and nNOS are constitutive forms and are always produced in low levels. Endothelial NOS is required for the maintenance of normal vascular tone, but iNOS is induced by inflammatory mediators such as TNF, IL-1, and free radicals. High levels of iNOS and resulting nitric oxide are induced as part of the inflammatory response and also have negative inotropic effects. Circulating nitric oxide is elevated in people and cats with cardiac disease and in some studies of dogs with cardiac disease (although another study showed reduced concentrations in dogs with MMVD) (de Laforcade et al. 2003; Freeman et al. 2003a; Pedersen et al. 2003; Cunningham et al. 2012). But while iNOS is upregulated in CHF, producing high circulating levels of nitric oxide, eNOS is actually downregulated, thus reducing endothelium-dependent vasodilation (Kubo et al. 1991). Endothelial dysfunction occurs as a result and contributes to exercise intolerance and poor quality of life in humans with CHF (Katz 1995). Arginine supplementation has been proposed as a possible approach to improving endothelial dysfunction in people with CHF. Nitric oxide is difficult to measure, but noninvasive techniques to assess endothelial function have been validated (Puglia

et al. 2006; Jones et al. 2010), and studies in dogs with CHF have shown an attenuated reactive hyperemia response (Cunningham et al. 2012; Jones et al. 2012). Studies are needed to determine whether nutritional interventions can alter this response in dogs with CHF.

Advanced Congestive Heart Failure (ACVIM Stage D)

In advanced CHF, dogs become refractory to routine drug therapy and typically require higher doses or additional medications. In this stage, greater restriction of dietary sodium may be beneficial, but this must be balanced with ensuring adequate calorie and protein intake. This can be a challenge, as anorexia, hyporexia, and especially dysrexia are very common in advanced CHF. Owners should be warned that these are common issues and be provided with strategies to help manage them. Owners also should be educated that anorexia or sudden worsening in food intake in an animal that has been eating can be an early sign of worsening disease or the need for medication adjustment, and should trigger a reevaluation. In addition to optimization of medical therapy for the underlying cardiac disease, capromorelin (Entyce®) can be used an appetite stimulant chronically in dogs with CHF. In terms of nutrition, the authors recommend multiple choices for appropriate pet foods so owners can rotate through different appropriate diet options, considering a nutritionally balanced home-cooked diet (formulated by a veterinary nutritionist) or even single food items (e.g. unsalted home-cooked meat, low-sodium breakfast cereal; https://heartsmart.vet.tufts.edu) that can increase calorie intake without exacerbating the underlying disease. Palatability enhancers (see earlier) and encouraging the owner to try offering foods at different temperatures may increase food intake in some animals (e.g. warmed vs. room temperature vs. cold). Supplementation with n-3 fatty acids also can be beneficial in some animals whose appetite is poor. Other tips that may increase food intake include providing smaller, more frequent meals; feeding the recommended diet from a dinner plate; or putting the recommended diet into a treat jar.

Additional Supplements for Dogs with Cardiac Disease

Supplementation of certain nutrients, either in the diet or in the form of dietary supplements, may have benefits for all dogs and cats with cardiac disease. The use of dietary supplements is more common in dogs, as there are more recommendations in this species and because pills are more easily administered to dogs than to cats. Although some studies have been conducted on these nutrients, the supporting data are not yet robust enough to make firm recommendations for most of these nutrients. However, because many of these have potential benefits and/or are already being used by owners, they are discussed here. With dietary supplements, both the cost and number of medications and supplements that are administered should be considered in order to maximize compliance. In addition, it is important for both the veterinarian and the owner to be aware of issues of safety, efficacy, and quality control for dietary supplements (see Chapter 5). Veterinarians should always specifically ask owners of dogs (and cats) with cardiac disease if they are administering dietary supplements, as this information is rarely volunteered by the owner. Nevertheless, it is estimated that 31% of dogs and 13% of cats with cardiac disease receive dietary supplements (Freeman et al. 2003b; Torin et al. 2007). While supplement use might be more common in dogs with DCM, some supplements might have use in dogs with DCM or MMVD, as noted later.

Taurine

While taurine is an essential nutrient for cats (i.e. they require dietary taurine), dogs are thought to be able to synthesize adequate amounts of taurine endogenously, so it is not classified as an essential nutrient for dogs. Dog breeds at high risk for DCM (e.g. Doberman pinschers, boxers) typically do not have taurine deficiency, although it can occur in certain situations (see later; Kramer et al. 1995). However, taurine deficiency has been documented in some dogs with DCM of certain breeds, such as the American cocker spaniel, Newfoundland, Portuguese water dog, Irish wolfhound, and golden retriever (Alroy et al. 2005; Backus et al. 2003, 2006; Fascetti et al. 2003; Freeman et al. 2001; Kittleson et al. 1997; Kramer et al. 1995). Taurine deficiency may occur more commonly in certain breeds because of higher requirements, breed-specific metabolic abnormalities, or low metabolic rate, but diet also may play a role (Ko et al. 2007). Very low-protein diets, certain lamb meal and rice diets, and some high-fiber diets have been associated with taurine deficiency, although the exact role of diet is not yet known (Backus et al. 2003, 2006; Delaney et al. 2003; Fascetti et al. 2003; Freeman et al. 2001; Kittleson et al. 1997; Ko et al. 2007; Kramer et al. 1995; Sanderson et al. 2001; Spitze et al. 2003; Torres et al. 2003). Other ingredients (e.g. beet pulp) and preparation techniques (e.g. cooking) also may increase risk of taurine deficiency (Ko and Fascetti 2016; Spitze et al. 2003).

Although at least one small study has shown some improvements in clinical or echocardiographic parameters in taurine-deficient dogs supplemented with taurine and L-carnitine, the response generally is not as dramatic as is seen in cats with taurine deficiency–induced DCM (Kittleson et al. 1997). Ongoing research in this area will help veterinarians to better understand this disease and to make better recommendations in the future; however, the authors currently recommend measuring plasma and whole blood taurine concentrations in all dogs with DCM (see Sidebar 18.1). Although the extent of benefits of supplementation in dogs with DCM is not yet clear, the authors recommend taurine supplementation until plasma and whole blood taurine concentrations are available. The optimal dose of taurine for correcting a deficiency in dogs with DCM has not been determined, although a dose of 250–1000 mg q8–12 h has been recommended. It also is important to recommend a specific taurine supplement of known good quality, since the quality control and disintegrative properties of taurine supplements vary widely (Bragg et al. 2009).

l-Carnitine
L-Carnitine is a vitamin-like compound synthesized from the amino acids lysine and methionine that is critical for myocardial energy production. In people, L-carnitine deficiency syndromes can be associated with primary myocardial disease, and carnitine deficiency was also reported in a family of boxers (Keene 1992). Since that time, L-carnitine is sometimes supplemented in some dogs with DCM, but no blinded prospective studies have been conducted in dogs. Even if primary carnitine deficiency is not present, a secondary deficiency of carnitine may develop in CHF. This has been demonstrated in a rapid-pacing model of CHF in dogs (McEntee et al. 2001; Pierpont et al. 1993). In this case, supplementation still may be beneficial by improving myocardial energy metabolism. This may be the reason for benefits shown in some, but not all, human studies.

L-Carnitine supplementation has few side effects, but it is a relatively expensive dietary supplement and supplements vary widely in quality control (Bragg et al. 2009). Some commercial cardiac diets also are enriched in carnitine. The authors offer the option of L-carnitine supplementation to owners of dogs with DCM, especially boxers, but do not consider it essential. However, there also is a rationale for using it in dogs with CHF due to MMVD to aid in myocardial energy metabolism. The minimum or optimal dose of L-carnitine necessary to replete a dog with low

myocardial carnitine concentrations is not known, but the dose that has been recommended is 50–100 mg/kg PO q8 h.

Coenzyme Q10
Coenzyme Q10 is a coenzyme for multiple mitochondrial enzymes and so is involved in myocardial energy production. This, in addition to its antioxidant properties, has made it a compound of interest for CHF, particularly for DCM but also for MMVD. Purported benefits of supplementation include correction of a coenzyme Q10 deficiency, improved myocardial metabolic efficiency, and increased antioxidant protection. Although no controlled studies evaluating supplementation of coenzyme Q10 are published in dogs with naturally occurring heart disease, a meta-analysis showed that human heart failure patients had lower mortality and improved exercise capacity, but no difference in cardiac function (Lei and Liu 2017). One study of dogs with rapid-pacing induced CHF (Harker-Murray et al. 2000) showed that serum or myocardial coenzyme Q10 concentrations were not reduced in dogs with CHF, nor did coenzyme Q10 supplementation increase myocardial concentrations or improve cardiac measurements (although serum concentrations did increase; Harker-Murray et al. 2000). Another study in dogs with naturally occurring congenital and acquired heart diseases of varying severity showed that coenzyme Q10 concentrations were not different compared to healthy controls (Svete et al. 2017). Controlled prospective studies will be necessary to accurately judge the efficacy of this supplement. The current recommended (but empirical) dose in dogs with heart disease is 30–90 mg PO twice a day (BID), depending on the size of the dog, but the optimal dose also depends on the form of coenzyme Q10 used (e.g. ubiquinone vs. ubiquinol).

Vitamin D
Vitamin D plays an important role in regulating bone and calcium metabolism, but also is associated with other body systems and disease

conditions. Vitamin D has cardioprotective effects, including reducing RAS activation, endothelial dysfunction, myocardial hypertrophy, and pro-inflammatory cytokines. Intracellular calcium handling and cardiac contractility also are improved through activation of cardiac vitamin D receptors. Recent human studies have shown associations between vitamin D status and cardiovascular diseases, including hypertension and CHF, as well as associations between vitamin D deficiency and disease progression and poor prognosis. Supplementation studies in humans, however, have had mixed results.

Two studies have been reported on vitamin D status in dogs with cardiac disease. In one study of with CHF secondary to DCM or MMVD (Kraus et al. 2013), vitamin D concentrations (as assessed by 25-hydroxyvitamin D) were significantly lower in dogs with CHF compared to unaffected dogs, but were not different when compared per kg of metabolic body weight. However, low vitamin D concentrations were associated with poor outcome (Kraus et al. 2013). In another study of dogs with varying stages of MMVD (Osuga et al. 2015), dogs with ACVIM Stages B2 and C/D had significantly lower 25-hydroxyvitamin D, but there were no significant differences between dogs with Stages B2 and C/D (Osuga et al. 2015). Whether or not vitamin D supplementation has any benefits in dogs with cardiac disease is currently unknown.

Hypertension

As with cats, low-sodium diets have been recommended for dogs with hypertension. Medical and nutritional treatment of the underlying disease is a priority for dogs with hypertension secondary to other diseases (e.g. chronic kidney disease). The focus of primary hypertension in dogs should be nutritional medical therapy, but until more research in this population is available, the authors recommending avoiding high-sodium diets, including treats, table food, foods used to administer medications, and other components of the diet.

General Nutritional Issues for Dogs and Cats with Cardiac Disease

No single diet is ideal for every animal with cardiac disease, and it is important to take each patient's individual characteristics into consideration. Animals may be asymptomatic or present for coughing, restless sleeping, or exercise intolerance. The nutritional modifications (and medications) selected will vary depending on the clinical signs exhibited. Physical examination findings also are important. An obese animal will require a different caloric intake than one that has weight loss, while a dog with ascites or other signs of active congestion requires greater sodium restriction than a dog that is asymptomatic. Diagnostic test results also help to determine the optimal nutrient modifications. For example, a biochemistry profile might demonstrate azotemia, hypo- or hyperkalemia, or hypoalbuminemia, all of which would affect diet selection. If thoracic radiographs show pulmonary edema or pleural effusion, more sodium restriction is indicated. Echocardiographic and electrocardiographic results also are important in designing the optimal medical and nutritional therapy. Concurrent diseases affect 61% of dogs and 56% of cats with heart disease and may affect diet choice (e.g. a dog with gastrointestinal disease and CHF may require a different diet than one with CHF alone; Freeman et al. 2003b; Torin et al. 2007). Finally, owner expectations and individual animal taste preferences will affect the diet that will be optimal for a given animal.

Based on these patient parameters, one or more diets can be selected for the individual patient (https://heartsmart.vet.tufts.edu). These can be diets designed specifically for patients with cardiac disease, a veterinary diet designed for another disease, or an over-the-counter diet with the properties desired for an individual patient. The authors try to offer a choice of diets so that the owner can determine which is most palatable to the pet. Having a number of choices is particularly beneficial for animals with severe CHF, in whom dysrexia is common.

All dietary changes should be done gradually over a period of at least 3–5 days. Dietary changes should not be attempted in animals with acute CHF or in those with complications from medications (e.g. digoxin toxicity or azotemia due to overzealous diuretic use), as this may induce food aversions. In these patients, the goal should be to encourage food intake while avoiding high-sodium diets. Once a patient has been stabilized (usually at the time of the recheck visit 7–10 days later), a gradual change to the selected diet(s) can be instituted. It also is important to instruct the owner to notify the veterinarian if the patient does not eat adequate amounts of the new food so that other options can be devised.

One of the keys to achieving optimal dietary intake is to be aware that sodium intake (or intake of any other nutrient, for that matter) comes from a number of sources: pet food, treats, table food, rawhides, dental products, and foods used to administer medications. Therefore, addressing each of these with the owner is important. It is estimated that 92% of dogs and 33% of cats with cardiac disease receive daily treats or table food (Freeman et al. 2003b; Torin et al. 2007). Treats and table food are often very high in sodium, so this can be a significant source of sodium for some animals. Another significant source of sodium and other nutrients is the method used for medication administration. Some 57% of dogs with cardiac disease are administered their medications or dietary supplements in food, mostly high-sodium foods such as cheese, peanut butter, or deli meats (Freeman et al. 2003). The percentage of cats with cardiac disease whose medications are administered in foods is lower (34%), but this can still be a significant source of sodium, as the foods used were typically high-sodium foods (e.g. cheese, baby food; Torin et al. 2007). Most owners are unaware of the sodium content of pet foods and table foods and need very specific instructions regarding appropriate pet foods, acceptable low-sodium treats, and methods for administering medications. Owners also should be counseled on specific foods to avoid (https://heartsmart.vet.tufts.edu).

While dogs and cats with cardiac disease can be a challenge to treat, they can be managed successfully when both medical and nutritional aspects of the case are addressed and when the treatment is individualized to the patient (Sidebar 18.2).

Sidebar 18.2   Nutrients of Concern to Consider in Cardiac Disease

- Calories
- Protein
- Amino acids (taurine, arginine)
- Fat (n-3 fatty acids)
- Sodium
- Magnesium
- Potassium
- B vitamins
- Other nutrients (e.g. l-carnitine, antioxidants, coenzyme Q10)

Summary

- Cardiac disease is one of the most common diseases in dogs and cats and optimal nutrition may reduce the medication an animal requires, reduce complications, improve quality of life, and slow the progression of the disease.
- No single diet is ideal for every animal with cardiac disease, and it is important to take each patient's individual characteristics into consideration.
- Concurrent diseases are very common in animals with cardiac disease, and nutritional modifications will vary depending on the clinical signs exhibited.
- Numerous other nutrients such as taurine, L-carnitine, arginine, coenzyme Q10, n-3 fatty acids, and antioxidants may have a role in managing cardiac disease. There is more evidence for some of the supplements than others.

- Mild sodium restriction and the maintenance of an optimal body condition score (BCS) are the two main goals in animals with asymptomatic cardiac disease.
- As cardiac disease progresses and congestive heart failure develops, dogs and cats begin to lose muscle (cardiac cachexia) even if they have a normal or even overweight BCS. Managing patients with cardiac cachexia can be challenging, but is more successful when identified and addressed early in the process. Early identification can be achieved by assessing muscle condition score, along with body weight and BCS, in every patient at every visit.

- Anorexia or, more commonly, hyporexia and dysrexia are often seen in dogs and cats with heart failure. Clinicians should be proactive in identifying and addressing these conditions through nutritional and pharmacologic approaches.
- It is important to recognize that sodium and other nutrient intake comes from a number of sources – pet food, treats, table food, and foods used to administer medications. Obtaining a complete diet history will help the clinician develop dietary recommendations to meet each individual animal's needs.

References

Adin, D., DeFrancesco, T.C., Keene, B. et al. (2019). Echocardiographic phenotype of canine dilated cardiomyopathy differs based on diet type. *J. Vet. Cardiol.* 21: 1–9.

Adin, D., Freeman, L., Stepien, R. et al. (2021). Effect of type of diet on blood and plasma taurine concentrations, cardiac biomarkers, and echocardiograms in 4 dog breeds. *J. Vet. Intern. Med.* 35: 771–779.

Adin, D.B., Haimovitz, D., Freeman, L.M., and Rush, J.E. (2022). Untargeted global metabolomic profiling of healthy dogs grouped on the basis of grain inclusivity of their diet and of dogs with subclinical cardiac abnormalities that underwent a diet change. *Am. J. Vet. Res.* 83: ajvr.22.03.0054.

Aldahl, M., Jensen, A.C., Davidsen, L. et al. (2017). Associations of serum potassium levels with mortality in chronic heart failure patients. *Eur. Heart J.* 38: 2890–2896.

Alroy, J., Rush, J.E., and Sarkar, S. (2005). Infantile dilated cardiomyopathy in Portuguese water dogs: correlation of the autosomal recessive trait with low plasma taurine at infancy. *Amino Acids* 28: 51–56.

Anker, S.D., Ponikowski, P., Varney, S. et al. (1997). Wasting as independent risk factor for mortality in chronic heart failure. *Lancet* 349: 1050–1053.

Atkins, C.E., Gallo, A.M., Kurzman, I.D., and Cowen, P. (1992). Risk factors, clinical signs, and survival in cats with a clinical diagnosis of hypertrophic cardiomyopathy: 74 cases (1985–1989). *J. Am. Vet. Med. Assoc.* 201: 613–618.

Backus, R.C., Cohen, G., Pion, P.D. et al. (2003). Taurine deficiency in Newfoundlands fed commercially available complete and balanced diets. *J. Am. Vet. Med. Assoc.* 239: 1441–1451.

Backus, R.C., Ko, K.S., Fascetti, A.J. et al. (2006). Low plasma taurine concentration in Newfoundland dogs is associated with low plasma methionine and cyst(e)ine concentrations and low taurine synthesis. *J. Nutr.* 136: 2525–2533.

Bakke, A.M., Wood, J., Salt, C. et al. (2022). Responses in randomized groups of healthy, adult Labrador retrievers fed grain-free diets with high legume inclusion for 30 days display commonalities with dogs with suspected dilated cardiomyopathy. *BMC Vet. Res.* 18: 157.

Bauer, J.E. (2011). Therapeutic uses of fish oils in companion animals. *J. Am. Vet. Med. Assoc.* 231: 1657–1661.

Bragg, R.R., Freeman, L.M., Fascetti, A.J., and Yu, Z. (2009). Composition, disintegrative properties, and labeling compliance of commercially available taurine and carnitine dietary products. *J. Am. Vet. Med. Assoc.* 234: 209–213.

Brown, S.A., Atkins, C., Bagley, R. et al. (2007). Guidelines for the identification, evaluation, and management of systemic hypertension in dogs and cats. *J. Vet. Intern. Med.* 21: 542–558.

Buchanan, J.W. (1999). Prevalence of cardiovascular disorders. In: *Textbook of Canine and Feline Cardiology*, 2e (ed. P.R. Fox, D. Sisson and N.S. Moise), 457–470. Philadelphia, PA: W.B. Saunders.

Buranakarl, C., Mathur, S., and Brown, S.A. (2004). Effects of dietary sodium chloride intake on renal function and blood pressure in cats with normal and reduced renal function. *Am. J. Vet. Res.* 65: 620–627.

Cavanaugh, S.M., Cavanaugh, R.P., Gilbert, G.E. et al. (2021). Short-term amino acid, clinicopathologic, and echocardiographic findings in healthy dogs fed a commercial plant-based diet. *PLoS One* 16: 0258044.

Chetboul, V., Reynolds, B.S., Trehiou-Sechi, E. et al. (2014). Cardiovascular effects of dietary salt intake in aged healthy cats: a 2-year prospective randomized, blinded, and controlled study. *PLoS One* 9: e97862.

Cote, E., Manning, A.M., Emerson, D. et al. (2004). Assessment of the prevalence of heart murmurs in overtly healthy cats. *J. Am. Vet. Med. Assoc.* 225: 384–388.

Cowgill, L.D., Segev, G., Bandt, C. et al. (2007). "Effects of dietary salt intake on body fluid volume and renal function in healthy cats" (abstract). *J. Vet. Intern. Med.* 21: 600.

Cunningham, S.M., Rush, J.E., and Freeman, L.M. (2012). Systemic inflammation and endothelial dysfunction in dogs with congestive heart failure. *J. Vet. Intern. Med.* 26: 547–557.

De Laforcade, A.M., Freeman, L.M., and Rush, J.E. (2003). Serum nitrate and nitrite in dogs with spontaneous cardiac disease. *J. Vet. Intern. Med.* 17: 315–318.

Delaney, S.J., Kass, P.H., Rogers, Q.R., and Fascetti, A.J. (2003). Plasma and whole blood taurine in normal dogs of varying size fed commercially prepared food. *J. Anim. Physiol. Anim. Nutr.* 87: 236–244.

Fascetti, A.J., Reed, J.R., Rogers, Q.R., and Backus, R.C. (2003). Taurine deficiency in dogs with dilated cardiomyopathy: 12 cases (1997–2001). *J. Am. Vet. Med. Assoc.* 223: 1137–1141.

FDA (2018a). FDA investigating potential connection between diet and cases of canine heart disease. US Food and Drug Administration. https://wayback.archive-it.org/7993/20201222194256/https://www.fda.gov/animal-veterinary/cvm-updates/fda-investigating-potential-connection-between-diet-and-cases-canine-heart-disease (accessed 03 January 2023).

FDA (2018b). FDA investigation into potential link between certain diets and canine dilated cardiomyopathy – February 2019 update. https://www.fda.gov/animal-veterinary/news-events/fda-investigation-potential-link-between-certain-diets-and-canine-dilated-cardiomyopathy-february.

FDA (2019). FDA investigation into potential link between certain diets and canine dilated cardiomyopathy – February 2019 update. US Food and Drug Administration. https://www.fda.gov/animal-veterinary/news-events/fda-investigation-potential-link-between-certain-diets-and-canine-dilated-cardiomyopathy-february (accessed 03 January 2023).

Finn, E. et al. (2010). The relationship between body weight, body condition, and survival in cats with heart failure. *J. Vet. Intern. Med.* 24: 1369–1374.

Fox, P.R. (1999). Feline cardiomyopathies. In: *Textbook of Canine and Feline Cardiology*, 2e (ed. P.R. Fox, D. Sisson and N.S. Moise), 621–678. Philadelphia, PA: W.B. Saunders.

Freeman, L.M. (2010). Beneficial effects of omega-3 fatty acids in cardiovascular disease. *J. Small Anim. Pract.* 51: 462–470.

Freeman, L.M. (2012). Cachexia and sarcopenia: emerging syndromes of importance in dogs and cats. *J. Vet. Intern. Med.* 26: 3–17.

Freeman, L.M., Rush, J.E., Cunningham, S.M. (2014). Bulmer BJ. A randomized study assessing the effect of diet in cats with hypertrophic cardiomyopathy. *J Vet Intern Med* 28: 847–856.

Freeman, L.M., Ruhs, J.E., Feugier, A., van Hoek, I. (2015). Relationship of body size to metabolic markers and left ventricular hypertrophy in cats. *J Vet Intern Med* 29: 150–156.

Freeman, L.M., Rush, J.E., Kehayias, J.J. et al. (1998). Nutritional alterations and the effect of fish oil supplementation in dogs with heart failure. *J. Vet. Intern. Med.* 12: 440–448.

Freeman, L.M., Rush, J.E., Meurs, K.M., Bulmer, B.J. and Cunningham, S.M. (2013). Body size and metabolic differences in Maine Coon cats with and without hypertrophic cardiomyopathy. *J Feline Med Surg* 15: 74–80.

Freeman, L.M., Brown, D.J., and Rush, J.E. (1999). Assessment of degree of oxidative stress and antioxidant concentrations in dogs with idiopathic dilated cardiomyopathy. *J. Am. Vet. Med. Assoc.* 215: 644–646.

Freeman, L.M., Rush, J.E., Brown, D.J., and Roudebush, P. (2001). Relationship between circulating and dietary taurine concentrations in dogs with dilated cardiomyopathy. *Vet. Therap.* 2: 370–378.

Freeman, L.M., McMichael, M.A., de Laforcade, A.M. et al. (2003a). Indirect determination of nitric oxide in cats with cardiomyopathy and arterial thromboembolism. *J. Vet. Emerg. Crit. Care* 13: 71–76.

Freeman, L.M., Rush, J.E., Cahalane, A.K. et al. (2003b). Dietary patterns in dogs with cardiac disease. *J. Am. Vet. Med. Assoc.* 223: 1301–1305.

Freeman, L.M., Rush, J.E., Milbury, P.E., and Blumberg, J.B. (2005). Antioxidant status and biomarkers of oxidative stress in dogs with congestive heart failure. *J. Vet. Intern. Med.* 19: 537–541.

Freeman, L.M., Rush, J.E., and Markwell, P.J. (2006). Effects of dietary modification in dogs with early chronic valvular disease. *J. Vet. Intern. Med.* 20: 1116–1126.

Freeman, L., Rush, J., Adin, D. et al. (2022). Prospective study of dilated cardiomyopathy in dogs eating nontraditional or traditional diets and in dogs with subclinical cardiac abnormalities. *J. Vet. Intern. Med.* 36: 451–463.

Freid, K.J., Freeman, L.M., Rush, J.E. et al. (2021). Retrospective study of dilated cardiomyopathy in dogs. *J. Vet. Intern. Med.* 35 (1): 58–67.

Gray, C.M., Sellon, R.K., and Freeman, L.M. (2004). Nutritional adequacy of two vegan diets for cats. *J. Am. Vet. Med. Assoc.* 225: 1670–1675.

Greco, D.S., Lees, G.E., Dzendzel, G., and Carter, A.B. (1994). Effects of dietary sodium intake on blood pressure measurements in partially nephrectomized dogs. *Am. J. Vet. Res.* 55: 160–165.

Haimovitz, D., Vereb, M., Freeman, L. et al. (2022). Effect of diet change in healthy dogs with subclinical cardiac biomarker or echocardiographic abnormalities. *J. Vet. Intern. Med.* 36: 1057–1065.

Hall, D.J., Freeman, L.M., Rush, J.E., and Cunningham, S.M. (2014). Comparison of serum fatty acid concentrations in cats with hypertrophic cardiomyopathy and healthy controls. *J. Fel. Med. Surg.* 16: 631–636.

Hanninen, S.A., Darling, P.B., Sole, M.J. et al. (2006). The prevalence of thiamin deficiency in hospitalized patients with congestive heart failure. *J. Am. Coll. Cardiol.* 47: 354–361.

Hansen, B., DiBartola, S.P., Chew, D.J. et al. (1992). Clinical and metabolic findings in dogs with chronic renal failure fed two diets. *Am. J. Vet. Res.* 53: 326–334.

Harker-Murray, A.K., Tajik, A.J., Ishikura, F. et al. (2000). The role of coenzyme Q10 in the pathophysiology and therapy of experimental congestive heart failure in the dog. *J. Cardiac. Fail.* 6: 233–242.

Hohenhaus, A.E., Simantov, R., Fox, P.R. et al. (2000). "Evaluation of plasma homocysteine and B vitamin concentrations in cardiomyopathic cats with congestive heart failure and arterial thromboembolism" (abstract). *Comp. Cont. Ed. Pract. Vet.* 22 (9A): 89.

Hutchinson, D., Freeman, L.M., Schreiner, K.E., Terkla, D.G. (2011). Survey of opinions about nutritional requirements of senior dogs and analysis of nutrient profiles of commercially available diets for senior dogs. *International J Appl Res Vet Med* 9: 68–79.

Johnson, L.N. and Freeman, L.M. (2017). Recognizing, describing, and managing reduced food intake in dogs and cats. *J. Vet. Intern. Med.* 251: 1260–1266.

Jones, I.D., Fuentes, V.L., Fray, T.R. et al. (2010). Evaluation of a flow-mediated vasodilation measurement technique in healthy dogs. *Am. J. Vet. Res.* 71: 1154–1161.

Jones, I.D., Fuentes, V.L., Boswood, A. et al. (2012). Ultrasonographic measurement of flow-mediated vasodilation in dogs with chronic valvular disease. *J. Vet. Cardiol.* 14: 203–210.

Jones, J., Carey, L., and Palmer, L.A. (2020). FDA update on dilated cardiomyopathy: Fully and partially recovered cases. https://www.ksvdl. org/resources/documents/dcm-forum/ FDA_KSU-Science-Forum-slides_09-29-2020. pdf (accessed 03 January 2023).

Kaplan, J.L., Stern, J.A., Fascetti, A.J. et al. (2018). Taurine deficiency and dilated cardiomyopathy in golden retrievers fed commercial diets. *PLoS One* 13: e0209112.

Karp, K.I., Freeman, L.M., Rush, J.E. et al. (2022). Dilated cardiomyopathy in cats: survey of veterinary cardiologists and retrospective evaluation of a possible association with diet. *J. Vet. Cardiol.* 39: 22–34.

Katz, S.D. (1995). The role of endothelium-derived vasoactive substances in the pathophysiology of exercise intolerance in patients with congestive heart failure. *Prog. Cardiovasc. Dis.* 38: 23–50.

Keene, B.W. (1992). L-carnitine deficiency in canine dilated cardiomyopathy. In: *Current Veterinary Therapy XI* (ed. R.W. Kirk and J.D. Bonagura), 780. Philadelphia, PA: W.B. Saunders.

Kirk, C.A., Jewell, D.E., and Lowry, S.R. (2006). Effects of sodium chloride on selected parameters in cats. *Vet. Therap.* 7: 333–346.

Kittleson, M.D. and Kienle, R.D. (1998). Hypertrophic cardiomyopathy. In: *Small Animal Cardiovascular Medicine* (ed. M.D. Kittleson and R.D. Kienle), 347–362. St. Louis, MO: Mosby.

Kittleson, M.D., Keene, B., Pion, P.D. et al. (1997). Results of the multicenter spaniel trial (MUST). *J. Vet. Intern. Med.* 11: 204.

Kittleson, M.D., Meurs, K.M., and Harris, S.P. (2015). The genetic basis of hypertrophic cardiomyopathy in cats and humans. *J. Vet. Cardiol.* 17 (Suppl 1): S53–S73.

Ko, K.S. and Fascetti, A.J. (2016). Dietary beet pulp decreases taurine status in dogs fed low protein diet. *J. Anim. Sci. Technol.* 58: 29.

Ko, K.S., Backus, R.C., Berg, J.R. et al. (2007). Differences in taurine synthesis rate among dogs relate to differences in their maintenance energy requirement. *J. Nutr.* 137: 1171–1175.

Kramer, G.A., Kittleson, M.D., and Fox, P.R. (1995). Plasma taurine concentrations in normal dogs and dogs with heart disease. *J. Vet. Intern. Med.* 9: 253–258.

Kraus, M.S., Rassnick, K.M., Wakshlag, J.J. et al. (2013). Relation of vitamin D status to congestive heart failure and cardiovascular events in dogs. *J. Vet. Intern. Med.* 28: 109–115.

Kubo, S.H., Rector, T.S., Bank, A.J. et al. (1991). Endothelium-dependent vasodilation is attenuated in patients with heart failure. *Circulation* 84: 1589–1596.

Lei, L. and Liu, Y. (2017). Efficacy of coenzyme Q10 in patients with heart failure: a meta-analysis of clinical trials. *BMC Cardiovasc. Disord.* 17: 196.

Levine, B., Kalman, J., Mayer, L. et al. (1990). Elevated circulating levels of tumor necrosis factor in severe chronic heart failure. *N. Engl. J. Med.* 323: 236–241.

Lund, E.M., Armstrong, P.J., Kirk, C.A. et al. (1999). Health status and population characteristics of dogs and cats examined at private practices in the United States. *J. Am. Vet. Med. Assoc.* 214: 1336–1341.

MacDonald, K. (2010). Myocardial disease: feline. In: *Textbook of Veterinary Internal Medicine*, 7e (ed. S. Ettinger and E. Feldman), 1328–1341. St. Louis, MO: Saunders Elsevier.

Mallery, K.F., Freeman, L.M., Harpster, N.K., and Rush, J.E. (1999). Factors contributing to the euthanasia decision in dogs with congestive heart failure. *J. Am. Vet. Med. Assoc.* 214: 1201–1204.

Mann, D.L. (2002). Inflammatory mediators and the failing heart: past, present, and the foreseeable future. *Circ. Res.* 91: 988–998.

Markovich, J.E., Freeman, L.M., and Heinze, C.R. (2014). Analysis of thiamine concentrations in commercial canned foods formulated for cats. *J. Am. Vet. Med. Assoc.* 244: 175–179.

McEntee, K., Flandre, T., Dessy, C. et al. (2001). Metabolic and structural abnormalities in dogs with early left ventricular dysfunction induced by incessant tachycardia. *Am. J. Vet. Res.* 62: 889–894.

McMichael, M.A., Freeman, L.M., Selhub, J. et al. (2000). Plasma homocysteine, B vitamins, and amino acid con centrations in cats with cardiomyopathy and arterial thromboembolism. *J. Vet. Intern. Med.* 14: 507–512.

Meurs, K.M., Fox, P.R., Miller, M.W. et al. (2002). Plasma concentrations of tumor necrosis factor-alpha in cats with congestive heart failure. *Am. J. Vet. Res.* 63: 640–642.

Nguyen, P.B., Reynolds, J.Z. et al. (2017). Sodium in feline nutrition. *J. Anim. Physiol. Anim. Nutr.* 101: 403–420.

Ontiveros, E.S., Whelchel, B.D., Yu, J. et al. (2020). Development of plasma and whole blood taurine reference ranges and identification of dietary features associated with taurine deficiency and dilated cardiomyopathy in golden retrievers: a prospective, observational study. *PloS One* 15 (5): e0233206.

Osuga, T., Nakamura, K., Morita, T. et al. (2015). Vitamin D status in different stages of disease severity in dogs with chronic valvular disease. *J. Vet. Intern. Med.* 29: 1518–1523.

Owens, E.J., LeBlanc, L.L., Freeman, L.M., and Scollan, K.F. (2022). Comparison of echocardiographic measurements and cardiac biomarkers in healthy dog eating non-traditional or traditional diets. *J. Vet. Intern. Med.* https://doi.org/10.1111/jvim.16606.

Oyama, M.A., Rush, J.E., O'Sullivan, M.L. et al. (2008). Perceptions and priorities of owners of dogs with heart disease regarding quality versus quantity of life for their pets. *J. Am. Vet. Med. Assoc.* 233: 104–108.

Paige, C.F., Abbot, J.A., Elvinger, F. et al. (2009). Prevalence of cardiomyopathy in apparently healthy cats. *J. Am. Vet. Med. Assoc.* 234: 1398–1403.

Paine, J.R., Brodbelt, D.C., and Luis Fuentes, V. (2015). Cardiomyopathy prevalence in 780 apparently healthy cats in rehoming centres (the CatScan study). *J. Vet. Cardiol.* 17 (Suppl 1): S244–S257.

Pedersen, H. (1996). Effects of mild mitral valve insufficiency, sodium intake, and place of blood sampling on the reninangiotensin system in dogs. *Acta. Vet. Scand.* 37: 109–118.

Pedersen, H.D., Schutt, T., Sondergaard, R. et al. (2003). Decreased plasma concentrations of nitric oxide metabolites in dogs with untreated mitral regurgitation. *J. Vet. Intern. Med.* 17: 178–184.

Pensinger, R. (1964). Dietary control of sodium intake in spontaneous congestive heart failure in dogs. *Vet. Med.* 59: 752–784.

Pierpont, M.E., Foker, J.E., and Pierpont, G.L. (1993). Myocardial carnitine metabolism in congestive heart failure induced by incessant tachycardia. *Basic. Res. Cardiol.* 88: 362–370.

Pion, P.D., Kittleson, M.D., Rogers, Q.R. et al. (1987). Myocardial failure in cats associated with low plasma taurine: a reversible cardiomyopathy. *Science* 237: 764–768.

Puglia, G.D., Freeman, L.M., Rush, J.E. et al. (2006). Use of a flow-mediated vasodilation technique to assess endothelial function in dogs. *Am. J. Vet. Res.* 67: 1533–1540.

Quest, B.W., Leach, S.B., Garimella, S. et al. (2022). Incidence of canine dilated cardiomyopathy diagnosed at referral institutes and grain-free pet food store sales: a retrospective survey. *Front. Anim. Sci.* 3: https://doi.org/10.3389/fanim.2022.846227.

Quilliam, C. (2021). Effects of feeding pulse-based, grain-free diets on digestibility, glycemic response, and cardiovascular health in domestic dogs. Master of Science thesis, University of Saskatchewan, Saskatoon, Canada. https://harvest.usask.ca/bitstream/handle/10388/13720/QUILLIAM-THESIS-2021.pdf?sequence=1 (accessed 03 January 2023).

Reimann, M.J., Haggstrom, J., Moller, J.E. et al. (2017). Markers of oxidative stress in dogs with myxomatous mitral valve disease are influenced by sex, neuter status, and serum cholesterol concentration. *J. Vet. Intern. Med.* 31: 295–302.

Rush, J.E., Freeman, L.M., Brown, D.J. et al. (2000). Clinical, echocardiographic, and neurohormonal effects of a low sodium diet in dogs with heart failure. *J. Vet. Intern. Med.* 14: 513–520.

Rush, J.E., Freeman, L.M., Fenollosa, N., and Brown, D.J. (2002). Population and survival characteristics of cats with hypertrophic cardiomyopathy: 260 cases (1990–1999). *J. Am. Vet. Med. Assoc.* 220: 202–207.

Sanderson, S.L., Gross, K.L., Ogburn, P.N. et al. (2001). Effects of dietary fat and L-carnitine on plasma and whole blood taurine concentrations and cardiac function in healthy dogs fed protein-restricted diets. *Am. J. Vet. Res.* 62: 1616–1623.

Slupe, J.L., Freeman, L.M., and Rush, J.E. (2008). The relationship between body weight, body condition, and survival in dogs with heart failure. *J. Vet. Intern. Med.* 22: 561–565.

Smith, C.E., Freeman, L.M., Rush, J.E. et al. (2007). Omega-3 fatty acids in boxer dogs with arrhythmogenic right ventricular cardiomyopathy. *J. Vet. Intern. Med.* 21: 265–273.

Smith, C.E., Parnell, L.D., Lai, C. et al. (2021). Investigation of diets associated with dilated cardiomyopathy in dogs using foodomics analysis. *Sci. Rep.* 11: 15881.

Spitze, A.R., Wong, D.L., Rogers, Q.R., and Fascetti, A.J. (2003). Taurine concentrations in animal feed ingredients: cooking influences taurine content. *J. Anim. Physiol. Anim. Nutr.* 87: 251–262.

Svete, A.N., Verk, B., Seliskar, A. et al. (2017). Plasma coenzyme Q10 concentration, antioxidant status, and serum N-terminal pro-brain natriuretic peptide concentration in dogs with various cardiovascular diseases and the effect of cardiac treatment on measured variables. *Am. J. Vet. Res.* 78: 447–457.

Tilley, L.P. (1975). Cardiomyopathy and thromboembolism in the cat. *Feline Pract.* 5: 32–41.

Tilley, L.P. and Weitz, J. (1977). Pharmacologic and other forms of medical therapy in feline cardiac disease. *Vet. Clin. North Am. Small Anim. Pract.* 7: 415–429.

Torin, D.S., Freeman, L.M., and Rush, J.E. (2007). Dietary patterns of cats with cardiac disease. *J. Am. Vet. Med. Assoc.* 230: 862–867.

Torres, C.L., Backus, R.C., Fascetti, A.J., and Rogers, Q.R. (2003). Taurine status in normal dogs fed a commercial diet associated with taurine deficiency and dilated cardiomyopathy. *J. Anim. Physiol. Anim. Nutr.* 87: 359–372.

Verk, B., Svete, A.N., Salobir, J. et al. (2017). Markers of oxidative stress in dogs with heart failure. *J. Vet. Diagnostic. Invest.* 29: 636–644.

Walker, A.L., DeFrancesco, T.C., Bonagura, J.D. et al. (2022). Association of diet with clinical outcomes in dogs with dilated cardiomyopathy and congestive heart failure. *J. Vet. Cardiol.* 40: 99–109.

World Small Animal Veterinary Association Nutritional Assessment Guidelines Task Force (2011). Nutritional Assessment Guidelines. *J. Small Anim. Pract.* 52: 385–396.

Xu, H., Laflamme, D.P., and Long, G.L. (2009). Effects of dietary sodium chloride on health parameters in mature cats. *J. Feline Med. Surg.* 11 (6): 435–441.

Yang, V.K., Freeman, L.M., Rush, J.E. (2008). Comparisons of morphometric measurements and serum insulin-like growth factor concentration in healthy cats and cats with hypertrophic cardiomyopathy. *Am J Vet Res* 69: 1061–1066.

19

Nutritional Management of Oncologic Diseases
Glenna E. Mauldin

Cancer is common in pet cats and dogs. Effective treatments including chemotherapy, radiotherapy, and surgery are available for many tumor types, and treated animals can enjoy prolonged survival with excellent quality of life. Nutrition always plays a central role in the successful and comprehensive management of cats and dogs with neoplastic disease. However, differences in tumor biology as well as wide individual variations in pre-existing nutritional status mean that no single diet is appropriate for every animal with cancer. This chapter will first review what is known about the complex relationship between nutritional status and cancer in people, cats, and dogs. Practical recommendations regarding selected nutritional requirements in individual cats and dogs will then be discussed. Finally, a systematic method that can be used to evaluate novel nutritional claims for cats and dogs with cancer will be presented. The primary purpose of this chapter is to provide practical techniques that will assist the pet owner and the veterinary healthcare team in providing optimal, individualized nutrition for cats and dogs with malignant disease.

Cancer-Associated Malnutrition

Weight Loss and Cachexia in Humans with Cancer

The unique form of protein-calorie malnutrition seen in people with cancer is called "cancer cachexia." This syndrome is characterized clinically by weight loss, fatigue, anemia, and loss of lean body mass, with variable loss of fat stores (Fearon et al. 2011). Cancer cachexia is common in humans, and its prevalence varies with tumor type (DeWys et al. 1980). While it occurs less frequently in people with relatively treatment-responsive tumors such as lymphoma, it is seen in over 80% of people with tumors of the stomach or pancreas. Regardless of the underlying tumor type, however, cancer-associated weight loss is clinically important, because it has a negative effect on quality of life and prognosis (Muscaritoli et al. 2014; Akbulut 2011; Fearon et al. 2001; Langer et al. 2001). Cancer cachexia causes weakness that compromises the ability to perform simple daily functions; it changes the pharmacokinetics and pharmacodynamics of chemotherapy drugs, increasing treatment-related toxicity and decreasing the patient's

Applied Veterinary Clinical Nutrition, Second Edition. Edited by Andrea J. Fascetti, Sean J. Delaney, Jennifer A. Larsen, and Cecilia Villaverde.

ability to tolerate aggressive treatment; and it is associated with shorter survival times and is a common immediate cause of death in people (Fearon et al. 2001; Holder 2003; Langer et al. 2001; Martin et al. 2015; Muscaritoli et al. 2014).

Objective clinical criteria that can be used to define and classify cancer cachexia in people have recently been published. An international consensus statement defines cancer cachexia as a multifactorial syndrome characterized by loss of more than 5% of current body weight, or loss of more than 2% of body weight in cases where there is pre-existing weight loss or sarcopenia (Fearon et al. 2011). Cancer cachexia is proposed to develop progressively through stages from pre-cachexia to cachexia to refractory cachexia, and is classified based on the degree of depletion of energy stores and lean body mass combined with the severity of ongoing weight loss. A significant association between the current cachexia classifications and prognosis has been documented (Blum et al. 2014). However, the intent is that this classification framework will evolve over time, resulting in improved clinical utility. For instance, it has been proposed that objective assessment of appetite and food intake as well as markers of inflammation such as C-reactive protein (CRP) should be included, in part so that less severely affected individuals with pre-cachexia and minimal or no weight loss are still identified and receive timely and effective therapy (Blum et al. 2014; Muscaritoli et al. 2014; Solheim et al. 2014). Regardless, the goal is for evolving but standardized criteria to facilitate improved clinical study design and allow the development of optimal and consistent strategies for clinical management based on stage and severity for people with cancer cachexia.

Cancer cachexia has been divided by underlying cause into two major categories, primary and secondary (Strasser and Bruera 2002). Affected individuals likely have a combination of contributing pathologies that vary with treatment and cancer progression. Secondary cancer cachexia is caused by any one of a variety of functional abnormalities that are not necessarily specific to the underlying neoplastic disease itself. For instance, tumors that involve the gastrointestinal tract can interfere physically with food intake, digestion, or absorption. Radiation and chemotherapy can also decrease nutrient utilization by changing taste and smell perception, by inducing nausea and vomiting, or by causing lethal injury to cells of the gastrointestinal epithelium. In contrast, primary cancer cachexia is a complex paraneoplastic syndrome that has been described in both people and animals with malignant disease. Unlike secondary cancer cachexia, it cannot be reversed through increased food intake or assisted feeding (Brennan 1977). This is because tumor-induced changes force the inefficient use of energy through altered intermediary metabolism of fat, protein, and carbohydrate. This in turn leads to the depletion of lean body mass and fat stores that are characteristic of cancer cachexia. No matter what the quantity of nutrients fed or how they are provided, it is impossible to meet the patient's requirements (Fearon et al. 2001; Strasser and Bruera 2002).

Numerous studies now show that primary cancer cachexia is most likely caused by interrelated changes in inflammatory mediators that have wide-ranging effects on energy and protein metabolism. Interleukin-1α (IL-1α), IL-1β, IL-6, tumor necrosis factor-α (TNF-α), interferon-γ (IFN-γ), and various eicosanoids have all been implicated in this scenario, and they are believed to be ultimately responsible for producing the physiologic and biochemical abnormalities considered typical of primary cancer cachexia (Fearon et al. 2012; McCarthy 2003; Mondello et al. 2015; Tisdale 1999; Wang and Ye 2015). Many characteristic metabolic alterations have been identified and studied over the years, including hyperlactatemia, accelerated gluconeogenesis from lactate and amino acids, increased whole-body protein turnover, glucose intolerance, hyperinsulinemia, and increased lipolysis. Ongoing work has identified some of the underlying defects responsible for these classic alterations, including increased protein degradation mediated by nuclear factor-κB (NF-κB)–related activation of the ubiquitin-dependent proteasome pathway in skeletal muscle; increased ability of catecholamines and natriuretic peptides to activate lipolysis through amplified expression of hormone-sensitive lipase and adipose triglyceride lipase; and induction of brown adipocytes within white adipose tissue (so-called browning) with uncoupling of oxidative phosphorylation in the mitochondrion and resultant energy "wasting" through increased thermogenesis (Argilés et al. 2014; Arner and Langin 2014; Fearon et al. 2012; Freeman 2012; Petruzzelli et al. 2014; de Vos-Geelen et al. 2014; Wang and Ye 2015). Such changes should cause increased energy expenditure in the tumor-bearing host, which is hypothesized to be the fundamental reason for weight loss in primary cancer cachexia (Wang and Ye 2015).

However, while the predicted increase in energy expenditure can be documented among weight-losing people with cancer in some studies, it is normal or even decreased in others (Akbulut 2011; Dev et al. 2015; Fearon et al. 2001; Langius et al. 2012; Strasser and Bruera 2002; Tisdale 1999; Vazeille et al. 2017; de Vos-Geelen et al. 2014). It seems likely that energy expenditure varies widely between populations, individuals, and even different time points in the same individual, depending on underlying cancer diagnosis, stage of disease, concurrent complicating conditions, and type of therapy pursued. Further work is still needed to better define the relationship between characteristic metabolic abnormalities and defects, energy expenditure, and primary cancer cachexia in people.

Weight Loss and Cachexia in Cats and Dogs with Cancer

The common occurrence of cancer cachexia and its negative impact on quality of life and survival are well accepted in humans. However, even though some of the biochemical changes considered characteristic of primary cancer cachexia can be present in dogs with naturally occurring tumors, a specific and significant association between these abnormalities, documented weight loss, and clinical outcome remains largely unproven. Overall, the weight loss necessary for a legitimate diagnosis of cancer cachexia appears to be less common and less severe in tumor-bearing dogs than it is in people. In one study conducted in 100 dogs treated at a referral oncology practice, only 4% of cases were cachectic based on body condition score, while 29% were obese; 15% of the dogs had clinically significant muscle wasting. Weight loss was documented in 68% of the dogs, but it represented less than 5% of the pre-cancer body weight in 31% of cases (Michel et al. 2004). The authors of a more recent retrospective case review reported similar findings in over 300 dogs with lymphoma and osteosarcoma: only 5.5% of the dogs in this study were underweight, while 40.4% were overweight at the time of their cancer diagnosis (Romano et al. 2016). The distribution of body condition scores among dogs with a variety of types of cancer has also been investigated and compared to dogs without cancer in a much larger study (Weeth et al. 2007). These authors found that dogs with malignant tumors were somewhat less likely to be overweight compared to dogs without neoplastic disease, but there was no difference in the prevalence of underweight or very thin dogs between dogs with cancer and controls. This study also showed that age, breed, neuter status, tumor type, and a history of corticosteroid administration are important confounding factors that affect nutritional status among dogs with cancer. Finally, investigators studying dogs receiving carboplatin chemotherapy for osteosarcoma found not only that these animals gained a small amount of weight over the course of their treatment, but also that changes in weight did not affect clinical outcome (Story et al. 2017).

Characteristic metabolic changes that have been specifically documented in dogs with naturally occurring tumors have included increased serum lactate (McQuown et al.

2018; Vail et al. 1990) and insulin concentrations (Vail et al. 1990); increased serum lactate and insulin concentrations after an intravenous glucose tolerance test (Ogilvie et al. 1997); altered lipoprotein profiles (Ogilvie et al. 1994); increased urinary nitrogen excretion and whole-body glucose flux with concurrently decreased whole-body protein synthetic rates (Mazzaferro et al. 2001); and increased blood beta-hydroxybutyrate concentrations (McQuown et al. 2018). Resting energy expenditure has variably been measured as increased, unchanged, or decreased compared to controls (Mazzaferro et al. 2001; Ogilvie et al. 1993, 1996). However, the drawbacks associated with studying all of these parameters in isolation from documented weight loss and clinical outcome are highlighted by work showing that the most common cause of hyperlactatemia in tumor-bearing dogs is hypoperfusion, and not metabolic abnormalities caused by primary cancer cachexia at all (Touret et al. 2010, 2012). Thus, it is important to recognize that isolated changes such as hyperlactatemia and glucose intolerance in tumor-bearing dogs cannot be used as reliable surrogates for a diagnosis of "cancer cachexia." Additional studies are clearly needed to demonstrate an association between such metabolic abnormalities, weight loss, and prognosis in dogs with malignant disease.

Fewer data that evaluate nutritional status in cats with cancer are available. In one study, body condition score was examined for its effect on prognosis in cats with neoplastic disease (Baez et al. 2007). These investigators found that unlike the dog, almost half of the cats they evaluated were underweight or very thin, and over 90% of them had evidence of muscle wasting (see Figure 19.1). Their data also showed that body condition score was strongly correlated with survival time and prognosis: cats with decreased body condition scores had much shorter survival times. These same investigators also showed in a later study that weight loss had a negative effect on survival times among cats receiving chemotherapy for large cell

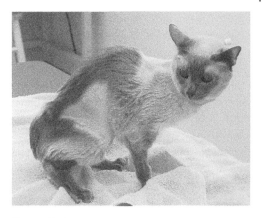

Figure 19.1 A cat with gastrointestinal lymphoma and an esophagostomy tube for assisted enteral feeding. Cats with cancer are likely to have weight loss, which has a negative impact on prognosis.

lymphoma (Krick et al. 2011). However, preliminary data suggest that sick cats are more likely to experience weight loss than sick dogs, regardless of whether they have cancer or not (Daniel et al. 1999). Further investigation is needed to determine if the weight loss observed in cats with cancer is the specific result of underlying neoplastic disease, or whether it is simply part of a typical feline response to critical illness.

Obesity in Humans with Cancer

Despite the classic link between weight loss and cancer, a strong association between obesity and cancer is now widely accepted in people as well. Obese individuals have a significantly increased risk of developing epithelial malignancies in a variety of anatomic locations, including the esophagus, stomach, pancreas, gallbladder, colon, liver, endometrium, breast, and kidney (Lauby-Secretan et al. 2016); rates of multiple myeloma, non-Hodgkin's lymphoma, and some types of leukemia are higher in this population as well (Renehan et al. 2008). Several different mechanisms have been proposed to explain the increased cancer risk in obese people. Obesity-related insulin resistance with hyperinsulinemia and increased production of insulin-like growth factor 1 (IGF-1) is believed to support the development and progression of malignant disease by stimulating cell proliferation, inhibiting programmed cell death (apoptosis), and promoting angiogenesis (Iyengar et al. 2015; Samani et al. 2007). Increased production of estrogen by adipose tissue appears to increase cancer risk by disrupting normal cellular growth and differentiation and also inhibiting apoptosis (Calle and Kaaks 2004; Cleary and Grossmann 2009; Iyengar et al. 2015). Synthesis of the antiproliferative adipokine adiponectin decreases with increasing adiposity, which reduces its protective role in tumor development (Iyengar et al. 2015). At the same time, the polypeptide hormone leptin is synthesized in increased quantities by adipose tissue, opposing and further limiting the potential tumor-suppressive effect of adiponectin and promoting tumor development by stimulating cell proliferation and again inhibiting apoptosis (Garofalo and Surmacz 2006; Iyengar et al. 2015). Finally, obesity causes a chronic systemic inflammatory response through alteration of the production and function of a variety of cytokines and other mediators of inflammation, in particular IL-6. Such changes have been proposed to increase cancer risk by establishing a more favorable environment for tumor development (Calle and Kaaks 2004; Mauer et al. 2015). This hypothesis is supported by a recent large, prospective study that documented a significantly decreased risk of obesity-related cancers in people who used non-steroidal anti-inflammatory drugs (Shebl et al. 2014).

Besides increasing cancer risk, obesity has a significant negative impact on multiple aspects of the management of cancer in people (Ligibel et al. 2014; Tao and Lagergren 2013). Ultimately, this leads to shorter survival; higher all-cause, cancer-specific, and cardiovascular death rates for multiple tumor types (Calle et al. 2003; Campbell et al. 2012; Ligibel et al. 2014); and decreased health-related quality of life (Tao and Lagergren 2013). Cancer is less likely to be diagnosed early in obese individuals, in part because they are reluctant to participate in cancer screening programs; even when they do, excess adipose tissue can make accurate assessment difficult (Clarke et al. 2018; Tao and Lagergren 2013). Obesity has been suggested to decrease measured concentrations of tumor biomarkers such as prostate-specific antigen (PSA) and carcinoembryonic antigen (CEA), presumably because of increased plasma volume and hemodilution. This could lead to false-negative or equivocal screening test results (Park et al. 2010; Pater et al. 2012). In addition, the quality of ultrasound, computed tomographic (CT), and magnetic resonance imaging (MRI) images can be compromised by excessive adipose tissue, making both the initial cancer diagnosis as well as ongoing monitoring more difficult (Tao and Lagergren 2013).

Obesity can significantly complicate the treatment of malignant disease as well. Important co-morbidities such as hypertension, cardiovascular disease, and type 2 diabetes mellitus are common. The dosing of chemotherapeutics can be challenging, with clinicians being understandably inclined to make chemotherapy dose adjustments in obese patients because of the relatively narrow therapeutic index of many of these agents. However, studies examining frequency of chemotherapy dose reductions as well as incidence and severity of treatment-related side effects such as myelosuppression suggest that obese people receiving chemotherapy are often undertreated (Griggs et al. 2005; Poikonen et al. 2001). The efficacy of chemotherapy may then be further impacted by obesity's effect on the pharmacokinetics of some chemotherapy agents, where important factors such as volume of drug distribution and hepatic drug metabolism may be altered (Tao and Lagergren 2013).

Finally, obesity can compromise the effective delivery of local cancer treatments such as surgery and radiation therapy. Although major complications and short-term mortality do not appear to be increased, minor complications are reported to be more likely after cancer surgery in obese people in some but not all studies

(Al-Refaie et al. 2010; Ejaz et al. 2015). The precise patient positioning necessary for delivery of technologically advanced types of radiation therapy such as intensity-modulated radiotherapy (IMRT) and stereotactic radiotherapy (SRT) can be also difficult in obese individuals. This can be the result of one or more factors, including increased skin mobility, movement of intra-abdominal organs within abdominal fat, and obscured bony landmarks (Tao and Lagergren 2013).

Obesity in Cats and Dogs with Cancer

The association between obesity and cancer is not nearly as well defined in cats and dogs as it is in people. Although several survey studies in dogs with cancer have revealed a high prevalence of obesity in this population (Michel et al. 2004; Romano et al. 2016; Weeth et al. 2007), this finding on its own does not prove a cause-and-effect relationship. Many potentially confounding factors are present in these studies, including age, neuter status, concurrent breed predispositions to both overweight and common tumor types studied, and medication history (Weeth et al. 2007). However, there are two canine cancers for which objective data exist supporting obesity as a risk factor for tumor development: transitional cell carcinoma of the urinary bladder (Glickman et al. 1989), and malignant mammary tumor (Alenza et al. 1998; Lim et al. 2015a; Sonnenschein et al. 1991).

Existing work also shows that some of the endocrine and inflammatory changes believed to be involved in the pathogenesis of malignant disease in obese people are also present in obese cats and dogs. For instance, serum or plasma leptin concentrations are increased in obese cats and dogs, as they are in people (Appleton et al. 2000; Bjornvad et al. 2014; Ishioka et al. 2007; Radin et al. 2009), while circulating concentrations of the anti-inflammatory adipokine adiponectin are decreased (Ishioka et al. 2009; Muranaka et al. 2011; Radin et al. 2009; Tvarijonaviciute et al. 2012). Canine

adipocytes possess the genes needed to synthesize the pro-inflammatory cytokine IL-6, and obese dogs have been shown to have increased serum concentrations of TNF-α and IGF-1 (Badman and Flier 2007; Gayet et al. 2004); furthermore, a significant decrease in plasma TNF-α concentration has been documented after weight loss in obese dogs (German et al. 2009). However, evidence of significant and persistent systemic inflammation or immunosuppression could not be confirmed in a group of laboratory beagles studied over a year of induced weight gain (Van de Velde et al. 2013). So far, investigators have been unable to demonstrate a convincing association between these types of obesity-associated changes and cancer risk in overweight cats or dogs with neoplastic disease. In one study, no difference was found in blood insulin or IGF-1 concentrations between dogs with lymphoma and age-, sex-, and weight-matched healthy controls (McQuown et al. 2018). Although overall it seems very possible that underlying pathogenic mechanisms as well as the negative impact on cancer diagnosis and treatment are similar in obese people, cats, and dogs, further work is needed to confirm these hypotheses.

Canine Mammary Tumors and Obesity

One of the cancers in small animals that has been evaluated most carefully for links between obesity and tumor risk is canine mammary neoplasia. A case–control study investigated the effect of body condition and diet on the development of mammary cancer in dogs and found that risk was decreased in both spayed and unspayed dogs that had been thin at 9–12 months of age (Sonnenschein et al. 1991). A similar study found that obesity at 12 months of age was associated with increased mammary tumor risk (Alenza et al. 1998). The authors of a third study were unable to find an association between survival and obesity in dogs with malignant mammary tumors, but they did not specifically evaluate the impact of historical obesity on tumor development later in life (Philibert et al. 2003). The results of these studies suggest that the impact of obesity on mammary tumor risk in dogs may be greatest early in life, at the same time when exposure to ovarian hormones can cause the greatest damage (Sorenmo et al. 2011). Obesity is believed to increase breast cancer risk in postmenopausal women because of increased estrogen production in peripheral adipose tissues, as well as adipose and tumor tissues within the breast itself (Cleary and Grossmann 2009). The results of existing canine studies suggest that a similar interaction between obesity, estrogen production, and tumor development may occur in young bitches.

Recent work has begun to correlate obesity and various factors secreted by adipocytes with mammary tumor development and prognosis in dogs. In one study, insulin receptor expression was significantly decreased in canine mammary carcinoma tissue compared to normal mammary gland as well as benign lesions, while there was no difference in IGF-1 receptor expression. The mRNA expression of IGF-1 and IGF-2 was significantly decreased in both benign and malignant tissues. Together these findings suggest that insulin and IGF-1 could act to stimulate cell proliferation early in canine mammary tumor development, but they may not play a role once cancer is established (Klopfleisch et al. 2010). Another group has shown that obese dogs are more likely to develop high-grade mammary tumors with histologic evidence of tumor invasion into lymphatics, and they do so at an earlier age. Overweight or obese dogs also have higher tumor expression of aromatase, the enzyme complex that is responsible for local estrogen synthesis, with a concurrent increase in hormone receptors. Finally, these same investigators have documented correlation of decreased tumor expression of adiponectin, an antiproliferative factor that is produced by adipose tissue in quantities that are inversely proportional to degree of adiposity, with histologically higher-grade tumors and lymphatic invasion

(Lim et al. 2015a, b). Additional work in this area is ongoing, but existing data already support intriguing parallels between the impact of obesity in dogs with mammary tumors and postmenopausal women with breast cancer.

Nutritional Management of Cats and Dogs with Cancer

Energy

The target food intake for a cat or dog with cancer is dictated by the animal's energy requirements. A complete and balanced ration is the most convenient way to provide nutrition because, except for water, basic requirements for all essential nutrients, including vitamins and minerals, are met when the quantity of food necessary to meet daily caloric needs is consumed. A food that has passed AAFCO (Association of American Feed Control Officials) feeding trial testing is preferred. Regardless of the ration chosen, water intake and fluid balance must be monitored carefully; supplements to correct specific nutrient deficiencies (i.e. potassium, phosphorus, vitamin K) are occasionally indicated.

Many different equations have been used to estimate maintenance energy requirements (MERs) in healthy cats and dogs, but there is no consensus regarding which one is most accurate (see Chapter 3). Furthermore, the effect of underlying neoplastic disease on MERs in small animals is largely unknown, and altered energy expenditure is certainly possible in some animals. Despite these factors, calculation of MERs remains the most practical way to estimate individual energy requirements for a self-supportive and weight-stable cat or dog with cancer in the home environment. Serial nutritional assessments are then used to decide whether adjustments in food intake are needed to maintain optimal body condition.

The energy needs of hospitalized animals with cancer are similarly incompletely defined.

Typically, the resting energy requirement (RER) is used as an approximation of the calories needed by a critically ill small animal (see Chapter 3) (Saker and Remillard 2010). Some authors also multiply the RER by an illness factor, which is intended to individualize energy intake based on the severity of underlying disease: requirements are believed to be higher in people and animals with more critical illnesses (Bartges 1996; Richardson and Davidson 2003; Saker and Remillard 2010). In general, however, conservative illness factors (between 1.0 and 1.4) are safest, because they are less likely to lead to the metabolic complications that can result from overfeeding. Once again, the animal's clinical response to the initial level of intake should be carefully monitored through repeated nutritional assessment so that adjustments to food intake can be made as indicated.

As already discussed, many cats and dogs with neoplastic disease are overweight or obese and the nutritional management of these animals can be challenging (see Figure 19.2). The health risks of obesity in otherwise normal small animals are well established and include induction or exacerbation of musculoskeletal disease, congestive heart failure, diabetes mellitus, and immunosuppression, among many other conditions (Toll et al. 2010). Dogs that are maintained in optimal body condition live longer than dogs that are overweight (Lawler et al. 2005). These facts

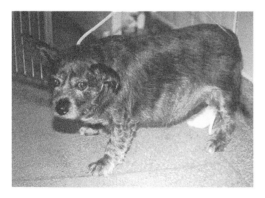

Figure 19.2 A dog with metastatic neoplastic disease. Many dogs with cancer are overweight or obese.

suggest that weight loss would also be beneficial in obese cats and dogs with neoplastic disease, although this will be true only for animals whose expected cancer survival times are long enough to justify the time and effort necessary to achieve a leaner body condition. It also seems likely that "metabolically healthy obesity" occurs in cats and dogs, as it does in people (Lin et al. 2017). Not only are people with metabolically healthy obesity less likely to derive short-term benefits from weight reduction (Lin et al. 2017; Tao and Lagergren 2013), their increased energy stores may in fact confer a paradoxical survival advantage when they are diagnosed with cancer (Greenlee et al. 2017; Lee et al. 2015; Weiss et al. 2014).

If weight reduction is undertaken in a cat or dog with underlying neoplasia, the protocols that are routinely used in otherwise healthy animals are not necessarily suitable in all cases. A conservative reduction in caloric intake below the calculated MER at ideal body weight is probably most appropriate for overweight cats and dogs that are clinically stable and self-supportive: The goal is simply to gradually achieve a more ideal body condition score and nutritional status.

For some obese cats and dogs with cancer, it may also be reasonable to stop planned weight loss at a somewhat overweight but still healthier body condition than previous. Aggressive weight-loss programs are contraindicated during critical illness, even in cats and dogs that are very obese. Severe caloric restriction in a sick animal could contribute to clinically significant protein-calorie malnutrition, with hypoproteinemia, loss of lean body mass, delayed wound healing, immunosuppression, and compromised organ function. Stabilization of the animal's medical condition is the priority, and weight reduction should be postponed until this has been achieved. The specific steps involved in designing a successful weight-loss program for an obese cat or dog are discussed in Chapter 9 and have been previously described (Brooks et al. 2014; Toll et al. 2010).

Calorie Sources

A change in diet is not automatically indicated in every cat or dog with cancer. Each animal must be carefully and individually evaluated, and those that are already maintaining good body condition on a high-quality complete and balanced food that is well tolerated and accepted may remain on this ration until there is an objective reason to change. In cases where a diet change is being considered, one of the most important factors to take into account is distribution of calories between protein, fat, and carbohydrate. Optimal caloric distribution is determined by the results of nutritional assessment, the type of cancer being treated, and the presence and severity of concurrent diseases. Since these factors vary from animal to animal, it is not possible to recommend a single ration or even ration type that will provide optimal nutrition in all cases. Instead, every animal should undergo a thorough and standardized nutritional assessment. Dietary recommendations are made only after this process is complete.

The commercial rations often recommended for cats and dogs with neoplastic disease and normal liver and kidney function deliver 30–35% of calories as protein, contain relatively fewer carbohydrate calories, and are high in fat. The commercial rations most likely to fit this profile are prescription critical care products, performance rations, and puppy or kitten foods. The high protein content of these products could help to preserve lean body mass and prevent the deleterious effects of protein-calorie malnutrition. In addition, their high-fat and low-carbohydrate content has several potential advantages. Fat provides more calories per gram (8.5–9 kcal/g) than protein (3.5–4 kcal/g) or carbohydrate (3.5–4 kcal/g). The increased energy density of a high-fat ration is helpful when voluntary food intake is decreased, and during tube feeding as well. In addition, high-fat rations are more palatable, which may improve food intake in some animals. Most cats and dogs can tolerate as much as 60–65% of their total energy requirement as fat, especially if they are permitted a period of adaptation (Reynolds et al. 1994; Saker and Remillard 2010).

A final consideration is that this type of caloric distribution theoretically takes advantage of some metabolic differences between tumor and normal host cells. Since neoplastic cells seem to prefer using glucose to produce the adenosine triphosphate (ATP) they need through aerobic glycolysis (the Warburg effect) and generally oxidize less fat (Vander Heiden et al. 2009), a high-fat, low-carbohydrate diet has been proposed as a way to preferentially supply energy to host tissues while avoiding inadvertent "feeding" of the tumor. However, it is increasingly clear that there is much more plasticity in the metabolic pathways used by cancer cells than historically believed: for example, depending on the situation and environment, cancer cells can and do use much of the glucose they consume for anabolism, they use glutamine to refill the Krebs (aka tricarboxylic acid, TCA) cycle, and they readily uptake and oxidize fatty acids when necessary (Carracedo et al. 2013; Corbet and Feron 2017). Although a high-fat ration appeared to normalize carbohydrate metabolism and prolong survival times in a subset of dogs with lymphoma in one study, this diet was also enriched with other nutrients including n-3 fatty acids and arginine (Ogilvie et al. 2000). More work is needed to confirm the clinical advantage of high-fat, low-carbohydrate diets across a variety of stages and types of cancer in cats and dogs, as well as to determine which specific dietary component or components were responsible for the observed benefit in this one particular study.

Despite potential advantages, it is also important to recognize that a high-fat, high-protein diet is contraindicated in many cats and dogs with cancer. Animals with a history of dietary fat intolerance should continue to have their dietary fat intake restricted whether they have underlying neoplastic disease or not. High-fat diets also make it more difficult to maintain optimal body condition in the substantial proportion of animals with cancer that are overweight or obese. Switching to a high-protein diet for a cat or dog with cancer that also has concurrent and significant renal or hepatic insufficiency may precipitate clinical decompensation that is difficult to reverse. Carbohydrate calories can be substituted in any of these situations where protein or fat intake must be restricted, although it makes sense to use complex rather than simple sugars to the greatest degree possible to avoid sharp spikes in blood glucose concentration. Regardless of their effect on tumor cells, carbohydrates may not be used efficiently by tumor-bearing animals because of insulin resistance and glucose intolerance (Ogilvie et al. 1997).

Once the optimal distribution of calories for an individual cat or dog with cancer has been identified, the commercial rations that meet these criteria are identified. Complete and balanced products that have been AAFCO feeding trial tested are preferred. A final selection is made after considering factors such as digestibility, fiber content, palatability, necessity for tube feeding, cost, and owner convenience. Historical episodes of food intolerance as well as strong preferences by the animal for certain diet formulations (dry, canned, or semi-moist) or flavors should also be taken into account (see Figure 19.3).

Protein and Amino Acids

As already discussed, a generous protein intake is usually recommended for cats and dogs with cancer. The goal is to support anabolic processes to the greatest degree possible, and in so doing prevent loss of lean body mass. However, providing dietary protein at levels above the animal's needs is expensive and offers little benefit. Protein requirements are dictated by requirements for essential amino acids that cannot be synthesized endogenously. Many studies in numerous species indicate that these requirements are increased during critical illness regardless of etiology (Bartges 1996; Richardson and Davidson 2003), and it is essential that sufficient protein be provided to meet them. Since it is difficult to determine exactly what the protein requirements are in an individual cat or dog with cancer, the most practical approach is to supply protein at a level that meets all anticipated needs and also incorporates an additional generous increment that will meet any unrecognized requirements. As described previously, providing protein at 30–35% of total calories will achieve this goal in most animals; repeated nutritional assessment should still be used to re-evaluate patient response and make any needed adjustments. However, once anabolic pathways (i.e. hepatic albumin synthesis) are operating at maximal capacity, it is not possible to force increased rates of activity by feeding ever higher quantities of protein. Amino acids supplied in excess of known plus unknown requirements will either be directly oxidized as an unnecessarily metabolically expensive source of energy, or deaminated and metabolized to glucose. Azotemia can result in some cases. If both the amino acid and total energy requirements of the animal are exceeded, then unneeded amino acids will eventually be stored as fat. None of these scenarios is desirable in a cat or dog with cancer.

Individual amino acids such as glutamine and arginine are often promoted as providing particular benefit for animals and people with neoplastic disease. Supplementation may be recommended, although the most appropriate doses and methods of administration in cats and dogs with cancer are largely unknown. Glutamine is the most abundant free amino acid in both plasma and intracellular pools. Although it is strictly defined as a non-essential amino acid, it plays an important role in many metabolic pathways and is "conditionally essential" during critical illness. Glutamine has two nitrogen groups, which allows it to function as a major means of nitrogen transport between tissues (Smith 1990). It is a primary substrate for ammonia synthesis in the kidney, and participates in the synthesis of nucleotides and many other molecules,

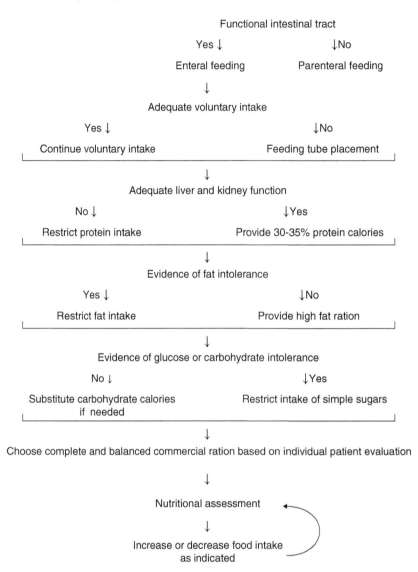

Functional intestinal tract

Yes ↓   ↓No

Enteral feeding   Parenteral feeding

↓

Adequate voluntary intake

Yes ↓   ↓No

Continue voluntary intake   Feeding tube placement

↓

Adequate liver and kidney function

No ↓   ↓Yes

Restrict protein intake   Provide 30-35% protein calories

↓

Evidence of fat intolerance

Yes ↓   ↓No

Restrict fat intake   Provide high fat ration

↓

Evidence of glucose or carbohydrate intolerance

No ↓   ↓Yes

Substitute carbohydrate calories   Restrict intake of simple sugars
if needed

↓

Choose complete and balanced commercial ration based on individual patient evaluation

↓

Nutritional assessment

↓

Increase or decrease food intake
as indicated

Figure 19.3   Flowchart outlining the clinical decision-making process involved in making a diet change for a cat or dog with cancer.

including nicotinamide adenine dinucleotide (NAD) and glutathione. Glutamine serves as a critical energy substrate for enterocytes, and it is also required by lymphocytes and other rapidly dividing cell populations (Morris et al. 2017; Smith 1990).

Substantial decreases in plasma and free intracellular glutamine concentrations occur in skeletal muscle in critically ill people. Intracellular glutamine represents a vital storage pool of carbon and nitrogen that can be mobilized to quickly meet the needs of many tissues (Rennie et al. 1989; Smith 1990). A high intake of glutamine helps prevent subsequent loss of lean body mass by supporting muscle protein synthesis and decreasing muscle protein catabolism (Hammarqvist et al. 1990; Yoshida et al. 2001). Glutamine also functions as a signaling molecule that enhances the expression of stress-induced heat shock proteins that augment the ability of cells to survive a variety of insults (Wischmeyer 2002). Potentially even more important is the central role played by glutamine in maintaining normal gastrointestinal and immune system function during illness (Remillard et al. 1998; Souba et al. 1990). Glutamine supplementation has been associated with decreased infectious complications and shorter hospital stays in human surgical patients, and decreased complications and reduced mortality in hospitalized, critically ill people (Novak et al. 2002). Glutamine has also been suggested to accelerate healing of acute radiotherapy side effects involving the oral mucosa in dogs (Khanna et al. 1995), and to decrease the severity of oral mucositis in people receiving chemotherapy for esophageal cancer when used in combination with an elemental diet (Tanaka et al. 2016). In addition, it appears in some studies to protect gut immunity and integrity in individuals receiving radiotherapy or chemotherapy (Nitenberg and Raynard 2000; Yoshida et al. 2001).

However, not all studies support a convincing benefit for glutamine supplementation: one meta-analysis showed that glutamine did not prevent radiation therapy-induced diarrhea in people receiving pelvic radiotherapy (Lawrie et al. 2018). Likewise, there was no survival advantage when people undergoing autologous stem cell transplantation for hematologic malignancies received prophylactic parenteral nutrition supplemented with glutamine (Sykorova et al. 2005). Furthermore, based on the results of recent ^{13}C tracer studies, it appears that tumor cells use glutamine to fuel the Krebs (TCA) cycle, especially in the presence of hypoxia (Corbet and Feron 2015). It is interesting to speculate that aggressive glutamine supplementation might inadvertently provide substrate to malignant cells, especially when there is advanced, systemic involvement. However, it also seems likely that the benefits of glutamine with respect to gut function and immunity and preservation of lean body mass outweigh any theoretic risk, particularly when it is administered enterally to individuals with localized disease undergoing anticancer therapy. Additional randomized, controlled studies are clearly needed to better define the potential benefits and drawbacks of glutamine supplementation for cats and dogs with cancer.

Assisted Feeding

Voluntary intake is the most practical and efficient way to meet the energy and other nutrient needs of cats and dogs with cancer. However, for this approach to be successful, the animal's caloric requirement must be calculated, and the daily quantity of food consumed must be measured as accurately as possible. If the amount of food eaten is consistently less than what is needed to meet requirements, then assisted feeding is indicated. There are three basic techniques for assisted feeding, and they can be used singly or in combination: pharmacologic appetite stimulation, assisted enteral feeding (see Chapter 20), and assisted parenteral feeding (see Chapter 21).

Pharmacologic appetite stimulation can be convenient and cost effective, but it is essential to confirm drug efficacy through careful measurement of actual food intake. Failure to take this step can result in a prolonged delay in the initiation of more appropriate and effective methods of assisted feeding (Baron 2000). Historically, the appetite stimulants used most commonly in cats and dogs with cancer have probably been cyproheptadine and mirtazapine (Agnew and Korman 2014). Objective data supporting the clinical efficacy of cyproheptadine in cats and dogs with any disease are scarce; however, mirtazapine has been shown to significantly increase food intake in cats with chronic kidney disease (Quimby and Lunn 2013). Megestrol acetate has been used more often in people with cancer (Alesi and del Fabbro 2014; Cuvelier et al. 2014; McQuellon et al. 2002; Ruiz Garcia et al. 2013), but there are no controlled trials confirming the safety and efficacy of this drug in anorexic cats or dogs with neoplastic disease. Megestrol acetate has been associated with the development of diabetes mellitus (Middleton and Watson 1985) and mammary adenocarcinoma in the cat (Misdorp 1991; Tomlinson et al. 1984), so caution is warranted when it is used in this species. A newer option for cats and dogs with cancer-associated anorexia is the ghrelin receptor agonist capromorelin; this drug has been shown to significantly improve appetite in client-owned dogs with anorexia due to various causes compared to placebo (Johannes and Musser, 2019; Zollers et al. 2016). More work is needed to define the role of appetite stimulants in the management of cats and dogs with cancer.

For a cat or dog with cancer that is not able to meet its energy and other nutrient requirements through voluntary intake, assisted feeding can be provided enterally or parenterally. Enteral or tube feeding is almost always preferred in small animals as well as people, because it maintains gut health and function and allows nutrients to be metabolized through normal pathways (Akbulut 2011; Bozzetti et al. 2009; Chan 2017; Cohen and Lefor 2001; Mercadante 1998; Qin et al. 2002; Remillard and Saker 2010; Remillard et al. 1998). Enteral support is usually easier to administer than parenteral nutrition, and it is also associated with fewer complications and shorter, less expensive hospital stays in people with cancer (Akbulut 2011; Chow et al. 2016; Peng et al. 2016; Roth et al. 2013; Zhao et al. 2016). An additional potential advantage of enteral feeding for cats and dogs with cancer is that older work suggests that parenteral feeding may stimulate the progression of neoplastic disease in people and rodent models (Mercadante 1998; Torosian and Donoway 1991), although authors of a more recent review of the existing literature were unable to confirm that such an effect exists (Bossola et al. 2011). Indwelling tubes that can be used to deliver enteral support in cats and dogs with cancer include nasoesophageal, esophagostomy, gastrostomy, and jejunostomy tubes. The indications, surgical techniques for placement, and use of these tubes are discussed in Chapter 20 and are also described in detail elsewhere (Davidson 2018; Marks 2017; Saker and Remillard 2010).

Assisted parenteral feeding is sometimes indicated in cats, dogs, and people with cancer. It is the only option available when the gastrointestinal tract is completely non-functional. It can also be used to help treat inflammatory intestinal conditions because it permits complete bowel rest. Parenteral feeding may be considered as well in selected cases where hemodynamic instability or coagulopathy would make general anesthesia for surgical placement of a feeding tube too risky (Remillard and Saker 2010). Despite these apparent indications and advantages, however, studies suggest that parenteral feeding has a negative impact on outcome when it is used in humans with neoplastic disease. People with cancer who receive parenteral nutrition have more complications, marginal improvement in nutritional status, and trends toward decreased survival (Akbulut 2011; Chow et al. 2016; Fearon et al. 2001; Mercadante 1998; Peng et al. 2016; Roth et al. 2013; Zhao et al. 2016). It seems likely that this is related at least in part to the compromised gut function that can occur during parenteral feeding. Lack of ingesta within the intestinal tract leads to intestinal mucosal atrophy, compromised gut immunity, and increased rates of bacterial translocation (Alverdy et al. 1985; Mercadante 1998; Qin et al. 2002; Remillard and Saker 2010; Remillard et al. 1998).

A combination of parenteral nutrition and enteral support should always be considered for animals that will tolerate it: even very small amounts of food within the intestinal tract help to maintain gut health. The techniques involved in assisted parenteral feeding for cats and dogs are discussed in detail in Chapter 21 and elsewhere (Chan 2017; Remillard and Saker 2010).

Initiation of assisted enteral or parenteral feeding is necessary and lifesaving for many cats and dogs with malignant disease. It improves the ability to tolerate aggressive antineoplastic therapy and speeds recovery from critical illness. However, the indications for nutritional support and the individual animal's long-term prognosis with respect to its underlying cancer should both be carefully considered before assisted feeding is implemented. Nutritional support does not improve nutritional or functional status in people with cancer who have a very short life expectancy (Akbulut 2011; Angus and Burakoff 2003; Brard et al. 2006; Chen et al. 2013; Niv and Abuksis 2002; Torelli et al. 1999), and the same is likely to be true in cats and dogs with terminal disease. When all treatment options have been exhausted and there is no reasonable probability of restoring an acceptable quality of life, nutritional support may only serve to prolong an uncomfortable death. The pet owner must obviously be involved in deciding whether to use assisted feeding techniques in their animal, but it is important for the clinician to be very clear and realistic about what can be achieved. Assisted feeding should provide tangible benefit to every patient that receives it (McKinlay 2004; Simmonds 2010).

Other Nutrients for Cats and Dogs with Cancer

Omega-3 (n-3) Fatty Acids

Many health benefits have now been associated with the consumption of long-chain n-3 fatty acids in people. Recent studies have shown that plasma docosahexaenoic acid (DHA) concentrations are inversely associated with all-cause mortality (Miura et al. 2016), and that higher combined intake of n-3 fatty acids from both fish and supplements is associated with decreased risk of coronary heart disease mortality (Lentjes et al. 2017). With specific respect to cancer, n-3 fatty acid–related mechanisms including modulation of cyclooxygenase-2 (COX2) activity, alterations in cell surface receptor function, and changes in gene expression are all believed to be responsible for decreased tumor-specific mortality in people with colorectal cancer (Song et al. 2017), decreased risk of brain tumors (Lian et al. 2017), decreased risk of estrogen receptor–negative breast cancers (Hidaka et al. 2017), and

decreased overall risk of cancer-related death (Nagata et al. 2017). N-3 fatty acid supplementation has also been proposed to specifically suppress the development of obesity-related cancers in people (Khatib et al. 2016), presumably through decreased systemic inflammation.

Based in part on extrapolation from these types of outcomes in people, therapeutic pet diets used in cats and dogs with cancer may be enriched with n-3 fatty acids. Additional supplementation above the level supplied in the diet is also recommended in many cases, even though the appropriate doses, methods of administration, and indications for n-3 fatty acids are not yet well defined. Regardless, marine oils are the preferred dietary source of long-chain n-3 fatty acids in both cats and dogs, since they are unable to efficiently convert the shorter-chain n-3 fatty acids contained in vegetable oils such as flax.

Changing the dietary ratio of n-6 to n-3 fatty acids alters the fatty acid composition of cell membranes throughout the body (Stoeckel et al. 2011), and this in turn impacts cell membrane eicosanoid production, cytokine synthesis, and the inflammatory cascade. Specifically, series 4 leukotrienes and series 2 prostaglandins are derived from the n-6 fatty acid arachidonic acid and are pro-inflammatory, while series 5 leukotrienes and series 3 prostaglandins are synthesized from the long-chain n-3 fatty acids eicosapentaenoic acid (EPA) and DHA and are less potent stimulators of inflammation. Studies have confirmed that the eicosanoids produced during inflammation in the dog vary with the dietary n-6 to n-3 fatty acid ratios, and that the inflammatory response can be attenuated by n-3 fatty acid supplementation in conditions such as atopy (Scott et al. 1997; Vaughn et al. 1994).

Ultimately, n-3 fatty acid interaction with eicosanoid production most likely affects the inflammatory response by altering synthesis of cytokines such as IL-1, TNF-α, and IL-6 (Endres et al. 1989; LeBlanc et al. 2008). It is therefore reasonable to hypothesize that inflammatory conditions such as primary cancer cachexia or obesity might be ameliorated through n-3 fatty acid supplementation. Added n-3 fatty acids have in fact been demonstrated to decrease synthesis of pro-inflammatory cytokines, improve immune function, and stabilize body condition in multiple studies of humans with pancreatic and gastrointestinal cancers (Barber et al. 2001; Fearon et al. 2003; Gärtner et al. 2015; Yu et al. 2017). In another study, people with advanced neoplastic disease who received n-3 fatty acid supplements also had prolonged survival compared to unsupplemented controls (Gogos et al. 1998). People with esophageal cancer have decreased incidence of chemotherapy-induced stomatitis when they receive n-3 fatty acid–enriched enteral nutrition during treatment (Miyata et al. 2017). Finally, although they did not have concurrent weight loss, some abnormalities in carbohydrate metabolism resolved in dogs with lymphoma that were fed a test diet enriched with both n-3 fatty acids and arginine (Ogilvie et al. 2000).

Despite these benefits, there are potential risks associated with excessive intake of n-3 fatty acids in people and animals. There is some recent evidence that very high dietary intake of long-chain n-3 fatty acids in people could increase the risk of some cancers, especially prostatic carcinoma (Serini and Calviello 2018), although this may not be a relevant observation for cats and dogs because of species differences in the biology of prostatic neoplasia. Another consideration is that increased intake of n-3 fatty acids causes decreased synthesis of thromboxane A_2 and increased production of prostaglandin I_3 in people, leading to decreased platelet aggregation and vasoconstriction (Kristensen et al. 1989). While this effect might inhibit metastasis and has also been suggested as the reason for the decreased incidence of atherosclerotic disease observed among fish-eating Inuit peoples, it could predispose some individuals to hemorrhage. However, no evidence of increased bleeding risk or significant changes in coagulation parameters were found in a recent large analysis of n-3 fatty acid–supplemented people (Jeansen et al. 2018), and investigators have been unable to demonstrate this to be a clinically significant problem in the dog either (Boudreaux et al. 1997; McNeil et al. 1999). Results are thus far mixed in cats: while platelet function remained normal among cats supplemented with n-3 fatty acids in one study (Bright et al. 1994), it was decreased in another (Saker et al. 1998).

Another area of concern is that consumption of diets containing high levels of n-3 fatty acids also appears to compromise normal immune function. Decreased lymphocyte proliferation has been documented in humans and dogs (LeBlanc et al. 2007; Meydani et al. 1991), and suppression of cell-mediated immunity has been observed in n-3 fatty acid–supplemented dogs (Wander et al. 1997). Increased tissue membrane lipid peroxidation caused by the ingestion of large quantities of polyunsaturated fatty acids has been suggested as the factor responsible for these alterations in immune function. Some authors have also speculated that relative vitamin E deficiency in the face of n-3 fatty acid supplementation may play a role (Meydani et al. 1991; Wander et al. 1997), although at least one investigator was unable to confirm this in dogs (LeBlanc et al. 2008).

Finally, n-3 fatty acids have been implicated as potential inhibitors of wound healing. However, histologic evidence of such an effect could not be demonstrated in the dog (Mooney et al. 1998). Additional studies are needed to define the best indications for the use of n-3 fatty acids in cats and dogs with cancer, including the method of supplementation (i.e. as a dietary component or administered separately), as well as dose.

Vitamin D

Vitamin D's central role in calcium homeostasis and metabolism in both people and animals has been recognized since the early twentieth century. However, it was not until 1980 that investigation into the link between vitamin D status and cancer risk in people really began (Mohr 2009). The mechanisms underlying vitamin D's antineoplastic effect are believed to include inhibition of cell proliferation and angiogenesis as well as promotion of cell differentiation and apoptosis, often through modulation of inflammation. Calcitriol inhibits COX2 activity and decreases prostaglandin E2 production. It inhibits NF-κB signaling as well, which in turn decreases production of cytokines including TNF-α and IL8. Calcitriol also suppresses the production of other cytokines and factors that are either proinflammatory or tumor promoting, including IL1β, IL6, IL17, and TGFβ1 (van Harten-Gerritsen et al. 2015).

One of the first tumor types examined in people for an association with vitamin D status was colorectal cancer, and a number of studies now support an inverse relationship between cancer risk and serum 25(OH)D for this disease. A recent meta-analysis showed that people with serum 25(OH)D concentrations greater than 35 ng/ml had a 40% lower risk of colorectal cancer than people with serum 25(OH)D concentrations less than 15 ng/ml (Garland and Gorham 2017). Another large meta-analysis revealed a similar association between the risk of not only colorectal cancer, but all types of invasive cancer (excluding skin cancer) in women, with a 67% lower risk when serum 25(OH)D was greater than 40 ng/ml, compared to when it was less than 20 ng/ml (McDonnell et al. 2016). Vitamin D status also appears to impact prognosis and outcome for men with prostatic carcinoma, who are more likely to have histologically more malignant and clinically more advanced disease when their serum 25(OH)D concentrations are low (Murphy et al. 2014; Nyame et al. 2016). However, the complex relationship between vitamin D and tumor development is not yet completely understood. For instance, based on the results of a large, randomized clinical trial in healthy postmenopausal women, it does not appear that simply supplementing with vitamin D3 necessarily decreases cancer risk. In this study, the risk of all types of cancer was not statistically different after four years in women who took a vitamin D supplement compared to those who received a placebo (Lappe et al. 2017).

The relationship between vitamin D status and cancer in cats and dogs has also been explored by a number of investigators, and, with the exception of one study where no difference was found between serum 25(OH)D concentrations in dogs with osteosarcoma and controls (Willcox et al. 2016), for the most part serum 25(OH)D concentrations seem to be decreased in cats and dogs with a variety of cancers. Labrador retrievers with mast cell tumors were found to have lower serum 25(OH)D concentrations compared to healthy Labrador retrievers (Wakshlag et al. 2011). Cats with inflammatory bowel disease and intestinal small cell lymphoma were shown to have significantly lower serum 25(OH)D concentrations compared to cats hospitalized because of other diseases or controls (Lalor et al. 2014); similar findings have been reported for dogs with inflammatory bowel disease (Gow et al. 2011). Dogs with *Spirocerca lupi*–induced sarcomas had significantly lower serum 25(OH)D concentrations than dogs that were infected with *S. lupi* but did not have cancer, as well as normal controls (Rosa et al. 2013). Dogs with low serum 25(OH)D concentrations (<40 ng/ml) had an approximately fourfold increase in relative risk of hemoabdomen and splenic cancer compared to normal controls in another study; these authors also used their data to predict that serum 25(OH)D concentrations of 100–120 ng/ml represented vitamin D sufficiency in the dog (Selting et al. 2016).

Finally, investigators studying dogs with lymphoma, osteosarcoma, and mast cell tumor constructed a more complex model including not only plasma 25(OH)D, but also dietary vitamin D intake, serum ionized calcium concentrations, and plasma 24,25(OH)$_2$D. They concluded that there was indeed a significant association between the presence of neoplastic disease and vitamin D metabolism, but that it was not as straightforward as dogs with cancer simply having lower plasma 25(OH)D concentrations: they found that plasma 25(OH)D concentrations increased as serum ionized calcium concentrations also increased among their dogs with cancer, while plasma 25(OH)D concentrations decreased as serum ionized calcium concentrations increased in their healthy controls (Weidner et al. 2017).

Based on the existing veterinary studies, it is certainly tempting to consider supplementing vitamin D in cats and dogs with cancer. However, insufficient data currently exist to support the routine use of vitamin D as a prevention or treatment for cancer in this population. The optimal dose of vitamin D is unknown, and authors disagree on the criteria that should be used to assess sufficiency in tumor-bearing small animals. It is also unclear whether supplementation that does not begin until after a diagnosis of cancer is made will necessarily have a positive impact on outcome. Additional studies are needed that confirm the normal range for serum 25(OH)D concentrations among cats and dogs with cancer, document the efficacy and long-term safety of a range of vitamin D doses, and objectively assess impact on tumor progression and prognosis before a confident recommendation for supplementation can be made.

Antioxidants

People who eat large quantities of fruits and vegetables have a significantly decreased risk of certain types of cancers, including carcinomas of the lung, head and neck, and gastrointestinal tract (Johnson 2004; Llewellyn et al. 2004; Makarem et al. 2015; Rao et al. 1994). Nutrients that could be responsible for this protective effect include antioxidants such as beta-carotene; lutein; selenium; and vitamins A, C, and E (Mandelker 2008a). These nutrients, among others, are added to many commercial pet foods and may also be recommended for additional supplementation beyond what is present in the diet. Marketing may suggest to the consumer that the added antioxidants will help prevent cancer in animals that consume these products.

There are three potential scenarios in which antioxidant supplementation could be considered for the cat or dog with cancer. First, antioxidants could be administered long term as a cancer preventive. Chronic oxidative stress with formation of reactive oxygen species is hypothesized to be one of the basic mechanisms causing cancer (Griffiths et al. 2016; Mandelker 2008b). Oxidative injury causes DNA damage and eventually this can lead to malignant transformation, with establishment of a neoplastic cell population. This process is more likely to occur when antioxidant capacity is marginal or inadequate, so appropriate supplementation could theoretically prevent it.

Preliminary work shows that dogs with mammary tumors and lymphoma do have systemic evidence of oxidative stress (Szczubiał et al. 2004; Winter et al. 2009), but for what duration or if these abnormalities are even present prior to tumor development has not been investigated. An increased degree of lipid peroxidation has been demonstrated in canine mammary tumor tissue compared to adjacent normal tissues, suggesting the possibility of a role for oxidative damage in the development of these lesions (Karayannopoulou et al. 2013; Kumaraguruparan et al. 2005). However, concurrently increased antioxidant activity was also found within the tumors assayed in one of these studies, making it unclear whether increased intake of antioxidants in these animals could have a protective effect (Kumaraguruparan et al. 2005). Finally, in two other studies, relatively short-term (seven months' duration) selenium supplementation within an optimal range above deficiency but below excess appeared to decrease DNA damage and prevent possible progression to tumor in non-neoplastic prostatic epithelial cells in geriatric laboratory beagles (Waters et al. 2003, 2005), but none of the dogs in these studies actually had definitively diagnosed prostatic neoplasia.

Unfortunately, then, none of these studies provides the objective data needed to assess the potential antineoplastic effect of long-term dietary antioxidant supplementation in pet cats and dogs. Which antioxidants might be most effective, at what dietary concentration or dose, and over what period are unknown. Various antioxidant cocktails that could play a role in preventing cancer are often advertised as one of the benefits of rations intended for use in "senior" cats and dogs, but, given the hypothesized mechanism of this protective effect, a legitimate question is whether the age of 7 or 8 (the age at which senior diets are typically recommended) might be too late for intervention. If oxidative stress with the potential to eventually induce malignant transformation is present over the lifetime of the animal, then antioxidant supplementation might be even more beneficial if it is provided over the same period. Regardless, the studies that would be needed to answer these questions are probably prohibitively complex and costly. Large groups of cats and dogs would have to be fed standardized diets containing different concentrations of various antioxidants beginning at different ages, so that potential differences in the incidence of neoplastic disease depending on the type and duration of antioxidant supplementation could be documented.

A second situation in which antioxidant supplementation may be considered is during cancer treatment, with the primary intention of reducing the severity of some of the side effects of therapy. This is an area of considerable controversy in human oncology (D'Andrea 2005; Marian 2017). Some types of chemotherapy and radiation therapy injure and kill cells through oxidative damage and generation of free radicals. The difficulty is that while this is a desired effect with respect to targeted cancer cells, the same process often leads to serious side effects when it occurs in normal host tissues. Many mainstream human cancer treatment centers currently advise individuals undergoing therapy to avoid taking high doses of any antioxidants, in order to maximize the efficacy of their cancer treatment (see the Memorial Sloan Kettering Cancer Center website page "About Herbs, Botanicals & Other Products," http://www.mskcc.org/mskcc/html/11570.cfm). However, other authors disagree and use the contradictory results of published studies in this area to support their point of view (Simone et al. 2007). More well-designed, prospective studies are needed to resolve these questions in humans; not surprisingly, no such studies exist for cats and dogs undergoing chemotherapy or radiotherapy. Until more specific information becomes available, the best recommendation is probably the same for cats and dogs as it is in people: high-level antioxidant supplementation should be avoided during cancer treatment.

A final situation where antioxidants could play a role is in prevention of tumor recurrence after completion of anticancer therapy. This has been examined in several large studies and meta-analyses in people. Unfortunately, the results have often been disappointing. First of all, it is not clear that taking antioxidants as supplements provides the same benefits as consumption of the same vitamins and minerals in their naturally occurring forms in whole foods (Johnson 2004). Furthermore, significantly increased rates of primary tumor recurrence or second primary cancers have actually been observed during supplementation with beta-carotene, vitamin A, and vitamin E (Bairati et al. 2005; Bjelakovic et al. 2007; Narita et al. 2018; Omenn et al. 1996). While there can be no doubt that there are numerous, clear benefits associated with adequate antioxidant intake in cats, dogs, and people, whether they have underlying cancer or not, more work remains to be done before antioxidant supplementation can be confidently recommended for tumor chemoprevention or management of cancer therapy side effects in any of these species.

Nutritional Fads

Supplements and Nutraceuticals

The diet history of every cat or dog with cancer should always include specific information about current and former medications and nutritional supplements. Dedicated human companions frequently make significant changes to their feeding practices and may also add a wide variety of supplements and nutraceuticals to their animal's diet after a diagnosis of cancer has been made. Their goal is simply to take advantage of every possible intervention that may benefit their pet, but these changes and additions are often made without veterinary advice. Some clients view veterinarians as poor sources of unbiased nutritional information, while others just want to avoid engaging a skeptical veterinarian in an uncomfortable and negative discussion about alternative or complementary therapies. It is important for clinicians to recognize that even though large-scale clinical trials documenting the clinical efficacy of many supplements and nutraceuticals are currently lacking, an expanding body of objective data outlines the potential mechanisms of action and benefits of such compounds for cats, dogs, and people with malignant disease (Dorai and Aggarwal 2004; Levine et al. 2016; Marian 2017). To provide the best recommendation for each individual animal, it is essential that the veterinarian remain objective, well informed, and nonjudgmental, and willing to engage in discussion.

A systematic approach to the evaluation of nutritional supplements, nutraceuticals, and novel feeding practices is the best way to ensure that the most appropriate advice is always given. A particularly valuable source of objective information that can be used throughout this process is the "About Herbs, Botanicals & Other Products" section of the Memorial Sloan Kettering Cancer Center website (http://www. mskcc.org/mskcc/html/11570.cfm). This site is constantly updated and provides citations for further reading where they are available. It is also separated into areas for healthcare professionals and patients, and so it can be confidently recommended to clients as a source of reliable and readily understandable information.

Ultimately, the following four basic questions must be answered in every case:

- **Does the product or practice work?** To answer this question, a logical scientific hypothesis supporting the benefit of the supplement or practice should be clearly apparent. This should include knowing specifically what the active compounds or advantageous qualities of a particular product are, as well as having access to studies published in the peer-reviewed scientific literature that describe the objective and consistent beneficial effects in controlled clinical trials. Ideally, these studies should be performed in cats and dogs with cancer; this is particularly true in the cat because of its numerous metabolic and nutritional peculiarities. However, data collected in human trials may also be helpful.
- **Is the product or practice safe?** To answer this question, reliable information from controlled studies investigating both the short- and long-term safety of the product at the proposed dose or doses to be used in cats and dogs (or at least people) should be available.
- **Will the product or practice interfere with the efficacy of cancer therapy?** It is particularly important in small animals with cancer to consider possible interactions and contraindications of supplements and nutraceuticals with anticancer therapy. Common contraindications include the risk that supplements with significant antioxidant activity will compromise the ability of chemotherapy and radiation therapy to injure and kill cancer cells through oxidative damage; the potential for gastrointestinal side effects that may be difficult to distinguish from complications related to ongoing conventional cancer therapy; and the possibility that some supplements could actually stimulate cancer progression. For example, the herb ginseng (*Panax ginseng*) appears to have

estrogenic activity (Lee et al. 2003), so would be contraindicated in cats or dogs with estrogen receptor–positive mammary cancers.

- **Is the product or products being used of acceptable quality?** To answer this final question, there should be some means of objective assurance that the specific product or products being used is of good quality: this includes consistent concentration and availability of the active ingredients, as well as lack of contamination.

Feeding Raw Foods to Cats and Dogs with Cancer

The feeding of raw foods to cats and especially dogs is increasingly popular (Dinallo et al. 2017; Morgan et al. 2017). These diets are intended to mimic the diet of wild cats and dogs and are believed by their proponents to provide nutrition that is superior to traditional cooked pet foods. Proposed benefits of raw food diets include improved nutrient digestibility and absorption, increased health of coat and skin, decreased incidence of obesity and improved lean body mass, improved immune function, resolution of various degenerative diseases, and increased lifespan. Detractors point to the increased likelihood of nutritional imbalance, higher incidence of gastrointestinal foreign bodies because of the ingestion of bones, and the potential contamination of the diet with pathogens that may cause disease in both the pet and its owner.

While controlled, long-term studies that objectively compare the advantages and disadvantages of the two approaches and definitively prove that one is better than the other do not yet exist, raw foods do pose one very significant concern for cats and dogs with cancer. Several studies show that raw pet foods and the ingredients used to prepare them can be contaminated with pathogenic organisms, including *Salmonella* spp. (van Bree et al. 2018; Fauth et al. 2015; Finley et al. 2007; Giacometti et al. 2017; Joffe and Schlesinger 2002; Stiver et al. 2003), *Listeria monocytogenes* (van Bree et al. 2018),

Campylobacter spp. (Bojanić et al. 2017), and *Toxoplasma gondii* (van Bree et al. 2018; Lopes et al. 2011; Nash et al. 2005). Cats and dogs with cancer can be significantly immunosuppressed, both by their disease and by its treatment, making life-threatening infections a legitimate risk when raw or undercooked foods are fed. For this reason, the owners of cats and dogs undergoing cancer treatment should be specifically counseled against the use of raw foods.

Summary

- Clinically significant loss of lean body mass and fat stores in an individual with cancer is called cancer cachexia.
- Weight loss decreases prognosis in cancer patients.
- Individualized nutritional assessment is essential for all cats and dogs with cancer:
  - Dogs are often overweight or obese.
  - Cats are more likely to have weight loss.
- Optimal food intake is dictated by energy requirements.
- Complete and balanced commercial pet foods that are relatively high in fat, low in carbohydrates, and provide ample protein are often used in cats and dogs with cancer.
- Dietary changes are not indicated in all cases:
  - Many animals can safely remain on their regular diet.
  - High-protein, high-fat diets are contraindicated in some animals with neoplastic disease.
- Sufficient evidence exists to recommend supplementing dogs (not cats) that have cancer with long-chain n-3 fatty acids, but the optimal dose and method of administration are unknown.
- Antioxidant supplements should not be administered to cats and dogs undergoing chemotherapy or radiation therapy.
- All supplements and novel nutritional therapies should be objectively and systematically evaluated before they are recommended for use in cats and dogs with cancer.

References

Agnew, W. and Korman, R. (2014). Pharmacological appetite stimulation: rational choices in the inappetant cat. *J. Feline Med. Surg.* 16: 749–756.

Akbulut, G. (2011). New perspective for nutritional support of cancer patients: enteral/parenteral nutrition. *Exp. Ther. Med.* 2: 675–684.

Alenza, D.P., Rutteman, G.R., Peña, L. et al. (1998). Relation between habitual diet and canine mammary tumors in a case-control study. *J. Vet. Intern. Med.* 12: 132–139.

Alesi, E.R. and del Fabbro, E. (2014). Opportunities for targeting the fatigue-anorexia-cachexia symptom cluster. *Cancer J.* 20: 325–329.

Al-Refaie, W.B., Parsons, H.M., Henderson, W.G. et al. (2010). Body mass index and major cancer surgery outcomes: lack of association or need for alternative measurement of obesity? *Ann. Surg. Oncol.* 17: 2264–2273.

Alverdy, J.C., Chi, H.S., and Sheldon, G.F. (1985). The effect of parenteral nutrition on gastrointestinal immunity. The importance of enteral stimulation. *Ann. Surg.* 202: 681–684.

Angus, F. and Burakoff, R. (2003). The percutaneous endoscopic gastrostomy tube: medical and ethical issues in placement. *Am. J. Gastroenterol.* 98: 272–277.

Appleton, D.J., Rand, J.S., and Sunvold, G.D. (2000). Plasma leptin concentrations in cats: reference range, effect of weight gain and relationship with adiposity as measure by dual energy x-ray absorptiometry. *J. Feline Med. Surg.* 2: 191–199.

Argilés, J.M., Busquets, S., Stemmler, B. et al. (2014). Cancer cachexia: understanding the molecular basis. *Nat. Rev. Cancer* 14: 754–762.

Arner, P. and Langin, D. (2014). Lipolysis in lipid turnover, cancer cachexia, and obesity-induced insulin resistance. *Trends Endocrinol. Metab.* 25: 255–262.

Badman, M.K. and Flier, J.S. (2007). The adipocyte as an active participant in energy balance and metabolism. *Gastroenterologist* 132: 103–115.

Baez, J.L., Michel, K.E., Sorenmo, K. et al. (2007). A prospective investigation of the prevalence and prognostic significance of weight loss and changes in body condition in feline cancer patients. *J. Feline Med. Surg.* 9: 411–417.

Bairati, I., Meyer, F., Gélinas, M. et al. (2005). A randomized trial of antioxidant vitamins to prevent second primary cancers in head and neck cancer patients. *J. Natl. Cancer Inst.* 97: 481–488.

Barber, M.D., Fearon, K.C.H., Tisdale, M.J. et al. (2001). Effect of a fish oil-enriched nutritional supplement on metabolic mediators in patients with pancreatic cancer cachexia. *Nutr. Cancer* 40: 118–124.

Baron, M. (2000). Appetite stimulants: the unsolved truth. *Health Care Food Nutr. Focus* 16: 5–7.

Bartges, J.W. (1996). Nutritional support. In: *Complications in Small Animal Surgery: Diagnosis, Management, Prevention* (ed. A.J. Lipowitz), 35–72. Baltimore, MD: Williams and Wilkins.

Bjelakovic, G., Nikolova, D., Gluud, L.L. et al. (2007). Mortality in randomized trials of antioxidant supplements for primary and secondary prevention: systematic review and meta-analysis. *JAMA* 297: 842–857.

Bjornvad, C.R., Rand, J.S., Tan, H.Y. et al. (2014). Obesity and sex influence insulin resistance and total and multimer adiponectin levels in adult neutered domestic shorthair client-owned cats. *Domest. Anim. Endocrinol.* 47: 55–64.

Blum, D., Stene, G.B., Solheim, T.S. et al. (2014). Validation of the consensus-definition for cancer cachexia and evaluation of a classification model – a study based on data from an international multicenter project (EPCRC-CSA). *Ann. Oncol.* 25: 1635–1642.

Bojanić, K., Midwinter, A.C., Marshall, J.C. et al. (2017). Isolation of *Campylobacter* spp. from client-owned dogs and cats, and retail raw meat pet food in the Manawatu, New Zealand. *Zoonoses Public Health* 64: 438–449.

Bossola, M., Pacelli, F., Rosa, F. et al. (2011). Does nutrition support stimulate tumor growth in humans? *Nutr. Clin. Pract.* 26: 174–180.

Boudreaux, M.K., Reinhart, G.A., Vaughn, D.M. et al. (1997). The effects of varying dietary n-6 to n-3 fatty acid ratios on platelet reactivity, coagulation screening assays, and antithrombin III activity in dogs. *J. Am. Anim. Hosp. Assoc.* 33: 235–243.

Bozzetti, F., Arends, J., Lundholm, K. et al. (2009). ESPEN guidelines on parenteral nutrition: non-surgical oncology. *Clin. Nutr.* 28: 445–454.

Brard, L., Weitzen, S., Strubel-Lagan, S.L. et al. (2006). The effect of total parenteral nutrition on the survival of terminally ill ovarian cancer patients. *Gynecol. Oncol.* 103: 176–180.

van Bree, F.P.J., Bokken, G.C.A.M., Mineur, R. et al. (2018). Zoonotic bacteria and parasites found in raw meat-based diets for cats and dogs. *Vet. Rec.* 182: 50.

Brennan, M.F. (1977). Uncomplicated starvation versus cancer cachexia. *Cancer Res.* 37: 2359–2364.

Bright, J.M., Sullivan, P.S., and Melton, S.L. (1994). The effects of n-3 fatty acid supplementation on bleeding time, plasma fatty acid composition, and in vitro platelet aggregation in cats. *J. Vet. Intern. Med.* 8 (247): 252.

Brooks, D., Churchill, J., Fein, K. et al. (2014). 2014 AAHA weight management guidelines for dogs and cats. *J. Am. Anim. Hosp. Assoc.* 50: 1–11.

Calle, E.E. and Kaaks, R. (2004). Overweight, obesity and cancer: epidemiological evidence and proposed mechanisms. *Nat. Rev. Cancer* 4: 579–591.

Calle, E.E., Rodriguez, C., Walker-Thurmond, K. et al. (2003). Overweight, obesity, and mortality from cancer in a prospectively studied cohort of US adults. *N. Engl. J. Med.* 348: 1625–1638.

Campbell, P.T., Newton, C.C., Dehal, A.N. et al. (2012). Impact of body mass index on survival after colorectal cancer diagnosis: the Cancer Prevention Study-II Nutrition Cohort. *J. Clin. Oncol.* 30: 42–52.

Carracedo, A., Cantley, L.C., and Pandolfi, P.P. (2013). Cancer metabolism: fatty acid oxidation in the limelight. *Nat. Rev. Cancer* 13: 227–232.

Chan, D.L. (2017). Critical care nutrition. In: *Textbook of Veterinary Internal Medicine*, 8e (ed. S.J. Ettinger, E.C. Feldman and E. Côté), 786–792. St. Louis, MO: Elsevier.

Chen, C.J., Shih, S.C., Wang, H.Y. et al. (2013). Clinical application of total parenteral nutrition in patients with peritoneal carcinomatosis. *Eur. J. Cancer Care* 22: 468–473.

Chow, R., Bruera, E., Chiu, L. et al. (2016). Enteral and parenteral nutrition in cancer patients: a systematic review and meta-analysis. *Ann. Palliat. Med.* 5: 30–41.

Clarke, M.A., Fetterman, B., Cheung, L.C. et al. (2018). Epidemiologic evidence that excess body weight increases risk of cervical cancer by decreased detection of precancer. *J. Clin. Oncol.* 36: 1184–1191.

Cleary, M.P. and Grossmann, M.E. (2009). Obesity and breast cancer: the estrogen connection. *Endocrinology* 150: 2537–2542.

Cohen, J. and Lefor, A.T. (2001). Nutrition support and cancer. *Nutrition* 17: 698–699.

Corbet, C. and Feron, O. (2015). Metabolic and mind shifts: from glucose to glutamine and acetate addictions in cancer. *Curr. Opin. Clin. Nutr. Metab. Care* 18: 346–353.

Corbet, C. and Feron, O. (2017). Emerging roles of lipid metabolism in cancer progression. *Curr. Opin. Clin. Nutr. Metab. Care* 20: 254–260.

Cuvelier, G.D.E., Baker, T.J., Peddie, E.F. et al. (2014). A randomized, double-blind, placebo-controlled clinical trial of megestrol acetate as an appetite stimulant in children with weight loss due to cancer and/or cancer therapy. *Pediatr. Blood Cancer* 61: 672–679.

D'Andrea, G.M. (2005). Use of antioxidants during chemotherapy and radiotherapy should be avoided. *CA Cancer J. Clin.* 55: 319–321.

Daniel, H.L., Mauldin, G.E., and Mauldin, G.N. (1999). Body condition scoring in dogs and cats with and without malignant disease. In: *Proceedings of the 19th Annual Conference of the Veterinary Cancer Society*. Veterinary Cancer Society: Woods Hole, MA, 36 (13–16 November 1999).

Davidson, J.R. (2018). Feeding tubes. In: *Veterinary Surgery: Small Animal*, 2e (ed. S.A. Johnston and K.M. Tobias), 1901–1917. St. Louis, MO: Elsevier.

Dev, R., Hui, D., Chisholm, G. et al. (2015). Hypermetabolism and symptom burden in advanced cancer patients evaluated in a cachexia clinic. *J. Cachexia. Sarcopenia Muscle* 6: 95–98.

DeWys, W.D., Begg, C., Lavin, P.T. et al. (1980). Prognostic effect of weight loss prior to chemotherapy in cancer patients. *Am. J. Med.* 69: 491–497.

Dinallo, G.K., Poplarski, J.A., Van Deventer, G.M. et al. (2017). A survey of feeding, activity, supplement use and energy consumption in North American agility dogs. *J. Nutr. Sci.* 6: e45.

Dorai, T. and Aggarwal, B.B. (2004). Role of chemopreventive agents in cancer therapy. *Cancer Lett.* 215: 129–140.

Ejaz, A., Spolverato, G., Kim, Y. et al. (2015). Impact of body mass index on perioperative outcomes and survival after re for gastric cancer. *J. Surg. Res.* 195: 74–82.

Endres, S., Ghorbani, R., Kelley, V.E. et al. (1989). The effect of dietary supplementation with n-3 polyunsaturated fatty acids on the synthesis of interleukin-1 and tumor necrosis factor by mononuclear cells. *N. Engl. J. Med.* 320: 265–270.

Fauth, E., Freeman, L.M., Cornjeo, L. et al. (2015). Salmonella bacteriuria in a cat fed a Salmonella-contaminated diet. *J. Am. Vet. Med. Assoc.* 247: 525–530.

Fearon, K.C.H., Barber, M.D., and Moses, A.G.W. (2001). The cancer cachexia syndrome. *Surg. Oncol. Clin. N. Am.* 10: 109–126.

Fearon, K.C., Von Meyenfeldt, M.F., Moses, A.G. et al. (2003). Effect of a protein and energy dense n-3 fatty acid enriched oral supplement on loss of weight and lean tissue in cancer cachexia: a randomised double blind trial. *Gut* 52: 1479–1486.

Fearon, K.C.H., Strasser, F., Anker, S.D. et al. (2011). Definition and classification of cancer cachexia: an international consensus. *Lancet* 12: 489–495.

Fearon, K.C.H., Glass, D.J., and Guttridge, D.C. (2012). Cancer cachexia: mediators, signaling, and metabolic pathways. *Cell Metab.* 16: 153–166.

Finley, R., Ribble, C., Aramini, J. et al. (2007). The risk of salmonellae shedding by dogs fed *salmonella*-contaminated commercial raw food diets. *Can. Vet. J.* 48: 69–75.

Freeman, L.M. (2012). Cachexia and sarcopenia: emerging syndromes of importance in dogs and cats. *J. Vet. Intern. Med.* 26: 3–17.

Garland, C.F. and Gorham, E.D. (2017). Dose-response of serum 25-hydroxyvitamin D in association with risk of colorectal cancer: a meta-analysis. *J. Steroid Biochem. Mol. Biol.* 168: 1–8.

Garofalo, C. and Surmacz, E. (2006). Leptin and cancer. *J. Cell. Physiol.* 207: 12–22.

Gärtner, S., Krüger, J., Aghdassi, A.A. et al. (2015). Nutrition in pancreatic cancer: a review. *Gastrointest. Tumors* 2: 195–202.

Gayet, C., Baihache, E., Dumon, H. et al. (2004). Insulin resistance and changes in plasma concentrations of TNFα, IGF1, and NEFA in dogs during weight gain and obesity. *J. Anim. Physiol. Anim. Nutr.* 88: 157–165.

German, A.J., Hervera, M., Hunter, L. et al. (2009). Improvement in insulin resistance and reduction in plasma inflammatory adipokines after weight loss in obese dogs. *Domest. Anim. Endocrinol.* 37: 214–226.

Giacometti, F., Magarotto, J., Serraino, A. et al. (2017). Highly suspected cases of salmonellosis in two cats fed with a commercial raw meat-based diet: health risks to animals and zoonotic implications. *BMC Vet. Res.* 13: 224.

Glickman, L.T., Schofer, F.S., McKee, L.J. et al. (1989). Epidemiologic study of insecticide exposure, obesity, and risk of bladder cancer in household dogs. *J. Toxicol. Environ. Health* 28: 407–414.

Gogos, C.A., Ginopoulos, P., Salsa, B. et al. (1998). Dietary omega-3 polyunsaturated fatty acids plus vitamin E restore immunodeficiency and prolong survival for severely ill patients with generalized malignancy: a randomized control trial. *Cancer* 82: 395–402.

Gow, A.G., Else, R., Evans, H. et al. (2011). Hypovitaminosis D in dogs with inflammatory bowel disease and hypoalbuminemia. *J. Small Anim. Pract.* 52: 411–418.

Greenlee, H., Unger, J.M., LeBlanc, M. et al. (2017). Association between body mass index (BMI) and cancer survival in a pooled analysis of 22 clinical trials. *Cancer Epidemiol. Biomarkers Prev.* 26: 21–29.

Griffiths, K., Aggarwal, B.B., Singh, R.B. et al. (2016). Food antioxidants and their anti-inflammatory properties: a potential role in cardiovascular diseases and cancer prevention. *Diseases* 4: 28.

Griggs, J.J., Sorbero, M.E., Lyman, G.H. et al. (2005). Undertreatment of obese women receiving breast cancer chemotherapy. *Arch. Intern. Med.* 165: 1267–1273.

Hammarqvist, F., Wernerman, J., von der Decken, A. et al. (1990). Alanyl-glutamine counteracts the depletion of free glutamine and the postoperative decline in protein synthesis in skeletal muscle. *Ann. Surg.* 212: 637–644.

van Harten-Gerritsen, A.S., Balvers, M.G.J., Witkamp, R.F. et al. (2015). Vitamin D, inflammation, and colorectal cancer progression: a review of mechanistic studies and future directions for epidemiological studies. *Cancer Epidemiol. Biomarkers Prev.* 24: 1820–1828.

Hidaka, B.H., Kimler, B.F., Fabian, C.J. et al. (2017). An empirically derived dietary pattern associated with breast cancer risk is validated in a nested case-control cohort from a randomized prevention trial. *Clin. Nutr. ESPEN* 17: 8–17.

Holder, H. (2003). Nursing management of nutrition in cancer and palliative care. *Br. J. Nurs.* 12: 667–674.

Ishioka, K., Hosoya, K., Kitagawa, H. et al. (2007). Plasma leptin concentration in dogs: effects of body condition score, age, gender and breeds. *Res. Vet. Sci.* 82: 11–15.

Ishioka, K., Omachi, A., Sasaki, N. et al. (2009). Feline adiponectin: molecular structure and plasma concentrations in obese cats. *J. Vet. Med. Sci.* 71: 189–194.

Iyengar, N.M., Hudis, C.A., and Dannenberg, A.J. (2015). Obesity and cancer: local and systemic mechanisms. *Annu. Rev. Med.* 66: 297–309.

Jeansen, S., Witkamp, R.F., Garthoff, J.A. et al. (2018). Fish oil LC-PUFAs do not affect blood coagulation parameters and bleeding manifestations: analysis of 8 clinical studies with selected patient groups on omega-3-enriched medical nutrition. *Clin. Nutr.* 37: 948–957.

Joffe, D.J. and Schlesinger, D.P. (2002). Preliminary assessment of the risk of Salmonella infection in dogs fed raw chicken diets. *Can. Vet. J.* 43: 441–442.

Johannes, C.M. and Musser, M.L. (2019). Anorexia and the cancer patient. *Vet. Clin. North Am. Small Anim. Pract.* 49: 837–854.

Johnson, I.T. (2004). Micronutrients and cancer. *Proc. Nutr. Soc.* 63: 587–595.

Karayannopoulou, M., Fytianou, A., Assaloumidis, N. et al. (2013). Markers of lipid peroxidation and α-tocopherol levels in the blood and neoplastic tissue of dogs with malignant mammary gland tumors. *Vet. Clin. Pathol.* 42: 323–328.

Khanna, C., Klausner, J.S., Walter, P. et al. (1995). A randomized clinical trial of glutamine versus placebo in the prevention of radiation-induced mucositis in dogs. In: *Proceedings of the 15th Annual Conference of the Veterinary Cancer Society*. Veterinary Cancer Society: Tucson, AZ, 46–47 (21–24 October 1995).

Khatib, S.A., Rossi, E.L., Bowers, L.W. et al. (2016). Reducing the burden of obesity-associated cancers with anti-inflammatory long-chain omega-3 polyunsaturated fatty acids. *Prostaglandins Other Lipid Mediat.* 125: 100–107.

Klopfleisch, R., Hvid, H., Klose, P. et al. (2010). Insulin receptor is expressed in normal canine mammary gland and benign adenomas but decreased in metastatic canine mammary carcinomas similar to human breast cancer. *Vet. Comp. Oncol.* 8: 293–301.

Krick, E.L., Moore, R.H., Cohen, R.B. et al. (2011). Prognostic significance of weight changes during treatment of feline lymphoma. *J. Feline Med. Surg.* 13: 976–983.

Kristensen, S.D., Schmidt, E.B., and Dyerberg, J. (1989). Dietary supplementation with n-3 polyunsaturated fatty acids and human platelet function: a review with particular emphasis on implications for cardiovascular disease. *J. Intern. Med. Suppl.* 731: 141–150.

Kumaraguruparan, R., Balachandran, C., Manohar, B.M. et al. (2005). Altered oxidant-antioxidant profile in canine mammary tumours. *Vet. Res. Commun.* 29: 287–296.

Lalor, S., Schwartz, A.M., Titmarsh, H. et al. (2014). Cats with inflammatory bowel disease and intestinal small cell lymphoma have lower serum concentrations of 25-hydroxyvitamin D. *J. Vet. Intern. Med.* 28: 351–355.

Langer, C.J., Hoffman, J.P., and Ottery, F.D. (2001). Clinical significance of weight loss in cancer patients: rationale for the use of anabolic agents in the treatment of cancer-related cachexia. *Nutrition* 17: S1–S20.

Langius, J.A., Kruizenga, H.M., Uitdehaag, B.M. et al. (2012). Resting energy expenditure in head and neck cancer patients before and during radiotherapy. *Clin. Nutr.* 31: 549–554.

Lappe, J., Watson, P., Travers-Gustafson, D. et al. (2017). Effect of vitamin D and calcium supplementation on cancer incidence in older women: a randomized clinical trial. *JAMA* 317: 1234–1243.

Lauby-Secretan, B., Scoccianti, C., Loomis, D. et al. (2016). Body fatness and cancer – viewpoint of the IARC working group. *N. Engl. J. Med.* 375: 794–798.

Lawler, D.F., Evans, R.H., Larson, B.T. et al. (2005). Influence of lifetime food restriction on causes, time, and predictors of death in dogs. *J. Am. Vet. Med. Assoc.* 226: 225–231.

Lawrie, T.A., Green, J.T., Beresford, M. et al. (2018). Interventions to reduce acute and late adverse gastrointestinal effects of pelvic radiotherapy for primary pelvic cancers. *Cochrane Database Syst. Rev.* 1: CD012529. https://doi.org/10.1002/14651858. CD012529.pub2.

LeBlanc, C.J., Dietrich, M.A., Horohov, D.W. et al. (2007). Effects of dietary fish oil and vitamin E supplementation on canine lymphocyte proliferation evaluated using a flow cytometric technique. *Vet. Immunol. Immunopathol.* 119: 180–188.

LeBlanc, C.J., Horohov, D.W., Bauer, J.E. et al. (2008). Effects of dietary supplementation with fish oil on *in vivo* production of inflammatory mediators in clinically normal dogs. *Am. J. Vet. Res.* 69: 486–493.

Lee, Y., Jin, Y., Lim, W. et al. (2003). A ginsenoside-Rh1, a component of ginseng saponin, activates estrogen receptor in human breast carcinoma MCF-7 cells. *J. Steroid Biochem. Mol. Biol.* 84: 463–468.

Lee, H.W., Jeong, B.C., Seo, S.I. et al. (2015). Prognostic significance of visceral obesity in patients with advanced renal cell carcinoma undergoing nephrectomy. *Int. J. Urol.* 22: 455–461.

Lentjes, M.A.H., Keogh, R.H., Welch, A.A. et al. (2017). Longitudinal associations between marine omega-3 supplement users and coronary heart disease in a UK population-based cohort. *BMJ Open* 7: e017471.

Levine, C.B., Bayle, J., Biourge, V. et al. (2016). Effects and synergy of feed ingredients on canine neoplastic cell proliferation. *BMC Vet. Res.* 12: 159–169.

Lian, W., Wang, R., Xing, B. et al. (2017). Fish intake and the risk of brain tumor: a meta-analysis with systematic review. *Nutr. J.* 16: 1.

Ligibel, J.A., Alfano, C.M., Courneya, K.S. et al. (2014). American Society of Clinical Oncology position statement on obesity and cancer. *J. Clin. Oncol.* 31: 3568–3575.

Lim, H.-Y., Im, K.-S., Kim, N.-H. et al. (2015a). Effects of obesity and obesity-related molecules on canine mammary gland tumors. *Vet. Pathol.* 52: 1045–1051.

Lim, H.-Y., Im, K.-S., Kim, N.-H. et al. (2015b). Obesity, expression of adipocytokines, and macrophage infiltration in canine mammary tumors. *Vet. J.* 203: 326–331.

Lin, H., Zhang, L., Zheng, R. et al. (2017). The prevalence, metabolic risk and effects of lifestyle intervention for metabolically healthy obesity: a systematic review and meta-analysis. *Medicine* 96 (47): e8838.

Llewellyn, C.D., Linklater, K., Bell, J. et al. (2004). An analysis of risk factors for oral cancer in young people: a casecontrol study. *Oral Oncol.* 40: 304–313.

Lopes, A.P., Santos, H., Neto, F. et al. (2011). Prevalence of antibodies to *Toxoplasma gondii* in dogs from northeastern Portugal. *J. Parasitol.* 97: 418–420.

Makarem, N., Lin, Y., Bandera, E.V. et al. (2015). Concordance with World Cancer Research Fund/American Institute for Cancer Research (WCRF/AICR) guidelines for cancer prevention and obesity-related cancer risk in the Framingham Offspring cohort (1991–2008). *Cancer Causes Control* 26: 277–286.

Mandelker, L. (2008a). Cellular effects of common antioxidants. *Vet. Clin. North Am. Small Anim. Pract.* 38: 199–211.

Mandelker, L. (2008b). Introduction to oxidative stress and mitochondrial dysfunction. *Vet. Clin. North Am. Small Anim. Pract.* 38: 1–30.

Marian, M.J. (2017). Dietary supplements commonly used by cancer survivors: are there any benefits? *Nutr. Clin. Pract.* 32: 607–627.

Marks, S.L. (2017). Nasoesophageal, esophagostomy, gastrostomy and jejunal tube placement techniques. In: *Textbook of Veterinary Internal Medicine*, 8e (ed. S.J. Ettinger, E.C. Feldman and E. Côté), 323–332. St. Louis, MO: Elsevier.

Martin, L., Senesse, P., Gioulbasanis, I. et al. (2015). Diagnostic criteria for the classification of cancer-associated weight loss. *J. Clin. Oncol.* 33: 90–99.

Mauer, J., Denson, J.L., and Brüning, J.C. (2015). Versatile functions for IL-6 in metabolism and cancer. *Trends Immunol.* 36: 92–101.

Mazzaferro, E.M., Hackett, T.B., Stein, T.P. et al. (2001). Metabolic alterations in dogs with osteosarcoma. *Am. J. Vet. Res.* 62: 1234–1239.

McCarthy, D.O. (2003). Rethinking nutritional support for persons with cancer cachexia. *Biol. Res. Nurs.* 5: 3–17.

McDonnell, S.L., Baggerly, C., French, C.B. et al. (2016). Serum 25-hydroxyvitamin D concentrations ≥40 ng/mL are associated with >65% lower cancer risk: pooled analysis of randomized trial and prospective cohort study. *PLoS One* 11 (4): e0152441.

McKinlay, A.W. (2004). Nutritional support in patients with advanced cancer: permission to fall out? *Proc. Nutr. Soc.* 63: 431–435.

McNeil, E.A., Ogilvie, G.K., Mallinckrodt, C. et al. (1999). Platelet function in dogs treated for lymphoma and hemangiosarcoma and supplemented with dietary n-3 fatty acids. *J. Vet. Intern. Med.* 13: 574–580.

McQuellon, R.P., Moose, D.B., Russell, G.B. et al. (2002). Supportive use of megestrol acetate (Megace) with head/neck and lung cancer patients receiving radiation therapy. *Int. J. Radiat. Oncol. Biol. Phys.* 52: 1180–1185.

McQuown, B., Burgess, K.E., and Heinze, C.R. (2018). Preliminary investigation of blood concentrations of insulin-like growth factor, insulin, lactate and β-hydroxybutyrate in dogs with lymphoma as compared with matched controls. *Vet. Comp. Oncol.* 16: 262–267.

Mercadante, S. (1998). Parenteral versus enteral nutrition in cancer patients: indications and practice. *Support. Care Cancer* 6: 85–93.

Meydani, S.N., Endres, S., Woods, M.M. et al. (1991). Oral (n-3) fatty acid supplementation suppresses cytokine production and lymphocyte proliferation: comparison between young and older women. *J. Nutr.* 121: 547–555.

Michel, K.E., Sorenmo, K., and Shofer, F.S. (2004). Evaluation of body condition and weight loss in dogs presented to a veterinary oncology service. *J. Vet. Intern. Med.* 18: 692–695.

Middleton, D.J. and Watson, A.D.J. (1985). Glucocorticoid intolerance in cats given short-term therapies of prednisolone and megestrol acetate. *Am. J. Vet. Res.* 46: 2653–2625.

Misdorp, W. (1991). Progestagens and mammary tumors in dogs and cats. *Acta Endocrinol.* 125 (Suppl 1): 27–31.

Miura, K., Hughes, M.C.B., Ungerer, J.P. et al. (2016). Plasma eicosapentaenoic acid is negatively associated with all-cause mortality among men and women in a population-based prospective study. *Nutr. Res.* 36: 1202–1209.

Miyata, H., Yano, M., Yasuda, T. et al. (2017). Randomized study of the clinical effects of ω-3 fatty acid-containing enteral nutrition support during neoadjuvant chemotherapy on chemotherapy-related toxicity in patients with esophageal cancer. *Nutrition* 33: 204–210.

Mohr, S.B. (2009). A brief history of vitamin D and cancer prevention. *Ann. Epidemiol.* 19: 79–83.

Mondello, P., Mian, M., Aloisi, C. et al. (2015). Cancer cachexia syndrome: pathogenesis, diagnosis, and new therapeutic options. *Nutr. Cancer* 67: 12–26.

de Vos-Geelen, J., Fearon, K.C.H., and Schols, A.M.W. (2014). The energy balance in cancer cachexia revisited. *Curr. Opin. Clin. Nutr. Metab. Care* 17: 509–514.

Mooney, M.A., Vaughn, D.M., Reinhart, G.A. et al. (1998). Evaluation of the effects of omega-3 fatty acid-containing diets on the inflammatory stage of wound healing in dogs. *Am. J. Vet. Res.* 59: 859–863.

Morgan, D.K., Willis, S., and Shepherd, M.L. (2017). Survey of owner motivations and veterinary input of owners feeding diets containing raw animal products. *PeerJ* 5: e3031.

Morris, C.R., Hamilton-Reeves, J., Martindale, R.G. et al. (2017). Acquired amino acid deficiencies: a focus on arginine and glutamine. *Nutr. Clin. Pract.* 32: 30S–47S.

Muranaka, S., Mori, N., Hatano, Y. et al. (2011). Obesity induced changes to plasma adiponectin concentration and cholesterol lipoprotein composition profile in cats. *Res. Vet. Sci.* 91: 358–361.

Murphy, A.B., Nyame, Y., Martin, I.K. et al. (2014). Vitamin D deficiency predicts prostate biopsy outcomes. *Clin. Cancer Res.* 20: 2289–2299.

Muscaritoli, M., Molfino, A., Lucia, S. et al. (2014). Cachexia: a preventable comorbidity of cancer. A T.A.R.G.E.T. approach. *Crit. Rev. Oncol. Hematol.* 94: 251–259.

Nagata, M., Hata, J., Hirakawa, Y. et al. (2017). The ratio of serum eicosapentaenoic acid to arachidonic acid and risk of cancer death in a Japanese community: the Hisayama study. *J. Epidemiol.* 27: 578–583.

Narita, S., Saito, E., Sawada, N. et al. (2018). Dietary consumption of antioxidant vitamins and subsequent lung cancer risk: the Japan Public Health Center-based prospective study. *Int. J. Cancer* 142: 2441–2460.

Nash, J.Q., Chissel, S., Jones, J. et al. (2005). Risk factors for toxoplasmosis in pregnant women in Kent, United Kingdom. *Epidemiol. Infect.* 133: 475–483.

Nitenberg, G. and Raynard, B. (2000). Nutritional support of the cancer patient: issues and dilemmas. *Crit. Rev. Oncol. Hematol.* 34: 137–168.

Niv, Y. and Abuksis, G. (2002). Indications for percutaneous endoscopic gastrostomy insertion: ethical aspects. *Dig. Dis.* 20: 253–256.

Novak, F., Heyland, D.K., Avenell, A. et al. (2002). Glutamine supplementation in serious illness: a systematic review of the evidence. *Crit. Care Med.* 30: 2022–2029.

Nyame, Y.A., Murphy, A.B., Bowen, D.K. et al. (2016). Associations between serum vitamin D and adverse pathology in men undergoing radical prostatectomy. *J. Clin. Oncol.* 34: 1345–1349.

Ogilvie, G.K., Fettman, M.J., Mallinckrodt, C.H. et al. (2000). Effect of fish oil, arginine, and doxorubicin chemotherapy on remission and survival time for dogs with lymphoma: a double-blind, randomized placebo-controlled study. *Cancer* 88: 1916–1928.

Ogilvie, G.K., Ford, R.B., Vail, D.M. et al. (1994). Alterations in lipoprotein profiles in dogs with lymphoma. *J. Vet. Intern. Med.* 8: 62–66.

Ogilvie, G.K., Walters, L.M., Fettman, M.J. et al. (1993). Energy expenditure in dogs with lymphoma fed two specialized diets. *Cancer* 71: 3146–3152.

Ogilvie, G.K., Walters, L.M., Salman, M.D. et al. (1996). Resting energy expenditure in dogs with nonhematopoietic malignancies before and after excision of tumors. *Am. J. Vet. Res.* 57: 1463–1467.

Ogilvie, G.K., Walters, L., Salman, M.D. et al. (1997). Alterations in carbohydrate metabolism in dogs with nonhematopoietic malignancies. *Am. J. Vet. Res.* 58: 277–281.

Omenn, G.S., Goodman, G.E., Thornquist, M.D. et al. (1996). Effects of a combination of beta carotene and vitamin A on lung cancer and cardiovascular disease. *N. Engl. J. Med.* 334: 1150–1155.

Park, J.S., Choi, G.S., Yang, Y.S. et al. (2010). Influence of obesity on the serum carcinoembryonic antigen value in patients with colorectal cancer. *Cancer Epidemiol. Biomarkers Prev.* 19: 2461–2468.

Pater, L.E., Hart, K.W., Blonigen, B.J. et al. (2012). Relationship between prostate-specific antigen, age, and body mass in a prostate cancer screening population. *Am. J. Clin. Oncol.* 35: 490–492.

Peng, J., Cai, J., Niu, Z.X. et al. (2016). Early enteral nutrition compared with parenteral nutrition for esophageal cancer patients after esophagectomy: a meta-analysis. *Dis. Esophagus* 29: 333–341.

Petruzzelli, M., Schweiger, M., Schreiber, R. et al. (2014). A switch from white to brown fat increases energy expenditure in cancer-associated cachexia. *Cell Metab.* 20: 433–447.

Philibert, J.C., Snyder, P.W., Glickman, N. et al. (2003). Influence of host factors on survival in dogs with malignant mammary gland tumors. *J. Vet. Intern. Med.* 17: 102–106.

Poikonen, P., Blomqvist, C., and Joensuu, H. (2001). Effect of obesity on the leukocyte nadir in women treated with adjuvant cyclophosphamide, methotrexate and fluorouracil dosed according to body surface area. *Acta Oncol.* 40: 67–71.

Qin, H.L., Su, Z.D., Hu, L.G. et al. (2002). Effect of early intrajejunal nutrition on pancreatic pathological features and gut barrier function in dogs with acute pancreatitis. *Clin. Nutr.* 21: 469–473.

Quimby, J.M. and Lunn, K.F. (2013). Mirtazipine as an appetite stimulant and anti-emetic in cats with chronic kidney disease: a masked placebo-controlled crossover clinical trial. *Vet. J.* 197: 651–655.

Radin, M.J., Sharkey, L.C., and Holycross, B.J. (2009). Adipokines: a review of biological and analytical principles and an update in dogs, cats and horses. *Vet. Clin. Pathol.* 38: 136–156.

Rao, D.N., Ganesh, B., Rao, R.S. et al. (1994). Risk assessment of tobacco, alcohol, and diet in oral cancer: a case-control study. *Int. J. Cancer* 58: 469–473.

Remillard, R.L., Guerino, F., Dudgeon, D.L. et al. (1998). Intravenous glutamine or limited enteral feeding in piglets: amelioration of small intestinal disuse atrophy. *J. Nutr.* 128: 2723S–2726S.

Remillard, R.L. and Saker, K.E. (2010). Parenteral-assisted feeding. In: *Small Animal Clinical Nutrition*, 5e (ed. M.S. Hand, C.D. Thatcher, R.L. Remillard, et al.), 478–498. Topeka, KS: Mark Morris Institute.

Renehan, A.G., Tyson, M., Egger, M. et al. (2008). Body-mass index and incidence of cancer: a systematic review and meta-analysis of prospective observational studies. *Lancet* 371: 569–578.

Rennie, M.J., MacLennan, P.A., Hundal, H.S. et al. (1989). Skeletal muscle glutamine transport, intramuscular glutamine concentration, and muscle-protein turnover. *Metabolism* 8 (Suppl): 47–51.

Reynolds, A.J., Fuhrer, L., Dunlap, H.L. et al. (1994). Lipid metabolite responses to diet and training in sled dogs. *J. Nutr.* 124: 2754S–2750S.

Rhodes, L., Zollers, B., Wofford, J.A., and Heinen, E. (2017). Capomorelin: a ghrelin receptor agonist and novel therapy for stimulation of appetite in dogs. *Vet. Sci.* 4 (1): 3–16.

Richardson, R.A. and Davidson, H.I.M. (2003). Nutritional demands in acute and chronic illness. *Proc. Nutr. Soc.* 62: 777–781.

Romano, F.R., Heinze, C.R., Barber, L.G. et al. (2016). Association between body condition score and cancer prognosis in dogs with lymphoma and osteosarcoma. *J. Vet. Intern. Med.* 30: 1179–1186.

Rosa, C.T., Schoeman, J.P., Berry, J.L. et al. (2013). Hypovitaminosis D in dogs with spirocercosis. *J. Vet. Intern. Med.* 27: 1159–1164.

Roth, B., Birkhäuser, F.D., Zehnder, P. et al. (2013). Parenteral nutrition does not improve postoperative recovery from radical cystectomy: results of a prospective randomized trial. *Eur. Urol.* 63: 475–482.

Ruiz Garcia, V., López-Briz, E., Sanchis, R.C. et al. (2013). Megestrol acetate for treatment of anorexia-cachexia syndrome. *Cochrane Database Syst. Rev.* (3): CD004310. https://doi.org/10.1002/14651858. CD004310.pub3.

Saker, K., Eddy, A., Thatcher, C. et al. (1998). Manipulation of dietary (n-6) and (n-3) fatty acids alters platelet function in cats. *J. Nutr.* 128: 2645S–2647S.

Saker, K.E. and Remillard, R.L. (2010). Critical care nutrition and enteral-assisted feeding. In: *Small Animal Clinical Nutrition*, 5e (ed. M.S. Hand, C.D. Thatcher, R.L. Remillard, et al.), 439–476. Topeka, KS: Mark Morris Institute.

Samani, A.A., Yakar, S., LeRoith, D. et al. (2007). The role of the IGF system in cancer growth and metastasis: overview and recent insights. *Endocr. Rev.* 28: 20–47.

Scott, D.W., Miller, W.H., Reinhart, G.A. et al. (1997). Effect of an omega-3/omega-6 fatty acid-containing commercial lamb and rice diet on pruritis in atopic dogs: results of a single-blinded study. *Can. J. Vet. Res.* 61: 145–153.

Selting, K.A., Sharp, C.R., Ringold, R. et al. (2016). Serum 25-hydroxyvitamin D concentrations in dogs – correlation with health and cancer risk. *Vet. Comp. Oncol.* 14: 295–305.

Serini, S. and Calviello, G. (2018). Long-chain omega-3 fatty acids and cancer: any cause for concern? *Curr. Opin. Clin. Nutr. Metab. Care* 21: 83–89.

Shebl, F.M., Hsing, A.W., Park, Y. et al. (2014). Non-steroidal anti-inflammatory drugs use is associated with reduced risk of inflammation-associated cancers: NIH-AARP study. *PLoS One* 9: e114633.

Simmonds, N.J. (2010). Ethical issues in nutrition support: a view from the coalface. *Frontline Gastroenterol.* 1: 7–12.

Simone, C.B. II, Simone, N.L., Simone, V. et al. (2007). Antioxidants and other nutrients do not interfere with chemotherapy or radiation therapy and can increase kill and increase survival. Part I. *Altern. Ther. Health Med.* 13: 40–47.

Smith, R.J. (1990). Glutamine metabolism and its physiologic importance. *J. Parenter. Enteral Nutr.* 14: 40S–44S.

Solheim, T.S., Blum, D., Fayers, P.M. et al. (2014). Weight loss, appetite loss and food intake in cancer patients with cancer cachexia: three peas in a pod? – analysis from a multicenter cross sectional study. *Acta Oncol.* 53: 539–546.

Song, M., Zhang, X., Meyerhardt, J.A. et al. (2017). Marine omega-3 polyunsaturated fatty acid intake and survival after colorectal cancer diagnosis. *Gut* 66: 1790–1796.

Sonnenschein, E.G., Glickman, L.T., Goldschmidt, M.H. et al. (1991). Body conformation, diet, and risk of breast cancer in pet dogs: a case-control study. *Am. J. Epidemiol.* 133: 694–703.

Sorenmo, K.U., Rasotto, R., Zappulli, V. et al. (2011). Development, anatomy, histology, lymphatic drainage, clinical features, and cell differentiation markers of canine mammary gland neoplasms. *Vet. Pathol.* 48: 85–97.

Souba, W.W., Klimberg, V.S., Plumley, D.A. et al. (1990). The role of glutamine in maintaining a healthy gut and supporting the metabolic response to injury and infection. *J. Surg. Res.* 48: 383–391.

Stiver, S.L., Frazier, K.S., Mauel, M.J. et al. (2003). Septicemic salmonellosis in two cats fed a raw-meat based diet. *J. Am. Anim. Hosp. Assoc.* 39: 538–542.

Stoeckel, K., Nielsen, L.H., Fuhrmann, H. et al. (2011). Fatty acid patterns of dog erythrocyte membranes after feeding of a fish-oil based DHA-rich supplement with a base diet low in n-3 fatty acids versus a diet containing added n-3 fatty acids. *Acta Vet. Scand.* 53: 57.

Story, A.L., Boston, S.E., Kilkenny, J.J. et al. (2017). Evaluation of weight change during carboplatin therapy in dogs with appendicular osteosarcoma. *J. Vet. Intern. Med.* 31: 1159–1162.

Strasser, F. and Bruera, E.D. (2002). Update on anorexia and cachexia. *Hematol. Oncol. Clin. North Am.* 16: 589–617.

Sykorova, A., Horacek, J., Zak, P. et al. (2005). A randomized, double blind comparative study of prophylactic parenteral nutritional support with or without glutamine in autologous stem cell transplantation for hematological malignancies – three years' follow-up. *Neoplasma* 52: 476–482.

Szczubiał, M., Kankofer, M., Łopuszyński, W. et al. (2004). Oxidative stress parameters in bitches with mammary gland tumors. *J. Vet. Med. A Physiol. Pathol. Clin. Med.* 51: 336–340.

Tanaka, Y., Takahashi, T., Yamaguchi, K. et al. (2016). Elemental diet plus glutamine for the prevention of mucositis in esophageal cancer patients receiving chemotherapy: a feasibility study. *Support. Care Cancer* 24: 933–941.

Tao, W. and Lagergren, J. (2013). Clinical management of obese patients with cancer. *J. Nat. Rev. Clin. Oncol.* 10: 519–533.

Tisdale, M.J. (1999). Wasting in cancer. *J. Nutr.* 129: 243S–246S.

Toll, P.W., Yamka, R.M., Schoenherr, W.D. et al. (2010). Obesity. In: *Small Animal Clinical Nutrition*, 5e (ed. M.S. Hand, C.D. Thatcher, R.L. Remillard, et al.), 501–584. Topeka, KS: Mark Morris Institute.

Tomlinson, M.J., Barteaux, L., Ferns, L.E. et al. (1984). Feline mammary carcinoma: a retrospective evaluation of 17 cases. *Can. Vet. J.* 25: 435–439.

Torelli, G.F., Campos, A.C., and Meguid, M.M. (1999). Use of TPN in terminally ill cancer patients. *Nutrition* 15: 665–667.

Torosian, M.H. and Donoway, R.B. (1991). Total parenteral nutrition and tumor metastasis. *Surgery* 109: 597–601.

Touret, M., Boysen, S.R., and Nadeau, M.E. (2010). Prospective evaluation of clinically relevant type B hyperlactatemia in dogs with cancer. *J. Vet. Intern. Med.* 24: 1458–1461.

Touret, M., Boysen, S.R., and Nadeau, M.E. (2012). Retrospective evaluation of potential causes associated with clinically relevant hyperlactatemia in dogs with lymphoma. *Can. Vet. J.* 53: 511–517.

Tvarijonaviciute, A., Ceron, J.J., Holden, S.L. et al. (2012). Obesity-related metabolic dysfunction in dogs: a comparison with human metabolic syndrome. *BMC Vet. Res.* 8: 147–154.

Vail, D.M., Ogilvie, G.K., Wheeler, S.L. et al. (1990). Alterations in carbohydrate metabolism in canine lymphoma. *J. Vet. Intern. Med.* 4: 8–11.

Van de Velde, H., Janssens, G.P.J., Rochus, K. et al. (2013). Proliferation capacity of T-lymphocytes is affected transiently after a long-term weight gain in Beagle dogs. *Vet. Immunol. Immunopathol.* 152: 237–244.

Vander Heiden, M.G., Cantley, L.C., and Thompson, C.B. (2009). Understanding the Warburg effect: the metabolic requirements of cell proliferation. *Science* 324 (5930): 1029–1033.

Vaughn, D.M., Reinhart, G.A., Swaim, S.F. et al. (1994). Evaluation of effects of dietary n-6 to n-3 fatty acid ratios on leukotriene B synthesis in dog skin and neutrophils. *Vet. Dermatol.* 5 163–172.

Vazeille, C., Jouinot, A., Durand, J.P. et al. (2017). Relation between hypermetabolism, cachexia and survival in cancer patients: a prospective study in 390 cancer patients before initiation of anticancer therapy. *Am. J. Clin. Nutr.* 105: 1139–1147.

Wakshlag, J.J., Rassnick, K.M., Malone, E.K. et al. (2011). Cross-sectional study to investigate the association between vitamin D status and cutaneous mast cell tumours in Labrador retrievers. *Br. J. Nutr.* 106: S60–S63.

Wander, R.C., Hall, J.A., Gradin, J.L. et al. (1997). The ratio of dietary (n-6) to (n-3) fatty acids influences immune system function, eicosanoid metabolism, lipid peroxidation and vitamin E status in aged dogs. *J. Nutr.* 127: 1198–1205.

Wang, H. and Ye, J. (2015). Regulation of energy balance by inflammation: common theme in physiology and pathology. *Rev. Endocr. Metab. Disord.* 16: 47–54.

Waters, D.J., Shen, S., Cooley, D.M. et al. (2003). Effects of dietary selenium supplementation on DNA damage and apoptosis in canine prostate. *J. Natl. Cancer Inst.* 95: 237–241.

Waters, D.J., Shen, S., Glickman, L.T. et al. (2005). Prostate cancer risk and DNA damage: translational significance of selenium supplementation in a canine model. *Carcinogensis* 26: 1256–1262.

Weeth, L.P., Fascetti, A.J., Kass, P.H. et al. (2007). Prevalence of obese dogs in a population of dogs with cancer. *Am. J. Vet. Res.* 68: 389–398.

Weidner, N., Woods, J.P., Conlon, P. et al. (2017). Influence of various factors on circulating 25(OH) vitamin D concentrations in dogs with cancer and healthy dogs. *J. Vet. Intern. Med.* 31: 1796–1803.

Weiss, L., Melchardt, T., Habringer, S. et al. (2014). Increased body mass index is associated with improved overall survival in diffuse large B-cell lymphoma. *Ann. Oncol.* 25: 171–176.

Willcox, J.L., Hammett-Stabler, C., and Hauck, M.L. (2016). Serum 25-hydroxyvitamin D concentrations in dogs with osteosarcoma do not differ from those of age- and weight-matched control dogs. *Vet. J.* 217: 132–133.

Winter, J.L., Barber, L.G., Freeman, L. et al. (2009). Antioxidant status and biomarkers of oxidative stress in dogs with lymphoma. *J. Vet. Intern. Med.* 23: 311–316.

Wischmeyer, P.E. (2002). Glutamine and heat shock protein expression. *Nutrition* 18: 225–228.

Wofford, J.A., Zollers, B., Rhodes, L. et al. (2018). Evaluation of safety of daily administration of Capromorelin in cats. *J. Vet. Pharmacol. Ther.* 41 (2): 324–333.

Yoshida, S., Kaibara, A., Ishibashi, N. et al. (2001). Glutamine supplementation in cancer patients. *Nutrition* 17: 766–768.

Yu, J., Liu, L., Zhang, Y. et al. (2017). Effects of omega-3 fatty acids on patients undergoing surgery for gastrointestinal malignancy: a systematic review and meta-analysis. *BMC Cancer* 17: 271.

Zhao, X.F., Wu, N., Zhao, G.Q. et al. (2016). Enteral nutrition versus parenteral nutrition after major abdominal surgery in patients with gastrointestinal cancer: a systematic review and meta-analysis. *J. Invest. Med.* 64: 1061–1074.

Zollers, B., Wofford, J.A., Heinen, E. et al. (2016). A prospective, randomized, masked, placebo-controlled clinical study of capromorelin in dogs with reduced appetite. *J. Vet. Intern. Med.* 30: 1851–1857.

20

Enteral Nutrition and Tube Feeding

Jennifer A. Larsen

Preventing or reversing malnutrition in hospitalized patients or those with chronic debilitating disease should be an important goal of all clinicians. In human medicine, it is known that malnutrition is associated with increased mortality and longer hospital stays, and this is a common problem in the elderly, young, and chronically ill (Groleau et al. 2014; Rahman et al. 2015; Alvarez-Hernandez et al. 2012; Corkins et al. 2014). While providing nutritional support by either parenteral or enteral routes has been beneficial, it is becoming apparent that utilizing the gastrointestinal tract whenever possible is important.

The Case for Enteral Feeding

The human medical literature supports that enteral feeding is more cost effective and results in overall significant decreases in complications with more positive outcomes in people (Gramlich et al. 2004; McClave et al. 2006; Jeejeebhoy 2007). In the veterinary literature, it has been shown in dogs with induced pancreatitis that parenteral nutrition (compared to enteral nutrition) has a negative impact on gut barrier function and is associated with decreased intestinal villus height, mucosal thickness, and total protein and DNA content, and that this occurs within just seven days (Qin et al. 2002). Similarly, other studies have demonstrated the tolerance of early implementation of enteral feeding, as well as showing benefits including shorter hospital stays and improved gastrointestinal function (Kawasaki et al. 2009; Mansfield et al. 2011; Liu et al. 2012). It is clear that the provision of adequate nutrition, administered enterally where possible, can be a powerful tool in the management of patients with a wide variety of disease conditions.

Nutritional Support of Veterinary Patients

Many articles have described techniques for successfully providing enteral nutrition in veterinary patients (Abood and Buffington 1991; Bright 1993; Marks 1998; Waddell and Michel 1998; Daye et al. 1999; Stevenson et al. 2000; von Werthern and Wess 2001). Despite these resources, data from different institutions have agreed that hospitalized dogs and cats uncommonly achieve caloric intake that meets predicted requirements (Remillard et al. 2001; Brunetto et al. 2010; Molina et al. 2018). In addition, these studies also reported a significant correlation between caloric intake and outcome. Reasons for failure to provide adequate nutritional support may include inadequate feeding orders, specific orders to withhold food, and patient's refusal

Applied Veterinary Clinical Nutrition, Second Edition. Edited by Andrea J. Fascetti, Sean J. Delaney, Jennifer A. Larsen, and Cecilia Villaverde.
© 2024 John Wiley & Sons, Inc. Published 2024 by John Wiley & Sons, Inc.

to eat. There is evidence that animals with diseases that have been traditionally managed with "nil per os" (NPO) orders, such as pancreatitis and parvoviral enteritis, may actually benefit from early enteral feeding (Qin et al. 2002; Mohr et al. 2003; Mansfield et al. 2011; Harris et al. 2017). In other critically ill patients, or after gastrointestinal surgery, early enteral feeding is tolerated and may support improved outcomes (Hoffberg and Koenigshof 2017; Kawasaki et al. 2009; Liu et al. 2012). Additionally, solving problems that involve poor order writing and encouraging proactive patient management that is inclusive of nutritional needs is perhaps simpler than overcoming a patient's anorexia.

There are different ways to accomplish enteral feeding, including voluntary intake. If an animal will eat adequate amounts of an appropriate diet for any disease states that may be present, intervention is not necessary. Voluntary intake can be encouraged with the utilization of various measures of altering diet palatability as well as managing the home or hospital environment (Delaney 2006). While pharmacologic appetite stimulants such as cyproheptadine, prednisone, benzodiazepines, propofol, megestrol acetate, and even dronabinol have been utilized with varied success in the short term in veterinary patients, these measures are often not feasible for long-term use, as they usually do not result in the consumption of adequate amounts of calories on a sustained basis. The most successful agents to date are mirtazapine and capromorelin (Quimby and Lunn 2013; Wofford et al. 2018; Zollers et al. 2015, 2016). Regardless, use of any appetite stimulant does not preclude monitoring of food intake and serial body weights to ensure consumption of adequate calories.

For partially or fully anorexic patients, other options include forced feeding with a syringe or other method, or placement of an enteral feeding device. Forced or "assisted" feeding is a commonly utilized method that usually involves the placement of a food bolus in the rear of the oral cavity. The animal either swallows the bolus by reflex or because the mouth is held closed. Obviously, this is not ideal, since it can be a stressful process for both the patient and hospital staff, and the method is not feasible in the long term. Additionally, forced feeding can lead to choking or aspiration as well as the development of food aversions and other undesirable responses in some patients (such as aggression or fear). Placement and use of an enteral feeding device are the preferred method of providing adequate amounts of an appropriate diet, and this can be accomplished on a long-term basis with many tube types (Figure 20.1).

When to Intervene

Nutritional support should be provided as soon as malnutrition is recognized or anticipated to occur. In some cases, this need will be identified and addressed at or very soon after the initial presentation. Animals with a longer history of suboptimal intakes and/or with chronic diseases in poor body condition are obvious candidates for early intervention; however, obesity is not a contraindication for nutritional support (Figure 20.2). Other cases will require medical stabilization prior to establishing nutritional support (trauma or other emergent cases). Regardless, intervention is indicated if anorexia has been documented for longer than 3–5 days (including the days before presentation, identified via a thorough diet history) or if a patient is not expected to eat within 2–3 days (such as those with significant orofacial trauma or in need of extensive orofacial surgery).

If the need can be anticipated, it is important to initiate a discussion with the client regarding potential feeding tube use early in the course of the disease. Feeding tubes are currently a standard treatment in some common diseases, such as feline hepatic lipidosis, and they are increasingly utilized for other conditions such as chronic kidney disease, pancreatitis, and trauma. The use of most types of

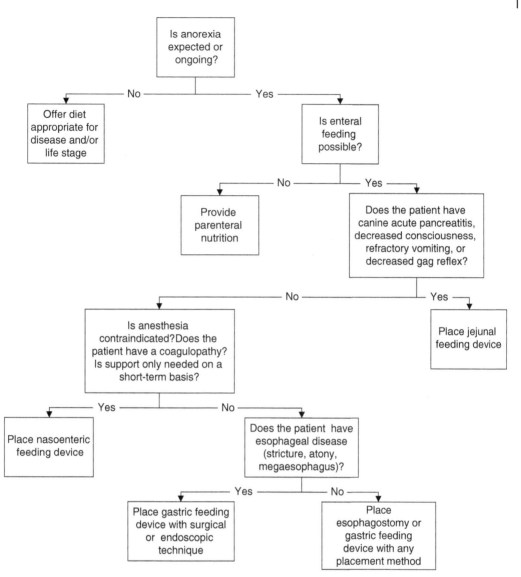

Figure 20.1 Decision-making process for addressing expected or ongoing anorexia in patients already under any indicated treatments for underlying diseases and with inadequate response to appetite stimulants and other support.

enteral feeding devices allows for care to continue at home even on a long-term basis, compared to parenteral nutrition, which must be administered in the hospital. However, client perceptions about feeding tubes strongly influence their acceptance of an enteral feeding device for their pet. Most people have at least a general awareness, if not first- or second-hand experience, of feeding tube use in human medicine. In most cases, clients will be aware of feeding tube use for people in vegetative states or for end-of-life situations. The general public tends to be less aware of feeding tube use for shorter-term management, such as in the case of severe acute pancreatitis, surgical procedures to repair orofacial trauma, or adverse effects of radiation therapy of head and neck tumors. Because of this negative

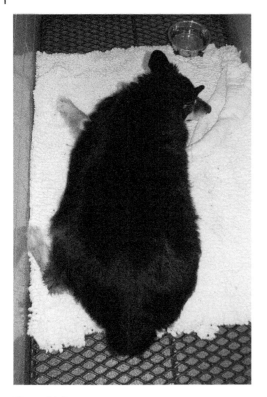

Figure 20.2 Consideration of nutritional needs should be part of the management of every patient, regardless of body condition. Loss of lean body mass can be difficult to assess in obese patients in particular.

association, clients may not be willing to accept the placement and use of a feeding tube in their pet. They may feel that taking this step represents a point of no return or that they are giving up. People often take a unique pleasure in preparing and eating meals, and food is a large part of family and cultural identity. Most owners also enjoy feeding their pets and giving treats, and they may resist a change to what they perceive is a medical procedure, similar to administering medications. Other people may feel uncomfortable with the idea of having such a device physically associated with their pet. In this case, it may be helpful to introduce the client to patients with similar devices, or to encourage them to discuss these issues with other clients who have been through the experience.

It is especially important to impress upon the client the benefits of feeding tube placement. Many sick pets are willing to eat, but they will not consume enough calories to maintain their body weight, or they will not consume a diet that is appropriate for their disease. Chronic kidney disease is a very common example, and a waxing and waning appetite is often observed in such patients. In addition to the direct physiologic and physical effects of hypergastrinemia and uremia on the gastrointestinal tract, other alterations in metabolism (such as electrolyte abnormalities, altered hormonal milieu, increases in cytokines, acid–base derangements, and dehydration) can significantly impact appetite. Azotemia can also be expected to affect taste and smell perception in veterinary patients, as has been reported in people (Ng et al. 2004). Additionally, many medications are known to alter smell and taste in people and this should be considered in animals as well (Bromley 2000). Many animals with chronic kidney disease will readily consume very high-protein diets, such as only meats. However, restriction of protein to control the blood concentrations of uremic toxins and manage proteinuria, as well as to limit dietary phosphorus, is a major feature of nutritional therapy for these patients. Also, many animals with renal disease develop hypertension and/or fat intolerance, which can necessitate the use of an even less palatable diet restricted in protein, sodium, and fat. Provision of an appropriate diet for these patients can positively impact quality of life and improve prognosis. Additionally, feeding tube placement can facilitate the administration of extra fluids as well as medications without necessitating their oral administration, a process that many owners and pets find unpleasant or difficult.

General Contraindications

Although it is clear that providing adequate nutritional support and administering it enterally if possible is of benefit in managing many cases, most enteral feeding devices are generally contraindicated in patients with an increased risk of aspiration. Risk can be increased in patients that have uncontrolled vomiting, a reduced gag reflex, or a reduced level of consciousness (due to head trauma or the need to be anesthetized for assisted ventilation). Regurgitation is not uncommon in critically ill patients, and decisions regarding the safety of enteral feeding should be based on risk assessments of the specific situation (Hopper et al. 2007). Accomplishing enteral feeding with devices that terminate in the jejunum is a viable option for some patients with an increased risk of aspiration (Shike and Latkany 1998). It is also important to consider whether frequent anesthesia or sedation may be necessary (due to bandage changes or other procedures). In this case, consideration should be given to using an enteral feeding technique that facilitates meal feeding (together with measures to promote gastrointestinal motility, including therapeutics as well as walking the patient if possible), or that terminates in the jejunum.

Enteral Feeding Devices

Enteral feeding devices include tubes that pass through the nares and end anywhere from the esophageal lumen to the jejunum (nasoenteral), pharyngostomy tubes, esophagostomy tubes, gastrostomy tubes, duodenostomy tubes, and jejunostomy tubes. Placement of any of these tubes requires the ability to confirm correct placement into the appropriate location in the gastrointestinal tract rather than into the airway, subcutaneous space, or peritoneum. For surgically, fluoroscopically, or endoscopically placed gastrostomy, duodenostomy, or jejunostomy tubes, this confirmation can be accomplished during the placement procedure.

For other types of tubes and placement procedures, few methods can confirm correct placement without doubt, particularly for tubes that terminate in the esophagus cranial to the carina. Nasoenteral or esophagostomy tube placement

can be confirmed radiographically if termination is in the stomach; the tube can then be partly withdrawn into the esophagus if desired. However, radiographic interpretation of correct placement is not always confirmatory (Rodriguez-Diaz et al. 2021). In addition, no method is feasible for confirming continued correct placement over the long term. Some instances of tube displacement can be difficult to identify, such as gastrostomy tube dislodgment into the peritoneal cavity (Elliott et al. 2000). However, with experience and the use of multiple confirmatory methods, the risks of feeding through an incorrectly placed device can be reduced. Radiography can be useful; other methods to determine correct tube placement into the esophagus or stomach rather than the bronchus include the injection of air or sterile water while observing for coughing or ausculting for borborygmi. Details and excellent instructions for tube placement are available elsewhere (Marks 1998; Seim and Willard 2002; Han 2004; Jergens et al. 2007; Herring 2016). Technical aspects of enteral feeding devices will only be discussed generally here.

Nasoenteral Feeding Tubes

Nasoesophageal, nasogastric, and nasojejunal tubes are typically small-diameter (5–8 French), polyurethane, polyvinylchloride, or silicone flexible tubes. Their advantages include the ability to place the tube without anesthesia or specialized equipment. These tubes can be irritating to the patient since they need to be attached to the face with suture or staples, making an Elizabethan collar necessary for the duration of use (Figure 20.3). Nasoenteral tubes are not generally an option for at-home use and are best utilized for short-term provision of nutrients (i.e. less than one week; for example, in the interim between medical stabilization and placement of a more permanent tube). These tubes can also be a good option for pets with coagulopathy because no incision is necessary. While epistaxis has been reported as a potential

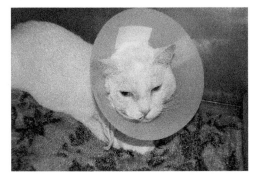

Figure 20.3 To avoid premature removal, an Elizabethan collar or similar barrier must be worn by patients with nasoenteral tubes.

complication during the placement of nasal tubes, refined techniques have resulted in a lower incidence (Abood and Buffington 1991) (Figure 20.4). Because general anesthesia is usually not necessary for nasoenteric tube placement, water and/or food can be administered immediately.

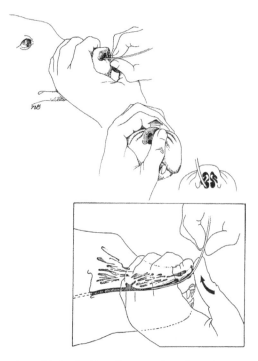

Figure 20.4 Pushing the nares dorsally and introducing the tube at a ventromedial angle facilitates proper placement. *Source:* Reproduced with permission from Abood and Buffington (1991).

Pharyngostomy Feeding Tubes

Pharyngostomy tubes are sometimes used in human medicine in lieu of nasogastric tubes and are most often used for gastric decompression rather than enteral feeding in some settings (Garza-Castillon et al. 2018). Although they appear to have a low complication rate (Meehan et al. 1984; Patil et al. 2006; Garza-Castillon et al. 2018), fatal hemorrhage has been reported due to dissection of the superior thyroid artery (Edge and Langdon 1991) and their use has been discouraged (Vanek 2003). In veterinary medicine, pharyngostomy tube placement has no advantages over esophagostomy tube placement and can potentially result in more serious complications (Crowe and Downs 1986). Additionally, placement of a pharyngostomy tube may demand more technical skill due to the proximity of critical surrounding structures. The two tube types are similar in their indications, disadvantages, and tube sizes. For these reasons, pharyngostomy tubes have fallen out of common use.

Esophagostomy Feeding Tubes

Esophagostomy tubes are very popular in both dogs and cats. The disadvantages include the need for anesthesia for placement. However, no special equipment is necessary, and placement is usually inexpensive, quick, and simple (Levine et al. 1997; Han 2004). These tubes are generally very well tolerated (Figure 20.5). Only a protective neck wrap is usually necessary, with both plain and decorative options being commercially available as well (Figure 20.6). There is little danger of serious complications if the tube is removed prior to stoma formation. They are useful for home use by the client; however, care must be taken to clean and maintain the stoma site to minimize the risk of infection (Figure 20.7). In one survey, most owners reported little difficulty with using the tube to feed their cats, and they became quite comfortable with the process with experience (Ireland et al. 2003). Complications are usually

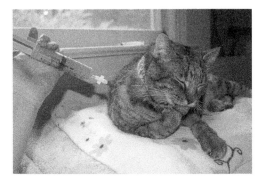

Figure 20.5 Esophagostomy tubes are generally well tolerated and are easily used in the home environment.

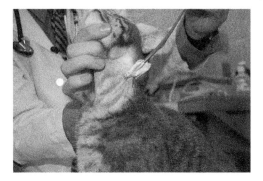

Figure 20.7 The area around the stoma for a feeding tube must be kept clean and dry to reduce local skin irritation and prevent cellulitis.

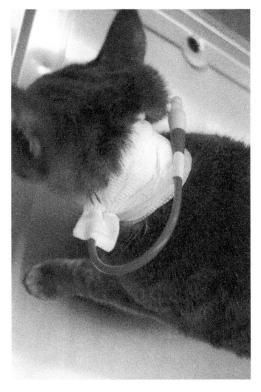

Figure 20.6 A properly wrapped esophagostomy tube.

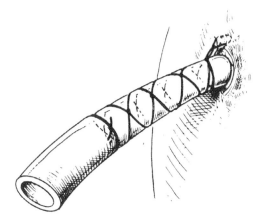

Figure 20.8 A loosely tied anchor suture is attached to the friction suture and allows for tube replacement without repuncturing the skin. *Source:* Reproduced with permission from Crowe (1986).

relatively minor, and include patient removal; irritation, infection, or leakage around the stoma site; obstruction of the tube with food, medications, or kinking; and vomition of the tube (Levine et al. 1997; Devitt and Seim 1997; Crowe and Devey 1997; Breheny et al. 2019; Perondi et al. 2021; Brunet et al. 2022).

Typical tube types used for esophagostomy tube feeding include those composed of polyvinylchloride, polyurethane, silicone, or red rubber. Depending on tube composition these tubes can be maintained for up to 6–8 weeks; however, with regular replacement enteral feeding can be accomplished for months to years. Tube replacement is facilitated with the use of a guide wire (which can be used if the blind end of the tube has been removed), as well as by using anchor suture that can be used to attach the new tube with a friction suture without repuncturing the skin (Figure 20.8). Polyethylene tubes appear to be quite irritating when compared to silicon tubes and should be avoided (Balkany et al. 1977). Tube sizes of 12–14 French are adequate for cats and small dogs, while sizes 14–18 French are adequate for larger dogs. Placement of tubes too large for the patient may result in adverse effects and likely impart no more than minimal benefit over more appropriately sized tubes. A size 18-French tube caused a head tilt and circling, which resolved immediately with tube removal in one cat, while in several other instances similar tubes in cats resulted in signs of discomfort and nausea (repeated swallowing, lip licking), which also resolved with tube removal (S.J. Delaney, personal communication). After esophagostomy tube removal, the stoma site typically heals uneventfully by second intention.

Gastrostomy Feeding Tubes

Gastrostomy tubes are particularly useful in the management of chronic diseases requiring long-term nutritional support (Figure 20.9). One study reported canine veterinary patients being fed through gastrostomy tubes for up to 6 years or more (Campbell et al. 2006). The tubes are typically latex or silicon and both traditional-length mushroom-tipped tubes as well as low-profile versions are available from a variety of manufacturers. Low-profile devices can be placed with the aid of an endoscope and may be more esthetically pleasing to owners,

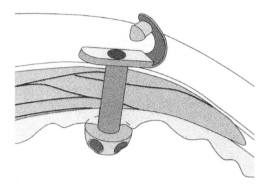

Figure 20.10 Low-profile gastrostomy tubes may be more esthetically pleasing for owners. *Source:* Reproduced with permission from Marks (2005).

while reducing the risks of clogging and chewing on the tube by the pet (Campbell et al. 2006) (Figure 20.10). Except in the smallest patients, they are large tubes (18–24 French).

With appropriate adaptors, a wide variety of diets can be fed, including puréed human food combinations as well as commercially available canned and dry diets blended with water. However, in some instances the diameter of the feeding adapter may be much smaller and may require adjustment. Gastrostomy tubes can be placed either endoscopically (percutaneous endoscopic gastrostomy [PEG] tube), surgically (including tube gastropexy), or with a transoral rigid tube introducer (the "blind" technique). Recent reports have described novel placement methods that expand clinical options (Hlusko et al. 2019; Griffin et al. 2020). Which method is used to achieve tube placement depends on the availability of specific equipment (such as endoscopes or rigid tube introducers), the skill and training of the clinician, and patient factors. Animals with esophageal disorders, including megaesophagus and strictures, should not undergo blind placement procedures using tube introducers due to the risk of perforation or other damage to the esophagus.

The disadvantages of gastrostomy tubes include the need for anesthesia for placement and the need for specialized equipment in some cases (for endoscopic and blind

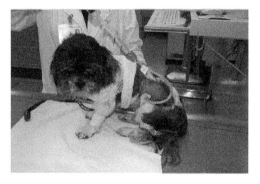

Figure 20.9 A gastrostomy tube is an excellent method of administering enteral nutritional support on a long-term basis.

placements). Most owners reported little diffi- culty using PEG tubes in their cats, and with experience most became comfortable with the procedure (Ireland et al. 2003). For dog owners surveyed regarding home use of a low-profile gastrostomy tube, most reported that the device was easy to use and maintain, and that the tube improved their pet's quality of life and positively impacted their lifespan (Yoshimoto et al. 2006; Campbell et al. 2006). One study reported no difference in PEG tube complica- tion rate and severity when compared to esophagostomy tubes in cats (Ireland et al. 2003). Overall, complications of gastros- tomy tubes range from minor to serious and include gastric bleeding during placement; improper tube placement; vomiting; irritation, infection, or leakage around the stoma site; aspiration pneumonia; premature tube removal by the patient; and peritonitis due to displacement of the tube into the abdomen (Glaus et al. 1998; Elliott et al. 2000; Hansen et al. 2019; Stevenson et al. 2000; Campbell et al. 2006; Elmenhorst et al. 2020). Although the total complication rate is high in some studies, most problems were minor and easily manageable.

Jejunal Feeding Tubes

Nasojejunal, gastrojejunostomy, and jejunos- tomy tubes enable postgastric feeding. Although there are no specific indications for one intestinal location over another, place- ment of duodenostomy tubes is also possible (Swann et al. 1998; Novo et al. 2001). Although the location of the stoma can be in the distal duodenum or in the proximal jejunum, the tube should terminate in the jejunum as far cranial as practical to maximize the absorptive surface area distal to the point of food intro- duction. The maximum recommended period for jejunal feeding device use depends partly on the tubing material. There are reports of clinical patients maintained with polyvinyl or polyurethane enterostomy tubes for up to four weeks (Novo et al. 2001). Another study

reported the maintenance of low-profile enter- ostomy tubes in healthy experimental dogs for 10 months (Swann et al. 1998).

Postgastric feeding is useful for providing nutritional support to patients in which gastric feeding is contraindicated due to pancreatitis, severe and/or diffuse structural or physiologic disease of the stomach, decreased level of con- sciousness, proximal obstruction, delayed gas- tric emptying, or intractable vomiting. A study in people with severe acute pancreatitis com- pared nasogastric and nasojejunal tube feed- ing; no differences were found in adverse effects or clinical outcomes (Kumar et al. 2006). However, because gastric emptying is often delayed secondary to pancreatitis, postgastric feeding is often a feasible alternative (Meier et al. 2006). Also, stimulation of pancreatic secretion is significantly decreased in healthy people in response to a liquid meal infusion into the jejunum compared to into the stom- ach, probably secondary to a reduced and delayed hormonal response (gastrin and chol- ecystokinin; Czakó et al. 1999). Similar results have been found in dogs: gastric and duodenal nutrient infusions caused an increase in pan- creatic secretion, while jejunal infusions did not (Ragins et al. 1973). When parenteral nutrition was compared with jejunal nutrition in a dog model of severe acute pancreatitis, enteral feeding was associated with decreased endotoxin and bacterial translocation and did not cause worsening of pancreatic pathology (Qin et al. 2002). In people with pancreatitis, early enteral feeding via the jejunal route is safe and is recommended in this context due to cost effectiveness compared to parenteral nutrition (McClave et al. 1997). Whenever pos- sible, it is advisable to provide nutritional sup- port enterally in veterinary patients with pancreatitis, and if needed this can be deliv- ered jejunally to reduce pancreatic stimulation.

It may be a challenge to achieve delivery of full caloric targets in many cases, which is likely due not only to the typical severity of ill- ness in these patients, but also to the usually short period of use and gradual increase in the rate of administration (Tsuruta et al. 2016). It remains unconfirmed if provision of any food is better than none; however, it has been shown that energy provision is positively associated with outcome in critically ill veterinary patients (Brunetto et al. 2010). The use of hypocaloric feeding (also known as trickle feeding, trophic feeding, or permissive underfeeding) is debated in the human critical care literature (Van Zanten et al. 2015; Patel et al. 2018), and a clear positive impact on outcomes of mortality and hospital discharge has not been definitively demonstrated. However, this practice even when intentional appears to have no risk per se, and may be of benefit in maintaining normal intestinal function as well as other more global parameters. Regardless, provision of energy and nutrients in amounts that satisfy metabolic needs should remain the goal.

Nasojejunal tubes are typically size 5–8 French polyurethane tubes with or without weighted tips. One advantage of nasojejunal tubes is that sedation or anesthesia is usually not necessary for placement. Verification of correct placement can be accomplished with fluoroscopic guidance (Wohl 2006), or with attempts to aspirate insufflated air (Harrison et al. 1997). Choosing a tube that includes a radio-opaque marker is useful for facilitating the verification of correct placement and for monitoring potential tube migration; however, this can also be accomplished with the injection of contrast material.

Gastrojejunostomy tubes consist of smaller-diameter tubes (12 French) fed through larger-bore gastrostomy tubes (Figure 20.11). General anesthesia is required for the placement of gastrojejunostomy tubes and generally also for enterostomy tubes; however, one study reported successful placement of duodenostomy tubes with only sedation in a small number of animals (Novo et al. 2001). Esophagojejunostomy tubes placed with endoscopy have also been used successfully (Hinden et al. 2020). Purpose-made products are available, and clinicians may also create

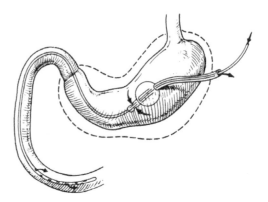

Figure 20.11 A small-gauge tube terminating in the small intestine can be placed through a larger gastrostomy tube. *Source:* Reproduced with permission from Crowe and Downs (1986).

suitable gastrojejunostomy devices from other tube types (Risselada et al. 2018). Gastrojejunostomy tubes can be useful in cases that initially require postgastric feeding but that may benefit from transition to enteral feeding directly into the stomach (Jennings et al. 2001). Also, if endoscopy or a blind technique is used to place this type of dual tube, surgery can be avoided (Jergens et al. 2007).

Enterostomy tubes are usually red rubber or silastic feeding tubes, although low-profile devices are also available (Swann et al. 1997, 1998). Jejunostomy tubes can be successfully placed with either surgical or laparoscopic techniques (Hewitt et al. 2004) (Figure 20.12). As human patients are likely less mobile than critically ill veterinary patients, migration may be a greater issue in dogs and cats. Also, tubes in veterinary patients are maintained in a more horizontal position even during activity. Some types of jejunal feeding devices have weighted tips to help achieve correct tube placement and to discourage retrograde movement. However, a prospective trial in humans showed that unweighted nasoenteral tubes traversed the pylorus into the intestine more often and more rapidly than weighted tubes (Lord et al. 1993). Also, a study investigating gastrojejunostomy tubes in dogs reported that correct placement of the distal catheter tip was important to avoid retrograde

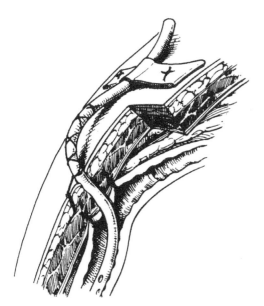

Figure 20.12 After a purse-string suture is placed in the intestinal serosa, the enterostomy site is attached to the abdominal wall. A technique for creating a serosal foldover to create an elongated pocket for tunneling of the tube prior to exiting the body wall has also been described (Delany et al. 1973). *Source:* Reproduced with permission from Crowe and Downs (1986).

movement when using unweighted tubes (Jergens et al. 2007). It appears that weighted tips are not necessarily critical either for self-advancing nasojejunal tube placement or for maintenance of proper positioning of jejunal tubes. Reported complications of jejunal feeding include premature tube removal, retrograde tube movement, diarrhea, vomiting, focal cellulitis, leakage of gastrointestinal contents, and tube obstruction (Swann et al. 1997, 1998; Wohl 2006; Jergens et al. 2007; Tsuruta et al. 2016).

Beginning Enteral Feeding

An initial first meal for veterinary patients with an enteral feeding device will be a liquid diet or a slurry of canned food, dry food, or human foods (such as a combination of cottage cheese and rice). With nasoenteric tubes placed without general anesthesia, feeding can be commenced immediately. For esophagostomy and gastrostomy tubes, water and food can be introduced via the new tube as soon as the patient is fully recovered from anesthesia. Typically, water is introduced first to ensure the patient's tolerance prior to feeding a first meal. For gastrostomy tubes, it has been commonly advised that food and water be given only after a period of 12–24 hours (Han 2004). Presumably the rationale is that the placement procedure may interfere with normal gastric motility, increasing the risk of aspiration or leakage. However, controlled studies in people have shown that initiation of feeding within four hours of PEG tube placement is not associated with increased morbidity compared to the traditional protocol of waiting for up to 24 hours (Choudhry et al. 1996; McCarter et al. 1998; Dubagunta et al. 2002), even in critically ill patients (Stein et al. 2002). There are no such published comparison studies in animals; however, successful tube feeding three hours after gastrostomy tube placement is reported (Elmenhorst et al. 2020). In addition, it is known that the presence of a gastrostomy tube does not slow the gastric emptying rate in healthy cats measured at one day post placement (Smith et al. 1998). Unlike human patients, veterinary patients must be anesthetized for the placement of such devices. There appears to be no reason to wait related to the gastrostomy device itself; however, depending on the anesthetic protocol and the patient, full recovery may take up to 24 hours.

In more debilitated patients, and perhaps in cases where tube placement proves difficult and is prolonged, it may be best to initiate feeding in a more conservative fashion. In these patients, 25–33% of the daily caloric requirement should be fed the first day over 4–6 meals, then 50–67% the second day, and so on. This helps allow for assessment of patient tolerance of the diet and volume. Alternatively, nasoenteric, esophagostomy, or gastrostomy tube feeding can be accomplished with a constant-rate infusion as in jejunal feeding; both methods result in delivery of adequate energy without gastrointestinal complications (Campbell et al 2010; Holahan et al. 2010). Of course, the rate of increasing to full caloric requirements will vary with underlying disease, body condition, length of anorexia, risk of refeeding syndrome, and level of patient-monitoring abilities. In many cases, it is best if the patient can stay in the hospital long enough to assess tolerance of feeding the entire amount of the daily caloric requirement. This is also a good time to teach the owner about feeding tube care and to encourage participation in some or all of the feedings. The owner should understand the importance of initially feeding at a slow rate to reduce the incidence of nausea and vomiting.

Some hospitalized patients may show volume intolerance in response to assisted enteral feeding. Most dogs and cats will tolerate meal sizes of 5–10 ml/kg body weight (BW) after a period of fasting (Remillard et al. 2000). The rate and/or volume should be decreased if drooling, retching, swallowing, or vomiting is noted during a feeding. If necessary, promotility agents can be administered in some cases to facilitate successful tube feeding (e.g. erythromycin, ranitidine, cisapride, metoclopramide). In people, such medications are recommended only for patients with evidence of intolerance of enteral feeding (Kreymann et al. 2006). Over time, the patient should begin to tolerate larger and less frequent meals; this can usually accommodate a reasonable feeding schedule at home.

Diet Choices

There is no one best diet for use with enteral feeding devices, and there are many options. Factors to be considered when choosing a diet include not only tube size and location, but also caloric density, macronutrient distribution, particle size, osmolarity, ingredients, cost, and availability. It is important as well to consider the expected period of feeding and whether the diet chosen is complete and balanced for the individual patient. For many patients, the underlying disease will limit the choices to diets that incorporate specific, appropriate modifications (renal or hepatic disease, fat intolerance). In some cases, tube size will limit diet choices to those of a particular viscosity (i.e. liquid diets for nasoenteric or enterostomy tubes). If possible, providing a complete and balanced commercially available diet is preferable. This includes slurries of puréed canned or dry diets; however, both commercially available and home-prepared options are available.

A wide range of both canned and dry foods can be fed enterally. For slurries of commercially available diets, it may be necessary to experiment with different water ratios to achieve the desired consistency that will easily flow through the selected tube. Maintaining a supply of different tube types and sizes for testing is recommended. This will help avoid tube obstructions and aid in calculation of the caloric density of specific diet slurries. The mixture should be puréed for a sufficient time to achieve a smooth consistency. Due to the time needed for this process and the potential for incorporation of some air into the slurry, as well as the effect of mechanical forces on the diet viscosity (thixotropy), the caloric density can only be accurately calculated by measuring the volume of the final slurry (i.e. the total volume may not be additive from the volume of diet and water).

It is helpful for the clinician to have a basic understanding of the characteristics of a range of different veterinary therapeutic diets. For example, knowing which options are lowest in fat in the categories of diets formulated for management of chronic kidney disease or of adverse food responses can be useful. Note that pet food manufacturers are frequently developing new products or modifying the formulations of existing diets, and it may be difficult for practitioners to remain up to date on current information. In general, an appropriate diet may be chosen on the basis of the caloric distribution (percent of calories from fat, protein, and carbohydrate), micronutrient levels (phosphorus or sodium restriction, profile compared to patient's requirements), and ingredient source. Consider commercially available pet food options and human enteral formulas as well as homemade diets. For fat-intolerant animals, cottage cheese and rice slurries are useful for tube feeding, and can be supplemented with a linoleic acid source and micronutrients as necessary for longer-term feeding. Likewise, homemade uncommon and limited-ingredient diets for patients with specific needs can be used; for example, a slurry of canned crab and pasta can be used for fat-intolerant patients with food-responsive enteropathy or lymphangiectasia.

Liquid diets are available that are marketed both for human and veterinary patients. They are the sole option for patients with small-diameter feeding tubes (nasoenteric and jejunal tubes). Such diets are generally well tolerated and can provide adequate nutrients to facilitate weight maintenance in hospitalized patients. Additionally, some animals will voluntarily consume a liquid diet while rejecting solids. Despite a range of variables (including patient disease state and life stage, method of administration, and consumption of various other diets), one prospective uncontrolled study of hospitalized dogs and cats reported few complications and a satisfactory success rate with the use of commercially available liquid diets (Crowe et al. 1997). The use of human products is not recommended for feline patients due to the lower protein content. In addition, liquid diets tend to be expensive, especially in larger patients, and it is important to note that many commonly used products do not meet every currently known nutrient requirement of dogs and cats, even veterinary products. One study found that of seven feline enteral diets analyzed for a limited number of nutrients using laboratory methods, all were found to be below recommended allowances in at least one essential nutrient, despite four of the products claiming to be complete and balanced (Prantil et al. 2016).

Liquid diets can be classified as monomeric (elemental) or polymeric (nonelemental). Monomeric formulations contain amino acids and/or short peptides (typically hydrolysates of protein isolates) in addition to highly digestible carbohydrates. Polymeric formulations contain longer peptide chains or complete proteins as well as more complex carbohydrates (starches). In order to provide a reasonable caloric density, liquid veterinary diets are generally high in fat (up to 51% of calories). High-fat diets are contraindicated in some cases (i.e. pancreatitis, lymphangiectasia, or other intestinal diseases). However, some human enteral formulations provide comparable energy while still restricting fat; these are acceptable alternatives for fat-intolerant canine patients (Table 20.1). For feline patients, note that many human enteral liquid diets are not supplemented with essential amino acids and some contain fructose, high concentrations of which should be avoided in cats due to resultant fructosuria (Droucher and Muller-Schlosser 1980).

In addition to liquid diet options, balanced critical care diets are available for both dogs and cats that have larger tubes or are willing to eat voluntarily (Table 20.2). These are good options for many cases able to tolerate complex diets composed of typical pet food ingredients. The advantages of these diets are that they meet the known nutrient requirements of dogs and cats, are generally cost effective, and are energy dense. However, they are high in fat and should not be used in patients with documented or suspected fat intolerance, such as those with pancreatitis, hyperlipidemia, or protein-losing enteropathy.

Immunomodulating Nutrients

Enteral formulas are increasingly supplemented with nutrients purported to promote gut health, speed healing, and/or modulate immune and inflammatory responses. There are several nutrients with a proposed direct

Table 20.1 Comparisons of selected veterinary and human liquid diet products available in the United States with National Research Council Recommended Allowances for fat and protein.

	Feline adult allowance	Canine adult allowance	Ensure Original Shake[a]	Vivonex Plus[b]	Royal Canin Veterinary Health Nutrition Recovery Liquid canine/feline[c]	Royal Canin Veterinary Health Nutrition Renal Support Liquid – canine[d]	Royal Canin Veterinary Health Nutrition Renal Support Liquid – feline[d]	Royal Canin Veterinary Health Nutrition Gastrointestinal Low Fat Liquid – canine[e]
Energy density (kcal/ml)			0.90	1.00	0.90	1.30	0.90	0.90
Calorie profile								
Protein %			17	18	32	13	26	35
Fat %			25	6	48	51	50	19
Carbohydrate %			58	76	20	36	24	46
Protein (g/1000 kcal)	50	25	41	45	90.9	36.7	74.6	101.2
Fat (g/1000 kcal)	22.5	13.8	27	6.7	56.8	59.8	59	22

[a] Ensure® Original Nutrition Shake; Abbott Nutrition, Columbus, OH, USA. Liquid product for humans; can be used in dogs for <2 weeks; not appropriate for feline patients.
[b] Vivonex® Plus; Nestlé HealthCare Nutrition, Gland, Switzerland. Liquid product for humans; can be used in dogs for <2 weeks; not appropriate for feline patients.
[c] Royal Canin USA, A division of MARS, Inc., St. Charles, MO, USA. Liquid product formulated to meet Association of American Feed Control Officials (AAFCO) Nutrient Profiles for maintenance of adult dogs and cats.
[d] Liquid product formulated for intermittent or supplemental feeding only.
[e] Liquid product formulated to meet AAFCO Nutrient Profiles for maintenance of adult dogs only.
Source: NRC (2006).

Table 20.2 Comparisons of commonly used critical care diets available in the United States with National Research Council recommended allowances for fat and protein.

	Feline adult allowance	Canine adult allowance	Hill's Prescription Diet a/d canine/feline[a]	Royal Canin Veterinary Health Nutrition feline and canine recovery[b]	Purina Pro Plan Veterinary Diets CN critical nutrition canine and feline formula[c]
Energy density (kcal/kg)			1175	986	1325
Energy density (kcal/ml)			1.2	1.0	1.35
Calorie profile					
Protein %			32	38	28.8
Fat %			58	58	62.6
Carbohydrate %			10	4	8.6
Protein (g/1000 kcal)	50	25	90	107	82.3
Fat (g/1000 kcal)	22.5	13.8	36	63.2	73.6

[a] Hill's Pet Nutrition, Topeka, KS, USA. Canned product formulated for intermittent or supplemental feeding of dogs and cats.
[b] Royal Canin USA, A division of MARS, Inc., St. Charles, MO, USA. Canned product formulated to meet Association of American Feed Control Officials (AAFCO) Nutrient Profiles for all life stages of dogs and cats.
[c] Nestlé Purina Petcare, St. Louis, MO, USA. Canned product formulated to meet AAFCO Nutrient Profiles for maintenance of adult dogs and cats.
Source: NRC (2006).

benefit to the intestinal tract, including glutamine, arginine, taurine, omega-3 fatty acids, and short-chain fatty acids. Such diets have been associated with improved outcomes in people (Wu et al. 2001; Song et al. 2015). Although these nutrients have been the focus of intense investigation in the human medical literature (including the use of rodent and canine models), there remains a dearth of scientific investigation of the possible benefits and adverse effects of these nutrients in dogs and cats with naturally occurring disease, as well as a lack of investigation into potential medication interactions.

Glutamine

Glutamine is a dispensable amino acid that has important metabolic roles. It serves as a vehicle of nitrogen transport, a precursor of glucose and glycogen, and is a substrate in the urea cycle and in nucleotide synthesis.

Glutamine is also used preferentially by enterocytes as an energy source, and under states of catabolic stress it is considered conditionally essential. It has been demonstrated that glutamine may be important for preventing bacterial or endotoxin translocation, reducing villus blunting and destruction, and maintaining normal enterocyte function when administered orally or parenterally to animal models (O'Dwyer et al. 1989; Chen et al. 1994; Houdijk et al. 1998; Boza et al. 2001). Some studies have shown that glutamine supplementation of enteral formulas for human patients is safe and even beneficial in terms of overall morbidity and mortality (Wischmeyer et al. 2001; Garrel et al. 2003). However, enteral glutamine supplementation has not been consistently demonstrated to improve overall outcomes in human intensive care unit patients (Conejero et al. 2002; Schulman et al. 2005), and a recent review has suggested an overall lack of significant benefit in most cases (Oldani et al. 2015; van Zanten et al. 2015). Additionally, a prospective study in cats with experimentally induced enteritis did not show a superior protective effect of glutamine supplementation (Marks et al. 1999). Due to the inconclusive body of evidence for the benefits of glutamine supplementation for gastrointestinal disease in people, routine use has not been recommended (Lochs et al. 2006).

While routine use of glutamine supplementation in certain diseases is discouraged in human medicine due to a lack of convincing efficacy data, the practice generally appears to be safe. However, in patients with renal or hepatic disease, it must be considered that additional glutamine at sometimes pharmacologic doses will contribute a significant nitrogen load and should be avoided. Free glutamine is unstable in solution, which precludes its use in many parenteral and enteral formulations; however, glutamine dipeptides such as alanyl-glutamine in parenteral formulas have been shown to be equally efficacious at maintaining nitrogen balance, plasma glutamine levels, villus area, and intestinal mucosal thickness in rats and dogs (Jiang et al. 1993). Glutamine dipeptides are increasingly present in both parenteral and enteral human formulations (Zheng et al. 2006; Lima et al. 2007).

Arginine

Arginine is an essential amino acid for dogs and cats. In people, it is considered conditionally essential in growing infants and during critical illness, being important for connective tissue repair as well as immune function and other fundamental processes. Supplementation of human enteral formulations with arginine is not uncommon, so the use of these products in dogs typically does not require enrichment. While still controversial, arginine supplementation has been demonstrated to help maintain immune function and improve wound healing in some circumstances (Stechmiller et al. 2005; Marin

et al. 2006). Because it is also important as a precursor of nitric acid, some research has explored its potential benefit in shock resuscitation (Yan et al. 2007). Data regarding the use of arginine together with omega-3 fatty acids in human patients seem to suggest a definitive benefit for specific populations (Marik and Zaloga 2010). There has been some work in using arginine therapeutically for neoplasia (Ma et al. 2010), and a systematic review found overall decreased infectious complications with various arginine-supplemented diets with no effect on mortality; however, there was a reduced hospital stay for patients undergoing non-gastrointestinal surgery (Drover et al. 2011).

Investigations of the use of arginine in clinical veterinary medicine are lacking. One study in dogs with lymphoma suggests that high concentrations of arginine fed in combination with omega-3 fatty acids increased survival times (Ogilvie et al. 2000); however, another study of human breast cancer patients suggests that supplemental arginine may increase protein synthesis within tumor cells (Park et al. 1992). When given parenterally, one study showed that arginine decreased survival and worsened shock in a dog model of *Escherichia coli* peritonitis (Kalil et al. 2006), and supplementation in human patients with sepsis remains controversial. Additionally, due to competition for transport processes between these two basic amino acids, excessive arginine supplementation may lead to increased urinary losses of lysine. Due to the lack of specific conclusive evidence of safety and efficacy, supplementation should be done with caution, especially in sepsis (Wilmore 2004; Patel et al. 2016). Until more convincing data are published to support the safe and efficacious use of high-dose arginine in the treatment of animal disease, supplementation beyond satisfaction of requirements cannot be recommended in all critically ill veterinary patients.

Other Nutrients

There are several other nutrients of interest in the management of critical illness in animals and people. These include omega-3 fatty acids, short-chain fatty acids, taurine, choline, nucleotides, various antioxidants, and other compounds. There are excellent reviews of the therapeutic use of many of these nutrients elsewhere (LeLeiko and Walsh 1996; Hickman 1998; Michel 1998; Simpson 1998). Despite some promising data from human trials and rodent models, there remain some concerns regarding safety (Hofman et al. 2016), and there is no definitive evidence for a beneficial therapeutic effect for most of these nutrients in naturally occurring clinical diseases of veterinary patients. Probably the most convincing data are from investigations of the effects of short-chain fatty acids on intestinal health (i.e. butyrate, propionate, and acetate). Sources of these compounds include those considered to be fermentable and/or soluble fibers such as fructooligosaccharides, beta-glucans, pectins, and gums. These are likely to impact both the small and large intestines due to increases in intestinal content viscosity and alterations in intestinal motility and nutrient absorption. Because of this, small amounts of fermentable fibers are typically included in critical care diets.

Calculation of Energy Requirements

It is believed that sick patients have increased requirements for energy and other nutrients. It has been demonstrated that critically ill dogs catabolize significant amounts of endogenous protein (i.e. lean body mass; Michel et al. 1997). Physiologic stress from trauma and illness enhances skeletal muscle breakdown by several mechanisms (Hasselgren and Fischer 2001). Because of this, animals that are anorexic due to disease are likely to become malnourished to a greater degree in a shorter time than healthy animals deprived of food. Although illness factors have been used in the past to account for these increased needs, these may overestimate the requirements of convalescing, recumbent, and inactive veterinary patients (Walton et al. 1996; Chan 2004). There are potentially adverse consequences to overfeeding, and there is general agreement that this should be avoided in veterinary patients despite few published scientific investigations. One study showed similar outcomes in hospitalized dogs and cats that were provided higher amounts of energy compared to approximately basal requirements (Brunetto et al. 2010). Although randomized prospective clinical trials have not yet been conducted in people, the European Society for Clinical Nutrition and Metabolism Guidelines on Enteral Nutrition advise against providing more than approximately basal energy requirements, especially in the acute phase of critical illness (Kreymann et al. 2006). This is partly because some evidence shows that achieving caloric intakes below calculated target values may improve outcomes in some patients (Krishnan et al. 2003).

The true energy requirements of veterinary patients are often not known, so the calculated needs can over- or underestimate actual requirements. To avoid overfeeding hospitalized patients with potentially wide variations in true requirements, it is best to start with resting energy requirement (RER: $BW_{kg}^{0.75} \times 70$), monitor body weight, and adjust the amount fed if necessary (Table 20.3). This approach avoids the potentially adverse effects of hyperalimentation while allowing for assessment of patient tolerance of the diet, volume, and route of administration.

Complications

Complications of assisted enteral feeding include those in the categories of mechanical (tube obstruction, leakage, or displacement), metabolic (refeeding syndrome, local infection or abscess), and gastrointestinal (vomiting and diarrhea).

Table 20.3 Example calculations for feeding a hospitalized canine patient.

20 kg canine patient with esophagostomy tube
RER $= 20^{0.75} \times 70 = 662$ kcal/d
Desired diet provides 1.25 kcal/ml when adequately blended for tube feeding
Volume to feed at full RER: 662 kcal/day/1.25 kcal/ml = 530 ml/d
Volume per meal when feeding 4 meals per day: 530 ml/d / 4 meals/day = 133 ml/meal
Day 1: Start at 25% of RER (166 kcal) Feed 33 ml/meal over 4 meals for a total of 133 ml/d
Day 2: Increase to 50% of RER (331 kcal) Feed 66 ml/meal over 4 meals for a total of 266 ml/d
Day 3: Increase to 75% of RER (497 kcal) Feed 99 ml/meal over 4 meals for a total of 398 ml/d
Day 4: Increase to 100% of RER (662 kcal) Feed 133 ml/meal over 4 meals for a total of 530 ml/d
Monitor body weight and adjust amount fed as needed to achieve target condition
Account for water requirements if patient cannot or will not consume water voluntarily
Water sources include diet, water for puréeing in the blender or food processor, and water for flushing tube
Patient requires 662 ml water/d for maintenance requirements, estimated using RER equation: $20^{0.75} \times 70 = 662$ ml/d
Example diet is 80% moisture and provides 1500 kcal/kg as fed
662 kcal/d/1500 kcal/kg = 0.441 kg/d
Patient requires 441 g as fed per day to meet energy needs
441 g of diet provides 353 g (353 ml) water
441 g * 80% = 353 g = 353 ml
For adequate puréeing, example diet requires 25 ml water/441 g For tube flushing, use 10 ml after each feeding
Water from diet (353 ml + 25 ml/d) + water from flushing (40 ml/d) = 418 ml/d Deficit of 244 ml/d (662 ml − 418 ml) must be provided through the tube
Monitor hydration status by checking urine specific gravity, skin turgor, and mucus membrane character, and adjust as needed

RER, resting energy requirement.

Mechanical Complications

Smaller-diameter and more flexible tubes (silicon) are more prone to obstruction due to food or medication clogs or kinking. Liquid diets are necessary for feeding through nasoenteral and enterostomy tubes due to their small inner lumen. Feeding other types of diets through these devices will increase the risk of tube obstruction. Commercial or homemade diets fed as purées through tubes should be appropriate texture for the specific tube used.

When creating purées for specific patients, testing the viscosity in a tube the same diameter, length, and material is advised. To prevent tube clogging in meal-fed patients, water should be flushed through the tube after feeding or administration of medication. The tube end should be capped or closed to ensure that a water column is left in the tube lumen. It is important to know how much water is necessary to thoroughly flush the tube, and to account for this added water when calculating the total amount of water needed by and given to the patient. If a clog occurs, gentle repeated suction and aspiration should be attempted initially. To clear more stubborn obstructions, infusion of a carbonated nonalcoholic beverage, pancreatic enzyme product, or meat tenderizer has been suggested to break up the coagulated material in the tube lumen (Marcuard and Stegall 1990; Marks 1998; Seim and Willard 2002). When tested with simulated clogs with critical care diets, the most successful solution was a combination of 0.25 tsp pancreatic enzyme plus 325 mg sodium bicarbonate in 5 ml water, and plain water was more successful than carbonated beverages or cranberry juice (Parker and Freeman 2013). Another option is to carefully introduce a guide wire or endoscopy forceps through the tube to physically dislodge the clogged material. If these attempts fail, tube replacement is necessary.

Leakage of gastric secretions or food out of the tube can occur. It is important to keep the area around the stoma clean and dry to prevent skin irritation and the development of cellulitis. Owners using enteral feeding devices at home should be counseled regarding maintenance and monitoring of the stoma site. Topical antibiotic ointments are usually applied to the stoma during healing; however, oral antibiotics and/or tube removal may be necessary if cellulitis or an abscess develops.

The displacement of an enteral feeding device can have a range of potential consequences. A nasoenteric tube pulled out of the nares can simply be replaced if necessary. If an esophagostomy tube is inadvertently removed from the outside, consequence to the patient is minimal even if an esophageal stoma has not yet formed. However, a potentially disastrous outcome can occur if a nasoenteric or esophagostomy tube is vomited out through the mouth (Seim and Willard 2002; Han 2004) (Figure 20.13). The animal can sever the end of the tube and swallow or aspirate it, necessitating a surgical or endoscopic procedure. An esophagostomy tube should be replaced under

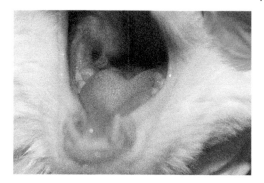

Figure 20.13 Vomition and severing of an esophagostomy tube warrant determination of a potential gastric foreign body due to swallowing of tube fragments. *Source:* Courtesy of Dr. Karl Jandrey.

heavy sedation or anesthesia to avoid positioning the tube in the subcutaneous space or in the mediastinum (Han 2004). Displacements of gastrostomy or enterostomy feeding devices may lead to peritonitis if this occurs soon after tube placement. Clearly, such tubes must be protected from damage by the patient or by other animals. Determined pets and/or inattentive hospital staff or owners can create a potentially life-threatening situation. The use of Elizabethan collars, wrap bandages, stockinettes, and similar barrier devices is required, at least initially.

To avoid the risk of peritonitis, a mature fistulous tract is required for removal of the feeding device. Animals with impaired ability to heal (severe debilitation, hypoproteinemia, hyperadrenocorticism, immunosuppressive medications) may take more time for the formation of a complete stoma. In people, inadvertent removal of the tube within seven days of placement is an indication for immediate laparotomy or endoscopic tube replacement; however, when the tube is no longer needed, the stoma is typically left to mature for up to three months prior to removal (Galat et al. 1990; Blocksom et al. 2004). In veterinary patients, formal guidelines for minimum intervals before gastrostomy tube removal have not been developed. Typical recommendations are usually to avoid tube removal for at least 7–14 days (Marks 1998; Han 2004). Because the consequences of gastric content spillage into the peritoneal space are serious, a conservative approach is advised for voluntary tube removal. However, some dogs and cats will remove their tubes despite the judicious use of barriers such as Elizabethan collars. If the tube is chewed, a portion of the tube may be left in the gastric lumen and pose a risk for intestinal obstruction. These patients must undergo endoscopy or laparotomy to remove this foreign body before obstruction occurs. Emergency surgery is clearly indicated in all animals if the tube is removed by the patient in the first 7–10 days following placement. If the tube is removed during the interval between this initial period and several weeks, the potential consequences are less clear.

Injection of contrast material into the feeding tube or through the fistula is a noninvasive way to confirm leakage into the peritoneal space with radiography. One study reported "complete but thin" gastrocutaneous fistulas found on necropsy of 4 out of 12 healthy cats as far out as 49–63 days post placement, although other cats in the study had adequate adhesions as early as 11 days post placement (Stevenson et al. 2000). The authors postulated that increased movement of the device resulting from the animal's activity may have delayed maturation of the fistula, especially the portion adjacent to the abdominal wall. Another study investigating fistulous tract formation in dogs reported that closer apposition of the serous surface of the stomach to the abdominal wall resulted in more complete fistulas (Mellinger et al. 1991). Thus, it appears that correct stem length and tube sizing as well as stabilization of the device may be important for allowing timely tract maturation. When sizing the tube to the patient, care must be taken to avoid either a tight fit (which can lead to pressure necrosis) or a loose fit (which may lead to inadvertent tube removal or delayed tract maturation), while expecting and accommodating mild to moderate postsurgical swelling.

Metabolic Complications

Refeeding syndrome can occur during the provision of either enteral or parenteral nutrition. During starvation, homeostasis preserves extracellular concentrations of electrolytes, glucose, and other metabolic mediators despite whole body depletion. Refeeding syndrome occurs upon reintroduction of nutrients during this physiologic state of starvation. Insulin is released in response to the sudden influx of carbohydrate, and a shift from the use of fatty acids and ketone bodies for energy. Insulin acts on peripheral cells to take up and utilize glucose, with subsequent increased intracellular movement and utilization of potassium, phosphorus, magnesium, and thiamin. The result is hypokalemia, hypophosphatemia, hypomagnesemia, and relative thiamin deficiency.

Refeeding syndrome is a well-recognized problem in human medicine during the management of anorexia nervosa and other causes of malnutrition and starvation (Crook et al. 2001; Kraft et al. 2005). This problem can be serious and life threatening; however, even in the human medical literature, there is a dearth of published scientific investigations. Although many individual case reports have been published, prospective or retrospective studies of treatments, risk factors, and outcomes are lacking, especially in the context of critical illness. It appears that more severe consequences may occur in humans compared to animals, with profound water balance derangements, seizures, and cardiac failure frequently reported (Havala and Shronts 1990; Crook et al. 2001; Kraft et al. 2005). However, there are reports of apparent refeeding syndrome (hypophosphatemia and hemolytic anemia) in dogs that were fed with an enteral device after starvation (Silvis et al. 1980) and in cats provided with enteral nutritional support during the course of several different diseases (Justin and Hohenhaus 1995). Case reports describe the management and outcomes of cats with refeeding syndrome (Armitage-Chan et al. 2006; DeAvilla and Leech 2016; Cook et al. 2021). It is unknown to what extent and for how long starvation must occur to elicit refeeding syndrome; however, it is likely to vary with individual animal factors. The extent of individual adaptation to the starvation state probably influences the manifestation of refeeding syndrome. It is likely to occur much sooner or with a higher rate of adverse consequences if the starvation was complete and prolonged rather than partial and brief. Additionally, patients that already have metabolic and hormonal derangements are likely at increased risk.

Local infection of the stomal site secondary to wound infection or due to constant drainage of food or gastric secretions can occur. Again, diligence in tube maintenance and monitoring is important for prevention and for early recognition of signs of infection. Severe problems such as abscessation or cellulitis may necessitate tube removal.

Gastrointestinal Complications

Tube placement can be associated with gastrointestinal complications. For example, there are concerns that nasoenteric tubes that must pass through the lower esophageal sphincter (LES), such as nasogastric and nasojejunal tubes, which may lead to irritation and potentially reflux or aspiration. However, one small study reported no difference in complications, including regurgitation or aspiration, in dogs with nasoesophageal tubes and those with nasogastric tubes (Yu et al. 2013). Several factors are likely responsible for increased reflux and aspiration risks; nevertheless, LES irritation does not appear to be a major cause of aspiration in humans, partly because tube size is not correlated with rates of aspiration (Gomes et al. 2003). A study in healthy dogs established that the use of size 14-French polyethylene esophagostomy tubes that terminated in the gastric lumen resulted in only minor complications (small abscess formation) in 3 out of 14 dogs, with no reports of reflux or aspiration (Cavalcanti et al. 2005). However, one

study involving the use of pharyngostomy tubes that terminated in the gastric lumen reported complications that included mucosal erosions of the caudal esophagus and vomiting that resolved when the tube was repositioned (Crowe and Downs 1986). A study of healthy dogs with pharyngostomy tubes reported distal esophageal erosions and/or ulcerations in 3 out of 6 subjects; evidence of inflammation (perivascular lymphocyte infiltration) was noted in all but one dog (Lantz et al. 1983). Unfortunately, the study was not only uncontrolled but also employed tubing made of irritating polyvinylchloride.

In addition, it appears that the presence of a tube into or traversing the pharynx may play a significant role in the occurrence of gastric reflux. In fact, a study in humans found that the presence of a catheter in the pharynx was adequate stimulation to cause a significant increase in the frequency of LES relaxation, suggesting that local stimulation of the pharyngeal area may be involved (Mittal et al. 1992). Further, stimulation of mechanoreceptors due to distension of the stomach causes relaxation of the LES in both dogs and humans (Franzi et al. 1990; Allocca et al. 2002; Penagini et al. 2004). This implies that simply feeding a patient may increase the risk of gastric reflux.

Esophagostomy tubes can also be positioned so that the termination is in the gastric lumen. A small controlled study in healthy dogs investigated the effects of two cervical esophagostomy tubing types (silicon and polyethylene) and two levels of tube termination (gastric lumen and mid-esophagus) on radiographic evidence of reflux and on gross and histopathologic features on the esophagus and stomach (Balkany et al. 1977). The study found no effect of tubing material or length on contrast fluoroscopic evaluation. Also, abnormalities of the esophageal and/or gastric mucosa were most pronounced in the long polyethylene tube group (severe ulcerative esophagitis in 3 out of 4 dogs) and absent in the short polyethylene tube group (0 out of 2 dogs); however, excessive granulation tissue was noted at the mucosal stoma site of 4 of 6 dogs with polyethylene tubes. For dogs with silicon tubes, inflammation was noted at the distal esophagus in 2 of 2 dogs with long tubes and 2 of 4 dogs with short tubes. Overall, 5 of 6 dogs with tubes that terminated in the gastric lumen showed evidence of adverse effects secondary to gastric reflux, compared to 2 of 6 dogs with tubes that terminated in the esophagus. However, even dogs with short silicon tubes showed evidence of reflux. Also, tube sizes were not reported. Interpretation of the data from this small study is difficult, and more definitive investigations are needed.

It is clear that multiple factors may be involved in LES competence, and the role that enteral feeding devices may play is far from obvious. Also, placing a nasoenteric tube such that it terminates in the gastric lumen rather than in the distal esophagus allows for confirmation of correct placement with radiography, but also facilitates the evaluation of gastric residuals if indicated as well as the relief of gastric gas distension (Crowe 1986). Nevertheless, in patients with normal esophageal function, there are no disadvantages to terminating the tube in the distal esophagus, and until further investigations have been done, clinical judgment and experience will suffice as guidance for the management of individual patients.

Enteral feeding intolerance can be manifested as a gastrointestinal complication. There have been reports of intolerance of early enteral feeding in people, including functional obstructions and delayed gastric emptying (Dedes et al. 2006; Nguyen et al. 2007). Although caution should also be exercised when feeding a patient with suspected severe gastrointestinal malfunction (such as severe ileus or malabsorption), evidence from the human literature indicates that early enteral feeding can facilitate a faster return of intestinal motility following gastrointestinal surgery (Ng and Neill 2006). A study of dogs with hemorrhagic gastroenteritis of unknown etiology reported increased survival in patients administered both parenteral and enteral nutrition compared to those provided only parenteral

nutritional support, although vomiting was a severe problem in the former group (Will et al. 2005). In any case, signs of gastrointestinal intolerance (i.e. vomiting, diarrhea, or discomfort with feeding) are unpleasant for both the patient and staff, and indicate that the administration volume and rate should be decreased.

The prevalence of vomiting and diarrhea in enterally fed veterinary patients is unknown, but it is believed to be high and of considerable consequence (Marks 1998). It is important to consider that many diseases will cause these clinical signs independent of enteral feeding, and patients with such clinical signs are likely to require nutritional support. However, feeding with an enteral device can predispose a patient to vomiting and/or diarrhea if the feeding is too fast, overly voluminous, or if the diet selected is inappropriate (i.e. high osmolarity, high fat). Food aversions can develop if patients experience nausea and vomiting associated with feeding specific diets.

Regurgitation is also a common complication in addition to being a frequent occurrence in critically ill patients. Although regurgitation severity and frequency may be a marker of high gastric residual volumes (GRVs), the value of their routine measurement is unclear. Findings from recent human clinical trials and systematic reviews has put the usefulness of monitoring GRV into question (Kuppinger et al. 2013; Elke et al. 2015; Ozen et al. 2016). Due to a lack of standardized methods and procedures for obtaining and measuring GRV, evidence of lack of benefit (Poulard et al. 2010; Reignier et al. 2013), a lack of guidelines for interpretation, and the potential complications such as clogging of feeding tubes with gastric material (Powell et al. 1993), current guidelines for provision of enteral nutrition in people advise against the routine monitoring of GRV in human patients (Taylor et al. 2016).

Management of enterally fed patients should include consideration of both rate and volume of food for either bolus or constant-rate infusion methods. Care should be taken to select appropriate diets for the disease process, and evaluation of the diet characteristics is indicated if intolerance is noted. For instance, diets high in fat will slow the rate of gastric emptying; a lower-fat formulation may be necessary to promote gastric emptying (together with other measures to enhance motility). Higher-fat diets should also be used cautiously in animals with malabsorptive diseases, as clinical experience has shown that many cases can only tolerate restricted-fat diets. If enteral feeding intolerance is severe enough to impair recovery of the patient or is causing additional problems (e.g. electrolyte and fluid imbalances, further weight loss), the use of parenteral nutrition should be considered as a complementary modality or as the sole source of nutritional support.

Transitioning Patients to Voluntary Intake

While some patients will require feedings through enteral devices on a long-term and even lifelong basis (such as those with severe and permanent orofacial or esophageal disease or with chronic kidney disease), others need tubes only temporarily. As underlying conditions improve or resolve with time and medical management, appetite may be restored and interest in food will resume. At this point, the patient can be offered the diet before scheduled feedings when they should be hungry. If some or all of the diet is not consumed voluntarily, it can be administered through the tube. Transitioning away from tube feeding is often successful with this strategy, and is beneficial when the enteral diet incorporates strategies

specific to the patient, such as a low-fat, novel, home-cooked diet slurry for animals with adverse food reaction and pancreatitis.

Other patients will have alternative options for longer-term diets, as there are many products with similar nutritional profiles appropriate for a variety of conditions. In these cases, a different diet than the one routinely fed through the tube may be accepted voluntarily, especially if food aversion occurred. Of course, for many situations the diet choice will be driven by the needs of the specific patient. For instance, animals with fiber-responsive diarrhea, chronic pancreatitis, adverse food reactions, or other conditions will require diets with specific modifications. Ultimately, options for long-term diets and transition to voluntary intake will vary according to the underlying conditions and are dependent on the individual patient.

Summary

- Hospitalized patients as well as those with trauma or chronic diseases are often malnourished or are consuming inadequate diets. Proactive nutritional assessment for all patients is indicated in order to identify those with actionable risk factors.
- Unless contraindicated, feeding enterally is preferred in order to provide energy and nutrients that support the function of the gastrointestinal tract.
- Enteral feeding devices are excellent options for providing adequate amounts of appropriate diets to patients with a wide range of needs.
- Enteral feeding devices can be readily and inexpensively utilized in any practice setting.

References

Abood, S.K. and Buffington, C.A. (1991). Improved nasogastric intubation technique for administration of nutritional support in dogs. *J. Am. Vet. Med. Assoc.* 199 (5): 577–579.

Allocca, M., Mangano, M., and Penagini, R. (2002). Effect of prolonged gastric distension on motor function of LES and of proximal stomach. *Am. J. Physiol. Gastrointest. Liver Physiol.* 283 (3): G677–G680.

Álvarez-Hernández, J., Planas Vila, M., León-Sanz, M. et al. (2012). Prevalence and costs of malnutrition in hospitalized patients; the PREDyCES study. *Nutr. Hosp.* 27 (4): 1049–1059.

Armitage-Chan, E.A., O'Toole, T., and Chan, D.L. (2006). Management of prolonged food deprivation, hypothermia, and refeeding syndrome in a cat. *J. Vet. Emerg. Crit. Care* 216 (2): S34–S41.

Balkany, T.J., Baker, B.B., Bloustein, P.A., and Jafek, B.W. (1977). Cervical esophagostomy in dogs: endoscopic, radiographic, and histopathologic evaluation of esophagitis induced by feeding tubes. *Ann. Otol. Rhinol. Laryngol.* 86 (5 Pt 1): 588–593.

Blocksom, J.M., Sugawa, C., Tokioka, S., and Field, E. (2004). Endoscopic repair of gastrostomy after inadvertent removal of percutaneous endoscopic gastrostomy tube. *Surg. Endosc.* 18 (5): 868–870.

Boza, J.J., Turini, M., Moennoz, D. et al. (2001). Effect of glutamine supplementation of the diet on tissue protein synthesis rate of glucocorticoid-treated rats. *Nutrition* 17 (1): 35–40.

Breheny, C.R., Boag, A., Le Gal, A. et al. (2019). Esophageal feeding tube placement and the associated complications in 248 cats. *J. Vet. Intern. Med.* 33 (3): 1306–1314.

Bright, R.M. (1993). Percutaneous endoscopic gastrostomy. *Vet. Clin. N. Am. Small Anim. Pract.* 23 (3): 531–545.

Bromley, S.M. (2000). Smell and taste disorders: a primary care approach. *Am. Fam. Physician* 61 (2): 427–438.

Brunet, A., Bouzouraa, T., Cadore, J.L. et al. (2022). Use of feeding tubes in 112 cats in an internal medicine referral service (2015–2020). *J. Feline Med. Surg.* 24 (10): e338–e346.

Brunetto, M.A., Gomes, M.O.S., Andre, M.R. et al. (2010). Effects of nutritional support on hospital outcome in dogs and cats. *J. Vet. Emerg. Crit. Care* 20 (2): 224–231.

Campbell, S.J., Marks, S.L., Yoshimoto, S.K. et al. (2006). Complications and outcomes of one-step low-profile gastrostomy devices for long-term enteral feeding in dogs and cats. *J. Am. Anim. Hosp. Assoc.* 42 (3): 197–206.

Campbell, J.A., Jutkowitz, L.A., Santoro, K.A. et al. (2010). Continuous versus intermittent delivery of nutrition via nasoenteric feeding tubes in hospitalized canine and feline patients: 91 patients (2002–2007). *J. Vet. Emerg. Crit. Care* 20 (2): 232–236.

Cavalcanti, C.A., Andreollo, N.A., and Santos, W.A. (2005). Cervical esophagostomy using indwelling catheter for analysis of gastric physiology in dogs. *Acta Cir. Bras.* 20 (5): 405–407.

Chan, D.L. (2004). Nutritional requirements of the critically ill patient. *Clin. Tech. Small Anim. Pract.* 19 (1): 1–5.

Chen, K., Okuma, T., Okamura, K. et al. (1994). Glutamine-supplemented parenteral nutrition improves gut mucosa integrity and function in endotoxemic rats. *J. Parenter. Enteral Nutr.* 18 (2): 167–171.

Choudhry, U., Barde, C.J., Markert, R., and Gopalswamy, N. (1996). Percutaneous endoscopic gastrostomy: a randomized prospective comparison of early and delayed feeding. *Gastrointest. Endosc.* 44 (2): 164–167.

Conejero, R., Bonet, A., Grau, T. et al. (2002). Effect of a glutamine-enriched enteral diet on intestinal permeability and infectious morbidity at 28 days in critically ill patients with systemic inflammatory response syndrome: a randomized, single-blind, prospective, multicenter study. *Nutrition* 18 (9): 716–721.

Cook, S., Whitby, E., Elias, N. et al. (2021). Retrospective evaluation of refeeding syndrome in cats: 11 cases (2013–2019). *J. Feline Med. Surg.* 23 (10): 883–891.

Corkins, M.R., Guenter, P., DiMaria-Ghalili, R.A. et al.; American Society for Parenteral and Enteral Nutrition(2014). Malnutrition diagnoses in hospitalized patients: United States, 2010. *J. Parenter. Enteral Nutr.* 38 (2): 186–195.

Crook, M.A., Hally, V., and Panteli, J.V. (2001). The importance of the refeeding syndrome. *Nutrition* 17 (7–8): 632–637.

Crowe, D.T. Jr. (1986). Use of a nasogastric tube for gastric and esophageal decompression in the dog and cat. *J. Am. Vet. Med. Assoc.* 188 (10): 1178–1182.

Crowe, D.T. Jr. and Devey, J.J. (1997). Esophagostomy tubes for feeding and decompression: clinical experience in 29 small animal patients. *J. Am. Anim. Hosp. Assoc.* 33 (5): 393–403.

Crowe, D.T. Jr. and Downs, M.O. (1986). Pharyngostomy complications in dogs and cats and recommended technical modifications: experimental and clinical investigations. *J. Am. Anim. Hosp. Assoc.* 22: 493–503.

Crowe, D.T. Jr., Devey, J., Palmer, D.A. et al. (1997). The use of polymeric liquid enteral diets for nutritional support in seriously ill or injured small animals: clinical results in 200 patients. *J. Am. Anim. Hosp. Assoc.* 33 (6): 500–508.

Czakó, L., Hajnal, F., Németh, J. et al. (1999). Effect of a liquid meal given as a bolus into the jejunum on human pancreatic secretion. *Pancreas* 18 (2): 197–202.

Daye, R.M., Huber, M.L., and Henderson, R.A. (1999). Interlocking box jejunostomy: a new technique for enteral feeding. *J. Am. Anim. Hosp. Assoc.* 35 (2): 129–134.

DeAvilla, M.D. and Leech, E.B. (2016). Hypoglycemia associated with refeeding syndrome in a cat. *J. Vet. Emerg. Crit. Care* 26 (6): 789–803.

Dedes, K.J., Schiesser, M., Schafer, M., and Clavien, P.A. (2006). Postoperative bezoar ileus after early enteral feeding. *J. Gastrointest. Surg.* 10 (1): 123–127.

Delaney, S.J. (2006). Management of anorexia in dogs and cats. *Vet. Clin. N. Am. Small Anim. Pract.* 36 (6): 1243–1249, vi.

Delany, H.M., Carnevale, N.J., and Garvey, J.W. (1973). Jejunostomy by a needle catheter technique. *Surgery* 73 (5): 786–790.

Devitt, C.M. and Seim, H.B. 3rd (1997). Clinical evaluation of tube esophagostomy in small animals. *J. Am. Anim. Hosp. Assoc.* 33 (1): 55–60.

Droucher, W. and Muller-Schlosser, S. (1980). Digestibility and tolerance of various sugars in cats. In: *Nutrition of the Dog and Cat* (ed. R.S. Anderson), 101–111. London: Pergamon Press.

Drover, J.W., Dhaliwal, R., Weitzel, F. et al. (2011). Perioperative use of arginine-supplemented diets: a systematic review of the evidence. *J. Am. Coll. Surg.* 212 (3): 385–399.

Dubagunta, S., Still, C.D., Kumar, A. et al. (2002). Early initiation of enteral feeding after percutaneous endoscopic gastrostomy tube placement. *Nutr. Clin. Pract.* 17 (2): 123–125.

Edge, C.J. and Langdon, J.D. (1991). Complications of pharyngostomy. *Br. J. Oral Maxillofac. Surg.* 29: 237–240.

Elke, G., Felbinger, T.W., and Heyland, D.K. (2015). Gastric residual volume in critically ill patients: a dead marker or still alive? *Nutr. Clin. Pract.* 30 (1): 59–71.

Elliott, D.A., Riel, R.L., and Rogers, Q.R. (2000). Complications and outcomes associated with use of gastrostomy tubes for nutritional management of dogs with renal failure: 56 cases (1994–1999). *J. Am. Vet. Med. Assoc.* 217 (9): 1337–1342.

Elmenhorst, K., Pérez López, P., Belch, A. et al. (2020). Retrospective study of complications associated with surgically-placed gastrostomy tubes in 43 dogs with septic peritonitis. *J. Small Anim. Pract.* 61 (2): 116–120.

Franzi, S.J., Martin, C.J., Cox, M.R. et al. (1990). Response of canine lower esophageal sphincter to gastric distension. *Am. J. Physiol.* 259 (3 Pt 1): G380–G385.

Galat, S.A., Gerig, K.D., Porter, J.A., and Slezak, F.A. (1990). Management of premature removal of the percutaneous gastrostomy. *Am. Surg.* 56 (11): 733–736.

Garrel, D., Patenaude, J., Nedelec, B. et al. (2003). Decreased mortality and infectious morbidity in adult burn patients given enteral glutamine supplements: a prospective, controlled, randomized clinical trial. *Crit. Care Med.* 31 (10): 2444–2449.

Garza-Castillon, R. Jr., Berger, J., Andrade, R. et al. (2018). The pharyngostomy tube:

indications, technique, efficacy, and safety in modern surgical practice. *Thorac. Cardiovasc. Surg.* 66 (5): 390–395.

Glaus, T.M., Cornelius, L.M., Bartges, J.W., and Reusch, C. (1998). Complications with non-endoscopic percutaneous gastrostomy in 31 cats and 10 dogs: a retrospective study. *Small Anim. Pract.* 39 (5): 218–222.

Gomes, G.F., Pisani, J.C., Macedo, E.D., and Campos, A.C. (2003). The nasogastric feeding tube as a risk factor for aspiration and aspiration pneumonia. *Curr. Opin. Clin. Nutr. Metab. Care* 6 (3): 327–333.

Gramlich, L., Kichian, K., Pinilla, J. et al. (2004). Does enteral nutrition compared to parenteral nutrition result in better outcomes in critically ill adult patients? A systematic review of the literature. *Nutrition* 20 (10): 843–848.

Griffin, M.A., Culp, W.T.N., Garcia, T.C. et al. (2020). Percutaneous radiologically guided gastrostomy tubes: procedural description and biomechanical comparison in a canine model. *Vet. Surg.* 49 (7): 1334–1342.

Groleau, V., Thibault, M., Doyon, M. et al. (2014). Malnutrition in hospitalized children: prevalence, impact, and management. *Can. J. Diet. Pract. Res.* 75 (1): 29–34.

Han, E. (2004). Esophageal and gastric feeding tubes in ICU patients. *Clin. Tech. Small Anim. Pract.* 19 (1): 22–31.

Hansen, S.C., Hlusko, K.C., Matz, B.M. et al. (2019). Retrospective evaluation of 24 cases of gastrostomy tube usage in dogs with septic peritonitis (2009–2016). *J. Vet. Emerg. Crit. Care* 29 (5): 514–520.

Harris, J.P., Parnell, N.K., Griffith, E.H., and Saker, K.E. (2017). Retrospective evaluation of the impact of early enteral nutrition on clinical outcomes in dogs with pancreatitis: 34 cases (2010–2013). *J. Vet. Emerg. Crit. Care* 27 (4): 425–433.

Harrison, A.M., Clay, B., Grant, M.J. et al. (1997). Nonradiographic assessment of enteral feeding tube position. *Crit. Care Med.* 25 (12): 2055–2059.

Hasselgren, P.O. and Fischer, J.E. (2001). Muscle cachexia: current concepts of intracellular mechanisms and molecular regulation. *Ann. Surg.* 233 (1): 9–17.

Havala, T. and Shronts, E. (1990). Managing the complications associated with refeeding. *Nutr. Clin. Pract.* 5 (1): 23–29.

Herring, J.M. (2016). A novel placement technique for nasogastric and nasoesophageal tubes. *J. Vet. Emerg. Crit. Care* 26 (4): 593–597.

Hewitt, S.A., Brisson, B.A., Sinclair, M.D. et al. (2004). Evaluation of laparoscopic-assisted placement of jejunostomy feeding tubes in dogs. *J. Am. Vet. Med. Assoc.* 225 (1): 65–71.

Hickman, M.A. (1998). Interventional nutrition for gastrointestinal disease. *Clin. Tech. Small Anim. Pract.* 13 (4): 211–216.

Hinden, S.E., Schweighauser, A., and Francey, T. (2020). Evaluation of a novel non-surgical post-pyloric feeding technique in dogs with severe acute kidney injury. *J. Vet. Emerg. Crit. Care (San Antonio)* 30 (4): 384–395.

Hlusko, K.C., Hansen, S.C., Matz, B. et al. (2019). Description of a novel technique for surgical placement of gastrostomy tubes in dogs. *J. Vet. Emerg. Crit. Care* 29 (5): 564–567.

Hoffberg, J.E. and Koenigshof, A. (2017). Evaluation of the safety of early compared to late enteral nutrition in canine septic peritonitis. *J. Am. Anim. Hosp. Assoc.* 53 (2): 90–95.

Hofman, Z., Swinkels, S., and van Zanten, A.R.H. (2016). Glutamine, fish oil, and antioxidants in critical illness: MetaPlus trial post hoc safety analysis. *Ann. Intensive Care* 6 (1): 119.

Holahan, M., Abood, S., Hauptman, J. et al. (2010). Intermittent and continuous enteral nutrition in critically ill dogs: a prospective randomized trial. *J. Vet. Intern. Med.* 24 (3): 520–526.

Hopper, K., Haskins, S.C., Kass, P.H. et al. (2007). Indications, management, and outcome of long-term positive-pressure ventilation in dogs and cats: 148 cases (1990–2001). *J. Am. Vet. Med. Assoc.* 230: 64–75.

Houdijk, A.P., Rijnsburger, E.R., Jansen, J. et al. (1998). Randomised trial of glutamine-enriched enteral nutrition on infectious morbidity in patients with multiple trauma. *Lancet* 352 (9130): 772–776.

Ireland, L.M., Hohenhaus, A.E., Broussard, J.D., and Weissman, B.L. (2003). A comparison of owner management and complications in 67 cats with esophagostomy and percutaneous endoscopic gastrostomy feeding tubes. *J. Am. Anim. Hosp. Assoc.* 39 (3): 241–246.

Jeejeebhoy, K.N. (2007). Enteral nutrition versus parenteral nutrition – the risks and benefits. *Nat. Clin. Pract. Gastroenterol. Hepatol.* 4 (5): 260–265.

Jennings, M., Center, S.A., Barr, S.C. et al. (2001). Successful treatment of feline pancreatitis using an endoscopically placed gastrojejunostomy tube. *J. Am. Anim. Hosp. Assoc.* 37 (2): 145–152.

Jergens, A.E., Morrison, J.A., Miles, K.G. et al. (2007). Percutaneous endoscopic gastrojejunostomy tube placement in healthy dogs and cats. *J. Vet. Intern. Med.* 21 (1): 18–24.

Jiang, Z.M., Wang, L.J., Qi, Y. et al. (1993). Comparison of parenteral nutrition supplemented with L-glutamine or glutamine dipeptides. *J. Parenter. Enteral Nutr.* 17 (2): 134–141.

Justin, R.B. and Hohenhaus, A.E. (1995). Hypophosphatemia associated with enteral alimentation in cats. *J. Vet. Intern. Med.* 9 (4): 228–233.

Kalil, A.C., Sevransky, J.E., Myers, D.E. et al. (2006). Preclinical trial of l-arginine monotherapy alone or with N-acetylcysteine in septic shock. *Crit. Care Med.* 34 (11): 2719–2728.

Kawasaki, N., Suzuki, Y., Nakayoshi, T. et al. (2009). Early postoperative enteral nutrition is useful for recovering gastrointestinal motility and maintaining the nutritional status. *Surg. Today* 39 (3): 225–230.

Kraft, M.D., Btaiche, I.F., and Sacks, G.S. (2005). Review of the refeeding syndrome. *Nutr. Clin. Pract.* 20 (6): 625–633.

Kreymann, K.G., Berger, M.M., Deutz, N.E. et al. (2006). ESPEN guidelines on enteral nutrition: intensive care. *Clin. Nutr.* 25 (2): 210–223.

Krishnan, J.A., Parce, P.B., Martinez, A. et al. (2003). Caloric intake in medical ICU patients: consistency of care with guidelines and relationship to clinical outcomes. *Chest* 124 (1): 297–305.

Kumar, A., Singh, N., Prakash, S. et al. (2006). Early enteral nutrition in severe acute pancreatitis: a prospective randomized controlled trial comparing nasojejunal and nasogastric routes. *J. Clin. Gastroenterol.* 40 (5): 431–434.

Kuppinger, D.D., Rittler, P., Hartl, W.H., and Rüttinger, D. (2013). Use of gastric residual volume to guide enteral nutrition in critically ill patients: a brief systematic review of clinical studies. *Forum Nutr.* 29 (9): 1075–1079.

Lantz, G.C., Cantwell, H.D., VanVleet, J.F. et al. (1983). Pharyngostomy tube induced esophagitis in the dog: an experimental study. *J. Am. Anim. Hosp. Assoc.* 19: 207–212.

LeLeiko, N.S. and Walsh, M.J. (1996). The role of glutamine, short-chain fatty acids, and nucleotides in intestinal adaptation to gastrointestinal disease. *Pediatr. Clin. N. Am.* 43 (2): 451–470.

Levine, P.B., Smallwood, L.J., and Buback, J.L. (1997). Esophagostomy tubes as a method of nutritional management in cats: a retrospective study. *J. Am. Anim. Hosp. Assoc.* 33 (5): 405–410.

Lima, N.L., Soares, A.M., Mota, R.M. et al. (2007). Wasting and intestinal barrier function in children taking alanyl-glutamine-supplemented enteral formula. *J. Pediatr. Gastroenterol. Nutr.* 44 (3): 365–374.

Liu, D.T., Brown, D.C., and Silverstein, D.C. (2012). Early nutritional support is associated with decreased length of hospitalization in dogs with septic peritonitis: a retrospective study of 45 cases (2000–2009). *J. Vet. Emerg. Crit. Care* 22 (4): 453–459.

Lochs, H., Dejong, C., Hammarqvist, F. et al. (2006). ESPEN guidelines on enteral nutrition: gastroenterology. *Clin. Nutr.* 25 (2): 260–274.

Lord, L.M., Weiser-Maimone, A., Pulhamus, M., and Sax, H.C. (1993). Comparison of weighted vs. unweighted enteral feeding tubes for efficacy of transpyloric intubation. *J. Parenter. Enteral Nutr.* 17 (3): 271–273.

Ma, Q., Wang, Z., Zhang, M. et al. (2010). Targeting the L-arginine-nitric oxide pathway for cancer treatment. *Curr. Pharm. Des.* 16 (4): 392–410.

Mansfield, C.S., James, F.E., Steiner, J.M. et al. (2011). A pilot study to assess tolerability of early enteral nutrition via esophagostomy tube feeding in dogs with severe acute pancreatitis. *J. Vet. Intern. Med.* 25 (3): 419–425.

Marcuard, S.P. and Stegall, K.S. (1990). Unclogging feeding tubes with pancreatic enzyme. *J. Parenter. Enteral Nutr.* 14 (2): 198–200.

Marik, P.E. and Zaloga, G.P. (2010). Immunonutrition in high-risk surgical patients: a systematic review and analysis of the literature. *J. Parenter. Enteral Nutr.* 34 (4): 378–386.

Marin, V.B., Rodriguez-Osiac, L., Schlessinger, L. et al. (2006). Controlled study of enteral arginine supplementation in burned children: impact on immunologic and metabolic status. *Nutrition* 22 (7–8): 705–712.

Marks, S.L. (1998). The principles and practical application of enteral nutrition. *Vet. Clin. N. Am. Small Anim. Pract.* 28 (3): 677–708.

Marks, S.L. (2005). Nasoesophageal, esophagostomy, and gastrostomy tube placement techniques. In: *Textbook of Veterinary Internal Medicine: Diseases of the Dog and Cat*, 6e (ed. S.J. Ettinger and E.C. Feldman), 329–336. St. Louis, MO: Elsevier Saunders.

Marks, S.L., Cook, A.K., Reader, R. et al. (1999). Effects of glutamine supplementation of an amino acid-based purified diet on intestinal mucosal integrity in cats with methotrexate-induced enteritis. *Am. J. Vet. Res.* 60 (6): 755–763.

McCarter, T.L., Condon, S.C., Aguilar, R.C. et al. (1998). Randomized prospective trial of early versus delayed feeding after percutaneous endoscopic gastrostomy placement. *Am. J. Gastroenterol.* 93 (3): 419–421.

McClave, S.A., Greene, L.M., Snider, H.L. et al. (1997). Comparison of the safety of early enteral vs parenteral nutrition in mild acute pancreatitis. *J. Parenter. Enteral Nutr.* 21 (1): 14–20.

McClave, S.A., Chang, W.K., Dhaliwal, R. et al. (2006). Nutrition support in acute pancreatitis: a systematic review of the literature. *J. Parenter. Enteral Nutr.* 30 (2): 143–156.

Meehan, S.E., Wood, R.A., and Cuschieri, A. (1984). Percutaneous cervical pharyngostomy. A comfortable and convenient alternative to protracted nasogastric intubation. *Am. J. Surg.* 148 (3): 325–330.

Meier, R., Ockenga, J., Pertkiewicz, M. et al. (2006). ESPEN guidelines on enteral nutrition: pancreas. *Clin. Nutr.* 25 (2): 275–284.

Mellinger, J.D., Simon, I.B., Schlechter, B. et al. (1991). Tract formation following percutaneous endoscopic gastrostomy in an animal model. *Surg. Endosc.* 5 (4): 189–191.

Michel, K.E. (1998). Interventional nutrition for the critical care patient: optimal diets. *Clin. Tech. Small Anim. Pract.* 13 (4): 204–210.

Michel, K.E., King, L.G., and Ostro, E. (1997). Measurement of urinary urea nitrogen content as an estimate of the amount of total urinary nitrogen loss in dogs in intensive care units. *J. Am. Vet. Med. Assoc.* 210 (3): 356–359.

Mittal, R.K., Stewart, W.R., and Schirmer, B.D. (1992). Effect of a catheter in the pharynx on the frequency of transient lower esophageal sphincter relaxations. *Gastroenterology* 103 (4): 1236–1240.

Mohr, A.J., Leisewitz, A.L., Jacobson, L.S. et al. (2003). Effect of early enteral nutrition on intestinal permeability, intestinal protein loss, and outcome in dogs with severe parvoviral enteritis. *J. Vet. Intern. Med.* 17 (6): 791–798.

Molina, J., Hervera, M., Manzanilla, E.G. et al. (2018). Evaluation of the prevalence and risk factors for undernutrition in hospitalized dogs. *Front. Vet. Sci.* 5: 205.

National Research Council (NRC), Ad Hoc Committee on Dog and Cat Nutrition (2006). *Nutrient Requirements of Dogs and Cats*. Washington, DC: National Academies Press.

Ng, W.Q. and Neill, J. (2006). Evidence for early oral feeding of patients after elective open colorectal surgery: a literature review. *J. Clin. Nurs.* 15 (6): 696–709.

Ng, K., Woo, J., Kwan, M. et al. (2004). Effect of age and disease on taste perception. *J. Pain Symptom Manage.* 28 (1): 28–34.

Nguyen, N.Q., Fraser, R.J., Chapman, M.J. et al. (2007). Feed intolerance in critical illness is associated with increased basal and nutrient-stimulated plasma cholecystokinin concentrations. *Crit. Care Med.* 35 (1): 82–88.

Novo, R.E., Churchill, J., Faudskar, L., and Lipowitz, A.J. (2001). Limited approach to the right flank for placement of a duodenostomy tube. *J. Am. Anim. Hosp. Assoc.* 37 (2): 193–199.

O'Dwyer, S.T., Smith, R.J., Hwang, T.L., and Wilmore, D.W. (1989). Maintenance of small bowel mucosa with glutamine-enriched parenteral nutrition. *J. Parenter. Enteral Nutr.* 13 (6): 579–585.

Ogilvie, G.K., Fettman, M.J., Mallinckrodt, C.H. et al. (2000). Effect of fish oil, arginine, and doxorubicin chemotherapy on remission and survival time for dogs with lymphoma: a double-blind, randomized placebo-controlled study. *Cancer* 88 (8): 1916–1928.

Oldani, M., Sandini, M., Nespoli, L. et al. (2015). Glutamine supplementation in intensive care patients: a meta-analysis of randomized clinical trials. *Medicine (Baltimore)* 94 (31): e1319.

Ozen, N., Tosun, N., Yamanel, L. et al. (2016). Evaluation of the effect on patient parameters of not monitoring gastric residual volume in intensive care patients on a mechanical ventilator receiving enteral feeding: a randomized clinical trial. *J. Crit. Care* 33: 137–144.

Park, K.G., Heys, S.D., Blessing, K. et al. (1992). Stimulation of human breast cancers by dietary L-arginine. *Clin. Sci. (Lond.)* 82 (4): 413–417.

Parker, V.J. and Freeman, L.M. (2013). Comparison of various solutions to dissolve critical care diet clots. *J. Vet. Emerg. Crit. Care* 23 (3): 344–347.

Patel, J.J., Miller, K.R., Rosenthal, C., and Rosenthal, M.D. (2016). When is it appropriate to use arginine in critical illness? *Nutr. Clin. Pract.* 31 (4): 438–444.

Patel, J.J., Martindale, R.G., and McClave, S.A. (2018). Controversies surrounding critical care nutrition: an appraisal of permissive underfeeding, protein, and outcomes. *J. Parenter. Enteral Nutr.* 42 (3): 508–515.

Patil, P.M., Warad, N.M., Patil, R.N., and Kotrashetti, S.M. (2006). Cervical pharyngostomy: an alternative approach to enteral feeding. *Oral Surg. Oral Med. Oral Pathol. Oral Radiol. Endod.* 102 (6): 736–740.

Penagini, R., Carmagnola, S., Cantu, P. et al. (2004). Mechanoreceptors of the proximal stomach: role in triggering transient lower esophageal sphincter relaxation. *Gastroenterology* 126 (1): 49–56.

Perondi, F., Stefanescu, A., Marchetti, V. et al. (2021). Oesophagostomy tube complications in azotaemic dogs: 139 cases (2015 to 2019). *J. Small Anim. Pract.* 62 (3): 194–199.

Poulard, F., Dimet, J., Martin-Lefevre, L. et al. (2010). Impact of not measuring residual gastric volume in mechanically ventilated patients receiving early enteral feeding: a prospective before-after study. *J. Parenter. Enteral Nutr.* 34: 125–130.

Powell, K.S., Marcuard, S.P., Farrior, E.S., and Gallagher, M.L. (1993). Aspirating gastric residuals causes occlusion of small-bore feeding tubes. *J. Parenter. Enteral Nutr.* 17: 243–246.

Prantil, L.R., Markovich, J.E., Heinze, C.R. et al. (2016). Nutritional analysis and microbiological evaluation of commercially available enteral diets for cats. *J. Vet. Emerg. Crit. Care* 26 (2): 254–261.

Qin, H.L., Su, Z.D., Gao, Q., and Lin, Q.T. (2002). Early intrajejunal nutrition: bacterial translocation and gut barrier function of severe acute pancreatitis in dogs. *Hepatobiliary Pancreat. Dis. Int.* 1 (1): 150–154.

Quimby, J.M. and Lunn, K.F. (2013). Mirtazapine as an appetite stimulant and anti-emetic in cats with chronic kidney disease: a masked placebo-controlled crossover clinical trial. *Vet. J.* 197 (3): 651–655.

Ragins, H., Levenson, S.M., Signer, R. et al. (1973). Intrajejunal administration of an elemental diet at neutral pH avoids pancreatic stimulation. Studies in dog and man. *Am. J. Surg.* 126 (5): 606–614.

Rahman, A., Wu, T., Bricknell, R. et al. (2015). Malnutrition matters in Canadian hospitalized patients: malnutrition risk in hospitalized patients in a tertiary care center using the malnutrition universal screening tool. *Nutr. Clin. Pract.* 30 (5): 709–713.

Reignier, J., Mercier, E., Le Gouge, A.A. et al. (2013). Effect of not monitoring residual gastric volume on risk of ventilator-associated pneumonia in adults receiving mechanical ventilation and early enteral feeding: a randomized controlled trial. *J. Am. Med. Assoc.* 309: 249–256.

Remillard, R.L., Armstrong, P.J., and Davenport, D.J. (2000). Assisted feeding in hospitalized patients: enteral and parenteral nutrition. In: *Small Animal Clinical Nutrition*, 4e (ed. M.S. Hand, C.D. Thatcher, R.L. Remillard and P. Roudebush), 351–400. Topeka, KS: Mark Morris Institute.

Remillard, R.L., Darden, D.E., Michel, K.E. et al. (2001). An investigation of the relationship between caloric intake and outcome in hospitalized dogs. *Vet. Ther.* 2 (4): 301–310.

Risselada, M., Griffith, E., Kapler, M. et al. (2018). Evaluation of various gastrojejunostomy tube constructs for enteral support of small animal patients. *J. Am. Vet. Med. Assoc.* 252 (10): 1239–1246.

Rodriguez-Diaz, J., Sumner, J.P., and Miller, M. (2021). Fatal complications of nasogastric tube misplacement in two dogs. *J. Am. Anim. Hosp. Assoc.* 57 (5): 242–246.

Schulman, A.S., Willcutts, K.F., Claridge, J.A. et al. (2005). Does the addition of glutamine to enteral feeds affect patient mortality? *Crit. Care Med.* 33 (11): 2501–2506.

Seim, H.B. III and Willard, M.D. (2002). Postoperative care if the surgical patient. In:

Small Animal Surgery, 2e (ed. T.W. Fossum), 70–91. St. Louis, MO: Mosby.

Shike, M. and Latkany, L. (1998). Direct percutaneous endoscopic jejunostomy. *Gastrointest. Endosc. Clin. N. Am.* 8 (3): 569–580.

Silvis, S.E., DiBartolomeo, A.G., and Aaker, H.M. (1980). Hypophosphatemia and neurological changes secondary to oral caloric intake: a variant of hyperalimentation syndrome. *Am. J. Gastroenterol.* 73 (3): 215–222.

Simpson, J.W. (1998). Diet and large intestinal disease in dogs and cats. *J. Nutr.* 128 (12 Suppl): 2717S–2722S.

Smith, S.A., Ludlow, C.L., Hoskinson, J.J. et al. (1998). Effect of percutaneous endoscopic gastrostomy on gastric emptying in clinically normal cats. *Am. J. Vet. Res.* 59 (11): 1414–1416.

Song, G.M., Tian, X., Zhang, L. et al. (2015). Immunonutrition support for patients undergoing surgery for gastrointestinal malignancy: preoperative, postoperative, or perioperative? A Bayesian network meta-analysis of randomized controlled trials. *Fortschr. Med.* 94 (29): e1225.

Stechmiller, J.K., Childress, B., and Cowan, L. (2005). Arginine supplementation and wound healing. *Nutr. Clin. Pract.* 20 (1): 52–61.

Stein, J., Schulte-Bockholt, A., Sabin, M. et al. (2002). A randomized prospective trial of immediate vs. next-day feeding after percutaneous endoscopic gastrostomy in intensive care patients. *Intensive Care Med.* 28 (11): 1656–1660.

Stevenson, M.A., Stiffler, K.S., and Schmiedt, C.W. (2000). One-step placement of a percutaneous nonendoscopic low-profile gastrostomy port in cats. *J. Am. Vet. Med. Assoc.* 217 (11): 1636–1641.

Swann, H.M., Sweet, D.C., and Michel, K. (1997). Complications associated with use of jejunostomy tubes in dogs and cats: 40 cases (1989–1994). *J. Am. Vet. Med. Assoc.* 210 (12): 1764–1767.

Swann, H.M., Sweet, D.C., Holt, D.E. et al. (1998). Placement of a low-profile duodenostomy and jejunostomy device in five dogs. *J. Small Anim. Pract.* 39 (4): 191–194.

Taylor, B.E., McClave, S.A., Martindale, R.G. et al. (2016). Guidelines for the provision and assessment of nutrition support therapy in the adult critically ill patient: Society of Critical Care Medicine (SCCM) and American Society for Parenteral and Enteral Nutrition (A.S.P.E.N.). *Crit. Care Med.* 44 (2): 390–438.

Tsuruta, K., Mann, F.A., and Backus, R.C. (2016). Evaluation of jejunostomy tube feeding after abdominal surgery in dogs. *J. Vet. Emerg. Crit. Care* 26 (4): 502–508.

Van Zanten, A.R., Dhaliwal, R., Garrel, D., and Heyland, D.K. (2015). Enteral glutamine supplementation in critically ill patients: a systematic review and meta-analysis. *Crit. Care* 19: 294.

Vanek, V.W. (2003). Ins and outs of enteral access: Part 2 – Long-term access – esophagostomy and gastrostomy. *Nutr. Clin. Pract.* 18 (1): 50–74.

Von Werthern, C.J. and Wess, G. (2001). A new technique for insertion of esophagostomy tubes in cats. *J. Am. Anim. Hosp. Assoc.* 37 (2): 140–144.

Waddell, L.S. and Michel, K.E. (1998). Critical care nutrition: routes of feeding. *Clin. Tech. Small Anim. Pract.* 13 (4): 197–203.

Walton, R.S., Wingfield, W.E., Ogilvie, G.K. et al. (1996). Energy expenditure in 104 postoperative and traumatically injured dogs with indirect calorimetry. *J. Vet. Emerg. Crit. Care* 6 (2): 71–79.

Will, K., Nolte, I., and Zentek, J. (2005). Early enteral nutrition in young dogs suffering from haemorrhagic gastroenteritis. *Vet. Med. A Physiol. Pathol. Clin. Med.* 52 (7): 371–376.

Wilmore, D. (2004). Enteral and parenteral arginine supplementation to improve medical outcomes in hospitalized patients. *J. Nutr.* 134 (10 Suppl): 2863S–2867S.

Wischmeyer, P.E., Lynch, J., Liedel, J. et al. (2001). Glutamine administration reduces Gram-negative bacteremia in severely burned patients: a prospective, randomized, double-blind trial versus isonitrogenous control. *Crit. Care Med.* 29 (11): 2075–2080.

Wofford, J.A., Zollers, B., Rhodes, L. et al. (2018). Evaluation of the safety of daily administration of capromorelin in cats. *J. Vet. Pharmacol. Ther.* 41 (2): 324–333.

Wohl, J.S. (2006). Nasojejunal feeding tube placement using fluoroscopic guidance: technique and clinical experience in dogs. *J. Vet. Crit. Care* 16 (S1): S27–S33.

Wu, G.H., Zhang, Y.W., and Wu, Z.H. (2001). Modulation of postoperative immune and inflammatory response by immune-enhancing enteral diet in gastrointestinal cancer patients. *World J. Gastroenterol.* 7 (3): 357–362.

Yan, H., Peng, X., Huang, Y. et al. (2007). Effects of early enteral arginine supplementation on resuscitation of severe burn patients. *Burns* 33 (2): 179–184.

Yoshimoto, S.K., Marks, S.L., Struble, A.L., and Riel, D.L. (2006). Owner experiences and complications with home use of a replacement low profile gastrostomy device for long-term enteral feeding in dogs. *Can. Vet. J.* 47 (2): 144–150.

Yu, M.K., Freeman, L.M., Heinze, C.R. et al. (2013). Comparison of complication rate in dogs with nasoesophageal versus nasogastric feeding tubes. *J. Vet. Emerg. Crit. Care* 23 (3): 300–304.

Zheng, Y.M., Li, F., Zhang, M.M., and Wu, X.T. (2006). Glutamine dipeptide for parenteral nutrition in abdominal surgery: a meta-analysis of randomized controlled trials. *World J. Gastroenterol.* 12 (46): 7537–7541.

Zollers, B., Allen, J., Kennedy, C., and Rhodes, L. (2015). Capromorelin, an orally active ghrelin agonist, caused sustained increases in IGF-1, increased food intake and body weight in cats. *J. Vet. Intern. Med.* 29 (4): 1122–1256.

Zollers, B., Wofford, J.A., Heinen, E. et al. (2016). A prospective, randomized, masked, placebo-controlled clinical study of capromorelin in dogs with reduced appetite. *J. Vet. Intern. Med.* 30 (6): 1851–1857.

21

Parenteral Nutrition
Sally C. Perea

There is an increasing awareness among veterinarians of the importance of nutritional support in hospitalized patients. Previous studies have demonstrated that nutritional support improves patient outcomes, and there remains an opportunity for significant improvement in the nutritional support provided to hospitalized veterinary patients. In one study, the caloric intakes and outcomes of 276 dogs over 821 days of hospitalization at four veterinary referral hospitals were retrospectively evaluated. Their findings revealed that caloric intake had a significant positive effect on patient outcome. However, the dogs in this study were also shown to be in a negative energy balance during the majority of the time of hospitalization (73% of the total days) (Remillard et al. 2001). In another study that included 467 dogs and 55 cats, energy intake was again shown to be positively associated with hospital discharge (Brunetto et al. 2010). Finally, a prospective study of 500 hospitalized dogs found that inadequate calorie intake was common and was associated with increased risk of death (Molina et al. 2018). Generally, the preferred first line of assisted feeding in anorectic patients is via the enteral route (Finck 2000). For patients in which enteral feeding is not tolerated, parenteral nutrition (PN) can be an essential tool to deliver nutritional needs.

History

Blood transfusions can be considered one of the first forms of PN, and they were reported experimentally in dogs as early as 1667 (Levenson et al. 1984). In 1873, when blood was unavailable, a physician by the name of Dr. E.M. Hodder took a bold step with one of the first reported uses of milk for intravenous infusion in a human patient with Asiatic cholera (Hodder 1873). This patient's condition was considered to be end stage and fatal, giving Hodder the opportunity to try his experimental therapy. While Hodder's colleagues did not support his pursuit (three of four were reported to have left the building), the patient tolerated the treatment and went on to recover.

Over time, the various components of current PN admixtures were introduced. Protein hydrolysates and glucose mixtures were reported to have been used intravenously as early as 1889 and 1896, respectively (Levenson et al. 1984). One of the first reports of intravenous injection of a fat emulsion was in 1915, when a 3% emulsion of lard was administered to two dogs (Levenson et al. 1984). Metabolic utilization of the fat was verified with a decrease in the respiratory quotient from 0.85 to 0.73, and a concurrent rise in heat production. The various components were refined

Applied Veterinary Clinical Nutrition, Second Edition. Edited by Andrea J. Fascetti,
Sean J. Delaney, Jennifer A. Larsen, and Cecilia Villaverde.

over time, and eventually combined to provide a three-in-one PN admixture providing all three of the major macronutrients.

The dog was a common experimental model in many of these early investigations, including one ground-breaking study that used PN as the sole nutrient source for normal growth in six 12-week-old Beagle puppies for up to 256 days (Dudrick et al. 1968). The use of PN in veterinary patients did not emerge until much later and the practice still lacks large randomized case-controlled prospective clinical studies. Our current knowledge of PN in dogs and cats is mainly limited to studies of healthy research animals, retrospective case series, clinical experience, and extrapolation from human literature.

Assessment of Nutritional Status and Patient Selection

The first criterion to consider when evaluating a candidate for PN is the patient's nutritional status. One of the most important aspects of the nutritional assessment is a thorough diet history. It is important to determine not only the length of complete anorexia, but also the duration of inadequate nutritional intake. The current energy intake should be quantified and compared to the patient's calculated energy requirement. It is also important to inquire about the feeding of commercial pet foods as well as treats and human foods, including those that may be used to administer medications. Many of these extra treats and foods provide additional calories, but are not typically complete and balanced. As such, if they comprise larger proportions of the overall intake, there is an increased risk of nutrient deficiencies and imbalances.

In addition to diet history, other components of the history should be considered, including presence of vomiting, diarrhea, and underlying disease. Vomiting and diarrhea reflect the presence of maldigestion, malabsorption, and the loss of essential nutrients (i.e. protein, fat,

and electrolytes) via the gastrointestinal tract. Other conditions that result in excess protein loss, such as open abdomen or large wounds or burns, also negatively impact nutritional status. Finally, many metabolic diseases negatively impact nutritional status, particularly chronic diseases that can lead to anorexia and cachexia such as chronic renal disease and congestive heart failure.

The next important tool for a complete nutritional assessment is the physical exam. Body weight, body condition score, and muscle mass should be evaluated in all patients. Recent and historical trends in these parameters can be informative. For example, the change in body weight is often more insightful than the patient's current body weight, as many patients may appear to have a healthy body weight and body condition, but have undergone recent unintentional weight loss. A history of weight loss at presentation has been shown to double the risk of mortality in feline PN patients (Pyle et al. 2004). Any unintentional weight loss is a concern, but scope and rate should be considered. Weight loss greater than 2% of the body weight per week is considered severe (Remillard 2000). Assessment of muscle mass is also an important component of the physical exam. Muscle wasting commonly occurs secondary to hypercatabolism in critically ill patients and may be present in patients who have normal or even high body condition scores (Michel et al. 1997; Chan 2004). A three-point muscle condition scoring system has been described, with three out of three being normal muscle mass, and one out of three representing severe muscle wasting (Buffington et al. 2004). Other evaluations assess animals as either having normal muscle mass or mild, moderate, or severe loss. Assessment of muscle mass should be made by palpation over the temporal bones, ribs, lumbar vertebrae, and pelvic bone, and visual assessment of bony prominences from a distance.

Finally, some hematologic markers can be helpful when assessing nutritional status. Although not specific, changes in serum concentrations of albumin, potassium, and red blood cell and lymphocyte counts can reflect nutritional status (Fascetti et al. 1997; Remillard 2000; Freeman and Chan 2006). Serum potassium concentrations reflect changes on a day-to-day basis, while albumin, red blood cell, and hemoglobin concentrations reflect changes in nutritional status over weeks to months. Although albumin is one of the main hematologic markers referenced to assess nutritional status, its concentration is dependent on a number of variables (including body water status, liver function, and renal losses), making it an unspecific marker. However, in human medicine albumin concentration has been demonstrated to correspond to overall health status and mortality rate (DeLegge and Drake 2007; Leite et al. 2016). Albumin concentration has also been shown to correlate with mortality rate in feline patients prior to and 96 hours after starting PN support (Pyle et al. 2004). Therefore, while albumin concentration may not always directly correspond to nutritional status, it can be a useful prognostic indicator in critically ill patients (Mehl et al. 2005).

After assessing the patient's history, physical exam, and hematologic status, consideration must also be given to the expected course of the patient's illness. For those patients with acute injuries (e.g. hit by a car) or elective surgeries, if their nutritional status at presentation is generally good, the period of withholding of food and/or anorexia is expected to be short (1–3 days). For these patients, voluntary intake is expected to resume within a short time period, and it is reasonable to delay nutritional support. However, animals with chronic illnesses are more likely to have a poor nutritional status at presentation and may have an extended period where voluntary food intake is expected to be reduced or absent. For these patients, nutritional support should be implemented as soon as possible.

Unlike in human medicine, standardized illness scores and specific guidelines for implementation of assisted feeding have not been established for veterinary patients. Table 21.1 provides a list of considerations that can serve as a guideline for assigning patients into categories of low, moderate, or high risk for malnutrition. This list is by no means exhaustive, but can serve as a starting place for clinicians in the decision-making process. Each patient should undergo nutritional assessment, taking into consideration the wide range of individual variables, rather than setting an arbitrary cutoff point for when assisted feeding should be implemented. When a patient has two or more high-risk factors for malnutrition, it is likely that that the patient is already in a malnourished state, and assisted feeding should be implemented as soon as possible (cardiovascular and electrolyte stability is a priority and must be established prior to nutritional intervention). Cats with or at risk for hepatic lipidosis should also receive prompt nutritional support. Patients with two or more moderate-risk factors should be carefully monitored, and assisted feeding should be implemented within 2–3 days of hospitalization if the condition does not significantly improve. Patients with only low-risk factors should also be carefully monitored to ensure that their nutritional status does not decline during hospitalization.

In human medicine there have been contrasting recommendations for the optional time to implement PN. This controversy has primarily been in the context of supplementing EN with PN in those patients that are not able to achieve desired energy delivery with EN alone. One school of thought is that PN should be implemented early when EN provision is less than 60% (European guidelines), while the opposing view recommends that PN not be initiated until day 8 in those patients with a body mass index (BMI) of 17 or greater (American and Canadian guidelines) (Preiser et al. 2015). One randomized, multicenter trial compared these two approaches, and found that late initiation of PN was associated with faster recovery and fewer complications (Casaer et al. 2011). It should be noted that the

Table 21.1 Nutritional assessment guidelines.

	Low risk	Moderate risk	High risk
History			
Intake < RER for <3 d	√		
Intake < RER for 3–5 d		√	
Intake < RER for >5 d			√
Anorexia <3 d		√	
Anorexia >3 d			√
Weight loss			√
Vomiting/diarrhea[a]		√	√
Other factors (may be low, moderate, or high risk)			
Physical exam			
BCS < 4/9			√
Muscle wasting present			√
Other factors (may be low, moderate, or high risk)			
Hematologic parameters			
Hypoalbuminemia[a]		√	√
Electrolyte abnormalities[a]		√	√
Anemia[a]		√	√
Lymphopenia[a]		√	√
Expected course of illness			
<2 d	√		
2–3 d		√	
>3 d			√

Patients with two or more high-risk factors should receive nutritional support as soon as they are appropriately stabilized. Patients with two or fewer moderate-risk factors should be carefully monitored, and assisted feeding should be implemented within 2–3 days of hospitalization if the condition does not significantly improve. Patients with only low-risk factors should also be carefully monitored to ensure that their nutritional status does not decline during hospitalization.
[a] The degree of clinical signs and hematologic abnormalities will dictate moderate- to high-risk assignment.
BCS, body condition score; RER, resting energy requirement.

differences were relatively modest with only a 1.06 hazard ratio, representing a 6.3% increase in the likelihood of being discharged from the intensive care unit (ICU) and from the hospital. However, the reduced healthcare costs in addition to relative reductions of days required for mechanical ventilation (two days) and renal replacement therapy (three days) are significant and raise questions about the philosophy of early implementation. One study in dogs found no difference in early PN versus early EN, but either route was associated with shorter hospitalization stays in dogs with septic peritonitis (Liu et al. 2012). Additional research is required in canine and feline patients to understand the optimal time for initiating PN, particularly when used to supplement EN.

Following the nutritional assessment, the decision must then be made as to what route of nutritional support is the most appropriate for the patient. Enteral nutrition is preferred over PN when the gastrointestinal tract is functional (see Figure 21.1). Indications for PN include intractable vomiting and/or diarrhea; anesthesia or lack of a gag reflex; recovery from severe gastric or intestinal resection; poor anesthetic candidate for proper feeding tube placement; or inability to meet full energy requirements via the enteral route. Patients with severe chylothorax may also be candidates for PN, as parenteral administration of lipids bypasses the lymphatic system and thoracic duct (Suddaby and Schiller 2004).

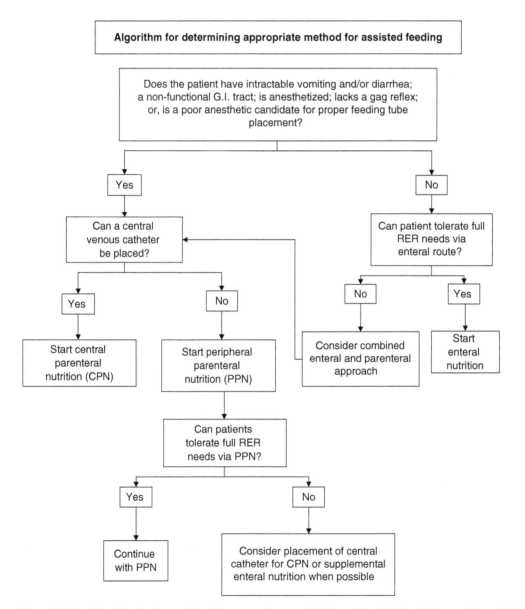

Figure 21.1 Algorithm for determining the appropriate method for assisted feeding. G.I., gastrointestinal; RER, resting energy requirement.

Successful reduction in triglyceride content of effusion from 1188 to 29 mg/dl has been reported with PN treatment in one veterinary chylothorax patient (Lippert et al. 1993).

The most commonly reported condition in veterinary patients that require PN is pancreatitis (Lippert et al. 1993; Pyle et al. 2004; Chan et al. 2006; Queau et al. 2011; Gajanayake et al. 2013), followed by gastrointestinal disease (Reuter et al. 1998), trauma (Olan and Prittie 2015), and hepatic diseases/hepatic lipidosis (Crabb et al. 2006). Enteral feeding is the preferred feeding method in patients with pancreatitis, and has been shown to be well tolerated and improve patient outcomes in dogs with pancreatitis (Harris et al. 2017). Therefore, while PN has commonly been leveraged for patients with pancreatitis that are not surgical candidates for placement of jejunostomy tubes, recent evidence supports additional consideration for EN in this population. For a complete discussion of enteral feeding, see Chapter 20.

Nomenclature

PN can be classified by the route of administration (central or peripheral) or by the degree of nutrition provided (total or partial). The term "total parenteral nutrition" (TPN) implies that the patient's complete nutritional needs are provided by the parenteral solution, which is not common practice in short-term (days to weeks) parenteral solutions administered to veterinary patients. The average duration of PN in dogs and cats from eight comprehensive retrospective studies is approximately 4 days, with a range of 3 hours to 25 days (Lippert et al. 1993; Reuter et al. 1998; Chan et al. 2002; Pyle et al. 2004; Crabb et al. 2006; Queau et al. 2011; Gajanayake et al. 2013; Olan and Prittie 2015). PN solutions used in veterinary medicine do not commonly provide all essential minerals and fat-soluble vitamins and are, therefore, not truly TPN solutions. Some define TPN as providing total energy needs, while partial parenteral nutrition provides only partial energy needs. Using this definition, TPN solutions are generally administered centrally, while partial parenteral solutions are generally administered peripherally. However, it is possible to provide the total target calories peripherally when utilizing high-fat solutions, while it can also be common practice to administer only partial energy needs centrally. Because of the discrepancies in nomenclature, this discussion will use the terms "central parenteral nutrition" (CPN) and "peripheral parenteral nutrition" (PPN), focusing on the characteristics of the solution that determine the route of administration.

Determination of Administration Route

PN may be administered via central or peripheral venous access. While peripheral venous access is easier to establish, central venous access provides more flexibility in the formulation of the parenteral solution. The primary limitation of peripheral solutions is the lower osmolarity that is required to prevent thrombophlebitis. Recommendations for maximum osmolarity of peripheral solutions range from 600 to 750 mOsmol/l, while central solutions can be as high as 1400 mOsmol/l (Delaney et al. 2006; Campbell et al. 2006; Olan and Prittie 2015). Based on the author's clinical experience, the more conservative end of this range is preferred for peripheral solutions, especially in patients with hypercoagulable conditions. To achieve reduced osmolarity, the parenteral solution must be formulated with a less concentrated dextrose solution, which decreases the energy density of the final solution. To help offset this effect, the calories provided by fat can be increased. Lipid solutions have low osmolarity and high energy density, and therefore help reduce the osmolarity and increase the energy density of the final solution. Most patients can tolerate these higher-fat solutions (Remillard 2000; Queau et al. 2011); however, those with preexisting hyperlipidemia or who develop hyperlipidemia while on parenteral nutrition may require a lower-fat approach in the form of CPN to deliver complete energy needs.

When central venous access is obtainable, CPN is generally preferred due to fewer restrictions in solution formulation, easier ability to meet full energy requirements, and reduced incidence of thrombophlebitis. In addition, one study identified PPN versus CPN as a risk factor for septic complications (Queau et al. 2011). However, successful administration of PPN in dogs and cats has been described (Zsombor-Murray and Freeman 1999; Chan et al. 2006; Gajanayake et al. 2013) and may be a more practical tool for practitioners who do not routinely place central catheters. Shorter durations of PN administration and the use of lipid-containing admixtures can also help reduce the incidence of thrombophlebitis (Chandler et al. 2000; Chandler and Payne-James 2006). In larger patients with neck injuries, or any size patient with coagulopathy, peripheral catheters may be required or preferred, therefore making PPN the method of choice for nutritional support.

Independent of the route of PN elected, it is important to continually reevaluate the patient and consider the introduction of enteral nutrition. Although most patients who are initially started on PN are not candidates for enteral nutrition, many may tolerate gradual initiation of enteral nutrition or even just a small proportion of their energy and nutrient needs simultaneously administered by the enteral route, also known as "trickle feeding." This concurrent implementation of enteral feeding may help to maintain intestinal integrity as well as immune and gut-barrier functions (Heidegger et al. 2007). One retrospective study evaluating partial PN in dogs and cats demonstrated improved survival in patients receiving concurrent enteral nutrition (Chan et al. 2002), providing further support for a combined approach and/or weaning to EN as soon as it can be tolerated.

Catheter Selection and Placement

Appropriate selection and management of peripheral catheters can help to minimize the risk of thrombophlebitis. Teflon catheters are associated with a high incidence of thrombophlebitis, while thrombophlebitis is reduced with the use of silicon and polyurethane catheters (Reynolds et al. 1995). Polyurethane catheters have a higher internal gauge with the same external diameter when compared to silicon catheters and have been shown to result in fewer occlusions (Culebras et al. 2004; Plusa et al. 1998). The use of small-diameter catheters, proper catheter care, and frequent catheter replacement can also reduce the incidence of thrombophlebitis (Chandler et al. 2000).

Multilumen polyurethane catheters are commonly utilized for CPN administration (Figure 21.2). Multilumen catheters provide the advantage of having a dedicated port for PN administration, with additional ports for blood draws, and crystalloid fluid and drug administration. These catheters are typically available in a wide range of diameters (4.5–8.5 Fr.) and lengths (8–60 cm). The shorter lengths are generally used for jugular placement, while the longer catheters can be used for peripherally inserted central venous catheters (centrally placed via the medial saphenous vein; much less commonly the femoral or cephalic veins). Central placement can be

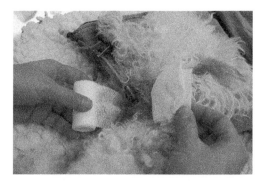

Figure 21.2 Placement of a multilumen polyurethane catheter in a dog for central parenteral nutrition administration.

radiographically verified and is highly recommended for peripherally inserted central venous catheters. In humans, peripherally inserted central venous catheters have been associated with higher rates of thrombophlebitis, particularly when used for PN administration (Cowl et al. 2000; Hammes et al. 2015). Although this has not been evaluated in dogs and cats, it is the author's clinical experience that complications associated with thrombophlebitis are more commonly seen with peripherally inserted central venous catheters. Because of this, jugular placement of central venous catheters is preferred when possible.

Parenteral Nutrition Components

Protein

Protein needs for patients receiving PN are provided by amino acid solutions, which are usually available in 8.5% and 10% concentrations. Amino acid solutions with a concentration of 8.5% have an energy density of 0.34 kcal/ml and osmolarity of 706–880 mOsmol/l. Therefore, compared to the lipid and dextrose components, the amino acid solution contributes relatively low energy density and moderately high osmolarity (Table 21.2).

Because parenterally administered amino acids are essentially 100% bioavailable, protein requirements that are established for oral feeding of commercial pet foods likely overestimate needs for parenteral administration. One study evaluated nitrogen balance in healthy dogs receiving different protein concentrations over a seven-day period (Mauldin et al. 2001). A control group received crystalloid fluids only, and the remaining three groups received infusions of 0, 1.36, or 2.04 g amino acid/kg body weight, with the remainder of their maintenance energy requirement (MER) provided by 50% lipid and 50% dextrose on a caloric basis. The study demonstrated that satisfying energy needs with carbohydrate and fat had a protein-sparing effect, with a greater negative nitrogen balance in dogs administered only crystalloid fluids compared to those administered the protein-free lipid and dextrose solution. All dogs had negative nitrogen balance, and calculations based on a linear relationship between nitrogen balance and amino acid administration estimated a requirement of 2.3 g protein/kg/d to achieve nitrogen balance. The dogs in this study averaged approximately 10 kg in body weight, with a calculated MER of 766 kcal/d. Therefore, this minimum protein requirement is equivalent to 3.0 g/100 kcal (12% protein on a metabolizable energy [ME] basis). This is lower than guidance established by the Association of American Feed Control Officials (AAFCO) for commercial diets formulated for adult canine maintenance (4.5 g/100 kcal), but is greater than both the minimum requirement and the recommended allowance established by the National Research Council (NRC) for adult canine maintenance (2.0 and 2.5 g/100 kcal, respectively).

The protein requirements in critically ill animals are likely different from those in healthy animals, as elevations in endogenous corticosteroids, catecholamines, and inflammatory cytokines promote a hypercatabolic state (Chan 2004; Preiser et al. 2014). An evaluation of urinary nitrogen excretion in critically ill dogs demonstrated losses that are two to six times the obligatory nitrogen excretion that is reported in healthy dogs (Michel et al. 1997). A healthy animal under conditions of starvation will adapt by decreasing muscle breakdown, converting primarily to the use of fatty acids and ketones for energy. However, in critically ill patients, muscle catabolism is not appropriately downregulated. In ill animals, the amino acids generated from muscle breakdown are primarily used for gluconeogenesis and production of acute-phase proteins, while synthesis of other selected proteins (such as albumin, transferrin, prealbumin, retinol-binding protein, and fibronectin) is actually decreased (Biolo et al. 1997; Thiessen et al. 2017).

As in veterinary medicine, there is also limited research in the human field to describe

Table 21.2 Commonly used solutions and supplements for parenteral nutrition.

Ingredient	Energy density and key nutrient contents	Osmolarity
Amino acid solutions		
Travasol 8.5%[a]	0.34 kcal/ml	880 mOsmol/l
Travasol 10%[a]	0.4 kcal/ml	998 mOsmol/l
Aminosyn II 8.5%[b]	0.34 kcal/ml	706 mOsmol/l
FreAmine 10%[c]	0.4 kcal/ml	950 mOsmol/l
Lipid solutions		
Intralipid 10%[a]	1.1 kcal/ml	260 mOsmol/l
	0.015 mmol PO_4/ml	
Intralipid 20%[a]	2 kcal/ml	260 mOsmol/l
	0.015 mmol PO_4/ml	
Liposyn II 10%[b]	1.1 kcal/ml	276 mOsmol/l
Liposyn II 20%[b]	2 kcal/ml	258 mOsmol/l
Dextrose solutions		
Dextrose 5%	0.17 kcal/ml	253 mOsmol/l
Dextrose 50%	1.7 kcal/ml	2525 mOsmol/l
Dextrose 70%	2.38 kcal/ ml	3640 mOsmol/l
Ready-made amino acid and carbohydrate solutions		
ProcalAmine (3% amino acid and 3% glycerol)[c]	0.25 kcal/ml	735 mOsmol/l
	24.5 mmol/l (24.5 mEq/l) K	
	41 mmol/l (41 mEq/l) Cl	
	35 mmol/l (35 mEq/l) Na	
	0.75 mmol/l (3 mEq/l) Ca	
	2.5 mmol/l (5 mEq/l) Mg	
	3.5 mmol/l (7 mEq/l) PO_4	
Electrolytes		
Potassium chloride	2 mEq K/ml	4000 mOsmol/l
Potassium phosphate	4.4 mEq K/ml	7357 mOsmol/l
	3 mmol PO_4/ml	
Magnesium sulfate 50%	4.06 mEq Mg/ml	4060 mOsmol/l
Sodium chloride 23.4%	4 mEq Na/ml	8000 mOsmol/l
Sodium chloride 14.6%	2.5 mEq Na/ml	5000 mOsmol/l
Vitamins and minerals		
Vitamin B complex[d]	Thiamine	Variable; 380–390 mOsmol/l
	Niacin	
	Pyridoxine	
	Pantothenic acid	
	Riboflavin	
	± Cyanocobalamin	

[a] Baxter Healthcare, Clintec Nutrition Division, Deerfield, IL, USA.
[b] Hospira Worldwide, Lake Forest, IL, USA.
[c] Braun Medical, Bethlehem, PA, USA.
[d] Various manufacturers; individual products contain different vitamin concentrations.

protein needs and optimal feeding practices. Studies involving human ICU patients have shown that protein intake is associated with multiple benefits including reduced infections, ventilation duration, time to discharge, and mortality (Heyland et al. 2017). However, other studies have shown mixed results, and additional studies are required to define the optimal amount of protein, influence of enteral versus parenteral delivery, and impacts on longer-term outcomes (Heyland et al. 2017).

The standard recommendation for protein concentrations in PN formulations is 4–5 g/100 kcal (16–20% protein on an ME basis) for dogs and 6 g/100 kcal (24% protein on an ME basis) for cats (Freeman and Chan 2006; Thomovsky et al. 2007; Queau et al. 2011). One goal of PN support should be providing adequate protein in order to minimize muscle breakdown and maintain lean body mass. Like energy, excessive protein should be avoided, as attempts to promote tissue anabolism through high-energy/high-protein PN administration may lead to complications such as azotemia and cholestasis (Klein et al. 1998). Protein concentrations are also dependent on individual patient needs and disease states. Animals with renal disease and hepatic encephalopathy should be provided PN solutions with reduced protein concentrations, while growing animals and patients with significant protein losses may require increased amounts to meet their needs.

Fat

Fat, provided by lipid emulsions, is an important component of PN, supplying both energy and essential fatty acids. The most commonly utilized lipid emulsions are 20% solutions, providing 2 kcal/ml with an osmolarity of 260 mOsmol/l. The lipid component of PN provides beneficial qualities to the final admixture, helping to temper the high osmolarity of the dextrose solution while enhancing the overall energy density. Recommended fat levels in PN formulations range from 30% to 80%

of total calories (Remillard 2000; Delaney et al. 2006; Freeman and Chan 2006). Higher fat levels (60–90% of nonprotein calories) have been reported to be well tolerated clinically in over 500 patients over a five-year period (Remillard 2000). Because animals that have been without food for over three days are utilizing primarily endogenous fat for energy, these higher-fat solutions may be more physiologically appropriate. Lower fat concentrations may be needed in animals with pre-existing hyperlipidemia, or who develop persistent lipemia while on PN. Although fat restriction is recommended for oral feeding in patients with pancreatitis, intravenous fat does not stimulate exocrine pancreatic secretion (Fried et al. 1982; Stabile et al. 1984); therefore, fat restriction is not necessary in PN formulations for patients with pancreatitis.

Lipid emulsions available within the United States are generally soybean oil and/or safflower oil based, with additional egg yolk phospholipids, glycerin, and water. Elimination and long-term (91-day) administration studies of lipid emulsions have been conducted in dogs (Cotter et al. 1984; Izzo et al. 1984). No significant differences were found in the maximum elimination capacity or fractional elimination rates of 10% Intralipid® (Baxter Healthcare, Deerfield, IL, USA) at bolus injection doses of 300 g/kg body weight or with continuous infusion doses of 3 or 6 g/kg body weight, indicating that the elimination mechanism had not been saturated. The researchers did note, however, that some of the data did not fit their model at the 6 g/kg level, suggesting individual variability in the ability to tolerate the lipid at higher administration rates. This finding reflects what is seen clinically, with some patients requiring reduced fat concentrations in PN solutions due to persistent hyperlipidemia during PN administration.

While soybean and safflower oil–based emulsions have been the mainstay of parental formulas in recent decades, recent research has suggested benefits of alternative lipid sources (blends including olive oil, fish oil, and medium-chain triglycerides). These mixtures may have fewer inflammatory properties, show immune benefits, and improve outcomes in some groups of patients (Raman et al. 2017). Soybean and safflower oil–based emulsions are composed of primarily omega-6 fatty acids and have been shown to inhibit lymphocyte proliferation and neutrophil chemotaxis and migration (Granato et al. 2000). These suppressive effects on the granulocyte and reticuloendothelial cell systems have raised concerns of immunosuppressive effects of high lipid-containing PN solutions. However, when different proportions of energy were supplied with a soybean oil-based emulsion during two-hour infusions in healthy research dogs, the function of polymorphonuclear neutrophils was only impacted by the highest infusion rate, which would be much more than is used in veterinary PN administration (Kang and Yang 2008).

One study reported an ex vivo investigation of the impact of a soybean oil-based emulsion on hemolysis in blood samples of healthy dogs and those with inflammatory leukograms (Behling-Kelly and Wakshlag 2018). The lipid doses used in the blood sample mixtures (1%, 3%, and 5% lipid solution) were extrapolated from predicted concentrations near a PN infusion site. Hemolysis was noted in blood samples from both groups, although samples from ill dogs were more affected only by the 5% lipid solution (16.4% vs. 25% hemolysis, respectively, as measured by optical density of supernatant). This study also investigated the impacts of the 5% lipid solution on thromboelastography in blood samples of healthy dogs (Behling-Kelly and Wakshlag 2018). An impact on clot formation was seen in both the vehicle-only and the lipid-treated samples; however, the addition of 5% lipid emulsion resulted in accelerated clot formation overall. The clinical significance of these potential effects is unknown and has yet to be evaluated in dogs and cats administered PN in the hospital setting.

In humans, the use of alternative lipids has been shown to reduce or eliminate some of these negative immunosuppressive effects (Chao et al. 2000; Sala-Vila et al. 2007; Wanten and Calder 2007; Raman et al. 2017). There is a dearth of similar investigations in veterinary patients. One study evaluated the use of parenteral infusions of soybean oil-based versus fish oil-based emulsions for three hours post-ovariohysterectomy in healthy dogs (Tsuruta et al. 2017). While apparently safe, the fish oil-based emulsion was not associated with any benefits with regard to plasma C-reactive protein concentration and leukocyte cytokine production. More research is needed to more fully evaluate various types of lipid emulsions in dogs and cats in order to guide future recommendations for clinical applications.

Carbohydrate

Dextrose solutions, ranging in concentrations from 5% to 70%, are utilized in PN solutions to provide carbohydrate calories. One of the most commonly used concentrations for CPN formulation is 50% dextrose, providing 1.7 kcal/ml, with an osmolarity of 2525 Osmol/l. For PPN formulations, 5% dextrose is commonly substituted, providing a 10-fold lower osmolarity of 253 Osmol/l, and a correspondingly lower energy density of 0.17 mOsmol/l. Some institutions and compounding pharmacies may utilize a higher dextrose solution and sterile water for peripheral PN formulations, titrating to an appropriate osmolarity for peripheral venous administration.

Recommended carbohydrate levels for PN solutions range from 20% to 50% on an ME basis (Delaney et al. 2006; Queau et al. 2011). Concentrations as high as 62% of the total calories have been well tolerated in healthy dogs over a nine-day period, although moderate hyperglycemia was present during the first few days of administration (Zentek et al. 2003). In order to avoid complications associated with hyperglycemia, some have recommended that rates of administration should not exceed 4 mg/kg/min (Freeman and Chan 2006). This rate is extrapolated from human data, where rates exceeding this level resulted in hyperglycemia in nondiabetic patients. Dextrose provides 0.034 kcal/mg; therefore, 4 mg/kg/min is equivalent to 0.136 kcal from dextrose/min/kg. For a 10 kg animal receiving resting energy requirement (RER; 393 kcal/day) over a 24-hour period, total kcal/min administration would be approximately 0.03 kcal/kg/min. Since only a portion of the total energy is provided by dextrose, these maximum dextrose infusion rates are not typically reached during routine PN administration. However, hyperglycemia is the most common metabolic complication seen with PN administration in dogs and cats (Lippert et al. 1993; Reuter et al. 1998; Chan et al. 2002; Pyle et al. 2004; Crabb et al. 2006; Queau et al. 2011); therefore, avoiding high concentrations of dextrose and ensuring frequent monitoring during PN administration are recommended.

Higher concentrations are sometimes unavoidable in patients that require protein and/ or fat restriction for other disease conditions. Lower levels may be beneficial in diabetic patients and animals that develop persistent or worsening hyperglycemia during PN administration. While dogs may successfully adapt to high dextrose infusions after one or two days of PN administration (Reuter et al. 1998; Zentek et al. 2003), cats have been reported to have persistent hyperglycemia after three days of PN administration (Pyle et al. 2004). Therefore, lower-carbohydrate formulations may be more appropriate for cats and/or they may require lower infusion rates and/or necessitate management with exogenous insulin.

Electrolytes and Trace Minerals

Potassium and phosphorus are the most commonly added electrolytes to PN admixtures for dogs and cats. Hypokalemia and hypophosphatemia can occur with refeeding syndrome and are routinely added to PN solutions (see the discussion under complications). For patients that are normokalemic, potassium phosphate should be added to provide 20–30 mEq K^+/l (Remillard 2000). Phosphorus is commonly provided by both the lipid solution and the additional potassium phosphate solution. Although no specific guidelines have been published for phosphorus content of canine and feline PN solutions, recommendations for human PN solutions range from 20 to 40 mM/l (Mirtallo 2001). For patients with pre-existing hyperphosphatemia and/or hyperkalemia (such as is commonly seen in patients with renal disease), potassium chloride can be substituted or omitted. It is recommended that any additional electrolyte abnormalities be corrected through crystalloid fluid supplementation, as the risk of solution instability and mineral precipitation is greater with additions to PN admixtures. Additionally, if further adjustments in electrolyte concentrations are required, this is more easily done via modifications to crystalloid fluids, given the cost of replacement of the PN solution.

Recommendations for the addition of trace minerals to PN admixtures in veterinary medicine are highly variable. Some institutions do not routinely include trace minerals (Pyle et al. 2004; Queau et al. 2011), while others may add trace minerals (chromium, copper, manganese, and zinc; Crabb et al. 2006), or routinely add zinc only (Michel 2007). For most clinical PN use, duration of administration is typically up to several days, and supplementing trace minerals into the PN admixtures is not necessary due to the low likelihood that a nutrient deficiency will develop. For patients on PN for longer than two weeks, the addition of trace minerals should be considered.

When adding electrolytes and/or trace minerals to PN admixtures, it is important to recognize the potential risks of instability and precipitation within the solution. Mineral stability within the nutrient admixture can vary based on the form used, pH of the solution, the ambient temperature, and the concentrations of amino acids, dextrose, and other electrolytes within the solution (Allwood and Kearney 1998). In general, monovalent ions are stable within PN admixtures, while di- and trivalent ions are more likely to form insoluble complexes. The most commonly reported precipitate within PN admixtures is calcium phosphate (Allwood and Kearney 1998). This has primarily been a problem in human infant PN admixtures, which require higher concentrations of calcium and phosphorus than adult formulations (Parikh et al. 2005).

There is little information about the stability of trace minerals within PN admixtures. Chromium, copper, manganese, and zinc have been shown to be both stable and compatible in PN admixtures for up to 48 hours at an ambient temperature (Allwood and Kearney 1998). However, formation of copper and iron precipitates has been reported within solutions containing sulfur amino acids (Allwood et al. 1998; Hardy et al. 1998). Precipitates can be difficult to visualize due to the opaque nature of the lipid-containing PN solutions. The use of inline filters can help to provide protection from precipitates that are not grossly visible, and should be strongly considered for PN administration lines regardless of the addition of trace minerals.

Vitamins

Because of their relatively rapid turnover rates and essential roles as cofactors in energy metabolism, B vitamins are important components of the PN solution. Most veterinary commercial B vitamin complexes contain thiamin, niacin, pyridoxine, pantothenic acid, and riboflavin, with some also including cyanocobalamin. Folic acid is not compatible with riboflavin and is therefore not included in B complex solutions. Cobalamin (vitamin B12) is generally the limiting B vitamin in terms of the amount needed to achieve minimum nutrient requirements; when added separately the amount can be more precise. The amount added to the PN solution should be sufficient to meet established nutrient requirements (see Box 21.1).

Because of their relatively slow turnover rates, fat-soluble vitamins are not routinely added to PN solutions for short-term administration in dogs and cats. For patients with specific nutrient concerns, such as vitamin K deficiency in patients with hepatic or hepatobiliary disease, parenteral supplementation may be administered separately. Additionally, for patients with long-term fat malabsorption, it has been recommended to give a one-time intramuscular administration of a vitamin A, D, and E complex (Vital E-A + D, Schering-Plow Animal Health, Kenilworth, NJ, USA), which will provide the needed nutrients for up to three months (Remillard 2000).

Box 21.1   Step-by-Step Calculations for Parenteral Formulations

Step 1	**Determine energy requirement**
kcal/day	Resting energy requirement (RER) = $70 \times (\text{body weight in kg})^{0.75}$
Step 2	**Determine macronutrient volumes**
Protein	____% ME × ____ RER (kcal/day) = ____ $\text{protein}_{\text{kcal}}$
	____ $\text{protein}_{\text{kcal}}$ ÷ ____ kcal/ml amino acid solution
	= ____ **ml amino acid solution**
Fat	____% ME × ____ RER (kcal/day) = ____ fat_{kcal}
	____ fat_{kcal} ÷ ____ kcal/ml lipid solution
	= ____ **ml lipid solution**
Carbohydrate	____% ME × ____ RER (kcal/day) = ____ $\text{carbohydrate}_{\text{kcal}}$
	____ $\text{carbohydrate}_{\text{kcal}}$ ÷ ____ kcal/ml dextrose solution
	= ____ **ml dextrose solution**

Step 3

Potassium level desired should be determined by patient's serum potassium concentration

Determine volume of potassium supplement

mEq K^+ needed = ___mEq/l K^+ desired × ___total macronutrient volume/100

volume KPO_4 = ___mEq K^+ needed ÷ 4.4 mEq/ml = **_____ ml KPO_4**

OR, for patients with hyperphosphatemia, use potassium chloride:

Volume KCl = ___mEq K^+ needed ÷ 2 mEq/l = **_____ ml KCl**

Step 4

Check total phosphorus and add supplementation if needed

Calculate total phosphorus

___ml lipid solution × ___mmol P/ml = ___mmol phosphorus

___ml KPO_4 × ___mmol P/ml = ___mmol phosphorus

_____total mmol phosphorus

Step 5

Add B vitamin complex (± separate vitamin B12 if not included) at amount needed to meet the following requirements

Calculate volume of B vitamin complex

Thiamin – 0.29 mg/1000 kcal solution

Riboflavin – 0.63 mg/1000 kcal solution

Niacin – 3.3 mg/1000 kcal solution

Pantothenic acid – 2.9 mg/1000 kcal solution

Pyridoxine – 0.29 mg/1000 kcal solution

Cyanocobalamin – 6.0 mcg/1000 kcal solution

Step 6

Calculate total volume and osmolarity

_____ ml amino acid solution × ___mOsm/ml = _____mOsmol

_____ ml lipid solution × ___mOsm/ml = _____mOsmol

_____ ml dextrose solution × ___mOsm/ml = _____mOsmol

_____ ml KCl or KPO_4 × ___mOsm/ml = _____mOsmol

_____ ml B vitamin complex × ___mOsm/ml = _____mOsmol

_____ total volume _____total mOsmol

Total mOsmol/l = total mOsmol/total volume

Step 7

Calculate energy density of solution

Energy density = ___total kcals (RER) ÷ ___ml total volume

= **___kcal/ml**

Energy Requirements

The goal of PN support is to provide an appropriate level of energy to sustain critical physiologic processes (such as immune function and wound healing) and maintain lean body mass, without overly stressing the patient's metabolic system with excessive nutrients. Many critically ill patients are underweight or trending down, and there is a tendency to desire weight gain in these animals. However, overfeeding is a common complication with PN and may contribute to problems such as cholestasis, hepatic lipidosis, and respiratory failure (Mauldin et al. 2001). Overfeeding may also contribute to hyperglycemia, which has been shown to be a negative prognostic indicator in critically ill human and feline patients receiving PN (Pyle et al. 2004; Cheung et al. 2005; Lin et al. 2007; Krinsley et al. 2017).

Energy needs can vary from patient to patient, and the ideal situation would be to measure individual patient needs via indirect calorimetry, as is commonly utilized in human hospitals (Boullata et al. 2007). However, these measurements are costly and unavailable in most veterinary hospital settings; therefore, calculation of predicted requirements is the most practical tool to estimate energy needs.

During hospitalization, patients are generally estimated to require energy levels equivalent to their calculated RER. There are multiple equations to estimate RER; exponential equations utilizing the patient's metabolic body weight are preferred in order to best meet the needs of the wide range of body sizes in veterinary medicine. Linear equations are not recommended due to likely overestimation of true needs for small and larger animals. Adjustment of energy provision targets based on the disease process is no longer recommended for hospitalized patients, as multiplying RER by illness factors generally results in overestimation of true energy needs (O'Toole et al. 2004). The amount fed should initially be gradually increased, starting at approximately 25% of RER, followed by additional increments of 25% RER every 8–12 hours until full RER is reached. The rate of increase can be modified based on patient tolerance. Once full RER has been reached, the patient may be reassessed to determine if increased levels are warranted. In the author's clinical experience, energy levels above RER are rarely needed, and maintaining more conservative rates helps reduce the risk of metabolic complications associated with overfeeding.

It is the author's preference to include all nutrients (protein, fat, and carbohydrate) for energy calculations, although some veterinary nutritionists prefer to consider protein needs separately, with the caloric needs met by fat and carbohydrate alone. However, not accounting for protein calories has been argued to be a potential cause for complications associated with overfeeding in veterinary patients receiving PN (Crabb et al. 2006). Additionally, one prospective study in healthy cats demonstrated

detrimental effects on hepatic function only in cats receiving PN doses that did not account for protein calories, compared to those for whom calories were accounted from all three macronutrients (Lippert et al. 1989). However, all cats in this study received doses of 1.4 times their calculated RER, which could have also contributed to the complications seen with overfeeding. The calculations presented in this chapter will account for protein calories. Independent of the method used, the primary conclusion is that overfeeding should be avoided.

Formulation Calculations

Step-by-step calculations for PN formulations are outlined in Box 21.1. First calculate the energy needs of the patient, using the calculation for RER. As already mentioned, illness energy factors are not recommended due to concerns of overfeeding. However, body weight should be monitored, and individual variations in energy needs should be considered after feeding at full RER is achieved. Steps 2–4 require selection of the desired energy distribution (percentage protein, percentage fat, and percentage carbohydrate on an ME basis) and electrolyte concentrations. These values will be determined on an individual patient basis, as discussed earlier. Table 21.2 outlines the energy density of commonly utilized components to aid in these calculations. Step 5 requires the calculation of the needed volume of B vitamin complex. The volume of B vitamin complex required will vary based on the product used and should be provided in amounts necessary to meet the patient's established requirements. B vitamins have a wide margin of safety, so it is common practice to provide excesses compared to minimum requirements. This also provides a safety buffer for expected ultraviolet (UV) degradation. Finally, the total volume, osmolarity, and energy density of the solution are calculated in Steps 6 and 7.

Compounding

Because lipid-containing PN solutions are supportive of bacterial and fungal growth, preparation must be conducted with careful, aseptic techniques. Preparation within a laminar flow hood has been the minimum standard for many years. However, the United States Pharmacopeia (USP) has established guidelines for the preparation of sterile compounding that are adopted by most state pharmacy boards and are enforceable by the US Food and Drug Administration. The relevant statutes describe procedures and requirements for compounding sterile preparations and apply to all settings, including those related to veterinary drugs. Compliance helps ensure patient safety and promotes high-quality care. PN is classified as a medium-risk formulation, and compounding should be conducted within an International Organization for Standardization (ISO) Class 5 environment (≤ 352000 particles of $0.5\,\mu m$ or larger size per m^3), such as a clean room or mobile isolation chamber.

The PN components may be mixed using manual or automatic methods. Manual compounding uses gravity flow of individual components, feeding into an empty sterile PN bag or glass bottle (Figures 21.3 and 21.4). While the manual method does not require expensive automatic compounding equipment, it is slow, is prone to inaccuracies, requires multiple manipulations, and has an increased likelihood of contamination (Mirtallo 2001). Automated

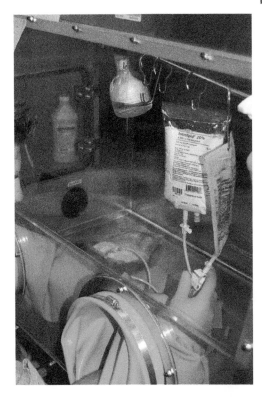

Figure 21.4 Manual parenteral nutrition solution compounding within a mobile isolation chamber at the University of California, Davis Veterinary Medical Teaching Hospital.

compounding devices help to eliminate these increased risks of human error and contamination, but are more expensive and may not be available in some areas (Figures 21.5–21.7).

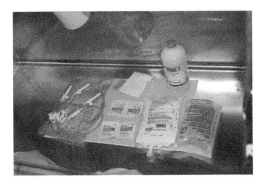

Figure 21.3 Individual components for manual parenteral nutrition solution compounding.

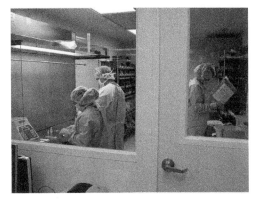

Figure 21.5 Clean room for automated parenteral nutrition compounding at the University of California, San Diego Medical Center.

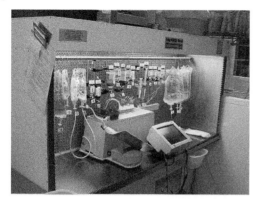

Figure 21.6 An automated compounder used for preparing parenteral nutrition solutions at the University of California, San Diego Medical Center.

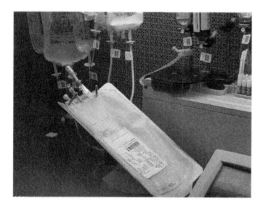

Figure 21.7 Automated parenteral nutrition solution compounding at the University of California, San Diego Medical Center.

For either method of compounding, it is important to ensure that appropriate mixing procedures are followed. The sequence of mixing the various ingredients affects solution stability. Of particular concern is the stability of the fat emulsion, as multiple factors, including pH, glucose, amino acid, and divalent-cation concentrations, can impact the fat emulsion stability (Allwood 2000). Procedural protocols have been developed to help reduce the likelihood of incompatibilities within the formulation. First, all trace elements and electrolytes (except phosphorus) should be added to the dextrose solution; second, any phosphorus additives should be mixed with the amino acid solution; third, the

amino acid and dextrose solution should be mixed; fourth, the lipid emulsion should be added to the dextrose and amino acid mixture; and finally, any addition of other medications or components should be considered in accordance with verified stability information (Campbell et al. 2006). Regular visual inspection and monitoring of the quality of the admixture should also be performed, assessing for precipitates and coalescence of fat particles.

While many teaching institutions regularly compound PN solutions, most veterinary practices do not have the appropriate equipment and/or facilities for proper PN compounding. Compounding pharmacies that are equipped for human PN preparation will generally also compound veterinary formulations. Alternatively, large veterinary referral hospitals or human hospitals in the area may compound PN solutions and will also work with local veterinarians. Finally, some university veterinary medical teaching institutions offer nutrition support services that provide individual PN formulations, compounding, and delivery.

Initiating Parenteral Nutrition

PN products should only be administered through a dedicated catheter or dedicated port. The administration line should also be dedicated for PN administration only, and should include a 1.2 μm inline filter to help prevent inadvertent administration of lipid globules or precipitates. To ensure the sterility of the line, it should not be disconnected during PN administration (including for patient walks). To help remind clinic staff not to disconnect the line and to prevent the line from becoming disconnected by the patient, it is helpful to tape the line at the connection ports (Figure 21.8). It is generally recommended to cover the PN bag to prevent degradation of B vitamins by UV light. The PN must be discarded after 24–48 hours of hanging, and the administration line should be discarded and replaced with each new bag of PN.

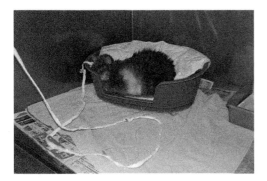

Figure 21.8 Feline patient at the University of California, Davis Veterinary Medical Teaching Hospital receiving central parenteral nutrition. Note that the administration line has been taped to help remind clinic staff not to disconnect the line and to prevent the line from becoming disconnected by the patient.

The PN should be administered by constant-rate infusion over a 24-hour period with the use of a calibrated fluid pump. Infusion of daily energy needs over a 10-hour period has been reported in healthy dogs (Zentek et al. 2003). Successful administration of partial energy needs via PPN over a 10–12-hour period has also been reported in hospitalized dogs (Chandler and Payne-James 2006). It has been suggested that higher-fat solutions may be better tolerated than high dextrose-containing solutions for shorter, more rapid rates of infusion (Zentek et al. 2003). Further research in this area is needed and could open up new avenues for more practical uses of PN in veterinary hospitals where 24-hour monitoring is unavailable.

The goal rate of PN administration is determined by the patient's daily energy requirement and the energy density of the solution. The total volume to be administered over the 24-hour period should be equivalent to the patient's calculated RER. The patient should be slowly increased to the PN goal rate, starting with 25% and increasing by 25% increments every 8–24 hours. The rate of increase will be dependent on the individual patient response, including the presence of hyperglycemia, hyperlipidemia, and/or electrolyte abnormalities. Guidelines for blood glucose monitoring during

the introduction period are outlined in Table 21.3. Patients who have been without food for an extended period of time are at an increased risk of developing electrolyte abnormalities upon refeeding (see discussion in the complications section). These patients may require slower increases, with more time at each incremental step and more frequent monitoring.

Monitoring Guidelines

Careful monitoring is essential during PN administration, especially during the period that amounts are being increased to the goal rate. The guidelines in Table 21.3 give minimum monitoring recommendations. The frequency at which specific parameters should be measured will be driven by the status of the patient. Patients with a poor nutritional status and in a more critical state of illness will require more frequent monitoring. Monitoring frequency may also be increased if faster time to achieve the goal rate is desired.

Complications

Complications associated with PN are classified as metabolic, mechanical, and septic. Metabolic complications are the most common, followed by mechanical and then septic. There have been several retrospective studies reporting complications associated with PN in dogs and/or cats (Lippert et al. 1993; Reuter et al. 1998; Chan et al. 2002; Pyle et al. 2004; Crabb et al. 2006; Queau et al. 2011; Gajanayake et al. 2013; Olan and Prittie 2015). Collectively, these studies provide an overview of the types of solutions administered as well as common complications associated with PN in dogs and cats.

Metabolic Complications

Hyperglycemia is the most common metabolic complication reported in both dogs and cats. Hyperglycemia was reported in 75% of cats and

Table 21.3 Parenteral nutrition monitoring guidelines.

---

1) Measure and record body weight, temperature, pulse, and respiration rate daily.

2) Measure blood glucose (BG) every 4 h until the goal rate of administration is reached. Start parenteral nutrition (PN) administration at 25% of the goal rate (determined by patient's daily resting energy requirement [RER]).

   a) If BG <250 mg/dl, increase the rate of administration by 25% of the goal rate until goal rate is reached.

   b) If BG 250–300 mg/dl, maintain the present rate of infusion during the weaning-on period. If infusing at 100% of goal rate and glucose level continues over two measurements at 4 h intervals, consider insulin administration, decrease the rate of infusion by 25%, or decrease the dextrose content of the solution.

   c) If BG >300 mg/dl, consider insulin administration, decrease the rate of infusion by 25%, or decrease the dextrose content of the solution.

3) Measure packed cell volume (PCV) and total solids (TS), and examine for lipemic and hemolytic serum daily.

4) Measure serum potassium and phosphorus concentrations within 12 h of starting PN infusion. Continue to measure at a frequency of no less than once daily during the weaning-on period, and no less than once every other day when at goal rate of infusion for 24 h.

5) Measure ionized magnesium within 24 h of starting PN infusion. Repeat within 48 h if hypomagnesemia is measured.

6) Measure complete chemistry panel within 24 h of starting PN infusion, and then no less than once every 2–3 d.

7) Measure serum triglycerides if lipemic serum is present for two or more consecutive measurements at 4 h intervals.

8) Perform thoracic radiographs if respiratory distress develops any time during administration.

9) Evaluate catheter site twice daily for evidence of infection and/or thrombophlebitis.

10) Perform catheter tip and/or blood cultures if sepsis is suspected.

Source: Adapted from Delaney et al. (2006).

31% of dogs in the Lippert study; 32% of dogs in the Reuter study; 12.5% of dogs and 44.7% of cats in the Chan study; 47% of cats in the Pyle study; 23% of cats in the Crabb study; 84% of cats and 61% of dogs in the Queau study; 28% of dogs in the Gajanayake study; and 11% of dogs in the Olan and Prittie study. The Queau study reported serum glucose concentrations of 146 ± 32.6 mg/dl in dogs and 213 ± 69.8 mg/dl in cats when hyperglycemia was first recognized after PN initiation, and the maximal concentration of 347 mg/dl in dogs and 489 mg/dl in cats. The increase in serum glucose concentration was lower in animals that were hyperglycemic before PN ($110 \pm 28.5\%$ in dogs and $132 \pm 38.2\%$ in cats) compared with those that were normo- or hypoglycemic before PN ($144 \pm 55.3\%$ in dogs and $182 \pm 56.4\%$ in cats; animals receiving insulin were excluded) (Queau et al. 2011).

Hyperglycemia has been a major topic of interest in both human and veterinary critical care patients in recent years. In the Pyle study, the risk of mortality was increased by greater than fivefold in cats that developed hyperglycemia after the first 24 hours of PN (odds ratio of 5.66). Similar increased risks of mortality have been demonstrated in human patients who develop hyperglycemia associated with PN administration during ICU hospitalization (Cheung et al. 2005; Lin et al. 2007; Krinsley et al. 2017). Other veterinary studies have not shown the same negative risk associated with hyperglycemia and outcome, but differences in hyperglycemia definitions as well as proactive monitoring and interventions, including insulin therapy, may help explain these inconsistencies (Chan et al. 2002; Queau et al. 2011).

Hyperglycemia is not limited to patients receiving PN, and it has been documented as a relatively common finding in both human and veterinary critically ill patients (Chan et al. 2006; Hafidah et al. 2007). An evaluation of cats that presented to an emergency service at a large referral hospital reported a 40% incidence of hyperglycemia at presentation (Chan et al. 2002). Hyperglycemic cats in this study were significantly more likely to die or be euthanized than those without hyperglycemia. Further evaluation by this same group of researchers revealed that critically ill cats have significantly higher glucose, lactate, cortisol, glucagon, and norepinephrine concentrations, and significantly lower insulin concentrations when compared to controls (Chan et al. 2006). These findings are consistent with those from human studies that have demonstrated higher concentrations of counter-regulatory hormones and insulin resistance in critically ill patients (Marik and Raghavan 2004; Zauner et al. 2007).

Further research in this area is needed to determine the most appropriate management strategies for hyperglycemic veterinary patients. However, closer monitoring and maintaining tighter glycemic control in patients receiving PN may aid in improving patient outcome. Patients who develop hyperglycemia in the initial phases of PN administration should be more slowly increased to the target administration rates. For those patients who are persistently hyperglycemic, insulin therapy should be implemented, or the PN solution should be reformulated to provide a lower carbohydrate concentration.

Hyperlipidemia is also a commonly reported metabolic complication seen in 46% of the dogs and cats in the Lippert study; 7% of the dogs in the Reuter study; 12.5% of the dogs and 19% of the cats in the Chan study; and 15% of the cats in the Crabb study. In contrast,

hyperlipidemia was also one of the reported metabolic corrections seen while on PN in the Reuter study. Similarly, in the Pyle study, 24% of cats had hyperlipidemia prior to starting PN, and this value decreased to 19% of cats after 24 hours, and 15% of cats after 96 hours of PN administration. The presence of hyperlipidemia prior to PN administration was not reported in the Lippert, Chan, or Crabb studies. The reason for the differences seen between these studies is unclear. However, in the Reuter and Pyle studies, patients with pre-existing hyperlipidemia likely reflected those with increased mobilization of fat in response to prolonged anorexia and illness (Wolfe et al. 1983). Hyperlipidemia is also a complication of poorly regulated diabetes mellitus (Michel 2005). Of the cats in the Pyle study, 17% had diabetes mellitus, but the association between the presence of diabetes mellitus and hyperlipidemia was not evaluated. In addition to the hyperglycemia commonly documented in critically ill cats, elevations in nonesterified fatty acids (NEFA) have also been reported (Chan et al. 2006). In those cases, refeeding may help reverse the catabolic state, decrease mobilization of adipose stores, and actually improve or resolve hyperlipidemia. Management of hyperlipidemia that develops or worsens during administration of PN includes decreasing the rate of administration or reformulation of the parenteral solution to provide a lower fat concentration.

A wide range of electrolyte abnormalities, including hyponatremia, hypokalemia, hypocalcemia, hypophosphatemia, and hypochloremia, were reported in seven of the eight retrospective studies (Lippert et al. 1993; Reuter et al. 1998; Pyle et al. 2004; Crabb et al. 2006; Queau et al. 2011; Gajanayake et al. 2013; Olan and Prittie 2015). Electrolyte abnormalities are commonly associated with "refeeding syndrome," a term commonly used to describe the metabolic abnormalities that can occur upon refeeding a patient following an extended period of anorexia (Crook et al. 2001). Due to lack of intake and/or obligatory or excessive losses, these patients often have an intracellular depletion of electrolytes that may not be recognized by evaluation of serum electrolytes. When nutrients are delivered, by either enteral or parenteral routes, there is an increased need for electrolytes (such as phosphorus and magnesium) to drive metabolic pathways as substrate and cofactors for adenosine triphosphate (ATP) synthesis. This increased intracellular need, in conjunction with cotransport of potassium into the cell with insulin-driven glucose uptake, results in an inward rectification of serum phosphorus, magnesium, and potassium.

In addition to the electrolyte abnormalities, the Gajanayake study also reported hyperkalemia as one of the common metabolic complications, and found this complication to be associated with a poor outcome (euthanasia or death). This study evaluated a lipid-free readymade PN solution that included 20 mEq/l potassium. Because of the small study population, it was difficult for the authors to determine if the hyperkalemia was an independent risk factor or a surrogate marker for a more severe underlying metabolic condition; however, it raised attention to the fact that patients receiving this type of ready-made solution should be monitored closely for this potential complication.

Hyperbilirubinemia is another common complication reported in patients on PN. Hyperbilirubinemia was seen in 24% of dogs in the Reuter study, and in 4% of the dogs and 6% of the cats in the Chan study. Hyperbilirubinemia was not reported in the Lippert, Pyle, Crabb, Queau, Gajanayake, or Olan and Prittie studies. Cholestasis and fatty infiltration of hepatic parenchyma have been associated with PN and may have contributed to the hyperbilirubinemia seen in these studies. Although high levels of fat in parenteral solutions can be responsible for this complication, high-carbohydrate infusions have also been associated with high activity of hormone-sensitive lipase (resulting in endogenous fatty acid release) and can be a contributing factor (Klein et al. 1998).

Azotemia has been reported in association with PN, seen in 17% of the dogs and cats in the Lippert study; 5% of the dogs in the Reuter study; 1.3% of the dogs in the Chan study; and 7.5% of the cats in the Crabb study. Hypercreatininemia in dogs independently of chronic kidney disease was reported in eight dogs (2.5%) in the Queau study. Azotemia was not a reported complication seen with PN in cats in the Chan and Pyle studies. Azotemia seen with PN administration has been attributed to a combined effect of endogenous (muscle catabolism) and exogenous (PN) amino acids that are rapidly cleared by the liver in critically ill and injured patients (Klein et al. 1998). Animals with pre-existing renal disease or who develop azotemia while on PN should be administered or switched to a parenteral solution with a reduced protein level.

Although they have not yet been reported in veterinary patients, respiratory complications associated with hypercapnia secondary to high caloric and high carbohydrate administration have been reported in human ventilatory patients (Askanazi et al. 1981; Jannace et al. 1988; Liposky and Nelson 1994; Tappy et al. 1998). The metabolism of carbohydrate generates more carbon dioxide than the metabolism of protein or fat and therefore contributes to the hypercapnia seen in these patients. Carbohydrate concentrations that resulted in the complications seen in human studies are higher than those generally used in veterinary PN solutions (80–100% of non-protein calories). Although evaluations have not yet been made in dogs and cats, overfeeding and high-carbohydrate solutions should be avoided in patients requiring ventilatory support.

Mechanical Complications

Mechanical complications are the second most frequent type of complication seen with PN. Mechanical complications are reported to occur in 9–46% of dogs and 9–28% of cats receiving PN. Common mechanical complications include broken or chewed lines, occluded catheter and/or lines, catheter dysfunction or dislodgment, jugular vein thrombosis, perivascular infiltration, and cellulitis (Lippert et al. 1993; Reuter et al. 1998; Chan et al. 2002; Pyle et al. 2004; Crabb et al. 2006; Queau et al. 2011; Gajanayake et al. 2013; Olan and Prittie 2015). Mechanical complications are typically assumed to be more common in dogs compared to cats due to a higher number of complications associated with chewing or breaking the line. Some of these complications can be avoided by careful monitoring of the patient, utilization of restrictive collars, and/or taping of the administration line (Figure 21.9).

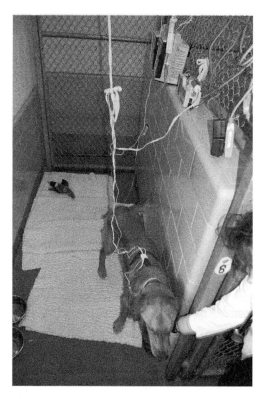

Figure 21.9 Canine patient at the University of California, Davis Veterinary Medical Teaching Hospital receiving central parenteral nutrition. Note that the administration line is hung and secured to a harness to help prevent mechanical complications.

Septic Complications

Although they are generally the least frequent type of complication, septic complications can have severe consequences and are therefore a concern during PN administration. Catheter-related septic complications and contamination of lipid-containing parenteral solutions with microorganisms are two of the primary concerns with PN administration. However, other factors contribute to the septic risks, including the underlying disease of the patient and gastrointestinal bacterial translocation (Harvey et al. 2006).

Despite these many concerns, reports of septic complications with PN administration have been fairly low. Studies evaluating animals receiving lipid-containing PN solutions report frequencies of septic complications ranging from 2.5% to 7% in dogs and 4% to 5% in cats. These percentages reflect cases that had positive blood or catheter tip cultures, local inflammation of the site of the catheter, and/or leukocytosis with a left shift. Additionally, the Pyle and Crabb studies had 8% and 12.5% of cats, respectively, that developed a fever after PN was initiated, but the PN per se could not be specifically implicated in any of these cases. In the Queau study, dogs had a higher risk of developing a septic complication when receiving peripheral versus centrally administered PN (odds ratio of 5.89). The Gajanayake study of dogs receiving a ready-made lipid-free PN solution confirmed that septic complications were noted in 7% of dogs. In this study 66% of the dogs received PPN, while the other 44% received CPN via a jugular catheter; however, no association was found between the development of septic complications and the type of catheter (central vs. peripheral). The different findings associated with peripheral versus central administration and septic complications could be a result of study size (the Queau study was much larger), or the type of PN solution administered (lipid containing versus lipid free).Other contributing factors to the septic complications seen in these studies included the patient chewing through the administration line, the catheter used for fluid and medication administration prior to use for PN, the catheter being placed by an inexperienced operator, poor nutritional status of the patient, and a severe underlying disease state. Septic complications can be decreased by practicing aseptic techniques during catheter placement, careful maintenance of an aseptic administration line and catheter insertion site, restrictive collars, or 24-hour monitoring, and may help to ensure that patients do not disrupt the administration line. Appropriate catheter care and replacement protocols, as well as frequent catheter monitoring, may help to prevent and/or identify problems at an early stage (Ukleja and Romano 2007). Finally, early transition to enteral nutrition, or providing a portion of nutritional needs via the enteral route, may help to reduce the occurrence of villous atrophy and bacterial translocation if bacteremia is from the gastrointestinal tract (Qin et al. 2002).

Discontinuing Parenteral Nutrition

Transition to enteral or oral feeding should be initiated as soon as can be tolerated by the patient (Figure 21.10). PN has been shown to reduce sham feeding in dogs by 50%, with the mechanism of action likely through peptide YY and neuropeptide Y (NPY) receptor–mediated events (Lee et al. 1997). Therefore, when transitioning to oral feeding, decreasing the rate of PN administration may be required to restore the patient's full appetite. Abrupt discontinuation of PN should be avoided, as this can result in rebound hypoglycemia. In order to ensure adequate adaptation as continuous PN is discontinued, the rate of administration should be slowly decreased in 25% increments over a 4–12-hour time frame while monitoring glycemia.

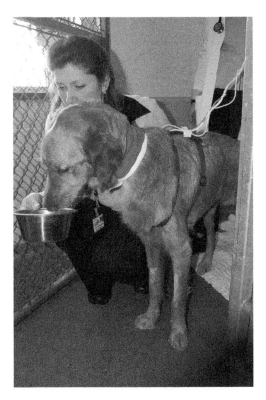

Figure 21.10 Canine patient at the University of California, Davis Veterinary Medical Teaching Hospital being offered oral feedings for transition off central parenteral nutrition.

Summary

- All hospitalized patients require assessment of nutritional status and consideration of when assisted feeding should be implemented.
- Parenteral nutrition (PN) is indicated in patients with intractable vomiting and/or diarrhea; anesthesia or lacking a gag reflex; recovery from severe gastric or intestinal resection; poor anesthetic candidate for proper feeding tube placement; or inability to meet full energy requirements via the enteral route.
- PN may be delivered via central or peripheral venous access.
- Central delivery of PN allows for greater osmolarity, providing more flexibility in formulations and typically a greater energy density of the solution.

- Caloric distribution of parenteral solutions should be determined on an individual patient basis, taking into consideration individual tolerance of protein, fat, and carbohydrate, and any underlying disease states.
- Metabolic complications are common, requiring frequent monitoring and adjustments.

- Many mechanical and septic complications can be avoided with appropriate monitoring and aseptic techniques.
- Transition to enteral or oral feeding should be initiated as soon as can be tolerated by the patient.

References

Allwood, M.C. (2000). Pharmaceutical aspects of parenteral nutrition: from now to the future. *Nutrition* 16 (7/8): 615–618.

Allwood, M.C. and Kearney, M.C.J. (1998). Compatibility and stability of additives in parenteral nutrition admixtures. *Nutrition* 14 (9): 697–706.

Allwood, M.C., Martin, H., Greenwood, M. et al. (1998). Precipitation of trace elements in parenteral nutrition mixtures. *Clin. Nutr.* 17 (5): 223–226.

Askanazi, J., Nordenstrom, J., Rosenbaum, S.H. et al. (1981). Nutrition for the patient with respiratory failure: glucose vs. fat. *Anesthesiology* 54 (5): 373–377.

Behling-Kelly, E.L. and Wakshlag, J. (2018). A commercial soy-based phospholipid emulsion accelerates clot formation in normal canine whole blood and induces hemolysis in whole blood from normal and dogs with inflammatory leukograms. *J. Emerg. Crit. Care* 28 (3): 252–260.

Biolo, G., Toigo, G., Ciocchi, B. et al. (1997). Metabolic response to injury and sepsis: changes in protein metabolism. *Nutrition* 13 (9S): 52S–57S.

Boullata, J., Williams, J., Cottrell, F. et al. (2007). Accurate determination of energy needs in hospitalized patients. *J. Am. Dietetic Assoc.* 107 (3): 393–401.

Brunetto, M.A., Gomes, M.O.S. et al. (2010). Effects of nutritional support on hospital outcome in dogs and cats. *J. Emerg. Crit. Care* 20 (2): 224–231.

Buffington, T., Holloway, C., and Abood, S. (2004). Nutritional assessment. In: *Manual of Veterinary Dietetics* (ed. T. Buffington, C. Holloway and S. Abood), 1–7. St. Louis, MO: Elsevier Saunders.

Campbell, S.J., Karriker, M.J., and Fascetti, A.J. (2006). Central and peripheral parenteral nutrition. *Waltham Focus* 16 (3): 2–10.

Casaer, M.P., Mesotten, D., Hermans, G. et al. (2011). Early versus late parenteral nutrition in critically ill adults. *N. Engl. J. Med.* 365: 506–517.

Chan, D.L. (2004). Nutritional requirements of the critically ill patient. *Clin. Tech. Small Anim. Pract.* 19 (1): 1–5.

Chan, D.L., Freeman, L.M., Labato, M.A. et al. (2002). Retrospective evaluation of partial parenteral nutrition in dogs and cats. *J. Vet. Intern. Med.* 16: 440–445.

Chan, D.L., Freeman, L.M., Rozanski, E.A. et al. (2006). Alterations in carbohydrate metabolism in critically ill cats. *J. Vet. Emerg. Crit. Care* 16 (S1): S7–S13.

Chandler, M.L., Guilford, W.G., and Payne-James, J. (2000). Use of peripheral parenteral nutritional support in dogs and cats. *J. Am. Vet. Med. Assoc.* 216 (5): 669–673.

Chandler, M.L. and Payne-James, J. (2006). Prospective evaluation of a peripherally administered three-in-one parenteral nutrition product in dogs. *J. Small Anim. Pract.* 47: 518–523.

Chao, C.Y., Yeh, S.L., Lin, M.T. et al. (2000). Effects of parenteral infusion with fish-oil or safflower-oil emulsion on hepatic lipids, plasma amino acids, and inflammatory mediators in septic rats. *Nutrition* 16: 284–288.

Cheung, N.W., Zaccaria, C., Napier, B. et al. (2005). Hyperglycemia is associated with adverse outcomes in patients receiving total parenteral nutrition. *Diabetes Care* 28 (10): 2367–2371.

Cotter, R., Martis, L., Cosmas, F. et al. (1984). Comparison of the elimination and metabolism of 10% Travamulsion and 10% Intralipid lipid emulsion in the dog. *J. Parenteral Enteral Nutr.* 8 (2): 140–145.

Cowl, C.T., Weinstock, J.V., AL-Jurf, A. et al. (2000). Complications and cost associated with parenteral nutrition delivered to hospitalized patients through either subclavian or peripherally inserted central catheters. *Clin. Nutr.* 19 (4): 237–243.

Crabb, S.E., Chan, D.L., and Freeman, L.M. (2006). Retrospective evaluation of total parenteral nutrition in cats: 40 cases (1991–2003). *J. Vet. Emerg. Crit. Care* 16 (S1): S21–S26.

Crook, M.A., Hally, V., and Panteli, J.V. (2001). The importance of the refeeding syndrome. *Nutrition* 17: 632–637.

Culebras, J.M., Martin-Peña, G., Garcia-de-Lorenzo, A. et al. (2004). Practical aspects of peripheral parenteral nutrition. *Curr. Opin. Clin. Nutr. Metab. Care* 7: 303–307.

Delaney, S.J., Fascetti, A.J., and Elliott, D.A. (2006). Critical care nutrition of dogs. In: *Encyclopedia of Canine Clinical Nutrition* (ed. P. Pibot, V. Biourge and D. Elliott), 426–447. Italia: Aniwas SAS.

DeLegge, M.H. and Drake, L.M. (2007). Nutritional assessment. *Gastroenterol. Clin. North Am.* 36: 1–22.

Dudrick, S.J., Wilmore, D.W., Vars, H.M. et al. (1968). Long-term total parenteral nutrition with growth, development, and positive nitrogen balance. *Surgery* 64: 134–142.

Fascetti, A.J., Mauldin, G.E., and Mauldin, G.N. (1997). Correlation between serum creatine kinase activities and anorexia in cats. *J. Vet. Intern. Med.* 11 (1): 9–13.

Finck, C. (2000). Enteral versus parenteral nutrition in the critically ill. *Nutrition* 16: 393–394.

Freeman, L.M. and Chan, D.L. (2006). Total parenteral nutrition. In: *Fluid Therapy in Small Animal Practice*, 3e (ed. S. DiBartola), 584–601. St. Louis, MO: Elsevier Saunders.

Fried, G.M., Ogden, W.D., Rhea, A. et al. (1982). Pancreatic protein secretion and gastrointestinal hormone release in response to parenteral amino acids and lipid in dogs. *Surgery* 92 (5): 902–905.

Gajanayake, I., Wylie, C.E., and Chan, D.L. (2013). Clinical experience with a lipid-free, ready-made parenteral nutrition solution in dogs: 70 cases (2006–2012). *J. Emerg. Crit. Care* 23 (3): 305–313.

Granato, D., Blum, S., Rössle, C. et al. (2000). Effects of parenteral lipid emulsions with different fatty acid composition on immune cell functions *in vitro*. *J. Parenteral Enteral Nutr.* 24 (2): 113–118.

Hafidah, S.A., Reuter, M.D., Chassels, L.J. et al. (2007). Effect of intravenous insulin therapy on clinical outcomes in critically ill patients. *Am. J. Med. Sci.* 333 (6): 354–361.

Hammes, M., Desai, A., Pasupneti, S. et al. (2015). Central venous catheters: incidence and predictive factors of venous thrombosis. *Clin. Nephrol.* 84 (1): 21–28.

Hardy, G., Ball, P., and McElroy, B. (1998). Basic principles for compounding all-in-one parenteral nutrition admixtures. *Curr. Opin. Clin. Nutr. Metab. Care* 1 (3): 291–296.

Harris, J.P., Parnell, N.K., Griffith, E.H. et al. (2017). Retrospective evaluation of the impact of early enteral nutrition on clinical outcomes in dogs with pancreatitis: 3 cases (2010–2013). *J. Vet. Emerg. Crit. Care* 27 (4): 425–433.

Harvey, R.B., Andrews, K., Droleskey, R.E. et al. (2006). Qualitative and quantitative comparison of gut bacterial colonization in enterally and parenterally fed neonatal pigs. *Curr. Issues Intestinal Microbiol.* 7 (2): 61–64.

Heidegger, C.P., Romand, J.A., Treggiari, M.M. et al. (2007). Is it now time to promote mixed enteral and parenteral nutrition for the critically ill patient? *Intensive Care Med.* 33: 963–969.

Heyland, D.K., Weijs, P.H., Cross-Bu, J.A. et al. (2017). Protein delivery in the intensive care unit: optimal or suboptimal? *Nutr. Clin. Pract.* 32 (1): 58S–71S.

Hodder, E.M. (1873). Transfusion of milk in cholera. *Practitioner* 10: 14–16.

Izzo, R.S., Larcker, S., Remis, W. et al. (1984). The effects on beagles of long-term administration of 20% Travamulsion fat emulsion. *J. Parenteral Enteral Nutr.* 8 (2): 160–168.

Jannace, P.W., Lerman, R.H., Dennis, R.C. et al. (1988). Total parenteral nutrition-induced cyclic hypercapnia. *Crit. Care Med.* 16 (7): 727–728.

Kang, J.H. and Yang, M.P. (2008). Effect of a short-term infusion with soybean oil-based lipid emulsion on phagocytic responses of canine peripheral blood polymorphonuclear neutrophilic leukocytes. *J. Vet. Intern. Med.* 22 (5): 1166–1173.

Klein, C.J., Stanek, G.S., and Wiles, C.E. (1998). Overfeeding macronutrients to critically ill adults: metabolic complications. *J. Am. Dietetic Assoc.* 98 (7): 795–806.

Krinsley, J.S., Maurer, P., Holewinski, S. et al. (2017). Glucose control, diabetes status, and mortality in critically ill patients. *May Clin. Proc.* 92 (7): 1019–1029.

Lee, M.C., Mannon, P.J., Grand, J.P. et al. (1997). Total parenteral nutrition alters NPY/PYY receptor levels in the rat brain. *Physiol. Behav.* 62 (6): 1219–1223.

Leite, H.P., Rodrigues da Silva, A.V., de Oliveira Iglesias, S.B. et al. (2016). Serum albumin is an independent predictor of clinical outcomes in critically ill children. *Pediatr. Crit. Care Med.* 17 (2): e50–e57.

Levenson, S.M., Hopkins, B.S., Waldron, M. et al. (1984). Early history of parenteral nutrition. *Fed. Proc.* 43: 1391–1406.

Lin, L.Y., Lin, H.C., Lee, P.C. et al. (2007). Hyperglycemia correlates with outcomes in patients receiving total parenteral nutrition. *Am. J. Med. Sci.* 333 (5): 261–265.

Liposky, J.M. and Nelson, L.D. (1994). Ventilatory response to high caloric loads in critically ill patients. *Crit. Care Med.* 22 (5): 796–802.

Lippert, A.C., Faulkner, J.E., Evans, A.T. et al. (1989). Total parenteral nutrition in clinically normal cats. *J. Am. Vet. Med. Assoc.* 194 (5): 669–676.

Lippert, A.C., Fulton, R.B., and Parr, A.M. (1993). A retrospective study of the use of total parenteral nutrition in dogs and cats. *J. Vet. Intern. Med.* 7: 52–64.

Liu, D.T., Brown, D.C., and Silverstein, D.C. (2012). Early nutritional support is associated with decreased length of hospitalization in dogs with septic peritonitis: a retrospective study of 45 cases (2000–2009). *J. Vet. Emerg. Crit. Care* 22 (4): 453–459.

Marik, P.E. and Raghavan, M. (2004). Stress-hyperglycemia, insulin and immunomodulation in sepsis. *Intensive Care Med.* 30 (4): 748–756.

Mauldin, G.E., Reynolds, A.J., Mauldin, N. et al. (2001). Nitrogen balance in clinically normal dogs receiving parenteral nutrition solutions. *Am. J. Vet. Res.* 62 (6): 912–920.

Mehl, M.L., Kyles, A.E., Hardie, E.M. et al. (2005). Evaluation of ameroid ring constrictors for treatment for single extrahepatic portosystemic shunts in dogs: 168 cases (1995–2001). *J. Am. Vet. Med. Assoc.* 226 (12): 2020–2030.

Michel, K.E. (2005). Nutritional management of endocrine disease. In: *Textbook of Veterinary Internal Medicine*, 6e (ed. S.J. Ettinger and E.C. Feldman), 577–578. St. Louis, MO: Elsevier Saunders.

Michel, K.E. (2007). Parenteral nutrition. In: *Clinical Veterinary Advisor Dogs and Cats* (ed. E. Côté), 1296–1298. St. Louis, MO: Mosby Elsevier.

Michel, K.E., King, L.G., and Ostro, E. (1997). Measurement of urinary urea nitrogen content as an estimate of the amount of total urinary nitrogen loss in dogs in intensive care units. *J. Am. Vet. Med. Assoc.* 210 (3): 356–359.

Mirtallo, J.M. (2001). Parenteral formulas. In: *Clinical Nutrition: Parenteral Nutrition* (ed. J.L. Rombeau and R.H. Rolandelli), 118–139. Philadelphia, PA: WB Saunders.

Molina, J., Hervera, M., Manzanilla, E.G. et al. (2018). Evaluation of the prevalence and risk factors for undernutrition in hospitalized dogs. *Front. Vet. Sci.* 5: 205.

Olan, N.V. and Prittie, J. (2015). Retrospective evaluation of ProcalAmine administration in a population of hospitalized ICU dogs: 36 cases (2010–2013). *J. Vet. Emerg. Crit. Care* 25 (3): 405–412.

O'Toole, E., Miller, G.W., Wilson, B.A. et al. (2004). Comparison of the standard predictive equation for calculation of resting energy expenditure with indirect calorimetry in hospitalized and healthy dogs. *J. Am. Vet. Med. Assoc.* 225 (1): 58–64.

Parikh, M.J., Dumas, G., Silvestri, A. et al. (2005). Physical compatibility of neonatal total parenteral nutrient admixtures containing organic calcium and inorganic phosphate salts. *Am. J. Health-Syst. Pharm.* 62 (11): 1177–1183.

Plusa, S.M., Horsman, R., Kendall-Smith, S. et al. (1998). Fine-bore cannulas for peripheral intravenous nutrition: polyurethane or silicone? *Ann. R. Coll. Surgeons Engl.* 80 (2): 154–156.

Preiser, J.C., Ichai, C., Orban, J.C. et al. (2014). Metabolic response to the stress of critical illness. *Br. J. Anaesth.* 113 (6): 945–954.

Preiser, J.C., vanZanten, A.R.H., Berger, M.M. et al. (2015). Metabolic and nutritional support of critically ill patients: concensus and controversies. *Crit. Care* 19: 35–46.

Pyle, S.C., Marks, S.L., and Kass, P.H. (2004). Evaluation of complications and prognostic factors associated with administration of total parenteral nutrition in cats: 75 cases (1994–2001). *J. Am. Vet. Med. Assoc.* 225 (2): 242–250.

Qin, H.L., Su, Z.D., Hu, L.G. et al. (2002). Effect of early intrajejunal nutrition on pancreatic pathological features and gut barrier function in dogs with acute pancreatitis. *Clin. Nutr.* 21 (6): 469–473.

Queau, Y., Larsen, J.A., Kass, P.H. et al. (2011). Factors associated with adverse outcomes during parenteral nutrition administration in dogs and cats. *J. Vet. Intern. Med.* 25: 446–452.

Raman, M., Almutairdi, A., Mulesa, L. et al. (2017). Parenteral nutrition and lipids. *Nutrients* 9: 388–399.

Remillard, R.L. (2000). Parenteral nutrition. In: *Fluid Therapy in Small Animal Practice*, 2e (ed. S.P. DiBartola), 465–482. Philadelphia, PA: WB Saunders.

Remillard, R.L., Darden, D.E., Michel, K.E. et al. (2001). An investigation of the relationship between caloric intake and outcome in hospitalized dogs. *Vet. Ther.* 2 (4): 301–310.

Reuter, J.D., Marks, S.L., Rogers, Q.R. et al. (1998). Use of total parenteral nutrition in dogs: 209 cases (1988–1995). *J. Vet. Emerg. Crit. Care* 8 (3): 201–213.

Reynolds, J.V., Walsh, K., Ruigrok, J. et al. (1995). Randomised comparison of silicone versus Teflon cannulas for peripheral intravenous nutrition. *Ann. R. Coll. Surgeons Engl.* 77 (6): 447–449.

Sala-Vila, A., Barbosa, V.M., and Calder, P.C. (2007). Olive oil in parenteral nutrition. *Curr. Opin. Clin. Nutr. Metab. Care* 10: 165–174.

Stabile, B.E., Borzatta, M., Stubbs, R.S. et al. (1984). Intravenous mixed amino acids and fats do not stimulate exocrine pancreatic secretion. *Am. J. Physiol.* 246 (3): G274–G280.

Suddaby, E.C. and Schiller, S. (2004). Management of chylothorax in children. *Pediatr. Nurs.* 30 (4): 290–295.

Tappy, L., Schwarz, J.M., Schneiter, P. et al. (1998). Effects of isoenergetic glucose-based or lipid-based parenteral nutrition on glucose metabolism, de novo lipogenesis, and respiratory gas exchanges in critically ill patients. *Crit. Care Med.* 26 (5): 860–867.

Thiessen, S.E., Derde, S., Derese, I. et al. (2017). Role of glucagon in catabolism and muscle wasting of critical illness and modulation by nutrition. *Am. J. Respir. Crit. Care Med.* 196 (9): 1131–1143.

Thomovsky, E., Backus, R., Reniker, A. et al. (2007). Parenteral nutrition: formulation, monitoring, and complications. *Compendium* 29: 88–102.

Tsuruta, K., Backus, R.C., DeClue, A.E. et al. (2017). Effects of parenteral fish oil on plasma nonesterified fatty acids and systemic inflammatory mediators in dogs following ovariohysterectomy. *J. Emerg. Crit. Care* 27 (5): 512–523.

Ukleja, A. and Romano, M.M. (2007). Complications of parenteral nutrition. *Gastroenterol. Clin. North Am.* 36: 23–46.

Wanten, G.J.A. and Calder, P.C. (2007). Immune modulation by parenteral lipid emulsions. *Am. J. Clin. Nutr.* 85: 1171–1184.

Wolfe, R.R., Shaw, J.H., and Durkot, M.J. (1983). Energy metabolism in trauma and sepsis: the role of fat. *Prog. Clin. Biol. Res.* 111: 89–109.

Zauner, A., Nimmerrichter, P., Anderwald, C. et al. (2007). Severity of insulin resistance in critically ill medical patients. *Metab. Clin. Exp.* 56 (1): 1–5.

Zentek, J., Stephan, I., Kramer, S. et al. (2003). Response of dogs to short-term infusion of carbohydrate- or lipid-based parenteral nutrition. *J. Vet. Med. Ser. A* 50 (6): 313–321.

Zsombor-Murray, E. and Freeman, L.M. (1999). Peripheral parenteral nutrition. *Compendium* 21 (6): 1–11.

22

Abridged Clinical Nutrition Topics for Companion Avian Species
Elizabeth Koutsos and Brian Speer

Companion avian species that are commonly maintained under human care include birds from the orders Psittaciformes, Passeriformes, Galliformes, and Anseriformes. Of these orders, the most common companion bird species are included in the order Psittaciformes (Forshaw and Cooper 1989). The order Psittaciformes is represented by 80 genera and approximately 360 different species. Of these, there are approximately 100–150 species most often represented in the pet trade.

There have been numerous publications addressing the topic of comparative and companion avian nutrition (Klasing 1998; Koutsos et al. 2001a; Koutsos 2016), although research in this area is limited for a variety of reasons, discussed in this chapter. This review will summarize the current knowledge in the field of companion avian nutrition and the role that nutritional status plays in clinical diseases, and provide some recommendations for future research areas.

Animals require certain concentrations of essential nutrients as well as the building blocks for the de novo synthesis of other nutrients. They require these nutrients in concentrations that vary depending on life stage, physiologic status, current plane of nutrition, and environment. Between species, requirements vary due to differences in gastrointestinal (GI) physiology, nutrient metabolism pathways (activity and expression), body size, and likely other factors that are yet undetermined.

The precise requirement for a nutrient is often not known due to the complexity of these factors, and because empirical data to establish specific requirements are costly, invasive, and thus limited for many companion avian species. However, research data are quite extensive in agriculturally relevant species. Information from poultry may be used as a baseline for guiding nutrient concentrations in many companion avian species, particularly those for whom granivory (seed-eating) is a wild-type feeding strategy. From these baseline data, limited empirical data, and field studies on natural feeding habits, recommendations may be made for appropriate nutrient concentrations.

Water

Water is the most essential nutrient, in that most animals can survive much longer under conditions without food than without water (Cade and Dybas 1962). Water can be derived from free water sources (e.g. drinking water), free water in food sources, and metabolic water – the water produced during oxidation of other organic compounds in the body. The water requirements of birds are generally lower than of similar-sized mammals due to their higher metabolic rate, and thus higher rate of

Applied Veterinary Clinical Nutrition, Second Edition. Edited by Andrea J. Fascetti, Sean J. Delaney, Jennifer A. Larsen, and Cecilia Villaverde.
© 2024 John Wiley & Sons, Inc. Published 2024 by John Wiley & Sons, Inc.

production of metabolic water. Additionally, nitrogen excretion via uric acid (as opposed to urea in mammals) requires less water (Bartholomew and Cade 1963).

Water requirements are proportionally higher in younger birds than in older birds, particularly in newly hatched chicks. In cockatiel chicks (*Nymphicus hollandicus*), water requirements are greater than 80% of their total intake needs for the first few days of life and gradually reduce over time (Roudybush and Grau 1986). In wild scarlet macaw chicks (*Ara macao*), 28–60 days post hatch, average crop moisture content was ~53%, was highest in younger chicks, and reduced over time (Brightsmith et al. 2010).

Evaporative water losses decline with body mass, such that very small birds (e.g. less than 50 g) can lose up to 25% of body weight as water per day (Bartholomew and Cade 1963). For example, the zebra finch (*Taeniopygia castanotis*), averaging 11 g body weight, produces ~1.0 g of water from oxidative processes, but loses ~2.1 g water per day through evaporation at room temperature (Bartholomew and Cade 1963). Likely because of this higher rate of loss in smaller birds, the ad libitum water intake of smaller birds is proportionally greater than that of larger birds. The 25–30 g house sparrow (*Passer domesticus*) consumes ~35% of its body weight in water per day, while birds weighing more than 40 g generally consume 5–10% of their body weight in water per day (Bartholomew and Cade 1963). Adult parrots are reported to require ~2.5% of their body weight in water per day (MacMillen and Baudinette 1993). The commonly kept budgerigar (*Melopsittacus undulatus*) is an exception to this inverse body mass to water requirement relationship, in that this relatively small bird (~30 g) consumes only ~5% of its body weight in water per day, which is likely an evolutionary adaptation to the very arid conditions of its native habitat (Bartholomew and Cade 1963).

Warmer environmental conditions also increase water demands, as evaporative heat loss can deplete the avian body of up to 40–50%

of its water (Bartholomew and Cade 1963), and requirements for water increase by as much as 12-fold in hot environments, as seen in monk parakeets (*Myiopsitta monachus*) (Weathers and Caccamise 1975). Specific needs for water vary by body weight (with an allometric scaling factor of 0.636 in wild habitats) and with wild-type feeding strategy. Specifically, nectarivores have higher water flux, insectivores and carnivores are intermediate, and granivores and omnivores have the lowest flux of water and there may be a direct correlation with high dietary water content (Song and Beissinger 2020).

Clinical and Welfare Considerations Associated with Water

A well-hydrated chick is evident by plumpness of skin, as opposed to a dehydrated chick, in which the skin is generally tight and dry in appearance (Abramson et al. 1995). Providing nutrition (e.g. vitamins) via the water is not advised, due to the considerable variation in intake observed in many birds (Koutsos et al. 2001b). Similarly, delivery of medication via the water should be limited to those medications for which pharmacokinetic data are available to support this method of administration (Powers et al. 2000). In addition to its importance for the maintenance and clinical needs already mentioned, water serves an important role in enrichment of maintenance behaviors, including bathing, feather care, and social interaction (Sibley et al. 2001).

Energy

Energy is created from nutrients to drive biochemical processes. Energy requirements are determined at the most basic level as the energy needed to maintain a basal metabolic rate (BMR) and for thermoregulation. The latter component can increase energy needs by 4–8 times BMR in cold environments and 1–2 times BMR in hot (Klasing 1998; McNab 2009). Beyond BMR and thermoregulation, additional energy is needed for activities including movement, perching, preening, eating, bathing, and singing/calling. These activities can increase energy requirements only nominally (e.g. resting while perching), or up to as high as 6–11 times BMR for sustained flight (Goldstein 1988). Finally, growth, reproduction, and molting all increase energy needs. Energy requirements for growth can be up to twice BMR for altricial chicks in the very early days post hatch, and over the course of the growing period generally account for a 25% increase in energy requirement compared to maintenance (Goldstein 1988; Klasing 1998). Monk parakeet chicks are known to have their highest energy requirements during the second half of pre-fledging growth and require ~1.4 times maintenance energy requirements (Petzinger 2015). Energetic costs of reproduction are highest for hens laying large numbers of eggs on a regular basis and can increase energy requirements 0.4–1.8-fold (Ricklefs 1974). Energetic costs of molting can be high due to inefficient protein utilization to supply the high amount of cyst(e)ine needed for feather protein formation.

In general, birds have a higher energy expenditure than mammals (Rezende et al. 2002), and smaller birds have higher energy requirements than larger birds (Goldstein 1988). Passerines have higher energy requirements than non-passerines, and parrots fall in an intermediate position in the general equations (Table 22.1) (Aschoff and

Pohl 1969; McNab 2009). Finally, carnivorous birds have higher energy requirements than do omnivorous or granivorous birds, resulting in predicted metabolic rates of carnivores like insectivorous birds and piscivorous penguins at ~60% and ~30% higher than that of granivorous psittacines, respectively (Nagy et al. 1999).

Sources of Energy

Energy can be derived from dietary proteins, lipids, or carbohydrates. In general, the wild-type feeding strategy of the bird (e.g. carnivore, omnivore, or herbivore) reflects the preferred energy substrate. Because of these adaptations, efficiency of energy production from non-preferred substrates may be lower. For example, starch may not be a readily available energy source for carnivorous birds (Earle and Clarke 1991; Underwood et al. 1991). Ideally, the appropriate energy substrate will be provided to birds maintained under human care. Due to the variation in efficiency of utilization of different substrates for energy, the use of gross energy values is not recommended when assessing the energy potential of food items. If data are not available on the energy value of a particular diet item for the species in question, the use of Association of American Feed Control Officials (AAFCO) metabolizable energy (ME) calculation based on modified Atwater factors is a reasonable starting point: ME per kg = $((3.5 \times \text{crude protein } \%) + (8.5 \times \text{crude fat } \%) + (3.5 \times \text{nitrogen-free extract } \%)) \times 10$.

Clinical Issues Associated with Energy Imbalance: Obesity

Obesity is a significant concern in captive avian species (Speer et al. 2016) (Figure 22.1). Although it is a common clinical problem associated with numerous other degenerative and metabolic conditions, the prevalence and incidence of this problem in captively maintained avian species are not quantitatively known. As discussed earlier, the energy requirements of captive birds are greatly reduced compared with

Table 22.1 Predicted BMR for passerines, non-passerines, and parrots.

Taxonomic group	BMR (kcal/d)
Passerine	$0.744 \times (\text{BW in g})^{0.713}$
	$114.7 \times (\text{BW in kg})^{0.73}$
Non-passerine	$0.510 \times (\text{BW in g})^{0.724}$
	$73.6 \times (\text{BW in kg})^{0.73}$
Psittacine	$0.697 \times (\text{BW in g})^{0.705}$

Source: Adapted from Aschoff and Pohl 1969; McNab 2009.

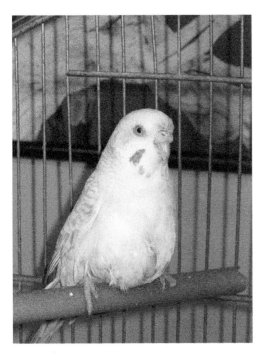

Figure 22.1 Marked obesity in a budgerigar (*Melopsittacus undulatus*).

their wild counterparts. The two most common activities by free-living birds are feeding/foraging and actively perching (as opposed to sleeping on a perch), and although the proportion of each of these in a day varies with season and by species, the combination of these activities can take up as much as 56–90% of daytime activity (Goldstein 1988). Instead, captive birds spend a significant proportion of the day dedicated to feeding without foraging, such that energy intake is greater than energy expenditure, resulting in obesity. Specific nutritional causes of obesity have also been examined in addition to overconsumption of energy. For example, sulfur amino acid deficiency (methionine or cyst(e)ine) has also been associated with fatty liver and obesity (Butler 1976; Harrison and McDonald 2006), and is commonly seen in South American psittacine species that are fed high-fat seed- and nut-based diets that are deficient in methionine (Harrison and McDonald 2006).

Methods to prevent or reduce obesity generally include caloric restriction, but care must be taken to provide other activities to compensate for the reduced time eating or foraging, or stereotypic behaviors will likely result (see food-based enrichment). Caloric restriction should not be too great or impaired immune function may result (Glick et al. 1983). Additionally, birds should have food available daily on a continual basis; complete food restriction is not recommended (Kalmar et al. 2010). Other interventions include ensuring that the diet is nutritionally balanced to begin with to prevent incidences of nutrient deficiencies or imbalances (resulting in obesity independent of excess caloric intake). L-carnitine has also been used as a therapeutic treatment for obesity. Lipomas, associated anecdotally with obesity, were reduced in size in budgerigars fed commercial pellets supplemented with L-carnitine (1000 mg/kg pellets) compared with birds fed unsupplemented pellets or seeds (De Voe et al. 2004). In general, any weight loss strategy should result in gradual weight loss, recommended at no more than 1% body weight loss per week (Stahl and Kronfeld 1998).

Food-Based Enrichment

Many aspects of enrichment, particularly through an emphasis on foraging activities, are accomplished by including weight management and nutritional balance plans as a part of the overall welfare management of birds. Foraging is a necessary form of enrichment, especially for animals in captivity, and can be utilized to redirect a bird's attention and behavior, to enrich the welfare of the birds themselves. Working for food by means of searching through toys or puzzles and shredding or chewing through paper or cardboard are great ways to keep birds busy. Many birds will need to be taught these behaviors, since they are not innate and are oftentimes very limited in the lifestyles of many companion birds. This may be particularly the case when some natural chewing behaviors are considered a nuisance by the human companion and discouraged.

Beginning foraging behaviors and shredding can be taught by demonstration and continued at home. These food-acquisition activities can range from very simple hidden treats in half-covered bowls to very complex puzzles and time-consuming boxes to untie or open. By increasing foraging in daily activities, often-times human companions can eliminate or lessen undesired behaviors, and quality of life can be enhanced (Speer and Hennigh 2017).

Amino Acids and Protein

Protein "requirements" are more accurately described by the total requirements for "essential" amino acids – those that cannot be synthesized by the body; "conditionally essential" amino acids – those that may not be synthesized in adequate quantities during certain times; and "non-essential" amino acids – those that can be synthesized de novo. Twelve amino acids are considered essential or conditionally essential for birds (i.e. phenylalanine, valine, threonine, methionine, alanine, tryptophan, histidine, isoleucine, leucine, lysine, glycine, and proline) and must be supplied in the diet. Additionally, adequate nitrogen must be supplied to support synthesis of non-essential amino acids.

It is generally thought that larger birds have higher protein requirements than do smaller birds (Klasing 1998; Kris-Etherton et al. 2008). Not surprisingly, growth and reproduction require higher concentrations of amino acids and nitrogen. In the wild (and likely in captive breeding colonies), protein availability appears to be a cue for breeding (Sailaja et al. 1988; Williams 1996). This information can be utilized to support reproductive success in captively managed populations; an increase in dietary protein is often recommended at least 30 days before the onset of lay is expected/desired.

Wild-type feeding strategy impacts protein/amino acid needs. Fruit- and nectar-eating species have lower rates of nitrogen loss compared to seed-eating birds, resulting in lower protein requirements (Frankel and Avram 2001; Pryor et al. 2001; Pryor 2003). In contrast, carnivorous birds have higher protein needs due to obligatory oxidation of protein as an energy and glucose source and they cannot adapt to lower dietary protein concentrations (NRC 1994). The underlying metabolic capacity to adapt to different concentrations of dietary protein should be considered when recommending and modifying avian diets.

Clinical Issues with Protein/Amino Acids

Deficiency or imbalance of protein/amino acids during growth reduces growth rates and feather production. If this restriction occurs during times of feather growth, "stress" bars may be visible on feathers, or other feather abnormalities may occur (Murphy et al. 1988) (Figure 22.2).

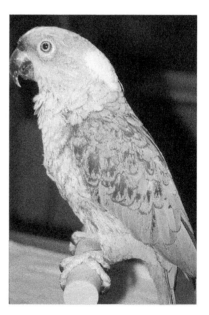

Figure 22.2 Abnormal colors (green to black change) of many contour feathers and some mild suggestion of barb and barbule deformities in some individual feathers suggest malnourishment in this yellow-naped Amazon parrot (*Amazona auropalliata*). In this case there was a delayed molt, secondary to malnutrition and obesity, with increased wear of the exposed contour feathers.

Excess protein is often referenced in relation to gout concerns, but in granivorous cockatiels very high protein concentrations (up to 70% as fed) were tolerated with no clinical pathology as birds upregulated enzymes for amino acid catabolism and excretion (Koutsos et al. 2001b). Thus, it is likely that non-carnivorous birds may be very capable of adapting to varying dietary protein concentrations. However, it is important to allow for a transition time when moving between dietary protein concentrations, be it low protein to high protein or vice versa. This allows for metabolic adaptations to occur to allow a bird to appropriately utilize the new concentration of dietary protein. In cases of renal disease, nutritional management may include increasing water consumption via various dietary interventions, reducing dietary protein to concentrations most appropriate for the feeding strategy of the bird in question, in addition to other interventions (Cojean et al. 2020).

Essential Fatty Acids and Lipids

Fatty acids are essential for energy production, cell membrane synthesis, intracellular signaling, and hormone production. In the diet, fatty acids are generally supplied in the form of lipids (e.g. triglycerides comprised of three fatty acids), but also can be supplied as free fatty acids or short- or medium-chain triglycerides, with the latter often considered in situations of poor digestive capacity. More unsaturated fatty acids (more double bonds in the hydrocarbon chain), termed polyunsaturated fatty acids (PUFAs), tend to be required in the diet, while most saturated fatty acids and many monounsaturated fatty acids can be synthesized de novo. Omega-3 and omega-6 fatty acids, characterized by the location of the first double bond on the carbon chain, have received considerable attention for their varying impacts on physiology, discussed further later. Since research on the requirements of non-poultry species is lacking, the poultry guidelines of 1% as fed linoleic acid (18:2, an omega-6 fatty acid) and 4–5% as fed total dietary fat are generally used as a reference for all avian species (NRC 1994). More carnivorous or piscivorous birds may also require alpha-linolenic acid (aka ALA or 18:3, a shorter-chain omega-3 fatty acid) and potentially long-chain omega-3 fatty acids (e.g. EPA and DHA), although further research is warranted to clarify this hypothesis and the safety of very low ratios of n:6 to n:3.

Clinical Issues Associated with Lipid Nutrition: Atherosclerosis

Atherosclerosis is likely an underlying factor or at least a component of the majority of non-infectious cardiovascular diseases of birds and has been described in almost all orders of birds. It is the most common lesion of the cardiovascular system identified post mortem in companion psittacine birds (Fitzgerald and Beaufrère 2015). Reported prevalence of atherosclerosis in psittacines varies widely (1.9–91.8%), with the highest prevalence in Amazon and gray parrots (*Psittacus erithacus*; Beaufrère 2013). Most recently, prevalence, risk factors, and epidemiology of clinically relevant atherosclerotic lesions (types IV–VI) were investigated by review of over 7600 psittacine cases representing five genera (Beaufrère et al. 2013). An overall prevalence of 6.8% was reported, but a significantly higher prevalence of advanced lesions was found for gray parrots (having 275% the odds compared to other genera), Amazon parrots (having 183% the odds), and cockatiels (having 146% the odds); cockatoos (*Cacatua* spp.) and macaws (*Ara* spp.) appeared to be less susceptible. There was a positive association in this study between advanced atherosclerosis and (i) increasing age, (ii) female sex, (iii) reproductive disease (predominantly female), (iv) hepatic disease, and (v) concurrent myocardial fibrosis. In addition, (vi) high-calorie and -fat diets, (vii) dyslipidemia (e.g. hypercholesterolemia), and (viii) limited physical activity were risk factors also identified.

The association between fatty acid nutrition and atherosclerosis has clinical significance. Diets rich in saturated fatty acids increased plasma cholesterol in gray parrots, while diets with similar fat concentrations, but composed of more PUFAs, did not increase plasma cholesterol (Bavelaar and Beynen 2004). More recently, the effects of omega-3 fatty acid nutrition have been examined in psittacines. Higher tissue concentrations of ALA were correlated with reduced severity of atherosclerosis (Bavelaar and Beynen 2003). Dietary ALA is reflected in the blood of parrots, demonstrating successful absorption of this fatty acid (Petzinger et al. 2014a). Further, higher blood concentrations of ALA were associated with higher blood concentrations of the longer-chain omega-3 PUFAs, eicosapentaenoic acid (EPA) and docosahexaenoic acid (DHA), demonstrating some capacity for elongation and desaturation of ALA (Heinze et al. 2012; Petzinger et al. 2014b). However, supplementation of ALA did not impact blood cholesterol or triglycerides in cockatiels or monk parrots, while fish oil (a source of EPA and DHA) did lower blood triglycerides and cholesterol (Heinze et al. 2012; Petzinger et al. 2014b). Thus, omega-3 fatty acids, and particularly EPA and DHA, may present a good dietary intervention strategy for psittacines at risk for atherosclerosis (Petzinger et al. 2010).

Most companion avian diets are highly enriched in omega-6 fatty acids and limited in omega-3 fatty acids of any kind. Domesticated foodstuffs used to make complete pellets, such as corn and soybean meal, are composed predominantly of omega-6 fatty acids (primarily linoleic acid). Flaxseed is a source of ALA, but is less commonly used in feed manufacturing because of susceptibility to oxidative rancidity. Many seeds and nuts commonly fed to psittacines have not been tested for fatty acid profiles, but for those that have been tested, ALA content is relatively low (Kris-Etherton et al. 2000). Some commonly fed food items have modest amounts of ALA (e.g. flax, chia, walnuts [also very high in linoleic acid, an n-6], kale,

strawberries). Sources of the longer-chain omega-3 fatty acids EPA and DHA are limited to fish and other marine products and algal-based sources, and palatability and stability of these sources may be an issue when considering supplementation.

An association between plasma lipid values, particularly plasma total cholesterol and high-density lipoprotein (HDL), and prevalence of atherosclerosis among certain psittacine genera has been shown, but the diagnostic value of a plasma lipid profile in assessing the relative atherosclerosis risk for an individual has not been established. At the present time, however, hypercholesterolemia itself is neither necessary nor sufficient for a diagnosis of atherosclerosis, as birds with normal plasma cholesterol may have atherosclerotic disease, while those with hypercholesterolemia may not (Fitzgerald and Beaufrère 2015). Reference lipid profiles have been published for a variety of captive Amazon parrots (Ravich et al. 2014) and for orange-winged Amazons (*Amazona amazonica*; Vergneau-Grosset et al. 2016), which may better inform interpretation of diagnostics in certain companion avian species.

In addition to modifying dietary fatty acid profiles, other dietary strategies have been considered to mitigate the risk of atherosclerosis, but data are limited and/or unsupportive of dietary intervention. For example, dietary fiber, which effectively modulates cholesterol absorption and excretion in mammals, has been investigated in birds with little impact; psyllium did not affect plasma cholesterol concentration of gray parrots (Bavelaar and Beynen 2003). Dietary pectin has been shown to reduce the incidence of atherosclerotic plaques in chickens. The mechanism is likely due to modified energy intake, as pectin can increase the rate of passage and likely reduce the absorption of calories. Feed-restriction strategies may also mitigate atherosclerosis risk, but may also induce behavioral issues that are undesirable (Petzinger and Bauer 2013).

Vitamins

Vitamins are organic molecules that function as co-factors, hormones, and other components of normal metabolism. Most vitamins are water soluble (i.e. B vitamins and vitamin C). The B vitamins are integral in many metabolic pathways and are easily excreted, but also not stored in very significant concentrations. Thus, more regular dietary access to "B" vitamins is generally required. Vitamin C is specifically involved in antioxidant systems and is not essential for some avian species for which de novo synthesis meets requirements (e.g. many granivores), while others have inadequate synthesis rates to meet their needs (e.g. Passeriformes) (Klasing 1998). Four vitamins are fat soluble: vitamins A, D, E, and K. These vitamins present a higher risk of toxicity due to the complexity of excretion of these compounds compared to the excretion of water-soluble vitamins in uric acid. Vitamin A is critical for vision and cellular differentiation via the induction of genes that regulate these processes. Vitamin D is critical for normal calcium metabolism and bone mineralization and likely is involved in immune function, as demonstrated in mammalian species. Vitamin D should be provided as vitamin D3 (aka cholecalciferol), as no evidence yet suggests that D2 (aka ergocalciferol) is a bioactive source in avian species (Klasing 1998). Vitamin D may be synthesized from ultraviolet (UV) B exposure, as demonstrated in gray parrots (Stanford 2004) and marabou storks (*Leptoptilos crumeniferus*) (Schaftenaar and van Leeuwen 2015), but this synthesis will be dependent on latitude, the time of exposure, and the level of feathering and pigmentation that may reduce UV transmission to the skin. Vitamin E is an antioxidant and works in conjunction with other antioxidant systems to reduce the impact of free radical damage on cellular integrity and gene expression. Vitamin K is involved in blood clotting and bone mineralization. These vitamins, as already noted, are often the most challenging to provide in appropriate amounts without concern for toxicity.

Clinical Issues Associated with Vitamin Nutrition

Vitamin A deficiency and toxicosis are both reported in companion birds. For those birds fed seed-based diets, vitamin A deficiency is of concern, as most seeds that are commercially available contain no vitamin A and little to no pro-vitamin A compounds (Bauck 1998). Insectivorous birds are also at risk for vitamin A deficiency from the negligible concentrations of vitamin A in commercially available insects such as crickets and mealworms (Finke 2002, 2013). Clinical signs of vitamin A deficiency may include keratinization of epithelial cells, particularly mucous membranes and salivary glands, anorexia, and impaired immune responses. Night blindness may also occur, but is reversible if treated early with supplemental vitamin A (Orosz 2014).

Vitamin A toxicosis is also a concern and occurs rapidly in response to high doses. Lorikeets (*Trichoglossus moluccanus*) have been reported to be susceptible to vitamin A toxicity, resulting in reduced fertility, increased embryonic deaths, high hatchling mortality, and compromised feather condition (McDonald 2004; Park 2006). In cockatiels, 100 000 IU vitamin A/kg diet resulted in toxicosis signs in under nine months, and even those fed 10 000 IU vitamin A/kg diet had impaired immunity and modified behavior (Koutsos et al. 2003). The more moderate concentration (10 000 IU/kg diet) of vitamin A is not unusually high for companion bird diets and certainly not for supplements, and thus caution should be applied when evaluating the complete diet. Finally, when birds have been fed appropriate concentrations of vitamin A, they are relatively insensitive to vitamin A depletion. Cockatiels, previously maintained on adequate vitamin A concentrations and then fed diets with no vitamin A source, maintained reasonable liver vitamin A concentrations for two years, demonstrating the degree to which vitamin A is conserved. However, these birds did have impaired antibody responses prior to any other clinical signs of vitamin A deficiency (Koutsos et al. 2003).

Beta-carotene (and several other carotenoids) can serve as a precursor to vitamin A (Green and Fascetti 2016), and because conversion of beta-carotene to vitamin A is regulated, this compound is considered a safer alternative to pre-formed vitamin A for species that have evolved to eat plant-based diets (Koutsos and Klasing 2005). The ability of carnivorous birds to utilize beta-carotene has not been determined, although it is likely that insect-eating species utilize carotenoids as vitamin A sources given the low/negligible concentration of retinol in wild insects (Finke 2002). Carotenoids can also serve as antioxidants and as a source of pigmentation, and are found in the circulation of most bird species studied, including birds of prey (Slifka et al. 1999; Ingram et al. 2017).

Minerals

By proportion of estimated dietary requirement, the essential minerals include calcium and phosphorus (critical for bone mineralization and eggshell synthesis), sodium, potassium, magnesium, and chloride (critical for maintenance of acid–base balance), and iron, zinc, copper, manganese, cobalt, and selenium (critical for a variety of metabolic functions including oxygen transport, gene expression, and antioxidant function). The requirement for dietary minerals is generally not known precisely for companion avian species, but requirements for poultry are usually considered to meet or exceed those of companion species.

Clinical Issues Associated with Mineral Nutrition

Calcium is the primary mineral of concern in companion avian diets as deficiencies are common in birds fed seed- or insect-based diets, which are a poor source of calcium (Stanford 2004, 2006). Further, many insects (although not all) have an inverted calcium-to-phosphorus ratio, exacerbating the impact of deficient calcium (Finke 2013). Calcium deficiency may lead to egg binding in females, impaired bone development in juveniles, and low bone density in adults (Murphy et al. 1988; Bauck 1995) (Figure 22.3).

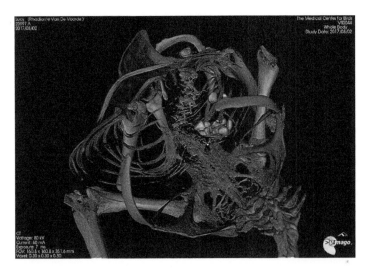

Figure 22.3 Metabolic bone disease in a duck. Note marked bony deformities in the spine on this 3D rendering.

When balancing diets for calcium, caution is needed when choosing the supplemental source. Some plant-based calcium sources like spinach also contain oxalate, which reduces calcium bioavailability (Weaver et al. 1987). Insects may be supplemented via gut loading or dusting, but for either method the time for which the insect is exposed to the supplement (gut loading) or the time from supplement addition to consumption of the insect by the bird (dusting) is critical to ensure proper calcium intake (Finke 2003). For the former, gut-loading supplementation generally requires 24–48 hours to be effective and must be provided when the insect is actively feeding. In contrast, dusting supplementation onto insects requires rapid feeding to the bird to avoid the insect grooming off the topical calcium supplements.

Zinc is commonly discussed in relation to companion bird nutrition, because toxicosis can occur by acute or chronic ingestion of excessive zinc from the diet or the housing environment (Romagnano et al. 1995). Acute and chronic zinc toxicoses have been described in cockatiels in one experimental study (Howard 1992). In acute toxicosis, signs included lethargy, dullness (birds left the perch and spent most of their time sitting on floor with feathers partly erect and eyes closed), shallow respiration, anorexia, dark green moist droppings, rapid weight loss, reluctance to move, recumbency, ataxia, and/or death. With acute toxicosis, mortality increased with increased concentrations of zinc consumed. In chronic toxicosis, birds showed variable, intermittent signs including lethargy/dullness, periodic dysphagia, and rapid weight loss. Many recovered spontaneously, but a few in one study developed recumbency and ataxia and were euthanized (Howard 1992). Plasma zinc concentration can be drastically altered by either dietary zinc or physiologic status, and responds homeostatically to a dietary zinc load, in that elevations are transient and return to within normal limits quickly. Diagnosis of zinc intoxication in birds is challenging and is rarely established with plasma zinc testing alone.

Treatment for zinc toxicosis typically is often supportive, and does not always require chelation (Fudge and Speer 2001). Parenteral fluid administration, gastroprotectants, and analgesia if indicated are common supportive treatments. Chelation may be indicated in more severely affected individuals.

Iron is a concern for avian species that are susceptible to iron storage disease (ISD), including many frugivorous species like toucans and tanagers and some frugivore/insectivore species like mynahs and starlings (Klasing et al. 2012). In these species, it appears there is limited ability to downregulate mechanisms of iron absorption such that dietary iron is rapidly absorbed and stored in the liver, followed by clinical ISD signs including weight loss, abdominal distension, ascites, and enlargement of the liver, heart, and spleen. Typically, hematology and serum biochemistry provide little diagnostic value unless ferritin and iron-binding capacity are carefully examined. Diets containing low concentrations of total iron (25–50 mg/kg diet or lower) can delay or prevent ISD in susceptible species, although these dietary iron concentrations may be too low for laying females and growing chicks. Adding compounds that decrease iron bioavailability such as tannins has been tried with some success, but these compounds may also reduce bioavailability of other minerals and should be used with caution. Organic acids such as citric acid and vitamin C (ascorbic acid) theoretically enhance iron absorption and so foods high in these compounds should be avoided or fed at times when food items that are higher in iron are not provided (Klasing et al. 2012).

Other Clinical Nutrition Issues

Nutrition and Feather-Damaging Behaviors

Self-inflicted feather damage is a common problem in companion bird species (Seibert 2006; van Zeeland et al. 2009). Often "boredom" is cited as a cause for feather-damaging behaviors, and although the underlying basis is multifactorial, there are several nutritional components that may impact feather-damaging behaviors. First, as mentioned in relation to obesity, foraging behaviors are natural for birds in their wild environment and generally limited in captivity. Not only is the provision of a balanced diet essential, but the manner of how these food items are acquired is of equal importance. Feather-damaging behaviors in some birds may result from a lack of foraging opportunities and may be improved with enrichment in the form of foraging opportunities and physical cage complexity, as demonstrated in orange-winged Amazons (Meehan et al. 2003). The use of food-based enrichment may also improve stereotypic behavior, as discussed earlier.

Frank nutrient deficiency or toxicosis may also be implicated in some feather-damaging behaviors. For example, vitamin A deficiency results in dermatologic clinical signs, including rough scaly skin and poor feather quality (Burgmann 1995), which may lead to excess grooming behaviors and feather-damaging behaviors. Deficiencies of other nutrients including niacin, riboflavin, zinc, pantothenic acid, biotin, salt, sulfur-containing amino acids, arginine, and folic acid can cause dry flaky skin that may induce feather-damaging behaviors (Burgmann 1995; Harrison and McDonald 2006).

Appropriate Diets for Birds and Their Role in Animal Well-Being

Historically, companion birds (generally granivores) were fed exclusively seed-based diets. This evolved to diets that included supplements and/or diets based on human foods. More recently, the use of commercially manufactured diets for birds has become more common (Harrison 1998). Unfortunately, for many companion birds globally, malnutrition remains a key contributor to many of the health problems that are seen (Speer et al. 2016).

Each of the aforementioned diet items comes with pros and cons. Seeds and insects are often preferred food items, but are generally deficient or imbalanced in essential nutrients, including amino acids, fatty acids, minerals, and vitamins (Peron and Grosset 2014). Those available commercially are generally quite dissimilar nutritionally to native diet items. Similarly, foods that have been selected for human domestication and consumption have often been heavily selected for sugar content and omega-6 fatty acids, and thus generally do not reflect avian wild-type diet items either. Commercially manufactured avian diets are limited in ingredient choices to those readily available human ingredients and do not provide the sensory variation that would be common in avian wild-type diets. Thus, it is likely ideal for diets of companion avian species to incorporate some combination of the diet items mentioned, and the balance will be based on availability, cost, and preference of both bird and human companion purchaser.

A common method of diet presentation is to offer a variety of food items and allow for selection by the bird. This can be problematic in that birds generally do not exhibit "nutritional wisdom" in diet item selection, particularly as it relates to micronutrients (Ullrey 1989; Ullrey et al. 1991; Hess et al. 2002; Carciofi et al. 2006; Brightsmith 2012). A better solution is to offer a diet with a mixture of items, but provided at specific dietary proportions, and potentially offered at varying times to ensure complete consumption of critical diet items. Current dietary recommendations for companion granivorous birds are 40–80% pellets and 20–60% produce and other food items (Reid and Perlberg 1998; Brightsmith 2012). Providing a mixture of food items, in a specific ratio, both provides both nutritional benefits (i.e. a complete and balanced diet to the best of our current knowledge) and benefits to well-being (i.e. a diverse sensory experience). Carnivorous and insectivorous species should incorporate appropriate meat- and/or insect-derived diet components in lieu of produce, and more herbivorous birds should have higher dietary fiber-based produce components.

Specific food-based enrichment opportunities may also be used in an effort to increase the amount of time a bird spends foraging to more closely mimic wild-type behaviors and potentially prevent or reduce undesired behaviors like feather picking (Lumeij and Hommers 2008; van Zeeland et al. 2009). Food-based enrichment may include offering large food particles, which have been demonstrated to increase the time spent foraging and feeding in orange-winged Amazons (Rozek et al. 2010; Rozek and Millam 2011), scattering food items around enclosures, and hiding certain food items to encourage activity. It is imperative that sanitation of enclosures is maintained to prevent pest infestation or undesirable growth of bacterial or fungal pathogens on old or uneaten foodstuffs. Non-food-based enrichment is also highly encouraged to promote natural behaviors and increase energy expenditure (Bauck 1998).

Conclusions

Avian nutrition is well understood regarding commercially relevant poultry species. Comparative avian nutrition is less well defined due to the diversity of species and the complexity of conducting such research. Thus, extrapolations and assumptions will remain a major component of comparative and companion avian nutrition. Using the fundamental knowledge of poultry nutrition, combined with an understanding of the GI physiology, wild-type diet, life stage, and health status of the bird(s) in question, informed recommendations can be made not only about the quantity but also the source of nutrients that will be most appropriate. These recommendations should be applied as a component of a comprehensive dietary, lifestyle, and welfare management program that incorporates a variety of food items in ways that encourage proper nutrition and appropriate feeding and foraging behaviors.

References

Abramson, J., Speer, B.L., and Thomsen, J.B. (1995). *The Large Macaws: Their Care, Breeding and Conservation*. Ft. Bragg, CA: Raintree Publications.

Aschoff, J. and Pohl, H. (1969). Rhythmic variations in energy metabolism. *Fed. Proc.* 29 (4): 1541–1552.

Bartholomew, G.A. and Cade, T.J. (1963). The water economy of land birds. *Auk* 80 (4): 504–539.

Bauck, L. (1995). Nutritional problems in pet birds. *Semin. Avian Exotic Pet Med.* 4 (1): 3–8.

Bauck, L. (1998). Psittacine diets and behavioral enrichment. *Semin. Avian Exotic Pet. Med.* 7 (3): 135–140.

Bavelaar, F. and Beynen, A. (2003). Severity of atherosclerosis in parrots in relation to the intake of α-linolenic acid. *Avian Dis.* 47 (3): 566–577.

Bavelaar, F. and Beynen, A. (2004). Atherosclerosis in parrots. A review. *Vet. Q.* 26 (2): 50–60.

Beaufrère, H. (2013). Avian atherosclerosis: parrots and beyond. *J. Exotic Pet Med.* 22 (4): 336–347.

Beaufrère, H., Ammersbach, M., Reavill, D.R. et al. (2013). Prevalence of and risk factors associated with atherosclerosis in psittacine birds. *J. Am. Vet. Med. Assoc.* 242 (12): 1696–1704.

Brightsmith, D.J. (2012). Nutritional levels of diets fed to captive Amazon parrots: does mixing seed, produce, and pellets provide a healthy diet? *J. Avian Med. Surg.* 26 (3): 149–160.

Brightsmith, D.J., McDonald, D., Matsafuji, D., and Bailey, C.A. (2010). Nutritional content of the diets of free-living scarlet macaw chicks in southeastern Peru. *J. Avian Med. Surg.* 24 (1): 9–23.

Burgmann, P.M. (1995). Common psittacine dermatologic diseases. *Semin. Avian Exotic Pet. Med.* 4 (4): 169–183.

Butler, E. (1976). Fatty liver diseases in the domestic fowl—a review. *Avian Pathol.* 5 (1): 1–14.

Cade, T.J. and Dybas, J.A. Jr. (1962). Water economy of the budgerygah. *Auk* 345–364.

Carciofi, A.C., Duarte, J.M.B., Mendes, D., and de Oliveira, L.D. (2006). Food selection and digestibility in yellow-headed conure (Aratinga jandaya) and golden-caped conure (Aratinga auricapilla) in captivity. *J. Nutr.* 136 (7): 2014S–2016S.

Cojean, O., Larrat, S., and Vergneau-Grosset, C. (2020). Clinical management of avian renal disease. *Vet. Clin.: Exotic Anim. Pract.* 23 (1): 75–101.

De Voe, R.S., Trogdon, M., and Flammer, K. (2004). Preliminary assessment of the effect of diet and L-carnitine supplementation on lipoma size and bodyweight in budgerigars (*Melopsittacus undulatus*). *J. Avian Med. Surg.* 18 (1): 12–18.

Earle, K.E. and Clarke, N.R. (1991). The nutrition of the budgerigar (*Melopsittacus undulatus*). *J. Nutr.* 121 (11 (Suppl)): 186S–192S.

Finke, M.D. (2002). Complete nutrient composition of commercially raised invertebrates used as food for insectivores. *Zoo Biol.* 21: 269–285.

Finke, M. (2003). Gut loading to enhance the nutrient content of insects as food for reptiles: a mathematical approach. *Zoo Biol.* 22: 147–162.

Finke, M.D. (2013). Complete nutrient content of four species of feeder insects. *Zoo Biol.* 32 (1): 27–36.

Fitzgerald, B. and Beaufrere, H. (2015). Cardiology. In: *Current Therapy in Avian Medicine and Surgery* (ed. B. Speer), 253–328. St. Louis, MO: Elsevier Health Sciences.

Forshaw, J.M. and Cooper, W.T. (1989). *Parrots of the World*. London: Blandford.

Frankel, T.L. and Avram, D.S. (2001). Protein requirements of rainbow lorikeets, Trichoglossus haematodus. *Aust. J. Zool.* 49: 435–443.

Fudge, A.M. and Speer, B. (2001). Selected controversial topics in avian diagnostic testing. *Semin. Avian Exotic Pet Med.* 10 (2): 96–101.

Glick, B., Taylor, R.L., Martin, D.E. et al. (1983). Calorie-protein deficiencies and the immune response of the chicken. II. Cell-mediated immunity. *Poult. Sci.* 62: 1889–1893.

Goldstein, D.L. (1988). Estimates of daily energy expenditure in birds: the time-energy budget as an integrator of laboratory and field studies. *Am. Zool.* 28 (3): 829–844.

Green, A.S. and Fascetti, A.J. (2016). Meeting the vitamin A requirement: the efficacy and importance of β-carotene in animal species. *ScientificWorldJournal* 2016: 7393620.

Harrison, G. (1998). Twenty years of progress in pet bird nutrition. *J. Am. Vet. Med. Assoc. (USA)* 212 (8): 1226–1230.

Harrison, G.J. and McDonald, D. (2006). Nutritional considerations section II. In: *Clinical Avian Medicine*, vol. 1 (ed. G.J. Harrison and T. Lightfoot), 108–140. Brenthwood, TN: Harrison's Bird Foods https://avianmedicine.net/wp-content/uploads/2013/03/04nutrition2.pdf (accessed October 7, 2022).

Heinze, C., Hawkins, M., Gillies, L. et al. (2012). Effect of dietary omega-3 fatty acids on red blood cell lipid composition and plasma metabolites in the cockatiel, Nymphicus hollandicus. *J. Anim. Sci.* 90 (9): 3068–3079.

Hess, L., Mauldin, G., and Rosenthal, K. (2002). Estimated nutrient content of diets commonly fed to pet birds. *Vet. Rec.* 150 (13): 399–404.

Howard, B. (1992). Health risks of housing small psittacines in galvanized wire mesh cages. *J. Am. Vet. Med. Assoc.* 200 (11): 1667–1674.

Ingram, T., Zuck, J., Borges, C.R. et al. (2017). Variations in native protein glycation and plasma antioxidants in several birds of prey. In: *Comp. Biochem. Physiol. B, Biochem. Mol. Biol.*, vol. 210, 18–28.

Kalmar, I.D., Janssens, G.P.J., and Moons, C.P.H. (2010). Guidelines and ethical considerations for housing and management of psittacine birds used in research. *Int. Lab. Anim. Res. J.* 51 (4): 409–423.

Klasing, K.C. (1998). *Comparative Avian Nutrition*. New York: CAB International.

Klasing, K.C., Dierenfeld, E.S., and Koutsos, E.A. (2012). Avian iron storage disease: variations on a common theme? *J. Zoo Wildl. Med.* 43 (3s): S27–S34.

Koutsos, E. (2016). *Foundations in Avian Nutrition*. St. Louis, MO: Elsevier Health Sciences.

Koutsos, E.A. and Klasing, K.C. (2005). Vitamin A nutrition of growing cockatiel chicks (Nymphicus hollandicus). *J. Anim. Physiol. Anim. Nutr.* 89 (11–12): 379.

Koutsos, E.A., Matson, K.D., and Klasing, K.C. (2001a). Nutrition of birds in the order Psittaciformes: a review. *J. Avian Med. Surg.* 15: 237–275.

Koutsos, E.A., Smith, J., Woods, L.W., and Klasing, K.C. (2001b). Adult cockatiels (Nymphicus hollandicus) metabolically adapt to high protein diets. *J. Nutr.* 131 (7): 2014–2020.

Koutsos, E.A., Tell, L.A., Woods, L.W., and Klasing, K.C. (2003). Adult cockatiels (Nymphicus hollandicus) at maintenance are more sensitive to diets containing excess vitamin A than to vitamin A-deficient diets. *J. Nutr.* 133 (6): 1898–1902.

Kris-Etherton, P.M. and Hill, A.M. (2008). N-3 fatty acids: food or supplements? *J. Am. Diet. Assoc.* 108 (7): 1125–1130.

Kris-Etherton, P., Taylor, D.S., Yu-Poth, S. et al. (2000). Polyunsaturated fatty acids in the food chain in the United States. *Am. J. Clin. Nutr.* 71 (1): 179S–188S.

Lumeij, J.T. and Hommers, C.J. (2008). Foraging "enrichment" as treatment for pterotillomania. *Appl. Anim. Behav. Sci.* 111 (1): 85–94.

MacMillen, R. and Baudinette, R. (1993). Water economy of granivorous birds: Australian parrots. *Funct. Ecol.* 704–712.

McDonald, D. (2004). Nutritional status of wild psittacines: optimizing the balance of fat-soluble vitamins. In: *Advances in Companion Bird Nutrition: from the Proceedings of the 2004 Avian Nutrition Seminar, Oberschleibheim*, Germany, 27. HBD's Avian Examiner https://avianmedicine.net/wp-content/uploads/2013/03/ae27.pdf (accessed October 7, 2022).

McNab, B.K. (2009). Ecological factors affect the level and scaling of avian BMR. *Comp. Biochem. Physiol. A Mol. Integr. Physiol.* 152 (1): 22–45.

Meehan, C.L., Millam, J.R., and Mench, J.A. (2003). Foraging opportunity and increased physical complexity both prevent and reduce psychogenic feather picking by young Amazon parrots. *Appl. Anim. Behav. Sci.* 80 (1): 71–85.

Murphy, M.E., King, J.R., and Lu, J. (1988). Malnutrition during the postnuptial molt of white-crowned sparrows: feather growth and quality. *Can. J. Zool.* 66 (6): 1403–1413.

Nagy, K.A., Girard, I.A., and Brown, T.K. (1999). Energetics of free-ranging mammals, reptiles, and birds. *Annu. Rev. Nutr.* 19 (1): 247–277.

NRC (National Research Council) (1994). *Nutrient Requirements of Poultry*. Washington, DC: National Academy Press.

Orosz, S.E. (2014). Clinical avian nutrition. *Vet. Clin.: Exotic Anim. Pract.* 17 (3): 397–413.

Park, F. (2006). Vitamin A toxicosis in a lorikeet flock. *Vet. Clinics: Exotic Anim. Pract.* 9 (3): 495–502.

Peron, F. and Grosset, C. (2014). The diet of adult psittacids: veterinarian and ethological approaches. *J. Anim. Physiol. Anim. Nutr. (Berl.)* 98 (3): 403–416.

Petzinger, C. (2015). Growth curves and their implications in hand-fed Monk parrots (*Myiopsitta monachus*). *Vet. Med. (Auckl)* 6: 321–327.

Petzinger, C. and Bauer, J.E. (2013). Dietary considerations for atherosclerosis in common companion avian species. *J. Exotic Pet Med.* 22 (4): 358–365.

Petzinger, C., Heatley, J.J., Cornejo, J. et al. (2010). Dietary modification of omega-3 fatty acids for birds with atherosclerosis. *J. Am. Vet. Med. Assoc.* 236 (5): 523–528.

Petzinger, C., Heatley, J., Bailey, C.A., and Bauer, J.E. (2014a). Lipid metabolic dose response to dietary alpha-linolenic acid in monk parrot (*Myiopsitta monachus*). *Lipids* 49 (3): 235–245.

Petzinger, C., Larner, C., Heatley, J. et al. (2014b). Conversion of α-linolenic acid to long-chain omega-3 fatty acid derivatives and alterations of HDL density subfractions and plasma lipids with dietary polyunsaturated fatty acids in monk parrots (*Myiopsitta monachus*). *J. Anim. Physiol. Anim. Nutr.* 98 (2): 262–270.

Powers, L.V., Flammer, K., and Papich, M. (2000). Preliminary investigation of doxycycline plasma concentrations in cockatiels (*Nymphicus hollandicus*) after administration by injection or in water or feed. *J. Avian Med. Surg.* 14: 23–30.

Pryor, G.S. (2003). Protein requirements of three species of parrots with distinct dietary specializations. *Zoo Biol.* 22 (2): 163–177.

Pryor, G.S., Levey, D.J., and Dierenfeld, E.S. (2001). Protein requirements of a specialized frugivore, Pesquet's parrot (*Psittrichas fulgidus*). *Auk* 118 (4): 1080–1088.

Ravich, M., Cray, C., Hess, L., and Arheart, K.L. (2014). Lipid panel reference intervals for Amazon parrots (Amazona species). *J. Avian Med. Surg.* 28 (3): 209–215.

Reid, R.B. and Perlberg, W. (1998). Emerging trends in pet bird diets. *J.Am. Vet. Med. Assoc.* 212 (8): 1236–1237.

Rezende, E.L., Swanson, D.L., Novoa, F.F., and Bozinovic, F. (2002). Passerines versus nonpasserines: so far, no statistical differences in the scaling of avian energetics. *J. Exp. Biol.* 205 (1): 101–107.

Ricklefs, R. (1974). Energetics of reproduction in birds. *Avian Energetics* 15: 152–192.

Romagnano, A., Grindem, C.B., Degernes, L., and Mautino, M. (1995). Treatment of a hyacinth macaw with zinc toxicity. *J. Avian Med. Surg.* 9: 185–189.

Roudybush, T.E. and Grau, C.R. (1986). Food and water interrelations and the protein requirement for growth of an Altricial bird, the cockatiel (*Nymphicus hollandicus*). *J. Nutr.* 116 (4): 552–559.

Rozek, J.C. and Millam, J.R. (2011). Preference and motivation for different diet forms and their effect on motivation for a foraging enrichment in captive Orange-winged Amazon parrots (*Amazona amazonica*). *Appl. Anim. Behav. Sci.* 129 (2–4): 153–161.

Rozek, J.C., Danner, L.M., Stucky, P.A., and Millam, J.R. (2010). Over-sized pellets naturalize foraging time of captive Orange-winged Amazon parrots (*Amazona amazonica*). *Appl. Anim. Behav. Sci.* 125 (1–2): 80–87.

Sailaja, R., Kotak, V.C., Sharp, P.J. et al. (1988). Environmental, dietary, and hormonal factors in the regulation of seasonal breeding in free-living female Indian rose-ringed parakeets (*Psittacula krameri*). *Horm. Behav.* 22 (4): 518–527.

Schaftenaar, W. and van Leeuwen, J.P. (2015). The influence of ultraviolet-B radiation on the growth of marabou stork (Leptoptilos crumeniferus) nestlings in relation to plasma calcium, phosphorus, and vitamin D3 concentrations. *J. Zoo Wildl. Med.* 46 (4): 682–690.

Seibert, L.M. (2006). Feather-picking disorder in pet birds. In: *Manual of Parrot Behavior* (ed. A.U. Luescher), 255–265. Ames, IA: Blackwell.

Sibley, D., Elphick, C.D., and John, B. (2001). *The Sibley Guide to Bird Life & Behavior*. New York: National Audubon Society.

Slifka, K.A., Bowen, P.E., Stacewicz-Sapuntzakis, M., and Crissey, S.D. (1999). A survey of serum and dietary carotenoids in captive wild animals. *J. Nutr.* 129: 380–390.

Song, S. and Beissinger, S.R. (2020). Environmental and ecological correlates of avian field metabolic rate and water flux. *Funct. Ecol.* 34 (4): 811–821.

Speer, B. and Hennigh, M. (2017). *High Impact Ways to Apply Behavioral Medicine in a Healthcare Setting*. Teaneck, NJ: Association of Avian Veterinarians.

Speer, B.L., Olsen, G.P., Doneley, R. et al. (2016). Common conditions of commonly held companion birds in multiple parts of the world. In: *Current Therapy in Avian Medicine and Surgery* (ed. B.L. Speer), 777–781. St. Louis, MO: Elsevier.

Stahl, S. and Kronfeld, D. (1998). Veterinary nutrition of large psittacines. *Semin. Avian Exotic Pet Med.* **7** (3): 128–134.

Stanford, M. (2004). Calcium metabolism in psittacine birds: The effects of husbandry. In: *Advances in Companion Bird Nutrition: from the Proceedings of the 2004 Avian Nutrition Seminar, Oberschleibheim*, Germany, 27. HBD's Avian Examiner https://avianmedicine. net/wp-content/uploads/2013/03/ae27.pdf (accessed October 7, 2022).

Stanford, M. (2006). Calcium metabolism. In: *Clinical Avian Medicine*, vol. 1 (ed. G.J. Harrison and T. Lightfoot), 141–151. Brenthwood, TN: Harrison's Bird Foods https://avianmedicine. net/publication_cat/clinical-avian-medicine (accessed October 7, 2022).

Ullrey, D.E. (1989). Nutritional wisdom. *J. Zoo Wildl. Med.* 20 (1): 1–2.

Ullrey, D.E., Allen, M.E., and Baer, D.J. (1991). Formulated diets versus seed mixtures for psittacines. *J. Nutr.* 121 (11 Suppl): S193–S205.

Underwood, M., Polin, D., O'Handley, P., and Wiggers, P. (1991). Short term energy and protein utilization by budgerigars (*Melopsittacus undulatus*) fed isocaloric diets of varying protein concentrations. *Proc. Assoc. Avian Vet.* 1991: 227–237.

Vergneau-Grosset, C., Polley, T., Holt, D.C. et al. (2016). Hematologic, plasma biochemical, and lipid panel reference intervals in orange-winged Amazon parrots (*Amazona amazonica*). *J. Avian Med. Surg.* 30 (4): 335–344.

Weathers, W.W. and Caccamise, D.F. (1975). Temperature regulation and water requirements of the monk parakeet, *Myiopsitta monachus. Oecologia* 18 (4): 329–342.

Weaver, C.M., Martin, B.R., Ebner, J.S., and Krueger, C.A. (1987). Oxalic acid decreases calcium absorption in rats. *J. Nutr.* 117 (11): 1903–1906.

Williams, T.D. (1996). Variation in reproductive effort in female zebra finches (Taeniopygia guttata) in relation to nutrient-specific dietary supplements during egg laying. *Physiol. Zool.* 1255–1275.

van Zeeland, Y.R.A., Spruit, B.M., Rodenburg, T.B. et al. (2009). Feather damaging behaviour in parrots: a review with consideration of comparative aspects. *Appl. Anim. Behav. Sci.* 121 (2): 75–95.

23

Nutrition for Small Mammalian Companion Herbivores and Carnivores

Jonathan Stockman and Olivia A. Petritz

In addition to domesticated companion animals such as dogs and cats, the popularity of small "exotic" or non-domestic mammals as companions is high in North America and across the world. For example, one survey estimated that over 6.7 million households in the United States have over 14 million small mammal pets (American Pet Product Association, www.americanpetproducts.org/press_industrytrends.asp). As a result of their popularity, herbivorous small mammals such as rabbits, chinchillas, guinea pigs, and carnivorous ferrets are frequently presented to veterinary practitioners, and clients often require guidance regarding species-specific nutrition requirements and husbandry in addition to veterinary care.

Most of the knowledge regarding the nutritional requirements for these species stems from production or laboratory animals, as information regarding the nutritional requirements of these species as companion animals is scarce. Further understanding of the requirements of small companion mammals is needed, as there are also important differences in the husbandry, longevity, and client expectations between production or laboratory animals and companion animals. Correct husbandry is paramount for the health and welfare of companion "exotic" mammals, and many health problems may stem from poor husbandry as well as inadequate nutrition. This chapter provides an overview on the nutritional physiology and nutrition-related pathology of companion herbivores – rabbits, chinchillas, guinea pigs, and carnivores such as ferrets. Not covered are the small mammalian omnivores such as hamsters (*Phodopus* spp.), rats (*Rattus* spp.), and mice (*Mus* spp.).

General Nutrition for Small Mammalian Companion Herbivores

Lagomorphs (Rabbits) and Caviomorphs (Chinchillas and Guinea Pigs)

Domestic rabbits *(Oryctolagus cuniculus)*, chinchillas (*Chinchilla laniger*), and guinea pigs *(Cavia porcellus)* are herbivores adapted to prehend, masticate, and digest vegetation. The gastrointestinal tracts of lagomorphs and caviomorph pet rodents are uniquely adapted to a diet high in fiber or roughage (Portsmouth 1977). Rabbits, chinchillas, and guinea pigs eat a wide variety of food, although they may select the more tender and succulent plants or plant parts.

As prey species, nighttime activity and feeding are common for rabbits and many rodents. The diet of these species is high in fiber, which is essential for normal peristalsis and a healthy gut microbiota. Due to their diets being less energy and nutrient dense, these animals also rely heavily on utilization of their gastrointestinal microbiota, and specifically hind-gut fiber fermentation, for several

Applied Veterinary Clinical Nutrition, Second Edition. Edited by Andrea J. Fascetti, Sean J. Delaney, Jennifer A. Larsen, and Cecilia Villaverde.
© 2024 John Wiley & Sons, Inc. Published 2024 by John Wiley & Sons, Inc.

essential nutrients. As hind-gut fermenters, the bacterial populations in the gastrointestinal tract have additional important roles in maintaining gastrointestinal health, and a disturbance to the intestinal microbiota may have severe health implications that can be life-threatening.

Gastrointestinal Physiology and Anatomic Features

The oral cavity in rabbits, chinchillas, and guinea pigs is small compared with many other mammals. The incisors, premolars, and molars are aradicular elondont, hypsodont teeth that grow continuously and never develop anatomic roots. These teeth are ideal for masticating high-roughage foods such as hays and grasses. Food fiber consistency is imperative for maintaining adequate teeth occlusion. Rabbits use their incisors in a vertical motion to chew large pieces of leaves or other parts of plants. Then horizontal motion is used to chew the leaf into smaller pieces by the molars and premolars (Vella and Donnelly 2012). A lack of adequate fiber in the diet can result in asymmetric dental wear patterns, leading to sharp points and malocclusions (Meredith et al. 2015).

The herbivorous small mammal gastrointestinal tract combines a simple stomach with a large cecum where much of dietary fiber fermentation occurs. In rabbits, chinchillas, and guinea pigs (as well as other herbivorous rodents), the role of cecal microbial digestion is highly important, as these species ingest feces of cecal origin, called cecotropes (commonly known as "night feces" or "night droppings," see more later), to optimize nutrient utilization. The relatively short gastrointestinal tract in these species requires a high food intake (65–80 g/kg body weight) and a relatively fast gastrointestinal transit time compared with larger herbivores (Irlbeck 2001).

The stomach of small herbivorous mammals including rabbits is relatively small and has a well-developed pyloric sphincter, but the wall of the stomach has a weak muscular layer

(Carabaño et al. 2010). The stomach continuously secretes acid; therefore the pH in the rabbit's stomach is very acidic, with a range between 1 and 5. As in other species, the next segment of the gastrointestinal tract is the small intestine, where much of the digestion and absorption occurs by both passive and active absorption. The most distal part of the small intestine is the ileum, which has an important role in absorption of many nutrients such as amino acids, starch, and vitamins.

The rabbit's cecum has a coiled structure and a thin and weak muscular layer, with **a** slightly acidic content, although it is less acidic than the stomach (pH 5.4–6.8) (García et al. 2002). The cecum has the volume capacity of almost half of the total digestive tract. The internal surface of the cecum is large, due to multiple mucosal folds over its circumference and a spiral fold running the length of the cecum and dividing it in two (Björnhag and Snipes 1999). The cecum contracts to mix the fermenting ingesta.

The normal fermentation process relies on a combination of a healthy diet and the composition of the microbiota. The predominant bacteria in the rabbit's cecum is *Bacteriodes* spp. In the cecum of chinchillas and guinea pigs, *Bacteriodes* spp., *Bifidobacterium* spp., and *Ruminococcus* spp. are prevalent (Worthington and Fulghum 1988; Takahashi et al. 2005). Anaerobic Gram-positive bacteria such as *Lactobacillus* spp., coliforms, and *Clostridium* spp. as well as yeast may also be present; however, these are not the dominant populations (Oglesbee and Jenkins 2012). Fermentation results in production of short-chain volatile fatty acids (i.e. acetic, formic, propionic, and butyric acids). These fatty acids may diffuse and absorb through the cecal mucosa or become incorporated into cecotropes and ingested after voiding (as further discussed later).

The anatomy of the proximal colon is different between rabbits and various rodent species. In rabbits, the most distal portion of the proximal colon leads to a short segment that connects the proximal and distal colon called the fusus coli, a densely innervated portion of the colon with thick continuous muscular layers. The fusus coli acts as a pacemaker for the production of hard feces. In caviomorph rodents, there are two opposing folds in the proximal colon with a longitudinal groove between them that holds bacteria, mucus, and food particles. In the rabbit, three muscular bands separate the haustra in the proximal part of the proximal colon, which are absent in the distal segment. In chinchillas and guinea pigs, the same arrangement of haustra is present throughout the proximal colon (Stan et al. 2014). The distal colon reaches a length of 80–100 cm in the rabbit, and it does not have many distinctive features in structure and function compared with other species (Snipes et al. 1982).

The colonic separation mechanism, which is responsible for allowing rapid transport of the larger, less digestible food particles down the digestive tract and retaining the smaller particles and associated microbiota in the cecum, exists in rabbits, guinea pigs, and chinchillas (Björnhag and Snipes 1999). This mechanism is important for sustaining the intestinal microbiota, as rapid gastrointestinal transport times may otherwise preclude sustaining stable microbiota. In rabbits, the colonic separation mechanism involves an anatomic structure in the proximal colon that allows a retrograde flow of small particles, liquid, and bacteria, whereas in rodents the mechanism relies on a colonic furrow that traps small particles and mucus that are transported back into the cecum (Björnhag and Snipes 1999).

The gut-associated lymphoid tissue (GALT) has an important role in developing mechanisms of tolerance for the normal microbiota while protecting against pathogens. The microbiota in turn plays an important role in the development of GALT, as the normal "flora" are required for developing the pre-immune antibody repertoire by promoting somatic diversification of immunoglobulin (Ig) genes in B cells that have migrated to the GALT. Goblet cells, which produce mucin, are found in the intestinal villi and crypts. The mucus produced has an important role as a defense against pathogens, and the goblet cells themselves are considered to be gatekeepers for presentation of antigens to the immune system (Pelaseyed et al. 2014).

Rabbits and caviomorph rodents rely on digestion of protein and vitamins of gut microbial origin through the production and subsequent ingestion of cecotropes, or "night feces" or "night droppings," which should be consumed by the animal post defecation. Typically, cecotropes have a distinct appearance, compared with "hard" feces, as cecotropes are softer, smaller, and enveloped in mucus. The hard feces should not be ingested, similar to other mammals. The mechanism of cecotrophy allows absorption of nutrients, produced by bacteria in the more distal large intestine, to occur in the more proximal intestinal tract. Cecotropes are high in protein, nitrogen, essential amino acids, short-chain fatty acids, potassium, sodium, B vitamins, and water. They are typically ingested directly from the anus. Thus, obesity, pelvic limb osteoarthritis, or pelvic limb paresis can impair a rabbit's ability to ingest its cecotropes from its anus. The amount of cecotrophy may vary between individuals and is dependent on diet, where a high-fiber diet typically increases cecotrophy.

Rabbit, Chinchilla, and Guinea Pig Normal Diet

Rabbits, chinchillas, and guinea pigs have their own unique nutritional requirements. Despite relying on nutrients synthesized by the gastrointestinal microbiota, food-sourced nutrients are also necessary to meet the nutritional requirements of these animals (NRC 1977) (Box 23.1).

Protein

Dietary protein of 12–16% (on a dry matter basis) is considered appropriate for pet rabbits (Snyder et al. 1976; NRC 1977). Nitrogen and

---

Box 23.1 Feeding the Healthy Rabbit, Chinchilla, and Guinea Pig[a]

Juveniles

- Diet of ad libitum high-quality grass (Timothy, oat, or orchard) hay or a mixture of alfalfa-grass hays plus controlled amounts of alfalfa-based concentrated food (aka pellets), dark leafy greens (e.g. chard, kale, collard, and mustard greens), and very small amounts of other vegetables (e.g. Brussels sprouts, bok choy, romaine lettuce, carrots) and rarely fruit (e.g. bell pepper, cucumber).
- Diet daily proportions (as is) should be ~75% hay, 15–20% pellets, up to 10% leafy greens, and <2.5% other vegetables and fruit.
- Any fresh food should be removed if uneaten after a few hours or soiled.

Adults

- Diet of ad libitum high-quality grass (Timothy, oat, or orchard) hay plus controlled amounts of grass hay pellets, dark leafy greens (e.g. chard, kale, collard, and mustard greens), and very small amounts of other vegetables (e.g. Brussels sprouts,

bok choy, romaine lettuce, carrots) and rarely fruit (e.g. bell pepper, cucumber).
- Diet daily proportions (as is) should be:
  70–75% hay
  15–20% pellets OR up to 1/3 cup (~80 ml) of pellets per 5 lb (~2.25 kg) body weight; reduce portion of pellets if undesired weight gain results
  10% leafy greens OR up to 2.5 chopped cups (~600 ml) per 5 lb (~2.25 kg) body weight
  <2.5% other vegetables and fruit OR up to 2.5 tablespoons (~37 ml) per 5 lb (~2.25 kg) body weight; these other vegetables and fruit are optional and should be avoided if undesired weight gain results
- Any fresh food should be removed if uneaten after a few hours or soiled.

[a] Guinea pigs require vitamin C in the diet at 20–25 mg/day for adult maintenance and 30–40 mg/day for reproduction. This requirement can be met with concentrated, fortified food (noting that it can degrade quickly due to oxidation), vitamin C tablets, and/or fresh food (e.g. kale, mustard greens, bell peppers). Vitamin C should not be added to water as it degrades too quickly to be an effective means of supplementation.

---

essential amino acid requirements are met by both food-sourced protein and bacterial synthesis of protein from fibrous ingesta in the cecum. The essential amino acids for these species are arginine, glycine, histidine, isoleucine, leucine, lysine, methionine (and cysteine), phenylalanine (and tyrosine), threonine, tryptophan, and valine (NRC 1977). Protein digestibility from forage is about 80%, partly due to cecotrophy.

Excess dietary protein may be detrimental to health. It can contribute to obesity and lead to an increase in cecal ammonia concentration, which alters acidity and can cause dysbiosis. Protein requirements are increased during growth and during reproduction. Higher protein ingredients such as legumes/pulses and alfalfa hay may be incorporated into the diet to

achieve a dietary protein concentration of 18–19% (as fed) (Campbell-Ward 2012) during these life stages.

Carbohydrate and Fiber

Simple carbohydrates such as high-sugar fruit and treats are often highly palatable for rabbits and rodents. In excess, simple carbohydrates may reach the cecum, cause shifts in the microbiota, and may lead to dysbiosis, gut stasis, and enterotoxemia. In addition, an excess of energy-dense sugars may lead to obesity and concurrent metabolic complications (Zhao et al. 2008). For this reason, energy-dense food items such as yogurt treats, fruit (fresh and dried), and seeds should be kept to a minimum.

Fiber should comprise a high proportion of the diet, with a recommended total dietary

Table 23.1 Nutrient comparison between different types of hay.

Averages	Western Timothy hay	Orchard grass hay	Oat grass hay	Organic meadow grass	Alfalfa hay
Crude protein (%)	10.5–11	12.5–13.5	9.5–10.5	9.5–10.5	18–19
Crude fat (%)	2.1–2.7	4.1–4.5	2.3–2.7	2.0–2.3	1.0–1.4
Crude fiber (%)	24.8–26.5	24.1–26	26.9–27.9	24–25.9	17.1–19.5
Acid detergent fiber (%)	29–30.5	27–28.5	29–30.3	29–30.4	27–28.4
Calcium (%)	0.45	0.47	0.4	0.59	1.6
Phosphorus (%)	0.22	0.28	0.22	0.18	0.27

fiber concentration of at least 20–25% as fed (Campbell-Ward 2012). Fiber is important for normal behavior, gut motility maintenance, and gut microbiota. Although fiber digestibility is generally low, its physical properties are important for gut motility, and it serves as a substrate for fermentation. For this reason, fiber length has importance. Pelleted food manufactured with finely ground hay and with short fiber length may not provide the same benefits for gastrointestinal health in rabbits that hay can provide. Rabbits that are fed primarily or exclusively pellets with short fiber length may experience decreased motility, longer gastrointestinal transit time, and higher incidence of gut dysbiosis (Irlbeck 2001). Ad libitum provision of lower calcium and protein hay such as Timothy grass hay (*Phleum pratense*) is recommended for rabbits, chinchillas, and guinea pigs. To ensure the hay is consumed and comprises the majority of the nutrition (70–75% as fed; Kohles 2014), other components of the diet such as pellets, vegetables, and treats should be limited, as they may be preferentially consumed despite their potential adverse effect on health when consumed in excess.

Hay and Other Plant Considerations
Grass hay such as Timothy, oat, and orchard hays are all acceptable options for rabbits, chinchillas, and guinea pigs. However, hay varies in its nutritional value, and the feeding of inappropriate hay may lead to adverse health outcomes. A comparison between different types of hay is presented in Table 23.1. Alfalfa hay is higher in protein calcium and phosphorus and lower in the percentage of crude fiber (Eastridge et al. 2009). It is recommended to limit alfalfa hay except for animals with high nutritional and metabolic needs, such as during reproduction or growth. If alfalfa hay is fed as a main source of hay, it may lead to various health concerns such as obesity, gut dysbiosis, and urinary tract disease. Similarly, other legume/pulse hays are also high in protein and are not recommended for maintenance.

To ensure that hay is consumed in sufficient amounts, it is recommended to provide hay in the cage ad libitum. Hay should be offered from weaning starting at 3 weeks of age. Changes in hay should be done gradually over 4–5 days to avoid stress and gastrointestinal signs that may occur as a result of abrupt changes. It is important to use fresh hay of good quality, clean of dust and any foreign material. Hay that is stored for prolonged periods of time will undergo vitamin degradation, including vitamins A and D. Mold may form if it is not stored appropriately in dry conditions. Hay palatability may also decrease with prolonged storage, potentially leading to selective eating of the other diet components, which may not be as optimal. Fresh, pesticide-free grass can be offered where available; however, lawn clippings are not recommended as they could be a source of contamination with infectious pathogens (Southard et al. 2013). Fresh grass also spoils quickly and may cause adverse reactions.

Hay-based pellets should only comprise 10–15% (as is) of the diet. Common commercial pellets contain Timothy and alfalfa hays. For rabbit, chinchilla, and guinea pig adult maintenance, Timothy pellets are recommended. Alfalfa pellets can be used in animals during growth and reproduction. It is important to avoid pellets in a mixture that also contains energy-dense foods such as dried fruit, sugary treats, oats, cereals, and nuts. Pellets should contain at least 18% as is total dietary fiber. As a rule of thumb, it has been suggested that up to one-third of a cup (~80 ml) of pellets per 5 lb (~2.25 kg) body weight can be provided to rabbits (Oglesbee and Jenkins 2012).

Fruit should be given sparingly as a rare treat and should not exceed 5% of the diet by volume. Small amounts (10% as is) of vegetables and greens (see earlier note about fresh grass) can be added for variety. These can provide some essential minerals and vitamins as well as added hydration. Since their fiber contribution is minimal, they should not be fed in excess. Some acceptable examples include dark leafy greens (e.g. chard, kale, collard, and mustard greens), bok choy, and romaine lettuce.

Fat

Fat should comprise a small percentage of the diet, and 2.5–4% (as fed) is a generally acceptable concentration (Campbell-Ward 2012). A diet lower in fat can result in clinical signs of deficiency in rabbits, manifested as hair loss, poor growth, and a negative effect on reproduction (Ahluwalia et al. 1967). Similarly, linoleic acid (a long-chain omega-6 polyunsaturated fatty acid [PUFA]) and eicosapentaenoic acid (a long-chain omega-3 PUFA) have both been shown to be essential for guinea pigs (Reid et al. 1964). Higher-fat diets are generally not recommended as these energy-dense diets will likely lead to obesity.

Vitamins and Minerals

While cecotrophy may meet the majority of the requirements for vitamins B and K, other essential vitamins and minerals need to be sourced from the diet.

The active form of vitamin A, retinol, may be derived from beta-carotene found in vegetables and grasses (Olson 1989). Although the efficiency of converting beta-carotene to active vitamin A is relatively high in lagomorphs and caviomorphs, beta-carotene only has about 40% of the molar efficiency of preformed vitamin A in these species (NRC 1995). Therefore, rabbits fed diets low in vitamin A may suffer from clinical signs of deficiency such as enteritis, poor growth, keratitis, and low fertility. Excessive vitamin A supplementation may also result in severe clinical signs such as coagulopathy and teratogenicity.

Vitamin C is essential for guinea pigs and must be provided in the diet (200 mg/kg diet as fed), as they lack L-gulonolactone oxidase activity, an enzyme required for endogenous vitamin C synthesis. Clinical signs of vitamin C deficiency or "scurvy" in guinea pigs include anemia, multiple hemorrhages as a result of impaired clotting, impaired collagen synthesis, and even death. Due to natural vitamin degradation from oxidation, vitamin C content in commercial diets may be reduced by up to 50% within three months, even with appropriate storage. Diets with "stabilized" vitamin C are commercially available, and those have a longer shelf life. Guinea pigs should be provided with the equivalent of 10 mg per kg body weight of vitamin C (or ascorbate) per day. The requirement may increase to 30 mg per kg body weight during reproduction (Harkness et al. 2010). Vitamin C supplementation is not essential for rabbits and chinchillas, but it can be provided in diets for its antioxidant properties if desired. As an acid, excessive vitamin C may have negative effects on the pH in the gastrointestinal tract, and may also become a pro-oxidant rather than an antioxidant.

Unlike dogs and cats, rabbits, chinchillas, and guinea pigs are capable, like humans, of synthesizing vitamin D in their skin when exposed to sunlight or UV radiation. It is generally accepted that rabbits are capable of absorbing calcium from their diet regardless of vitamin D; although this is primarily based on data in growing rabbits and reproducing does, similar data are not available for adult rabbits in maintenance (Chapin and Smith 1967). Calcium absorption was shown to increase when vitamin D concentrations were higher (Harcourt-Brown 1996). Similarly, guinea pigs are unlikely to develop clinical signs of vitamin D deficiency, even when fed diets low in vitamin D, if the diet is adequate in calcium and phosphorus concentrations and at an adequate calcium-to-phosphorus ratio (i.e. calcium 8–10 g Ca/kg as fed, phosphorus 4–7 g P/kg as fed; NRC 1995). Signs of vitamin D deficiency can occur when the dietary intake of these minerals is low or if the ratio of calcium to phosphorus is reduced. Excess dietary vitamin D may be detrimental in rabbits, similar to other species, where the subsequent hypercalcemia may lead to soft tissue mineralization and organ failure, especially affecting the kidneys.

Vitamin E is an essential antioxidant, and a deficiency can result in muscular dystrophy (Mackenzie and McCollum 1940) and reduced reproductive success. In guinea pigs, vitamin E and selenium deficiencies lead to a condition called nutritional muscular dystrophy, primarily observed in guinea pigs during reproduction (Hawkins and Bishop 2012). This condition is reversible, if diagnosed and treated with vitamin E supplementation, but ultimately it can be fatal.

As stated earlier, calcium absorption is highly efficient in rabbits, possibly even when vitamin D intake (and/or UV radiation exposure) is low. Typically companion rabbits will have elevated serum and urine calcium, compared to other mammals. In guinea pigs, and likely in chinchillas, calcium absorption is a reflection of the dietary calcium intake as well as the ratio between calcium and other minerals, primarily phosphorus and magnesium (NRC 1995). In general, a ratio of calcium:phosphorus of 1–2:1 is recommended to maintain calcium homeostasis. Excess dietary calcium is thought to result in renal disease and urolithiasis, although this relationship is uncertain.

The magnesium requirement has been demonstrated in weanling rabbits, where deficiency caused decreased growth and neurologic signs, which reversed following magnesium supplementation (NRC 1977). In guinea pigs, fluorine and potassium have a sparing effect on magnesium and may reverse clinical signs of magnesium deficiency, whereas phosphorus and calcium have the opposite effect. Therefore, the dietary magnesium requirement in guinea pigs is dependent on the ratios of the other minerals. In herbivores, dietary phosphorus is primarily in the form of phytates (i.e. the main phosphorus storage form in plants), which has low bioavailability in non-herbivores; however, rabbits have phytase activity throughout their gastrointestinal tract, primarily in the cecum, which allows dietary phytates to be a good source of phosphorus (Marounek et al. 2009).

Phosphorus deficiency may lead to rickets in growing animals, as demonstrated in rodents (Ko et al. 2016). Trace minerals such as iron, copper, manganese, zinc, iodine, and selenium are all considered essential and clinical signs of deficiency may occur, particularly in growing animals.

Water

Water should always be provided. It is important that water is fresh and clean, as unclean water may not be consumed, leading to dehydration. Water requirements are 10–12% of body weight per day. Water requirements may increase in dry or warm weather. Some authors have made recommendations to encourage water intake by providing water in a bowl rather than a bottle (Tschudin et al. 2011). Chinchillas are especially sensitive to high temperatures and should not be exposed to temperatures above 80 °F (26.7 °C).

General Warning about Energy-Dense Foods and Treats

Avoiding high-fat, high-protein, and high-sugar items is generally recommended, as these can lead to obesity and gastrointestinal disease. Some examples to avoid include breakfast cereals, sweets, dried fruit, nuts, seeds, yogurt "drops," cheese, meat, egg, and human table scraps that are not the vegetables noted earlier.

Nutrition-Related Diseases of Small Mammalian Companion Herbivores

Lagomorphs (Rabbits) and Caviomorphs (Chinchillas and Guinea Pigs)

Dental Disease and Malocclusion

Dental disease and malocclusion are very common in rabbits, chinchillas, and guinea pigs. This disease may manifest in a range of different clinical signs, such as ptyalism or excessive drooling during eating, selective eating of pellets or other food items that require less mastication, decreased eating (i.e. hyporexia or anorexia), dysphagia, and/or decreased defecation. The severity of this condition varies and generally increases in chronic cases. A complete description of dental disease diagnosis and treatment in rabbits and rodents is beyond the scope of this chapter, and the reader is directed to further information elsewhere (Capello and Lennox 2012).

While there are multiple etiologies for dental disease, it is widely recognized that a poor diet is a common cause. Diets deficient in fiber can cause dental disease, since dental wear during mastication of fiber has an important role in maintaining normal occlusion. As a vicious cycle, once malocclusion is present, mastication of long fibers may be avoided by the patient as this may result in pain and discomfort. Dental malocclusion seems to be a rare problem in wild chinchillas, whereas it is quite common in captive-bred chinchillas (Crossley and del Mar Miguélez 2001). This finding may have several possible explanations; however, the difference in diets fed to chinchillas in captivity is an important consideration. Diets for companion chinchillas are commonly composed primarily of soft hay and vegetation as well as pellets, fruit, and vegetables, whereas the diet for chinchillas in the wild would be composed of tougher plant parts higher in abrasive components such as phytoliths. However, the assertion that dietary fiber and diet abrasiveness are most impactful on dental wear has recently come into question, as some studies suggest that hay is mostly important for incisor wear, but not premolar or molar wear, in healthy guinea pigs (Müller et al. 2015).

In guinea pigs, vitamin C deficiency may result in periodontal disease as it affects periodontal collagen and the gingiva, and eventually leads to dental disease and malocclusion (Glickman 1948). This may be corrected with higher-dose vitamin C supplementation via parenteral or enteral supplementation (50–100 mg/guinea pig subcutaneously or orally; Quesenberry 1994).

In many cases, dental disease may progress to become a systemic and complicated condition. Secondary trauma to the tongue or cheeks and gingiva may lead to pain, inflammation, and secondary infection. Abscesses may form as a result of topical infection and inflammation, and in some cases lead to a life-threatening and systemic disease where supportive care is required to stabilize the patient. Once stabilized, further treatment would include surgical and medical treatment of the abscess and correcting the predisposing factors. An occlusal adjustment, or dental prophylaxis, is often required to reduce the crown height of the incisors, premolars, and molars to achieve as normal an occlusion as possible. These procedures typically need to be performed chronically over time due to the continuous growth of these teeth in these species, as many of the predisposing factors (such as genetic predisposition or permanent changes in occlusion from trauma) may not be possible to correct. The time interval between dental prophylaxis will vary between individuals, but it is likely that proactively correcting the diet, where it was previously inadequate in fibrous hay, will help increase the time where the patient is free from clinical signs of dental malocclusion and any associated discomfort.

Obesity

Obesity is an epidemic in companion animals, including small mammalian companion herbivores, just as it is in dogs and cats (Figure 23.1). Obese rabbits and rodents are at high risk for multiple metabolic diseases, including urinary tract disease, gastrointestinal dysbiosis, and orthopedic disease. Severely overweight animals may have difficulty grooming, which can lead to matted and unkempt hair and even myiasis (i.e. larvae or maggot infestation), as reproducing flies may be attracted to unclean hair and skin. Obese animals may also have trouble consuming cecotropes as they may not be able to reach their anus, and as a result may suffer from nutritional deficiencies. Obese animals may be at higher risk for dysbiosis, as an association between obesity and altered gut microbiota is well documented in many species, including

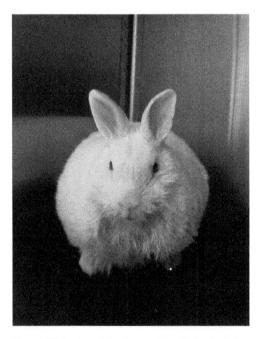

Figure 23.1 An adult obese rabbit. This rabbit had been fed an inappropriate diet of greens and yogurt. *Source:* Courtesy of Dr. Olivia Petritz.

rodents (Turnbaugh et al. 2006). In addition, excess adipose tissue may have an impact on gut motility and on inflammation. In companion rabbits, chinchillas, and guinea pigs, obesity is often the result of limited access to high-quality hay such as Timothy and grass hays, combined with high intake of high-fat and high-sugar food items such as fruit, grains including oats, sweets, and nuts, as well as limited physical activity. Excess feeding of commercial pellets with insufficient hay can also promote excessive weight gain. Correction of the diet and increasing opportunities for physical activity may have an enormous impact on health and quality of life.

A weight-loss diet should retain the optimal proportions of 75% good-quality non-legume/non-pulse hay, no more than 15% hay-based pellets, and 10% vegetables and greens. Treats and other food items should not be provided at all if possible, or should be reduced to a minimum. Hay can be fed ad libitum, but pellets and vegetables and greens limited to induce weight loss. Since rabbits and rodents feed/graze throughout the day, food amounts should not be restricted per se; however, many times increasing the proportion of hay in the diet and reducing treats can help the animal to lose weight.

Before starting a weight-loss plan, the need for dental malocclusion adjustment should be determined, and if needed performed to address any existing dental disease. Weight-loss rates greater than 2% of body weight per week should be avoided, and care taken to ensure that dental disease or discomfort is not the root cause of faster rates of loss. Transition to the optimal diet proportions, if not already fed, should be gradual over 5–7 days to allow for microbiota adjustment, minimizing gastrointestinal upset. Regular exercise should be encouraged, which may mean distribution of more palatable or higher-reward foods, like pellets and vegetables and greens, in numerous locations that need to be traversed multiple times a day, if possible in the home environment.

Gastrointestinal Stasis or Ileus

Decreased gastrointestinal motility, stasis, or ileus is a common presentation for small mammalian companion herbivores to seek veterinary care. Decreased motility can occur as a result of almost any underlying disease, as well as stress, dehydration, inadequate ambient temperatures, pain, inflammation, or gut dysbiosis. Since the gut microbiota are vital for health, decreased motility may disrupt the normal microbiota where potentially pathogenic bacteria such as *Clostridium* spp. and coliforms may overgrow. In addition, changes in the normal motility may impact the regular fermentation process and change the luminal pH, further impacting bacterial populations and potentially leading to diarrhea and enterotoxemia (Oglesbee and Jenkins 2012). On examination, patients may appear quieter than normal, but typically not overtly depressed. Auscultation and palpation of the gastrointestinal tract may reveal reduced or abnormal borborygmi and gastric or cecal gas dilation.

Treatment of ileus requires addressing the underlying condition such as pain or infection, as well as supportive care with pain management, fluids, and assisted (syringe/enteral) feeding (see later discussion). In cases where the animal is obtunded or suffers from severe dehydration, respiratory distress, or electrolyte imbalances, these conditions should be addressed first and further treatment postponed until the patient is stable.

Urolithiasis

Urolithiasis is a common presentation in rabbits and guinea pigs particularly, while in chinchillas it is less commonly reported (Martel-Arquette and Mans 2016). The location of calculi may be anywhere along the urinary tract. The causes of urolithiasis are not fully understood; however, nutrition, anatomy, and body condition are all likely involved. Rabbits are highly efficient in absorption of dietary calcium (Eckermann-Ross 2008), and as such their urine is typically high in excreted calcium carbonate. When the urine is highly saturated with the precursors for crystal formation (i.e. calcium) and when the conditions (i.e. higher urinary pH and lower concentration of inhibitors) support this process, crystals form. In affected patients, urine may be thick and gritty and over time a calculus may form. On presentation, patients may display depression, lethargy, bruxism (teeth grinding), anorexia, hematuria, and stranguria. The urinary bladder may be palpably enlarged and firm (particularly in rabbits). Abdominal ultrasonography or radiography confirms the diagnosis. Treatment of this condition varies according to location and severity at presentation; however, surgical treatment, such as cystotomy, is indicated for large cystic calculi. A non-surgical approach may be indicated when a calculus is present in the kidney or the ureter and is non-obstructive. This may include diuresis with intravenous fluids, manual expression of the bladder for several days, or cystoscopic removal (Wenger and Hatt 2015; Coutant et al. 2019).

By far the most common composition of urinary calculi in rabbits, chinchillas, and guinea pigs is calcium carbonate (Hawkins et al. 2009; Osborne et al. 2009). A thorough diet history may be needed to identify food items or supplements contributing to dietary calcium excess, although whether or not a high-calcium diet is a common cause of urolithiasis in these species remains controversial. If leafy greens and vegetables are provided, it is important to evaluate the calcium content in these foods. A recent study found that grass hay significantly reduced urinary calcium excretion compared with legume/pulse hay, and also increased total water intake (Clauss et al. 2012). Other causes that have been hypothesized to be related to rabbit and rodent urolithiasis include excess or deficiency in nutrients such as ascorbate and citrate. Therefore, an evaluation of vitamin supplementation should be performed in animals with a history of urolithiasis and in guinea pigs in particular (as they require vitamin C as an essential nutrient). Urinary dilution is important in the management of many types of uroliths, as urinary dilution reduces precursor supersaturation. Therefore, maintaining hydration is a key factor in prevention of urolith formation and efforts should be made to provide clean water in multiple locations. Dietary salt is not currently used to increase thirst in small mammalian companion herbivores. In areas where water hardness and mineral content are high, filtered water should be considered for use in high-risk patients or those with a previous history of urolithiasis to reduce the intake of calcium.

Clinical nutrition is a powerful tool in veterinary medicine that can be used to treat a variety of metabolic diseases. Use of veterinary therapeutic diets to nutritionally manage conditions and diseases in small mammalian companion herbivores is in its infancy. Several rabbit and rodent veterinary therapeutic diets formulated for specific diseases, such as obesity, gastrointestinal disease, and urinary tract disease, are now commercially available in the United States and Europe (Proença and Mayer 2014); however, additional clinical studies are required to better establish the efficacy and benefits of these diets.

Critical Care Nutrition for Small Mammalian Companion Herbivores

Dysrexia is an outcome in many disease processes affecting rabbits and rodents. Reduced food intake may have a detrimental impact on gut motility and the gut microbiota, leading to reduced defecation and discomfort, and may progress to hepatic lipidosis or severe intestinal disease, which may be life-threatening (Oglesbee and Jenkins 2012). This cascade may not be broken without subcutaneous and/or intravenous fluid administration and assisted feeding intervention. If the animal is dehydrated and/or there are blood electrolyte shifts, this needs to be corrected before nutritional intervention is attempted.

Unlike dogs and cats, rabbits, chinchillas, and guinea pigs generally tolerate assisted feeding with a syringe quite well. When this is done carefully and slowly, allowing the animal to chew and swallow, the risk of trauma and aspiration is low. Powdered foods (e.g. Oxbow Critical Care, Oxbow Animal Health, Murdock, NE, USA; EmerAid Herbivore, Lafeber's, Cornell, IL, USA) are formulated to be mixed with water and administered via a wide-tip (catheter-tip) syringe (Figure 23.2). Fine powdered diets (e.g. Critical Care Fine Grind, Oxbow Animal Health) may also be provided via slip-tip syringe or via feeding tubes with a narrow lumen in rabbits (14–22 French orogastric tube or 3.5–8 French nasogastric tube). When selecting a specific diet for a patient that

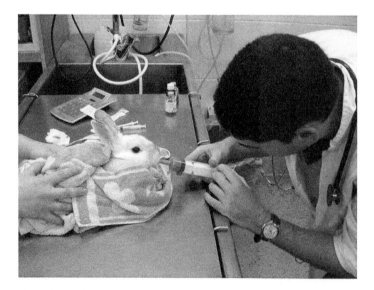

Figure 23.2 Syringe-assisted feeding in a rabbit. *Source:* Courtesy of Dr. Ady Gancz and Dr. Jonathan Stockman.

requires assisted feeding, it is recommended to choose a diet that provides the longest fiber possible with consideration to the animal's size and route of feeding. Very fine, powdered fiber is less likely to stimulate gastrointestinal motility, as it may enter the cecum and undergo fermentation instead of reaching the colon, whereas longer fiber promotes motility (Paul-Murphy 2007; Proença and Mayer 2014).

Use of nasogastric tubes is implemented in rabbits (mostly) as a temporary method to deliver nutrition. These are very narrow lumen tubes with a small outside diameter; therefore, a liquid food consistency is needed to avoid tube occlusion. Tube size may vary between 3.5 and 8 French rubber tubes, depending on the size of the patient's nasal cavity. Esophageal or pharyngeal tubes may also be considered, but are not commonly used as they require anesthesia and surgical placement. Delivering the patient's resting energy requirement (RER; see later calculation) is the goal, with either a constant-rate infusion (CRI) or small frequent (4–6 times/day) bolus feedings. The energy density of slurries may vary according to the formula and the tube used; however common formulas such as Oxbow Critical Care provides approximately 2 kcal/ml once reconstituted with 1:2 volume/volume powder to water. This concentration is usually sufficient to provide RER without resulting in volume intolerance. Signs of intolerance include refusal to ingest the food and resistance to feeding; however, animals that are sedated or are recovering from anesthesia should not be fed right away since aspiration of food may occur. Generally support is provided until the patient is hydrated and able to eat on their own when offered food before the next bolus feeding or after stopping any CRI for up to four hours, but the determination of when to stop with assisted feeding should also include the overall assessment of the patient, including assessment of overall alertness and behavior, improvement in borborygmi, and fecal production. The authors recommend continuing assisted feeding as needed until these clinical parameters improve sufficiently. An effort must also be made to correct the underlying problem (if one exists) that led to the dysrexia.

Parenteral nutrition is uncommon due to the requirement for fiber and food presence in the gastrointestinal tract and the small diameter and fragility of the blood vessels, given the hyperosmolarity of parenteral feeding solutions. Parenteral nutrition may be used to supplement other methods of feeding in cases where energy requirements cannot be solely met by enteral feeding. Similar rules of hygiene and aseptic catheter placement apply in rabbits, chinchillas, and guinea pigs, just as they do in other species such as dogs and cats.

Energy Calculations for Rabbits, Chinchillas, and Guinea Pigs

While many human companions feed ad libitum, as rabbits, chinchillas, and guinea pigs graze throughout the day, energy calculations become important when animals are in a critical state that requires intervention. The RER or the basal metabolic requirement is not different from other mammals and is calculated based on Kleiber's energy equation:

$$RER = 70 \times body\ weight\ (in\ kg)^{0.75}$$

Some authors (Proença and Mayer 2014) recommend adding a factor to this calculation to reflect the change in energy requirements in light of the animal's illness. These factors, which range from 0.5 to 3.0, are meant to address individual differences in energy requirements according to life stage (e.g. higher in growing animals) or disease. Practically, it should be noted that energy requirement prediction is rarely accurate, and patient assessment and adjustments are always necessary. Therefore, a caloric provision approximating a critical patient's RER may be a good starting point in many adult patients, and adjustments should be made according to tolerance of feeding, disease progression, and body weight shifts. A higher caloric intake as well as a higher frequency of feeding may be required in very young patients.

General Nutrition for Small Mammalian Carnivores

Ferrets

Ferrets (*Mustela putorious furo*) are very popular pets across the United States and Europe despite legal restrictions that exist in some states such as California and Hawaii. In the United States, ferrets are typically sold after being ovariohysterectomized or castrated and descented by the breeding facility before they are 6 weeks of age. Relatively few private breeders exist. Ferrets belong to the Mustelidae family, which also includes mink, weasels, badgers, and so on. They are descendants of the European polecat (*Mustela putorius*) and, like others in the Mustelidae family, they are obligate carnivores. Historically, companion ferrets have been fed diets formulated to meet the requirements for mink or cats; however, diets formulated for domestic ferrets are now widely available.

Digestive Physiology

The gastrointestinal tract of ferrets resembles that of other mammalian carnivores. Ferrets have a relatively short gastrointestinal tract with a simple stomach. The small intestine is about five times the length of the ferret's body (Johnson-Delaney 2014). Ferrets lack a cecum and an ileocolic valve, expediting gastric transit, which is around three hours in the adult (Powers and Brown 2012; Johnson-Delaney 2014). Due to the relatively short length of the intestinal tract, the rapid transit time, and the lower concentration of digestive enzymes on the intestinal brush border, the ferret's digestive process is considered inefficient compared with other species. Ferrets are spontaneous secretors of hydrochloric acid and, unlike some carnivores that eat few large meals in a day, ferrets eat small, frequent meals.

Nutrition-Related Diseases of Small Mammalian Companion Carnivores

Ferrets and Considerations for Mink

Marine Food Sources: Hypovitaminosis E/ Nutritional Steatitis, Thiamine Deficiency, and Salt Toxicity

Nutritional steatitis (i.e. adipose tissue inflammation, characterized by yellow discoloration) has been reported in ferrets that were fed diets high in PUFAs. These ferrets were being fed a blended diet consisting of 40% squid offal, with a total dietary PUFA concentration of 7.7% dry matter. Unfortunately, the vitamin E concentrations were not adequate for a higher PUFA diet, leading to pathology. As a consequence, squid is no longer recommended in any diet formulation for either ferrets or mink (Brooks et al. 1985). More significantly, ferrets' vitamin E requirement, like that of other species, is proportional to dietary PUFAs, and inadequate dietary vitamin E concentration can lead to steatitis.

Thiamine deficiency has been reported in farmed ferrets fed a diet high in thiaminase-containing fish (Fox and Marini 2014). Salt toxicity is a possible sequela of feeding ferrets a diet high in salted fish, such as tuna stored in brine. Reported clinical signs are similar to those seen in domestic swine, which include depression, seizures, and death 24–96 hours after ingestion (Fox and Marini 2014).

Considerations for Mink

Mink are also members of the Mustelidae family like ferrets, and are farmed for pelts. Despite their physiologic similarities, they are considered a production animal, and thus have a very different feeding strategy compared with the companion ferret. Many of the reported nutritionally related diseases of mink may not be applicable to the companion ferret that consumes a commercially prepared pelleted diet formulated for ferrets. However, some issues could potentially also be seen in companion ferrets fed unbalanced home-prepared diets, and as such are briefly shared here.

Experimentally induced biotin deficiency in mink has been described secondary to feeding a diet containing dried eggs. A glycoprotein, avidin, found in raw or not fully cooked egg whites can bind available biotin in the diet, and create a deficiency (Wehr et al. 1980). Mink fed a pyridoxine-deficient diet showed behavioral, neurologic, and reproductive (sterility) abnormalities similar to other mammals (Helgebostad et al. 1963). Iron-deficient diets have led to growth retardation, microcytic-hypochromic anemia, and achromotrichia in mink (Stout et al. 1960).

Nutrition-Related Diseases of Small Mammalian Carnivores

Ferrets

Compared to other "exotic" small companion mammals, the incidence of nutritional-related diseases in ferrets is low. This is likely due to the availability of complete formulated diets, unlike herbivorous small mammals that require a more complex diet consisting of multiple components (hay, greens, etc.; see earlier in chapter). Ferrets may thrive with diets that are formulated for cats as well as diets formulated specifically for ferrets; however, feline diets may not be adequate for ferrets who are stressed or when the metabolic needs are high, such as during reproduction (Johnson-Delaney 2014). In addition, the high variability in cat diets raises the question of whether any feline diet would be adequate for ferrets, therefore a diet formulated specifically for ferrets is a safer choice.

Obesity

The most common nutritional-related disease in ferrets seen in one author's (OP) practice is obesity. While weight gain may be seasonal and while male ferrets are typically larger and have more adipose tissue than females, it is important to identify ferrets that are obese. In many cases, affected ferrets are being fed ad libitum both a commercial pelleted diet as well as a combination of other supplemental food items, including homemade "duck or dook soup," canned cat food, and other treat items. Excessive administration of high-fat supplements, such as Ferretone (8-in-1, Spectrum Brands, Islandia, NY, USA), in addition to a high-quality ferret diet has also been associated with obesity (Johnson-Delaney 2014). Increasing the physical activity of ferrets by letting them play and explore larger spaces may help with weight loss, but the ability to do this may be limited for some human companions, as the area in which ferrets are allowed to roam freely must be ferret proofed. Decreasing or eliminating treats from the diet may help, as well as limiting the total amount of calories offered, although this may be more difficult when multiple ferrets are group housed. It should be noted that some seasonal weight gain during the cold months is expected and is a part of normal physiology, particularly in males.

It is unknown whether feline weight-loss diets can be used successfully in obese ferrets to induce weight loss; however, ferrets may not do clinically well on a high-fiber diet, as some weight-loss diets are (Johnson-Delaney 2014). Cutting back on high-fat treats and improving physical activity many times would suffice to achieve weight loss, and a general weight-loss rate of 1–2% of body weight per week, as recommended in dogs and cats, appears appropriate; however, this may be more difficult to achieve in some cases (for example, in a colder climate) (see Box 23.2).

Urolithiasis

Ferret diets high in plant-based proteins, such as yellow corn (*Zea mays*), are at risk of developing magnesium ammonium phosphate, otherwise known as struvite, urolithiasis (Figure 23.3). Metabolism of plant proteins produces more alkaline urine than the typical acidic urine of ferrets, which predisposes them

---

Box 23.2 Feeding the Healthy Ferret and Caloric Restriction for Weight Loss

Juveniles

- Ad libitum feeding of commercially prepared all-life-stage or growth ferret food.

Adults

- Meal feed commercially prepared all-life-stage or adult maintenance ferret food; cat food may not meet ferret requirements, likely being higher in carbohydrate calories as suggested later, so care should be taken in selecting a food designed for this separate obligate carnivore species.
- Lower-carbohydrate dog foods and home-made ferret food should be avoided due to likely nutrient deficiencies, unless

concurrently formulated to meet ferret nutritional needs.

- Suggested caloric distribution for adult ferret diet at maintenance: above 35% protein calories, above 40% fat calories, and under 25% carbohydrate calories (Chitty 2009).
- Treats should be limited to no more than 10% of daily caloric intake.
- Adult energy requirements are typically 200–300 kcal/kg body weight (Johnson-Delaney 2014).
- Weight loss in overweight/obese patients can be induced by eliminating high-fat treats and by caloric restriction (20% reduction initially, with monitoring and intake adjustment as needed).

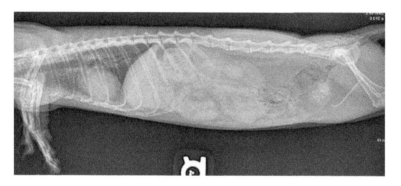

Figure 23.3 A lateral whole-body view radiograph of an adult male castrated ferret with multiple radiopaque cystoliths. *Source:* Courtesy of Dr. Olivia Petritz.

to the development of struvite uroliths. Cases of urolithiasis in ferrets have been associated with feeding a low-quality cat food or dog food to ferrets (Nguyen et al. 1979).

Bacterially induced struvite crystalluria is uncommon in ferrets, as it is in cats, although urine culture can help rule out an underlying bacterial infection. According to a retrospective analysis of the Minnesota Urolith Center, struvite uroliths were the most common stone type from ferrets between 1981 and 2009, comprising 66–67% of all submissions, followed by

cystine uroliths (15–16%) and calcium oxalate uroliths (10–11%) (Osborne et al. 2009; Nwaokorie et al. 2011, 2013). The latest reports from a recent large-scale retrospective survey show a significant increase in the prevalence of cystine urolithiasis in North American ferrets. Cystine uroliths represented 93% of the 1014 uroliths submitted between 2010 and 2018, with the most dramatic increase in the most recent years (Hanak et al. 2019, 2021). This increase is not as dramatic in Europe, where prevalence was 27% of analyzed uroliths. While the reasons for this shift are poorly understood, it is possible that changes in ferret nutrition to a higher–animal protein diet reduced the prevalence of struvite urolithiasis, or perhaps excessive inbreeding has increased the risk for cystine urolithiasis due to a change in genetics.

While the etiology of cystine urolithiasis in ferrets is not completely understood, some authors have reported an anecdotal relationship between feeding a high–legume protein diet and cystine urolithiasis. This suggested association may be puzzling, as legumes/pulses are generally limiting in sulfur amino acids (SAAs) including cystine; however, a small retrospective study showed that many of these diets are similar in SAA content to non-grain-free diets (Lamglait et al. 2021). A hereditary trait for impaired renal tubular reabsorption of cysteine is associated with increased urinary cystine supersaturation and cystine crystal and urolith formation in dogs and in people. Although a genetic predisposition may play a role in cystine urolithiasis in ferrets, this has not been extensively studied (Nwaokorie et al. 2013). Cystine supersaturation is increased with lower urinary pH; therefore, urine alkalization may be beneficial in ferrets with a history of cystine urolithiasis.

Data regarding the nutritional management of urolithiasis in ferrets are lacking. Attempts to feed a urinary therapeutic diet such as Royal Canin Veterinary Diet Feline Urinary SO (Royal Canin, St. Charles, MO, USA) or Hill's Prescription Diet c/d Feline (Hill's Pet Nutrition, Topeka, KS, USA) are generally not recommended, as these diets are not formulated to meet the nutritional requirements of ferrets, and strategies to prevent urolithiasis recurrence in cats may not apply to ferrets. Since highly concentrated urine is an important risk factor for urolithiasis and crystalluria of all types, maintaining adequate hydration to decrease urine concentration is a beneficial strategy that applies for the prevention of all uroliths. Use of high salt intake to increase drinking and thereby dilute urine, or increasing water intake by mixing water into the food, may have potential in urolithiasis prevention; however, there are no published data regarding the usefulness of these strategies in ferrets.

Ferret Pancreatic Islet Beta-Cell Tumor (Insulinoma)

Pancreatic islet beta-cell tumors, insulinomas, are the most commonly diagnosed neoplasm in ferrets, with a reported incidence of 22–25% (Bakthavatchalu et al. 2016). Unlike in domestic dogs, this disease often remains undiagnosed for prolonged periods of time, likely due in part to free-choice feeding strategies for ferrets compared with meal-fed dogs. A concurrent insulinoma and subsequent exacerbation of subclinical hypoglycemia are of greater concern in the dysrexic ferret. Signs of hypoglycemia in ferrets include lethargy, ptyalism, and weakness, while seizures are uncommon. Immediate glucose (or if not readily available, sucrose) supplementation, usually orally, does temporarily treat hypoglycemia; however, this also can stimulate insulin secretion from the tumor and lead to a repeated hypoglycemic episode (Bell 1999). Therefore, an oral supplement, high in glucose but also high in fat, such as Nutri-Cal (Tomlyn Nutri-Cal for Cats, Tomlyn, Fort Worth, TX, USA), has been recommended for immediate treatment of a hypoglycemic episode prior to intravenous dextrose administration (Bell 1999). In addition to other medical and surgical therapy, affected ferrets should be encouraged to eat every 2–4 hours and also before times of increased activity (Johnson-Delaney 2014). Food should be available 24 hours a day, which often allows a ferret to self-regulate its glucose needs in addition to any medical therapy, such as glucocorticoids.

Inflammatory Bowel Disease

Inflammatory bowel disease (IBD) is relatively common in ferrets (Burgess and Garner 2002). Similar to other species, the etiology of this condition is unknown. Typically, this disease in ferrets is characterized by lymphoplasmacytic infiltrates; however, without the use of immunohistochemistry severe IBD may sometimes be confused with enteric lymphoma (Watson et al. 2016). While the role of diet in the pathogenesis of this disease is unknown, some ferrets respond well to dietary change, and some "limited-ingredient" commercial diets may be trialed if novel to the patient (Totally Ferret Turkey-Venison-Lamb Meal Formula, Performance Foods, Broomfield, CO, USA). Consideration may be given to feeding limited-ingredient, novel antigen therapeutic cat diets if diets formulated for ferrets are not tolerated well by the patient. The role of dietary fiber in the management of clinical signs of IBD is controversial in ferrets. While plant fiber or animal fiber (such as hair or indigestible ligaments) may help support the gastrointestinal microbiota and stool consistency, these constituents decrease diet digestibility overall, which may exacerbate clinical signs. Since response to fiber supplementation may be idiosyncratic, gradual supplementation of dietary fiber may be attempted while monitoring for a response.

Critical Care Nutrition for Small Mammalian Companion Carnivores

Ferrets

Similar to other carnivores, such as the domestic cat, hepatic lipidosis also occurs in ferrets after a prolonged fasting period (Bjornvad et al. 2004). Immediate nutritional support with a high-protein, high-fat diet is highly recommended for any sick ferret. In the United States, there are several commercially available powdered diets for small mammalian companion carnivores that are readily accepted by most ferrets, including EmerAid Exotic Carnivore (Lafeber Company) and Carnivore Care (Oxbow Animal Health). Both of these formulations are appropriate for syringe feeding or administration via an esophagostomy tube. Energy needs are usually calculated as RER using the same equation as given earlier for herbivores. Despite ferrets being averse to novel food items, most will readily accept these diets, and some may even refuse to transition back to their normal diet.

References

Ahluwalia, B., Pincus, G., and Holman, R.T. (1967). Essential fatty acid deficiency and its effects upon reproductive organs of male rabbits. *J. Nutr.* 92 (2): 205–214.

Bakthavatchalu, V., Muthupalani, S., Marini, R.P., and Fox, J.G. (2016). Endocrinopathy and aging in ferrets. *Vet. Pathol.* 53 (2): 349–365.

Bell, J.A. (1999). Ferret nutrition. *Vet. Clin. North Am. Exot. Anim. Pract.* 2 (1): 169–192.

Björnhag, G. and Snipes, R.L. (1999). Colonic separation mechanism in lagomorph and rodent species—a comparison. *Zoosyst. Evol.* 75 (2): 275–281.

Bjornvad, C.R., Elnif, J., and Sangild, P.T. (2004). Short-term fasting induces intra-hepatic lipid accumulation and decreases intestinal mass without reduced brush-border enzyme activity in mink (Mustela vison) small intestine. *J. Comp. Physiol. B* 174 (8): 625–632.

Brooks, H.V., Rammell, C.G., Hoogenboom, J.J.L., and Taylor, D.E.S. (1985). Observations on an outbreak of nutritional steatitis (yellow fat disease) in fitch (Mustella putorius furo). *N. Z. Vet. J.* 33 (9): 141–145.

Burgess, M. and Garner, M.M. (2002). Clinical aspects of inflammatory bowel disease in ferrets. *Exot. DVM* 4 (2): 29–34.

Campbell-Ward, M.L. (2012). Gastrointestinal physiology and nutrition. In: *Ferrets, Rabbits, and Rodents*, 3e (ed. K.E. Quesenberry and J.W. Carpenter), 183–192. St. Louis, MO: Elsevier.

Capello, V. and Lennox, A.M. (2012). Small mammal dentistry. In: *Ferrets, Rabbits, and Rodents Clinical Medicine and Surgery*, 3e (ed. K.E. Quesenberry and J.W. Carpenter), 452–471. St. Louis, MO: Elsevier.

Carabaño, R., Piquer, J., Menoyo, D., and Badiola, I. (2010). The digestive system of the rabbit. In: *Nutrition of the Rabbit*, 2e (ed. C. De Blas and J. Wiseman), 1–18. Cambridge, MA.

Chapin, R.E. and Smith, S.E. (1967). The calcium tolerance of growing and reproducing rabbits. *Cornell Vet.* 57: 480–491.

Chitty, J. (2009). Ferrets: biology and husbandry. In: *BSAVA Manual of Rodents and Ferrets 2009* (ed. E. Keeble and A. Meredith), 193–204. Gloucester: BSAVA Library.

Clauss, M., Burger, B., Liesegang, A. et al. (2012). Influence of diet on calcium metabolism, tissue calcification and urinary sludge in rabbits (Oryctolagus cuniculus). *J. Anim. Physiol. Anim. Nutr.* 96 (5): 798–807.

Coutant, T., Dunn, M., Langlois, I., and Maccolini, E. (2019). Cystoscopic-guided lithotripsy for the removal of a urethral stone in a guinea pig. *J. Exotic Pet Med.* 28: 111–114.

Crossley, D.A. and del Mar Miguélez, M. (2001). Skull size and cheek-tooth length in wild-caught and captive-bred chinchillas. *Arch. Oral Biol.* 46 (10): 919–928.

Eastridge, M.L., Bucci, P.B., and Ribeiro, C.V. (2009). Feeding equivalent concentrations of forage neutral detergent fiber from alfalfa hay, grass hay, wheat straw, and whole cottonseed in corn silage based diets to lactating cows. *Anim. Feed Sci. Technol.* 150 (1-2): 86–94.

Eckermann-Ross, C. (2008). Hormonal regulation and calcium metabolism in the rabbit. *Vet. Clin. North Am. Exot. Anim. Pract.* 11 (1): 139–152.

Fox, J.G. and Marini, R.P. (ed.) (2014). *Biology and Diseases of the Ferret*, 3e. Ames, IA: Wiley.

García, J., Gidenne, T., Falcão-e-Cunha, L., and de BLAS, C. (2002). Identification of the main factors that influence caecal fermentation traits in growing rabbits. *Anim. Res.* 51 (2): 165–173.

Glickman, I. (1948). Acute vitamin C deficiency and periodontal disease: I. The periodontal tissues of the Guinea pig in acute vitamin C deficiency. *J. Dent. Res.* 27 (1): 9–23.

Hanak, E.B., Di Girolamo, N., DeSilva, U. et al. (2019). Composition of ferret uroliths in North America and Europe: 1055 Cases (2010–2018). Abstract, presented at Exotics Conference with American Association of Zoo Veterinarians, St. Louis, MO (30 September 2019).

Hanak, E.B., Di Girolamo, N., DeSilva, U. et al. (2021). Variation in mineral types of uroliths from ferrets (Mustela putorius furo) submitted for analysis in North America, Europe, or Asia over an 8-year period. *J. Am. Vet. Med. Assoc.* 259 (7): 757–763.

Harcourt-Brown, F.M. (1996). Calcium deficiency, diet and dental disease in pet rabbits. *Vet. Rec.* 139 (23): 567–571.

Harkness, J.E., Turner, P.V., VandeWoude, S., and Wheler, C.L. (2010). Introduction, general husbandry and disease prevention. In: *Harkness and Wagner's Biology and Medicine of Rabbits and Rodents*, 5e, 3–21. Ames, IA: Wiley.

Hawkins, M.G. and Bishop, C.R. (2012). Disease problems of Guinea pigs. In: *Ferrets, Rabbits, and Rodents Clinical Medicine and Surgery*, 3e (ed. K.E. Quesenberry and J.W. Carpenter), 295–310. St. Louis, MO: Elsevier.

Hawkins, M.G., Ruby, A.L., Drazenovich, T.L., and Westropp, J.L. (2009). Composition and characteristics of urinary calculi from Guinea pigs. *J. Am. Vet. Med. Assoc.* 234 (2): 214–220.

Helgebostad, A.R., Svenkerud, R., and Ender, F. (1963). Sterility in mink induced experimentally by deficiency of vitamin B6. *Acta Vet. Scand.* 4: 228–237.

Irlbeck, N.A. (2001). How to feed the rabbit (Oryctolagus cuniculus) gastrointestinal tract. *J. Anim. Sci.* 79 (E-Suppl): E343–E346.

Johnson-Delaney, C.A. (2014). Ferret nutrition. *Vet. Clin. North Am. Exot. Anim. Pract.* 17 (3): 449–470.

Ko, F.C., Martins, J.S., Reddy, P. et al. (2016). Acute phosphate restriction impairs bone formation and increases marrow adipose tissue in growing mice. *J. Bone Miner. Res.* 31 (12): 2204–2214.

Kohles, M. (2014). Gastrointestinal anatomy and physiology of select exotic companion mammals. *Vet. Clin. North Am. Exot. Anim. Pract.* 17 (2): 165–178.

Lamglait, B., Brieger, A., Rainville, M.P. et al. (2021). Retrospective case control study of pet ferrets with cystine urolithiasis in Quebec, Canada: epidemiological and clinical features. *J. Vet. Med. Surg.* 5, 31 (1).

Mackenzie, C.G. and McCollum, E.V. (1940). The cure of nutritional muscular dystrophy in the rabbit by alpha-tocopherol and its effect on creatine metabolism: four figures. *J. Nutr.* 19 (4): 345–362.

Marounek, M., Břeňová, N., Suchorská, O., and Mrázek, J. (2009). Phytase activity in rabbit cecal bacteria. *Folia Microbiol.* 54 (2): 111–114.

Martel-Arquette, A. and Mans, C. (2016). Urolithiasis in chinchillas: 15 cases (2007 to 2011). *J. Small Anim. Pract.* 57 (5): 260–264.

Meredith, A.L., Prebble, J.L., and Shaw, D.J. (2015). Impact of diet on incisor growth and attrition and the development of dental disease in pet rabbits. *J. Small Anim. Pract.* 56: 377–382.

Müller, J., Clauss, M., Codron, D. et al. (2015). Tooth length and incisal wear and growth in Guinea pigs (Cavia porcellus) fed diets of different abrasiveness. *J. Anim. Physiol. Anim. Nutr.* 99 (3): 591–604.

National Research Council (NRC) (1977). *Nutrient Requirements of Rabbits: 1977.* Washington, DC: National Academies Press.

National Research Council (NRC) (1995). *Nutrient Requirements of Laboratory Animals,* 4th rev. ed. Washington, DC: National Academies Press.

Nguyen, H.T., Moreland, A.F., and Shields, R.P. (1979). Urolithiasis in ferrets (Mustela putorius). *Lab. Anim. Sci.* 29: 243–245.

Nwaokorie, E.E., Osborne, C.A., Lulich, J.P. et al. (2011). Epidemiology of struvite uroliths in ferrets: 272 cases (1981–2007). *J. Am. Vet. Med. Assoc.* 239 (10): 1319–1324.

Nwaokorie, E.E., Osborne, C.A., Lulich, J.P., and Albasan, H. (2013). Epidemiological evaluation of cystine urolithiasis in domestic ferrets (Mustela putorius furo): 70 cases (1992–2009). *J. Am. Vet. Med. Assoc.* 242 (8): 1099–1103.

Oglesbee, B.L. and Jenkins, J.R. (2012). Gastrointestinal diseases. In: *Ferrets, Rabbits, and Rodents*, 3e (ed. K.E. Quesenberry and J.W. Carpenter), 193–204. St. Louis, MO: Elsevier.

Olson, J.A. (1989). Provitamin A function of carotenoids: the conversion of β-carotene into vitamin A. *J. Nutr.* 119 (1): 105–108.

Osborne, C.A., Albasan, H., Lulich, J.P. et al. (2009). Quantitative analysis of 4468 uroliths retrieved from farm animals, exotic species, and wildlife submitted to the Minnesota Urolith Center: 1981 to 2007. *Vet. Clin. North Am. Small Anim. Pract.* 39 (1): 65–78.

Paul-Murphy, J. (2007). Critical care of the rabbit. *Vet. Clin. North Am. Exot. Anim. Pract.* 10 (2): 437–461.

Pelaseyed, T., Bergström, J.H., Gustafsson, J.K. et al. (2014). The mucus and mucins of the goblet cells and enterocytes provide the first defense line of the gastrointestinal tract and interact with the immune system. *Immunol. Rev.* 260 (1): 8–20.

Portsmouth, J.I. (1977). The nutrition of rabbits. In: *Nutrition and the Climatic Environment* (ed. W. Haresign, H. Swan and D. Lewis), 93–111. London: Butterworths.

Powers, L.V. and Brown, S.A. (2012). Basic anatomy, physiology, and husbandry. In: *Ferrets, Rabbits, and Rodents Clinical Medicine and Surgery*, 3e (ed. K.E. Quesenberry and J.W. Carpenter), 1–12. St. Louis, MO: Elsevier.

Proença, L.M. and Mayer, J. (2014). Prescription diets for rabbits. *Vet. Clin. North Am. Exot. Anim. Pract.* 17 (3): 485–502.

Quesenberry, K.E. (1994). Guinea pigs. *Vet. Clin. North Am. Small Anim. Pract.* 24 (1): 67–87.

Reid, M.E., Bieri, J.G., Plack, P.A., and Andrews, E.L. (1964). Nutritional studies with the guinea pig: X. Determination of the linoleic acid requirement. *J. Nutr.* 82 (4): 401–408.

Snipes, R.L., Clauss, W., Weber, A., and Hörnicke, H. (1982). Structural and functional differences in various divisions of the rabbit colon. *Cell Tissue Res.* 225 (2): 331–346.

Snyder, W., Richmond, M., and Pond, W. (1976). Protein nutrition of juvenile cottontails. *J. Wildl. Manage.* 40 (3): 484–490.

Southard, T., Bender, H., Wade, S.E. et al. (2013). Naturally occurring Parelaphostrongylus tenuis-associated choriomeningitis in a guinea pig with neurologic signs. *Vet. Pathol.* 50 (3): 560–562.

Stan, F., Damian, A., Gudea, A. et al. (2014). Comparative anatomical study of the large intestine in rabbit and chinchilla. *Bull. UASVM Vet. Med.* 71 (1): 2014.

Stout, F.M., Oldfield, J.E., and Adair, J. (1960). Aberrant iron metabolism and the "cotton-fur" abnormality in mink. *J. Nutr.* 72 (1): 46–52.

Takahashi, T., Karita, S., Yahaya, M.S., and Goto, M. (2005). Radial and axial variations of bacteria within the cecum and proximal colon of guinea pigs revealed by PCR–DGGE. *Biosci. Biotechnol. Biochem.* 69 (9): 1790–1792.

Tschudin, A., Clauss, M., Codron, D. et al. (2011). Water intake in domestic rabbits (Oryctolagus cuniculus) from open dishes and nipple drinkers under different water and feeding regimes. *J. Anim. Physiol. Anim. Nutr.* 95 (4): 499–511.

Turnbaugh, P.J., Ley, R.E., Mahowald, M.A. et al. (2006). An obesity-associated gut microbiome with increased capacity for energy harvest. *Nature* 444 (7122): 1027.

Vella, D. and Donnelly, T.M. (2012). Basic anatomy, physiology, and husbandry. In: *Ferrets, Rabbits, and Rodents*, 3e (ed. K.E. Quesenberry and J.W. Carpenter), 157–173. St. Louis, MO: Elsevier.

Watson, M.K., Cazzini, P., Mayer, J. et al. (2016). Histology and immunohistochemistry of severe inflammatory bowel disease versus lymphoma in the ferret (Mustela putorius furo). *J. Vet. Diagn. Invest.* 28 (3): 198–206.

Wehr, N.B., Adair, J., and Oldfield, J.E. (1980). Biotin deficiency in mink fed spray-dried eggs 1. *J. Anim. Sci.* 50 (5): 877–885.

Wenger, S. and Hatt, J.M. (2015). Transurethral cystoscopy and endoscopic Urolith removal in female guinea pigs (Cavia porcellus). *Vet. Clin. North Am. Exot. Anim. Pract.* 18 (3): 359–367.

Worthington, J.M. and Fulghum, R.S. (1988). Cecal and fecal bacterial flora of the Mongolian gerbil and the chinchilla. *Appl. Environ. Microbiol.* 54 (5): 1210–1215.

Zhao, S., Chu, Y., Zhang, C. et al. (2008). Diet-induced central obesity and insulin resistance in rabbits. *J. Anim. Physiol. Anim. Nutr.* 92 (1): 105–111.

Index

Applied Veterinary Clinical Nutrition, Second Edition. Edited by Andrea J. Fascetti,
Sean J. Delaney, Jennifer A. Larsen, and Cecilia Villaverde.
© 2024 John Wiley & Sons, Inc. Published 2024 by John Wiley & Sons, Inc.